Massachusetts General Hospital

HANDBOOK OF
GENERAL HOSPITAL
PSYCHIATRY

Massachusetts General Hospital

HANDBOOK OF GENERAL HOSPITAL PSYCHIATRY

Eighth Edition

Theodore A. Stern, MD
Psychiatrist and Chief Emeritus
Avery D. Weisman Psychiatry Consultation Service,
Director
Thomas P. Hackett Center for Scholarship in
    Psychosomatic Medicine
Massachusetts General Hospital;
Ned H. Cassem Professor of Psychiatry in the Field of
    Psychosomatic Medicine/Consultation
Harvard Medical School
Boston, Massachusetts

Scott R. Beach, MD
Psychiatrist
Department of Psychiatry
Massachusetts General Hospital;
Associate Professor
Department of Psychiatry
Harvard Medical School
Boston, Massachusetts

Felicia A. Smith, MD
Associate Chief
Department of Psychiatry,
Chief
MGH Division of Psychiatry and Medicine
Massachusetts General Hospital;
Assistant Professor
Department of Psychiatry
Harvard Medical School
Boston, Massachusetts

Oliver Freudenreich, MD
Co-Director
MGH Psychosis Clinical and Research Program
Department of Psychiatry
Massachusetts General Hospital;
Professor of Clinical Psychiatry
Department of Psychiatry
Harvard Medical School
Boston, Massachusetts

Ana-Maria Vranceanu, PhD
Director
Center for Health Outcomes and
    Interdisciplinary Research (CHOIR)
Department of Psychiatry
Massachusetts General Hospital;
David T. Rovee PhD and Joanne V. Rovee Endowed
    Chair in Psychiatry,
Professor of Psychology
Department of Psychiatry
Harvard Medical School
Boston, Massachusetts

Maurizio Fava, MD
Psychiatrist-in-Chief
Department of Psychiatry,
Vice Chair
Executive Committee on Research,
Executive Director
Clinical Trials Network and Institute
Massachusetts General Hospital;
Associate Dean for Clinical and Translational Research
Slater Family Professor of Psychiatry
Harvard Medical School
Boston, Massachusetts

ELSEVIER

Elsevier
1600 John F. Kennedy Blvd.
Ste 1800
Philadelphia, PA 19103-2899

MASSACHUSETTS GENERAL HOSPITAL HANDBOOK OF GENERAL HOSPITAL   ISBN: 978-0-443-11895-1
PSYCHIATRY, EIGHTH EDITION

Notice

Practitioners and researchers must always rely on their own experience and knowledge in evaluating and using any information, methods, compounds or experiments described herein. Because of rapid advances in the medical sciences, in particular, independent verification of diagnoses and drug dosages should be made. To the fullest extent of the law, no responsibility is assumed by Elsevier, authors, editors or contributors for any injury and/or damage to persons or property as a matter of products liability, negligence or otherwise, or from any use or operation of any methods, products, instructions, or ideas contained in the material herein.

Previous editions copyrighted 2018, 2010, 2004, 1997, 1991, 1987 and 1978.

Content Strategist: Mary Hegeler
Content Development Specialist: Lisa Barnes
Publishing Services Manager: Deepthi Unni
Senior Project Manager: Beula Christopher
Book Designer: Ryan Cook

Printed in India

Last digit is the print number: 9 8 7 6 5 4 3 2 1

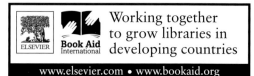

To our students, our colleagues, and our mentors and on behalf of the patients who suffer, we hope this edition improves the detection and treatment of psychiatric problems and brings much-needed relief.

Theodore A. Stern
Scott R. Beach
Felicia A. Smith
Oliver Freudenreich
Ana-Maria Vranceanu
Maurizio Fava

CONTRIBUTORS

ANNAH N. ABRAMS, MD
Chief
Division of Pediatric Psychooncology
Department of Pediatric Hematology and Oncology,
Staff
Pediatric Psychiatry Consultation-Liaison Service
Department of Child Psychiatry
Massachusetts General Hospital;
Assistant Professor
Department of Psychiatry
Harvard Medical School
Boston, Massachusetts
*38 Psychiatric Consultation to Children and
Adolescents*

MENEKSE ALPAY, MD
Psychiatrist
Department of Psychiatry
Massachusetts General Hospital;
Instructor
Department of Psychiatry
Harvard Medical School
Boston, Massachusetts
17 Pain

JONATHAN E. ALPERT, MD, PHD
Chair
Department of Psychiatry and Behavioral
  Sciences
Montefiore Medical Center and Albert Einstein
  College of Medicine;
Professor
Department of Psychiatry, Neuroscience, and
  Pediatrics
Albert Einstein College of Medicine
Bronx, New York
37 Psychopharmacology in the Medical Setting

MIRZA BAIG, MD
Resident Physician
Department of Psychiatry
Massachusetts General Hospital
Boston, Massachusetts;
Resident Physician
McLean Hospital
Belmont, Massachusetts;
Clinical Fellow in Psychiatry
Harvard Medical School
Boston, Massachusetts
*49 Approaches to Collaborative Care and Behavioral
Health Integration*

ASHIKA BAINS, MD
Psychiatrist
Department of Psychiatry
Massachusetts General Hospital;
Instructor
Department of Psychiatry
Harvard Medical School
Boston, Massachusetts
13 Substance Use Disorders
28 HIV Infection and AIDS
32 Burns, Trauma, and Intensive Care Unit Treatment

AMANDA WATERS BAKER, PHD
Psychologist
Department of Psychiatry
Massachusetts General Hospital;
Associate Professor
Department of Psychiatry
Harvard Medical School
Boston, Massachusetts
12 Pharmacotherapy of Anxiety Disorders

Scott R. Beach, MD
Psychiatrist
Department of Psychiatry
Massachusetts General Hospital;
Associate Professor
Department of Psychiatry
Harvard Medical School
Boston, Massachusetts
14 Somatic Symptom and Related Disorders and Functional Somatic Syndromes
15 Factitious Disorders and Malingering
21 Catatonia, Neuroleptic Malignant Syndrome, and Serotonin Syndrome
24 The Psychiatric Management of Patients With Cardiac Disease
29 COVID-19 Infection

BJ Beck, MSN, MD, BFA, MFA
Psychiatrist
Private Practice
Sonoma, California
49 Approaches to Collaborative Care and Behavioral Health Integration
50 Community Psychiatry

Noor Beckwith, MD
Hospitalist
Department of Psychiatry
Royal Columbian Hospital
New Westminster, British Columbia, Canada;
Clinical Instructor
Department of Psychiatry
Faculty of Medicine
University of British Columbia
Vancouver, British Columbia, Canada
9 Delirium

Eugene V. Beresin, MD, MA
Executive Director
The Clay Center for Young Healthy Minds;
Psychiatrist,
Director
Division of Professional and Public Mental Health Education
Department of Psychiatry
Massachusetts General Hospital;
Professor of Psychiatry
Harvard Medical School
Boston, Massachusetts
2 The Doctor-Patient Relationship
3 The Psychiatric Interview

Suzanne A. Bird, MD
Director
Acute Psychiatry Service
Massachusetts General Hospital;
Assistant Professor
Department of Psychiatry
Harvard Medical School
Boston, Massachusetts
42 Care of the Patient With Thoughts of Suicide
43 Emergency Psychiatry

Mark A. Blais, PsyD
Associate Chief of Psychology
Department of Psychiatry
Massachusetts General Hospital;
Associate Professor of Psychology
Department of Psychiatry
Harvard Medical School
Boston, Massachusetts
6 Psychological and Neuropsychological Assessment in the Medical Setting

Marie D. Bomm, MD, PhD
Resident Psychiatrist
Department of Psychiatry
Massachusetts General Hospital;
Clinical Fellow in Psychiatry
Harvard Medical School
Boston, Massachusetts
29 COVID-19 Infection

RAHEL BOSSON, MD
Medical Director
Program of Assertive Community Treatment
McLean Hospital;
Associate Program Director
Adult Psychiatry Residency Training Program
Massachusetts General Hospital/McLean Hospital;
Instructor
Department of Psychiatry
Harvard Medical School
Boston, Massachusetts
51 Global Psychiatry and Mental Healthcare Delivery

REBECCA WEINTRAUB BRENDEL, MD, JD
Director
Center for Bioethics,
Associate Professor
Psychiatry and Global Health and Social Medicine
Harvard Medical School
Boston, Massachusetts
48 Legal Aspects of Psychiatric Consultation

ERIC BUI, MD, PHD
Professor
Department of Psychiatry
University of Caen Normandy
Caen, France
12 Pharmacotherapy of Anxiety Disorders

JOAN A. CAMPRODON, MD, MPH, PHD
Chief
Division of Neuropsychiatry
Department of Psychiatry,
Director
Laboratory for Circuit Neuroscience and
   Neuromodulation,
Director
Transcranial Magnetic Stimulation Clinical Service
Department of Psychiatry
Massachusetts General Hospital;
Associate Professor
Department of Psychiatry
Harvard Medical School
Boston, Massachusetts
*5 Functional Neuroanatomy and the Neurologic
Examination*
*36 Device Neuromodulation and Brain Stimulation
Therapies*

JASON P. CAPLAN, MD
Chair
Department of Psychiatry
St. Joseph's Hospital and Medical Center
Phoenix, Arizona;
Professor
Department of Psychiatry
Creighton University School of Medicine
Phoenix, Arizona
9 Delirium

PAOLO CASSANO, MD, PHD
Director of Photobiomodulation
Division of Neuropsychiatry and
   Neuromodulation
Department of Psychiatry
Massachusetts General Hospital;
Associate Professor
Department of Psychiatry
Harvard Medical School
Boston, Massachusetts
8 Mood Disorders: Depression and Bipolar Disorder

CHRISTOPHER M. CELANO, MD
Associate Director
Cardiac Psychiatry Research Program
Department of Psychiatry
Massachusetts General Hospital;
Associate Professor
Department of Psychiatry
Harvard Medical School
Boston, Massachusetts
*24 The Psychiatric Management of Patients With
Cardiac Disease*
*49 Approaches to Collaborative Care and Behavioral
Health Integration*

PRANGTHIP CHAROENPONG, MD, MPH
Assistant Professor
Department of Pulmonary and Critical Care Medicine
Louisiana State University Health Sciences Center at
   Shreveport
Shreveport, Louisiana;
Assistant Professor
Department of Pulmonary and Critical Care Medicine
Baylor College of Medicine
Houston, Texas
31 Pulmonary Disease

ZEINA CHEMALI, MD, MPH
Director
Neuropsychiatry Clinics and Education
Department of Psychiatry,
Director, McCance Center for Brain Health
Department of Neurology
Massachusetts General Hospital;
Associate Professor
Departments of Neurology and Psychiatry
Harvard Medical School
Boston, Massachusetts
51 Global Psychiatry and Mental Healthcare Delivery

JUSTIN A. CHEN, MD, MPH
Vice Chair of Ambulatory Services,
Vice Chair of Health Justice,
Associate Professor of Clinical Psychiatry
Department of Psychiatry
Weill Cornell Medicine/New York-Presbyterian
New York, New York
47 Culture and Psychiatry
*49 Approaches to Collaborative Care and Behavioral
Health Integration*

AMIT CHOPRA, MBBS
Psychiatrist
Massachusetts General Hospital;
Assistant Professor
Department of Psychiatry
Harvard Medical School
Boston, Massachusetts
22 Patients With Disordered Sleep

JONAH N. COHEN, PhD
Psychologist
Department of Psychiatry
Massachusetts General Hospital;
Assistant Professor
Department of Psychiatry
Harvard Medical School
Boston, Massachusetts
*34 Coping With Medical Illness and Psychotherapy of
the Medically Ill*

LEE S. COHEN, MD
Director
Ammon-Pinizzotto Center for Women's Mental
   Health
Massachusetts General Hospital;
Edmund and Carroll Carpenter Professor of Psychiatry
Department of Psychiatry
Harvard Medical School
Boston, Massachusetts
*46 Psychiatric Illness During Pregnancy and the
Postpartum Period*

MARY KATHRYN COLVIN, PhD, ABPP
Director
Learning and Emotional Assessment Program
Department of Psychiatry
Massachusetts General Hospital;
Assistant Professor of Psychology
Department of Psychiatry
Harvard Medical School
Boston, Massachusetts
*6 Psychological and Neuropsychological Assessment in
the Medical Setting*

NKECHI T. CONTEH, MBBS, MPH
Psychiatrist
Boston Medical Center;
Program Director
Psychiatry Residency Program
Boston University Medical Center;
Instructor in Psychiatry
Department of Psychiatry
Boston Medical Center
Boston, Massachusetts
51 Global Psychiatry and Mental Healthcare Delivery

M. CORNELIA CREMENS, MD, MPH
Geriatric Psychiatrist
Department of Psychiatry
Massachusetts General Hospital;
Assistant Professor
Department of Psychiatry
Harvard Medical School
Boston, Massachusetts
44 Geriatric Psychiatry
45 Care at the End of Life

CRISTINA CUSIN, MD
Psychiatrist
Department of Psychiatry
Massachusetts General Hospital;
Associate Professor
Department of Psychiatry
Harvard Medical School
Boston, Massachusetts
36 Device Neuromodulation and Brain Stimulation Therapies

ABIGAIL L. DONOVAN, MD
Director
Child Psychiatry Emergency Services,
Associate Director
Acute Psychiatry Service,
Director
First Episode and Early Psychosis Program
Massachusetts General Hospital;
Assistant Professor
Department of Psychiatry
Harvard Medical School
Boston, Massachusetts
11 Patients With Psychosis
35 Resilience, Wellness, and Coping With the Rigors of Psychiatric Practice
42 Care of the Patient With Thoughts of Suicide
43 Emergency Psychiatry

DARIN D. DOUGHERTY, MD, MSc
Director
Division of Neurotherapeutics
Department of Psychiatry
Massachusetts General Hospital;
Associate Professor
Department of Psychiatry
Harvard Medical School
Boston, Massachusetts
36 Device Neuromodulation and Brain Stimulation Therapies

KAMRYN T. EDDY, PhD
Co-Director
Eating Disorders Clinical and Research Program
Massachusetts General Hospital;
Associate Professor
Department of Psychiatry
Harvard Medical School
Boston, Massachusetts
16 Eating Disorders

ANASTASIA B. EVANOFF, MD
Psychiatrist
Department of Psychiatry
McLean Hospital;
Instructor
Department of Psychiatry
Harvard Medical School
Boston, Massachusetts
29 COVID-19 Infection

A. EDEN EVINS, MD, MPH
Director
Center for Addiction Medicine
Department of Psychiatry
Massachusetts General Hospital;
William Cox Family Professor of Psychiatry in the Field of Addiction Medicine
Harvard Medical School
Boston, Massachusetts
39 Chronic Disease and Unhealthy Lifestyle Behaviors: Behavioral Management

MAURIZIO FAVA, MD
Psychiatrist-in-Chief
Department of Psychiatry,
Vice Chair
Executive Committee on Research,
Executive Director
Clinical Trials Network and Institute
Massachusetts General Hospital;
Associate Dean for Clinical and Translational Research
Slater Family Professor of Psychiatry
Harvard Medical School
Boston, Massachusetts
7 Diagnostic Rating Scales, Procedures, and Laboratory Tests
8 Mood Disorders: Depression and Bipolar Disorder
37 Psychopharmacology in the Medical Setting

CARLOS G. FERNANDEZ-ROBLES, MD, MBA
Chief
Department of Psychiatry
Brigham and Women's Faulkner Hospital
Jamaica Plain, Massachusetts;
Vice Chair of Faulkner Psychiatry
Department of Psychiatry
Brigham and Women's Hospital;
Assistant Professor
Department of Psychiatry
Harvard Medical School
Boston, Massachusetts
30 Patients With Cancer
36 Device Neuromodulation and Brain Stimulation
Therapies

CHRISTINE T. FINN, MD
Medical Director and Vice Chair for Clinical Services
Department of Psychiatry
Dartmouth Hitchcock Medical Center;
Associate Professor
Department of Psychiatry
Geisel School of Medicine
Lebanon, New Hampshire
33 Patients With Genetic Syndromes

ALICE W. FLAHERTY, MD, PhD
Attending Physician
Department of Neurology
Massachusetts General Hospital;
Associate Professor
Departments of Neurology and Psychiatry
Harvard Medical School
Boston, Massachusetts
19 Patients With Abnormal Movements

ELIZABETH PEGG FRATES, MD
Director of Wellness Programming
Physical Medicine and Rehabilitation
Spaulding Rehabilitation Hospital
Charlestown, Massachusetts;
Assistant Professor, Part-time
Department of Physical Medicine and Rehabilitation
Harvard Medical School
Boston, Massachusetts
39 Chronic Disease and Unhealthy Lifestyle Behaviors:
Behavioral Management

MARLENE P. FREEMAN, MD
Associate Director
Perinatal and Reproductive Psychiatry Program,
Professor
Department of Psychiatry
Harvard Medical School
Boston, Massachusetts
46 Psychiatric Illness During Pregnancy and the
Postpartum Period

OLIVER FREUDENREICH, MD
Co-Director
MGH Psychosis Clinical and Research Program
Department of Psychiatry
Massachusetts General Hospital;
Professor of Clinical Psychiatry
Department of Psychiatry
Harvard Medical School
Boston, Massachusetts
11 Patients With Psychosis
19 Patients With Abnormal Movements

GREGORY L. FRICCHIONE, MD
Associate Chief
Department of Psychiatry,
Director
Benson-Henry Institute for Mind-Body Medicine;
Director Emeritus
Division of Psychiatry and Medicine
Massachusetts General Hospital;
Professor
Department of Psychiatry
Harvard Medical School
Boston, Massachusetts
21 Catatonia, Neuroleptic Malignant Syndrome, and
Serotonin Syndrome
39 Chronic Disease and Unhealthy Lifestyle Behaviors:
Behavioral Management
51 Global Psychiatry and Mental Healthcare Delivery

JENNIFER R. GATCHEL, MD, PhD
Assistant Psychiatrist
Department of Psychiatry
Massachusetts General Hospital/McLean Hospital;
Assistant Professor
Department of Psychiatry
Harvard Medical School
Boston, Massachusetts
10 Patients With Neurocognitive Disorders

Bizu Gelaye, PhD, MPH
Associate Professor
Department of Psychiatry
Harvard Medical School;
Associate Professor
Department of Epidemiology
Harvard T.H. Chan School of Public Health
Boston, Massachusetts
51 Global Psychiatry and Mental Healthcare Delivery

Anna M. Georgiopoulos, MD
Consulting Psychiatrist
Cystic Fibrosis Program
Massachusetts General Hospital;
Associate Professor
Department of Psychiatry
Harvard Medical School
Boston, Massachusetts
31 Pulmonary Disease

Sharmin Ghaznavi, MD, PhD
Psychiatrist
Department of Psychiatry,
Associate Director and Director of Cognitive
    Neuroscience
The Center for the Neuroscience of Psychedelics
Massachusetts General Hospital;
Instructor
Department of Psychiatry
Harvard Medical School
Boston, Massachusetts
8 Mood Disorders: Depression and Bipolar Disorder

Taha Gholipour, MD
Neurologist
Departments of Neurology and Neurosurgery
The George Washington University Epilepsy Center
Washington, District of Columbia
*18 Neuropsychiatric Conditions: Seizures, Headaches,
Stroke Syndromes, and Traumatic Brain Injuries*

Alexandra K. Gold, PhD
Clinical Fellow in Psychology
Department of Psychiatry
Massachusetts General Hospital;
Clinical Fellow
Department of Psychiatry
Harvard Medical School
Boston, Massachusetts
8 Mood Disorders: Depression and Bipolar Disorder

Christopher D. Gordon, MD
Psychiatrist
Department of Psychiatry
Massachusetts General Hospital;
Associate Professor
Department of Psychiatry
Harvard Medical School
Boston, Massachusetts
2 The Doctor-Patient Relationship
3 The Psychiatric Interview

Donna B. Greenberg, MD
Psychiatrist
Department of Psychiatry
Massachusetts General Hospital;
Associate Professor
Department of Psychiatry
Harvard Medical School
Boston, Massachusetts
*14 Somatic Symptom and Related Disorders and
Functional Somatic Syndromes*
15 Factitious Disorders and Malingering
30 Patients With Cancer

Joseph A. Greer, PhD
Co-Director
Cancer Outcomes Research and Education
    Program
Massachusetts General Hospital;
Associate Professor of Psychology
Department of Psychiatry
Harvard Medical School
Boston, Massachusetts
30 Patients With Cancer

James E. Groves, MD
Psychiatrist
Department of Psychiatry
Massachusetts General Hospital;
Associate Professor
Department of Psychiatry
Harvard Medical School
Boston, Massachusetts
41 Difficult Patients

VICTORIA A. GRUNBERG, MS, PhD
Clinical Psychologist
Department of Psychiatry
Massachusetts General Hospital;
Assistant Professor of Psychology
Department of Psychiatry
Harvard Medical School
Boston, Massachusetts
53 Building Interdisciplinary Collaborations Across Healthcare Settings

G. KYLE HARROLD, MD
Assistant in Neurology
Department of Neurology
Massachusetts General Hospital;
Clinical Instructor
Department of Neurology
Brigham and Women's Hospital;
Instructor
Department of Neurology
Harvard Medical School
Boston, Massachusetts
20 Infectious or Inflammatory Neuropsychiatric Impairment

ERIC P. HAZEN, MD
Director
Pediatric Psychiatry Consultation Service
Department of Psychiatry
Massachusetts General Hospital;
Assistant Professor
Department of Psychiatry
Harvard Medical School
Boston, Massachusetts
38 Psychiatric Consultation to Children and Adolescents

MICHAEL E. HENRY, MD
Director
Somatic Therapy Service
Department of Psychiatry
Massachusetts General Hospital;
Associate Professor
Department of Psychiatry
Harvard Medical School
Boston, Massachusetts
36 Device Neuromodulation and Brain Stimulation Therapies

CHARLOTTE S. HOGAN, MD
Psychiatrist
Department of Psychiatry
Massachusetts General Hospital;
Instructor
Department of Psychiatry
Harvard Medical School
Boston, Massachusetts
7 Diagnostic Rating Scales, Procedures, and Laboratory Tests
46 Psychiatric Illness During Pregnancy and the Postpartum Period

JULIA E. HOOKER, PhD
Clinical Fellow in Psychology
Department of Psychiatry
Massachusetts General Hospital;
Clinical Fellow in Psychology
Department of Psychiatry
Harvard Medical School
Boston, Massachusetts
53 Building Interdisciplinary Collaborations Across Healthcare Settings

JEFFERY C. HUFFMAN, MD
Director
Clinical Services
Department of Psychiatry,
Director
Cardiac Psychiatry Research Program
Department of Psychiatry
Massachusetts General Hospital;
Professor
Department of Psychiatry
Harvard Medical School
Boston, Massachusetts
18 Neuropsychiatric Conditions: Seizures, Headaches, Stroke Syndromes, and Traumatic Brain Injuries
21 Catatonia, Neuroleptic Malignant Syndrome, and Serotonin Syndrome
24 The Psychiatric Management of Patients With Cardiac Disease

KELLY EDWARDS IRWIN, MD, MPH
Director
Collaborative Care and Community Engagement
  Program
Center for Psychiatric Oncology and Behavioral Sciences
Massachusetts General Hospital;
Assistant Professor
Department of Psychiatry
Harvard Medical School
Boston, Massachusetts
30 Patients With Cancer

ANA IVKOVIC, MD
Psychiatrist
Department of Psychiatry
Massachusetts General Hospital;
Assistant Professor
Department of Psychiatry
Harvard Medical School
Boston, Massachusetts
25 Patients With Kidney Disease
40 Complementary Medicine and Natural Medications
43 Emergency Psychiatry

JAMIE M. JACOBS, PhD
Program Director
Center for Psychiatric Oncology and Behavioral Sciences
Massachusetts General Hospital Cancer Center;
Assistant Professor of Psychology
Department of Psychiatry
Harvard Medical School
Boston, Massachusetts
30 Patients With Cancer

FELIPE A. JAIN, MD
Psychiatrist and Director
Healthy Aging Studies
Depression Clinical and Research Program
Department of Psychiatry
Massachusetts General Hospital;
Member of the Faculty
Health Sciences and Technology
Harvard-Massachusetts Institute of Technology;
Assistant Professor
Department of Psychiatry
Harvard Medical School
Boston, Massachusetts
35 Resilience, Wellness, and Coping With the Rigors of
Psychiatric Practice

GRETA JANKAUSKAITE, MA, MS
Clinical Fellow
Department of Psychiatry
Massachusetts General Hospital;
Clinical Fellow
Harvard Medical School
Boston, Massachusetts
30 Patients With Cancer

JAMES L. JANUZZI, JR., MD
Physician
Department of Cardiology
Massachusetts General Hospital;
Hutter Family Professor of Medicine
Harvard Medical School;
Chief Scientific Officer
Baim Institute for Clinical Research
Boston, Massachusetts
24 The Psychiatric Management of Patients With
Cardiac Disease

KATE N. JOCHIMSEN, PhD, ATC
Researcher
Center for Health Outcomes and Interdisciplinary
  Research
Massachusetts General Hospital;
Member of the Faculty
Department of Psychiatry
Harvard Medical School
Boston, Massachusetts
53 Building Interdisciplinary Collaborations Across
Healthcare Settings

MASOUD KAMALI, MD
Psychiatrist
Department of Psychiatry
Massachusetts General Hospital;
Assistant Professor
Department of Psychiatry
Harvard Medical School
Boston, Massachusetts
8 Mood Disorders: Depression and Bipolar Disorder

TAMAR C. KATZ, MD, PhD
Attending in Neuropsychiatry
Boston Children's Hospital;
Instructor
Department of Psychiatry
Harvard Medical School
Boston, Massachusetts
33 Patients With Genetic Syndromes

ALEX S. KEUROGHLIAN, MD, MPH
Associate Chief
Public and Community Psychiatry
Michele and Howard J. Kessler Chair and
    Director
MGH Division of Public and Community
    Psychiatry
Massachusetts General Hospital;
Associate Professor of Psychiatry
Department of Psychiatry
Harvard Medical School
Boston, Massachusetts
50 Community Psychiatry
52 Care of LGBTQIA+ Patients

HYUN-HEE KIM, MD
Psychiatrist
Department of Psychiatry
Massachusetts General Hospital;
Instructor
Department of Psychiatry
Harvard Medical School
Boston, Massachusetts
50 Community Psychiatry
52 Care of LGBTQIA+ Patients

YOUNGJUNG RACHEL KIM, MD, PhD
Psychiatrist
Department of Psychiatry
Massachusetts General Hospital;
Instructor
Department of Psychiatry
Harvard Medical School
Boston, Massachusetts
16 Eating Disorders

FRANKLIN KING IV, MD
Psychiatrist
Department of Psychiatry
Massachusetts General Hospital;
Instructor
Department of Psychiatry
Harvard Medical School
Boston, Massachusetts
10 Patients With Neurocognitive Disorders
41 Difficult Patients

KATHERINE A. KOH, MD, MSc
Psychiatrist
Department of Psychiatry
Massachusetts General Hospital;
Assistant Professor
Department of Psychiatry
Harvard Medical School
Boston, Massachusetts
42 Care of the Patient With Thoughts of Suicide

SAMUEL I. KOHRMAN, MD
Psychiatrist and Medical Director
Inpatient Psychiatric Service
Department of Psychiatry
Massachusetts General Hospital;
Instructor
Department of Psychiatry
Harvard Medical School
Boston, Massachusetts
18 Neuropsychiatric Conditions: Seizures, Headaches,
Stroke Syndromes, and Traumatic Brain Injuries
25 Patients With Kidney Disease
26 Patients With Gastrointestinal Disease

NICHOLAS KONTOS, MD
Program Director
Fellowship in Consultation–Liaison Psychiatry
Department of Psychiatry
Massachusetts General Hospital;
Assistant Professor
Department of Psychiatry
Harvard Medical School
Boston, Massachusetts
4 Limbic Music
14 Somatic Symptom and Related Disorders and
Functional Somatic Syndromes
15 Factitious Disorders and Malingering

CAROL LIM, MD, MPH
Medical Director
MGH Clozapine Clinic
Department of Psychiatry
Massachusetts General Hospital;
Instructor
Department of Psychiatry
Harvard Medical School
Boston, Massachusetts
11 Patients With Psychosis

JENNY J. LINNOILA, MD, PHD
Neurologist
Department of Neurology
Division of Neuroimmunology and Multiple Sclerosis
University of Pittsburgh Medical Center;
Associate Professor
Department of Neurology
University of Pittsburgh School of Medicine
Pittsburgh, Pennsylvania
20 Infectious or Inflammatory Neuropsychiatric Impairment

JAMES LUCCARELLI, MD, DPHIL
Psychiatrist
Massachusetts General Hospital;
Instructor
Department of Psychiatry
Harvard Medical School
Boston, Massachusetts
36 Device Neuromodulation and Brain Stimulation Therapies

ELIZABETH N. MADVA, MD
Psychiatrist
Massachusetts General Hospital;
Instructor
Department of Psychiatry
Harvard Medical School
Boston, Massachusetts
26 Patients With Gastrointestinal Disease

HEENA R. MANGLANI, PHD
Psychologist
Department of Psychiatry
Massachusetts General Hospital;
Instructor
Department of Psychiatry
Harvard Medical School
Boston, Massachusetts
53 Building Interdisciplinary Collaborations Across Healthcare Settings

THOMAS H. MCCOY, JR., MD
Director of Research
Center for Quantitative Health
Massachusetts General Hospital;
Assistant Professor
Departments of Psychiatry and Medicine
Harvard Medical School
Boston, Massachusetts
9 Delirium

KATHERINE A. MCDERMOTT, PHD
Clinical Research Fellow
Department of Psychiatry
Massachusetts General Hospital;
Clinical Fellow
Department of Psychiatry
Harvard Medical School
Boston, Massachusetts
53 Building Interdisciplinary Collaborations Across Healthcare Settings

DAVID MISCHOULON, MD, PHD
Psychiatrist and Director
Depression Clinical and Research Program
Department of Psychiatry
Massachusetts General Hospital;
Joyce R. Tedlow Professor of Psychiatry
Harvard Medical School
Boston, Massachusetts
7 Diagnostic Rating Scales, Procedures, and Laboratory Tests
8 Mood Disorders: Depression and Bipolar Disorder
37 Psychopharmacology in the Medical Setting
40 Complementary Medicine and Natural Medications

ALEJANDRA ELIZABETH MORFIN RODRIGUEZ, MD
Fellow in Consultation-Liaison Psychiatry
Massachusetts General Hospital;
Clinical Fellow
Department of Psychiatry
Harvard Medical School
Boston, Massachusetts
14 Somatic Symptom and Related Disorders and Functional Somatic Syndromes

SHAMIM H. NEJAD, MD, FASAM
Medical Director
Addiction Medicine and Psychiatry Consultation Services
Department of Psychiatry
University of Washington Medicine Valley Medical Center
Renton, Washington
17 Pain

AMY L. NEWHOUSE, MD
Psychiatrist
Department of Psychiatry,
Internist
Department of Medicine
Massachusetts General Hospital;
Instructor
Department of Psychiatry
Harvard Medical School
Boston, Massachusetts
29 COVID-19 Infection

ANDREW A. NIERENBERG, MD
Director
Dauten Family Center for Bipolar Clinic and Research
    Program,
Associate Director
Depression Clinical and Research Program
Massachusetts General Hospital;
Thomas P. Hackett, MD Professor of Psychiatry
Harvard Medical School
Boston, Massachusetts
8 Mood Disorders: Depression and Bipolar Disorder

MLADEN NISAVIC, MD
Director
Burns and Trauma Psychiatry
Department of Psychiatry
Massachusetts General Hospital;
Instructor
Department of Psychiatry
Harvard Medical School
Boston, Massachusetts
13 Substance Use Disorders
32 Burns, Trauma, and Intensive Care Unit Treatment

RUTA NONACS, MD, PhD
Psychiatrist
Department of Psychiatry
Massachusetts General Hospital;
Instructor
Department of Psychiatry
Harvard Medical School
Boston, Massachusetts
*46 Psychiatric Illness During Pregnancy and the
Postpartum Period*

MICHAEL J. OSTACHER, MD, MPH, MMSc
Director
Bipolar and Depression Research Program
Department of Psychiatry
VA Palo Alto Health Care System
Palo Alto, California;
Professor
Department of Psychiatry and Behavioral
    Sciences
Stanford University School of Medicine
Stanford, California
8 Mood Disorders: Depression and Bipolar Disorder

GEORGE I. PAPAKOSTAS, MD
Psychiatrist and Scientific Director
Clinical Trials Network,
Institute Director of Treatment-Resistant Depression
    Studies
Department of Psychiatry
Massachusetts General Hospital;
Professor
Department of Psychiatry
Harvard Medical School
Boston, Massachusetts
8 Mood Disorders: Depression and Bipolar Disorder

ELYSE R. PARK, PhD, MPH
Director
Behavioral Health Research
MGH Benson-Henry Mind-Body Medicine;
Director
Behavioral Sciences
MGH Tobacco Treatment and Research Center;
Department of Psychiatry
Massachusetts General Hospital and Mongan
    Institute;
Professor
Department of Psychiatry
Harvard Medical School
Boston, Massachusetts
*39 Chronic Disease and Unhealthy Lifestyle Behaviors:
Behavioral Management*

CELESTE PEAY, MD, JD
Assistant Professor
Department of Psychiatry
University of Southern California Keck School of
    Medicine
Los Angeles, California
48 Legal Aspects of Psychiatric Consultation

ADERONKE BAMGBOSE PEDERSON, MD
Psychiatrist
Department of Psychiatry
Massachusetts General Hospital;
Assistant Professor
Department of Psychiatry
Harvard Medical School
Boston, Massachusetts
47 Culture and Psychiatry

ROY H. PERLIS, MD, MSC
Director
Center for Quantitative Health
Massachusetts General Hospital;
Professor
Department of Psychiatry
Harvard Medical School
Boston, Massachusetts
8 Mood Disorders: Depression and Bipolar Disorder

AMY T. PETERS, PHD
Psychologist
Department of Psychiatry
Massachusetts General Hospital;
Assistant Professor of Psychology
Department of Psychiatry
Harvard Medical School
Boston, Massachusetts
8 Mood Disorders: Depression and Bipolar Disorder

LAURA M. PRAGER, MD
Chief
Child and Adolescent Psychiatry,
Vice Chair
Department of Psychiatry
Boston Medical Center;
Senior Psychiatrist
Department of Psychiatry
Boston Children's Hospital
Boston, Massachusetts
27 Organ Failure and Transplantation
43 Emergency Psychiatry

NATHAN PRASCHAN, MD, MPH
Psychiatrist
Department of Psychiatry
Brigham and Women's Hospital;
Psychiatrist
Department of Psychiatry
Massachusetts General Hospital;
Instructor
Department of Psychiatry
Harvard Medical School
Boston, Massachusetts
*21 Catatonia, Neuroleptic Malignant Syndrome, and
Serotonin Syndrome*

JEFFERSON B. PRINCE, MD
Director
Child Psychiatry,
Vice-Chair
Department of Psychiatry
Massachusetts General Brigham Salem Hospital
Salem, Massachusetts;
Psychiatrist
Department of Child Psychiatry
Massachusetts General Hospital;
Instructor
Department of Psychiatry
Harvard Medical School
Boston, Massachusetts
38 Psychiatric Consultation to Children and Adolescents

JULIA M. PROBERT, MD
Fellow
Consultation-Liaison Psychiatry
Department of Psychiatry
Massachusetts General Hospital;
Clinical Fellow
Department of Psychiatry
Harvard Medical School
Boston, Massachusetts
29 COVID-19 Infection

MARIA C. PROM, MD
Assistant Director
Training Development and Research
The Chester M. Pierce, MD Division of Global Psychiatry
Massachusetts General Hospital;
Instructor
Department of Psychiatry
Harvard Medical School
Boston, Massachusetts
51 Global Psychiatry and Mental Healthcare Delivery

DIANA PUNKO, MD, MS
Psychiatrist
Department of Psychiatry
Massachusetts General Hospital;
Instructor
Department of Psychiatry
Harvard Medical School
Boston, Massachusetts
43 Emergency Psychiatry

GIUSEPPE J. RAVIOLA, MD, MPH
Associate Director
The Chester M. Pierce, MD Division of Global Psychiatry
Department of Psychiatry
Massachusetts General Hospital;
Director
The Program in Global Mental Health and Social Change
Department of Global Health and Social Medicine,
Director
Mental Health Partners In Health;
Associate Professor
Department of Psychiatry
Harvard Medical School
Boston, Massachusetts
51 Global Psychiatry and Mental Healthcare Delivery

ELLEN M. ROBINSON, RN, PHD, HEC-C, FAAN
Nurse Ethicist
Patient Care Services, Institute for Patient Care;
Co-Chair
MGH Optimum Care (Ethics) Committee
Department of Medicine
Massachusetts General Hospital;
Nurse Scientist
Yvonne L. Munn Nursing Research Center
Massachusetts General Hospital
Boston, Massachusetts
45 Care at the End of Life

JOSHUA L. ROFFMAN, MD, MMSc
Co-Director
Mass General Neuroscience,
Director
Mass General Early Brain Development Initiative
Department of Psychiatry
Massachusetts General Hospital;
Associate Professor
Department of Psychiatry
Harvard Medical School
Boston, Massachusetts
7 Diagnostic Rating Scales, Procedures, and Laboratory Tests

DAVID H. RUBIN, MD
Director
Division of Professional and Public Education
Department of Psychiatry
Massachusetts General Hospital;
Dean
Continuing Education and Professional Development
Massachusetts General Hospital Institute of Health Professions
Charlestown, Massachusetts;
Executive Director
MGH Psychiatry Academy and MGH Visiting
Department of Psychiatry
Massachusetts General Hospital;
Assistant Professor
Department of Psychiatry
Harvard Medical School
Boston, Massachusetts
38 Psychiatric Consultation to Children and Adolescents

CHRISTINA L. RUSH, PHD
Psychologist
Department of Psychiatry
Massachusetts General Hospital;
Instructor
Department of Psychiatry
Harvard Medical School
Boston, Massachusetts
53 Building Interdisciplinary Collaborations Across Healthcare Settings

STEVEN C. SCHLOZMAN, MD
Division Chief
Child and Adolescent Psychiatry,
Associate Professor
Department of Psychiatry
University of Vermont
Burlington, Vermont
34 Coping With Medical Illness and Psychotherapy of the Medically Ill

RONALD SCHOUTEN, MD, JD
Director
Forensic Psychiatry Fellowship Program
Saint Elizabeth's Hospital
Washington, District of Columbia;
Associate Professor
Department of Psychiatry
Harvard Medical School
Boston, Massachusetts;
Affiliate Professor
Department of Psychiatry and Behavioral Sciences
Howard University College of Medicine
Washington, District of Columbia
48 Legal Aspects of Psychiatric Consultation

LINDA C. SHAFER, MD
Psychiatrist
Department of Psychiatry
Massachusetts General Hospital;
Assistant Professor
Department of Psychiatry
Harvard Medical School
Boston, Massachusetts
23 Sexual Disorders and Sexual Dysfunction

JENNIFER SHEETS, PsyD
Psychologist
Hematology/Oncology
Lahey Hospital and Medical Center
Burlington, Massachusetts;
Psychologist
Acute Psychiatry Service
Massachusetts General Hospital;
Instructor in Psychology
Department of Psychiatry
Harvard Medical School
Boston, Massachusetts
35 Resilience, Wellness, and Coping With the Rigors of Psychiatric Practice

YELIZAVETA SHER, MD
Director
Psychiatric and Psychological Services
Stanford Adult Cystic Fibrosis Program,
Clinical Professor
Psychiatry and Behavioral Sciences
Stanford University Medical Center
Stanford, California
31 Pulmonary Disease

JANET C. SHERMAN, PhD
Psychologist and Clinical Director
Psychology Assessment Center
Department of Psychiatry
Massachusetts General Hospital;
Associate Professor
Department of Psychiatry
Harvard Medical School
Boston, Massachusetts
6 Psychological and Neuropsychological Assessment in the Medical Setting
7 Diagnostic Rating Scales, Procedures, and Laboratory Tests

FELICIA A. SMITH, MD
Associate Chief
Department of Psychiatry,
Chief
MGH Division of Psychiatry and Medicine
Massachusetts General Hospital;
Assistant Professor
Department of Psychiatry
Harvard Medical School
Boston, Massachusetts
7 Diagnostic Rating Scales, Procedures, and Laboratory Tests
14 Somatic Symptom and Related Disorders and Functional Somatic Syndromes
15 Factitious Disorders and Malingering
18 Neuropsychiatric Conditions: Seizures, Headaches, Stroke Syndromes, and Traumatic Brain Injuries
19 Patients With Abnormal Movements
28 HIV Infection and AIDS
29 COVID-19 Infection
40 Complementary Medicine and Natural Medications
54 Management of a Psychiatric Consultation Service

EMILY M. SORG, MD
Psychiatrist
Center for Psychiatric Oncology and Behavioral Sciences
Massachusetts General Cancer Center;
Instructor
Department of Psychiatry
Harvard Medical School
Boston, Massachusetts
30 Patients With Cancer

THEODORE A. STERN, MD
Psychiatrist and Chief Emeritus
Avery D. Weisman Psychiatry Consultation Service,
Director
Thomas P. Hackett Center for Scholarship in
    Psychosomatic Medicine
Massachusetts General Hospital;
Ned H. Cassem Professor of Psychiatry in the Field of
    Psychosomatic Medicine/Consultation
Harvard Medical School
Boston, Massachusetts
*1 Approach to Psychiatric Consultation in the General
Hospital*
*7 Diagnostic Rating Scales, Procedures, and Laboratory
Tests*
8 Mood Disorders: Depression and Bipolar Disorder
9 Delirium
12 Pharmacotherapy of Anxiety Disorders
*18 Neuropsychiatric Conditions: Seizures, Headaches,
Stroke Syndromes, and Traumatic Brain Injuries*
*21 Catatonia, Neuroleptic Malignant Syndrome, and
Serotonin Syndrome*
22 Patients With Disordered Sleep
*24 The Psychiatric Management of Patients With
Cardiac Disease*
25 Patients With Kidney Disease
*34 Coping With Medical Illness and Psychotherapy of
the Medically Ill*
*35 Resilience, Wellness, and Coping With the Rigors of
Psychiatric Practice*
37 Psychopharmacology in the Medical Setting
42 Care of the Patient With Thoughts of Suicide
54 Management of a Psychiatric Consultation Service

JOAN M. STOLER, MD
Clinical Geneticist
Division of Genetics and Genomics
Boston Children's Hospital;
Associate Professor
Department of Pediatrics
Harvard Medical School
Boston, Massachusetts
33 Patients With Genetic Syndromes

LOUISA G. SYLVIA, PHD
Psychologist and Associate Director
Dauten Family Center for Bipolar Treatment Innovation
Department of Psychiatry,
Director
Office for Women's Careers
Massachusetts General Hospital;
Associate Professor
Department of Psychiatry
Harvard Medical School
Boston, Massachusetts
8 Mood Disorders: Depression and Bipolar Disorder

JOHN B. TAYLOR, MD, MBA
Psychiatrist
Acute Psychiatry Service
Avery D. Weisman Psychiatry Consultation Service
Massachusetts General Hospital;
Assistant Professor
Department of Psychiatry
Harvard Medical School;
Vice President,
Population Health and Executive,
Medical Director
Author Health
Boston, Massachusetts
54 Management of a Psychiatric Consultation Service

ROBYN P. THOM, MD
Psychiatrist
Lurie Center for Autism,
Co-Director
MGH Williams Syndrome Program
Department of Psychiatry
Massachusetts General Hospital;
Assistant Professor
Department of Psychiatry
Harvard Medical School
Boston, Massachusetts
38 Psychiatric Consultation to Children and Adolescents

EMMA M. TILLMAN, PHARMD, PHD
Research Associate Professor
Department of Medicine
Indiana University
Indianapolis, Indiana
31 Pulmonary Disease

NHI-HA TRINH, MD, MPH
Psychiatrist
Department of Psychiatry
Massachusetts General Hospital;
Associate Professor
Department of Psychiatry,
Associate Director
Hinton Society
Harvard Medical School
Boston, Massachusetts
47 Culture and Psychiatry

ANA-MARIA VRANCEANU, PHD
Director
Center for Health Outcomes and Interdisciplinary
    Research (CHOIR)
Department of Psychiatry
Massachusetts General Hospital;
David T. Rovee PhD and Joanne V. Rovee Endowed
    Chair in Psychiatry,
Professor of Psychology
Department of Psychiatry
Harvard Medical School
Boston, Massachusetts
*53 Building Interdisciplinary Collaborations Across
Healthcare Settings*

BETTY WANG, MD
Psychiatrist
Department of Psychiatry
Massachusetts General Hospital;
Instructor
Department of Psychiatry
Harvard Medical School
Boston, Massachusetts
*46 Psychiatric Illness During Pregnancy and the
Postpartum Period*

KHADIJAH BOOTH WATKINS, MD, MPH
Director
Child and Adolescent Psychiatry Residency Training,
Associate Director
The Clay Center for Young Healthy Minds
Department of Psychiatry
Massachusetts General Hospital/Harvard Medical School;
Instructor
Department of Psychiatry
Harvard Medical School
Boston, Massachusetts
38 Psychiatric Consultation to Children and Adolescents

MARC S. WEINBERG, MD, PHD
Psychiatrist
Department of Psychiatry
Massachusetts General Hospital;
Instructor
Department of Psychiatry
Harvard Medical School
Boston, Massachusetts
10 Patients With Neurocognitive Disorders

SYLVIE J. WEINSTEIN, BA
Clinical Research Assistant II
Center for Anxiety and Depression Research
McLean Hospital
Belmont, Massachusetts
31 Pulmonary Disease

ILSE R. WIECHERS, MD, MPP, MHS
Deputy Executive Director
VHA Office of Mental Health and Suicide
    Prevention
Department of Veterans Affairs
Washington, District of Columbia;
Associate Professor of Clinical Psychiatry
Department of Psychiatry and Behavioral
    Sciences
UCSF School of Medicine
San Francisco, California;
Associate Professor Adjunct of Psychiatry
Department of Psychiatry
Yale University School of Medicine
New Haven, Connecticut
10 Patients With Neurocognitive Disorders

JOHN W. WINKELMAN, MD, PHD
Chief
Sleep Disorders Clinical Research Program
Departments of Psychiatry and Neurology
Massachusetts General Hospital;
Professor
Department of Psychiatry
Harvard Medical School
Boston, Massachusetts
22 Patients With Disordered Sleep

ALBERT S. YEUNG, MD, ScD
Psychiatrist and Associate Director
Depression Clinical and Research Program
Massachusetts General Hospital;
Professor of Psychiatry, Part-time
Department of Psychiatry
Harvard Medical School
Boston, Massachusetts
47 Culture and Psychiatry
49 Approaches to Collaborative Care and Behavioral Health Integration

JULIANA ZAMBRANO, MD, MPH
Resident Physician
Department of Psychiatry
Massachusetts General Hospital;
Clinical Fellow
Department of Psychiatry
Harvard Medical School
Boston, Massachusetts
24 The Psychiatric Management of Patients With Cardiac Disease

PREFACE

This eighth edition, revised, updated, and substantially expanded, was put together by a stalwart group of general hospital psychiatrists and psychologists. Our collective efforts culminated in this 54-chapter book; although it was written by more than 100 authors (most from the Massachusetts General Hospital [MGH] Department of Psychiatry) it reads as though it has one "voice." New chapters (i.e., on COVID-19 Infection; Pulmonary Disease; Resilience, Wellness, and Coping With Burnout; Community Psychiatry; Global Psychiatry and Mental Healthcare Delivery; Care of LGBTQIA+ Patients; and Interdisciplinary Collaborations Across Healthcare Settings) have been added. This volume was designed to help practitioners care for their patients on medical and surgical floors and in outpatient practices filled with patients with co-morbid medical and psychiatric illness. As a result, our chapters were intended to be practical and were crafted for readability. Clinical vignettes have been placed throughout the book to act as a nidus around which clinical pearls would grow.

Consultation psychiatry, formerly known as "psychosomatic medicine," typically requires the rapid recognition, evaluation, and treatment of psychiatric problems in medical settings. Practitioners in this subspecialty must manage psychiatric reactions to medical illness, psychiatric complications of medical illness and its treatment, and psychiatric illness in those who suffer from medical or surgical illness. Because clinicians who work in general hospitals face problems related to the affective, behavioral, and cognitive (the "ABCs") realms of dementia, depression, anxiety, substance use disorders, disruptive personalities, and critical illness, an emphasis has been placed on successful management strategies that can be implemented by consultants and by the physicians of record to whom they consult.

To understand more about where the field is going, it is helpful to see where it began. Therefore we offer an historical context for the practice of consultation psychiatry and its growth at the MGH and beyond.

Psychosomatic medicine grew out of the long-recognized relationship between the psyche and the soma; certain ancient physicians (such as Hippocrates) have been eloquent on the subject. However, the search for the precise origins of psychosomatic medicine is a difficult undertaking unless one chooses to focus on the first use of the term itself. Johann Heinroth appears to have coined the term *psychosomatic* in reference to certain causes of insomnia in 1818.[1] The word *medicine* was added to *psychosomatic* first by the psychoanalyst Felix Deutsch in the early 1920s.[2] Deutsch later emigrated to the United States with his wife Helene, and both worked at the MGH for a time in the 1930s and 1940s.

Three streams of thought flowed into the area of psychosomatic medicine, providing fertile ground for the growth of general hospital and consultation psychiatry.[3,4] The psychophysiologic school, perhaps represented by the Harvard physiologist, Walter B. Cannon, emphasized the effects of stress on the body.[5] The psychoanalytic school, best personified by the psychoanalyst Franz Alexander, focused on the effects that psychodynamic conflicts had on the body.[6] The organic synthesis point of view was ambitiously pursued by Helen Flanders Dunbar, who tried with limited success to unify the physiologic and psychoanalytic approaches.[7] George Engel's biopsychosocial model[8] sought and seeks to apply not just these approaches but all branches of knowledge to health-related considerations. It has perhaps had more impact on medical education than on practice.[9] More recently, a higher overall profile for mind-body investigations practices has been evident in mainstream medicine.

The history of general hospital psychiatry in the United States in general,[10] and in consultation psychiatry,[11] has been extensively reviewed by Lipowski.[12-17]

In 2003 the American Board of Medical Specialties unanimously approved the American Board of Psychiatry and Neurology's (ABPN's) issuance of Subspecialty Certification in psychosomatic medicine.[18] The first certifying examinations were administered in 2005. As of 2009 the completion of an American Board of Medical Specialties–certified fellowship in psychosomatic medicine became mandatory for all who wish to sit for that examination. The achievement of subspecialty status for psychosomatic medicine was the product of nearly 75 years of clinical work by psychiatrists on medical-surgical units, an impressive accumulation of scholarly work contributing to the psychiatric care of general medical patients and determined intellectual and organizational efforts by the Academy of Psychosomatic Medicine (APM), now called the Academy of Consultation-Liaison Psychiatry.

Before 1975 scant attention was given to the work of psychiatrists in general hospitals. Consultation topics were seldom presented at the national meetings of the American Psychiatric Association. Even the American Psychosomatic Society, which has many strong links to consultation work, rarely gave more than a nod of acknowledgment to presentations or panels discussing this aspect of psychiatry. Residency training programs, in general, were not much better. Today, consultation-liaison (C-L) training is mandated by the ABPN as part of general adult psychiatry training.

Several factors account for the growth of C-L psychiatry in the last quarter of the 20th century. One was the leadership of Dr. James Eaton, former director of the Psychiatric Education Branch of the National Institute of Mental Health (NIMH). Eaton provided the support and encouragement that enabled the creation of C-L programs throughout the United States. Another reason for this growth was the burgeoning interest in primary care, which required skills in psychiatric diagnosis and treatment. Finally, parallel yet related threats to the viability of the psychiatric profession from third-party payers and non-physician providers were an incentive to (re-)medicalize the field. For these reasons and because of expanding knowledge in neuropsychiatry, consultation work enjoyed a renaissance.

The origins of organized interest in the mental lives of patients at the MGH dates to 1873, when James Jackson Putnam, a young Harvard neurologist, returned from his grand tour of German Departments of Medicine to practice his specialty. He was awarded a small office under the arch of one of the famous twin flying staircases of the Bulfinch Building. The office was the size of a cupboard and was designed to house electrical equipment. Putnam was given the title of "electrician." One of his duties was to ensure the proper function of various galvanic and faradic devices that were then used to treat nervous and muscular disorders. It is no coincidence that his office came to be called the "cloaca maxima" by Professor of Medicine George Shattuck. This designation stemmed from the fact that patients whose maladies defied diagnosis and treatment—in short, referred to as the "crocks"—were referred to young Putnam. With such a beginning, it is not difficult for today's consultation psychiatrist to relate to Putnam's experience and mission. Putnam eventually became a Professor of Neuropathology and practiced both neurology and psychiatry, treating medical and surgical patients who developed mental disorders. Putnam's distinguished career, interwoven with the acceptance of Freudian psychology in the United States, is chronicled elsewhere.[19]

In the late 1920s, Dr. Howard Means, Chief of Medicine, appointed Boston psychiatrist William Herman to study patients who developed mental disturbances in conjunction with endocrine disorders. Herman's studies are hardly remembered today, although he was honored by having a conference room at the MGH named after him.

In 1934 the Department of Psychiatry took shape when Stanley Cobb was given the Bullard Chair of Neuropathology and granted some money by the Rockefeller Foundation to establish a ward for the study of psychosomatic conditions. Under Cobb's tutelage, the Department expanded and became known for its eclecticism and for its interest in the mind-brain relationship. Several European emigrants fled Nazi tyranny and were welcomed to the department by Cobb. Felix and Helene Deutsch, Edward and Grete Bibring, and Hans Sachs were early arrivals from the continent. Erich Lindemann came in the mid-1930s and worked with Cobb on a series of projects, the most notable being his study of grief, which came as a result of his work with victims of the 1942 Cocoanut Grove nightclub fire.

When Lindemann became Chief of the Psychiatric Service in 1954, the Consultation Service had not yet been established. Customarily, the resident assigned to night call in the emergency department saw all medical and surgical patients in need of psychiatric evaluation. This was regarded as an onerous task, and such calls were often set aside until after supper in the hope that the disturbance might quiet in the intervening hours. Notes in the chart were terse and often impractical. Seldom was there any follow-up. As a result, animosity toward psychiatry grew. To remedy this, Lindemann officially established the Psychiatric Consultation Service under the leadership of Avery Weisman in 1956. Weisman's resident, Thomas Hackett, divided his time between doing consultations and learning outpatient psychotherapy. During the first year of the consultation service, 130 consultations were performed. In 1958 the number of consultations increased to 370, and an active research program was organized that later became one of the cornerstones of the overall operation and part of its legacy of scholarship.

By 1960 a rotation through the Consultation Service had become a mandatory part of the MGH's psychiatric residency. Second-year residents were each assigned two wards. Each resident spent 20 to 30 hours a week on the Consultation Service for 6 months. Between 1956 and 1960 the service attracted the interest of fellowship students, who contributed postgraduate work on psychosomatic topics. Medical students also began to choose the Consultation Service as part of their elective in psychiatry during this period. From our work with these fellows and medical students, collaborative research studies were initiated with other services. Examples of these early studies are the surgical treatment of intractable pain,[20,21] the compliance of patients with duodenal ulcer with their medical regimen,[22] post-amputation depression in the elderly patient,[23] emotional maladaptation in the surgical patient,[24-27] and the psychological aspects of acute myocardial infarction.[28,29]

By 1970 Hackett, then Chief of the Consultation Service, had one full-time (postgraduate year [PGY]-IV) chief resident and six half-time (PGY-III) residents to see consultations from the approximately 400 house beds. A private Psychiatric Consultation Service was begun to systematize consultations for the 600 private beds of the hospital. A Somatic Therapies Service was created; it offered electroconvulsive therapy to treat refractory conditions. Three fellows and a full-time faculty member were added to the roster in 1976. Edwin (Ned) Cassem became Chief of the Consultation Service, and George Murray was appointed director of a new fellowship program in psychosomatic medicine. In 1995 Theodore A. Stern was named Chief of the Avery Weisman Psychiatric Consultation Service, followed by Felicia A. Smith in 2017. Now, fellows and residents take consultations in rotation from throughout the hospital. Our Child Psychiatry Division, composed of residents, fellows, and attending physicians, provides full consultation to the 50 beds of the MGH Hospital for Children.

In July 2002 Gregory Fricchione was appointed director of the new Division of Psychiatry and Medicine, with a mission to integrate the various inpatient and outpatient medical-psychiatry services at the MGH and its affiliates, while maintaining the diverse characteristics and strengths of each unit. The Division, now also directed by Felicia A. Smith since 2017, includes the Avery D. Weisman Psychiatric Consultation Service; the MGH Center for Psychiatric Oncology and Behavioral Sciences at the MGH Cancer Center; the Transplant Psychiatry Consultation Service; the Trauma and Burns Psychiatry Service; the HIV and Infectious Disease Psychiatry Service; the Primary Care Psychiatry Service; the Pain Center Psychiatry Service; the Cardiovascular Disease Prevention Center Service; and the Spaulding Rehabilitation Hospital's Behavioral and Mental Health Service.

THE CONSULTATION SERVICE

The three functions provided by any consultation service are patient care, teaching, and research.

Patient Care

At the MGH, between 11% and 13% of all inpatients are followed by a Psychiatric Consultation Service psychiatrist; more than 3500 initial consultations are performed each year. The service includes subspecialty inpatient consultation teams specific to psycho-oncology, burns, and trauma surgery. An additional 10% of inpatients with substance-related problems are seen by the Addictions Consultation Team. The problems discovered reflect the gamut of conditions listed in the *Diagnostic and Statistical Manual of Mental Disorders,* fifth edition[30]; however, the most common reasons for consultation are related to affective, behavioral, and cognitive problems (often associated with depression, delirium, anxiety, substance use disorders, character pathology, dementia, or medically unexplained symptoms) and the evaluation of capacity.

Patients are seen in consultation only at the request of another physician, who must write an order for the consultation. When performing a consultation, the psychiatrist, like any other physician, is expected to provide a diagnosis and treatment recommendations. This includes defining the reason for the consultation; reading the chart; gathering information from nurses and family members when indicated; interviewing the patient; performing the appropriate physical and neurologic examinations; writing a clear consultation note in the electronic medical record with a clinical impression and treatment plan; ordering or suggesting laboratory tests, procedures, and medications; speaking with the referring physician when indicated; and making follow-up visits until the patient's problems are resolved, the patient is discharged, or the patient dies.

The interviewing style, individual to begin with, is further challenged and refined in the consultation arena, where the psychiatrist is frequently presented with patients who typically did not ask to be seen and who are often put off by the very idea that a psychiatrist has been called. In addition, the lack of privacy in many patient care areas and the threat of acute illness often cause patients to be less forthcoming than under usual circumstances. The stigma of mental illness and the fear of illness are universal; they are part of every physician's territory, and each psychiatrist learns to deal with them in a unique way. Residents learn to coax cooperation from such patients by trial and error, by self-understanding, and by observing role models. Essential, however, are interest in the patient's medical situation and an approach that is comparable to that used by a rigorous and caring physician in any specialty. Each consultation can thus be viewed as an opportunity to provide care, to de-stigmatize mental illness, and to de-stigmatize psychiatry by personally representing it, via manner, tone, and examination, as a proper medical specialty.

Teaching

Teaching psychiatry to medical and surgical house officers on a formal basis can be challenging. More than 50 years ago, Lindemann, to educate medical house officers about the emotional problems of their patients, enlisted the help of several psychiatric luminaries from the Boston area. A series of biweekly lectures was announced, in which Edward and Grete Bibring, Felix and Helene Deutsch, Stanley Cobb, and Carl Binger, among others, shared their knowledge and skills. In the beginning, approximately one-fifth of the medical house officers attended. Attendance steadily dwindled in subsequent sessions until finally the psychiatry residents were required to attend to infuse the lecturers with enough spirit to continue. This might be alleged to illustrate disinterest or intimidation on the part of the non-psychiatric staff, but we think that such didactics were simply too far removed (geographically and philosophically) from their day-to-day work.

We believe that teaching, to be most effective and reliable, is best done at the bedside on a case-by-case basis. Each resident and fellow is paired with an attending physician for bedside supervision, and all new patients are interviewed by our consultation attending staff. Residents teach as well. Medical students, neurology residents, and other visiting trainees are supervised by PGY-III residents, the chief resident, the fellows, and our attending staff. Twice weekly, rounds are held with attendings, the chief resident, and the rest of the service. New and ongoing cases are discussed in significant depth, with a focus as much on an approach to the differential diagnosis as on medical knowledge and problem-solving. We value safety and efficacy more than speed.

Each group of trainees begins their 4-month half-time rotation with 25 introductory discussions of practical topics (e.g., how to perform a consultation; how to write the note; how to perform the neurologic or neuropsychological examination; the nature of normal and maladaptive coping; ruling out organic causes of psychiatric symptoms; the interface of psychiatry and oncology; diagnosing and managing delirium and dementia; using psychotropic medications in the medically ill; assessing decisional capacity; geriatric psychiatry; performing hypnosis; identifying factitious disorders and malingering; assessment and management of depression; anxiety; posttraumatic stress disorder; pain; substance use/abuse/withdrawal; and managing functional somatic symptoms) in tandem with presentations of new cases. In concert with the orientation series, we provide residents with relevant articles, with an annotated bibliography,[31] and with updates in psychosomatic medicine.[32] The overall curriculum is much like the one recommended by the APM's Task Force on Residency Training in C-L Psychiatry.[33]

Fellows also attend the rounds with Nicholas Kontos (Director), as well as a "deep bench" of former fellows who preside three times per week. In addition to routine staffing of cases, fellows see patients at the bedside, with senior attending staff weekly. Fellows have an additional 2 hours each week of didactic sessions on advanced topics of psychosomatic medicine, neuropsychiatry, leadership, service delivery, and guided readings in psychodynamics; they also attend the Department's monthly Morbidity and Mortality Conference and a professionalism seminar.[34] The Fellowship Program in psychosomatic medicine, largely under the leadership of Murray, is approaching its 50th year; it has trained more than 135 fellows as of this writing. Many graduates have gone on to direct C-L services and Departments of Psychiatry across the United States.

Every resident and fellow delivers two formal presentations (i.e., reviews of the literature on topics chosen by the presenter and elaborated on by a senior discussant). These high-quality weekly Psychosomatic Conferences also enhance speaking skills, lead to publications, and serve to crystalize the interests and expertise of our trainees.[35–71]

Research

Research activity by the Consultation Service, besides answering important questions, builds bridges between medical specialties. When physicians from other services are involved in research planning and when there is co-authorship of published accounts, friendships are bonded, and cross-disciplinary obstacles disappear. Eventually, multi-site collaborations will become possible. The general hospital population provides such a cornucopia of academic material that a consultation service would be missing a golden opportunity if it did not take advantage of it. Examples include multi-site studies, reviews, case reports, and conceptual papers (cited here and in the chapters that follow).[72–80]

Small projects are the cornerstone of larger ones.[81–93] So long as generativity is held as a value, research need not be funded through federal or state agencies, and scholarship need not be confined to research. Medical students can also become involved during their

month-long rotation on the service. These endeavors can be the starting point for larger investigations and, sometimes, for a career.

Once the direction of the consultation team has been pointed toward research, scholarship, and publication, productivity usually follows. One of the distressing roadblocks to publication is the poor writing skills of many physicians. One or two experienced attendees can serve as guides and as editors. For almost 45 years, we have held a biweekly writing seminar, in which attendees submit drafts of papers that are reviewed by the seminar group and Dr. Stern. The late Eleanor Hackett was pivotal in co-founding and co-running this group. All efforts seem worthwhile once the printed or digital page ends up before the authors' eyes. The pride of accomplishment compounds the excitement of the research and stimulates renewed academic efforts intended for publication in a broad array of journals.

RECENT DIRECTIONS

Perhaps inevitably, sub-specialization has created clinical niches (e.g., burns and trauma, intensive care, rehabilitation, oncology, substance use, obstetrics, gastroenterology, infectious diseases).

Connected with this trend, fueled by robust literature,[94–96] and codified in the Accreditation Council for Graduate Medical Education requirements for C-L psychiatry fellowship training, is the provision of "outpatient consultation" to primary care settings. These endeavors expand academic opportunities and introduce new logistical challenges to the administration of consultation psychiatry and psychosomatic medicine services.

C-L psychiatry, by virtue of the premium it places on effective communication with other specialties and systems, as well as on population health promotion and illness prevention, is well suited to facilitating global mental health and empowering patients.[97–118] At the MGH, these principles are core components of the Chester M. Pierce, MD, Division of Global Psychiatry, and of the Benson-Henry Institute for Mind-Body Medicine.

Curious physicians have always investigated the mysteries of the mind-body relationship. The energy of this intellectual enterprise led to the growth of general hospital psychiatry, initially aided by Rockefeller Foundation funding in 1934, as well as the development of consultation psychiatry, supported through the funding of Eaton's NIMH program in the 1970s and 1980s. Since then, psychosomatic medicine has matured and the field has grown.

At each step along the way, the MGH Psychiatric Consultation Service has played an important role. This book, which reviews the essentials of general hospital psychiatry, is a testimony to the caring, creativity, and diligence of those who have come before us.

Theodore A. Stern, MD
Scott R. Beach, MD
Felicia A. Smith, MD
Oliver Freudenreich, MD
Ana-Maria Vranceanu, PhD
Maurizio Fava, MD

REFERENCES

1. Heinroth JC. *Lehrbuch der Storungen des Seelenlebens*. FCW Vogel; 1818.
2. Deutsch F. Der gesunde und der kranke korper in psychoanalytischer betrachtun. *Int Zeit Psa*. 1922;8:290.
3. Heldt TJ. Psychiatric services in general hospitals. *Am J Psychiatry*. 1939;95:865–871.
4. Henry GW. Some modern aspects of psychiatry in general hospital practice. *Am J Psychiatry*. 1929;86:481–499.
5. Cannon WB. *Bodily Changes in Pain, Hunger, Fear, and Rage: An Account of Recent Researches Into the Function of Emotional Excitement*. Appleton; 1915.
6. Alexander F. *Psychosomatic Medicine: Its Principles and Applications*. Norton; 1950.
7. Powell RC. Helen Flanders Dunbar (1902–1959) and a holistic approach to psychosomatic problems—II: The role of Dunbar's nonmedical background. *Psychiatr Q*. 1978;50:144–157.
8. Engel GL. The need for a new medical model: a challenge for biomedicine. *Science*. 1977;196:129–136.
9. Kontos N. Biomedicine—menace or straw man? Reexamining the biopsychosocial argument. *Acad Med*. 2011;86:509–515.
10. Summergrad P, Hackett TP. Alan Gregg and the rise of general hospital psychiatry. *Gen Hosp Psychiatry*. 1987;9:439–445.
11. Schwab JJ. Consultation-liaison psychiatry: a historical overview. *Psychosomatics*. 1989(3):245–254.
12. Lipowski ZJ. Review of consultation psychiatry and psychosomatic medicine—I: General principles. *Psychosom Med*. 1967;29:153–171.
13. Lipowski ZJ. Review of consultation psychiatry and psychosomatic medicine:—II: Clinical aspects. *Psychosom Med*. 1967;29:201–224.
14. Lipowski ZJ. Review of consultation psychiatry and psychosomatic medicine—III: Theoretical issues. *Psychosom Med*. 1968;30:395–421.
15. Lipowski ZJ. Consultation-liaison psychiatry: an overview. *Am J Psychiatry*. 1974;131:623–630.
16. Lipowski ZJ. Psychiatric consultation: concepts and controversies. *Am J Psychiatry*. 1977;134:523–528.
17. Lipowski ZJ. Consultation-liaison psychiatry: the first half century. *Gen Hosp Psychiatry*. 1986;8:305–315.
18. Gitlin DF, Levenson JL, Lyketsos CG. Psychosomatic medicine: a new psychiatric subspecialty. *Psychosomatics*. 2004;28:4–11.
19. Hale NG. *Freud and the Americans*. Oxford University Press; 1971.
20. White JC, Sweet WH, Hackett TP. Radiofrequency leukotomy for the relief of pain. *Arch Neurol*. 1960;2:317–330.
21. Mark VH, Hackett TP. Surgical aspects of thalamotomy in the human. *Trans Am Neurol Assoc*. 1959;84:92–94.
22. Hernandez M, Hackett TP. The problem of nonadherence to therapy in the management of duodenal ulcer recurrences. *Am J Dig Dis*. 1962;7:1047–1060.
23. Caplan LM, Hackett TP. Prelude to death: emotional effects of lower limb amputation in the aged. *N Engl J Med*. 1963;269:1166–1171.
24. Weisman AD, Hackett TP. Psychosis after eye surgery: establishment of a specific doctor–patient relation and the prevention and treatment of black patch delirium. *N Engl J Med*. 1958;258:1284–1289.
25. Weisman AD, Hackett TP. Predilection to death: death and dying as a psychiatric problem. *Psychosom Med*. 1961;23:232–257.
26. Hackett TP, Weisman AD. Psychiatric management of operative syndromes—I: The therapeutic consultation and the effect of noninterpretive intervention. *Psychosom Med*. 1960;22:267–282.
27. Hackett TP, Weisman AD. Psychiatric management of operative syndromes—II: Psychodynamic factors in formulation and management. *Psychosom Med*. 1960;22:356–372.
28. Olin HS, Hackett TP. The denial of chest pain in thirty-two patients with acute myocardial infarction. *JAMA*. 1964;190:977–981.
29. Cassem NH, Hackett TP. Psychiatric consultation in a coronary care unit. *Ann Int Med*. 1971;75:9–14.
30. American Psychiatric Association. *Diagnostic and Statistical Manual of Mental Disorders*. 5th ed. American Psychiatric Press; 2013.
31. Cremens MC, Calabrese LV, Shuster JL, et al. The Massachusetts General Hospital annotated bibliography for residents training in consultation-liaison psychiatry. *Psychosomatics*. 1995;36:217–235.
32. Freudenreich O, Huffman JC, Sharpe M, et al. Updates in psychosomatic medicine: 2014. *Psychosomatics*. 2015;56:445–459.
33. Gitlin DF, Schindler BA, Stern TA, et al. Recommended guidelines for consultation-liaison psychiatric training in psychiatry residency programs: a report from the Academy of Psychosomatic Medicine Task Force on psychiatric residency training in consultation-liaison psychiatry. *Psychosomatics*. 1996;37:3–11.
34. Freudenreich O, Kontos N. Professionalism, physicianhood, and psychiatric practice: conceptualizing and implementing a senior psychiatry resident seminar in reflective and inspired doctoring. *Psychosomatics*. 2019;60(3):246–254.
35. Stern TA. Munchausen's syndrome revisited. *Psychosomatics*. 1980;21:329–336.
36. Jenike MA. Obsessive-compulsive disorders. *Compr Psychiatry*. 1983;24:99–115.

37. Pollack MH, Rosenbaum JF. The treatment of antidepressant induced side effects. *J Clin Psychiatry.* 1987;43:3–8.

38. Fava M, Copeland PM, Schweiger V, et al. Neurochemical abnormalities of anorexia nervosa and bulimia nervosa. *Am J Psychiatry.* 1989;146:963–971.

39. Peterson B, Summergrad P. Binswanger's disease—II: Pathogenesis of subcortical arteriosclerotic encephalopathy and its relation to other dementing processes. *J Geriatr Psychiatry Neurol.* 1989;2:171–181.

40. Cohen LS, Heller VL, Rosenbaum JF. Treatment guidelines for psychotropic use in pregnancy. *Psychosomatics.* 1989;30:25–33.

41. Stern TA, Prager LM, Cremens MC. Autognosis rounds for medical housestaff. *Psychosomatics.* 1993;34:1–7.

42. Calabrese LV, Stern TA. Neuropsychiatric manifestations of systemic lupus erythematosus. *Psychosomatics.* 1995;36:344–359.

43. Leiter F, Nierenberg AA, Sanders KM, et al. Discontinuation reactions following sertraline discontinuation. *Biol Psychiatry.* 1995;38:694–695.

44. Goldstein LE, Sporn J, Brown S, et al. New-onset diabetes mellitus and diabetic ketoacidosis associated with olanzapine treatment. *Psychosomatics.* 1999;40:438–443.

45. Kim HG, Schmahmann J, Sims K, et al. A neuropsychiatric presentation of mitochondrial myopathy, encephalopathy, lactic acidosis, and stroke-like episodes. *Medicine + Psychiatry.* 1999;2:3–9.

46. Lagomasino IT, Stern TA. "Steroid psychosis": the neuropsychiatric complications of glucocorticoid use. *Psychiatry + Medicine.* 2001;4:35–43.

47. Groves JE, Dunderdale BA, Stern TA. Celebrity patients, VIPs, and potentates. *Prim Care Companion J Clin Psychiatry.* 2002;4:215–223.

48. Freudenreich O, Stern TA. Clinical experience with the management of schizophrenia in the general hospital. *Psychosomatics.* 2003;44:12–23.

49. Huffman JC, Stern TA. The diagnosis and treatment of Munchausen's syndrome. *Gen Hosp Psychiatry.* 2003;25:358–363.

50. Maytal G, Stern TA. The desire for death in the setting of terminal illness: a case discussion. *Prim Care Companion J Clin Psychiatry.* 2006;8:299–305.

51. Jacobsen JC, Maytal G, Stern TA. Demoralization in medical practice. *Prim Care Companion J Clin Psychiatry.* 2007;9:139–143.

52. Bhuvaneswar CG, Chang G, Epstein LA, et al. Alcohol use during pregnancy: its prevalence and impact. *Prim Care Companion J Clin Psychiatry.* 2007;9:455–460.

53. Bhuvaneswar CG, Chang G, Epstein LA, et al. Cocaine and opioid use during pregnancy: prevalence and management. *Prim Care Companion J Clin Psychiatry.* 2008;10:59–65.

54. Gross AF, Smith FA, Stern TA. Dread complications of catatonia: a case discussion and review of the literature. *Prim Care Companion J Clin Psychiatry.* 2008;10:153–155.

55. Politte LC, Huffman JC, Stern TA. Neuropsychiatric manifestations of multiple sclerosis. *Prim Care Companion J Clin Psychiatry.* 2008;10:318–324.

56. Quinn DK, McGahee SM, Politte LC, et al. Complications of carbon monoxide poisoning: a case discussion and review of the literature. *Prim Care Companion J Clin Psychiatry.* 2009;11:74–79.

57. Palmieri JJ, Stern TA. Lies in the doctor–patient relationship. *Prim Care Companion J Clin Psychiatry.* 2009;11:163–168.

58. Quinn DK, Stern TA. Linezolid and serotonin syndrome. *Prim Care Companion J Clin Psychiatry.* 2009;11:353–356.

59. Zimmerman DJ, Stern TA. Offensive language in the general hospital. *Psychosomatics.* 2010;51:377–385.

60. Viron MJ, Stern TA. The impact of serious mental illness on health and healthcare. *Psychosomatics.* 2010;51:458–465.

61. Wei MH, Querques J, Stern TA. Teaching trainees about the practice of consultation-liaison psychiatry in the general hospital. *Psychiatr Clin North Am.* 2011;34:689–707.

62. Silverman BC, Stern TW, Gross AF, et al. Lewd, crude, and rude behavior: the impact of manners and etiquette in the general hospital. *Psychosomatics.* 2012;53:13–20.

63. Dubovsky A, Arvikar S, Stern TA, et al. The neuropsychiatric complications of glucocorticoid use: steroid psychosis revisited. *Psychosomatics.* 2012;53:103–115.

64. Bauer LK, Baggett TP, Stern TA, et al. Caring for homeless persons with serious mental illness in general hospitals. *Psychosomatics.* 2013;54:14–21.

65. Johnson JM, Nachtigall LB, Stern TA. The effect of testosterone levels on mood in men: a review. *Psychosomatics.* 2013;54:509–514.

66. Gross AF, Stern TA. Neuropsychiatric conditions associated with anesthesia exposure. *Psychosomatics.* 2013;55:21–28.

67. Johnson JM, Stern TA. Preparing psychiatrists for leadership roles in healthcare. *Acad Psychiatry.* 2013;37:297–300.

68. Gerstenblith TA, Stern TA. Lyme disease: a review of its epidemiology, evaluation, and treatment. *Psychosomatics.* 2014;55:421–429.

69. Rustad JK, Cho T, Chemali Z, et al. The recognition and treatment of rabies: a case report and discussion. *Psychosomatics.* 2015;56:196–201.

70. Bhuvaneswar C, Burke B, Matthews J, et al. Psychiatric care of deaf patients in the general hospital: an overview. *Psychosomatics.* 2015;56:1–11.

71. Lokko HN, Stern TA. Confrontations with difficult patients: the good, the bad, and the ugly. *Psychosomatics.* 2015;56:556–560.

72. Dec GW, Stern TA, Welch C. The effects of electroconvulsive therapy on serial electrocardiograms and serum cardiac enzymes: a prospective study of depressed hospitalized inpatients. *JAMA.* 1985;253:2525–2529.

73. Stern TA, Mulley AG, Thibault GE. Life-threatening drug overdose: precipitants and prognosis. *JAMA.* 1984;251:1983–1985.

74. Stern TA, O'Gara PT, Mulley AG, et al. Complications after overdose with tricyclic antidepressants. *Crit Care Med.* 1985;13:672–674.

75. Mahoney J, Gross PL, Stern TA, et al. Quantitative serum toxic screening in the management of suspected drug overdose. *Am J Emerg Med.* 1990;8:16–22.

76. Wilens TE, Stern TA, O'Gara PT. Adverse cardiac effects of combined neuroleptic ingestion and tricyclic antidepressant overdose. *J Clin Psychopharmacol.* 1990;10:51–54.

77. Stern TA, Gross PL, Pollack MH, et al. Drug overdose seen in the emergency department: assessment, disposition, and follow-up. *Ann Clin Psychiatry.* 1991;3:223–231.

78. Sanders KM, Stern TA, O'Gara PT, et al. Delirium during intra-aortic balloon pump therapy. Incidence and management. *Psychosomatics.* 1992;33:35–44.

79. Sanders KM, Stern TA, O'Gara PT, et al. Medical and psychiatric complications associated with the use of the intraaortic balloon pump. *J Intensive Care Med.* 1992;7:154–160.

80. Kalantarian S, Stern TA, Mansour M, et al. Cognitive impairment associated with atrial fibrillation. *Ann Int Med.* 2013;158:338–346.

81. Celano CM, Healy B, Suarez L, et al. Cost-effectiveness of a collaborative care depression and anxiety treatment program in patients with acute cardiac illness. *Value Health.* 2016;19:185–191.

82. Celano CM, Millstein RA, Bedoya CA, et al. Association between anxiety and mortality in patients with coronary artery disease: a meta-analysis. *Am Heart J.* 2015;170:1105–1115.

83. Huffman JC, Beale EE, Celano CM, et al. Effects of optimism and gratitude on physical activity, biomarkers, and readmissions after an acute coronary syndrome: The Gratitude Research in Acute Coronary Events Study. *Circ Cardiovasc Qual Outcomes.* 2016;9:55–63.

84. Beach SR, Walker J, Celano CM, et al. Implementing collaborative care programs for psychiatric disorders in medical settings: a practical guide. *Gen Hosp Psychiatry.* 2015;37:522–527.

85. Huffman JC, Beale EE, Beach SR, et al. Design and baseline data from the Gratitude Research in Acute Coronary Events (GRACE) study. *Contemp Clin Trials.* 2015;44:11–19.

86. Beach SR, Kostis WJ, Celano CM, et al. Meta-analysis of selective serotonin reuptake inhibitor-associated QTc prolongation. *J Clin Psychiatry.* 2014;75:e441–e449.

87. Huffman JC, Mastromauro CA, Beach SR, et al. Collaborative care for depression and anxiety disorders in patients with recent cardiac events: the Management of Sadness and Anxiety in Cardiology (MOSAIC) randomized clinical trial. *JAMA Intern Med.* 2014;174:927–935.

88. Beach SR, Chen DT, Huffman JC. Attitudes and beliefs of trainees and nurses regarding delirium in the intensive care unit. *Acad Psychiatry.* 2013;37:436–438.

89. Beach SR, Januzzi JL, Mastromauro CA, et al. Patient Health Questionnaire-9 score and adverse cardiac outcomes in patients hospitalized for acute cardiac disease. *J Psychosom Res.* 2013;75:409–413.

90. Bauer LK, Caro MA, Beach SR, et al. Effects of depression and anxiety improvement on adherence to medication and health behaviors in recently hospitalized cardiac patients. *Am J Cardiol.* 2012;109:1266–1271.

91. Celano CM, Mastromauro CA, Lenihan EC, et al. Association of baseline anxiety with depression persistence at 6 months in patients with acute cardiac illness. *Psychosom Med.* 2012;74:93–99.

92. Celano CM, Freudenreich O, Fernandez-Robles C, et al. Depressogenic effects of medications: a review. *Dialogues Clin Neurosci.* 2011;13:109–125.

93. Traeger L, Greer JA, Fernandez-Robles C, et al. Evidence-based treatment of anxiety in patients with cancer. *J Clin Oncol.* 2012;30:1197–1205.

94. Katon WJ, Roy-Byrne P, Russo J, et al. Cost-effectiveness and cost offset of a collaborative care intervention for primary care patients with panic disorder. *Arch Gen Psychiatry.* 2002;59:1098–1104.

95. Unutzer J, Schoenbaum M, Druss BG, et al. Transforming mental health care at the interface with general medicine: report for the president's commission. *Psychiatr Serv.* 2006;57:37–47.

96. Huffman JC, Niazi SK, Rundell JR, et al. Essential articles on collaborative care models for the treatment of psychiatric disorders in medical settings: a publication by the Academy of Psychosomatic Medicine Research and Evidence-based Practice Committee. *Psychosomatics.* 2014;55:109–122.

97. Stern TA, Sekeres MA, eds. *Facing Cancer: A Complete Guide for People With Cancer, Their Families, and Caregivers.* McGraw Hill; 2004.

98. Beach Stern TA, Januzzi JL, eds. *Facing Heart Disease: A Guide for Patients and Their Families.* MGH Psychiatry Academy; 2018.

99. Wexler DJ, Celano CM, Stern TA, eds. *Facing Diabetes: A Guide for Patients and Their Families.* MGH Psychiatry Academy; 2018.

100. Stanford FC, Stevens JR, Stern TA, eds. *Facing Overweight and Obesity: A Complete Guide for Children and Adults.* MGH Psychiatry Academy; 2018.

101. Bolster MB, Stern TA, eds. *Facing Osteoporosis: A Guide for Patients and Their Families.* MGH Psychiatry Academy; 2020.

102. Bolster MB, Stern TA, eds. *Facing Scleroderma: A Guide for Patients and Their Families.* MGH Psychiatry Academy; 2020.

103. Bolster MB, Stern TA, eds. *Facing Lupus: A Guide for Patients and Their Families.* MGH Psychiatry Academy; 2020.

104. Bolster MB, Stern TA, eds. *Facing Rheumatoid Arthritis: A Guide for Patients and Their Families.* MGH Psychiatry Academy; 2020.

105. Kourosh AS, Stern TA, eds. *Facing Psoriasis: A Guide for Patients and Their Families.* MGH Psychiatry Academy; 2020.

106. Kourosh AS, Stern TA, eds. *Facing Eczema: A Guide for Patients and Their Families.* MGH Psychiatry Academy; 2020.

107. Kourosh AS, Stern TA, eds. *Facing Vitiligo: A Guide for Patients and Their Families.* MGH Psychiatry Academy; 2020.

108. Kourosh AS, Stern TA, eds. *Facing Acne: A Guide for Patients and Their Families.* MGH Psychiatry Academy; 2020.

109. Kourosh AS, Friedstat J, Stern TA, eds. *Facing Burns and Scars: A Guide for Patients and Their Families.* MGH Psychiatry Academy; 2020.

110. Sher Y, Georgiopoulos AM, Stern TA, eds. *Facing Cystic Fibrosis: A Guide for Patients and Their Families.* MGH Psychiatry Academy; 2020.

111. Reynolds KL, Cohen JV, Zubiri L, Stern TA, eds. *Facing Immunotherapy: A Guide for Patients and Their Families.* MGH Psychiatry Academy; 2020.

112. Sher Y, Stern TA, eds. *Facing Transplantation: A Guide for Patients and Their Families.* MGH Psychiatry Academy; 2020.

113. De EJB, Stern TA, eds. *Facing Pelvic Pain: A Guide for Patients and Their Families.* MGH Psychiatry Academy; 2021.

114. Wang JP, Tannyhill RJ, Stern TA, eds. *Facing Post-Operative Pain: A Guide for Patients and Their Families.* MGH Psychiatry Academy; 2020.

115. Chemali Z, Stern TA, eds. *Facing Memory Loss and Dementia: A Guide for Patients and Their Families.* MGH Psychiatry Academy; 2021.

116. Freudenreich O, Cather C, Stern TA. *Facing Serious Mental Illness: A Guide for Patients and Their Families.* MGH Psychiatry Academy; 2021.

117. Sher Y, Fishman J, Stern TA, eds. *Facing COVID-19: A Guide for Patients and Their Families.* MGH Psychiatry Academy; 2021.

118. Williams WW, Ivkovic A, Stern TA, eds. *Facing Chronic Kidney Disease: A Guide for Patients and Their Families.* MGH Psychiatry Academy; 2022.

ACKNOWLEDGMENTS

Without the contributions of so many physicians and related healthcare professionals, this book would never have been possible. We thank our chapter authors for their thoughtfulness and gifted writing, as well as their tolerance for our deadlines and edits. We thank our teachers and mentors for imbuing in us a sense of responsibility to educate, to write with rigor, and, most importantly, to provide exceptional care to our patients.

The eighth edition of this book would not have been possible without the steady hands of our editor, Mary Hegeler, and an experienced content development specialist, Lisa Barnes, both at Elsevier; to them we owe our deepest gratitude for overseeing the production of this book with grace and style.

CONTENTS

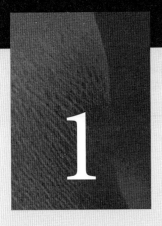

1

APPROACH TO PSYCHIATRIC CONSULTATIONS IN THE GENERAL HOSPITAL

THEODORE A. STERN, MD

■ ■

My emphasis to the residents is: 'Now that you've learned a lot about compassion and human dignity ... you must learn to be competent,' adding 'or else'. The goals for the trainee are specialty-competence, that is, some specific things about consultation: accountability, commitment, industry, discipline; these are the components that go into the make-up of a professional.

— Ned H. Cassem, MD[1]

This chapter provides a practical approach to the assessment of affective, behavioral, and cognitive problems experienced by general hospital patients. First we survey the landscape of consultation psychiatry and then identify six broad domains of psychiatric problems commonly encountered in medical settings. Next, we describe differences in the clinical approach, environment, interactive style, and use of language that distinguish psychiatry in general hospitals from practice in other venues. We then provide a step-by-step guide on how to conduct a psychiatric consultation. The chapter concludes with a review of treatment principles critical to caring for the medically ill. Throughout this chapter, we emphasize the hallmarks of competence identified by Cassem[1] nearly four decades ago: accountability, commitment, industry, and discipline.

CATEGORIES OF THE PSYCHIATRIC DIFFERENTIAL DIAGNOSIS IN GENERAL HOSPITALS

The borderland between psychiatry and medicine, where consultation psychiatrists ply their trade, can be visualized as the area shared by two intersecting ovals in a Venn diagram (Fig. 1.1). As depicted in the figure and consistent with the fundamental tenet of psychosomatic medicine (i.e., that mind and body are indivisible), the likelihood that either a psychiatric or a medical condition will have no impact on the other is incredibly slim. Within the overlapping area in the Venn diagram, the problems most commonly encountered on a consultation-liaison (C-L) service can be grouped into six categories (modified from Lipowski;[2] see Fig. 1.1). Examples of each classification follow.

Psychiatric Presentations of Medical Conditions

Case 1

An elderly man had an aneurysm of the anterior communicating artery clipped. Several days after his neurosurgical procedure, he became diaphoretic, confused, agitated, tachycardic, and hypertensive. Because of a long history of an alcohol use disorder, a diagnosis of alcohol withdrawal delirium was considered. Despite aggressive benzodiazepine treatment, he remained confused. Later, when he became febrile, a lumbar puncture was performed and his cerebrospinal fluid (CSF) analysis was consistent with a herpes simplex virus (HSV) infection. His sensorium cleared after a course of acyclovir.

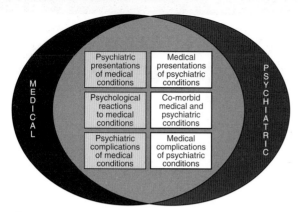

Fig. 1.1 ■ A representation of the overlap between medical and psychiatric care.

In this case, an infection of the central nervous system (CNS) by HSV was heralded by delirium.

Psychiatric Complications of Medical Conditions or Treatments

Case 2

A young man, without a history of a psychiatric illness, was diagnosed with human immunodeficiency virus (HIV) infection with a high viral load; he was started on efavirenz, a non-nucleoside reverse transcriptase inhibitor. Within several days, he experienced vivid nightmares, a known side effect of efavirenz. Over the next few weeks, his nightmares resolved. He continued to take his antiretroviral treatment; however, he became increasingly despondent and developed a full complement of neurovegetative symptoms of major depressive disorder.

A chronic, incurable viral illness—the treatment of which caused a neuropsychiatric complication—precipitated a depressive episode.

Psychological Reactions to Medical Conditions or Their Treatments

Case 3

A woman with a history of preeclampsia during her first pregnancy was admitted with hypertension in the 38th week of her second pregnancy. Preeclampsia was diagnosed, and she delivered a healthy baby.

As she prepared for hospital discharge, and despite her obstetrician's reassurance, she fretted that a hypertensive catastrophe was going to befall her at home.

Pathologic anxiety resulted from an acute obstetric condition.

Medical Presentations of Psychiatric Conditions

Case 4

A young female graduate student from another country, who for several years had habitually induced vomiting to relieve persistent abdominal pain, presented with generalized weakness and was found to have a low serum potassium level. Although she had a long history of bulimia nervosa, the current psychiatric consultant found no evidence for this disorder and instead diagnosed a conversion disorder, believing that her chronic abdominal pain was a converted symptom of psychological distress over leaving her family to study abroad.

In this case, a conversion disorder presented as persistent abdominal pain.

Medical Complications of Psychiatric Conditions or Treatments

Case 5

A man with schizophrenia was treated with olanzapine despite having a body mass index of 35; he gained an additional 30 pounds over the next 6 months. Repeated measurements of his fasting serum glucose were consistent with a diagnosis of diabetes mellitus.

Treatment with an atypical antipsychotic was complicated by an endocrine condition.

Comorbid Medical and Psychiatric Conditions

Case 6

A middle-aged man with long-standing obsessive-compulsive disorder (OCD) was effectively treated with high-dose fluoxetine; however, he presented to his primary care physician with a cough, dyspnea, and fever. A chest x-ray revealed a left lower-lobe infiltrate, consistent with pneumonia. His fever abated after several doses of an intravenous (IV) antibiotic, and he was discharged from the hospital so that he could complete his antibiotic course at home. His OCD remained in remission.

An infectious illness and a psychiatric condition co-occurred independently.

THE ART OF PSYCHIATRIC CONSULTATION IN THE GENERAL HOSPITAL

Determining where on the vast border between psychiatry and medicine a patient's signs and symptoms are located is one of the psychiatric consultant's fundamental tasks. Like any physician, their chief responsibility is to establish an accurate and timely diagnosis so that appropriate treatment can be initiated. The C-L psychiatrist (i.e., a practitioner of psychosomatic medicine) is aided in this enterprise by appreciation of four key differences between general hospital psychiatry and practice in other venues: clinical approach, the influence of the environment, interaction style, and the use of language.

Clinical Approach

A late senior psychiatrist at the Massachusetts General Hospital and the founding director of its Psychosomatic Medicine–Consultation Psychiatry Fellowship Program, Dr. George Murray, advised his trainees to think in three ways when consulting on patients: physiologically, existentially, and "dirty." Each element of this tripartite conceptualization is no more or less important than the other, and the most accurate formulation of a patient's problem will often prove elusive without attention to all three ways.

First, psychiatrists as physicians adhere to the medical model: altered bodily structures and functions lead to disease, and their correction through physical means leads to restoration of health. Although allegiance to this model may be impolitic in this era of biopsychosocial holism, the degree of morbidity

in general hospitals is ever more acute, and the technology brought to bear against it is increasingly more sophisticated.[3] Consultation psychiatrists who fail to keep pace with the knowledge base of their medical and surgical colleagues jeopardize their usefulness to physicians and patients alike.

In addition to the physiologic considerations, consultation psychiatrists must think existentially; that is, they must nurture a healthy curiosity about the meaning of illness to their patients (given their patients' lives and the circumstances in which their patients find themselves during their illness). For example, what does it mean to the woman presented in Case 3 that both of her pregnancies were complicated by preeclampsia? How might this meaning be connected to her unshakeable fear that she will become dangerously hypertensive at home? How does this fear impact her ability to care for her children, and how does it impact her husband? To be curious about such matters, the consulting psychiatrist must first *know* the details of the patient's situation, largely achieved by a careful reading of the medical record, and then *ask* the patient about it.

Consultation psychiatrists are wise to maintain a measured skepticism toward patients' and others' statements, motivations, and desires. In other words, they should consider the possibility that the patient (or another informant) is somehow distorting information to serve their own agenda. Providers of history can distort the truth in myriad ways, ranging from innocuous exaggeration to outright lies; their aims are equally diverse: money, revenge, convenience, and cover-up of infidelities or crimes. For example, the beleaguered mother of a young woman with borderline personality disorder embellished her daughter's suicidal comments to secure involuntary commitment for her daughter and respite for herself. By paying attention to their own countertransference—the personal interpretation of the limbic music[4] emanating from the mother-daughter dyad—the psychiatric consultant called in to assess the patient's suicidal thoughts ably detected the mother's self-serving distortion, thus avoiding unwitting collusion with it. This special case of distortion, aimed at removing a relative to a psychiatric facility, has been termed the *gaslight phenomenon*.[5-7] Although thinking dirty is merely a realization that people refract reality through the lens of their own personal experience, other health professionals—even some psychiatrists—bristle at even a consideration, let alone a suggestion, that patients and their families harbor unseemly ulterior motives. Consequently, this perspective does not make the consultation psychiatrist many friends; his or her thinking "dirty" may even earn him or her an unsavory reputation. However, neither an ever-widening social circle nor victory in popularity contests is the C-L psychiatrist's *raison d'être*—competent doctoring is.

Environment

The successful psychiatric consultant must be prepared to work in an atmosphere that is less formal, rigid, and predictable than what is typically found in an office or a clinic; flexibility and adaptability are crucial in this setting. Patients are often seen in two-bed rooms with nothing but a thin curtain providing only the appearance of privacy; roommates—as well as nurses, aides, dietary personnel, and other physicians—are frequent interlocutors.[8] Cramped quarters are the rule, with IV poles, tray tables, and one or two chairs, leaving little room for much else. When family members and other visitors are present, the physician may ask them to leave the room; alternatively, the physician may invite them to stay to "biopsy" the interpersonal dynamics among the family and friends, as was done in the case of the patient with borderline personality described previously. The various alarms and warning signals of medical equipment (e.g., IV pumps, cardiac monitors, ventilators) and assorted catheters and tubes traveling into and out of the patient's body add to the unique ambiance of the bedside experience, distinguishing it from the quiet comfort afforded by a private office. Perhaps off-putting at first, for the psychiatrist who, as Lewis Glickman in his book on consultation put it (as cited in Cassem[1]), loves medicine and is fascinated with medical illness, the exigencies of life and work in a modern hospital quickly become compelling.

Style of Interaction

The adaptability required by these environmental circumstances allows the psychiatric consultant to be more flexible in their relations with the patient. For example, psychiatric consultants should permit themselves to crouch at the bedside; lowering themselves to the recumbent patient's eye level can diminish apprehension and minimize the inherent power differential between doctor and patient. Shaking hands or otherwise laying on hands may achieve a similar effect. Performing a physical examination provides an excellent opportunity to allay anxiety and dramatically distinguishes consultation work from office-based psychiatry, where any touching of a patient—let alone physical examination—is considered taboo (rightly or wrongly). An offer to make the person more comfortable by adjusting the bed or getting the patient something to drink before beginning the interview goes a long way towards building rapport. When the patient is unable to do even these simple things unaided, it becomes a kind, humane gesture. When the patient tends to be cantankerous and irascible, concern for the patient's comfort may prevent the patient from expelling the consultant from the room. Finally, as a simple matter of respect, one should make every effort to leave the room as one found it (e.g., if towels and sheets are removed from a chair before sitting on it, they should be replaced on getting up).

Use of Language

The allowance for flexibility also extends to psychiatrists' use of language; in this setting, they can feel more free than they might in other practice settings to use humor, slang expressions, and perhaps even foul language.[9] All of these varieties of verbal expression create a temporarily jarring juxtaposition between the stereotypical image of the staid physician and the present one; defenses may be briefly disabled just long enough to connect with the truth and allow connection with the patient. For example, in a technique taught by Murray, the psychiatrist raised a clenched fist in front of an angry but anger-phobic patient and asked him, "If you had one shot, where would you put it?" In this case, the sight and sound of a "healer" in a boxer's pose inquiring about the placement of a "shot" creates a curious, even humorous, incongruity that disarms the patient's defenses and allows an otherwise intolerable emotion (anger) to emerge (if it is there in the first place). A variant of this maneuver, substitution of a verbal expression of anger for the physical one, is also possible.

Case 7

A 30-year-old man with leukemia, refractory to bone marrow transplantation, was admitted with graft-versus-host disease. His mother and sister kept a near-constant vigil at his bedside. When he refused to eat and to talk to his family and the nurses, the psychiatrist was summoned. Quickly sizing up the situation, the consultant said to the young man, "It must be a pain to have your mother constantly hovering over you." The patient grinned slightly and answered in the affirmative.

TABLE 1.1
Procedural Approach to Psychiatric Consultation

Speak directly with the referring clinician.

Review the current and pertinent past records.

Review the patient's medications.

Gather collateral data.

Interview and examine the patient.

Formulate a diagnosis and management plan.

Write a note.

Speak directly again with the referring clinician.

Provide periodic follow-up.

Lack of the formal arrangements of office-based psychiatric practice makes such techniques permissible in the general hospital, often to the delight of residents, who sometimes feel unnecessarily constrained in their interpersonal comportment and in whom even a little training unfortunately can do much to limit their natural spontaneity.

THE PROCESS OF PSYCHIATRIC CONSULTATION IN THE GENERAL HOSPITAL

With this general overview of the art of consultation, we next outline the step-by-step approach to the actual performance of a psychiatric consultation. Table 1.1 summarizes the key points elaborated in the following text.

Speak Directly With the Referring Clinician

The consultative process begins with the receipt of the referral. With experience, the thoughtful consultant begins to formulate preliminary hypotheses even at this early stage. For example, the consultant might realize that the referral originates from a certain unit within the hospital or from a physician who has previously requested consultations and recall their prior conversations. In addition, the consultant may discern a difference in the way this consultation request was communicated compared with those of previous requests. In a form of parallel process, this alteration in the usual routine—even if subtle and only in retrospect—often reflects something about the patient. Throughout the consultative process, these crude

preliminary hypotheses are refined and ultimately either accepted or rejected. The continual revision of previous theories as additional data become available is as fundamental to the practice of C-L psychiatry as it is to the whole of medicine.

The reason for the consultation, as stated in the request, might differ from the real reason for the consultation. The team may accurately sense a problem with the patient but fail to capture it precisely. In some cases, they may be quite far afield, usually when the real reason for the consultation involves management of a difficult patient.[10] It is up to the consultant to identify the core issue and ultimately address it in the consultation. Practically speaking, a special effort to contact the consultee is not usually required. In general, during the course of reading the chart or reviewing laboratory data, one encounters a member of the team and can inquire about the consultation request at that time.

Review the Current and Pertinent Past Records

A careful review of the current medical record is indispensable to a thorough and comprehensive evaluation of the patient. Perhaps no other element of the consultative process requires as much discipline as this one. The seasoned consultant can accomplish this task quite efficiently, knowing fruitful areas of the chart to mine. For example, nursing notes often contain behavioral data that is often lacking from the notes of those in other disciplines; a well-written consultation provided

by another service can provide a general orientation to
a case. However, in the current era of widespread use
of electronic medical records, when copying and past-
ing parts of previous notes often substitutes for crafting
new ones, the consultant must take care not to propagate errors by failing to check primary data personally. Other bountiful areas of the chart include notes
written by medical students (who tend to be the most
thorough of all), physical and occupational therapists
(for functional data), and speech pathologists (for cognitive data). In reading the chart, the focus of the psychiatric consultant's attention varies according to the
nature of the case and the reason for the consultation.
In cases where sensorium is altered, for example, it is
crucial to note changes in the patient's level of awareness, behavior, and cognition, especially as they relate
to changes in the medical condition and its treatment.

Review the Patient's Medications

Regardless of the case's particulars, a detailed evaluation of medications, paying special attention to those
recently initiated or discontinued, is always in order.
For example, in Case 2, knowledge that the HIV-
positive male had recently initiated treatment with
efavirenz was key to diagnosing the cause of his nightmares. Medications that the patient might have taken
before admission, including those on which he may
be physiologically dependent (e.g., benzodiazepines,
narcotic analgesics), might inadvertently have been
excluded from his current regimen. Patients who have
been transferred among various units in the hospital
may be at particular risk of such inadvertent omis-
sions. In cases in which mental status changes have
arisen, withdrawal phenomena often top the differential diagnosis; therefore a carefully constructed
timeline of the patient's use of psychoactive agents is
often the only way to identify the problem. In much
the same way as an infectious disease specialist charts
the administration of antibiotics in relation to culture
results, and dermatologists plot newly prescribed medications against the appearance of rashes, the psychiatric consultant should tabulate mental status changes,
vital signs, and dosages of psychoactive medications to
clarify the diagnostic picture. Such a procedure exemplifies the industry and discipline required for a competent consultant.

Gather Collateral Data

The gathering of collateral information from family,
friends, and outpatient treaters is no less important in
consultation work than in other psychiatric settings.
For several reasons (e.g., altered mental status, denial,
memory impairment, malingering), patients' accounts
of their history and current symptoms are often vague,
spotty, and unreliable. Although data from other
sources are vital, the astute psychiatrist recognizes that
their information, too, may be distorted by the same
factors and by selfish interests, as already described.
Consultation psychiatrists must guard against accepting any one party's version of events as the truth and
must maintain an open mind when constructing a history that is informed by multiple sources.

Interview and Examine the Patient

Next follows the interview of the patient and performance of a mental status examination, in addition to relevant portions of the physical and
neurologic examinations.

A detailed assessment of cognitive function is not
necessary for all patients. If there is no evidence that
a patient has a cognitive problem, a simple statement to the effect that no gross cognitive problem is
apparent is sufficient. However, even a slight whiff of
a cognitive disturbance should trigger performance
of a more formal screen. We recommend the Folstein
Mini-Mental State Examination (MMSE)[11] and the
Montreal Cognitive Assessment[12] for this purpose and
supplement these tests with others that specifically
target frontal executive functions (e.g., clock drawing, Luria maneuvers, and cognitive estimations).
Any abnormalities that arise on these bedside tests
should be comprehensively evaluated by formal neuropsychological testing. It is convenient if a psychologist—especially one trained in neuropsychology—is
affiliated with the consultation service. Conversely, if a
patient is obviously inattentive, the performance of the
MMSE (or similar tests) is not indicated because one
can predict a priori poor performance resulting from
the patient's general inattention to the required tasks.

The consultant should, at the very least, review the
physical examinations performed by other physicians.
This does not, however, preclude doing his or her own
examination of relevant systems, including the CNS,

which, unless the patient is on the neurology service or is known to have a motor or a sensory problem, has likely been left unexamined. Several physical findings can be discerned simply by observation: pupillary size (noteworthy with opioid withdrawal or intoxication); diaphoresis, either present (from fever, or from alcohol or benzodiazepine withdrawal) or absent (associated with anticholinergic intoxication); and adventitious motor activity (e.g., tremors, tremulousness, or agitation). Vital signs are especially relevant in cases of substance withdrawal, delirium, and other causes of agitation. Primitive reflexes (e.g., snout, glabellar, grasp), deep-tendon reflexes, extraocular movements, pupillary reaction to light, and muscle tone are among the key elements of the neurologic examination that the psychiatrist often checks.

Formulate a Diagnosis and Management Plan

Any physician's tasks are twofold: diagnosis and treatment. This dictum is no different for the psychiatrist, whether in the general hospital or elsewhere. To arrive at a diagnosis, laboratory testing comes after the history and examination. When a psychiatric consultation is requested, most hospitalized patients have already undergone extensive laboratory testing, including comprehensive metabolic panels and complete blood cell counts; these should be reviewed. In constructing the initial parts of a management plan, the psychiatric consultant should attend to diagnostics and specifically consider each of the tests listed in Table 1.2.

Toxicology screens of both serum and urine are required any time a substance use disorder is suspected and in cases of altered sensorium, intoxication, or withdrawal.

Well known by every student of psychiatry, syphilis, thyroid dysfunction, and deficiencies of vitamin B_{12} and folic acid are always included in an exhaustive differential diagnosis of virtually every neuropsychiatric disturbance. Although it is certainly possible that these conditions can *cause* any manner of psychiatric perturbation (e.g., dementia, depression, mania), more commonly these ailments often coexist with other conditions, which together *contribute* to psychiatric disturbances. Although blood tests can be analyzed and treatments for these diseases implemented relatively

TABLE 1.2
Laboratory Tests in Psychiatric Consultation

Toxicology
- Serum
- Urine

Serology
- Rapid plasma reagin
- VDRL test

Thyroid-stimulating hormone
Vitamin B_{12} (cyanocobalamin)
Folic acid (folate)
Electroencephalography
Cerebrospinal fluid analysis
Neuroimaging
- Head computed tomography
- Brain magnetic resonance imaging

VDRL, Venereal Disease Research Laboratory.

easily, these tests should not be recommended reflexively in every case; instead, they should be reserved for situations in which there is a specific reason for testing (e.g., vitamin testing for anemia).

For purposes other than the evaluation of an acute intracranial hemorrhage, cerebral magnetic resonance imaging (MRI) is preferred to computed tomography. MRI provides higher resolution and greater detail, particularly of subcortical structures of interest to the psychiatrist. A thorough consultation is incomplete without reading the actual radiology report of the study; merely reviewing the telegraphic summary in a house officer's progress note is insufficient because important findings are often omitted. For example, an MRI scan that shows no abnormalities other than periventricular white matter changes is invariably recorded as "normal" or as showing "no acute change." Although periventricular white matter changes are not acute, they are certainly not normal and should be documented in a careful psychiatric consultation note. They may be evidence of insults that form a substrate for depression or dementia and may be a predictive sign of a sensitivity to the usual dosages of psychotropic medications.

An electroencephalogram (EEG) can be particularly helpful to document the presence of generalized slowing in patients thought by their primary physicians to have a functional problem. Such indisputable evidence of an electric dysrhythmia often puts a sudden end to the primary team's skepticism. In cases of suspected complex partial seizures, depriving the patient of sleep the night before the EEG increases the test's sensitivity. Continuous EEG and video monitoring or ambulatory EEG monitoring may be necessary to capture aberrant electrical activity. As with neuroimaging reports, the consultant psychiatrist must read the EEG report themselves; non-psychiatrists commonly equate the absence of "organized electrographic seizure activity" with normality, even though focal slowing may be evidence of seizure activity.

CSF analysis is often overlooked by psychiatrists and other physicians. However, it should be considered in cases with an altered mental status in the context of fever, leukocytosis, or meningismus, and when causes of clouded consciousness are not obvious. In some cases (e.g., Case 1), some conditions initially considered causative are not, and the true culprit is identified only after a lumbar puncture is performed and the CSF analyzed.

Any suspicion of a somatic symptom disorder (especially a conversion disorder) should trigger referral for psychological testing using the Minnesota Multiphasic Personality Inventory (MMPI) or the shorter Personality Assessment Inventory. For example, the MMPI results of the young female graduate student in Case 4 may demonstrate the conversion (or psychosomatic) V pattern of marked elevations on the hypochondriasis and hysteria scales and a normal or slightly elevated score on the depression scale. These pencil-and-paper tests can also be useful in assessments of psychological contributions to pain. Projective testing (e.g., Rorschach inkblots) is more commonly obtained in outpatient venues.

Write a Note

The psychiatric consultant's note should serve as a model of clear and concise writing, with careful attention paid to specific, practical diagnostic and therapeutic recommendations. Several reviews of this topic are available.[13,14] If the stated reason for the consultation differs from the consultee's more fundamental concern, both should be addressed in the note. If the referring physician adopts the consultant's

recommendations, they should be able to transcribe them directly into computerized order-entry systems. "Note wars," criticism of the consultee, accusations of shoddy work, pejorative labels, and jargon should be avoided. If the consultee chooses a diagnostic or therapeutic course equally appropriate to the consultant's suggested choice, an indication of agreement is more prudent than rigid insistence on the psychiatrist's preference. The consultant should avoid prognostication (e.g., "This patient will probably have decision-making capacity after his infection has resolved" or "This patient will likely need psychiatric hospitalization after he recovers from tricyclic antidepressant [TCA] toxicity"). Such forecasts do not engender confidence in the consultant's skill if they prove inaccurate, may be invoked by the consultee even when they no longer apply, and are unnecessary if routine follow-up is provided.

Speak Directly Again With the Referring Clinician

The consultative process is not complete without further contact, either by phone or in person, with the referring physician or another member of the patient's team, especially if the diagnosis or recommended intervention warrants immediate attention.

Provide Periodic Follow-up

The committed consultant sees the patient as often as necessary to treat the patient competently, and the consultant holds themselves accountable for tracking the patient's clinical progress, following up on laboratory tests, refining earlier diagnostic impressions, and modifying diagnostic and treatment recommendations. The consultation comes to an end only when the problem for which the consultant was called resolves, any other concerns identified by the consultant are fully addressed, or the patient is discharged or dies. Rarely do any of these outcomes occur after a single visit, making repeated visits the rule and availability, even at inopportune times, crucial. However, the consultant is not obligated to continue consulting on a case if their recommendations are being ignored.[15] In these cases, it is appropriate to sign off. In some settings, psychiatric consultants may be expected to ensure that insurance coverage is available for psychiatric admissions and to locate available psychiatric beds.

PRINCIPLES OF PSYCHIATRIC TREATMENT IN THE GENERAL HOSPITAL

As in other practice settings, in the general hospital, psychiatric treatment proceeds on biological, psychological, and social fronts.

Biological Management

When prescribing psychotropics for medically ill patients who are taking other medications, the consultant must be aware of pharmacokinetic profiles, drug-drug interactions, and adverse effects, all of which are considered in depth in Chapter 37.

Pharmacokinetic Profiles

Pharmacokinetics refers to a drug's absorption, distribution, metabolism, and excretion. Because an acutely medically ill patient might not be able to take medications orally, absorption is a primary concern in the general hospital setting. Often in such situations (e.g., in an intubated patient), a nasogastric (NG) tube is in place, and medications can be crushed and administered through the NG tube. However, if one is not in place, the psychiatric consultant is obliged to consider medications that can be given intramuscularly, intravenously, or in suppository form. In addition, orally disintegrating formulations may be available (e.g., mirtazapine, olanzapine, risperidone); these formulations still work enterally.

Many psychotropic medications are metabolized by the liver and excreted through the kidneys. Thus impaired hepatic and renal function can lead to increased concentrations of parent compounds and pharmacologically active metabolites. This problem is readily overcome by using lower initial doses and increasing them slowly. However, concern for metabolic alterations in medically ill patients should not justify the use of homeopathic doses for an indeterminate duration, as most patients ultimately tolerate and require standard regimens.

Drug-Drug Interactions

Many psychotropics are metabolized by the cytochrome P450 isoenzyme system. Many also inhibit various isoforms in this extensive family of hepatic enzymes, and the metabolism of many is, in turn, inhibited by other classes of medications, thus creating fertile ground for drug-drug interactions in patients taking several medications. This topic is reviewed extensively in Chapter 37. Psychiatric consultants should also be aware that cigarette smoking induces the metabolism of many drugs. When patients are hospitalized and thus stop or curtail smoking, serum concentrations of these drugs (e.g., clozapine) increase, and the propensity for adverse effects thus also increases.

Adverse Effects

Depending on the practice venue, the profile of adverse effects of concern to the psychiatrist varies. For example, the likelihood that TCAs will cause dry mouth and sedation may be of more concern in the outpatient setting than in the general hospital, where concern about the cardiac conduction and gut-slowing effects will likely be of greater importance in patients recovering from myocardial infarction (MI) or bowel surgery. Traditional neuroleptics—often relegated to second-line status in otherwise healthy patients with psychosis—may be preferable to the atypical agents in general medical settings, where patients with obesity, diabetes mellitus, and dyslipidemia may be seen for the complications of these conditions (e.g., MI, stroke, diabetic ketoacidosis).

Psychological Management

Psychological management of the hospitalized medically ill individual begins—as does all competent treatment—with the diagnosis. That is, the psychiatric consultant first appraises the patient's psychological strengths and vulnerabilities. Armed with this psychological balance sheet, the psychiatrist then uses this information therapeutically in how they phrase questions and comments to the patient and describe the patient to the medical and nursing staff. Several schemas have been developed to aid in such a personality assessment.[10,16,17] Groves' formulation is reviewed in Chapters 34 and 41; Table 1.3 summarizes Kahana and Bibring's approach.[16]

The consultant should realize that the patient may find that the psychiatrist is the only outlet available to vent the patient's feelings about hospital treatment. This is an appropriate function of the consultant—and, in fact, it may be the tacit reason for the consultation. Relieved of the patient's feelings, often hostile and at odds with the team's treatment efforts, the patient is thus better able to work with the team.

TABLE 1.3
Personality Assessment and Management in the General Hospital

Personality Type	Major Traits	Reaction to Illness	Recommended Strategies
Dependent	Craves special attention Expects services on demand Requires constant reassurance	Perceived abandonment generates feeling of helplessness Increased anxiety prompts more demands	Express desire to provide comprehensive care Make minor concessions if possible
Obsessive	Values detail and order Becomes anxious with uncertain outcomes Well defended against fear and pain	Illness represents threat to self-control Need for certainty and control prevents questioning of staff, thus increasing anxiety	Provide ample information, using and defining medical terms Ally with patient's desire for mastery Allow patient to participate in medical decisions
Histrionic	Prematurely trusts others Uses repression, denial, and avoidance Dramatizes feelings	Illness represents threat to masculinity or femininity	Recognize patient's grace under pressure Omit details in reassuring patient
Masochistic	Plays the martyr role Seems to enjoy suffering Feels unappreciated	Illness represents deserved punishment Illness is welcomed as a form of suffering Lack of recognition of martyr status risks non-compliance	Appreciate patient's suffering Recommend treatment as an additional burden that will aid others
Paranoid	Is suspicious, wary, and guarded Readily feels slighted Bickers when feeling persecuted	Illness represents an external assault Medical interventions generate suspicions and fear of harm	Inform patient completely about tests and treatments Acknowledge difficulty of illness
Narcissistic	Requests and receives help with difficulty Strives to appear smart, strong, and superior Fears dependence	Illness challenges self-esteem and superior stance Efforts to appear effectual and strong are redoubled	Recognize patient's strengths and knowledge Allow patient to participate in medical decisions Expect gaps in history, because more illness connotes weakness
Schizoid	Is aloof, uninvolved, and detached Prefers solitary occupations	Illness requires contact with caregivers Rejection risk spurs greater withdrawal	Recognize preference for isolation Minimize intrusions Assure patient of interest and concern

Adapted from Shuster JL, Stern TA. Intensive care units. In: Wise MG, Rundell JR, eds. *The American Psychiatric Publishing Textbook of Consultation–Liaison Psychiatry: Psychiatry in the Medically Ill*. 2nd ed. American Psychiatric Publishing; 2002:753–770; Kahana RJ, Bibring GL. Personality types in medical management. In: Zinberg NE, ed. *Psychiatry and Medical Practice in a General Hospital*. International Universities Press; 1965:108–123; and Wool C, Geringer ES, Stern TA. The management of behavioral problems in the ICU. In: Rippe JM, Irwin RS, Alpert JS, et al., eds. *Intensive Care Medicine*. 2nd ed. Little, Brown; 1991:1906–1916.

Social Management

Psychiatric consultants may be called on to help make decisions about end-of-life care (e.g., do-not-resuscitate and do-not-intubate orders), disposition to an appropriate living situation (e.g., home with services, assisted-living residence, skilled nursing facility, or nursing home), short-term disability, probate guardianship for a patient deemed clinically unable to make medical decisions for himself or herself, and involuntary psychiatric commitment. For patients who are agitated and thereby placing themselves and others in harm's way, the consultant may recommend the use of various restraints (e.g., Posey vests, mitts [to prevent removing IV and other catheters], soft wrist restraints, and leather wrist and ankle restraints) and constant observation.

SUMMARY

Regardless of the practice setting, the basics of competent psychiatric care remain the diagnosis of affective, behavioral, and cognitive disturbances (the "ABCs") and their treatment by pharmacologic, psychological, and social interventions. The psychiatrist in the general hospital applies these fundamentals while remaining *accessible* to the consultee and to the patient, *adaptable* to the exigencies of the hospital environment, and *flexible* in one's clinical approach and interpersonal style. The consultation psychiatrist adheres to the tenets of competent doctoring, including accountability, commitment, industry, and discipline.

REFERENCES

1. Cassem NH. The consultation service. In: Hackett TP, Weisman AD, Kucharski A, eds. *Psychiatry in a General Hospital: The First Fifty Years.* PSG Publishing; 1987:34.
2. Lipowski ZJ. Review of consultation psychiatry and psychosomatic medicine: II. Clinical aspects. *Psychosom Med.* 1967;29:201–224.
3. Murray GB. The liaison psychiatrist as busybody. *Ann Clin Psychiatry.* 1989;1:265–268.
4. Murray GB, Kontos N. Limbic music. In: Stern TA, Fricchione GL, Cassem NH, eds. *Massachusetts General Hospital Handbook of General Hospital Psychiatry.* 6th ed. Saunders Elsevier; 2010:45–51.
5. Lund CA, Gardiner AQ. The gaslight phenomenon: an institutional variant. *Br J Psychiatry.* 1977;131:533–534.
6. Smith CG, Sinanan K. The "gaslight phenomenon" reappears: a modification of the Ganser syndrome. *Br J Psychiatry.* 1972;120:685–686.
7. Barton R, Whitehead TA. The gaslight phenomenon. *Lancet.* 1969;1:1258–1260.
8. Eshel N, Marcovitz DE, Stern TA. Psychiatric consultations in less-than-private places: challenges and unexpected benefits of hospital roommates. *Psychosomatics.* 2016;57:97–101.
9. Zimmerman DJ, Stern TA. Offensive language in the general hospital. *Psychosomatics.* 2010;51:377–385.
10. Groves JE. Taking care of the hateful patient. *N Engl J Med.* 1978;298:883–887.
11. Folstein MF, Folstein SE, McHugh PR. "Mini-Mental State": a practical method for grading the cognitive state of patients for the clinician. *J Psychiatr Res.* 1975;12:189–198.
12. Nasreddine ZS, Phillips NA, Bedirian V, et al. The Montreal Cognitive Assessment: a brief screening tool for mild cognitive impairment. *J Am Geriatr Soc.* 2005;358:695–699.
13. Alexander T, Bloch S. The written report in consultation-liaison psychiatry: a proposed schema. *Aust N Z J Psychiatry.* 2002;36:251–258.
14. Garrick TR, Stotland NL. How to write a psychiatric consultation. *Am J Psychiatry.* 1982;139:849–855.
15. Kontos N, Freudenreich O, Querques J, et al. The consultation psychiatrist as effective physician. *Gen Hosp Psychiatry.* 2003;25:20–23.
16. Kahana RJ, Bibring GL. Personality types in medical management. In: Zinberg NE, ed. *Psychiatry and Medical Practice in a General Hospital.* International Universities Press; 1965:108–123.
17. Bibring GL. Psychiatry and medical practice in a general hospital. *N Engl J Med.* 1956;254:366–372.

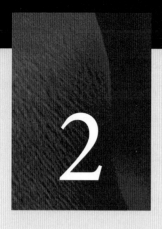

2

THE DOCTOR-PATIENT RELATIONSHIP

CHRISTOPHER D. GORDON, MD ▪ EUGENE V. BERESIN, MD, MA

OVERVIEW

Despite all the pressures of clinical productivity, algorithm-driven practice, insatiably demanding electronic medical records, and other teeth-gnashing bureaucracies, the patient-doctor relationship remains a profound partnership. Ideally, it is a sacred space in which a distressed person feels safe enough to reveal to another their innermost concerns in the hope of healing.[1,2] In this professional intimacy, when we earn our patient's trust, we can be privileged to learn about concerns that our patient may not have shared—or will ever share—with another living soul. For our part, we hope to bring to this relationship technical mastery of our craft, such wisdom as we have accumulated through study and experience, and humility about the limits of our own knowledge and the limitations of our beloved field of psychiatry. We commit to stand by our patients—that is, not to be driven away by any degree of pain, suffering, ugliness, or even death itself—through the course of their illness. We forswear our own gratification, beyond our professional satisfaction and reward, to put our patients' interests above our own. We also have a sober understanding that the medical space, and especially the psychiatric medical space, is inherently dangerous.[3] It is full of potentially stigmatizing and disempowering language and imbalanced power dynamics that can threaten patients' autonomy and agency. So, we are both our patient's partner and their advocate. We hope to co-create a healing relationship while working to do no harm.

In psychiatry, the patient-doctor relationship is one of the most potent aspects of care itself. Excellent clinical outcomes arise from relationships in which patients feel heard, understood, respected, and included in treatment planning.[4,5] Empowered patients tend to report higher satisfaction and to work effectively with their physicians. Patients are more likely to commit to treatment regimens they have co-created. Poor outcomes—including "non-adherence" with treatment plans, complaints to oversight boards, and malpractice actions—tend to arise when patients feel unheard, disrespected, or otherwise out of partnership with their doctors.[6,7] Collaborative care is also more efficient than non-collaborative care in achieving good outcomes.[8–12] The relationship matters.

An effective doctor-patient relationship may be especially important in psychiatry because psychiatric maladies can seem to blend with the sufferer's sense of personhood. In psychiatry, there is a sense that when the patient is ill, there is something wrong with the person, rather than that the person "has" or suffers from a discrete condition. Our language can aggravate this sense of personal defectiveness or deficiency in psychiatric illness. We tend to speak of "being depressed," "I am bipolar," or "he is a schizophrenic," as if these were qualities of the whole person rather than a condition to be dealt with. Even more hurtfully, we sometimes speak of people as "borderlines" or "schizophrenics," as if these diagnostic labels summed up the person. This language, together with the persistent stigma attached to mental illness in our culture, amplifies the risk of unintended shame, humiliation, and disempowerment that patients may experience in any doctor-patient interaction.[13,14] We physicians must work to create conditions of safety in the relationship.

In this chapter, we will discuss how to promote a collaborative doctor-patient relationship. We will then look more deeply at the elements of collaborative patient-centered care and how to build these concepts into the clinical encounter. We then present an example of the model for constructing a care path. Lastly, we turn to problems and obstacles that can arise and some ideas for addressing these difficulties.

THE OPTIMAL HEALING ENVIRONMENT: PATIENT-CENTERED CARE

Although cultural factors may limit the validity of this generalization, patients usually prefer care that acknowledges their own concerns, addresses their perspective about these concerns, uses language that is straightforward, promotes collaboration, and respects the patient as a fully empowered partner in decision-making.[15] This model of care may be well described by the term *patient-centered care*[8,16] or *relationship-centered care*. In *Crossing the Quality Chasm*, the Institute of Medicine identified person-centered practice as a key to achieving high-quality care that focuses on the unique perspective, needs, values, and preferences of the individual patient.[17] Person-centered care involves a collaborative relationship in which two experts— the practitioner and the patient—attempt to blend the practitioner's knowledge and experience with the patient's unique perspective, needs, values, and goals.[18]

In person-centered care, the patient's preferences and values are integral to every clinical decision, and outcomes are defined not only by evidence-based, disease-centered metrics but also by patient-reported and patient-defined functional outcomes.[19] One struggle for physicians is to balance the pressures to remain within the treatment path of evidence-based practice while providing truly individualized care, based on the patient's perspective and values—the "quintessential skill" of modern medicine.[20]

This shift from paternalism to collaboration can be particularly challenging in situations in which the patient's competence is in question. But even in situations in which the patient is incompetent, we should still make every effort to honor the person's preferences and values and to involve the person maximally in whatever way the patient can exercise choice.

The shift to patient-centered care reflects a sea change in our culture away from top-down doctorly directives toward mutually respectful dialogue. This shift owes a debt to feminism,[21] as women awakened the culture to the reality of disempowering and oppressing people through tyrannies of role and language. Moreover, feminism resulted in a paradigmatic shift in the healing professions, in which the perspectives of both patients and practitioners have equal claim to legitimacy and importance, and in which the relationship itself has deep value for the outcome of the clinical enterprise. The rise of consumerism and the wide dissemination of information on the internet have also contributed to the emergence of more empowered patients as consumers.[22] Health care has seen a shift from paternalistic practices to nurturing dialogues among health care providers, users of care, and their networks of support. Rapid shifts in insurance plans have led patients to change from one practitioner to another with greater frequency, reinforcing the "informed shopper" approach to patienthood. As Lazare and colleagues[22] presciently noted, patients increasingly view themselves as customers and seek value, which is always in the eye of the beholder.

Quill and Brody[18] described a model of doctor-patient interaction that they termed *enhanced autonomy*. They described a relationship in which the patient's autonomous right to make critical decisions regarding his or her own care is augmented by the physician's full engagement in a dialogue about these decisions (including the physician's input, recommendations, and open acknowledgment of bias, if present). Quill and Brody[18] pointed out that in purely autonomous decision-making, which they denoted as the "independent choice" model, there is a sort of perversion of patient-centeredness, in which the patient is essentially abandoned to make critical decisions without the benefit of the physician's counsel. In the independent choice model, physicians see their role as providing information, options of treatment, and odds of success; answering questions objectively; and eschewing recommendations (so as not to bias the patient or family).

In relationship-centered practice, the physician does not cede decision-making authority or responsibility to the patient and family, but rather enters into a real dialogue about the nature of the problem or the problems at hand; the various options for dealing with these problems, including the risks and benefits of each as well as of no intervention; the patient's and family's values, concerns, and preferences; and if asked, what options the physician recommends and why. Most patients and families seek a valued doctor's answer to the question (stated or not), "What would you want if this were your family member?"[23] This transparent and candid collaboration shares power rather than ceding it and conveys respect and concern. Enhanced autonomy involves a commitment to know the patient deeply and to respect the patient's wishes; to share information as openly and honestly as the patient desires; to involve others with the patient's direction; and to treat the patient as a full partner to the greatest extent possible. This relationship also requires that the physician be present in the relationship as a fully human, fallible, and embodied human being. This means tolerating the uncertainty inherent in many critical clinical decisions—such as whether to use a given medicine, for example—and being transparent about the uncertainty.[24]

In patient-centered care, the physician works to avoid inadvertently hurting, shaming, or humiliating the patient through careless use of language or other slights. When such hurt or other error occurs, the practitioner apologizes clearly and in a heartfelt way to restore the relationship.[25,26]

Patient-centered care involves six processes. First, the physician endeavors to create conditions of hospitality,[27] extending welcome, respect, and safety so that the patient can reveal their concerns and perspective. An almost essential goal of this phase is to engender rapport. Without rapport, the work will likely falter.[12] Second, the physician works to understand the patient deeply, listening to both the words and the "music" of what is communicated. Third, the physician checks, confirms, and demonstrates his or her understanding through direct, non-jargonistic language with the patient. Fourth, if the physician successfully establishes common ground on the nature of the problem as the patient perceives it, an attempt is made to synthesize these problems into workable diagnoses and problem lists. Fifth, using expertise, technical mastery, and experience, the physician envisions and shares possible paths toward the desired outcomes, developed with the patient. Finally, together, the physician and patient can then negotiate about which path makes the most sense for them.

Through all of this work, the physician models and cultivates a relationship that values candor, collaboration, and authenticity; it should be able to withstand conflict—even welcoming conflict as a healthy part of human relationships. In so doing, the physician-patient partnership forges a relationship that can stand the vicissitudes of the patient's illness, its treatment, and turbulence as it arises in the relationship itself.

Physician Qualities in Patient-Centered Care

Self-awareness, open-heartedness, and warmth promote partnership and collaboration and enrich the doctor's technical competence and cognitive mastery. One key to calm awareness and the capacity to tolerate difficult emotions without action is *mindfulness*,[28] a quality described by Messner,[29] as one acquired through a process of constant *autognosis,* or self-awareness. Mindfulness appreciates that a person's emotional life (i.e., both the physician's and the patient's) has meaning and importance, deserving our respect and attention. Mindfulness connotes a commitment to respectful monitoring of one's own feelings, as well as to the feelings of the patient, and acceptance of feelings in both parties without judgment and with the knowledge that feelings are separate from actions.

Mindfulness, which springs from roots in Buddhism,[30] has enriched the practice of psychotherapy (e.g., helping patients to tolerate unbearable emotions without action and helping clinicians to tolerate the sometimes horrific histories their patients share with them). Mindfulness enables us to attend to our feelings (with acceptance and compassion) and to those of our patients, without a compulsion to act on these feelings. Through mindful practice, the physician can be informed by the wealth of his or her inner emotional life without being driven to act on these emotions; this can serve as a model for the relationship with the patient.

Other personal qualities of the physician that promote healthy and vibrant relationships with patients include humility, genuineness, optimism, a belief in the value of living a full life, kindness, good humor, candor, and transparency in communication.[31]

Important communication skills include the ability to elicit the patient's perspective; help the patient feel understood; explain conditions and options in clear, non-technical language; generate input and consensus about paths forward in care; acknowledge the difficulty in the relationship without aggravating it; welcome input and even conflict; and work through difficulty to a mutually acceptable, win-win solution.[12,32,33]

SIX PERSPECTIVES ON THE WHOLE PERSON

In today's busy, often frenzied practice pace, it is hard to find the time and space to get to know the whole person.[34] In the consultation-liaison (C-L) setting, in which the physician may be a stranger meeting the patient for the first time, getting to know the whole person can be particularly challenging. The COVID-19 pandemic and the sudden expansion of telemedicine have posed new challenges to intimate conversations.[35] The electronic medical record keeps practitioners' eyes on monitors and on the relentless need for documentation and the justification of interventions that distract us from deep listening. But knowing the whole person remains paramount.[36] In this section, we will lay out the conceptual model that is "running in the background" of our minds when we meet a new patient. This is not an outline or sequence of interviewing; it is more like a grid that we keep in mind as we converse with a patient. As we will discuss, it is also a model that we share with patients when we get to the treatment planning stage of our meeting. More about that is below.

In our practice, we have found that thinking about a person from six perspectives yields a good portrait of the whole person. We build on the traditional bio-psycho-social model[37] by adding two additional axes and grounding these five perspectives on a sixth and critical dimension: a deliberate inventory and acknowledgment of the person's strengths, accomplishments, and capacities.[38]

The first lens we use is considering what social factors in current time might shed light on the person's difficulties (such as bereavement, marital turbulence,

and school troubles), with a focus on here-and-now challenges that may be overwhelming the person. We then expand the field to consider what may have happened and has remained problematic (such as unresolved grief). We start with this social dimension to keep top of mind the role of trauma in many patients' lives and the often critical role that social determinants of health play in their lives.[39] This frame of "what happened to you?" rather than the implied "what is wrong with you?" sets the problem in terms of coping with circumstances rather than necessarily positing a disease entity.[40]

Second, we consider psychological factors that might contribute to the current problem, using the paradigm that most psychological difficulties manifest in adult life as *recurrent patterns*, usually with a strong interpersonal component.[38] Examples of recurrent patterns suggestive of psychological issues could involve relationships that end when they begin to become too intimate or a pattern of bucking authority leading to repeated job losses. A corollary idea is that most patterns begin as *attempts to cope, which then morph into problems*. An accessible example of a solution that becomes a problem is substance misuse, which usually starts as a self-soothing effort before becoming problematic.

The third lens is in many ways most accessible to psychiatrists, that is, considering possible biological aspects of the person's difficulty. Naturally, much of our thinking involves recognizing and differentiating the rich field of psychiatric conditions that are either established or suspected to have biological etiologies or contributions. This is our special psychiatric expertise. Precision and accuracy of diagnosis are paramount. Very often, even when biological factors substantially account for the person's presenting problem, social and psychological factors often contribute to how the person responds to, or engages in, treatment, or otherwise critically influence the experience of illness and recovery.

In recent years, we have added two other lenses to the classic bio-psycho-social model. The first is to make room for spiritual/existential factors, such as a strong faith system or a compelling commitment to a set of values. For example, a person with strong religious faith may weather bereavement with less despair than someone without such faith; on the other hand, if a person with a strong faith in a just and caring God loses a child to cancer, their faith may be rattled, aggravating their grief. Lastly and most recently, we have added a category of "mystery"—as a way of acknowledging with humility that most of the time we simply do not know the full story behind why a person suffers, yet we still want to try to help, to keep our minds and hearts open as we get to know the patient in greater depth, and, in the meantime, to not make matters worse.

We have found that this bio-psycho-social-spiritual-"mystery" model, which is grounded on an explicit acknowledgment of people's strengths, is a useful way of conceptualizing what is troubling patients when they arrive for care. The model captures the multi-dimensional process of being a practicing psychiatrist and appreciating the whole person. Also, we have found this model to be an accessible and congenial way of talking with patients about their difficulties and designing care. The model has the benefit of using down-to-earth language and being non-pathologizing. Since it leads with the person's strengths, it promotes partnership. When we share this model as a way of inviting conversation about the nature of the problem and treatment options, most patients report feeling understood. Patients seem to appreciate the lens of "mystery." We will give an example of this model in practice below.

IN THE BEGINNING

When patients and doctors meet for the first time, it is easy to get off on the wrong foot. Whether the setting is a private office waiting room or a first meeting with a hospitalized patient coping with serious illness, the chances for missteps are ever-present. One of our great teachers, Aaron Lazare, advanced the idea of seeing patients as customers, which to some of us trainees struck a discordant note, using a commercial or business term to describe our sacred doctor-patient relationship. But he was more concerned about leveling the playing field and modifying the power dynamics of patienthood. He knew that smart business people treated customers like gold and worked hard to meet their needs, whereas patients, especially in lofty academic medical centers, can, at times, be taken for

granted. More and more hospital systems have seen the light and have begun to practice hotel-quality customer service. Many wise doctors do much the same.

It is always crucial to put yourself in the patient's shoes. For those of us who practice psychiatry every day and have for years, it is hard to remember how scary, threatening, and downright weird a first encounter can be with the mental health system. Patients bring with them all sorts of preconceptions and stereotypes ("Can he read my mind? Will she think I'm crazy?") and if we are aloof or cool, it can be easy to project negative attributions. Moreover, for those of us in academic or public sector settings, many people we meet for the first time have had a lot of experience with psychiatry, often quite negative. People who come for care may have had a variety of traumatic experiences, including involuntary treatment or simple disrespect. When this is the case, we are starting the relationship with two strikes against us. We must establish kindness, warmth, and respect for the person immediately.

One way to do this is to practice the principles of hospitality, treating the patient as an honored guest.[26] A warm greeting, a smile, and other simple signs of friendliness go a long way. If the person has been waiting, an apology is in order (not followed by a disqualifying "but," as in "I am sorry you had to wait so long, but we have been very busy."). Name symmetry is important; if you expect to be called by the honorific "doctor," then Mr. or Ms. is appropriate for adults. Making sure that the person is comfortable, if they are with children that the children's needs are met, and any other host-like concerns are important.

Early on, we try to give the patient an idea of how long our meeting will be and our general process. "We will talk about your situation for about 45 minutes, including if we can any relevant past issues and treatment and how it helped or didn't, and then we'll use the last 15 or so minutes to figure out what, if anything, we'll do next. This might mean that we'll meet again because we need to talk more about that before we make any plans. Does that sound OK?" During first encounters in C-L settings, it is usually helpful to be clear that the consultant is part of the larger medical/surgical team; one part of the consultant's role can be to function as a liaison/advocate with other team members.

COLLABORATING AROUND HISTORY-TAKING

One goal of an initial interview is to generate a database that will support a comprehensive differential diagnosis. However, there are other over-arching goals. These include demystifying and explaining the process of collaboration, finding out what is troubling and challenging to the patient, co-creating a treatment path to address these problems, understanding the person as a whole, encouraging the patient's participation, welcoming feedback, and modeling a mindful appreciation of the complexity of human beings (including our inner emotional life).[41] It is especially important to determine why the patient is coming for care at this particular moment, as well as find out what they are hoping for (and, perhaps, what they are afraid might happen). At the end of the history-taking, a conversation should be feasible about paths toward healing and the patient's and doctor's mutual roles in that process.

Effective Clinical Interviewing

We will deal comprehensively with clinical interviewing in the following chapter. Here we will touch on those aspects of the clinical interview that reflect important features of the doctor-patient relationship. Keys to effective clinical interviewing are friendliness, warmth, a capacity to help patients feel at ease in telling their stories, and an ability to engage the person in a mutual exploration of what is troubling them. We find that if we demystify the clinical encounter, we are more likely to achieve good interviews. Similarly, by pausing often to ask the patient if we are understanding clearly or by seeking the patient's input and questions, we promote real conversation (rather than a one-sided interrogation) that yields deeper information.[42]

We find that another useful technique is to offer to tell the patient what we already know about him or her. For example, "I wonder if it would be helpful if I told you what Dr. Smith mentioned to me when she called me to consult in your care? That way, if I have any information wrong, you could straighten it out from the start." This technique allows us to "show our cards" before we ask the patient to reveal information about himself or herself. Moreover, by inviting correction, we demonstrate right away that we honor the person's

input. Last, this technique allows us to put the person's story in neighborly, non-pathological language, setting the stage for the interview to follow.[43]

Having opened the interview, we then try to be quiet and make room for the person to tell his or her story, encouraging (with body language, open-ended questions, and other encouragement) the person to say more. We try to resist the temptation to jump too early on closed-ended symptom checklists. We try to listen deeply to both the words and the music.

After a reasonable period, we ask the patient if we can summarize what we have heard and see whether we understand accurately what the patient is trying to say.[44] Saying, "Would it be OK if I check to see if I understand what you are saying so far?" is a good way of moving on to this part of the interview.

Asking Permission to Summarize Shifts the Often-Skewed Power Dynamic in Favor of the Patient

In reflecting back to the patient our summary of what we have heard, it is important to use language carefully. Whenever possible, we avoid inflammatory or otherwise inadvertently hurtful language ("So, it sounds like you were hallucinating, and perhaps having other psychotic symptoms"), in favor of neighborly, neutral language ("Sounds like things were difficult—did I understand you to say you were hearing things that troubled you?"). Whenever possible, we use the exact words that the patient has used to describe their emotional state. For example, if the person says, "I have been feeling so tired, just so very, very tired—I feel like I have nothing left," and we say, "It sounds as if you have been exhausted," we may not convey to the person that we have understood them; but if we say, "You have been just so terribly tired," it is more likely that the person will feel understood.

The "Nod"

Rapport is the essential core of successful interviewing. One indicator of rapport comes from getting the "nod"—that is, simply noticing if in the early stages of the interview the patient is nodding in agreement and otherwise giving signs of feeling understood.[37] If the "nod" is absent, it is a signal that something is amiss—either we have missed something important, have inadvertently offended the person, have failed to explain our process, or have otherwise derailed the relationship. A clinical interview without the "nod" is an interview in peril. Offering to say first what you know, putting the problem in neighborly language, asking permission to summarize what you have heard, and using the patient's own words are useful techniques for winning the "nod." Even more important is the power of simple kindness, friendliness, and neighborliness in our words, tone, and body language. Similarly, a friendly acknowledgment of something in common ("Interesting—I grew up in Maryland, too!") can go a long, long way toward creating connection and rapport.

Having established a tone of collaboration, identified the problem, and been given the "nod," the next area of focus is the history of the present illness. In eliciting the history of present illness, it is important to let the person tell his or her story. For many people, it is a deeply healing experience merely to be listened to in an empathic and attuned way.[39] We find it best to listen actively (by not interrupting and by not focusing solely on establishing the right diagnosis) and to make sure one is "getting it right" from the patient's point of view. When the physician hypothesizes that the patient's problem may be more likely to be in the psychological or interpersonal realm, it is especially important to give the patient a chance to share what is troubling him or her in an atmosphere of acceptance and empathy.

In taking the history of the present illness, under the pressure of time, it can be an error to rely too quickly on symptom checklists or to ask a series of closed-ended questions to rule-in or rule-out a diagnosis (such as major depression). Doing this increases the risk of prematurely closing off important information that the patient might otherwise impart about the social or psychological aspects of the situation.

As we move to different sections of the history, we consider explaining what we are doing and why: "I'd like now to ask some questions about your past psychiatric history, if any, to see if anything like this has happened before." This guided interview tends to demystify what you are doing and to elicit collaboration.[42]

The next area of focus is the past psychiatric history. The past psychiatric history can further illuminate the present illness. The interviewer ascertains past episodes of similar or related suffering (e.g., past episodes of depression or periods of anxiety, how they were treated, and how the patient responded). Past experiences of psychiatric treatment—positive or negative—are golden opportunities to learn what the patient has experienced as helpful or hurtful and may be useful in not repeating another practitioner's mistakes or practices or following the lead of practitioners who were felt to be helpful ("I really like working with Dr. Smith—he didn't just sit there; he told me what he thought. I didn't always agree with him, but I knew where he stood.").

The interview should establish past episodes of unrelated psychiatric illness (such as problems with anxiety, phobias, fears, and obsessions). These episodes may point the way to a diathesis toward affective or anxiety disorders that would otherwise be obscure. It may be useful to inquire about past periods of emotional difficulty as distinct from psychiatric illness per se.

The past medical history is a critical part of the database for every patient, regardless of the nature of the person's complaint or concern. The principal reason for this recalls the six-model method of conceptualizing psychiatric conditions alluded to earlier. By the end of the evaluation, it is critical that the physician be able to consider a differential diagnosis that includes hypotheses using all models: biological, psychological, social, spiritual/existential, and "mystery." For the biological model, of course, the past medical history is essential.

If a history of substance abuse was not included in the past psychiatric history, it can be elicited here, including gross indices of abuse (such as a history of detoxifications, attempts to cut down on substances, or specific substances of abuse), as well as more subtle questions, and possibly the use of structured inquiry, such as the CAGE questionnaire (which addresses whether a person has ever felt the need to *cut down on* their drinking; been *annoyed* by others criticizing their drinking; felt *guilty* about drinking; or needed a drink first thing in the morning, i.e., an *eye opener*).[45]

The family psychiatric history can yield important clues about conditions that may have genetic significance (such as bipolar disorder, schizophrenia, mood disorders, anxiety disorders, and substance use disorders). This is also a convenient time to sketch a limited genogram, attend to birth order, and consider the current circumstances of family members.

The social and developmental history offers an opportunity for data gathering in the social and psychological realms. Where the person was raised, what family life was like, how far the person went in school, what subjects the person preferred, and what hobbies and interests the person has are all fertile lines of pursuit. Marital and relationship history, whether the person has been in love, whom the person admires most, and who has been most important in the person's life are even deeper probes into this aspect of the person's experience. A deep and rapid probe into a person's history can often be achieved by the simple question, "What was it like for you growing up in your family?" Spiritual orientation and practice (including whether the person ever had a spiritual practice, and if so, what happened to change it?) fit well into this section of the history.[46]

The formal mental status examination continues the line of inquiry that was begun in the history of the present illness (i.e., the symptom checklists to rule-in or rule-out diagnostic possibilities and to ask more about detailed signs and symptoms to establish pertinent positives and negatives in the differential diagnosis). We deal with this in detail in Chapter 3.

An extremely important area, and one all too frequently given short shrift in diagnostic evaluations, is the area of the person's strengths and capabilities. As physicians, we are trained in the vast nosology of disease and pathology, and we admire the most learned physician as one who can detect the most subtle or obscure malady; indeed, these are important physician strengths. But there is, regrettably, no comparable nosology of strengths and capabilities. Yet, in the long road to recovery, it is almost always the person's strengths that the physician relies on to make a partnership toward healing. It is vitally important that the physician note these strengths and let the person know that the physician sees them and appreciates them.[47]

Sometimes strengths are obvious (e.g., high intelligence in a young person with a first-break psychosis or a committed and supportive family surrounding a person with recurrent depression). At other times, strengths are more subtle, or even counter-intuitive—for example, seeing that a woman who cuts herself repeatedly to distract herself from the agony of remembering past abuse has found a way to live with the unbearable; viewed this way, self-injury rather than suicide is a strength. Notable, too, may be her strength to survive, her faith to carry on, and other aspects of her life (e.g., a history of playing a musical instrument, a loving concern for children, a righteous rage to make justice in the world). Whatever the person's strengths, we must note them, acknowledge them to the patient, and remember them. An inability to find strengths and capacities to admire in a patient (alongside other attributes perhaps far, far less admirable) is almost always a sign of countertransference malice; this bears careful thought and analysis.

Finally, a clinical diagnostic interview should always include an opportunity for the patient to offer areas for discussion: "Are there areas of your life that we have not discussed that you think would be good for me to know about?" or "Are there things we have mentioned that you'd like to say more about?" or "Is there anything I haven't asked you about that I should have?"

PLANNING THE PATH FORWARD: CREATING A CLINICAL FORMULATION

Having heard the patient's story, the next challenge is to formulate an understanding of the person that can lead to a mutually developed treatment path. A formulation is not the same as a diagnosis.[38] A diagnosis describes a condition that can be reasonably delineated and described to the person, which implies a relatively foreseeable clinical course and usually implies options for treatment. As important as a diagnosis is in clinical medicine, a diagnosis alone is insufficient for effective treatment planning, and it is an inadequate basis for work by the doctor-patient dyad.

As we have mentioned, our preferred model is an expanded version of the bio-psycho-social framework, with three added dimensions: explicitly cataloging strengths; spiritual/existential issues; and a dimension we demarcate as "mystery," which is a placeholder that reminds us that much, if not most, of the time we are uncertain about the why of people's suffering, so we should humbly acknowledge our uncertainty and still try to be helpful, while not making matters worse.[25]

Not only is this model very useful in organizing our thoughts about a patient, but it can also be an efficient and effective way of inviting patients to think with us about what is wrong and how we might work together.

For example, we might engage in a conversation like the following:

"Mr. Jones, we have been talking for about 35 minutes and of course we've barely scratched the surface of your life story, but I'd like to spend the next 15 minutes or so putting our heads together about what is wrong and what we might do to help. Would that be OK?"

If Mr. Jones agrees, then we would usually ask, "Before we shift gears, is there anything we missed that you want to be sure I understand, or anything you want to add?"

Sometimes this stimulates important additional information; however, the person usually demurs. We then continue as follows: "Mr. Jones, I wonder if it would be OK if I took a few minutes to share with you how I think about people? This is what I think about when I'm trying to figure out if I can be helpful to someone. Would that be OK?" Nearly everyone agrees.

"OK. Thanks. When I meet someone who's having difficulties, I try to think about that person from six points of view, to get a 360-degree view of the whole person. Does that make sense?

"I start with reminding myself of the person's strengths—their talents, skills, abilities, attributes—because I don't want to get swamped by problems, and these strengths will be resources in whatever work we do together. You, Mr. Jones, for example, are clearly very intelligent, and you are very accomplished in your field of law, so you must have a lot of grit and capacity for hard work. You also sound to me like a loving father and you've been married for 15 years. You are a skilled golfer, which I admire. Even though you are feeling low, I can see you have a sense of humor, which is a great gift, and you have long-time friends. In other words, lots and lots of strengths. [*These strengths, of course, are specific to the individual patient; it's important that they are specific, and true.*]

"Then I try to think about the problems the person is facing from five points of view. The first one I call social: is there anything going on in the person's life that for whatever reason is making them miserable, anxious, overwhelmed? Or, is there something like

that that happened, that didn't get dealt with well and that is still bothering the person. Like, for example, a death of a loved one where grief was interrupted by too many responsibilities, and so it got swept under the rug. That's the social perspective. [*If relevant, we cite social stressors here.*] Does that make sense?

"The second way I think about things is psychological, and it's a little more complicated. The idea is that practically everybody has issues, usually stemming from when we were young, and these issues manifest themselves as recurrent patterns in our lives. Somebody who can't stand authority, for example, or someone who's very uncomfortable with intimacy, or someone who somehow married three consecutive spouses who were unfaithful—these would be examples of recurrent patterns. Most of the time, these patterns started as attempts to cope or solve a problem, but then the solution became a problem. An example would be alcohol use, which often starts as a soothing solution, but for some people turns into a problem. Make sense? [*We usually do not cite possible psychological patterns here, but we may, depending on the patient.*]

"The third model is biological, the idea that some problems that bring people to psychiatrists have biological causes or aspects. Some forms of depression, anxiety, bipolar disorder, or schizophrenia could be examples. This is the area where psychiatrists are most trained. [*Here we may cite the array of symptoms, severity and/or family history or other factors suggesting a biological aspect of the person's difficulties.*] And we have many options for dealing with the biological aspects of these sorts of difficulties.

"The fourth lens is not relevant to everyone, but it's important for some people and that is spiritual. If a person has a strong faith, for example, and something shakes it, like the death of a child or some other grievous event, it can turn a person's world upside down. [*Here we mention either spiritual factors or acknowledge that they may not be relevant.*]

"And lastly, I use a lens I call "mystery." That's just a way of reminding myself that these models are fine, but really everyone is very complicated, and much of the time we don't know and can't know the cause of suffering, and if we are too certain about our ideas, we can cause a lot of mischief. And yet, we want to help and to not make matters worse.

"So, these are the five models: social, psychological, biological, spiritual, and mystery. Do you relate to them? Do they make sense to you?"

Over many years of practice, our experience has been that people like and relate to the bio-psycho-social-spiritual-"mystery" model. In general, it earns "the nod." People seem to think it is useful, and they can relate to it. We think it is non-pathologizing and non-stigmatizing.

Laying out the bio-psycho-social-spiritual-mystery model this way creates an opportunity to draw out the patient's perspective. "May I ask then which of these lenses, if any, do you think would be most useful in thinking about the problems you've been dealing with?" The answer is almost always a combination, with a rare endorsement of the spiritual model and a wide appreciation for the mystery model. Sometimes the answer is surprising, as when a person with recurrent, severe depressive episodes and several relatives with mood disorders does not endorse the biological lens, or a person with chronic self-injury does not endorse the psychological lens. These are important signals to proceed carefully, and being forewarned of a tender, sensitive issue can save a lot of hurt and misunderstanding.

Almost everyone finds the five models understandable and meaningful, and most people appreciate having their strengths acknowledged. Moreover, and importantly, these five models avoid using language that overly pathologizes the person, and they use language that tends to universalize the patient's experience. Together, the strengths plus five lenses yield a comprehensive, practical formulation to frame the primary diagnosis. This initial formulation can facilitate a more in-depth discussion of diagnostic possibilities. With this framework, for example, the differential diagnosis can be addressed from a biological perspective, and acute social stressors can be acknowledged. The diagnosis and treatment can be framed in a manner consistent with the person's spiritual orientation. Fleshing out the psychological aspects can be more challenging, but this framework creates a way to address psychological patterns in a person's life, his or her interest in addressing them, and their ability to address them.

We also find it helpful to emphasize as part of the mystery model, the very imperfect art and science of psychiatric diagnosis and prognosis—humbly acknowledging the limits of knowledge. We find this tempers the sometimes stinging hurt of a stigmatized psychiatric diagnosis.

TREATMENT PLANNING

Having a good formulation as a frame for a comprehensive differential diagnosis permits the doctor and the patient to look at treatment options (including different modalities or even alternative therapies or solutions not based on traditional medicine). It is possible from this vantage point to look together at the risks and benefits of various approaches, as well as the demands of different approaches (the time and money invested in psychotherapy, for example, or the side effects that are expected in many medication trials). The sequence of treatments, the location, the cost, and other parameters of care can all be made explicit and weighed together.

This approach is also effective in dealing with situations in which the physician's formulation and that of the patient differ, so that consultation and possibly mediation can be explored.[47] For example, the physician's formulation and differential diagnosis for a person might be that the person's heavy drinking constitutes alcohol misuse, or possibly dependence, and that cessation from drinking or harm reduction is a necessary part of the solution to the patient's chronic severe anxiety and depression. The patient, on the other hand, may feel that if the doctor were offering more effective treatment for his anxiety and depression, he would then be able to stop drinking. An explicit formulation enables the patient and the doctor to see where, and how, they disagree and to explore alternatives. For example, in the case cited, the physician could offer to meet with family members with the patient, so both could get family input into the preferred solution, or the physician could offer the patient a referral for expert psychopharmacological consultation to test the patient's hypothesis.

In either case, however, the use of an explicit formulation in this way can identify problems and challenges early in the evaluation and can help the physician avoid getting involved in treatment under conditions that are likely to fail. Mutual expectations can be made clear (e.g., the patient must engage in a 12-step program, get a sponsor, and pursue sobriety for the duration of the treatment together), or the physician and patient may agree not to work together.

The formulation and differential diagnosis are, of course, always in flux, as more information becomes available and the doctor and patient come to know each other more deeply.

OBSTACLES AND DIFFICULTIES IN THE DOCTOR-PATIENT RELATIONSHIP

Many problems in the doctor-patient relationship arise from a misalignment between what the patient thinks is wrong, and what should be done about it, on the one hand, and the doctor's diagnosis and treatment plan, on the other. Looking back, it is sometimes the case that these difficulties arose out of insufficient rapport at the start, a lack of "nodding" if you will. Other causes of such misalignment include not getting clear early on what the patient's hopes and expectations are (e.g., in the case above, the patient's expectation might be that the doctor would prescribe benzodiazepines for anxiety) and what the doctor's limits are (that prescription of benzodiazepines in the setting of active alcohol misuse is contraindicated). In that case, the expectations and limits can collide, often heatedly in urgent or emergency circumstances. It is much safer and more effective to have these issues arise before treatment commences, during the evaluation phase.

This example also highlights another common element in doctor-patient conflicts. Physicians may misunderstand a patient's readiness to change and may assume that once the doctor has identified a diagnosis or problem, the patient is prepared to work to change it. A patient may not even recognize the problem, much less be prepared to take serious action to change it. In fact, when we talk to patients about problems they do not own (despite what may be a mountain of evidence), the person usually responds with hostility and defensiveness. Clarity about where the patient is in the cycle of change[48,49] can illuminate such misunderstandings and help the physician direct his or her efforts at helping the patient become more ready to change, rather than fruitlessly urging change to which the patient is not committed. Similarly, physicians may underestimate social, psychological, or spiritual aspects of a person's suffering that complicates the

person's willingness or ability to partner with the physician toward change. A deeply depressed patient, for example, whose sense of shame and worthlessness is so profound that the person feels that they do not deserve to recover, may be uncooperative with a treatment regimen until these ideas are examined in an accepting and supportive relationship.

Conflict may also arise from the nature of the problem to be addressed. In general, patients are interested in their illness—how they experience their symptoms, how their health can be restored, and how to ameliorate their suffering—whereas physicians are often primarily concerned with making an accurate diagnosis of an underlying disease.[47] Moreover, physicians may erroneously believe that the patient's "chief complaint" is the one that the patient gives voice to first, whereas patients often approach their doctors warily, not leading with their main concern, which they may not voice at all unless conditions of safety and trust are established.[47] Any inadvertent shaming of the patient makes the emergence of the real concern all the less likely.[13]

Conflict and difficulty may arise from the physician's training, language, or office environment. Physicians who use overly technical, arcane, or obtuse language distance themselves and make communication difficult. Similarly, physicians may lose sight of how intimidating, unintelligible, and forbidding medical practice—perhaps especially psychiatry—can appear to the uninitiated, unless proactive steps toward demystification occur. More insidious may be assumptions regarding the supposed incapacity of psychiatric patients to be full partners in their own care. Hurtful, dismissive language or a lack of appreciation for the likelihood that a patient has previously experienced hurtful care may damage the relationship.[13] Overly brief, symptom-focused interviews that fail to address the whole person, as well as his or her preferences, questions, and concerns, are inadequate foundations for an effective relationship.

Conflict may arise, too, over the goals of the work. Increasingly, mental health advocates and patients promote "recovery" as a desired outcome of treatment, even for severe psychiatric illnesses. Working toward recovery from schizophrenia or bipolar disorder, which most psychiatrists will regard as life-long conditions that require ongoing management, may seem unrealistic or even disingenuous.[50]

It may be useful for physicians to be aware that the term *recovery* is often used in the mental health community to signify a state of being analogous to recovery from alcohol use disorder or other substance abuse. In this context, one is never construed to be a "recovered" alcoholic, but rather a "recovering" alcoholic—someone whose sobriety is solid, who understands their condition and vulnerabilities well, practices good self-care, and is ever alert to risks of relapse, to which the person is vulnerable for his or her entire life.

In a mental health context, "recovery" similarly connotes a process of reclaiming one's life, taking charge of one's options, and stepping out of the position of passivity and victimization that major mental illness can often involve, particularly if treatment has involved involuntary treatment, stigmatization, or downright oppression. From this perspective, recovery means moving beyond symptomatic control of the disease to having a full life of one's own design (including work, friends, sexual relationships, recreation, political engagement, spiritual involvement, and other aspects of a full and challenging life). Symptoms are sometimes reframed as meaningful and manageable aspects of life.[50]

Other sources of conflict in the doctor-patient relationship may include conflict over methods of treatment (a psychiatrist, perhaps, who emphasizes medication to treat depression to the exclusion of other areas of the patient's life, such as a troubled and depressing marriage); over the conditions of treatment (e.g., the frequency of appointments, length of appointments, or access to the physician after hours); or over the effectiveness of treatment (e.g., the psychiatrist believes that antipsychotic medications restore a patient's function, whereas the patient believes the same medications create a sense of being drugged and "not myself").[12]

In these examples, as in so many challenges on the journey of rendering care, an answer may lie neither solely in the doctor's offered treatment nor in the patient's "resistance" to change, but in the vitality, authenticity, and effectiveness of the relationship between them.

REFERENCES

1. Lipkin M. Sisyphus or Pegasus? The physician interviewer in the era of corporatization of care. *Ann Intern Med.* 1996;124:511–513.
2. Neuberger J. Internal medicine in the 21st century: the educated patient: new challenges for the medical profession. *J Intern Med.* 2000;247:6–10.
3. Steiner K. Time for a paradigm change: pervasiveness and dangers of the medical model in adolescent psychology. *Ethical Hum Psychol Psychiatry.* 2014;16(2):99–113.
4. Stewart M, Brown JB, Donner A, et al. The impact of patient-centered care on outcomes. *J Fam Pract.* 2000;49:796–804.
5. Stevenson FA, Barry CA, Britten N, et al. Doctor-patient communication about drugs: the evidence for shared decision making. *Soc Sci Med.* 2000;50:829–840.
6. Frances V, Korsch BM, Morris MJ. Gaps in doctor-patient communication: patient response to medical advice. *N Engl J Med.* 1969;280:535–540.
7. Gutheil TG, Bursztajn HJ, Brodsky A. Malpractice prevention through the sharing of uncertainty. Informed consent and the therapeutic alliance. *N Engl J Med.* 1984;311:49–51.
8. Stewart M. Towards a global definition of patient centered care. *BMJ.* 2001;322:444–445.
9. Levinson W, Roter D, Mullooly JP, et al. Physician-patient communication—the relationship with malpractice claims among primary care physicians and surgeons. *JAMA.* 1997;277(7):553–559.
10. Zolnierek KBH, Dimatteo MR. Physician communication and patient adherence to treatment: a meta-analysis. *Medical Care.* 2009;47(8):826–834.
11. Stewart MA. Effective physician-patient communication and health outcomes: a review. *Can Med Assoc J.* 1995;152(9):1423–1433.
12. McCabe R, Healey PGT. Miscommunication in doctor-patient communication. *Topics in Cogn Sci.* 2018;10:409–424.
13. Lazare A. Shame and humiliation in the medical encounter. *Arch Intern Med.* 1987;147:1653–1658.
14. Knaak S, Mantler E, Szeto A. Mental illness-related stigma in healthcare: barriers to access and care and evidence-based solutions. *Healthc Manage Forum.* 2017;30(2):111–116.
15. Bedell SE, Graboys TB, Bedell E, et al. Words that harm, words that heal. *Arch Intern Med.* 2004;164:1365–1368.
16. Deegan PE, Drake RE. Shared decision making and medication management in the recovery process. *Psychiatr Serv.* 2006;57:1636–1638.
17. Crossing the quality chasm: a new health system for the 21st century, Washington, DC, 2001, Committee on Quality of Health Care in America, Institute of Medicine, National Academies Press.
18. Quill TE, Brody H. Physician recommendations and patient autonomy: finding a balance between physician power and patient choice. *Ann Intern Med.* 1996;125:763–769.
19. Henbest RJ. Time for a change: new perspectives on the doctor-patient interaction. *S Afr Fam Pract.* 1989;10:8–15.
20. Reuben DB, Tinetti ME. Goal-oriented patient care—an alternative health outcomes paradigm. *N Engl J Med.* 2012;366(9):777–779.
21. Charles C, Whelan T, Gafni A. What do we mean by partnership in making decisions about treatment? *BMJ.* 1999;319:780–782.
22. Lazare A, Eisenthal S, Wasserman L. The customer approach to patienthood. Attending to patient requests in a walk-in clinic. *Arch Gen Psychiatry.* 1975;32:553–558.
23. Beach MC, Sugarman J. Realizing shared decision-making in practice. *JAMA.* 2019;322(9):811–812.

24. Adler DA, Erlich MD, Goldman B, et al. Psychiatry in the time of COVID: credibility, uncertainty, and self-reflection. *J Nerv Ment Dis*. 2021;209(11):779–782.

25. Lazare A. *On Apology*. Oxford University Press; 2004.

26. Nouwen HJM. *Reaching Out: the Three Movements of the Spiritual Life*. Doubleday; 1975.

27. Hunter-Jones P, Line N, Zhang JJ, et al. Visioning a hospitality-oriented patient experience (HHOPE) framework in healthcare. *J Service Management, Bingley*. 2020;5(31):869–888.

28. Santorelli S. *Heal Thy Self. Lessons on Mindfulness in Medicine*. Bell Tower; 1999.

29. Messner E. Autognosis: diagnosis by the use of the self. In: Lazare A, ed. *Outpatient Psychiatry: Diagnosis and Treatment*. Williams & Wilkins; 1979.

30. Suzuki S. *Zen Mind, Beginner's Mind*. Weatherhill; 1980.

31. Novack DH, Suchman AL, Clark W, et al. Calibrating the physician: personal awareness and effective patient care. *JAMA*. 1997;278:502–509.

32. Brendel RW, Brendel DH. Professionalism and the doctor-patient relationship in psychiatry. In: Stern TA, ed. *The Ten-minute Guide to Psychiatric Diagnosis and Treatment*. Professional Publishing Group; 2005.

33. Gabbard GO, Nadelson C. Professional boundaries in the physician-patient relationship. *JAMA*. 1995;273:1445–1449.

34. Beresin EV. The doctor-patient relationships in pediatrics. In: Kaye DL, Montgomery ME, Munson SW, eds. *Child and Adolescent Mental Health*. Lippincott Williams & Wilkins; 2002.

35. Menage J. Why telemedicine diminishes the doctor-patient relationship. *BMJ*. 2020;371:4348.

36. Charon R. Narrative medicine: a model for empathy, reflection, profession and trust. *JAMA*. 2001;286:1897–1902.

37. Sanneke DH. Bio-psycho-social interaction: an enactive perspective. *Int Rev Psychiatry*. 2021;33(5):471–477.

38. Gordon C, Riess H. The formulation as a collaborative conversation. *Harv Rev Psychiatry*. 2005;13:112–123.

39. Thompson KS, Tasman A. This is the water: the social determinants of mental health and the future of Psychiatr. *Psychiatric Times*. 2022;39(1):6.

40. Sweeney A, Filson B, Kennedy A, et al. A paradigm shift: relationships in trauma-informed mental health services. *BJPsych Advances*. 2018;24(5):319–333.

41. Platt FW, Coulehan JL, Fox L, et al. "Tell me about yourself:" the patient centered interview. *Ann Intern Med*. 2001;134:1079–1085.

42. Gordon C, Goroll A. Effective psychiatric interviewing in primary care medicine. In: Stern TA, Herman JB, Slavin PL, eds. *The MGH Guide to Primary Care Psychiatry*. 2nd ed. New York: McGraw-Hill; 2004.

43. Hak T, Campion P. Achieving a patient-centered consultation by giving feedback in its early phases. *Postgrad Med J*. 1999;75:405–409.

44. Coulehan JL, Platt FW, Egener B, et al. "Let me see if I have this right": words that help build empathy. *Arch Intern Med*. 2001;135:221–227.

45. McQuade WH, Levy SM, Yanek LR, et al. Detecting symptoms of alcohol abuse in primary care settings. *Arch Fam Med*. 2000;9:814–821.

46. Koenig HG. Religion, spirituality and medicine: application to clinical practice. *JAMA*. 2000;284:1708.

47. Walsh K. The gap between doctors' and patients' perceptions. *BMJ*. 2004;329:502.

48. Levinson W, Cohen MS, Brady D, et al. To change or not to change: "sounds like you have a dilemma". *Arch Intern Med*. 2001;135:386–391.

49. Prochaska J, DiClemente C. Toward a comprehensive model of change. In: Miller WR, ed. *Treating Addictive Behaviors*. Plenum Press; 1986.

50. Jacobson N, Greenley D. What is recovery: a conceptual model and explication. *Psychiatr Serv*. 2001;52:482–485.

3

THE PSYCHIATRIC INTERVIEW

EUGENE V. BERESIN, MD, MA ■ CHRISTOPHER D. GORDON, MD

OVERVIEW

The purpose of the initial psychiatric interview is to build a relationship and a therapeutic alliance with an individual or a family, as well as to collect, organize, and synthesize information about present and past thoughts, feelings, and behavior. The relevant data derive from several sources: observing the patient's behavior with the examiner and with others present; attending to the emotional responses of the examiner; obtaining pertinent medical, psychiatric, social, cultural, and spiritual history (using collateral resources, if possible); and performing a mental status examination (MSE). The initial evaluation should enable the practitioner to develop a clinical formulation that integrates biological, psychological, and social dimensions of a patient's life and establish provisional clinical hypotheses and questions—the differential diagnosis—that need to be tested empirically in future clinical work.

A collaborative review of the formulation and differential diagnosis can provide a platform for developing (with the patient) options and recommendations for treatment, accounting for the patient's amenability to therapeutic intervention.[1] Few medical encounters are more intimate and potentially frightening and shameful than the psychiatric examination.[2] Therefore it is essential for the examiner to establish a secure environment conducive to the intimate self-disclosure that is necessary.

Several methods of the psychiatric interview are examined in this chapter. These methods include promoting a healthy and secure attachment between the doctor and the patient that promotes self-disclosure and reflection, and lends itself to the creation of a coherent narrative of the patient's life; appreciating the context of the interview that influences the interviewer's clinical technique; establishing an alliance around the task at hand and fostering effective communication; collecting data necessary for creation of a formulation of the patient's strengths and weaknesses, a differential diagnosis, and recommendations for treatment, if necessary; educating the patient about the nature of emotional, behavioral, and interpersonal problems and psychiatric and medical illness (while preparing the patient for psychiatric interventions, if indicated and agreed on, and setting up arrangements for follow-up); using special techniques with children, adolescents, and families; understanding difficulties and errors in the psychiatric interview; and documenting the clinical findings for the medical record and communicating with other clinicians involved in the patient's care. Finally, the interview must generate a relationship both with the patient and with the primary medical or surgical team as the basis of future collaboration for treatment.

Case 1

Mr. C, a 96-year-old male, presented to the emergency department (ED) the day after he tripped and fell on his way to the bathroom the previous night in his assisted-living facility. There was no pain, no head injury, and no loss of consciousness. He had called his 65-year-old son (a physician) and they agreed that Mr. C could probably return to bed and that they would talk the next day.

25

The day after the fall, Mr. C called his primary care provider (PCP) and reported that he had not urinated that day. He was told to go to the ED. His son, who was notified, met him at the hospital. His medications included a diuretic for hypertension, metoprolol for an arrhythmia, and escitalopram for anxiety. He had been treated for prostate cancer 6 years earlier, with excellent results.

In the ED he was alert and articulate, and able to describe his medical, social, and psychiatric history. His son corroborated the history. The consultant frequently turned to the son to obtain parts of the history. Mr. C also had a 60-year-old daughter. His wife had died 10 years earlier from cancer. He said that he was dizzy and short of breath. His work-up revealed that his hematocrit had dropped from a baseline of 35.3 to 29, and he had a large hematoma in his left chest, with six fractured ribs. There was no pneumothorax. Mr. C received a blood transfusion.

In the ED, he became disoriented and agitated and began talking to his wife. His son informed the nurse and a psychiatric consultation was ordered. About 2 hours later, the psychiatric consultant arrived and noted that Mr. C was oriented (times three), that his recent and remote memory was intact, and his speech was normal in flow and form. His mood and affect were normal, and he did not recall having spoken with his deceased wife. He denied hallucinations, paranoia, or suicidal ideation. The psychiatrist's interview included a lengthy discussion of his passion for fishing, boating, and gourmet cooking. They talked about his life-long work as an entrepreneur, and the loving relationship he had with his late wife. They also talked about their mutual love for sushi. He made frequent jokes about the long wait for a bed, and the frantic pace in the ED. Given Mr. C's long wait in the ED, he thought it might be a good idea for the hospital to have room service and this might help in the financial problems in the healthcare system, and he suggested that the hospital leadership might consult him for advice. He noted that serving fish would be wonderful for raising everyone's omega-3 fatty acids.

After Mr. C was admitted to the medical floor, he again became disoriented, agitated, and needed restraint (as he was attempting to pull out his intravenous lines and to leave his bed). The psychiatrist returned to his bedside, noted the changes in his mental status, and suggested low-dose haloperidol for what appeared to be an episode of delirium.

Later that evening, the consultant returned to find the man much improved. On greeting him, the psychiatrist was asked how he was doing with establishing room service, particularly now that he was in his room. They talked about the terrible quality of the hospital food, and the need for changes to the healthcare system, as well as a sushi bar in the hospital.

Unfortunately, delirium recurred despite moderately increased doses of haloperidol. The consultant discussed the case with the psychiatric resident covering the consultation service. The resident asked the attending consultant if the recurrent delirium might be complicated by alcohol withdrawal. The resident, who spent considerable time alone with Mr. C, inquired about his daily use of alcohol and noted that he tended to drink up to a fifth of vodka nightly to aid a chronic sleep problem. The senior consultant realized that his history was deficient, largely because he did not ask about alcohol or substance use and reflected that his history was influenced by the presence of the patient's son, who was a physician. He appreciated that he inadvertently omitted sensitive, but essential, parts of the interview to avoid shaming the patient and his son. This appreciation resulted in ordering lorazepam and having a more detailed discussion of substance use and his sleep disturbance.

LESSONS FROM ATTACHMENT THEORY, NARRATIVE MEDICINE, AND MINDFUL PRACTICE

"I'm the spirit's janitor. All I do is wipe the windows a little bit so you can see for yourself."
Godfrey Chips, Lakota Medicine Man[3]

Healthy interactions with "attachment figures" in early life (e.g., parents) promote robust biological, emotional, and social development in childhood and throughout the life cycle.[4] The foundations for attachment theory are based on research findings in cognitive neuroscience, genetics, and brain development that indicate an ongoing and life-long dance between an individual's neural circuitry, genetic predisposition, brain plasticity, and environmental influences.[5] Secure attachments in childhood foster emotional resilience[6] and generate skills and habits of seeking out selected attachment figures for comfort, protection, advice, and strength. Relationships based on secure attachments lead to effective use of cognitive functions, emotional flexibility, enhancement of security, assignment of meaning to experiences, and effective self-regulation.[5] In emotional relationships of many sorts, including the student-teacher and doctor-patient relationships, there may be many features of attachment present (such as seeking proximity or using an individual as a "safe haven" for soothing and as a secure base).[7]

What promotes secure attachment in early childhood, and how can we learn from this to understand a therapeutic doctor-patient relationship and an effective psychiatric interview? The foundations for secure attachment for children (according to Siegel) include several attributes ascribed to parents[5] (Box 3.1).

BOX 3.1

ELEMENTS THAT CONTRIBUTE TO SECURE ATTACHMENTS

- Communication that is collaborative, resonant, mutual, and attuned to the cognitive and emotional state of the child.
- Dialogue that is reflective and responsive to the state of the child. This creates a sense that subjective experience can be shared, and it allows for the child to "be seen." It requires use of empathy, "mindsight," and an ability to "see," or be in touch with, the child's state of mind.
- Identification and repair of miscommunications and misunderstandings. When the parent corrects problems in communication, the child can make sense of painful disconnections. Repair of communication failures requires consistent, predictable, reflective, intentional, and mindful caregiving. The emphasis here is on mindfulness and reflection. Mindfulness in this instance is an example of a parent's ability for self-awareness, particularly in his or her emotional reactions to the child and the impact of his or her words and actions on the child.
- Emotional communication that involves sharing feelings that amplify the positive and mitigate the negative.
- Assistance in the child's development of coherent narratives that connect experiences in the past and present, creating an autobiographical sense of self-awareness (using language to weave together thoughts, feelings, sensations, and actions as a means of organizing and making sense of internal and external worlds).

Clinicians should avoid patronizing their patients and steer clear of paternalistic power dynamics that could be implied in analogizing the doctor-patient relationship to one between parents and children; nonetheless, if we substitute "doctor" for "parent" and similarly substitute "patient" for "child," we can immediately see the relevance to clinical practice. We can see how important each of these elements is in fostering a doctor-patient relationship that is open, honest, mutual, collaborative, respectful, trustworthy, and secure. Appreciating the dynamics of secure attachment also deepens the meaning of "patient-centered" care. The medical literature indicates that good outcomes and patient satisfaction involve physician relationship techniques that involve reflection, empathy, understanding, legitimization, and support.[8,9] Patients reveal more about themselves when they trust their doctors, and trust has been found to relate primarily to behavior during clinical interviews[9] rather than to any preconceived notion of competence of the doctor or behavior outside the office.

Particularly important in the psychiatric interview is the facilitation of a patient's narrative. The practice of narrative medicine involves the ability to acknowledge, absorb, interpret, and act on the stories and struggles of others.[10] Charon[10] describes the process of listening to patients' stories as a process of following the biological, familial, cultural, and existential threads of the situation. It encompasses recognizing the multiple meanings and contradictions in words and events; attending to the silences, pauses, gestures, and non-verbal cues; and entering the world of the patient, while simultaneously arousing the doctor's own memories, associations, creativity, and emotional responses—all of which are seen in some way by the patient.[10] Narratives, like all stories, are co-created by the teller and the listener. Storytelling is an age-old part of social discourse that involves sustained attention, memory, emotional responsiveness, non-verbal responses and cues, collaborative meaning-making, and attunement to the listener's expectations. It is a vehicle for explaining behavior. Stories and storytelling are pervasive in society as a means of conveying symbolic activity, history, communication, and teaching.[5] If a physician can assist the patient in telling his or her story effectively, reliable and valid data will be collected, and the relationship solidified. Narratives are facilitated by authentic, compassionate, and genuine engagement.

A differential diagnosis detached from the patient's narrative is arid; even if it is accurate it may not lead to an effective and mutually designed treatment path. By contrast, an accurate and comprehensive differential diagnosis that is supported by a deep appreciation of the patient's narrative is experienced by both the patient and the physician as more three dimensional, and more real, and it is more likely to lead to a mutually created and achievable plan, with which the patient is much more likely to "comply."

Creating the optimal conditions for a secure attachment and the elaboration of a coherent narrative requires mindful practice. Just as the parent must be careful to differentiate his or her emotional state and needs from the child's and be aware of conflicts and communication failures, so too must the mindful practitioner. Epstein[11] notes that mindful practitioners attend in a non-judgmental way to their own physical and mental states during the interview. Their critical self-reflection allows them to listen carefully to a patient's distress, recognize their own errors, make evidence-based decisions, and stay attuned to their own values so that they may act with compassion, technical competence, and insight.[11]

Self-reflection is critical in psychiatric interviewing. Reflective practice entails observing ourselves (including our emotional reactions to patients, colleagues, and illness); our deficits in knowledge and skill; our personal styles of communicating; our responses to personal vulnerability and failure; our willingness or resistance to acknowledge error, to apologize, and to ask for forgiveness; and our reactions to stress. Self-awareness allows us to be aware of our own thoughts, feelings, and actions while we are in the process of practicing. By working in this manner, a clinician enhances his or her confidence, competence, sensitivity, openness, and lack of defensiveness—all of which assist in fostering secure attachments with patients and helping them share their innermost fears, concerns, and problems.

THE CONTEXT OF THE INTERVIEW: FACTORS INFLUENCING THE FORM AND CONTENT OF THE INTERVIEW

All interviews occur in a context. Awareness of the context may require modification of interviewing techniques. There are four elements to consider: the setting, the situation, the subject, and the significance.[12]

The Setting

Patients are exquisitely sensitive to the environment in which they are evaluated. There is a vast difference between being seen in an ED, on a medical floor, on an inpatient or partial hospital unit, in a psychiatric outpatient clinic, in a private doctor's office, in a school, or in a court clinic. Each setting has its benefits and downsides, and these must be assessed by the evaluator. For example, in the ED or on a medical or surgical floor, space for private, undisturbed interviews is usually inadequate. Such settings are filled with action and drama; hospital personnel frequently race around. ED visits may require long waits, and these contribute to impersonal approaches to patients and negative attitudes toward psychiatric patients. For a patient with borderline traits who is in crisis, this can create extreme frustration and exacerbate chronic fears of deprivation, betrayal, abandonment, and aloneness, and precipitate regression.[13] For these and for higher-functioning patients, the public nature of the environment and the frantic pace of the emergency service may make it difficult for the patient to present personal, private material calmly. In other public places (such as community health centers or schools), patients may worry about being recognized by neighbors or friends. Whatever the setting, it is always advisable to ask the patient directly how comfortable he or she feels in the examining room and to try to ensure privacy and a quiet environment with minimal distractions.

The setting must be comfortable for the patient and the physician. If the patient is agitated, aggressive, or threatening, it is always important to calmly assert that the examination requires that everyone is safe and that words and not actions will be used during the interview. Hostile patients should be interviewed in a setting in which the doctor is protected. An office in which an aggressive patient can block the door and in which there is no emergency button or access to a phone to call for help should be avoided; in such situations, alternative settings should be arranged. In some instances, local security may be needed to ensure safety.

The COVID-19 pandemic has been traumatic to many children, adolescents, and adults; it has raised significant mental health challenges, particularly with patients who are unable to, or are advised not to, be seen in the hospital. This has prompted a surge in telepsychiatry. Although many clinicians and patients had concerns about using digital media for psychiatric treatment, for many it was a godsend; it functioned much like home visits that were plentiful before the pandemic and provided a superb foundation for consultation and collaborative care with PCPs.[14] Studies have shown that telepsychiatry is an effective means of delivering psychiatric care, with the advantages of equality of access and high degrees of satisfaction among patients and clinicians. Unfortunately, there is a paucity of studies on its cost-effectiveness, and on the legal, ethical, and professional obstacles, such as practicing across state borders.[15,16] In particular, a major consideration is whether physicians must be licensed in other states if their patients reside outside of the state in which the physician is practicing. The question is basically where is the care being provided? This situation is particularly challenging for child and adolescent psychiatrists, who have often seen their patients for many years and made sound attachments with them and with their families. However, if these young people go to college, graduate school, or work in a different state, many hospital systems say they must receive care in the state in which they are residing. Thus if a clinician does not have a license in that state, they may not treat the patient or prescribe medications for them. This threatens a breach in a trusting relationship and can interfere with continuity of care, as the patient cannot always arrange to meet with another clinician without a long wait. This remains an unsolved and complex problem that challenges the patient-doctor relationship.[16] Although this is the current model, exceptions are made for physicians who work within the Veterans Administration System or the Indian Health Service. They can work in any state in the United States while having a license in only one state.

In the case of inpatients, private settings for the psychiatric interview are not easy to arrange. Semi-private rooms are common and, at times, confidentiality cannot be ensured. It is critical for the examining psychiatrist (and all members of the team) to acknowledge and apologize for the unfortunate lack of privacy. Being explicit about this may reinforce trust and demonstrate empathy. Clearly, the downsides of taking a history when others are in earshot risks the disclosure of sensitive information, disruption due to noise from those on the other side of a dividing curtain, refusal of physical examinations, and shame, stress, and inhibition to disclose important information, such as substance use. However, on occasion, hospital roommates can provide support, combat loneliness and isolation, and keep a close watch on another patient's condition.[17]

The Situation

Many individuals seek psychiatric help because they are aware that they have a problem. This may be a second or third episode of a recurrent condition (such as a mood disorder). They may have been referred by their PCP or by a doctor encountered in other ways. Given the limitations placed on psychiatrists by managed care companies, it is not unusual for a patient to have called multiple psychiatrists, only to find that their practices are all filled. Many clinics have no room for patients or are constrained by their contracts with specific vendors. The frustrating process of finding a psychiatrist sets the stage for some patients to either disparage the field and the healthcare system or to idealize the psychiatrist who has made the time for the patient. In either case, much goes on before the first visit that may affect the initial interview. To complicate matters, the evaluator needs to understand the patient's experience with psychiatrists and psychiatric treatment. Sometimes a patient has had a negative experience with another psychiatrist—perhaps a mismatch of personalities, a style that was ineffective, a treatment that did not work, or another problem. Many will wonder about a repeat performance. In all cases, in the history and relationship building, it is propitious to ask about prior treatments, what worked, and what did not, and particularly how the patient felt about the psychiatrist. There should be reassurance that this information is confidential and that the interest is in understanding that the match between doctor and patient is crucial. Even at the outset, it might be mentioned that the doctor will do his or her best to understand the patient and the problem, but that when plans are made for treatment, the patient should consider what kind of professional and setting is desired.

Other patients come to care reluctantly or even with great resistance. Many arrive at the request or demand of a loved one, friend, colleague, or employer because of behaviors deemed troublesome. The patient may deny any problem, or simply be too terrified to confront a condition that is bizarre, unexplainable, or "mental." Some conditions are ego-syntonic, such as anorexia nervosa. A patient with this eating disorder typically sees the psychiatrist as the enemy—as a doctor who wants to make her "get fat." For resistant patients, it is often useful to address the issue at the outset. For example, with a patient with anorexia who was referred by her internist and brought in by family, one could begin by saying, "Hi, Ms. Jones. I know you really don't want to be here. I understand that your doctor and family are concerned about your weight. I assure you that my job is first and foremost to understand your point of view. Can you tell me why you think they wanted you to see me?" Another common situation with extreme resistance is the individual who uses alcohol excessively and who is brought for care by a spouse or friend, and who is not ready to stop drinking. In this case you might say, "Good morning, Mr. Jones. I heard from your wife that she is really concerned about your drinking, and your safety, especially when you are driving. First, let me tell you that neither I nor anyone else can stop you from drinking. That is not my mission today. I do want to know what your drinking pattern is, but more, I want to get the picture of your entire life to understand your current situation." Extremely resistant patients may be brought for care involuntarily to an emergency service, often in restraints, by police or ambulance, because they are considered dangerous to themselves or others. It is typically terrifying, insulting, and humiliating to be physically restrained. Regardless of the reasons for admission, unknown to the psychiatrist, it is often wise to begin the interview as follows: "Hi, Ms. Carter, my name is Dr. Beresin. I am terribly sorry you are strapped down, but the police and your family were very upset when you locked yourself in your car and turned on the ignition. They found a suicide note on the kitchen table. Everyone was really concerned about your safety. I would like to discuss what is going on and see what we can do together to figure things out."

Psychiatrists are often asked to perform evaluations on medical or surgical inpatients who have symptoms arising from their treatment. These patients may have no idea that they are going to be seen by a psychiatrist. This was never part of their agreement when they came into the hospital for surgery, and no one may have explained the risks of developing delirium. Some delirious patients are cognizant of their altered mental status and are extremely frightened. They may wonder whether the condition is going to persist. For example, if we know a patient has undergone abdominal surgery for colon cancer and has been agitated, sleepless, hallucinating, and delusional, a psychiatric consultant might begin, "Good morning, Mr. Harris. My name is Dr. Beresin. I heard about your surgery from Dr. Rand and understand that you have been having some strange or frightening experiences. Sometimes after surgery, people have a reaction to the procedure or the medications used, which leads to agitation, confusion, and difficulties with sleep. This is not unusual, and it is generally temporary. I would like to help you and your team figure out what is going on and what we can do about this." Other requests for psychiatric evaluation may require entirely different skills, such as when the medical team or emergency service seeks help for a family who has lost a loved one.

In each of these situations, the psychiatrist needs to understand the situation and account for it when conducting the evaluation. In the examples provided above, only the introduction was addressed. However, when we see the details (discussed next) about building a relationship and modifying communication styles and questions to meet the needs of each situation, other techniques might need to be employed to create a therapeutic alliance. It is always helpful to obtain as much ancillary information as possible before the interview begins. This may be done by talking with the PCP, looking in an electronic medical record, and talking with family, friends, or professionals (such as police or emergency medical technicians).

The Subject

Naturally, the clinical interview needs to account for features of the subject, including age, developmental level, sex, sex identity, preferred pronouns for being addressed, and cultural background. Moreover, one needs to determine "who" the patient is. In families, there may be an identified patient (e.g., a child with conduct disorder or a child with chronic abdominal pain). However, the examiner must keep in mind that psychiatric and medical syndromes do not develop in a vacuum. While the family has determined an "identified patient," the examiner should consider that when evaluating the child, all members of the environment need to be part of the evaluation. A similar situation occurs when an adult child brings in an elderly demented parent for an evaluation. It is incumbent on the evaluator to consider the home environment and caretaking, in addition to simply evaluating the elderly patient. In couples, one or both may identify the "other" as the "problem." An astute clinician needs to allow each person's perspective to be clarified, and the examiner will not "take sides."

Children and adolescents require special consideration. While they may, indeed, be the "identified patient," they are embedded in a home life that requires evaluation; the parent(s) or guardian(s) must help administer any prescribed treatment, psychotropic or behavioral. Furthermore, the developmental level of the child should be considered in the examination. Young children may not be able to articulate what they are experiencing. For example, an 8-year-old boy who has panic attacks may simply throw temper tantrums and display oppositional behavior when asked to go to a restaurant. Although he may be phobic about malls and restaurants, his parents may simply see his behavior as defiance. When asked what he is experiencing, he may be unable to describe palpitations, shortness of breath, fears of impending doom, or tremulousness. However, if he is asked to draw a picture of himself at the restaurant, he may draw himself with a scared look on his face, and with jagged lines all around his body. Then, when specific questions are asked, he can acknowledge many classic symptoms of panic disorder. For young children, the room should be equipped with toys, dollhouses, and materials to create pictures.

Evaluation of adolescents raises additional issues. While some adolescents are seen willingly, others are dragged to the assessment against their will. In this instance, it is important to identify and empathize with the teenager: "Hi, Tony. I can see this is the last place you want to be. But now that you have been hauled in here by your folks, we should make the best of it. Look, I have no clue what is going on, and don't even know if you are the problem! Why don't you tell me your story?" Teenagers may indeed feel like hostages. They may have bona fide psychiatric disorders or may be stuck in a terrible home situation. The most important thing the examiner must convey is that the teenager's perspective is important, and that this will be looked at, as well as the parent's point of view. It is also critical to let all patients know about the rules and limits of confidentiality. Many children think that whatever they say will be directly transmitted to their parents. Surely this is their experience in school. However, there are clear guidelines about adolescent confidentiality, and these should be delineated at the beginning of the clinical encounter. Confidentiality is a core part of the evaluation, and it will be honored for the adolescent; it is essential that this is communicated to them so they may feel safe in divulging sensitive and private information without fear of repercussion. Issues such as sexuality, sexually transmitted diseases, substance misuse, and issues in mental health are protected by state and federal statutes. There are, however, exceptions; one major exception is that if the patient or another is in danger by virtue of an adolescent's behavior, confidentiality is waived.[18]

The Significance

Psychiatric disorders are commonly stigmatized and subsequently are often accompanied by profound shame, anxiety, denial, fear, and uncertainty. Patients generally have a poor understanding of psychiatric disorders, either from myth, lack of information, or misinformation from the media (e.g., TV, radio, social media, and the Internet).[19] Many patients have preconceived notions of what to expect (bad or good), based on the experience of friends or family. Some patients, having talked with others or having searched online, may be certain or worried that they suffer from a certain condition, and this may color the information presented to an examiner. A specific syndrome or symptom may have significance to a patient, perhaps because a relative with a mood disorder was hospitalized for many years, before the de-institutionalization of mentally disordered individuals. Hence, he or she may be extremely wary of divulging any indication of severe symptoms lest life-long hospitalization result. Obsessions or compulsions may be seen as evidence of losing one's mind, having a brain tumor, or becoming like Aunt Jesse with a chronic psychosis.[12] Some patients (based on cognitive limitations) may not understand their symptoms. This may be normal, such as with the developmental stage of a school-age child, whereas others may be a function of congenital cognitive impairment, autism spectrum disorder, or cerebral lacunae secondary to multiple infarcts following embolic strokes.

Finally, there are cultural differences in the way mental health and mental illness are viewed. Culture may influence health-seeking and mental health–seeking behavior, the understanding of psychiatric symptoms, the course of psychiatric disorders, the efficacy of various treatments, or the kinds of treatments accepted.[20] Psychosis, for example, may be viewed as possession by spirits. Some cultural groups have much higher completion rates for suicide, and thus previous attempts on one's life in some individuals should be taken more seriously. Understanding the family structure may be critical to the negotiation of treatment; approval by a family elder could be crucial in the acceptance of professional help.

ESTABLISHING AN ALLIANCE AND FOSTERING EFFECTIVE COMMUNICATION

Studies of physician-patient communication have demonstrated that good outcomes flow from effective communication; developing a good patient-centered relationship is characterized by friendliness, courtesy, empathy, and partnership building, and by the provision of information. Positive outcomes have included benefits to emotional health, symptom resolution, and physiological measures (e.g., blood pressure, blood glucose level, and pain control).[21–24]

In 1999 leaders and representatives of major medical schools and professional organizations convened at the Fetzer Institute in Kalamazoo, Michigan, to propose a model for doctor-patient communication that would lend itself to the creation of curricula for medical and graduate medical education, and for the development of standards for the profession. The goals of the Kalamazoo Consensus Statement[25] were to foster a sound doctor-patient relationship and to provide a model for the clinical interview. The key elements of this statement are summarized in Box 3.2 and are applicable to the psychiatric interview.

In recent years, we have become more sensitive to the importance of trauma-informed care. Understanding the importance of trauma in an individual's life requires a sensitivity to adverse childhood experiences that may have a life-long influence on emotions, situational triggers, relationships, trust, and confidence in

---

BOX 3.2
BUILDING A RELATIONSHIP: THE FUNDAMENTAL TASKS OF COMMUNICATION

- Elicit the patient's story while guiding the interview by diagnostic reasoning.
- Maintain an awareness of the fact that feelings, ideas, and values of both the patient and the doctor influence the relationship.
- Develop a partnership with the patient and form an alliance in which the patient participates in decision-making.
- Work with patients' families and support networks.

OPEN THE DISCUSSION
- Allow the patient to express his or her opening statement without interruption.
- Encourage the patient to describe a full set of concerns.
- Maintain a personal connection during the interview.

GATHER INFORMATION
- Use both open- and closed-ended questions.
- Provide structure, clarification, and a summary of the information collected.
- Listen actively, using verbal and non-verbal methods (e.g., eye contact).

UNDERSTAND THE PATIENT'S PERSPECTIVE
- Explore contextual issues (e.g., familial, cultural, spiritual, age, sex, and socioeconomic status).
- Elicit beliefs, concerns, and expectations about health and illness.
- Validate and respond appropriately to the patient's ideas, feelings, and values.

SHARE INFORMATION
- Avoid technical language and medical jargon.
- Determine if the patient understands your explanations.
- Encourage questions.

REACH AGREEMENT ON PROBLEMS AND PLANS
- Welcome participation in decision-making.
- Determine the patient's amenability to following a plan.
- Identify and enlist resources and support.

PROVIDE CLOSURE
- Ask if the patient has questions or other concerns.
- Summarize and solidify the agreement with a plan of action.
- Review the follow-up plans.

others; this may also extend to physicians. Establishing effective communication with a trauma victim ultimately requires eliciting the precipitating event(s), as well as the resultant impact on thoughts, feelings, emotions, relationships, and behavior; however, this is usually not accomplished in the initial patient-doctor interview. It is critical that the interviewer acknowledge that a patient has experienced trauma and that if past or current trauma is occurring in some form, we need to identify a way to talk about this together. Addressing safety during the initial interview is essential. Thus initially asking about traumatic events, and inquiring about current threats to oneself or others is essential. It is also useful for us to say something like, "Ms. Jones, I understand you have been through a lot, and that you are continuing to struggle with the results of personal trauma. May we agree to continue this discussion in a way that is sensitive, respectful, and that covers areas that impact your life, in an ongoing way? Let's consider this a marathon and not a sprint. But for now, I just need to be sure you are safe. OK?"[26]

Motivational interviewing has been an effective tool for working with patients with addictions. It helps to build an alliance around the management of substance use but has broader applications in health care and is extremely valuable in eliciting, fostering, and maintaining the motivation for change. The fundamental principles of motivational interviewing involve a patient-centered approach that supports and encourages self-reflection and the desire for change while appreciating that there is more than a modicum of ambivalence in the effort to modify one's behavior.[27] The key technique of the provider is to know when to transition from reflective exploration of the balance between motivation for, and resistance to, change while building goals and a plan.

BUILDING THE RELATIONSHIP AND THERAPEUTIC ALLIANCE

All psychiatric interviews should begin with making a personal introduction and establishing the purpose of the interview; this helps to create an alliance around the initial examination. The interviewer should attempt to greet the person warmly and use words that demonstrate care, attention, and concern. Note taking and use of computers should be minimized, and if used, should not interfere with ongoing eye contact. The interviewer should indicate that this interaction is collaborative and that any misunderstandings on the part of the patient or physician should be clarified immediately. In addition, the patient should be instructed to ask questions, interrupt, and provide corrections or additions at any time. The time frame for the interview should be announced. In general, the interviewer should acknowledge that some of the issues and questions raised will be highly personal, and that if there are issues that the patient has real trouble with, he or she should let the examiner know. Confidentiality should be assured at the outset of the interview. These initial guidelines set the tone, quality, and style of the clinical interview. An example of a beginning is, "Hi, Mr. Smith. My name is Dr. Beresin. I am delighted you came in today. I would like to discuss some of the issues or problems you are dealing with so that we can both understand them better and figure out what kind of assistance may be available. I will need to ask you several questions about your life, about your past and the present, and if I need some clarification about your descriptions, I will ask for your help to be sure that I 'get it.' If you think I have missed the boat, please chime in and correct my misunderstanding. Some of the topics may be highly personal, and I hope that you will let me know if things get a bit too much. We will have about an hour to go through this, and then we'll try to come up with a reasonable plan together. I do want you to know that everything we say is confidential. Do you have any questions about our job today?" This should be followed with an open-ended question about the reasons for the interview.

One of the most important aspects of building a therapeutic alliance is helping the patient feel safe. Demonstrating warmth and respect is essential. In addition, the psychiatrist should display genuine interest and curiosity in working with a new patient. Preconceived notions about the patient should be eschewed. We need to be cognizant that every clinician has a certain degree of implicit bias: an unconscious awareness that leads to stereotypic, or at worst, devaluation of a patient, often based on race, ethnicity, sex identity, or sexual preference. It is incumbent on our healthcare system to work assiduously to help us make our biases conscious, and then through various means, disarm them.[28] Although implicit bias is unconscious, it is often identified by the patient, just as the implicit bias of the patient is perceived by the clinician. This mutual process is one of the most common forms of threatening a trusting relationship and it needs to be considered for each interview. If there are questions about the patient's cultural background or spiritual beliefs that may have an impact on the information provided, on the emotional response to symptoms, or on the acceptance of a treatment plan, the physician should note at the outset that if any of these areas are of central importance to the patient, he or she should feel free to speak about such beliefs or values. The patient should have the sense that both the doctor and the patient are exploring the history, life experience, and current symptoms together.

For many patients, the psychiatric interview is probably one of the most confusing examinations in medicine. The psychiatric interview is at once professional and profoundly intimate. We are asking patients to reveal parts of their life they may only have shared with extremely close friends, a spouse, clergy, or family if anyone. And they are coming into a setting in which they are supposed to do this with a total stranger. Being a doctor may not be sufficient to allay the apprehension that surrounds this situation; being a trustworthy, caring human being may help a great deal. It is vital to make the interview highly personal and to use techniques that come naturally. Beyond affirming and validating the patient's story with extreme sensitivity, some clinicians may use humor and judicious self-revelation. These elements are characteristics of healers.[29]

An example should serve to demonstrate some of these principles. A 65-year-old deeply religious female was seen for an evaluation of delirium following coronary artery bypass graft surgery. She told the psychiatric examiner in her opening discussion that she wanted to switch from her PCP, whom she had seen for over 30 years. As part of her post-operative delirium, she developed the delusion that he may have raped her during one of his visits with her. She felt that she could not possibly face him, her priest, or her family, and she was stricken with deep despair. While the examiner may have recognized this as a biological consequence of her surgery and post-operative course, her personal experience spoke differently. She would not

immediately accept an early interpretation or explanation that her brain was not functioning correctly. In such a situation, the examiner must verbally acknowledge her perspective, seeing the problem through her eyes, and helping her see that he or she "gets it." For the patient, this was a horrible nightmare. The interviewer might have said, "Mrs. Jones, I understand how awful you must feel. Can you tell me how this could occurred given your longstanding and trusting relationship with your doctor?" She answered that she did not know, but that she was really confused and upset. When the examiner established a trusting relationship, completed the examination, determined delirium was present, and explained the nature of this problem, they agreed on using haloperidol to improve sleep and "nerves." Additional clarifications could be made in a subsequent session after the delirium cleared.

As noted earlier, reliable mirroring of the patient's cognitive and emotional state and self-reflection of one's affective response to patients are part and parcel of establishing secure attachments. Actively practicing self-reflection and clarifying one's understanding help to model behavior for the patient, as the doctor and patient co-create the narrative. Giving frequent summaries to "check in" on what the physician has heard may be very valuable, particularly early in the interview, when the opening discussion or chief complaints are elicited. For example, a 22-year-old female gradually developed obsessive-compulsive symptoms over the past 2 years that led her to become housebound. The interviewer said, "So, Ms. Thompson, let's see if I get it. You have been stuck at home and cannot get out of the house because you must walk up and down the stairs for several hours. If you did not 'get it right,' something terrible would happen to one of your family members. You also noted that you were found walking the stairs in public places, and that even your friends could not understand this behavior, and they made fun of you. You mentioned that you had to 'check' on the stove and other appliances being turned off, and could not leave your car, because you were afraid it would not turn off, or that the brake was not fully on, and again, something terrible would happen to someone. And, you said to me that you were really upset because you knew this behavior was 'crazy.' How awful this must be for you! Did I get it right?" The examiner should be sure to see both verbally and non-verbally that this captured the patient's problem. If positive feedback did not occur, the examiner should attempt to see if there was a misinterpretation, or if the interviewer came across as judgmental or critical. One could "normalize" the situation and reassure the patient to further solidify the alliance by saying, "Ms. Thompson, your tendency to stay home, stuck, in the effort to avoid hurting anyone is totally natural given your perception and concern for others close to you. I do agree, it does not make sense, and appreciate that it feels bizarre and unusual. I think we can better understand this behavior, and later I can suggest ways of coping and maybe even overcoming this situation through treatments that have been quite successful with others. However, I do need to get some additional information. Is that OK?" In this way, the clinician helps the patient feel understood—that anyone in that situation would feel the same way, and that there is hope. But more information is needed. This strategy demonstrates respect and understanding, and provides support and comfort while building the alliance.

DATA COLLECTION: BEHAVIORAL OBSERVATION, THE MEDICAL AND PSYCHIATRIC HISTORY, AND THE MENTAL STATUS EXAMINATION

Behavioral Observation

There is a lot to be learned about patients by observing them before, during, and after the psychiatric interview. It is useful to see how the patient interacts with support staff of the clinic, and with family, friends, or others who accompany him or her to the appointment. In the interview one should take note of grooming, the style and state of repair of clothes, mannerisms, normal and abnormal movements, posture and gait, physical features (such as natural deformities, birthmarks, or cutting marks, scratches, tattoos, or piercings), skin quality (e.g., color, texture, and hue), language (including English proficiency, the style of words used, grammar, vocabulary, and syntax), and non-verbal cues (such as eye contact and facial expressions). All these factors contribute to clinical formulation.

The Medical and Psychiatric History

Box 3.3 provides an overview of the key components of the psychiatric history.

Presenting Problems

The interviewer should begin by presenting the problem using open-ended questions. The patient should be encouraged to tell his or her story without interruptions. Many times, the patient will turn to the doctor for elaboration, but it is best to let the patient know that he or she is the true expert and that only he or she has experienced this situation directly. It is best to use clarifying questions throughout the interview. For example, "I was really upset and worked up" may mean one thing to the patient and something else to an examiner. It could mean frustrated, anxious, agitated, violent, or depressed. Such a statement requires clarification. So, too, does a comment such as "I was really depressed." Depression to a psychiatrist may be very different for a patient. To some patients, depression means aggravated, angry, or sad. It might be a momentary agitated state or a chronic state. Asking more detailed questions not only clarifies the affective state of the patient but also transmits the message that he or she knows best and that a real collaboration and dialogue is the only way we will figure out the problem. In addition, once the patient's words are clarified it is very useful to use the patient's own words throughout the interview to verify that you are listening.[30]

When taking the history, it is vital to remember that the patient's primary concerns may not be the same as the physician's. For example, while the examiner may be concerned about bipolar disorder and escalating mania, the patient may be more concerned about her husband's unemployment and how this is making her agitated and sleepless. If this was the reason for the psychiatric visit, namely concern about coping with household finances, this should be validated. There will be ample time to get a detailed history to establish a diagnosis of mania, particularly if the patient feels the clinician and she are on the same page. It is always useful to ask, "What are you most worried about?"

In discussing the presenting problems, it is best to avoid checklist-type questions, but one should cover the bases to create a *Diagnostic and Statistical Manual of Mental Disorders, Fifth Edition (DSM-5)*, differential diagnosis. It is best to focus largely on the chief complaint and present problems and to incorporate other parts of the history around this. The presenting problem is the reason for a referral, and is probably most important to the patient, even though additional questions

BOX 3.3
THE PSYCHIATRIC HISTORY

IDENTIFYING INFORMATION

Name, address, phone number, and e-mail address
Insurance
Age, sex, marital status, occupation, children, ethnicity, and religion
For children and adolescents: primary custodians, school, and grade
Primary care physician
Psychiatrist, allied mental health providers
Referral source
Sources of information
Reliability

CHIEF COMPLAINT/PRESENTING PROBLEM(S)

History of Present Illness

Onset
Perceived precipitants
Signs and symptoms
Course and duration
Treatments: professional and personal
Effects on personal, social, and occupational or academic function
Co-morbid psychiatric or medical disorders
Psychosocial stressors: personal (psychological, medical), family, friends, work/school, legal, housing, and financial

PAST PSYCHIATRIC HISTORY

Previous Episodes of the Problem(s)

Symptoms, course, duration, and treatment (inpatient or outpatient)

Psychiatric Disorders

Symptoms, course, duration, and treatment (inpatient or outpatient)

Past Medical History

Medical problems: past and current
Surgical problems: past and current
Accidents
Allergies
Immunizations
Current medications: prescribed and over-the-counter (OTC) medications
Other treatments: acupuncture, chiropractic, homeopathic, yoga, and meditation
Tobacco: present and past use
Substance use: present and past use
Pregnancy history: births, miscarriages, and abortions
Sexual history: birth control, safe sex practices, and history of, and screening for, sexually transmitted infections

Past or present physical or sexual abuse
Assessment of pain (on a scale of 0–10)

REVIEW OF SYSTEMS

Family History

Family psychiatric history
Family medical history

PERSONAL HISTORY: DEVELOPMENTAL AND SOCIAL HISTORY

Early Childhood

Developmental milestones
Family relationships

Middle Childhood

School performance
Learning or attention problems
Family relationships
Friends
Hobbies
Media use

Adolescence

School performance (include learning and attention problems)
Friends and peer relationships
Family relationships
Psychosexual history
Dating and sexual history
Work history
Substance use
Problems with the law
Media use

Early Adulthood

Education
Friends and peer relationships
Hobbies and interests
Marital and other romantic partners
Occupational history
Military experiences
Problems with the law
Media use

Mid-life and Older Adulthood

Career development
Marital and other romantic partners
Changes in the family
Media use
Losses
Aging process: psychological and physical

Adapted from Beresin EV. The psychiatric interview. In: Stern TA, editor. *The Ten-minute Guide to Psychiatric Diagnosis and Treatment*. Professional Publishing Group; 2005.

about current function and the past medical or past psychiatric history may be more critical to the examiner. A good clinician, having established a trusting relationship, can always redirect a patient to ascertain additional information (such as symptoms not mentioned by the patient and the duration, frequency, and intensity of symptoms). In addition, it is important to ask how the patient has coped with the problem and what is being done personally or professionally to help him or her deal with it. One should ask if there are other problems or stressors, medical problems, or family issues that exacerbate the current complaint. Questions about extreme distress, including pain (on a scale of 0–10) must always be assessed. After a period of open-ended questions about the current problem, the interviewer should ask questions about mood, anxiety, and other behavioral problems and how they affect the presenting problem. A key part of the assessment of the presenting problem should be a determination of safety. Questions about suicide, homicide, domestic violence, other forms of trauma, and abuse should be included in a review of the current situation. If one is concerned about self-harm, the interviewer should ask about the possible means, including access to firearms in the home. Finally, one should ascertain why the patient came for help now, how motivated he or she is to get help, and how the patient is faring in their personal, family, social, and professional life. Without knowing more, since this is early in the interview, the examiner should avoid offering premature reassurance; instead, it is preferable to provide support and encouragement for therapeutic assistance that will be offered in the latter part of the interview.

Past Psychiatric History

After the opening phases of the interview, open-ended questions may shift to more focused questions. In the past psychiatric history, the interviewer should inquire about previous DSM-5 diagnoses (including the symptoms of each, partial syndrome, how they were managed, and how they affected the patient's life). A full range of treatments, including outpatient, inpatient, and partial hospital, should be considered. It is most useful to ask what treatments, if any, were successful, and if so, in what ways. By the same token, the examiner should ask about treatment failures. This, of course, will contribute to the treatment recommendations provided at the end of the interview. This may be a good time in the interview to get a sense of how the

patient copes under stress. What psychological, behavioral, and social means are employed in the service of maintaining equilibrium in the face of hardship? It is also wise to focus not just on coping skills, defenses, and adaptive techniques in the face of the psychiatric disorder but also on psychosocial stressors in general (e.g., births, deaths, loss of jobs, problems in relationships, and problems with children). Discerning a patient's coping style may be highly informative and contribute to psychiatric formulation. Does the patient rely on venting emotions, shutting affect off and wielding cognitive controls, using social supports, displacing anger onto others, or on finding productive distractions (e.g., plunging into work)? Again, knowing something about a person's style of dealing with adversity uncovers defense mechanisms, reveals something about personality, and aids in the consideration of treatment options. For example, a person who avoids emotion uses reason and sets about to increase tasks in hard times may be an excellent candidate for a cognitive-behavioral approach to a problem. An individual who thrives through venting emotions, turning to others for support, and working to understand the historical origins of his or her problems may be a good candidate for psychodynamic psychotherapy, either individual or group.

Past Medical History

Several psychiatric symptoms and behavioral problems are secondary to medical conditions, the side effects of medications, and to drug-drug interactions (including those related to OTC medications). The past medical history needs to be thorough and must include past and current medical and surgical conditions, past and current use of medications (including vitamins, herbs, and non-traditional remedies), use of substances (e.g., tobacco, alcohol, and other drugs [past and present]), immunization and travel history, pregnancies, menstrual history, a history of hospitalizations and day surgeries, accidents (including sequelae, if any), and sexual history (including use of contraception, abortions, history of sexually transmitted infections, and testing for the latter).

Review of Systems

By the time the examiner asks about the past medical history and the review of systems, checklist-type questioning is adopted in lieu of the previous format of interviewing. It is useful to elicit a complete review of systems following the medical history. Several undiagnosed medical disorders may be picked up in the course of the psychiatric interview. Many patients do not routinely see their PCP, and psychiatrists have a unique opportunity to consider medical conditions and their evaluation in the examination. While not a formal part of the interview, laboratory testing is a core part of the psychiatric examination. Though this chapter refers to the interview, the review of systems may alert the clinician to order additional laboratory tests and consult the PCP about the medical investigation.

Family History

The fact that many illnesses run in families requires an examiner to ask about the family history of medical, surgical, and psychiatric illnesses, along with their treatments.

Social and Developmental History

The developmental history is important for all psychiatric patients, but especially for children and adolescents, because prevention and early detection of problems may lead to interventions that can correct deviations in development. The developmental history for early and middle childhood and adolescence should include questions about developmental milestones (e.g., motor function, speech, growth, social and moral achievements), family relationships in the past and present, school history (including grade levels reached and any history of attention or learning disabilities), friends, hobbies, jobs, interests, athletics, substance use, and any legal problems. Questions about adult development should focus on the nature and quality of intimate relationships, friendships, relationships with children (e.g., natural, adopted, products of assisted reproductive technology, stepchildren), military history, work history, hobbies and interests, legal issues, and financial problems. Questions should always be asked about domestic violence (including a history of physical or sexual abuse in the past and present).

The social history should include questions about a patient's cultural background, including the nature of this heritage, how it affects family structure and function, belief systems, values, and spiritual practices. Questions should be asked about the safety of the community and the quality of the social supports in the neighborhood, the place of worship, or other loci in the community.

An important component of social and developmental history, particularly valuable for children and adolescents, is media history. The overwhelming amount, availability, and use of media have grown exponentially since television was introduced in the 1950s. Children 8 to 18 years old spend an average of 6.5 hours a day using media (if one considers the time involved with television, movies, video games, print, radio, and recorded music), much of it digital media; the time spent reaches 8 hours daily when simultaneous media are used. This takes up more time than any other activity for youth other than sleeping.[31] The impact of media, including violent media, on the growth and development of children, is under considerable debate. Studies have demonstrated that media significantly affects clinical symptoms, such as body image,[32] post-traumatic stress disorder (PTSD),[33] and potentially aggressive behavior.[34] Few parents know what their children are watching or even the content of their video games.[35] Further, media is used by adults for multiple purposes, including obtaining medical and psychiatric information. Many patients will come in for an evaluation with a preconceived notion of their problem, or even ask for a specific medication based on information they have found online. Conversely, others will refuse treatment recommendations based on information (or misinformation) posted online.

Given the influence of media, both positive and negative, on the health of our youth and our adult patients, it is highly advisable to include a media history in the psychiatric interview. Beyond taking stock of what types of media are used by family members and for what purposes, clinicians, allied health professionals, and parents should become more media literate, and understand the broad range of material and methods of transmission of information and communication.[35]

Use of Corollary Information

While many interviews of adults are conducted with just the patient, it is quite useful to obtain additional information from other important people in the patient's life (such as a spouse or partner, siblings, children, parents, friends, and clergy). For example, a patient who appears paranoid and mildly psychotic may deny such symptoms or not see them as problems. To understand the nature of the problem, its duration and intensity, and its impact on function, others may need to be contacted (with informed consent). This applies to many other conditions, particularly substance use disorders (SUDs), in which the patient may deny the quantity used and the frequency of effects of substances on everyday life.

Obtaining consent to contact others in a patient's life is useful not only for information gathering but also for the involvement of others in the treatment process, if needed. For children and adolescents, this is essential, as is obtaining information from teachers or other school personnel. Contacting the patient's PCP or therapist may be useful for objective assessment of the medical and psychiatric history, as well as for corroboration of associated conditions, doses of medications, and past laboratory values. Finally, it is always useful to review the medical record (if accessible, and with permission).

The Mental Status Examination

The MSE is part and parcel of any medical and psychiatric interview. Its traditional components are indicated in Box 3.4. Most of the data needed in this model can be ascertained by asking the patient about elements of the current problems. Specific questions may be needed for the evaluation of perception, thought, and cognition. Most of the information in the MSE is obtained by simply taking the psychiatric history

and by observing the patient's behavior, affect, speech, mood, thought, and cognition.

Perceptual disorders include abnormalities of sensory stimuli. There may be misperceptions of sensory stimuli, known as *illusions*, for example, micropsia or macropsia (objects that appear smaller or larger, respectively, than they are). Phenomena such as this include distortions of external stimuli (affecting the size, shape, intensity, or sound of stimuli). Distortions of stimuli that are internally created are hallucinations and may occur in any one or more of the following modalities: auditory, visual, olfactory, gustatory, or tactile.

Thought disorders may manifest with difficulties in the form or content of thought. Formal thought disorders involve the way ideas are connected. Abnormalities in form may involve the logic and coherence of thinking. Such disorders may herald neurological disorders, severe mood disorders (e.g., psychotic depression or mania), schizophreniform psychosis, delirium, or other disorders that impair reality testing. Examples of formal thought disorders are listed in Box 3.5.[36,37]

Disorders of the content of thought pertain to the specific ideas themselves. The examiner should always inquire about paranoid, suicidal, and homicidal

---

BOX 3.4
THE MENTAL STATUS EXAMINATION

General appearance and behavior: grooming, posture, movements, mannerisms, and eye contact
Speech: rate, flow, latency, coherence, logic, and prosody
Affect: range, intensity, lability
Mood: for example, euthymic, elevated, depressed, irritable, anxious
Perception: illusions and hallucinations
Thought (coherence and lucidity): form and content (illusions, hallucinations, and delusions)
Safety: suicidal and homicidal thoughts, self-injurious ideas, impulses, and plans
Cognition
- Level of consciousness
- Orientation
- Attention and concentration
- Memory (registration, recent and remote)
- Calculation
- Abstraction
- Judgment
- Insight

BOX 3.5
EXAMPLES OF FORMAL THOUGHT DISORDERS

- **Circumstantiality**: a disorder of association with the inclusion of unnecessary details until one arrives at the goal of the thought
- **Tangentiality**: use of oblique, irrelevant, and digressive thoughts that do not convey the central idea to be communicated
- **Loose associations**: jumping from one unconnected topic to another
- **Clang associations**: an association of speech without logical connection dictated by the sound of the words rather than by their meaning; it frequently involves using rhyming or punning
- **Perseveration**: repeating the same response to stimuli (such as the same verbal response to different questions) with an inability to change the responses
- **Neologism**: words made up; often a condensation of different words; unintelligible to the listener
- **Echolalia**: persistent repetition of words or phrases of another person
- **Thought blocking**: an abrupt interruption in the flow of thought, in which one cannot recover what was just said

thinking. Other indications of disorder of thought content include delusions, obsessions, and ideas of reference (Box 3.6).[37]

The cognitive examination includes an assessment of higher processes of thinking. This part of the examination is critical for a clinical assessment of neurological function and is useful for differentiating focal and global disorders, delirium, and dementia. The traditional model assesses a variety of dimensions (Box 3.7).[38]

Alternatively, the Mini-Mental State Examination[39] may be administered (Table 3.1). It is a highly valid and reliable instrument that takes about 5 minutes to perform and is very effective in differentiating depression from dementia.

BOX 3.6
DISORDERS OF THOUGHT CONTENT

- **Delusions**: fixed, false, unshakable beliefs
- **Obsessions**: persistent thought that cannot be extruded by logic or reasoning
- **Idea of reference**: misinterpretation of incidents in the external world as having special and direct personal reference to the self

---

BOX 3.7
CATEGORIES OF THE MENTAL STATUS EXAMINATION

- **Orientation**: to time, place, person, and situation, for example.
- **Attention and concentration**: for example, remembering three objects immediately, in 1 and 3 minutes; spelling "world" backward; performing digit span.
- **Memory**: registration; recent and remote memory. Registration is typically a function of attention and concentration. Recent and remote memory is evaluated by recalling events in the short and long term, for example, the names of the presidents provided backward.
- **Calculations**: evaluated typically by serially subtracting 7 from 100.
- **Abstraction**: assessed by the patient's ability to interpret proverbs or other complex ideas.
- **Judgment**: evaluated by seeing if the patient demonstrates an awareness of personal issues or problems and provides appropriate ways of solving them.
- **Insight**: an assessment of self-reflection and an understanding of one's condition or the situation of others.

There are several brief, valid, and reliable instruments that may be used in history and MSE. Since substance misuse is such a common problem, the clinician might include the CAGE* examination for alcohol abuse[40,41] for adults or the CRAFFT† examination for alcohol or substance abuse in teenagers aged 14 to 18 years.[42,43]

SHARING INFORMATION AND PREPARING THE PATIENT FOR TREATMENT

The conclusion of the psychiatric interview requires summarizing the symptoms and history and organizing them into a coherent narrative that can be reviewed and agreed on by the patient and the clinician. This involves recapitulating the most important findings and explaining their meaning to the patient. It is crucial to obtain an agreement on the clinical material and the way the story holds together for the patient. If the patient does not concur with the summary, the psychiatrist should return to the relevant portions of the interview in question and revisit the topics that are in dispute.

This part of the interview should involve explaining one or more diagnoses (their biological, psychological, and environmental etiology) to the patient, as well as providing a formulation of the patient's strengths, weaknesses, and style of managing stress. The latter part of the summary is intended to help ensure that the patient feels understood. The next step is to delineate the kinds of approaches that the current standards of care would indicate

---

*The CAGE assessment for alcohol use in adults, expanded is: Have you felt the need to Cut down on your drinking? Do you feel Annoyed by people complaining about your drinking? Do you ever feel Guilty about your drinking? Do you ever drink an Eye-opener in the morning to relive the shakes?.

†The CRAFFT examination for substance use in teenagers is part of an assessment tool for substance use and has a rating scale associated. The major questions include: Have you ever ridden in a CAR driven by someone (including yourself) who was "high" or had been using alcohol or drugs? Do you ever use alcohol or drugs to RELAX, feel better about yourself, or fit in? Do you ever use alcohol or drugs while you are by yourself, or ALONE? Do you ever FORGET things you did while using alcohol or drugs? Do your FAMILY or FRIENDS ever tell you that you should cut down on your drinking or drug use? Have you ever gotten into TROUBLE while you were using alcohol or drugs?.

TABLE 3.1
Mini-Mental State Examination

MEAN SCORES

Depression	9.7
Depression with impaired cognition	19.0
Uncomplicated depression	25.1
Normal	27.6

Maximum Score	Score	
		Orientation
5	( )	What is the (year) (date) (day) (month)?
5	( )	Where are we (state) (county) (town) (hospital) (floor)?
		Registration
3	( )	Name three objects: 1 second to say each. Then ask the patient all three after you have said them. Give 1 point for each correct answer. Then repeat them until the patient learns all three. Count trials and record.
Trials _____		
		Attention and Calculation
5	( )	Serial 7s: 1 point for each correct. Stop after five answers. Alternatively, spell "world" backward.
		Recall
3	( )	Ask for three objects repeated above. Give 1 point for each correct answer.
		Language
2	( )	Name a pencil and watch. (2 points)
1	( )	Repeat the following: "No ifs, ands, or buts." (1 point)
3	( )	Follow a three-stage command: "Take a piece of paper in your right hand, fold it in half, and put it on the floor." (3 points)
1	( )	Read and obey the following: "Close your eyes." (1 point)
1	( )	Write a sentence. It must contain a subject and a verb and be sensible. (1 point)
		Visual-Motor Integrity
1	( )	Copy design (two intersecting pentagons; all 10 angles must be present and 2 must intersect). (1 point)

Total score _____

Assess level of consciousness along a continuum:

Alert	Drowsy	Stupor	Coma

Reproduced from Folstein MF, Folstein SE, McHugh PE. The Mini-Mental State Exam: a practical method for grading the cognitive state of patients for the clinician. *J Psychiatr Res.* 1975;12:189–198.

are appropriate for treatment. If the diagnosis is uncertain, further evaluation should be recommended to elucidate the problem or co-morbid problems. This might require one or more of the following: further laboratory evaluation; medical, neurological, or pediatric referral; psychological or neuropsychological testing; use of standardized rating scales; or consultation with a specialist (e.g., a psychopharmacologist or a sleep disorders or SUD specialist).

Education about treatment should include reviewing the pros and cons of various options. This is a good time to dispel myths about psychiatric treatments, either pharmacotherapy or psychotherapy. Each of these domains has a significant stigma associated with them. For patients who are prone to shun pharmacotherapy (not wanting any "mind-altering" medications), it may be useful to "medicalize" the psychiatric disorder and note that common medical conditions involve attention to biopsychosocial treatment.[12] For example, few people would refuse medications for the treatment of hypertension, even though it may be clear that the condition is exacerbated by stress and lifestyle. The same may be said for the treatment of asthma, migraines, diabetes, and peptic ulcers. In this light, the clinician can refer to psychiatric conditions as problems of "chemical imbalances"—a neutral term—or as problems with the brain, an organ that people often forget about when talking about "mental" conditions. A candid dialogue in this way, perhaps describing how depression or panic disorder involves abnormalities in brain function, may help. It should be noted that this kind of discussion should in no way be construed or interpreted as pressure—rather as an educational experience. Letting the patient know that treatment decisions are collaborative and patient centered is essential in a discussion of this magnitude.

A similar educational conversation should relate to the use of psychotherapies. Some patients disparage psychotherapies as "mumbo jumbo," lacking scientific evidence. In this instance, the discussion can center around the fact that scientific research indicates that experience and the environment can affect biological function. An example of this involves talking about how early trauma affects child development, or how coming through an experience in war can produce PTSD, a significant dysfunction of the brain. Many parents will immediately appreciate how the experiences in childhood affect a child's mood, anxiety, and behavior, though they will also point out that children are born with certain personalities and traits. This observation is wonderful as it opens a door for a discussion of the complex and ongoing interaction among the brain, environment, and behavior.

THE EVALUATION OF CHILDREN AND ADOLESCENTS

Psychiatric disorders in children and adolescents will be discussed elsewhere in this book. In general, children and adolescents pose certain unique issues for the psychiatric interviewer. First, a complete developmental history is required. For younger children, most of the history is taken from the parents. Rarely are young children seen apart (initially) from their parents. Observation of the child is critical. The examiner should notice how the child relates to the parents or caregivers. Conversely, it is important to note whether the adult's management of the child is appropriate. Does the child seem age appropriate in terms of motor function and growth? Are there any observable neurological impairments? The evaluator should determine whether speech, language, cognition, and social function are age appropriate. The office should have an ample supply of toys (including a dollhouse and puppets for fantasy play, and building blocks or similar toys), board games (for older school-age children), and drawing supplies. Collateral information from the pediatrician and schoolteachers is critical to verify or amplify parental and child-reported data. For children with suspected attention-deficit/hyperactivity disorder (ADHD), a brief rating scale, such as the Conners or Vanderbilt[44] is a useful screening device. Remember, though "all that wheezes is not asthma," all that appears as distractibility is not necessarily ADHD; if this is a strong consideration, referral for comprehensive neuropsychological testing is warranted to consider other neurological or emotional underpinnings of poor attention.

Adolescents produce their own set of issues and problems for the interviewer.[45] A teenager may or may not be brought in by a parent. However, given the developmental processes that surround the quests for identity and separation, the interviewer must treat the teen with the same kind of respect and collaboration as with an adult. The issue and importance of ensuring confidentiality have been mentioned previously. The adolescent also needs to hear at the outset that the interviewer will need to obtain permission to speak with parents or guardians and that any information received from them will be faithfully transmitted to the patient.

Although all the principles of attempting to establish a secure attachment noted previously apply to the adolescent, the interview of the adolescent is quite different from that of an adult. Developmentally, teenagers are capable of abstract thinking and are developmentally becoming increasingly autonomous. At the same time, they are struggling with grandiosity that alternates with extreme vulnerability and self-consciousness and managing body image, sexuality and aggression, mood lability, and occasional regression to dependency—all of which make an interview and relationship difficult. Furthermore, with incomplete myelination, particularly of their frontal lobes, incomplete until the mid-20s, they are more prone to impulsivity, acting without considering consequences, and more prone to peer pressure. The interviewer must constantly consider what counts as normal adolescent behavior and what risk-taking behaviors, mood swings, and impulsivity are pathological. This is not easy, and typically teenagers need a few initial meetings for the clinician to feel capable of co-creating a narrative—albeit a narrative in progress. The stance of the clinician in working with adolescents requires moving in a facile fashion between an often-needed professional authority figure and a big brother or sister, camp counselor, and friend. The examiner must be able to know something about the adolescent's culture, use humor and exaggeration, be flexible, and be empathic in the interview, yet not attempt to be "one of them." It is essential to validate strengths and weaknesses and to inspire self-reflection and some philosophical thinking—all attendant with the new cognitive developments since earlier childhood.

DIFFICULTIES AND ERRORS IN THE PSYCHIATRIC INTERVIEW

Dealing With Sensitive Subjects

Several subjects are particularly shameful for patients. Such topics include sexual problems, substance misuse and other addictions, financial matters, impulsive behavior, bizarre experiences (such as obsessions and compulsions), domestic violence, histories of trauma and abuse, and symptoms of psychosis. Some patients will either deny or avoid discussing these topics. In this situation, non-threatening, gentle encouragement and acknowledgment of how difficult these matters are may help. If the issue is not potentially dangerous or life-threatening to the patient or to others, the clinician may omit some questions known to be important in the diagnosis or formulation. If it is not essential to obtain this information in the initial interview, it may be best for the alliance to let it go, knowing the examiner or another clinician may return to it as the therapeutic relationship grows.

In other situations that are dangerous (such as occur with suicidal, homicidal, manic, or psychotic patients), in which pertinent symptoms must be ascertained, questioning is crucial no matter how distressed the patient may become. In some instances when danger seems highly likely, hospitalization may be necessary for observation and further exploration of a serious disorder. Similarly, an agitated patient who needs to be assessed for safety may need sedation or hospitalization to complete a comprehensive evaluation, particularly if the cause of agitation is unknown and the patient is not collaborating with the evaluative process.

Disagreements About Assessment and Treatment

There are times when a patient disagrees with a clinician's formulation, diagnosis, and treatment recommendations. In this instance, it is wise to listen to the patient and hear where there is conflict. Then the evaluator should systematically review what was said and how he or she interpreted the clinical findings. The patient should be encouraged to correct misrepresentations. Sometimes clarification will help the clinician and patient reach an agreement. At other times, the patient may deny or minimize a problem. In this case, additional interviews may be necessary. It is sometimes useful to involve a close relative or friend if the patient allows this. If the patient is a danger to self or others, however, protective measures will be needed, short of any agreement. If there is no imminent danger, explaining one's clinical opinion and respecting the right of the patient to choose treatment must be observed.

Errors in Psychiatric Interviewing

Common mistakes made in the psychiatric interview are provided in Box 3.8.

BOX 3.8
COMMON ERRORS IN THE PSYCHIATRIC INTERVIEW

- Premature closure and false assumptions about symptoms
- False reassurance about the patient's condition or prognosis
- Defensiveness around psychiatric diagnoses and treatment, with arrogant responses to myths and complaints about psychiatry
- Omission of significant parts of the interview due to theoretical bias of the interview (e.g., mind-body splitting)
- Recommendations for treatment when diagnostic formulation is incomplete
- Inadequate explanation of psychiatric disorders and their treatment, particularly not giving the patient multiple options for treatment
- Minimization or denial of the severity of symptoms due to overidentification with the patient; countertransference phenomenon (e.g., as occurs with treatment of a "very important person" in a manner inconsistent with ordinary best practice, with a resultant failure to protect the patient or others)
- Inadvertently shaming or embarrassing a patient and not offering an apology

REFERENCES

1. Gordon C, Reiss H. The formulation as a collaborative conversation. *Harv Rev Psychiatry.* 2005;13:112–123.
2. Lazare A. Shame and humiliation in the medical encounter. *Arch Intern Med.* 1987;147:1653–1658.
3. Garrett M. *Walking on the Wind: Cherokee Teachings for Harmony and Balance.* Bear & Co; 1998:145.
4. Parkes CM, Stevenson-Hinde J, Marris P, eds. *Attachment Across the Life Cycle.* Routledge; 1991.
5. Siegel DJ. *The Developing Mind: How Relationships and the Brain Interact to Shape Who We Are.* 2nd ed. Guilford Press; 2012.
6. Rutter M. Clinical implications of attachment concepts: retrospect and prospect. In: Atkinson L, Zucker KJ, eds. *Attachment and Psychopathology.* Guilford Press; 1997.
7. Lieberman AF. Toddlers' internalization of maternal attribution as a factor in quality of attachment. In: Atkinson L, Zucker KJ, eds. *Attachment and Psychopathology.* Guilford Press; 1997.
8. Lipkin M, Frankel RM, Beckman HB, et al. Performing the medical interview. In: Lipkin M Jr, Putnam SM, Lazare A, eds. *The Medical Interview: Clinical Care, Education and Research.* Springer-Verlag; 1995.
9. Lipkin M Jr. Sisyphus or Pegasus? The physician interviewer in the era of corporatization of care. *Ann Intern Med.* 1996;124:511–513.
10. Charon R. Narrative medicine: a model for empathy, reflection, profession and trust. *JAMA.* 2001;286:1897–1902.
11. Epstein RM. Mindful practice. *JAMA.* 2004;291:2359–2366.
12. Beresin EV. The psychiatric interview. In: Stern TA, ed. *The Ten-Minute Guide to Psychiatric Diagnosis And Treatment.* Professional Publishing Group; 2005.
13. Beresin EV, Gordon C. Emergency ward management of the borderline patient. *Gen Hosp Psychiatry.* 1981;3:237–244.
14. Fortney JC, Haegerty PJ, Bauer AM, et al. Study to promote innovation in rural integrated telepsychiatry (SPIRIT): rational and design of a randomized comparative effectiveness trial of managing complex psychiatric disorders in rural primary care clinics. *Contemp Clin Trials.* 2020;90. https://doi.org/10.1016/j.cct.2019.105873.
15. Chakrabarti S. Usefulness of tele psychiatry: a critical evaluation of videoconferencing-based approaches. *World J Psychiatry.* 2015;22;5(3):286–304.
16. Mehrotra A, Nimgaonkar A, Richman B. Telemedicine and licensure - potential paths for reform. *N Engl J Med.* 2021;384:687–690.
17. Eshel N, Marcovitz DE, Stern TA. Psychiatric consultations in less-then private places: challenges an unexpected benefits of hospital roommates. *Psychosomatics.* 2016;57(1):97–101. https://doi.org/10.1016/j-psym.2015.09.007.
18. Ford C, English A, Sigman G. Confidential health care for adolescents: position paper of the Society for Adolescent Medicine. *J Adolesc Health.* 2004;35:160–167.
19. Butler JR, Hyler S. Hollywood portrayals of child and adolescent mental health treatment: implications for clinical practice. *Child Adolesc Psychiatr Clin N Am.* 2005;14:509–522.
20. Mintzer JE, Hendrie HC, Warchal EF. Minority and sociocultural issues. In: Sadock BJ, Sadock VA, eds. *Kaplan and Sadock's Comprehensive Textbook of Psychiatry.* Lippincott Williams & Wilkins; 2005.
21. Stewart MA. Effective physician–patient communication and health outcomes: a review. *CMAJ.* 1995;152:1423–1433.
22. Simpson M, Buckman R, Stewart M, et al. Doctor-patient communication: the Toronto consensus statement. *BMJ.* 1991;303:1385–1387.
23. Williams S, Weinman J, Dale J. Doctor-patient communication and patient satisfaction: a review. *Fam Pract.* 1998;15:480–492.
24. Ong LML, De Haes CJM, Hoos AM, et al. Doctor-patient communication: a review of the literature. *Soc Sci Med.* 1995;40:903–918.
25. Makoul G. Participants in the Bayer-Fetzer Conference on Physician-Patient Communication in Medical Education Essential elements of communication in medical encounters: the Kalamazoo Consensus Statement. *Acad Med.* 2001;76:390–393.
26. Knight C. Trauma informed practice and care: implications for field instruction. *Clin Social Work J.* 2019;47:79–89.
27. Rsnicow K, McMaster F. Motivational interviewing: moving from why to how with autonomy support. *Int J Behav Nutr Phys Act.* 2012;9:19.
28. Fitzgerald C, Hurst S. Implicit bias in healthcare professionals: a systematic review. *BMC Med Ethics.* 2017;18:19. https://doi.org/10.1186/s12910-017-0179-8.
29. Novack DH, Epstein RM, Paulsen RH. Toward creating physician-healers: fostering medical students' self-awareness, personal growth, and well-being. *Acad Med.* 1999;74:516–520.

30. Gordon C, Goroll A. Effective psychiatric interviewing to primary care medicine. In: Stern TA, Herman JB, Slavin PL, eds. *Massachusetts General Hospital Guide in Primary Care Psychiatry*. 2nd ed. McGraw-Hill; 2004.

31. Kaiser Family Foundation *Generation M: Media in the Lives of 8–18-Year-Olds*. Kaiser Family Foundation; 2005.

32. Wiseman CV, Sunday SR, Becker AE. Impact of media on body image. *Child Adolesc Psychiatric Clin N Am*. 2005;14:453–471. In: Beresin EV, Olson CK, editors: Child Psychiatry and the Media.

33. Fremont WP, Pataki C, Beresin EV. The impact of terrorism on children and adolescents: terror in the skies, terror on television. *Child Adolesc Psychiatric Clin N Am*. 2005;14:429–451. In: Beresin EV, Olson CK, editors: Child Psychiatry and the Media.

34. Gunter B. Media violence: is there a case for causality? *Am Behav Sci*. 2008;51(8):1061–1122.

35. Villani SV, Olson CK, Jellinek MS. Media literacy for clinicians and parents. *Child Adolesc Psychiatric Clin N Am*. 2005;14:523–553. In: Beresin EV, Olson CK, editors: Child Psychiatry and the Media.

36. Scheiber SC. The psychiatric interview, psychiatric history, and mental status examination. In: Hales RE, Yudofsky SC, eds. *The American Psychiatric Press Synopsis of Psychiatry*. American Psychiatric Press; 1996.

37. Sadock BJ. Signs and symptoms in psychiatry. In: Sadock BJ, Sadock VA, eds. *Kaplan and Sadock's Comprehensive Textbook of Psychiatry*. Lippincott Williams & Wilkins; 2005.

38. Silberman EK, Certa K. The psychiatric interview: settings and techniques. In: Tasman A, Kay J, Lieberman J, eds. *Psychiatry*. 2nd ed. John Wiley & Sons; 2004.

39. Folstein MF, Folstein SE, McHugh PE. The Mini-Mental State Exam: a practical method for grading the cognitive state of patients for the clinician. *J Psychiatr Res*. 1975;12:189–198.

40. Dhalla S, Kopec JA. The CAGE questionnaire for alcohol misuse: a review of reliability and validity studies. *Clin Invest Med*. 2007;30(1):33–41.

41. Ewing JA. Detecting alcoholism: the CAGE questionnaire. *JAMA*. 1984;252:1905–1907.

42. Knight JR, Sherritt L, Shrier LA, et al. Validity of the CRAFFT substance abuse screening test among adolescent patients. *Arch Pediatr Adolesc Med*. 2002;156(6):607–614.

43. Knight JR, Shrier LA, Bravender TD, et al. A new brief screen for adolescent substance abuse. *Arch Pediatr Adolesc Med*. 1999;153:591–596.

44. Gaba P, Giordanego M. Attention-deficit/hyperactivity disorder: screening and evaluation. *Am Family Physician*. 2019;99(11):712.

45. Beresin EV, Schlozman SC. Psychiatric treatment of adolescents. In: Sadock BJ, Sadock VA, eds. *Kaplan and Sadock's Comprehensive Textbook of Psychiatry*. Lippincott Williams & Wilkins; 2005.

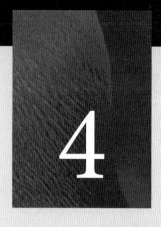

4

LIMBIC MUSIC

NICHOLAS KONTOS, MD

When you talk with the patient, you should listen, first, for what he wants to tell, secondly for what he does not want to tell, thirdly for what he cannot tell.
— L.J. Henderson 1935[1]

INTRODUCTION

First appearing in 1987 in an internally published collection of essays celebrating the 50th anniversary of the Massachusetts General Hospital Department of Psychiatry,[2] George Murray's "Limbic Music" is a rare example of medical literature producing actual *literature*. Its synthesis of neuroscience, philosophy, clinical wisdom, and engaging writing was, like Dr. Murray himself, unique. Subsequent versions of that essay appearing in the journal *Psychosomatics*,[3] and in every edition of this *Handbook*, inspired many psychiatrists' career paths and practice patterns.

With the publication of this chapter expected to occur within months of the 10th anniversary of Dr. Murray's death, readers are encouraged to track down and spend some time with one of his own iterations of it. Those who do will find much of (clinical, academic, and entertainment) value and little that is rendered obsolete by intervening developments in the fields of knowledge drawn on. As nicely argued recently by Pievani,[4] evolution does not necessarily build over the past (as some views of the "primitive" limbic system maintain). Instead, evolution often builds with what already exists, revising, integrating, and sometimes repurposing rather than discarding—as we do with our understanding of the brain and with the teachings and work of our mentors.

This chapter retains and works with several core themes from its pedigree. First, the limbic system concept is advanced here in a way that bucks against an intellectual bias that privileges "higher" (read:

"neocortical") cognitive functions over "lower" (read: "primitive" or "subcortical") emotional, conditioned, and instinctive functions in routine and aspirational human life. Second, important parts of our individual and shared existences go on outside of conscious awareness; it is helpful for psychiatrists to understand some of the anatomic, philosophical, and psychological ideas that expand this truth beyond (and enrich) important but more prosaic teaching about the "unconscious." Third, this knowledge presents opportunities to access the limbic domain and an imperative to respect it.

WHY LIMBIC MUSIC?

Why introduce, let alone carry forward, "Limbic Music" in this text? One cannot justify attention to the limbic system with a trite, "because it's there," since for more than four decades there has been debate over whether or not it is[5]—but more on that to come. Instead, the limbic system and the limbic music concept provide a site where philosophy, psychology, and biology can co-mingle in ways that are clinically practical. Make no mistake, though; while the limbic system is fertile scientific ground, its clinical usage in this chapter does not always reflect 100% established brain-behavior relationships.

Dr. Murray made no bones about his paper being "primarily heuristic."[3] Some aspects of limbic music stray into the realm of meta-psychology. Describing an emotionally detached, hyper-rationalized person as an "overgrown neocort" or a mercurial, shallow thinker as a "thin-layer neocort"[2] exemplifies the descriptive utility of indulging in neuroanatomic metaphor. However, couching meta-psychology in the jargon of neuroscience does not make it ipso facto real. Morse notes the flaws in claims sometimes staked by those willing to extrapolate from current neuroscience a complete lack of free will in those who suffer from addictions,[6] and Uttal[7] picks apart some of the definitional and neuroscientific impediments to abstract concepts (e.g., love) being ready for pedagogic prime time in psychiatry. On the other hand, some mobilize skepticism about neuroscientific claims in the ironic service of boosting their own proof-light, non-biologically referent meta-psychologies (e.g., psychodynamics).[8,9]

Limbic music favors neuroanatomically referenced explanations, does not shy away from potential accusations of "dualism," but also recognizes that brain-based explanations are meaningless unless attached to the outside world as understood through psychology and philosophy. Stretching the music metaphor, limbic music treats these occasionally adversarial ways of understanding like the treble and bass clefs. A holist might see them (correctly) as artificially dividing up the unity of musical notes. But it does not take a dualist to see that some instruments, not to mention our bodies, are constructed such that composition, performance, and appreciation demand that the clefs sometimes be cleft. The same goes for mind-body, bio-psycho-social, and other ways of thinking about, interacting with, and treating our patients.[10]

So why privilege the brain, let alone the limbic system? Because it is the target organ of our specialty, because the explanation of disease through biological theory is a distinguishing trait of the Western medical tradition of which psychiatry is part,[11] and because cognitive neuroscience is marching inexorably toward validating materialist, brain-based understandings of psychological phenomena (though the "hard problem" of experience shows no signs of being solved any time soon).[12] Some would argue that, for clinicians, this understanding can be achieved without using the brain as an intermediary. Those arguing otherwise need to be wary of pushing their luck further than contemporary neuroscience can support.[13] However, even (mis-guidedly) putting aside the neglected need for greater

neuropsychiatric competency among psychiatrists, an everyday, pragmatic biological model of unconscious processes, which is the essence of limbic music, does not get much airtime.

Most other models of mind that incorporate unconscious elements (e.g., ego psychology, object relations theory, self-psychology) are taught with reference to their respective psychotherapies. Infrequent exceptions do exist and, interestingly, tend to appear in the psychosomatic literature.[14,15] Limbic music fills a void that even these approaches to personality/coping categorization and life narratives cannot. That is, limbic music, like any music, need not serve a preconceived function or occur in a specific context or frame. It may, like other approaches, lead to a formulation or an intervention, but it is playing and can be played from the very start of a clinical interaction. Dr. Murray enjoyed using "limbic probes" (Table 4.1),[16,17] which can be employed to elicit "squelched" affect, test hunches, convey understanding, hold an emotional mirror up to the patient, demonstrate what cannot be tolerated if spoken aloud, comfort, or even strategically antagonize a patient. Mental health professionals often speak of using themselves as instruments; limbic music augments this idea by making the model itself an instrument. Not just that, it embraces the uncertainty principle by which that instrument simultaneously takes the measure of and influences (or, some would say, manipulates) the patient.

WHAT IS LIMBIC MUSIC?

As we will see later about the limbic system itself, Dr. Murray's definition of limbic music was simultaneously fuzzy edged and potent. "*Limbic music* is a term that denotes the existential, clinical raw feel emanating from the patient. It is a truer rendering of the patient's clinical state than is articulate speech."[3] It arises from processes that subserve, among other things, survival-related functions and exert their effects via neuroanatomic structures and pathways that bypass downstream association cortex.

This definition partially recalls Paul MacLean's initial proposals of the "visceral brain," for which he later coined the term "limbic system" (note: earlier usages of the term "limbic" by Willis and Broca referred to the border, or *limbus*, formed by the cingulate and para-hippocampal gyri around the corpus callosum and

TABLE 4.1
"Limbic Probe" Examples

Probe	Content	Goal
"The Frank Jones Story"	"I'm gonna tell you a story. Tell me what you think of it. I have a friend named Frank Jones. His feet are so big he has to put his pants on over his head" (said without humor). Patient responds. "Can he do it?"	Type 1 Response: Laugh. "No." Type 2: Laugh. "Yes" + implausible reason. Type 3: No laugh. "Yes" ± reason. Initially thought to discriminate between delirium and dementia based on the relative intactness of the limbic system vs. cortex. Does not do this, but it is a gross (and fun) brief screen for cognitive dysfunction.[16]
"The Cup Push"	"How do you feel about that (cup)?" Patient looks and responds quizzically. Move the cup a bit toward the edge of the table. "How about it now?" Patient less quizzical, more amused vs. annoyed vs. indifferent. Repeat until stopped or theatrically balance the cup half off the edge.	Screen for the obsessive character. Tolerance for loss of control is proportional to the distance the cup can be moved before annoyance (if any) occurs. Best response ever: Examiner moved the cup 1 inch. Patient instantly pushed it back where it was, stating "I liked it THERE!" But then was able to talk about why being in the hospital is so hard.
"The Fist"	"What's this?" (putting up a clenched fist and waving it about—not at the patient—with a pseudo-aggressive expression) Patient (eventually) gets your drift. "If you had one pop with this, where would you put it?"	Screen for direction and tolerance of suspected rage. "Oh my, no one. Never," in a sad tone.— "Ineluctable bepissment." "No one," sincerely—a saint "Myself," often in a sad tone—depression. "God," often with a guilty tone—demoralization. "That bastard, ____," with laughter and mock guilt—OK. "That bastard, ____," with glee—watch out.
Profanity	Casually but strategically use profanity as punctuation. The first time is the telling time. Must come naturally to you. Authenticity is important. If necessary, might ask first if the patient is offended by profanity. Do not use it if it feels inauthentic to you.	Catch an honest affective response in a "squelched" patient.

rostral brainstem). MacLean entertained the possibility that the limbic system is "not at all unconscious but rather eludes the grasp of the intellect because its animalistic and primitive structure makes it impossible to communicate in verbal terms." He connected the intellect with "the word brain."[18]

While agreeing in principle about a language-limbic disconnect, Dr. Murray bristled (or worse) at the depiction of the limbic system as "animalistic and primitive." He had disdain for an "Olympian"[3] view of humans as ideally and uniquely rational, language-based creatures who are at their best when suppressing their limbic processes. The lofty viewpoint finds some loose correspondence between MacLean's "triune brain," with its reptilian complex, paleomammalian complex (corresponding to his concept of the limbic system), and neomammalian complex[19] and Plato's tripartite soul with its appetitive, spirited, and rational parts[20] (and perhaps even Freud's id, ego, and superego).

Evolution and Western thought thus seem to grade our humanity and morality based on our respective rational:emotive ratios. However, this view comes under fire not solely from 30 years of "Limbic Music" but also from figures in contemporary philosophy, neuroscience, and psychology. Even Plato saw his tripartite soul as optimally operating in harmony with itself, not necessarily as a constant top-down hierarchy. Lakoff and Johnson,[21] in their book *Philosophy in the Flesh*, make a compelling case against a Western philosophical tradition that views conscious reason as the defining feature of humanity and the measuring stick of virtue. While "we think of our 'higher' (moral and rational) self in a struggle to get control over our 'lower' (irrational and amoral) self," they argue that "abstract reason builds on and makes use of forms of perceptual and motor inference present in 'lower' animals." Their work receives cross-disciplinary support from Pessoa[22] who, from a neuroscience perspective, argues against a sharp cognition-emotion divide or a "class-based view of the brain" that places the neocortex hierarchically as well as anatomically superior to subcortical and paralimbic areas. Hayles, writing about the cognitive non-conscious, reinforces Murray's reluctance to extol rational/linguistic idealism:

Higher consciousness, because it generates the verbal monologues that interpret the actions of the self, has a tendency to become imperialistic, to appropriate to itself the entirety of consciousness and even of cognition.[23]

Even ethology increasingly reveals the "primitive," largely limbic, brains of many non-human animals to be capable of symbol manipulation, relatedness, and self-awareness previously believed beyond them,[24] backing Murray's 1987 assertion that "as a psychiatric interviewer I learned as much from a 3-year residency with monkeys as I did in a 3-year residency with humans."[2] The "word brain" declares its own evolutionary, intellectual, and moral superiority, but perhaps we should not simply take its word for it.

This leveling of the neuropsychological playing field sees the barriers between cognition and emotion collapsing into a "cognitive-emotional" brain[25] where "a full-fledged emotion is a complex of sensory, motor, and cognitive processes."[26] The limbus of the limbic system, long past merely surrounding the brainstem and diencephalon, contains a domain of thought as well as feelings. Inside its borders are what lies outside of awareness.

The "psychological unconscious" as a major influencer of human behavior takes several forms, many, if not most, of which are subsumed under the functions of the limbic system. Khilstrom[27] identified many of these, bringing to light that the psychological unconscious can include some highly complex cognitive processes. Dehaene describes this as possible via the use of modules of neural networks, only achieving "ignition" and entry into conscious awareness when sufficient stimulus strength and/or attention occur in bottom-up or top-down fashions, respectively.[28] Along with the emotions traditionally thought of as limbic, these processes are thought to be constantly "prenoetically"[29] running like subroutines, yet able to nonetheless exert effects on behavior.[30]

The co-mingling and dissociability of non-conscious recognition are illustrated in cases of prosopagnosia, where some patients with downstream visual association cortex lesions or disconnection syndromes can still feel affective responses to faces they do not consciously recognize, likely due to preserved connections between (relatively) upstream visual association cortex and limbic and paralimbic areas. In "desynchrony," behavioral or physiological correlates of emotion are expressed without the agent being consciously aware of what is occurring.[27]

Moving from psychology and neuroscience to metapsychology, the prosopagnosia situation described above is not too far afield from transference reactions. We can easily view the latter as "limbic" responses to incomplete information with enough valence to activate the bypass connections described below and influence experience and behavior without one knowing why. Desynchrony is seen every day in what is often casually brushed aside by psychiatrists and patients as a "nervous laugh" (both parties conveniently not registering that these quick chuckles sometimes sound more sadistic than nervous). Most often bubbling up from the limbic depths when the conversation edges toward anger or fear (begging for speculation on the role of the amygdala), these laughs demand that the interviewer make quick decisions about whether to bring them to light and/or continue the line of inquiry that elicited them. "Higher"-level cortex may be your friend or enemy here, playing dumb or clamping down on a limbic system that has shown too much of its hand (a state, when persistent, referred to by Dr. Murray as "ineluctable bepissment" and signaling a smoldering, long-suffering state), surrendering to the gratification and peril of opening the floodgates of rage, or being guided to a state of Platonic harmony where balances between true feelings and "cortical squelch" and between rapid automatic cognitive processes and slow deliberation[31] can co-exist in a state of well-modulated honesty.

Habib Davanloo's Intensive Short-Term Dynamic Psychotherapy indirectly exemplifies many of the points just raised.[32] Davanloo's approach touches on neurophysiology, including involuntary motor responses and autonomic nervous system activity, in listening for limbic music (though he does not use the term) and making decisions about what to do with it. In his "central dynamic sequence," the patient's laughter (and, often, reflexive rationalization or apology) might be met with light pressure ("You just laughed while telling me how difficult your husband is. Did you notice that?") that is incrementally increased ("You just did it again. Do you always laugh when you are starting to get angry?" "And there it is again. Why are you putting up this wall?") or decreased depending on responses that range from modulated but honest emotion, to hyper-rationalization, to autonomic dyscontrol (e.g., have you ever had an emotionally intense consultation interrupted by borborygmi and the patient's departure to the bathroom?). In Davanloo's work, we see a model that, removed from its formal psychotherapeutic context and translated via the concept of limbic music, can be used in a multitude of ways in the interactions and assessments of routine consultation psychiatry. The same could be done with many other psychotherapeutic approaches.

WHERE DOES LIMBIC MUSIC COME FROM AND WHAT DOES IT WANT?

Limbic music emanates from the limbic system and conveys emotion; if only it were that easy. Table 4.2 is an over-simplified representation of the expansion of the limbic system from its humble beginnings as a grossly, then architectonically, defined "border zone" with mainly olfactory functions, to its current status as a functionally and connectivity-defined "system" or assembly of sub-systems with a range of functions.[33–35]

The idea that there is no limbic system was already mentioned. Generally credited as starting with Brodal[5]

in 1969, this argument hinges on the idea that the limbic system was even then incorporating and connecting to so much of the brain that its boundaries and status as a system would reach a point of meaninglessness. In his argument for a non-distinction or network-based entanglement of emotion and cognition in the brain, Pessoa argues that "although the term 'limbic system' is probably one of the most broadly used in neuroscience, the concept has proven to be too unwieldy and unstable to be scientifically useful."[22] Note that the limbic system described in Table 4.2 is cumulative, with few, if any, structures eliminated over time.

Heimer and co-workers suggested that "the limbic system is a concept in perpetual search for a definition," and that the "anatomical characterization of such a comprehensive functional system … may be impossible without enlisting practically the entire brain."[33] These same authors and others,[36] however, ultimately find utility and reality in the limbic system based on the robustness of its connections to the hypothalamus, neuromodulatory nuclei in the brainstem, and the cortical regions most affiliated with emotional functions. Simultaneously acknowledging and embracing the expansiveness of their "greater limbic lobe," Heimer and associates remark that "when the amygdala speaks, the entire brain listens."[33] While he draws a different conclusion, Pessoa also notes that "regions involved in emotional circuits are among the most widely connected in the brain, suggesting they play at times a 'quasi-global' communication role."[25]

Other neuroscientists who embrace a larger limbic system do so by dividing it into parts. Rolls,[34] for example, concludes that there are two limbic systems that are connected but double dissociated. One is organized around the orbitofrontal cortex and amygdala, involving (non-exclusively) anterior cingulate and parietal cortex as well as ventral striatum, hypothalamus, and brainstem nuclei. This limbic system, which loosely corresponds to Mesulam's olfacto-centric paralimbic belt,[37] is thought to subserve emotion, reward valuation/learning, and reward related decision-making; it overlaps with what has since incorporated the anterior insula into a separate "salience network."[25,38] Rolls' second limbic system is organized around the hippocampus, involving (non-exclusively) the entorhinal, parahippocampal, perirhinal, and posterior cingulate cortices as well as the connected fornix-mammillary bodies-anterior thalamus. This

TABLE 4.2
Anatomic Expansion of the Limbic System[33–41]

Investigator	Circa	Corticoid Areas and Subcortical Nuclei	Allocortical and Mesocortical Areas	Neocortical Areas	Brainstem/ Cerebellum
Willis	1664		Cingulate, parahippocampal gyrus		
Broca	1878		Same as Willis; expands concept		
Papez	1937	Hypothalamus, mammillary bodies, anterior thalamus, fornix	Hippocampus	Precuneus	
Yakovlev	1950	Amygdala	Medial orbitofrontal, olfactory cortex including part of the insula, temporal pole		
MacLean	1955+	Septum			Midbrain central gray, reticular activating system
Nauta	1958+	"Limbic forebrain"		Frontal neocortical connections	Raphe nuclei, ventral tegmental area
Heimer	1970+	Ventral striatum, ventral pallidum, extended amygdala, septal nuclei	Entire hippocampal/ parahippocampal complex, insula (greater portion)	Medial frontal, retrosplenial	
Nieuwenhuys	1996				Vagal-solitary complex, parabrachial nucleus, tegmental nuclei
Schmahmann	1997+				(Lateral) cerebellum
Connectivists (e.g., Sporns)	2010+			"Default Mode Network" including medial prefrontal, posterior cingulate, lateral prefrontal, retrosplenial, cortical midline (some mesocortical overlap)	

limbic system, which loosely corresponds to Mesulam's hippocampocentric paralimbic belt[37] and the well-known Papez circuit,[39] is thought to subserve episodic memory. This function of Rolls' second limbic system is affected by emotional states but is neither dependent on nor generative of them.

In another multiple-limbic-systems scheme, Catoni and colleagues[35] add a third system corresponding to the default mode network. This system is believed to involve (non-exclusively) anterior cingulate, other medial prefrontal, posterior cingulate, and retrosplenial cortices as well as the precuneus. Active mainly, but not only, in the resting state, the default mode network operates in a "mode of cognition that is directed internally rather than being externally driven and that is concerned with self and social context,"[40] thus subserving functions such as introspection, theory of mind, and working memory.[41]

These models of the limbic system(s) reiterate Dr. Murray's focus on the hippocampus and amygdala in "Limbic Music." They also illustrate the proliferation of brain areas thought to participate in limbic functions and the aforementioned proliferation of those functions to include not just emotion but forms of learning, reward valuation, episodic memory, introspection, empathy, and even some aspects of working memory. Neuroscience has clearly widened its scope to include more than even Dr. Murray's re-formulation, by way of Lazarus,[42] of the limbic "4-Fs" as pertaining to "gender role, territoriality, and bonding."[2]

The blurred and debatable boundary between emotion and cognition in the limbic system is anatomical as well as phenomenological, with the basal forebrain/ventral striatum funnel of the greater limbic lobe mirroring the subcortical paths of other cortical and cerebellar regions.[33] Uttal matter-of-factly refers frequently to "emotions and other cognitive functions," only stopping briefly to say it is "incontestable that emotional responses are at least a useful adjunct to higher level cognitive processes *if not another one of them*" [italics added].[7]

So where does this leave limbic music? Initially put forth by Dr. Murray as an expression of the limbic system as a mind-brain mediator, it now additionally emerges as a means of considering the mysteries of consciousness itself. This being a "handbook of general hospital psychiatry," we should avoid getting (further) bogged down in philosophy and neuroscience. Suffice it to say that the human brain, and its limbic system(s) in particular, is set up such that much or most of its processing goes on outside of our awareness. This non-conscious processing may occur through LeDoux's[43] "low road" cortical bypass, routing incompletely processed, high-priority, sensory information via the thalamus directly to the amygdala; through connections between limbic structures and upstream sensory cortex that "flavor" the way situational perception occurs using prior learning that may, in turn, have been acquired limbically[33]; through upstream unimodal association to paralimbic/limbic cortical and hypothalamic "shortcuts"[25,29,30,37,44]; through "bottom-up" interoceptive mechanisms (validating the James-Lange theory of emotion over a

century after its formulations)[45]; or through any of the many mechanisms of the aforementioned "psychological unconscious."

Each of these non-conscious goings-on influences behavior in ways that are similarly non-conscious (until we and/or helpful others attend to them). At the same time, they express our authentic selves as much or more than our deliberate choices and actions. Limbic music is playing constantly and warrants a close listen.

LIMBIC MUSIC APPRECIATION

Ultimately, like any other skill, limbic music appreciation is developed through experience. At the risk of introducing a heuristic within a heuristic, the concept of predictive processing offers a helpful perspective. In this model of brain, mind, and computation, we do not experience the world from outside in (or, interoceptively, from inside in), but rather the other way around, that is, as a prediction based on our learned "priors" or models of the world. These predictions are fed backward (perhaps from prefrontal areas) to upstream sensory areas, influencing and being matched against the incoming stimuli such that "only any unpredicted elements (in the form of residual 'prediction errors') propagate information forward."[46] According to this model, if you look out of your window right now, you only "see" what is actually there if something unexpected arises or you deliberately direct your attention to the details. Otherwise, you are seeing your predictive model of the view. Intrusions of the unexpected are experienced by the brain as "surprisal."

In a highly apt attempt to capture what "surprisal" might be like, Clark states that "the experiential impact of an unexpected omission (as when a note is missed out of a familiar sequence) can be every bit as perceptually striking and significant as the inclusion of an unexpected note."[46] For the latter, return to the Henderson epigraph at the beginning of this chapter and add to it, "fourthly, what he tells without intending." Murray's classic example is the smile or laugh, a human "limbic-ometer." Laughter's spontaneous form arises from a network of limbic system hubs distinct from the anatomy that produces its deliberate motor simulation.[47] It is the unexpected or incongruent limbic output (or omission) from the patient (or oneself) that catches the examiner's attention.

When this happens, one must either update one's model or adjust the world to fit one's existing model. Either of these may occur through closer scrutiny and assessment or through probes and questions by which the patient (or examiner) reveals themself more clearly. In one prediction-based theory of emotion, an increase in prediction error is associated with negative emotion and its reduction/resolution with positive emotion.[48] In addition to developing one's models over time, other educational tasks include acquiring the habit of noticing surprisal and skillfully deciding how to deal with it.

It might also be formulated that hospitalized patients, especially when undiagnosed or prognostically in the dark, are experiencing unresolvable uncertainty and the negative emotions that accompany their frustrated attempts to bring their strange new world into equilibrium with their old models.

CLINICAL EXAMPLES
Case 1

A 72-year-old, independently living female is admitted for a work-up of a lung mass. She is noted by staff to be "forgetful" during education and consent discussions. Psychiatry is consulted to assess for dementia. She performs poorly on the Montreal Cognitive Assessment when administered by the resident. She seems withdrawn and disinterested during subsequent interviewing by the attending psychiatrist, who suggests that "seeing me is not your number one priority, is it?" and requests "just one test and then I'll leave you alone." $1, $10, and $20 bills are each "hidden" in locations initially shown to the patient. Some jokes are made about her "pretending to forget where my money is ... don't let me leave without it." After 10 minutes of surprisingly permitted further interaction during which she acknowledged and discussed her fear of cancer, the patient is asked to "tell me where my money is." She readily recalls the denominations and their respective locations—six out of six items spanning verbal and visuo-spatial recent recall.

This female does not care about remembering random memory items on a cognitive screen. It is not hard to use one's own limbic system to hypothesize

about what is really distracting her. Some humor and empathy, along with the use of a limbically activating array of memory items that she might not have expected a "serious" doctor to employ (residents may need to borrow money to perform this "test"), led to a more genuine display of feelings and cognitive ability than were initially evident.

Case 2

A 50-year-old male, with a "diagnosis" of "unspecified mood disorder" and an electronic medical record history of over a dozen psychiatric hospitalizations for self-presentations with suicidal ideation never succeeded by follow-through with outpatient care, presents with suicidal ideation and chest pain. A cardiac origin is excluded that day. During psychiatric consultation for "placement," the patient is spontaneously effusive and detailed about his suicidal thinking but, seemingly inconsistent with a male seeking the relief of his stated suffering, will not describe other psychological experiences. He mentions having been recently assaulted by a male who is going to be tried for battery. The patient knows and intensely dislikes this male, briefly smiling and becoming incongruently animated about the subject when it initially came up. The interviewing psychiatrist returns to the topic later, asking the patient if he expects his assailant to "get what's coming to him" in court. Big smile and a nod; "he's on probation." The trial is revealed to be a week away. Asked if he plans to be there as a witness or to "just see him suffer," the patient replies in the emphatic affirmative. He is discharged despite a now-tepid reassertion of suicidal ideation and after his continued refusal to discuss what his actual needs might be and how they might be better addressed.

While perhaps manipulative, the psychiatrist in this case noted incongruities between this patient's "word brain" and limbic music. Through his own choice of words, the psychiatrist attempted to communicate with the patient's limbic system and obtained consistent and specific future orientation that belied the patient's assertions of suicidality. The patient's survival was confirmed by an almost identical presentation not long afterward.

CONCLUSION

Originally introduced by Dr. George Murray in 1987, "Limbic Music" is a concept with neuroanatomic, psychological, and philosophical aspects. It is sometimes discussed factually and sometimes metaphorically. In both instances, it utilizes a neuroscientific frame of reference, in the form of the limbic system. This framework is felt to not only make the limbic music concept informative but also more versatile in some situations than are theories of emotion bound to therapeutic interventions. The limbic system that "plays" limbic music and the functions attributed to it have expanded and become controversial over time. But so long as limbic music is rooted in the brain structures, emotions, and non-conscious forces that govern human lives, it will play tunes that psychiatrists would be well advised to listen to—in their patients and in themselves.

REFERENCES

1. Henderson LJ. Physician and patient as a social system. *N Engl J Med*. 1935;212:819–823.
2. Murray GB, et al. Limbic music. In: Hackett TP, Weisman AD, Kucharski A, eds. *Psychiatry in a General Hospital: The First Fifty Years*. PSG Publishing; 1987:101–110.
3. Murray GB. Limbic music. *Psychosomatics*. 1990;33:16–23.
4. Pievani T. *Imperfection: A Natural History*. MIT Press; 2022.
5. Brodal A. *Neurological Anatomy in Relation to Clinical Medicine*. Oxford University Press; 1969.
6. Morse SJ. The neuroscientific non-challenge to meaning, morals, and purpose. In: Caruso GD, Flanagan O, eds. *Neuroexistentialism: Meaning, Morals, and Purpose in the Age of Neuroscience*. Oxford University Press; 2018:333–357.
7. Uttal WR. *Mind and Brain: A Critical Appraisal of Cognitive Neuroscience*. MIT Press; 2011.
8. Watson BO, Michels R. Neuroscience in the residency curriculum: the psychoanalytic psychotherapy perspective. *Acad Psychiatry*. 2014;38:124–126.
9. Pulver SE. On the astonishing clinical irrelevance of neuroscience. *J Am Psychoanal Assoc*. 2001;51:1–18.
10. Kontos N. Biomedicine – menace or straw man? Reexamining the biopsychosocial argument. *Acad Med*. 2011;86:509–515.
11. Neve M, et al. Conclusion. In: Conrad LI, Neve M, Nutton V, eds. *The Western Medical Tradition: 800 BC to AD 1800*. Cambridge University Press; 1995:477–494.
12. Pennington BF. *Explaining Abnormal Behavior: A Cognitive Neuroscience Approach*. Guilford Press; 2014.
13. Salzman C. The importance of teaching neuroscience to psychiatric residents in the context of psychological formulations. *Asian J Psychiatr*. 2015;17:130.
14. Kahana RJ, Bibring GL. Personality types in medical management. In: Zinberg NE, ed. *Psychiatry and Medical Practice in a General Hospital*. International Universities Press; 1964.
15. Viederman M, Perry SW. 3rd: Use of a psychodynamic life narrative in the treatment of depression in the physically ill. *Gen Hosp Psychiatry*. 1980;2:177–185.
16. Bechtold KT, Horner MD, Labbate LA, et al. The construct validity and clinical utility of the Frank Jones story as a brief screening measure of cognitive dysfunction. *Psychosomatics*. 2001;42:146–149.
17. Frühholz S, Trost W, Grandjean D. The role of the medial temporal limbic system in processing emotions in voice and music. *Prog Neurobiol*. 2014;123:1–17.
18. MacLean PD. Psychosomatic disease and the "visceral brain": recent developments bearing on the Papez theory of emotion. *Psychosom Med*. 1949;11:338–353.
19. MacLean PD. *The Triune Brain in Evolution*. Plenum Press; 1990.
20. Callender JS. *Free Will and Responsibility: A Guide for Practitioners*. Oxford University Press; 2010.
21. Lakoff G, Johnson M. *Philosophy in the Flesh: The Embodied Mind and Its Challenge to Western Thought*. Basic Books; 1999.
22. Pessoa L. *The Entangled Brain*. MIT Press; 2022.
23. Hayles NK. *Unthought: The Power of the Cognitive Nonconscious*. The University of Chicago Press; 2017.
24. Despret V. *What Would Animals Say if We Asked the Right Questions?* University of Minnesota Press; 2016.
25. Pessoa L. *The Cognitive-Emotional Brain: From Interactions to Integration*. MIT Press; 2013.
26. Pennartz CMA. *The Brain's Representational Power: On Consciousness and the Integration of Modalities*. MIT Press; 2015.
27. Khilstrom JF. The psychological unconscious. In: John O, Robins R, Pervin L, eds. *Handbook of Personality: Theory and Research*. 3rd ed. Guilford; 2010:583–602.
28. Dehaene S. *Consciousness and the Brain: Deciphering How the Brain Codes Our Thoughts*. Penguin Books; 2014.
29. Gallagher S. Prenoetic effects on perception and judgment. In: Ramdan Z, ed. *Before Consciousness: In Search of the Fundamentals of Mind*. Imprint Academic; 2017:164–174.
30. Cleermans A. The mind is deep. In: Cleermans A, Allkhverdov V, Kuvaldina M, eds. *Implicit Learning: 50 Years On*. Routledge; 2019:41–70.
31. Reber PJ, Batterink LJ, Thompson KR, Rouveni B. Implicit learning: history and applications. In: Cleermans A, Allkhverdov V, Kuvaldina M, eds. *Implicit Learning: 50 Years On*. Routledge; 2019:41–70.
32. Davanloo H. *Unlocking the Unconscious: Selected Papers of Habib Davanloo*. John Wiley & Sons; 1990.
33. Heimer L, Van Hoesen GW, Trimble M, et al. *Anatomy of Neuropsychiatry: The New Anatomy of the Basal Forebrain and Its Implications for Neuropsychiatric Illness*. Elsevier; 2008.
34. Rolls ET. Limbic systems for emotion and for memory, but no single limbic system. *Cortex*. 2015;62:119–157.
35. Catoni M, Dell'Acqua F, Thiebaut de Schotten M. A revised limbic system model for memory, emotion and behaviour. *Neurosci Biobehav Rev*. 2013;37:1724–1737.
36. Banwinkler M, Theis H, Prange S, van Eimeren T. Imaging of the limbic system in Parkinson's disease – a review of limbic pathology and clinical symptoms. *Brain Sci*. 2022;12:1248.
37. Mesulam MM. Behavioral neuroanatomy: large scale networks, association cortex, frontal syndromes, the limbic system, and

hemispheric specializations. In: Mesulam MM, ed. *Principles of Behavioral and Cognitive Neurology*. 2nd ed. Oxford University Press; 2000.

38. Kandilarova S, St. Stoyanov D, Paunova R, et al. Effective connectivity between major notes of the limbic system, salience, and frontoparietal networks differentiates schizophrenia and mood disorders from healthy controls. *J Pers Med*. 2021;11:1110.

39. Papez JW. A proposed mechanism of emotion. *Arch Neurol Psychiatry*. 1937;38:725–744.

40. Sporns O. *Networks of the Brain*. MIT Press; 2011.

41. Raichle ME. The brain's default mode network. *Ann Rev Neurosci*. 2015;58:433–437.

42. Lazarus RS. Thoughts on the relations between emotion and cognitions. In: Scherer KR, Ekman P, eds. *Approaches to Cognition*. Lawrence Erlbaum Associates; 1984:271–291.

43. LeDoux JE. Emotion circuits in the brain. *Annu Rev Neurosci*. 2000;23:155–184.

44. Kamali A, Sherbaf FG, Rahmani F, et al. A direct visuosensory cortical connectivity of the human limbic system. Dissecting the trajectory of the pariety-occipito-hypothalamic tract in the human brain using diffusion weighted tractography. *Neurosci Letters*. 2020;728:134955.

45. Costadi M. *Body Am I: The New Science of Self-Consciousness*. MIT Press; 2022.

46. Clark A. *Surfing Uncertainty: Prediction, Action, and the Embodied Mind*. Oxford University Press; 2016.

47. Talami F, Vaudano AE, Meletti S. Motor and limbic system contribution to emotional laughter across the lifespan. *Cereb Cortex*. 2020;30:3381–3391.

48. Parr T, Pezzulo G, Friston KJ. *Active Inference: The Free Energy Principle in Mind, Brain, and Behavior*. MIT Press; 2022.

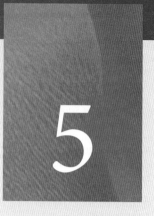

5

FUNCTIONAL NEUROANATOMY AND THE NEUROLOGIC EXAMINATION

JOAN A. CAMPRODON, MD, MPH, PHD

OVERVIEW

For the psychiatric consultant, the neurologic examination is an important component of every patient evaluation. By reviewing the main components of the standard examination and attempting to relate them to anatomic constructs, the consulting psychiatrist may gain a theoretical and pragmatic framework for the neurologic examination that can facilitate case formulation, differential diagnosis, and treatment planning.

FUNCTIONAL NEUROANATOMY

At its most basic level, our nervous system allows us to interact with external stimuli, serving as a bridge between the environment and our internal mental and physical worlds. In humans, there is a large evaluation step between stimulus and response, which allows for a carefully chosen (or programmed) response that is additionally influenced by an actual or perceived situational context. Using an information-processing model, we can map these concepts in three distinct steps: *input* of sensory information through perceptual modules, the internal integration and *evaluation* of this information, and the production of a *response*. These steps are carried out by four main anatomic systems in the brain: the *thalamus*, the *cortex*, the *medial temporal lobe*, and the *basal ganglia* (Fig. 5.1).

Sensory organs provide information about the physical attributes of incoming information. Details of physical attributes (e.g., temperature, sound frequency, and color) are conveyed through multiple segregated channels in each perceptual module. Information then passes through the thalamus, which serves as the gateway to cortical processing for all sensory data, except for olfaction. Specifically, it is the relay nuclei of the thalamus (ventral posterior lateral for somatosensory and pain, medial geniculate for auditory, and lateral geniculate for visual information) that convey sensory signals from the sensory organs to the appropriate area of the primary sensory cortex (i.e., S1, A1, or V1) (Fig. 5.2).

The first step in the integration and evaluation of incoming stimuli occurs in unimodal association areas of the cortex, where physical attributes of one sensory domain are linked together (e.g., shape, color, motion, and more complex object-specific features, such as object or facial characteristics). A second level of integration is reached in multi-modal association areas, including regions in the parietal lobe and prefrontal

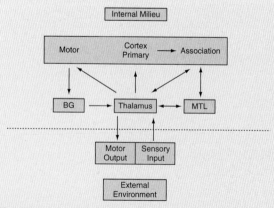

Fig. 5.1 ■ Basic circuitry of information processing. *BG*, Basal ganglia; *MTL*, medial temporal lobe.

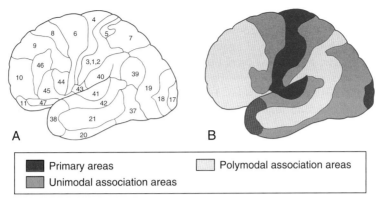

Primary areas	Polymodal association areas
Unimodal association areas	

Fig. 5.2 ■ **Functional role of areas in the human cerebral cortex.** (A) Map of cytoarchitectonic areas according to Brodmann. The parcellation of the cortical mantle into distinct areas is based on the microscopic analysis of neurons in the six layers of the cortex. (B) Map of functional areas according to Mesulam. The primary sensory areas (visual = area 17; auditory = areas 41, 43; somatosensory = areas 3, 1, 2) and the primary motor area 4 are indicated in *brown*. The association areas, dedicated to one stream of information processing (visual = areas 18, 19, 20, 37; auditory = area 42; somatosensory = areas 5, 7, 40; motor = areas 6, 44), are indicated in *tan*. The polymodal association areas, where all sensory modalities converge, are indicated in *beige*. The temporal pole is part of the paralimbic areas, which occupy large regions on the medial surface of the brain (i.e., cingulate cortex and parahippocampal cortex). (A, From Brodmann K. *Vergleichende lokalisationslehre der grosshirnrinde in ihren prinzipien dargestellt auf grund des zellenbaues.* JA Barth; 1909; B, From Mesulam M-M. *Principles of Behavioral Neurology.* FA Davis; 1985.)

cortex, which link together the physical attributes from different sensory domains. A third level of integration is provided by input from limbic and paralimbic regions of the brain, including the cingulate cortex and regions of the medial temporal lobe (hippocampus and amygdala). At this level of integration, the brain creates a representation of experience that has the spatiotemporal resolution and full complexity of the outside world, imbued with emotion and viewed in the context of prior experience. Evaluation and interpretation involve the comparison of new information with previously stored information and current expectations or desires, which allows the brain to classify information as new or old, or as threatening or non-threatening.

Based on the results of evaluation and interpretation, the brain then creates a response. The regions involved in generating, for example, motor responses, include the motor cortex, the basal ganglia, the motor nuclei of the thalamus, and the cerebellum. The basal ganglia, which include the striatum (made up of the caudate and the putamen) and the globus pallidus, are charged with integrating and coordinating this motor output. The striatum receives input from the motor cortex, projecting to the globus pallidus. The globus pallidus in turn relays the neo-striatal input to

the thalamus. The thalamus then projects back to the cortical areas that gave rise to the cortico-striatal projections, thereby closing the cortico-striato-pallido-thalamo-cortical (CSPTC) loop. This loop is thought to facilitate the enactment of motor control; damage to regions in this loop leads to disorders, such as Parkinson disease and Huntington disease. In addition to motor responses, the brain generates other types of outputs, such as cognitive decision-making, emotional reactions, or socially meaningful behavioral responses. These outputs also rely on similar frontal CSPTC loops, which start in non-motor areas of the frontal cortex, such as the dorsolateral prefrontal, the medial prefrontal, or the orbitofrontal cortices. Structural or physiologic lesions to these systems lead to the affective, behavioral, or cognitive signs and symptoms that constitute neuropsychiatric syndromes, including obsessive-compulsive or substance use disorders.

Case 1

Mr. H, a 43-year-old man, was brought to the emergency department after he was found wandering barefoot on the street; he was belligerent and disheveled. On presentation, his vital signs and a basic screening evaluation for intoxication or acute medical illness were normal. Psychiatry was consulted to assess his capacity to leave the hospital against medical advice. On interview, Mr. H was alert but disoriented; his mood was elevated, and he had grandiose, paranoid, and persecutory delusions. He was irritable, easily distracted, and angrily insisted that his health was "100% perfect."

On neurologic examination, his visual fields were full on confrontation, his extraocular movements were intact in all directions with smooth pursuit and no nystagmus, his face was symmetric, and his speech was slightly dysarthric. There was no evidence of myoclonus or asterixis, but perioral and bilateral upper extremity tremors were present. Muscle bulk, tone, and strength were normal and symmetric. Deep tendon reflexes were brisk and symmetric. There was no evidence of primitive reflexes; he had normal plantar responses. There was symmetric withdrawal of all four extremities to painful stimuli. There were no gross ataxic movements in the extremities or trunk. Gait had normal posture, stride, arm swing, and turns, but with a widened stance and he fell with tandem gait. The Romberg sign was present. These findings prompted a magnetic resonance imaging (MRI) scan of the brain with and without gadolinium, which revealed left greater than right mesial temporal and basal ganglionic inflammation. Additional serum studies, including human immunodeficiency virus, syphilis rapid plasma reagin (RPR), fluorescent treponemal antibody absorption test, and serum paraneoplastic antibodies, were negative. Lumbar puncture revealed a normal opening pressure. Cerebrospinal fluid (CSF) analysis revealed normal glucose, no leukocytosis, and an elevated total protein. CSF viral studies were negative, but the Venereal Disease Research Laboratory (VDRL) test was highly elevated. Treatment was initiated for the diagnosis of neurosyphilis with intravenous penicillin for 2 weeks. Mr. H had a gradual improvement in his mental status and was discharged to a physical rehabilitation hospital.

THE NEUROLOGIC EXAMINATION

The neurologic examination is designed to probe the input, integration and evaluation, as well as output

domains of information processing. Here, we provide an overview of the examination using this framework. For more complete details, see standard texts of neurology.

Input

Sensory information enters the central nervous system (CNS) by two routes: spinal nerves and cranial nerves. The former handle somatosensory information presented to the body, and the latter handle somatosensory information presented to the face and each of the remaining special senses (vision, hearing, smell, and taste).

Peripheral Sensory Examination

Peripheral sensation allows tactile exploration of our environment. The most thorough examiner could not test every square inch of the body for intact sensation, although it would not be necessary. Knowledge of the full sensory examination is important for the patient with a focal sensory complaint (see other texts for detailed information on peripheral nerve examination[1-10]). The main sensory modalities include the following:

> *Pain*: Tested by pinprick (using disposable sterile pins).
>
> *Temperature*: Tested by touching the skin with a cold metal object (e.g., a tuning fork).
>
> *Light touch*: Tested by simply brushing the patient's skin with your hand or a moving wisp of cotton.
>
> *Vibration sense*: Tested by applying a "buzzing" tuning fork to osseous prominences of the distal lower extremities.
>
> *Proprioception*: Efficiently tested by Romberg maneuver. Ask the patient to stand with the feet as close together as possible while still maintaining stability. Then ask the patient to close their eyes, assuring the patient that you will not let him or her fall. The patient with poor proprioception will begin to sway and lose balance after closing their eyes. Falling during the maneuver indicates the presence of the Romberg sign, a manifestation of severe proprioceptive sensory loss once postural compensation based on visual inputs is blocked.

Stereognosis: The ability to recognize objects using touch, which can be tested by placing common objects (e.g., a coin) in the patient's hand and asking the patient to name each item, with the eyes closed.

Graphesthesia: The ability to recognize numbers or letters traced on the skin, most often using the palm, with the patient's eyes closed. As with stereognosis, primary sensory modalities must be intact for this test to have meaning.

Sensory (I, II, VIII) and Sensorimotor (V, VII, IX, X) Cranial Nerves

Seven cranial nerves serve an input function and are known as sensory (I, II, VIII) or sensorimotor (V, VII, IX, X) cranial nerves to distinguish them from those that exclusively play a motor/output role (Table 5.1).

Olfactory Nerve (Cranial Nerve I). The first cranial nerve runs along the orbital surface of the frontal lobe. Lesions (e.g., a frontal lobe meningioma) in this area may produce behavioral dysregulation such as impulsivity (consistent with a cortical lesion), with or without unilateral anosmia (indicating a cranial nerve

lesion). In addition, anosmia can be an early sign of neurodegenerative conditions before the onset of cognitive (e.g., in Alzheimer disease) or motor (e.g., in Parkinson disease) symptoms. Routine testing of smell is therefore important. A small vial of coffee provides a simple and convenient method for testing smell, but olfaction can also be tested with an inexpensive smell identification test booklet. The nostrils should be tested separately.

Optic Nerve (Cranial Nerve II). The optic nerve and its posterior radiations run the entire length of the brain and produce different patterns of signs and symptoms depending on where they are compromised; therefore, a thorough evaluation can be quite informative. There are five components to the visual examination:

Funduscopy: Because the optic nerve is the only nerve that can be visualized directly with an ophthalmoscope, the funduscopic examination reveals much about its integrity, the systemic vascular system, and the presence of increased intracranial pressure.

Visual acuity: Poor vision can profoundly impair a person's ability to function or orient themselves

TABLE 5.1
The Cranial Nerves

Number	Name	Sensory (Input), Motor (Output), or Sensorimotor (Both)?	Function
I	Olfactory	Sensory	Olfaction
II	Optic	Sensory	Vision
III	Oculomotor	Motor	Innervation of extraocular musculature
IV	Trochlear	Motor	Innervation of extraocular musculature
V	Trigeminal	Sensorimotor	Facial sensation + innervation of muscles of mastication
VI	Abducens	Motor	Innervation of extraocular musculature
VII	Facial	Sensorimotor	Taste + innervation of muscles of facial expression
VIII	Vestibulocochlear	Sensory	Hearing + balance
IX	Glossopharyngeal	Sensorimotor	Taste + innervation of stylopharyngeus muscle
X	Vagus	Sensorimotor	Parasympathetic innervation + innervation to muscles of larynx and pharynx
XI	Spinal accessory	Motor	Innervation of the sternocleidomastoid and trapezius muscles
XII	Hypoglossal	Motor	Innervation of tongue

and is often reversible with corrective lenses or surgery. Acuity is easily assessed in each eye while the patient is wearing current corrective lenses.

Pupillary measurement: Pupillary size represents the delicate balance between sympathetic and parasympathetic input to the ciliary muscles of the eye. The presence of abnormally large or small pupils reflects an imbalance and may be an important sign of disease or toxicity. Similarly, an inequality in pupillary size (anisocoria) can be an important hallmark of a severe intracranial pathologic condition. Each pupil is measured in millimeters with measurements clearly documented for future reference, including whether measurement was performed in a light or dark room.

Pupillary reaction (direct and consensual): The direct and consensual pupillary reactions to light, and the near reaction (accommodation), assess any damage in the afferent and efferent pathways that compose the pupillary response. A penlight and close observation are all that are necessary.

Confrontational visual fields: Because the visual system runs from the retina to the occipital cortex, involving a substantial area of the CNS, lesions anywhere along this pathway lead to visual field deficits. Importantly, the patient is almost never aware of this abnormality of vision. Careful testing is therefore required. One can sit directly in front of the patient and have him or her look at a single point between your eyes. The eyes should be tested separately by bringing an object (e.g., a pin or a wiggling finger) into each visual quadrant while ensuring that the patient does not move their eyes. For the patient who is unable to cooperate in this fashion, having them count fingers displayed in each quadrant is another option. Assessing for blink to visual threat in each quadrant may be viable in more inattentive patients.

Trigeminal Nerve (Cranial Nerve V). The sensory component of the trigeminal nerve captures somatosensory information from the face via the ophthalmic (V_1), maxillary (V_2), and mandibular (V_3) branches. Testing light touch (by stroking the face with your fingers) or temperature sensitivity (using a cold metal tuning fork) is usually adequate. Simply asking, "Does this feel normal on both sides?" will detect any major abnormalities worthy of further investigation.

Facial Nerve (Cranial Nerve VII). The sensory component of the facial nerve (chorda tympani) transmits taste from the anterior two-thirds of the tongue. Testing this aspect of the facial nerve involves the application of a sweet, sour, or salty solution (via a cotton-tipped swab) to the outstretched tongue. The yield of this component of the examination without specific gustatory complaints is minimal.

Acoustic Nerve (Cranial Nerve VIII). In addition to its role in the maintenance of equilibrium (via the vestibular branch), cranial nerve VIII is the primary input channel for auditory information. Lesions in this nerve can be associated with vertigo, hearing loss, or both. One should ensure that the external ear canal is not occluded with cerumen. Rubbing your fingers together near the ear may bring out high-pitched hearing deficits, a finding typically associated with presbycusis that can exacerbate confusional states. More in-depth testing can include the Rinne test, which involves the use of a vibrating tuning fork (128–512 Hz) applied to the mastoid bone until it can no longer be heard. It is then placed next to the ear. This comparison determines whether hearing is better with air or bone conduction. Conduction hearing loss is characterized by hearing the sound better with the tuning fork applied to the mastoid than next to the ear. In sensorineural hearing loss, the sound is better perceived next to the ear than via the mastoid bone. The Weber test uses a tuning fork placed in the midline at the vertex or forehead to determine on which side the sound is heard best. Sound referred to an ear with decreased acuity indicates a conductive hearing loss. Sound referred to the opposite (unaffected) ear occurs with sensorineural hearing loss. These tests are crude compared to audiologic testing. Hearing loss can exacerbate auditory hallucinations and paranoia.

Glossopharyngeal and Vagus Nerves (Cranial Nerves IX and X). These two nerves innervate the palate, pharynx, and larynx and are important for speech and swallowing. The cranial nerve IX also conducts taste and touch sensations for the posterior third of the tongue. Lesions of these two nerves are clinically meaningful as they cause dysarthric or aphonic speech, dysphagia, and drooling (details are provided later in the text).

Integration and Evaluation

Automatic or reflexive responses (e.g., pupillary light reflex and corneal reflex in the sensory evaluation) can be tested, as can three sets of reflexes (proprioceptive, nociceptive, and primitive) commonly probed in a standard neurologic examination.

In addition, higher-level information processing also occurs in the brain. This is not a pre-programmed reflex but a flexible and adaptive output that is generally dependent on the environment (external and internal) leading to a wide range of affective, behavioral, and cognitive responses.[6] The mental status examination is the clinical tool to evaluate these functions.

Reflexes

Proprioceptive reflexes: Proprioceptive reflexes, also known as deep tendon reflexes (DTRs), are based on the simple reflex arcs that are activated by stretching or tapping. Because they are influenced by the descending corticospinal tracts, DTRs can provide important information on the integrity of this pathway at several levels. The reader is probably familiar with the methods used to elicit the five major DTRs: biceps, triceps, brachioradialis, quadriceps (knee), and Achilles (ankle) (Box 5.1 describes root levels tested by each DTR). The grading of each reflex is on a 4-point scale with a score of 2 (2+) designated as normal (see Box 5.2 for the full scoring scale), although special attention is placed on asymmetry in reflex strength (e.g., with a difference between upper versus lower extremities or left versus right).

Nociceptive reflexes: Nociceptive reflexes are based on reflex arcs located in the skin (rather than in the muscle tendons) and are therefore elicited by scratching or stroking. These include the abdominal, cremasteric, and ano-cutaneous reflexes, none of which is used extensively in the clinical examination. The major nociceptive reflex of clinical value is the plantar reflex.

BOX 5.1
ROOT LEVELS TESTED WITH DTRS

Biceps: C_5–C_6
Brachioradialis: C_6
Triceps: C_7–C_8
Quadriceps (knee): L_3–L_4
Achilles (ankle): S_1–S_2

BOX 5.2
GRADING OF REFLEXES

0: Absent
1+: Diminished
2+: Normal
3+: Increased without clonus
4+: Increased with clonus

Stroking the sole of the foot should elicit plantar flexion of the toes. Babinski sign, marked by an extensor response (i.e., dorsiflexion) of the toes, often with fanning of the toes and flexion of the ankle, is seen in pyramidal tract disease. Of note, a positive Babinski sign is normal (physiologic) in infants up to the age of 24 months.

Primitive reflexes (release reflexes): Primitive reflexes are also present at birth and disappear in early infancy. Their reappearance later in life is abnormal and reflects cortical disease, often attributed to (but not exclusively) the frontal lobes. They include the grasp reflex (stroking the patient's palm leads to an automatic clutching of your finger between his or her thumb and index finger); the glabellar reflex (cessation of the natural blink response in response to repetitive tapping on the forehead, also known as Meyerson sign); and the snout reflex (gentle tapping over the patient's upper lip causes a puckering of the lips). Note that this may also elicit a suck response or a turning of the head toward the stroking stimulus (rooting reflex).

The Mental Status Examination

The brains of higher mammals, particularly humans, have the added capacity to integrate sensory information across domains, evaluate this information, and react in a manner consistent with their experiences, the current context, or future expectations. The ability to use these higher level faculties is often considered part of the mental status examination (MSE). The MSE has been traditionally divided into the "psychiatric" portion of the MSE and the cognitive examination or "neurologic" portion of the MSE. While this distinction has a limited biological, psychological, pathophysiological, or clinical basis, we will use it for didactic purposes.

The "Psychiatric" Mental Status Examination

Box 5.3 provides a summary of the components of the psychiatric portion of the MSE.

General Appearance. This is similar to the "general" category that often starts the physical examination. The clinician will describe the patient's appearance with an emphasis on sex, ethnicity, body habitus, hygiene, clothing, and body art (e.g., tattoos, piercings).

Motor Behavior. This term is mostly descriptive and different from the motor component of the neurologic examination. Here we assess the degree of psychomotor depression or agitation, the presence of posturing or echopraxia, and abnormal movements (such as tremors, dyskinesias, dystonias, or akathisia). A comprehensive examination should always be followed by a motor neurologic examination with a focus on bulk, tone, and strength.

BOX 5.3
ELEMENTS OF THE PSYCHIATRIC MENTAL STATUS EXAMINATION

General appearance
Motor behavior
Attitude
Speech (rate, volume, prosody)
Mood and affect
Thought process
Thought content
- Suicidal ideation/homicidal ideation
- Obsessions
- Delusions: paranoia, ideas of reference, thought broadcasting
Perceptions
- Auditory, visual, olfactory, and tactile hallucinations; illusions
Insight and Judgment

Attitude. The assessment of the patient's attitude toward the examiner and overall demeanor is performed throughout the examination and should be reported in simple descriptive terms without equivocal jargon (e.g., avoid terms like "hysterical" or "borderline" that may have different meanings to different people). Note the patient's social graces, the degree of cooperation with the interview, and the quality of the eye contact.

Speech. Speech is the verbal output of language (it is therefore different from language). Clinicians will describe the quantity, volume, and rate of speech, as well as its rhythm or prosody. Additional variables can describe the flow, the pronunciation, and the presence of accents.

Mood and Affect. These terms are analogous to the symptoms (mood) and signs (affect) of emotional disturbance, respectively. Mood represents how the patient feels and is often reported as a direct quote between quotation marks. Affect is how the patient displays that mood to the world. A useful description of affect will provide a qualitative static description (e.g., sad) followed by a report of the dynamic qualities of displayed emotion (e.g., range and reactivity).

Thought Process. The expression of thought should be a goal-directed process in which thoughts are connected and presented in a logical manner. Abnormality of thought process lies on a continuum from subtle parenthetical comments to a complete lack of connection between ideas. Attention should be directed to the organization and linear structure of the patient's narrative, the presence of circumstantiality or tangentiality, loose associations, thought blocking, perseveration, and echolalia.

Thought Content. Our inner world of beliefs, convictions, and moment-to-moment ideas is hidden from even the savviest psychiatrist. Thought content can therefore be assessed only by direct inquiry ("What are you thinking about?"), an analysis of speech, or inference from behavior. Particular attention should be paid to content related to safety (such as suicidal thoughts, intentions and plans, self-injurious impulses, and homicidal or violent thoughts). In addition, psychotic content with an emphasis on delusions (including paranoid ideation, ideas of reference, thought insertion, thought withdrawal, and thought broadcasting), obsessions, and intrusive thoughts should be elicited.

Perceptions. A description of perceptions is sometimes framed under thought content, but it is useful to note them separately. Here the focus is on illusions and hallucinations with a review of different modalities (auditory, visual, somatosensory, olfactory, and less frequently taste).

Insight and Judgment. These are general measures that reflect the patient's insight into the illness and their judgment and decision-making abilities in the context of presenting symptoms.[10]

The Cognitive Examination or "Neurologic" Mental Status Examination

The cognitive examination is testing specific cognitive functions with relatively well-known neuroanatomical correlates. A thorough cognitive examination can involve hours or days of detailed neuropsychological testing, which may feel daunting or too complex to be performed by most clinicians. In this section, we will present the "bedside" cognitive examination, which is the first step to assess cognition and can be easily performed. This examination can lead to more specific testing, usually performed by a neuropsychologist, to reveal and quantify subtle deficits. Most tests are composites that assess more than a single cognitive function (e.g., drawing a clock will test executive and visuospatial functions, word recall will test short-term memory and language). When noting errors in a specific cognitive domain, one may want to perform more than a single test to isolate and clarify the deficit (e.g., test attention with digit span and also the spelling of the word WORLD backward). Unlike other features of the neurologic examination, it is important that the different components be done in order since certain basic functions (such as attention) must be intact in order to perform more complex tasks.

Level of Consciousness. Consciousness (i.e., arousal) lies on a continuum from full alertness to coma. While the two extremes are generally obvious, the middle ground can be subtle and caused by multiple etiologies (e.g., poor sleep, intoxication, mood disorder, delirium). It is important to note that we are providing a quantitative assessment of consciousness (i.e., more or less alert), not a qualitative report (e.g., perceptions or qualia). A standard measure of the level of consciousness is the Glasgow Coma Scale (Box 5.4), but one should not always be compelled to use it, as more descriptive terms (such as alert, somnolent, lethargic) derived from the observation of the general interview are acceptable. As a general rule for the whole neuropsychiatric examination, the greater the impairment, the greater the need for detailed quantification. The reader will note that some textbooks and authors talk of the level of consciousness and attention indistinguishably. These are related but different functions with segregated neuroanatomical systems sustaining them. Therefore, describing them separately is clearer and of greater diagnostic utility. Sustained alertness is required to participate in the assessment of other cognitive functions. Therefore, impairment of the level of consciousness may invalidate other results and should be assessed first.

BOX 5.4
GLASGOW COMA SCALE

EYES (4 POINTS)

1. No eye opening
2. Eye opening in response to pain
3. Eye opening in response to verbal command
4. Eye opening spontaneously

VERBAL (5 POINTS)

1. No verbal response
2. Incomprehensible sounds (moaning)
3. Inappropriate but discernible words
4. Confused conversation, but able to answer questions
5. Oriented

MOTOR (6 POINTS)

1. No motor response
2. Extension to pain (decerebrate response)
3. Flexion to pain (decorticate response)
4. Withdrawal in response to pain
5. Localizes pain (purposeful movements)
6. Obeys commands for movement
   Range: 3–15; Normal: 15; Mild: 13–14; Moderate: 9–12; Severe: 3–8.

Orientation. Clinicians will often test orientation to self, place, and time. Additionally, one can test orientation to circumstances (why the evaluation is being conducted). One may see findings usually reported as O x 3 or O x 4, but this is of limited value. Common to the whole neuropsychiatric assessment, it is preferable to be descriptive, as patients may be oriented to "hospital" but not to the specific hospital, city, or floor. Similarly, being oriented to the year, season, month, and day of the week conveys different levels of severity.

Attention. We are constantly being bombarded by stimuli from the external and internal environment that exceed the processing capacity of the brain. As a consequence, many stimuli are minimally processed by the brain and only a subset of those become conscious. Attention is the capacity to select specific stimuli to enter awareness for detailed processing. In the examination, we generally focus on volitional attention (our capacity to select what stimuli we want to examine and what to inhibit) but a related yet anatomically segregated function is stimulus-driven attention (e.g., responsible for the shift in focus and head turn when we hear a loud noise in the back of a quiet library). Intact attention is required to participate in further cognitive testing and should therefore be tested before most of the examination. A number of techniques can be used to test attention; we will describe some of the most common techniques.

Digit span. The examiner may have the patient repeat a randomly presented list of digits, starting with just a few numbers (two or three) and increasing the size of the list until two mistakes are made. The examiner should ask the patient to repeat the numbers in the same order they were presented (forward digit span) and once their limit of performance is reached, the same exercise will be repeated by asking the patient to repeat the list of numbers in reverse order; for example, if you say "1, 5, 3" they should say "3, 5, 1" (backward digit span). A normal capacity is between five to seven numbers forward and three to five numbers backward.

Serial 7s. The examiner may ask the patient to subtract 7 from 100 and then to continue serially subtracting 7 from the remainder; one can stop after five subtractions. This test is limited by its reliance on calculation, which may be more a function of education than attention.

Backward spelling/naming. The examiner may have the patient spell a five-letter word (e.g., WORLD) backward. Alternatively, the patient can name the days of the week or months of the year backward.

Executive Function. Executive function (i.e., frontal function) is computed in frontal cortico-subcortical circuits and allows us to solve problems. Complex and fundamental to adaptation, it consists of the capacity to choose a task, plan a strategy, develop the strategy, inhibit distractors, and assess performance by monitoring and correcting errors. Many of the tasks described in the cognitive examination require the appropriate use of executive function and intact fronto-subcortical circuits. Tests of attention and concentration (e.g., digit span, serial 7s), word-list generation, or complex visuospatial constructions require (and therefore test) executive function and the capacity to program a response. The following are commonly used tests for executive function.

Clock drawing. Already described above, this is a good approach to testing organizational and planning executive functions in the spatial domain.

Luria three-step command. Named after the famous Russian neuropsychologist, this test of frontal function shows the patient how to perform a three-step motor sequence and then asks for it to be repeated several times. The sequence traditionally starts with a light tap on the table of the right hand closed in a fist, followed by a second tap with the hand open and the palm facing medially, and finishes with a third tap with the hand open facing downwards. Patients with dysexecutive symptoms may be unable to perform this organized motor plan, may show rapid extinction with deterioration of the task over time, or may perseverate due to the inability to switch from one position to the other.

Complex sequence drawing. The patient is presented with a drawing that presents a repeating series of alternating triangles and squares and is asked to copy the drawing. Similar deficits due to disorganization or perseveration may be observed.

Memory. Memory function is generally divided into three components. It may be useful to test not only verbal but also non-verbal memory (e.g., spatial or procedural memory).

Working memory. Working memory is primarily an executive function that allows immediate recall of information (remembering a phone number given by the operator long enough to dial it). Registration and working memory are tested together by both digit span (described above) and phrase repetition (see section on Language). The examiner may ask the patient to immediately repeat three named items (e.g., red, table, honesty).

Short-term memory. Short-term memory involves the ability to store information for later use. Asking the patient to reproduce the three previously named items after a span of 3 to 5 minutes is a common test. A similar test for spatial memory involves hiding objects in three different locations in the room and then asking the patient where they are hidden after the same amount of time has elapsed. When deficits in short-term memory are identified, semantic or phonemic cues can be used (e.g., the word is a color or starts with the letter "r"). Correct responses after cues will separate amnestic (storage) from retrieval deficits: an amnestic patient never stored the information so cannot access it even with the help of cues, while a patient with a retrieval deficit can use the cue to access information that was properly stored.

Long-term memory. Long-term memory involves the recall of past events. This is nearly impossible to test accurately at the bedside since the examiner is rarely privy to details of remote events from the patient's life. Asking about well-known national events or people (e.g., How did JFK die?) is usually a good strategy although it is dependent on the age and educational background of the patient. Biographical information confirmed by trustworthy collateral sources (e.g., records, family members) can also be asked about.

Language. Language is the means by which we present our thoughts to each other. Like other cognitive functions, language can be extraordinarily complex, with entire texts of psycholinguistics and aphasiology dedicated to its study. The bedside clinical examination will assess four primary components of language that will test the integrity of the circuit: fluency, comprehension, repetition, and naming. These components should be assessed in oral and written language.

Is the language *fluent* or *non-fluent*? The analysis of spontaneous speech will determine if the patient can communicate with normal articulation and flow, using grammatical sentences with appropriate syntax and choosing words correctly. Verbal fluency can be formally tested with *word-list generation*, in which the patient is asked to name, in 1 minute, as many animals as possible (semantic fluency; 18 ± 6 is normal) or as many words starting with a certain letter, usually F, A, or S (phonemic fluency; 15 ± 5 is normal).

Is *comprehension* normal or abnormal? Does the patient seem to understand what you are saying? A request to complete a one- to three-step command (though complex commands may test more than just receptive language function) best assesses this. Asking simple "yes/no" questions (e.g., "Were you born in Mexico?" or "Are we in the kitchen?") is another common method.

Is *repetition* normal or abnormal? Having the patient repeat a phrase such as "no ifs ands or buts" is quite sensitive, given the difficulty of repeating conjunctions.

Can the patient *name* objects appropriately? Presenting the patient with a series of objects and asking him or her to name them (using high-frequency and low-frequency words such as "watch" and "face of the watch" respectively) is useful.

Reading and Writing. Because language is a meta-modal function (meaning that it is not based on a specific sensory modality but is a higher-order function that involves several modalities), one should test oral comprehension and speech as well as reading and writing. Asking the patient to follow a written command (such as, "close your eyes") and writing a sentence on a piece of paper are meaningful tasks.

Visuospatial Function. These components of the examination assess both visuospatial construction and spatial attention.

Figure drawing. Copying a three-dimensional (*cube*) of complex (*intersecting pentagons*) figure tests the capacity to organize spatial information.

Clock drawing. Having the patient fill in a circle with numbers in the form of a clock and then asking the patient to set the hands at 10 minutes to 2 (asking it as "ten to two" adds complexity). Abnormalities can occur in planning (poor spacing of numbers) or in positioning of the hands, which may belie frontal (executive) dysfunction. Absence of detail on one side of the clock (usually left) may represent a hemi-neglect syndrome, commonly though not exclusively associated with a (right) parietal lesion and deficit in spatial attention.

Line bisection. More specific to deficits in visual attention and neglect, this test presents a horizontal line and asks the patient to cross it with a vertical line exactly in the middle. Significant right-sided biases are seen in patients with left hemi-spatial neglect. For added complexity, one can present multiple horizontal lines in the four quadrants of the paper and assess not only if the vertical lines have a spatial bias but also if the horizontal lines in the left hemi-space are neglected or present even stronger spatial biases. For this test, it is important that the paper is presented well centered with respect to the patient.

Extinction. A related deficit of spatial attention, patients with extinction will identify individual stimuli in the left and right hemi-spaces, but when double stimuli are presented on both sides simultaneously they can only identify objects in the healthy ipsilesional side (usually the right side for the left hemi-spatial extinction). Because attention is also a multimodal function, one can identify deficits in extinction with visual (asking the patient to look to the examiner's nose and show fingers in left and/or right quadrants) and somatosensory stimuli (using light touch on the left and/or right extremities). Basic sensory functions (vision and touch) must be intact.

For the sake of not extending this section further, we will not describe the testing of other functions (such as calculation, praxis, object and face recognition, and right-left recognition). For more detailed descriptions, please see the suggested readings.[1–10]

Output

Although there are many potential responses to environmental stimuli, including subtle changes in the internal hormonal or neurochemical milieu, the response often involves some type of motor output. The examination of this output can be divided into a motor (or muscular) component and a coordination component.

Motor (III, IV, VI, XI, XII) and Sensorimotor (V, VII, IX, X) Cranial Nerves

These cranial nerves are responsible for motor function in the head and neck and are tested by examining the functionality of the muscles they subserve. For example, cranial nerves III, IV, and VI innervate the extraocular muscles that allow the eye to scan its environment. They are therefore tested by examining the range of eye movements in all directions by having the patient track one's finger or a salient object. Cranial nerve V can be assessed by applying an opposing force to the muscles of mastication; however, of greater importance is the assessment of cranial nerve VII, which innervates the facial muscles and can be tested by observing the face at rest (e.g., noting facial new-onset asymmetry, such as nasolabial fold flattening, or significant ptosis) or with action (i.e., asking the patient to raise their forehead, close their eyes tightly against opposition, smile, or puff their cheeks). Weakness related to cranial nerve IX can be noted by listening for dysarthria or dysphasia, which can be assessed by asking the patient to voluntarily cough, clear their throat, swallow, and, if safe, drink a sip of water while noting if there is a change in the quality of speech after swallowing. Cranial nerve XI can be tested by observation and confrontation with shoulder shrugging and horizontal head rotation. Cranial nerve XII can be assessed by asking the patient to protrude their tongue and have it push against the inside of their mouth while an opposing external force is applied.

Motor Examination

There are four aspects evaluated in the motor examination: abnormal movements, muscle tone, bulk, and strength. The four aspects may be affected separately.

Abnormal movements can be broadly classified as syndromes of movements that are decreased (hypokinetic signs, such as akinesia, bradykinesia, or hypomimia) or increased (hyperkinetic signs, such as tremors, tremulousness, fasciculation, myokymia, dyskinesia, dystonia, athetosis, chorea, asterixis, myoclonus, stereotypies, or simple and complex tics). Each movement is assessed first with passive observation, followed by changes in posture and action, such as arms and hands outstretched, or during ambulation.

A clear narrative description is most valuable. More structured elements to note for each movement include occurrence (e.g., at rest, with action, or with specific tasks or postures); character/phenotype (e.g., simple, complex, or patterned; rhythmic or irregular; tonic or clonic; high or low amplitude); rate (e.g., fast or slow frequency); and location (e.g., focal or diffuse; specific body parts involved; symmetry or laterality; synchronous or asynchronous).

Muscle tone refers to the resistance of a limb to passive movement through its normal range of motion. To examine for tone, one can have the patient relax the arms and legs fully to allow the physician to determine the degree of stiffness during passive motion. An increased level of tone (noted by rigidity or spasticity as can be seen in parkinsonism) is an important finding that may underlie an upper motor neuron or extrapyramidal lesion.

Assessment of *muscle bulk* can be extraordinarily challenging because of natural variation in body habitus and the role of weightlifting or exercise (i.e., "bulking up"), but it is important since muscle atrophy can indicate a lower motor neuron sign of neurodegenerative diseases, such as amyotrophic lateral sclerosis. Muscles that are unaffected by weightlifting or exercise (e.g., the facial muscles or the intrinsic muscles of the hand) may therefore provide the best estimate of overall muscle bulk.

When testing *muscle strength*, it is impractical (and unnecessary) to test each of the several hundred muscles in the human body. If the patient has a focal motor complaint, knowledge of major muscle groups in the proximal and distal limbs becomes important. Muscle strength is graded from 0 (no motion) to 5 (normal strength) (Box 5.5).

Observation of gait is an excellent screening test for the patient without focal weakness. If the patient can rise briskly and independently from a seated position and walk independently, gross motor deficits can be confidently ruled out. The ability to walk on one's heels and toes further ensures distal lower-extremity strength. Gait must be tested in all patients, particularly in older adults, for whom a fall can be a life-threatening event.

Table 5.2 summarizes examination findings in upper or primary versus lower or secondary motor neuron disease.

Coordination

Coordination reflects the ability to orchestrate and control movement, and it is crucial in the translation of movement into productive activity. Although the cerebellum plays a lead role in motor coordination, several other structures (e.g., the basal ganglia and red nucleus) are also involved.

The complexity of walking makes it an ideal screening test for coordination ability. Humans have a particularly narrow base when standing upright; with any degree of incoordination (ataxia), the patient needs to widen the base to remain upright. Balance becomes even more difficult when other sensory information is removed, forming the basis for the Romberg maneuver where the patient is asked to stand with their feet together and eyes closed. The Romberg sign is present if the patient begins to fall and it is absent if the patient only has mild postural instability. The sensitivity of screening is further increased by having the patient walk heel-to-toe (as on a tightrope). The ability to do this smoothly and quickly makes having a major impairment in coordination unlikely.

BOX 5.5
GRADING OF MUSCLE STRENGTH

0: No evidence of muscle contraction
1: Muscle contraction without movement of the limb
2: Muscle movement but not against gravity
3: Muscle movement against gravity
4: Muscle movement against partial resistance
5: Muscle movement against full resistance

TABLE 5.2
Upper Motor Neuron Versus Lower Motor Neuron Findings

Upper Motor Neuron Lesion	Lower Motor Neuron Lesion
▪ Spastic paralysis (increase tone)	▪ Flaccid paralysis (decreased tone)
▪ Hyperreflexia	▪ Areflexia
▪ Clonus	▪ No clonus
▪ Babinski sign	▪ No Babinski sign
▪ No fasciculations	▪ Fasciculations
▪ Atrophy (decreased use)	▪ Atrophy (denervation)

Diadochokinesia refers to the alternating movements made possible by the paired nature of agonist and antagonist muscle activity in coordinated limb movement. Abnormalities of this function are detected by several simple maneuvers, including rapid alternating movements (quick pronation or supination of the forearm, or finger/foot tapping). In tapping a rhythm in the context of cerebellar damage, the rhythm is poorly timed with incorrect emphases.

REFERENCES

1. LeBlond RF, Brown DD, DeGowin RL. *DeGowin's Diagnostic Examination*. 10th ed. McGraw-Hill; 2014.
2. Glick TH. *Neurologic Skills*. Blackwell Science; 1993.
3. Campbell WW. *DeJong's the Neurologic Exam*. 7th ed. Lippincott Williams & Wilkins; 2012.
4. Heimer L, Van Hoesen GW, Trimble M, et al. *Anatomy of Neuropsychiatry: The New Anatomy of the Basal Forebrain and Its Implications for Neuropsychiatric Illness*. Academic Press; 2007.
5. Lishman WA. *Organic Psychiatry*. 4th ed. Blackwell Science; 2012.
6. Mesulam MM. *Principles of Behavioral and Cognitive Neurology*. 2nd ed. Oxford University Press; 2000.
7. Ropper AH, Samuels MA, Klein JP. *Adams and Victor's Principles of Neurology*. 10th ed. McGraw-Hill; 2014.
8. Ropper AH, Samuels MA. *The Manual of Neurologic Therapeutics*. 8th ed. Lippincott Williams & Wilkins; 2010.
9. Samuels MA, Feske S, Livingstone C. *Office Practice of Neurology*. 2nd ed. Saunders; 2003.
10. Camprodon JA. The neurologic examination. In: Stern TA, Herman JB, Rubin DH, eds. *Massachusetts General Hospital Psychiatry Update and Board Preparation*. 4th ed. MGH Psychiatry Academy Publishing; 2018:407–418.

6

PSYCHOLOGICAL AND NEURO-PSYCHOLOGICAL ASSESSMENT IN THE MEDICAL SETTING

MARY KATHRYN COLVIN, PHD, ABPP ■ MARK A. BLAIS, PSYD ■ JANET C. SHERMAN, PHD

OVERVIEW

In the medical setting, psychological assessments are consultations in which the psychologist integrates information from a patient's clinical history, medical records, behavioral observations, and performance on standardized tests and questionnaires to answer specific clinical questions. These questions may relate to differential diagnosis, determining whether there has been a change in functioning from an estimated premorbid baseline or establishing a baseline from which to measure the efficacy of planned treatments or to monitor the course of a disease. Assessments can be performed at any stage of life, from infancy to very old age, and may be performed in the inpatient or outpatient setting. The evaluating psychologist often meets with the patient and their family to review the results of the testing and to offer recommendations, which are almost always formalized in a written report. Evaluations may be used to address legal questions (e.g., medico-legal liability, disability) and/or to determine eligibility for support services (e.g., special education services, guardianship); however, in the medical setting, these topics are not usually the primary reason for the referral. In this chapter, we focus on psychological and neuropsychological evaluations that are typically performed within a hospital setting. We provide cases to illustrate the methodology and potential findings and recommendations.

Broadly speaking, psychological evaluations characterize cognitive and emotional functioning, typically to better understand the nature of psychopathology a patient faces. Psychological assessments may help to characterize a mood or anxiety disorder, personality features, or how the overall level of cognitive functioning interacts with emotional functioning. Assessments typically combine symptom-based measures (e.g., questionnaires that patients or informants complete) and performance-based measures that are appropriate for the patient's age, cultural background, and the referral question. Information from assessments may assist both the patient and their healthcare provider (e.g., therapist, psychiatrist) to improve understanding of the patient's functioning and to facilitate the treatment process. The request for psychological testing might be framed as portrayed in Case 1.[1-4]

Case 1[1-4]

Please conduct a psychological assessment on Ms. B, a 28-year-old, right-handed, single attorney to help determine if her presentation represents depression with suicidality and/or atypical personality functioning.

Ms. B initially presented to the emergency department with complaints of extreme back pain. The physician noted mild confusion and disorientation, and Ms. B was admitted to the medical service for further evaluation. By the next morning, her mental status had improved. However, she continued to complain of extreme back pain and made vague suicidal statements. A pain work-up and psychiatric consultation were both ordered.

A review of the medical chart revealed that she had graduated from a prestigious university and law school and was employed at a large legal firm. She had developed severe back pain secondary to multiple equestrian injuries that occurred while riding competitively in college. She had received various diagnoses for her pain; there had been multiple unsuccessful interventions, including medication trials and surgery; and she made limited progress as a patient on an inpatient pain rehabilitation unit.

Ms. B completed a brief but comprehensive psychological assessment. The test battery included the Wechsler Abbreviated Scale of Intelligence—Second Edition (WASI-II)[1]; the Rorschach inkblot test[2]; four Thematic Apperception Test (TAT) cards[3]; and the Personality Assessment Inventory (PAI).[4] Ms. B's assessment was conducted in her semi-private room; while not ideal, hospital evaluations are commonly performed in this setting.

Impressions and Recommendations

Overall, the assessment strongly suggested the presence of clinical depression in the context of above-average intellectual functioning. Depression was likely masked to some extent by both the patient's focus on her physical function (back pain) and her inability or unwillingness to express her emotional pain. As a result, her depression was likely more significant and disruptive to her functioning than she reported, particularly given her personality functioning, which is likely to include an immature, self-centered view of the world and narcissistic traits. She did not appear to be actively suicidal on either the self-report or performance tests. However, given her emotionally overwhelmed and depressed state of being and her reduced coping ability, Ms. B should be considered at an increased risk (over and above being depressed) for impulsive self-harm. Her safety should be monitored closely.

Psychotherapy will be challenging given her personality style; nevertheless, it is recommended. The primary focus should be practical efforts to improve her coping skills and function. Once her functioning stabilizes, the focus of therapy might be expanded to include her interpersonal style. Medication to treat depression should also be considered.

Neuropsychological evaluations focus on relating an observed pattern of performances on measures of cognitive functioning to brain function; they are often most helpful when there are complex questions regarding the differential diagnosis, for example, at the interface of psychiatry and neurology. Referrals for neuropsychological evaluations are indicated when there are specific questions about the impact of a neurodevelopmental disorder (e.g., autism spectrum disorder [ASD], intellectual disability) or neurological condition (e.g., stroke, seizure, head injury, neurodegenerative disorder) on daily functioning. In addition to assessing intellectual and general psychological functioning, a complete neuropsychological assessment evaluates abilities within additional cognitive domains, including attention, executive functions, learning, memory, language functions, visuospatial functions, and higher-order motor and sensory functions. The request for neuropsychological testing might be framed as portrayed in Case 2.

Case 2

Mr. A, a 20-year-old, right-handed male with a childhood history of attention-deficit/hyperactivity disorder (ADHD) and a seizure disorder, developed psychotic symptoms approximately 4 years ago, and these prompted a recent psychiatric hospitalization for stabilization. A neuropsychological evaluation was requested to assess his current cognitive function, establish a baseline to monitor his future course, aid in differential diagnosis, and guide treatment. Assistance in determining the degree to which his presentation may reflect focal neurologic dysfunction was requested.

Mr. A was recently discharged from a psychiatric unit, where he was treated for symptoms of schizophrenia that included hallucinations (in multiple perceptual systems) and dysregulated behavior. Despite a long history of emotional and behavioral concerns (including a diagnosis of ADHD given at age 9, seizures that were clinically diagnosed at age 12, and visual hallucinations that first developed at age 16), there was no history of significant developmental delays or learning difficulties. He has completed some college courses. Since his diagnosis with a seizure disorder, he has been treated with antiepileptic drugs, and a variety of antidepressants and antianxiety agents were attempted in his mid- to late teens. Antipsychotics were started in the past year. Although he denied the use of substances within the past 4 months, he has a history of regular marijuana use.

Mr. A's evaluation included a review of medical records, an interview with him and his mother, and a discussion with his outpatient treaters. A comprehensive battery of neuropsychological and psychological measures was completed, and Mr. A cooperated fully with the evaluation. Performances on embedded measures of performance and symptom validity were within normal limits (i.e., all the psychological tests were valid and interpretively useful).

Salient Findings

- Overall intellectual functioning was estimated to fall at least in the average range of intellectual functioning.
- His profile was lateralizing. Verbal abilities (Verbal Comprehension Index) were stronger than non-verbal abilities (Perceptual Reasoning Index). The magnitude of the discrepancy between his verbal and non-verbal abilities was statistically significant, raising the possibility of relative right hemisphere inefficiency. Consistent with this, performances on measures of verbal memory were also stronger than on measures of visual memory. Dexterity (Grooved Pegboard Task) in his left (non-dominant) hand was borderline to low average and weaker than his average dexterity with his right (dominant) hand.
- On measures assessing visuospatial functions, performances were relatively weak, generally falling in the borderline impaired to low average range for age, including the construction of block designs (Wechsler Adult Intelligence Scale—Fourth Edition [WAIS-IV] Block Design) and mental rotation of "puzzle pieces" to identify an object (Hooper Visual Organization Test) or make an abstract pattern (WAIS-IV Visual Puzzles). His copy of the Rey Complex Figure was basically accurate, but notable for a piecemeal approach that did not indicate an appreciation of the overall gestalt.
- Receptive language skills were intact. Expressive language tasks indicated mild difficulties with

retrieval. On the Boston Naming Test, he correctly named 52 items (out of 60) spontaneously, which was below aptitude-based expectations. When provided with phonemic cues, his score improved to 58 (out of 60). Verbal fluency was also reduced; phonemic fluency fell in the borderline range (FAS phonemic fluency [letters F, A, S] = 20 words) while semantic fluency was slightly stronger and fell in the low average range for age (animals = 16 words). His ability to define the meaning of words and to describe similarities between words was average (WAIS-IV Vocabulary, WAIS-IV Similarities).

- Memory testing did not indicate a significant loss of information over time, suggesting that any inefficiency was likely due to reduced encoding (learning) or retrieval.
- There were difficulties with aspects of attention and executive function. His passive span of auditory attention was intact (WAIS-IV Digit Span Forward) but performances on measures of auditory working memory (reversal and sequencing of digits) were slightly reduced, falling in the low average range. Performance on a measure of sustained attention was notable for impulsivity and poor vigilance (Conners CPT). Processing speed fell in the low average to average range, and he was slower as task demands increased (WAIS-IV Coding; WAIS-IV Symbol Search). Consistent with this, performance on a straightforward visuomotor sequencing task and rapid naming task was low average to average (Trail Making Test Part A; Stroop Rapid Naming). When a set-shifting component was added to the sequencing task, he made three impulsive errors suggesting problems with inhibition of his behavior (Trail Making Test Part B). Sustained inhibition was low average (Stroop Color-Word Interference).
- The PAI profile was notable for elevations on the depression and schizophrenia scales. All three of the depression subscales (cognitive, affective, and physiological) were elevated (indicating a strong likelihood of major depression), as were all three schizophrenia subscales (psychotic experiences, social isolation, and thought disorder). Mr. A also reported having

a stimulus-seeking personality style and little motivation for psychological treatment. Each of these features will complicate his treatment.

Impressions

The neuropsychological evaluation revealed three principal findings: (1) given his reported developmental history, Mr. A's pre-morbid and current intellectual functioning likely falls in the average range for age; (2) his profile is lateralizing with test findings indicating that left hemisphere functions are stronger than right hemisphere functions; and (3) there are significant difficulties with aspects of attention and executive functions that contribute to weaknesses in cognitive efficiency, including his ability to learn and recall new information, and implicate dysfunction within networks involving the frontal lobes. Regarding the etiology, the degree of difficulty with attention and executive function is consistent with his psychiatric history, including ADHD, depression, and possibly an emerging schizophrenia-spectrum illness. The weaknesses in skills related to right hemisphere function are less likely to be fully accounted for by his current psychiatric symptoms. This may be related to developmental factors, including his seizure disorder. Given this, follow-up with neurology would be appropriate.

Although standardized tests may appear relatively straightforward to administer and score, it is important to emphasize that this is only one component of an evaluation; errors in data analysis and interpretation can lead to a significant risk of harm to the patient. The interpretation process requires an ability to assess the validity of the test data using knowledge of each test's psychometric principles, knowledge of the patient's behavior and background, as well as typical profiles for different psychiatric and neurological conditions. For these reasons, test materials are generally only available to psychologists who meet specific training requirements. Psychologists who specialize in conducting psychological assessments typically have a doctorate in clinical psychology, with additional postdoctoral training (residency) in assessment. Neuropsychologists have often undergone additional training in neuroscience and/or behavioral neurology.

Typically, psychologists train in either pediatrics or adult assessment, but a sizeable minority are qualified to perform assessments across the lifespan. Board certification in clinical neuropsychology is becoming more commonplace, especially for those who work in medical settings.[5]

In this chapter, we review the major domains of psychological and neuropsychological assessment. We include examples of the types of skills and abilities that may be evaluated, along with the names of common measures used for pediatric and adult populations. These measures have reasonable validity and reliability, but their appropriateness for each patient depends on multiple demographic factors, including the patient's age, educational background, and cultural background (e.g., dominant language). For a more comprehensive description of these tests and normative data, the reader is referred to Spreen and Strauss, or Lezak. [6,7]

Adjustments to the standardized assessment process may be needed when differences exist between the patient's background and the normative sample's background (e.g., use of a medical interpreter) or when there are concerns that a patient's performance does not accurately reflect their everyday abilities. Since the methods used for addressing the impact of these factors are beyond the scope of this chapter, our aim is to familiarize clinicians with the assessment process and the types of information that may be gathered, so that the maximal clinical benefit from referrals can be achieved.

Assessment of Intellectual Functioning

The conceptualization and assessment of intelligence have evolved over time. Current models of intelligence emphasize a dimensional approach, which combines performance on standardized tests (that assess different types of cognitive skills to estimate an individual's ability to perform in the everyday setting).[8] Valid interpretation of these measures requires knowledge of the patient's clinical history, cultural factors, normative data, and behavioral observations, especially when there are significant differences among the scores that assess different aspects of cognition (e.g., a significant discrepancy between verbal and non-verbal abilities). For those who are native English speakers and live in North America, common measures of intellectual functioning are listed in Table 6.1.[1,9–14]

TABLE 6.1
Common Measures of Intellectual Functioning[1,9–14]

Measure	Age Range
Wechsler Preschool and Primary Scale of Intelligence—Fourth Edition (WPPSI-IV)[9]	2–7
Wechsler Intelligence Scale for Children—Fifth Edition (WISC-V)[10]	6–16
Wechsler Adult Intelligence Scale—Fourth Edition (WAIS-IV)[11]	16–89
Wechsler Abbreviated Scale of Intelligence—Second Edition (WASI-II)[1]	6–89
Stanford-Binet Intelligence Scales—Fifth Edition (SB-5)[12]	2–85
Kaufman Brief Intelligence Test—Second Edition (KBIT-2)[13]	4–90
Differential Ability Scale—Second Edition (DAS-2)[14]	2–17

Tests of Personality, Psychopathology, and Psychological Function

Self-Report Measures

Objective psychological tests, also called *self-report tests*, are designed to clarify and quantify a patient's personality function and psychopathology. Objective tests use a patient's response to a series of true/false or multiple-choice questions to broadly assess psychological function. Scoring involves the use of standardized procedures and the application of frequently automated and appropriate normative data. Many computer-generated reports for psychometric tests that assess psychological functioning suggest making a *Diagnostic and Statistical Manual of Mental Disorders, Fifth Edition (DSM-5)* diagnosis, but these tests should not be used in isolation to create a psychiatric diagnosis. Computerized interpretations are not intended to replace psychologists, who are trained in the integration of multiple data sources in the evaluation process.

Symptom validity, the extent to which responses are likely to reflect an individual's functioning, is one factor that psychologists consider and often specifically measure. Validity scales are incorporated into all major objective tests to assess the degree to which a patient's response may have distorted the findings. The three main response styles that compromise test validity are careless or random responding (which may indicate

that someone is either not reading or understanding the test), attempting to "look good" by denying pathology, and attempting to "look bad" by over-reporting pathology (e.g., a cry for help or malingering). When these indices are atypical, the test results will need to be interpreted carefully, if at all.

The Minnesota Multiphasic Personality Inventory-2 (MMPI-2) is a 567-item true/false, self-report test of psychological function.[15] It was designed to provide an objective measure of abnormal behavior in adults, to separate subjects into two groups (normal and abnormal), and to further categorize the abnormal group into specific classes. The MMPI-2 contains 10 clinical scales (that assess major categories of psychopathology) and three validity scales (designed to assess test-taking attitudes). MMPI-2 validity scales are (L) lie, (F) infrequency, and (K) correction. The MMPI-2 clinical scales include (1) Hs, hypochondriasis; (2) D, depression; (3) Hy, conversion hysteria; (4) Pd, psychopathic deviate; (5) Mf, masculinity-femininity; (6) Pa, paranoia; (7) Pt, psychasthenia; (8) Sc, schizophrenia; (9) Ma, hypomania; and (10) Si, social introversion. More than 300 new or experiential scales have also been developed for the MMPI-2, which can help sharpen and individualize the clinical interpretation. The MMPI-2 is interpreted by determining the highest two or three scales, called a *code type*. For example, a 2-4-7 code type indicates the presence of depression (scale 2), impulsivity (scale 4), and anxiety (scale 7), along with the likelihood of a personality disorder.[15]

The Millon Clinical Multiaxial Inventory-IV (MCMI-IV) is a 195-item true/false, self-report questionnaire designed to identify personality patterns, clinical symptomatology, and response styles.[16] The MCMI-IV is composed of five validity scales, 15 personality scales, 45 facet scales, and 10 clinical syndrome scales, that allow for the simultaneous assessment of a wide variety of psychopathology. The most recent revision included updated norms, new test items, and the re-naming of scales to be more closely aligned with the updated DSM-5. Given its relatively short length (195 items vs. 567 for the MMPI-2), the MCMI-IV has an advantage in the assessment of patients who are agitated, whose stamina is significantly impaired, or who are sub-optimally motivated.

The Personality Assessment Inventory (PAI)[4] possesses outstanding psychometric features and is an ideal test for broadly assessing multiple domains of relevant psychological function.[17] The PAI includes 344 items and a 4-point response format (false, slightly true, mainly true, and very true) to create 22 non-overlapping scales. These 22 scales include 4 validity scales, 11 clinical scales, 5 treatment scales, and 2 interpersonal scales. There is a version for adolescents (Personality Assessment Inventory—Adolescent or PAI-A).[18] The PAI covers a wide range of psychopathology and other variables related to interpersonal function and treatment planning (including suicidal ideation, resistance to treatment, and aggression).

The Spectra: Indices for Psychopathology is a newer test that was developed to provide a tiered approach to the assessment of psychopathology.[19,20] It is theoretically grounded in research showing that there is a high degree or overlap (i.e., co-morbidity) among psychiatric disorders (e.g., with high rates of depression and anxiety).[21,22] The Spectra includes 96 items that assess 12 core clinical constructs, selected for their strong associations with the core higher-order dimensions of psychopathology (i.e., internalizing, externalizing, and reality impairing). These higher-order scales are combined to form an overarching general psychopathology dimension, commonly referred to as the "p-factor." The p-factor is conceptualized as representing the global psychiatric burden (e.g., illness severity, complexity, and impairment) experienced by a person.[23–25]

Performance-Based Measures

Performance tests (formerly known as projective tests) of psychological function differ from objective tests, in that they are less structured and require more effort on the part of the patient to make sense of, and to respond to, the test stimuli. As a result, the patient has a greater degree of freedom to demonstrate his or her own unique personality characteristics. Performance tests are more like problem-solving tasks, and they provide insights into a patient's style of perceiving, organizing, and responding to external and internal stimuli. When data from objective and performance tests are combined, they can provide a detailed picture or description of a patient's range of psychological function.

The Rorschach inkblot test assesses a patient's contact with reality and the quality of his or her thinking. The test consists of 10 cards that contain inkblots (five are black and white; two are black, red, and white; and three are various pastels), and the patient is asked to say what the inkblot might be. The examining psychologist reviews these codes rather than the verbal responses to interpret the patient's performance. Rorschach "scoring" has been criticized for being subjective; there are two standardized systems for interpretation, the Exner Comprehensive System (CS) and the Rorschach Performance Assessment System (R-PAS).

The CS system has demonstrated acceptable levels of reliability.[26] Using the scoring system, high inter-rater reliability coefficients can be obtained (e.g., kappa > 0.80) and are required for all Rorschach variables reported in research studies. In the CS, the test is administered in two phases. First, the patient is presented with the 10 inkblots one at a time and asked, "What might this be?" The patient's responses are recorded verbatim. In the second phase, the examiner reviews the patient's responses and inquires where on the card the response was seen (known as *location* in Rorschach language) and what about the blot made it look that way (known as the *determinants*).[26] For example, if a patient responds to Card V with "A flying bat." The practitioner asks, "Can you show me where you saw that?" The patient answers, "Here. I used the whole card." The practitioner asks, "What made it look like a bat?" The patient answers, "The color, the black made it look like a bat to me."

The Thematic Apperception Test (TAT) is helpful in revealing a patient's dominant motivations, emotions, and core personality conflicts.[3] The TAT consists of a series of 20 cards in which drawings depict people engaged in various interpersonal interactions. The cards were intentionally drawn to be ambiguous. The TAT is administered by presenting 8 to 10 of these cards, one at a time, with the following instructions: "Make up a story about this picture. Like all good stories, it should have a beginning, a middle, and an ending. Tell me how the people feel and what they are thinking." Although there is no standard scoring method for the TAT (making it more of a clinical technique than a psychological test), when enough cards are presented, meaningful information can be obtained. Psychologists typically assess TAT stories for emotional themes, the level of emotional and cognitive integration, the interpersonal relational style, and their view of the world (e.g., whether it is seen as a helpful or hurtful place). This type of data can be particularly useful in predicting a patient's response to psychotherapy. Recent research has shown that TAT narratives can be reliably scored to reveal a patient's level of personality organization, emotional regulation, identity integration, and social understanding.[27] The Children's Apperception Test is a related measure for pediatric patients.[28]

Overview of Neuropsychological Assessment Methods

A neuropsychological test battery is usually comprised of measures of intellectual and cognitive function that cover the major domains of cognitive functioning and are appropriate for the patient and the referral question. Patient characteristics are considered (e.g., age, native or primary language, educational attainment), along with the referral question. "Flexible" test batteries are typical to allow for greater depth of exploration based on behavioral observations and test data.[29] Patients' raw scores are converted to standard scores based on normative data for each test. These standard scores correspond to percentiles that are based on demographic factors and allow for comparisons across tests. Interpretation of neuropsychological test findings involves comparing patients' performances to an estimated baseline as well as normative data to determine whether the test data reveal a known pattern of cognitive dysfunction in developmental and acquired syndromes consistent with an identifiable etiology. The precise scores obtained from a neuropsychological evaluation also allow for monitoring of a patient's functioning.

Attention

Difficulties with attention and concentration are common cognitive complaints of patients who have neurological or psychiatric disorders. Attentional disturbances are often found in neurodevelopmental disorders (e.g., ADHD, ASD) and acquired disorders (e.g., traumatic brain injury [TBI]). Attentional regulation is highly complex and involves dissociable abilities, including orienting to a stimulus, filtering out extraneous information, and sustaining focus on a stimulus or activity. These abilities involve a widespread network of cortical and subcortical areas. Specific midbrain structures, such as the reticular activating system, play a fundamental role in alertness and arousal. Subcortical structures, such as certain thalamic nuclei, play a role

in selective attention, acting as a gatekeeper for both sensory and motor input. Limbic system structures, including the amygdala, also play an important role in designating the motivational significance of a stimulus. Finally, several cortical regions are involved in various aspects of attention, including spatial selective attention (inferior parietal cortex), behavioral initiation and inhibition (orbital frontal region), sustained attention (anterior cingulate region), task-shifting (dorsolateral prefrontal cortex), and visual search (frontal eye fields).[30]

Assessment of a patient's attentional capacity involves clinical observation, standardized testing, and questionnaires that are completed by the patient and/or informants (e.g., spouse, parents). In pediatric patients, it is important to consider what is typical for developmental stage. Across the lifespan, it is also important to consider whether there may be a combination of factors that contribute to observed or reported difficulties with attentional regulation (e.g., whether distractibility reflects symptoms of post-traumatic stress disorder or TBI, or both conditions simultaneously).

Common measures for the assessment of attentional abilities across the lifespan are listed in Table 6.2.[10,11,31–39] Measures to assess attention span, or attentional capacity, typically involve repetition of increasingly larger amounts of information (e.g., digits or spatial positions).[10,11,14,31] Working memory, a related construct, involves the brief manipulation of increasingly larger amounts of information (e.g., reversing or ordering sequences of digits, reversing a series of spatial positions, remembering a sequence of pictures in serial order).[10,11,14,31] The ability to orient to a stimulus in external space, particularly to the left side following right hemisphere damage, is frequently assessed through cancellation or line bisection tasks.[7] Vigilance, or sustained attention, is frequently assessed by asking the patient to monitor a series of stimuli over a longer period (e.g., counting how many letters are presented in a long auditory string of numbers and letters, responding when a target letter is presented in a long string of visually presented letters).[7]

Executive Functions

"Executive functions" is a term that has historically referred to a group of cognitive processes associated with the frontal lobes.[7] Broadly, these skills allow an

TABLE 6.2

Common Measures of Attentional Regulation[10,11,31–39]

Component Assessed	Measure	Test Example
Attentional capacity	Digit span forward	WAIS-IV[11]; WISC-V[10]
Short-term memory span	Spatial span forward	WMS-3 Spatial Span[31]; WRAML-3[32]
Working memory	Digit span backward	WAIS-IV[11]; WISC-V[10]
	Spatial span backward	WMS-3 Spatial Span[31]
	Letter-number sequencing	WAIS-IV[11]
Complex visual search and scanning	Symbol substitution	Coding (WAIS-IV,[11] WISC-V)[10]
	Visual search/symbol discrimination	Symbol Search (WAIS-IV,[11] WISC-V)[10]
	Visuomotor tracking	Trail Making Test Part A[33]
Sensory selective attention	Cancellation	Visual Search and Attention Test[34]; WPPSI-IV[9]
	Visuomotor tracking	Trail Making Test Part A[33]
	Line bisection	
Sustained attention and task vigilance	Cancellation	(see above)
	Vigilance	Conners' Continuous Performance Test (CPT-III or K-CPT)[35,36]
Selective/divided attention	Sustained and selective serial addition	Paced Auditory Serial Addition Test (PASAT)[37]
	Selective auditory tracking	Brief Test of Attention (BTA)[38]
	Selective attention and response inhibition	Stroop Color and Word Test[39]

WAIS-IV, Wechsler Adult Intelligence Scale—Fourth Edition; *WISC-V*, Wechsler Intelligence Scale for Children—Fifth Edition; *WMS-3*, Wechsler Memory Scale-III; *WPPSI-IV*, Wechsler Preschool and Primary Scale of Intelligence—Fourth Edition; *WRAML-3*, Wide Range Assessment of Memory and Learning—Third Edition.

individual to access and apply knowledge to meet current environmental demands. There are executive functions related to cognitive efficiency (including initiation, inhibitory control, set-shifting, and processing speed). There are also executive functions related to goal-directed behavior (including planning, organization, reasoning, problem-solving, and judgment). While traditionally conceptualized as cognitive processes, executive functions are also critically involved in emotional and social skills (e.g., responding appropriately to others and changing behavior given the circumstances). Indeed, some of the most dramatic changes in personality and behavioral functioning follow damage to frontal lobe networks (e.g., behavioral variant frontotemporal dementia [bvFTD], TBI) and executive dysfunction is associated with a wide range of psychiatric disorders (e.g., bipolar disorder).[40,41]

As with attentional regulation, assessment of executive functions involves clinical observation, standardized testing, and questionnaires completed by the patient and/or informants (e.g., spouse, parents). In pediatric patients, it is also important to consider that executive function skills emerge relatively slowly and in a hierarchical manner over the course of childhood and adolescence (e.g., reasoning skills may not be fully developed until late adolescence). Executive function skills can be dissociable (e.g., a patient may struggle with inhibitory control but have good organizational strategies), but also intertwined (e.g., showing a high number of perseverative [repetitive] responses/errors may indicate reduced flexibility and/or inhibitory control). As such, the pattern of test performances across the entire domain is important to consider, as is informant-derived data (e.g., from a parent or spouse) from standardized questionnaires that assess executive function skills (e.g., BRIEF-2, FrSBe), as cognitive measures may not always capture related emotional, behavioral, and social dysregulation.[42]

Common measures for the assessment of executive functions across the lifespan are listed in Table 6.3.[9–11,14,33,39,43–53] Initiation is frequently assessed by asking patients to generate novel material quickly (e.g.,

TABLE 6.3
Common Measures of Executive Functions[9-11,14,33,39,43-53]

Component Assessed	Measure	Example Test
Initiation and maintenance of a complex task set; generation of multiple response alternatives	Verbal fluency	Controlled Oral Word Association Test (COWAT)[43]; Delis-Kaplan Executive Function Systems (D-KEFS) Verbal Fluency Test[44]
	Design fluency	D-KEFS Design Fluency Test[44]
Cognitive flexibility	Set-shifting (alphanumeric sequencing)	Trail Making Test Part B[33]
	Card sorting	Wisconsin Card Sorting Test[45]
	Verbal fluency	D-KEFS Verbal Fluency Test[44]
Organization/planning	Spatial organization and planning	Rey-Osterrieth Complex Figure Test[46]; D-KEFS Tower Test[44]; Tower of London[47]
	Use of semantic clustering strategies on verbal learning tasks	California Verbal Learning Test (CVLT-3 or CVLT-C)[48,49]
Concept formation and reasoning	Proverb interpretation	D-KEFS Proverb Test[44]
	Verbal conceptualization	Similarities (WPPSI-IV, WISC-V, DAS-2, WAIS-IV)[9-11,14]
	Non-verbal concept formation	The Category Test[50]
	Matrix reasoning	Matrix Reasoning (WISC-V, WAIS-IV)[10,11]
	Card sorting	Wisconsin Card Sorting Test (WCST)[45]
Inhibitory control	Selective attention and response inhibition	Stroop Color and Word Test[39]; D-KEFS Color-Word Interference Test[44]; Go/no-go tasks
Decision-making	Balancing risk and reward	Iowa Gambling Task[51]
Self- and family observations	Behavioral ratings	Frontal Systems Behavior Scale (FrSBe)[52]; Behavior Rating Inventory of Executive Functions—Second Edition (BRIEF-2)[53]

fluency tasks). Cognitive flexibility, or the ability to adjust to changing demands, is often assessed by asking patients to alternate between two different response patterns or to integrate new information as it is being presented.[33] Inhibitory control tasks often require a patient to stop responding in a manner that is overly learned (e.g., to say the opposite of what is typical).[54,55] Processing speed is assessed through timed tasks that measure a patient's ability to quickly integrate and act on new information.[11,54,55] Organization and planning can be assessed through formal testing (e.g., building towers from concentric disks while following specific rules) and through process observations (e.g., whether there is an organized approach to copying a complex figure, to learning a list of words, or to generating block designs).[56,57] Concept formation and abstract reasoning can be assessed by asking a patient to identify similarities or ways of grouping novel information, or through pattern analysis and completion.[11] Effective decision-making that balances risk and reward can

also be assessed through computerized testing that adjusts contingencies based on performance.

Learning and Memory

Learning and memory for new information can be divided into three stages that involve different brain networks: (1) learning or acquisition; (2) storage or consolidation; and (3) retrieval or recognition. Learning or acquisition is closely aligned with attention and executive functions; it is subserved by networks that involve the frontal lobes. Indeed, many patients who have primary attention difficulties associated with a wide range of neurodevelopmental (e.g., ADHD), psychiatric (e.g., anxiety), or neurological (e.g., TBI) conditions will describe these as memory problems because they fail to register material as it is being presented to them. Weaknesses in executive functions, such as slow processing speed or difficulties making conceptual connections, may also contribute to shallow or inefficient learning. These same skills and brain networks are also involved in the retrieval of recently learned information. Thus, patients who have difficulty with learning and retrieval will often perform better on recognition tasks, because demands on initiation, association, and organization are reduced.

In contrast, memory storage is critically dependent on the medial temporal lobes, the hippocampus, and associated structures (e.g., the parahippocampal gyrus, entorhinal cortex, fornix, and amygdala). Anterograde amnesia, which is characterized by an inability to form and consciously recollect facts, events, images, and episodes, results from medial temporal damage.[58] Damage to regions with rich interconnections to the medial temporal lobes (e.g., the thalamus, basal forebrain) may also be associated with consolidation difficulties or rapid forgetting. This is the hallmark of Alzheimer disease, in which basal forebrain and hippocampal functioning are disrupted, but it can also be seen in a variety of neurological conditions that impact the medial temporal network (e.g., anoxic injuries, temporal lobe epilepsy [TLE], autoimmune or infectious encephalopathies). If dysfunction is lateralized, there may also be dissociations between different types of stimulus material (e.g., verbal or visual).

Common measures for the assessment of learning and memory across the lifespan are listed in Table 6.4.[31,32,46,48,49,54,59-64] Evaluation should include both verbal and visual memory measures, measure immediate and delayed recall, assess the pattern and rate of new learning, and explore differences between recognition (memory with a retrieval cue) and unaided recall. Encoding (learning) difficulties are identified by shallow learning curves and greater difficulty on tasks where material is presented "all at once" or in an unstructured manner. Storage difficulties (e.g., rapid forgetting may indicate anterograde amnesia) are identified by a loss of information that was present on immediate, but not on delayed, recall or recognition. Retrieval difficulties are identified by a discrepancy between delayed recall and recognition, with better performance on recognition.

While declarative memory is typically the focus of a neuropsychological assessment, it is important to note that there are other types of memory difficulties. Patients may manifest challenges with source memory (e.g., recalling when or where new information was presented, which can manifest as intrusions between similar tasks). When semantic access is disrupted,

---

TABLE 6.4
Common Measures of Learning and Memory[31,32,46,48,49,54,59-64]

Domain	Types of Measures	Example Test
Auditory-verbal memory	Recall and recognition of unrelated words presented over multiple trials	Rey Auditory-Verbal Learning Test[59]; Child and Adolescent Memory Profile (ChAMP)[60]; Wide Range Assessment of Memory and Learning—Third Edition (WRAML-3)[32]
	Recall and recognition of semantically related word presented over multiple trials	California Verbal Learning Test (CVLT-3 and CVLT-C) [48,49]
	Recall and recognition of word pairs over multiple trials	WMS-III Verbal Paired Associates Learning[31]
	Story recall	WMS-IV Logical Memory[54]; WRAML-3[32]
Visual memory	Recall and recognition of simple designs (drawing required)	WMS-IV Visual Reproduction[54]
	Recall and recognition of multiple designs presented over repeated trials (drawing required)	Brief Visuospatial Memory Test—Revised[61]
	Recall of complex visual information (drawing required)	Rey-Osterrieth Complex Figure Test[46]
	Learning of a spatial pattern (over multiple trials)	7-24 Spatial Recall Test[62]; WRAML-3[32]
	Face learning and recognition	WMS-III Face Recognition[31]
	Learning and recognition of abstract shapes or pictures	WRAML-3[32]; ChAMP[60]
Remote/long-term memory	Recall of facts	Wechsler Information
	Recall of public semantic knowledge	Transient Events Test [63]
	Autobiographical memory	Autobiographical Memory Interview[64]

there may also be challenges with fact retrieval, and remote memories. Loss of this information may occur in a temporally graded manner, with loss of more recent events first. Finally, challenges with autobiographical memories can be seen in association with dense anterograde amnesia or as an isolated impairment, and this is typically assessed through a semistructured interview with collateral verification (e.g., the Autobiographical Memory Interview).[64]

Language

Brain networks that subserve language function are widespread and typically associated with the left hemisphere, except in a minority of patients. The primary auditory cortex is in the superior temporal gyrus and surrounding temporal areas (including Wernicke area) and is associated with auditory comprehension and semantic knowledge. The arcuate fasciculus is a white matter pathway that forms the backbone of the language system by looping from the temporal lobes, through the parietal lobes, and into the frontal lobes. At the junction of the parietal and temporal cortex, there is a specialization for language-based academic skills (including reading, writing, and aspects of mathematics). The frontal lobes are important in language expression, including fluency and organization. Interestingly, some language processes related to social communication (e.g., interpretation of tone of voice or facial affect) may involve the right hemisphere.[65]

Assessment of language abilities should first consider acuity and attention and must account for the patient's cultural and educational background. Whenever possible, the patient should be tested in their dominant language. If this is not possible, then a medical interpreter should be used; standardized assessment practices do not permit the use of an untrained individual (e.g., a family member or friend) as an interpreter. Many standardized measures have been translated into other languages and have normative data available for populations in other parts of the world. For bilingual individuals, it may be important to consult multiple sets of normative data. Educational access should also be considered, especially when interpreting language-based academic skills (e.g., reading and writing). Similarly, language-based learning disabilities are common (e.g., dyslexia affects approximately

5%–7% of the general population) and may impact performance on language measures in adulthood; therefore this should be accounted for when assessing a decline in language abilities secondary to an acquired condition (e.g., TBI or a neurodegenerative disease).

After considering and/or addressing these factors, a thorough assessment of language considers speech patterns (e.g., rate, articulation, fluency, and prosody), expressive output (e.g., grammar, vocabulary, and clarity of expression), receptive skills (e.g., comprehension of words, phrases, and passages), and functional communication (e.g., ability to communicate effectively with others, including an appreciation of slang, metaphors, and non-literal language). Assessment of each of these aspects of language should be considered to identify potential dissociations between expression and comprehension (e.g., impaired fluency with spared comprehension as in Broca aphasia, spared fluency with impaired comprehension as in Wernicke aphasia), semantic knowledge and functional communication (e.g., a strong vocabulary but with poor pragmatic skills as in some with ASD), and between auditory comprehension and reading/writing (e.g., as in those with developmental dyslexia). When discrepancies arise, a more detailed evaluation of speech and language may also be needed. Common measures for the assessment of language functions across the lifespan are listed in Table 6.5.[66–79]

Higher-Order Visual Functions

A neuropsychological evaluation typically focuses on visual skills associated with cortical functioning; however, it should first consider acuity and attention when interpreting test findings. At the cortical level, the ventral visual stream is involved in analyzing and synthesizing information for object recognition and it spans occipitotemporal regions. This pathway is known as the "what" pathway because it processes an object's characteristics (e.g., color, shape, form) and there are specialized areas for some types of objects (e.g., faces, words). The pathway eventually connects with language areas in the temporal lobe, which are important in semantic processing (e.g., naming). In contrast, the dorsal ventral stream is involved in analyzing spatial orientation and location and it spans the occipitoparietal regions. This pathway is known as the "where" pathway and it eventually connects with motor and sensory

TABLE 6.5
Common Measures of Language Function[66–79]

Domain	Types of Measures	Sample Tests
Receptive language (spoken modality)	Word-picture matching	PPVT-5,[66] Expressive One-Word Picture Vocabulary Test—Fourth Edition (EOWPVT-4)[67]
	Word definition	Wechsler Vocabulary subtests, Clinical Evaluation of Language Fundamentals—Fifth Edition (CELF-5)[68]
	Following commands	BDAE Commands subtest,[69] NEPSY-II Comprehension of Instructions,[70] CELF-5[68]
	Sentence comprehension	BDAE Syntactic Processing subtest,[69] CELF-5[68]
Receptive language (written modality)	Word recognition	PALPA Visual Lexical-Decision Test[71]
	Word comprehension	BDAE Word-Identification Subtest[69]
	Sentence comprehension	PALPA Sentence-Picture matching (written version)[71]; CELF-5[68]
Expressive language (spoken modality)	Confrontation naming	Boston Naming Test[72]
	Repetition	BDAE Repetition of Words, Non-words, Sentences[69]; CELF-5[68]
	Sentence production	BDAE Action description subtest[69]; CELF-5[68]
	Conversational speech	BDAE Picture description Test[69]
Expressive language (written modality)	Writing to dictation	PALPA Spelling to Dictation subtest[71]; Wechsler Individual Achievement Test—Fourth Edition (WIAT-4)[73]
	Written picture naming	BDAE Written Picture Naming subtest[69]
	Narrative writing	BDAE Picture Description[69]; Test of Written Language—Fourth Edition (TOWL-4)[74]
Social communication	Non-literal language, multiple meanings, social scripts	CELF-5,[68] Wechsler Advanced Clinical Solutions[75]
Other language-based academic skills	Reading (phonemic decoding, oral reading fluency, reading comprehension)	Wechsler Individual Achievement Test—Fourth Edition (WIAT-4),[73] Woodcock Johnson Tests of Academic Achievement—Third Edition (WJA-3),[76] Kaufman Test of Educational Achievement—Third Edition (KTEA-3),[77] Test of Word Reading Efficiency—Second Edition (TOWRE-2),[78] Gray Oral Reading Test—Fifth Edition (GORT-5)[79]
	Calculation, math fluency	Wechsler Individual Achievement Test—Fourth Edition (WIAT-4),[73] Woodcock Johnson Tests of Academic Achievement—Third Edition (WJA-3),[76] Kaufman Test of Educational Achievement—Third Edition (KTEA-3)[77]

processing areas that are important for goal-directed action.[80] While both brain hemispheres are involved in basic perceptual processing, the right hemisphere tends to be more specialized for spatial and constructional skills.[81]

Common measures for the assessment of higher-order visual functions across the lifespan are listed in Table 6.6.[9-11,34,82-87] Basic visuoperceptual tasks assess shape, form, and object recognition associated with occipitotemporal areas (ideally), independently from motor skills. Spatial abilities (including mental rotation, judgment of line orientation, and appreciation of the overall gestalt or global structure) are more typically associated with the right parietal cortex. Constructional difficulties (e.g., difficulties with three-dimensional drawings or positioning writing on the page) may also be associated with right parietal damage, but these tasks involve other perceptual and motor skills that are likely represented bilaterally.

Higher-Order Sensory and Motor Functions

Disruption of higher-order sensory and motor functions can be important in identifying brain dysfunction and functional impairment, as they involve cortical (frontal and parietal areas) and subcortical networks (e.g., in the cerebellum, basal ganglia). These

TABLE 6.6
Common Measures of Visuospatial Skills[9-11,34,82-87]

Component Assessed	Measure	Example of Specific Test
Visuoperceptual abilities	Object recognition	Hooper Visual Organization Test[82]
	Face recognition	Benton Facial Recognition Test[83]
	Shape and form discrimination	Motor-Free Visual Perception Test—Fourth Edition (MVPT-4)[84]
Visuospatial abilities	Spatial orientation and location	Visual Object and Space Perception Battery (VOSP) subtests,[85] Motor-Free Visual Perception Test—Fourth Edition (MVPT-4)[84]
	Judgment of angular orientation	Benton Judgment of Line Orientation Test [86]
	Cancellation	Visual Search and Attention Test [34]
	Line bisection	
Visuoconstructional abilities	Drawing	Beery-Buktenica Developmental Test of Visual-Motor Integration[87]
	Block design	Block Design (WPPSI-IV, WISC-V, WAIS-IV)[9-11]

are usually thoroughly assessed as part of a neurological examination, but they may be further characterized in a neuropsychological evaluation, especially if there is a question of lateralization. Behavioral observations often provide crucial data. Difficulties with balance and coordination may indicate cerebellar dysfunction, while deficits in praxis, graphesthesia (e.g., an inability to identify symbols written on the patients' hands or fingertips), finger agnosia (e.g., an inability to name fingers), or challenges with left-right orientation are associated with parietal damage. The presence of tremors, rigidity, repetitive behaviors (e.g., tics, stereotypies, compulsions), and micrographia are signs and symptoms of subcortical involvement.

Formal testing may assess hand strength (e.g., with a hand dynamometer), speed (e.g., with finger tapping[6]), dexterity (e.g., with the Grooved Pegboard Test[88]), and praxis (e.g., with imitative tool use). Sensory tests may assess for loss of smell (e.g., the Smell Identification Test), finger localization abilities, and the ability to detect simultaneously presented touch (e.g., with Two-Point Discrimination, and a Simultaneous Extinction Test[6]). When interpreting results, it is important to account for attention, effort, and medical history (e.g., whether there is peripheral nerve damage or vision loss). If these factors are not contributory, then deficits on one side of the body may be associated with damage to the contralateral side of the brain, such that a discrepancy between the two sides of the body can indicate lateralization of a neurological disorder.

Neuropsychological Screening Instruments

Screening tools are designed to identify the possibility of a disorder. Because they are sensitive but not specific, they may have high false-positive rates and be unlikely to assist with complex differential diagnostic questions. Nonetheless, tests like the Mini-Mental State Examination [89] and the Montreal Cognitive Assessment, often used by neurologists, can help triage patients who need more comprehensive neuropsychological evaluations.[90]

Brief neuropsychological assessments can be helpful in specific situations, including inpatient settings, during acute recovery from a neurological event, for time-limited evaluations, and when rapid identification of a condition is needed to access treatment and services (e.g., intellectual disability, ASD, a neurodegenerative disorder), or when a patient's course is being closely tracked. These brief measures generally include tasks that assess the major areas of cognitive function (e.g., attention, executive functions, learning and memory, language, and visuospatial functions). For adolescents and adults, there is the Repeatable Battery for the Assessment of Neuropsychological Status (RBANS).[91] For older adults who present with a concern for a neurodegenerative disorder, the Addenbrooke's Cognitive Examination—Third Edition (ACE-3)[92] has been shown to be predictive of neuropsychological test performance.[93]

The Mattis Dementia Rating Scale, second edition (DRS-2) is sometimes used for older adults being evaluated for cognitive impairment and question of dementia.[94]

Integrating Psychological and Neuropsychological Assessments

Neuropsychologists often include psychological assessment tools, including those described earlier in this chapter, to formally assess a patient's emotional and behavioral functioning. Psychiatric disorders may present with cognitive challenges (e.g., a patient with ADHD or anxiety may complain of memory difficulties) that will be detected on neuropsychological tests. Likewise, neurological dysfunction may be manifest in symptoms of a possible psychiatric disorder, including changes in behavior, personality, emotional regulation, and mood. In addition, bvFTD is sometimes misdiagnosed initially as a psychiatric disorder, while TLE is also sometimes mistaken for a schizophreniform illness.[41] Right frontal damage may manifest as indifference, anosognosia, or inappropriate euphoria. Left anterior damage may manifest as catastrophic reactions, depression, agitation, and anxiety.[95] Psychiatric disorders may also emerge secondary to an individual living with a neurological condition (e.g., a brain tumor, stroke) or following a neurosurgical intervention (e.g., depression that follows deep brain stimulation [DBS]). Understanding the etiology of such psychological concerns is critically important when making treatment decisions and improving the patient's quality of life.

Common Neuropsychological Assessment Referral Questions for Psychiatrists

Neuropsychological evaluations are warranted when there is a question of an acute or subacute change in cognitive, emotional, or social functioning that is related to neurological function in either a child or an adult. In these cases, the precipitant may be known (e.g., TBI, brain tumor, seizure, stroke) or suspected (e.g., a neurodegenerative disease). Many chronic medical conditions are also associated with psychiatric symptoms and cognitive dysfunction, including autoimmune disorders (e.g., multiple sclerosis [MS]). The course of symptoms may be static, progressive, or waxing and waning, and the degree to which this can be characterized will assist the neuropsychologist in the creation of a differential diagnosis.

Neuropsychological evaluations also help when there is concern about a neurodevelopmental disorder (e.g., intellectual disability, ASD) or a genetic syndrome (e.g., Turner syndrome, 22q11 deletion syndrome) that impacts cognitive, emotional, and social development. In childhood and adolescence, neuropsychological testing can track the development of certain skills and can help with the creation of a differential diagnosis. For example, a psychiatrist who is treating a child for emotional and behavioral dysregulation may seek a neuropsychological evaluation to help determine whether the child has ADHD or another neurodevelopmental condition, such as ASD or a learning disability. Once a diagnosis has been determined, a neuropsychologist can make recommendations as to the most appropriate interventions and treatment and can also track the patient's progress over time to quantify the impact of interventions on behavior. The psychiatrist may also wish to refer their patient for a neuropsychological re-evaluation once the child has been treated with medications and psychotherapy (e.g., for ADHD) to determine the efficacy of those interventions and whether residual symptoms (e.g., anxiety) are interfering with cognitive functioning and need management.

At the other end of the lifespan, neuropsychological assessment helps to distinguish between cognitive difficulties that are caused by psychiatric disorders and difficulties caused by neurological disorders. One of the most common referral questions is whether an older individual's memory problems are due to depression or to an incipient neurodegenerative process. By evaluating the profile of deficits obtained across a battery of tests, a neuropsychologist can help to distinguish between these disorders. For example, depressed patients tend to have problems with attention, concentration, and memory (new learning and retrieval), whereas patients with early dementia of the Alzheimer type have problems with delayed recall (retention) and word-finding or naming problems, with relative preservation of attention.

Neuropsychological assessments can often aid in treatment planning for patients with moderate to severe psychiatric illness. Neuropsychological assessment informs treatment planning by providing objective data (a test profile) regarding the patient's cognitive skills (deficits and strengths). The availability of such data can help clinicians and family members develop more realistic expectations about the patient's functional capacity.[96] This can be particularly helpful for patients suffering from severe disorders. For example, the presence of neuropsychological deficits has been found to be more predictive of long-term outcomes in those with schizophrenia than positive or negative symptoms.[97]

OBTAINING AND UNDERSTANDING TEST REPORTS

Referring a patient for an assessment should be like referring a patient to any professional colleague. Psychological and neuropsychological testing cannot be done "blind." The psychologist will want to hear about relevant case information and may ask the referring practitioner to provide specific questions that need answers. Based on this case discussion and referral question(s), the psychologist will select an appropriate battery of tests designed to obtain the desired information. It is helpful if the referrer prepares the patient for the testing by reviewing why the consultation is desired and informing them that neuropsychological evaluations often take several hours to complete. The referrer should expect the psychologist to evaluate the patient in a timely manner and provide verbal feedback, a "wet read," quickly. The written report should follow shortly thereafter (inpatient reports are typically produced within 48 hours and outpatient reports are generally available within 2-3 weeks, although this may vary depending on the setting).

The psychological assessment report is the written statement of the psychologist's findings. It should be understandable and stated plainly; moreover, it should answer the referral question(s). The report should contain relevant background information, a list of the tests used in the consultation, a statement about the validity of the results and the confidence the psychologist has in the findings, a detailed integrated description of the patient, and clear recommendations. It should contain test data (e.g., intelligence quotient [IQ] scores) as appropriate to allow for meaningful follow-up testing. To a considerable degree, the quality of a report (and the assessment consultation) can be judged from the recommendations provided. The referrer should never read just the summary of a test report; this leads to the loss of important information because the whole report is really a summary of a very complex consultation process.

A neuropsychological evaluation report may be less integrated but should provide a summary that reviews and integrates the major findings, including implications for diagnosis and brain-behavior relationships. Test findings are typically reviewed for each major area of cognitive function (intelligence, attention, executive functions, learning and memory, language, higher-order visual skills, higher-order sensory and motor skills). These reports typically contain substantial amounts of data to allow for retesting comparison and they include useful and meaningful recommendations.

As with all professional consultations, the evaluating psychologist should meet with the patient to review the findings and if needed with the referrer. This is especially important as the information that is provided by psychological and neuropsychological evaluations can help with diagnostic questions, questions regarding further investigations that may be helpful, and recommendations regarding how to best move forward in terms of clinical management to enhance a patient's functioning.

REFERENCES

1. Wechsler D, Hsiao-Pin C. *WASI-II: Wechsler Abbreviated Scale of Intelligence*. Pearson; 2011.
2. Rorschach H. *Psychodiagnostics*. G. Stratton; 1942.
3. Murray HA. *Explorations in Personality*. Oxford University Press; 1938.
4. Morey LC. *Personality Assessment Inventory*. Routledge; 1991.
5. Sweet JJ, Klipfel KM, Nelson NW, et al. Professional practices, beliefs, and incomes of U.S. neuropsychologists: the AACN, NAN, SCN 2020 practice and "salary survey". *Clinical Neuropsychol*. 2021;35(1):7–80.
6. Spreen O, Strauss E. *A Compendium of Neuropsychological Tests: Administration, Norms, and Commentary*. Oxford University Press; 1998.
7. Lezak MD. *Neuropsychological Assessment*. Oxford University Press; 2004.
8. Carroll JB. *Human Cognitive Abilities: A Survey of Factor-analytical Studies*. Cambridge University Press; 1993.
9. Wechsler D. *Wechsler Preschool and Primary Scale of Intelligence*. 4th ed. Pearson; 2012.
10. Wechsler D. *Wechsler Intelligence Scale for Children*. 5th ed. Pearson; 2014.
11. Wechsler D, Coalson DL, Raiford SE. *WAIS-IV: Wechsler Adult Intelligence Scale*. Pearson; 2008.
12. Roid GH. *Stanford Binet Intelligence Scales*. 5th ed. Riverside Publishing; 2003.
13. Kaufman AS, Kaufman NL. *Kaufman Brief Intelligence Test*. 2nd ed. American Guidance Services; 2004.
14. Elliot CD. *Differential Ability Scales: Introductory and Technical Handbook*. 2nd ed. PsychCorp; 2007.

15. Greene RL. *The MMPI-2: An Interpretive Manual.* Allyn & Bacon; 2000.
16. Millon T, Grossman S, Millon C. *Millon Clinical Multiaxial Inventory-IV (MCMI-IV).* Pearson Assessments; 2015.
17. Siefert CJ, Sinclair SJ, Kehl-Fie KA, et al. An item level psychometric analysis of the personality assessment inventory clinical scales. *Assessment.* 2009;16:373–383.
18. Morey LC. *Personality Assessment Inventory-Adolescent (PAI-A).* Psychological Assessment Resources; 2007.
19. Blais MA, Sinclair SJ. *Spectra: Indices of Psychopathology.* Psychological Assessment Resources; 2018.
20. Blais MA, Sinclair SJ. *Introduction to the Spectra: Indices of Psychopathology: An Assessment Inventory Aligned With the Hierarchical-Dimensional Model of Psychopathology.* Psychological Assessment Resources (PAR); 2020.
21. Krueger RF. The structure of common mental disorders. *Arch Gen Psychiatry.* 1999;56:921–926.
22. Krueger RF, Derringer J, Markon KE, et al. Initial construction of a maladaptive personality trait model and inventory for DSM-5. *Psycholog Med.* 2012;42:1879–1890.
23. Blais MA, Sinclair SJ, Richardson LA, et al. External correlates of the SPECTRA: indices of psychopathology. *Clin Psychol Psychother.* 2021;28(4):929–938.
24. Blais MA, Stein MB, Sinclair SJ, et al. Exploring the *SPECTRA: indices of psychopathology's* (SPECTRA) hierarchical factor structure in a clinical sample. *Pers Individ Diff.* 2021;179 110946.
25. Blais MA, Baity MR. Exploring the psychometric properties and clinical utility of the Modified Mini-Mental State Examination (3MS) in a medical psychiatric sample. *Assessment.* 2005;12:1–7.
26. Exner JR. *The Rorschach: A Comprehensive System, Volume 1: Basic Foundations.* Wiley; 1993.
27. Stein MB, Slavin-Mulford J, Sinclair JS, et al. Exploring the construct validity of the social cognition and object relations scale in a clinical sample. *J Pers Assess.* 2012;94(5):533–540.
28. Bellak L, Bellak SS. *Children's Apperception Test.* 1949
29. Milberg WP, Hebben N, Kaplan E, et al. The Boston process approach to neuropsychological assessment. In: Grant I, Adams KM, eds. *Neuropsychological Assessment and Neuropsychiatric Disorders.* Oxford University Press; 2009:42–65.
30. Mesulam MM. *Principals of Behavioral Neurology.* FA Davis; 1985.
31. Wechsler D. *Wechsler Memory Scale (WMS-III).* Psychological Corporation; 1997.
32. Sheslow D, Adams W. *Wide Range Assessment of Memory and Learning.* 3rd ed. NCS Pearson, Inc; 2021.
33. Reitan RM. *Trail Making Test: Manual for Administration and Scoring.* Neuropsychology Laboratory; 1992.
34. Trenerry MR, Crosson B, DeBoe J, et al. *Visual Search and Attention Task.* Psychological Assessment Resources; 1990.
35. Conners KC. *Conners Continuous Performance Test.* 3rd ed. Multi-Health Systems; 2014.
36. Conners KC. *Conners' Kiddie Continuous Performance Test.* Multi-Health Systems; 2001.
37. Gronwall DM. Paced auditory serial addition task: a measure of recovery from concussion. *Percept Motor Skills.* 1997;44:367–373.
38. Schretlen D. *Brief Test of Attention Professional Manual.* Psychological Assessment Resources; 1997.
39. Golden CJ, Freshwater SM. *Stroop Color and Word Test: A Manual for Clinical and Experimental Uses.* Stoelting; 2002.
40. Cristofori I, Cohen-Zimerman S, Grafman J. Executive functions. *Handb Clin Neurol.* 2019;163:197–219. https://doi.org/10.1016/B978-0-12-804281-6.00011-2. PMID: 31590731.
41. Ducharme S, Dols A, Laforce R, et al. Recommendations to distinguish behavioural variant frontotemporal dementia from psychiatric disorders. *Brain.* 2020 Jun 1;143(6):1632–1650. https://doi.org/10.1093/brain/awaa018. Erratum in: Brain. 2020 Jul 1;143(7):e62.
42. Biederman J, Petty CR, Fried R, et al. Discordance between psychometric testing and questionnaire-based definitions of executive function deficits in individuals with ADHD. *J Atten Disord.* 2008 Jul;12(1):92–102.
43. Benton AL, Hamsher K, Rey GL, et al. *Multilingual Aphasia Examination.* 3rd ed. AJA Associates; 1994.
44. Delis DC, Kaplan E, Kramer JH. *Delis-Kaplan Executive Function System: Technical Manual.* Harcourt Assessment Company; 2001.
45. Heaton RK. *A Manual for the Wisconsin Card Sorting Test.* Western Psychological Services; 1981.
46. Meyers JE, Meyers KR. Rey Complex Figure Test and Recognition Trial: Professional Manual. Psychological Assessment Resource; 1995.
47. Culbertson WC, Zillmer EA. *The Tower of London, Drexel University, Research Version: Examiner's Manual.* Multi-Health Systems; 1999.
48. Delis DC, Kramer JH, Kaplan E, et al. *California Verbal Learning Test-Children's Version (CVLT-C).* The Psychological Corporation; 1994.
49. Delis DC, Kramer JH, Kaplan E, et al. *CVLT-3: California Verbal Learning Test-3.* 3rd ed. Psychological Corporation; 2000.
50. Halstead WC. *Brain and Intelligence: A Quantitative Study of the Frontal Lobes.* University of Chicago Press; 1947.
51. Bechara A. *Iowa Gambling Task Professional Manual.* Psychological Assessment Resources, Inc; 2007.
52. Grace J, Malloy PF. *Frontal Systems Behavior Scale. Professional Manual.* Psychological Assessment Resources; 2001.
53. Gioia GA, Isquith PK, Guy SC, et al. *Behavior Rating Inventory of Executive Function®, Second Edition (BRIEF®2).* PAR Inc; 2015.
54. Wechsler D. *Wechsler Memory Scale (WMS-IV).* Pearson; 2009.
55. Trenerry MR, Crosson B, DeBoe J, et al. *Stroop Neurological Screening Test.* Psychological Assessment Resources; 1989.
56. Stern RA, Singer EA, Duke LM, et al. The Boston qualitative scoring system for the Rey-Osterrieth complex figure: description and interrater reliability. *Clin Neuropsychol.* 1994;8(3):309–322.
57. Culbertson WC, Zillmer EA. *The Tower of London, Drexel University, Research Version: Examiner's Manual.* Multi-Health Systems; 1999.
58. Tulving E, Markowitsch HJ. Episodic and declarative memory: role of the hippocampus. *Hippocampus.* 1984;8:204–1998.
59. Schmidt M. *Rey Auditory Verbal Learning Test: A Handbook.* Western Psychological Services; 1996.

60. Sherman EMS, Brooks BL. *Child and Adolescent Memory Profile.* Psychological Assessment Resources; 2015.

61. Benedict RH. *Brief Visuospatial Memory Test–Revised: Professional Manual.* Psychological Assessment Resources; 1997.

62. Gontkovsky ST, Vickery CD, Beatty WW. Construct validity of the 7/24 spatial recall test. *Appl. Neuropsychol.* 2004;11:75–84.

63. O'Connor MG, Sieggreen MA, Bachna K, et al. Long-term retention of transient news events. *J Int Neuropsycholog Soc: JINS.* 2000;6(1):44–51.

64. Kopelman MD. The Autobiographical Memory Interview (AMI) in organic and psychogenic amnesia. *Memory.* 1994;2:211–235.

65. Blonder LX, Bowers D, Heilman KM. The role of the right hemisphere in emotional communication. *Brain.* 1991 Jun;114(Pt 3):1115–1127. Erratum in: Brain 1992 Apr;115(Pt 2): 645. PMID: 2065243.

66. Dunn DM, Dunn LM. *Peabody Picture Vocabulary Test: Manual.* Pearson; 2007.

67. Martin N, Brownell R. *Expressive One-Word Picture Vocabulary Test.* 4th ed. Academic Therapy Publications; 2011.

68. Wiig EH, Semel E, Secord WA. *Clinical Evaluation of Language Fundamentals (CELF-5).* 5th ed. Pearson; 2013.

69. Goodglass H, Kaplan E, Barresi B. *Boston Diagnostic Aphasia Examination.* 3rd ed. Lippincott Williams & Wilkins; 2001.

70. Korkman M, Kirk U, Kemp S. *NEPSY-II.* The Psychological Corporation; 2007.

71. Kay J, Lesser R, Coltheart M. *Psycholinguistic Assessments of Language Processing in Aphasia (PALPA).* Erlbaum; 1992.

72. Kaplan E, Goodglass H, Weintraub S. *Boston Naming Test.* Pro-ed; 2001.

73. NCS Pearson *Wechsler Individual Achievement Test.* 4th ed. NCS Pearson; 2020.

74. Hammill DD, Larsen SC. *Test of Written Language.* 4th ed. Pro-Ed; 2009.

75. Pearson NC. *Advanced Clinical Solutions for WAIS-IV and WMS-IV: Administration and Scoring Manual.* The Psychological Corporation; 2009.

76. Woodcock RW, McGrew KS, Mather N. *Woodcock-Johnson III Tests of Achievement.* Riverside Publishing; 2001.

77. Kaufman AS, Kaufman NL, Breaux K. *Technical & Interpretive Manual: Kaufman Test of Educational Achievement.* 3rd ed. NCS Pearson; 2014.

78. Torgesen JK, Wagner RK, Rashotte CA. *Test of Word Reading Efficiency.* 2nd ed. Pro-Ed; 2012.

79. Wiederholt JL, Bryant BR. *Gray Oral Reading Test: Examiner's Manual.* 5th ed. Pro-Ed; 2012.

80. Mishkin M, Ungerleider LG, Macko KA. Object vision and spatial vision: two cortical pathways. *Trends Neurosci.* 1983;6:414–417. https://doi.org/10.1016/0166-2236(83)90190-X.

81. Gazzaniga M. Forty-five years of split-brain research and still going strong. *Nat Rev Neurosci.* 2005;6:653–659.

82. Hooper HE. *Hooper Visual Organization Test.* Western Psychological Services; 1983.

83. Benton AL, Sivan AB, Hamsher KDS, et al. Facial Recognition: Stimulus and Multiple-Choice Pictures. Contribution to Neuropychological Assessment. Oxford University Press; 1983:30–40.

84. Colarusso R, Hammill D. *Motor-Free Visual Perception Test-4 (MVPT-4).* 4th ed. Academic Therapy Publications; 2015.

85. Warrington EK, James M. *The Visual Object and Space Perception Battery.* Thames Valley Test Company; 1991.

86. Benton AL, Varney N, Hamsher K. Visuospatial judgment: a clinical test. *Arch Neurol.* 1978;35:364–367.

87. Beery KE, Buktenica NA, Beery NA. *The Beery–Buktenica Developmental Test of Visual–Motor Integration: Administration, Scoring, and Teaching Manual.* 6th ed. Pearson; 2010.

88. Kløve H. *Grooved Pegboard.* Lafayette Instruments; 1963.

89. Folstein MF, Folstein SE, McHugh PR. "Mini-mental state": a practical method for grading the cognitive state of patients for the clinician. *J Psychiatr Res.* 1975;12(3):189–198.

90. Nasreddine ZS, Phillips NA, Bédirian V, et al. *Montreal Cognitive Assessment (MoCA).* APA PsycTests; 2005.

91. Randolph C. *Repeatable Battery for the Assessment of Neuropsychological Status (RBANS): Update.* Psychological Corporation; 2012.

92. Hsieh S, Schubert S, Hoon C, et al. Validation of the Addenbrooke's Cognitive Examination III in frontotemporal dementia and Alzheimer's disease. *Dement Geriatr Cogn Disord.* 2013;36:242–250.

93. Zarrella GV, Kay CD, Gettens K, et al. Addenbrooke's Cognitive Examination–Third Edition predicts neuropsychological test performance. *J Neuropsychiatry Clin Neurosci.* 2023;35(2): 178–183.

94. Jurica PJ, Mattis S, Leitten CL. *Dementia Rating Scale-2: DRS-2.* Psychological Assessment Resources; 2001.

95. Heilman KM, Bowers D, Valenstein E. Emotional disorders associated with neurological disease. In: Heilman KM, Valenstein E, eds. *Clinical Neuropsychology.* 3rd ed. Oxford University Press; 1993.

96. Keefe RS. The contribution of neuropsychology to psychiatry. *Am J Psychiatry.* 1995;152(1):6–15.

97. Harvey PD, Strassnig M. Predicting the severity of everyday functional disability in people with schizophrenia: cognitive deficits, functional capacity, symptoms, and health status. *World J Psychiatry.* 2012;11(2):73–79.

7

DIAGNOSTIC RATING SCALES, PROCEDURES, AND LABORATORY TESTS

FELICIA A. SMITH, MD ■ DAVID MISCHOULON, MD, PHD ■ JOSHUA L. ROFFMAN, MD, MMSC ■ CHARLOTTE S. HOGAN, MD ■ JANET C. SHERMAN, PHD ■ MAURIZIO FAVA, MD ■ THEODORE A. STERN, MD

OVERVIEW

Unlike other medical specialties, psychiatry relies largely on patient interviews and observation for diagnosis and treatment monitoring. Without well-established physical or biomarker findings in psychiatry, the mental status examination (MSE) represents our primary diagnostic instrument. The MSE provides a framework to collect information about affective, behavioral, and cognitive symptoms of psychiatric disorders and provides enough detail to categorize symptom clusters into recognized clinical syndromes and to initiate appropriate treatment.

However, the MSE alone is often insufficient to collect a complete inventory of symptoms or to yield a unifying diagnosis. For example, if a psychotic patient has symptoms of avolition, flat affect, and social withdrawal, it might be difficult to determine whether this reflects negative symptoms, co-morbid depression, or medication-induced akinesia. Performing a full MSE may also identify fewer patients compared to the use of an appropriate screening instrument.[1] Finally, MSEs are too subjective for use in research studies, in which multiple clinicians may be assessing subjects; without an objective, reliable diagnostic tool, subjects may be inadequately or incorrectly categorized, generating results that are difficult to interpret and generalize. By using diagnostic rating scales, clinicians can obtain more objective, and often quantifiable, information about symptoms. Rating scales may serve as an adjunct to the diagnostic interview, or as stand-alone measures

(as in research or screening milieus). The psychiatric diagnostic rating instruments reviewed here are versatile and varied, and can aid in symptom assessment, creation of a differential diagnosis, treatment planning, and treatment monitoring. Information is also provided on how to acquire copies of the rating scales discussed in this chapter.

GENERAL CONSIDERATIONS IN THE SELECTION OF DIAGNOSTIC RATING SCALES

Before describing the various rating scales in detail, several factors important to evaluating rating scale design and implementation will be considered (Table 7.1).

Reliability refers to the extent to which an instrument produces consistent measurements across different raters and testing milieus. Such a scale is said to have good *inter-rater reliability*, that is, several observers reach similar conclusions based on the same information.

The *validity* of a rating scale concerns whether it correctly detects the underlying condition. A scale that correctly rules out a disorder is said to produce a *true negative* result, and one that correctly rules in a disorder produces a *true positive* result (Table 7.1). When a false positive occurs, we call this a *type 1 error*, and the patient may have been incorrectly diagnosed. Conversely, a false negative represents a *type 2 error* in which the clinician misses the correct diagnosis. The

TABLE 7.1

Factors Used to Evaluate Diagnostic Rating Scales

Reliability	For a given subject, are the results consistent across different evaluators, test conditions, and test times?
Validity	Does the instrument truly measure what it is intended to measure? How well does it compare to the gold standard?
Sensitivity	If the disorder is present, how likely is it that the test is positive?
Specificity	If the disorder is absent, how likely is it that the test is negative?
Positive predictive value	If the test is positive, how likely is it that the disorder is present?
Negative predictive value	If the test is negative, how likely is it that the disorder is absent?
Cost- and time-effectiveness	Does the instrument provide accurate results in a timely and inexpensive way?
Administration	Are ratings determined by the patient or the evaluator? What are the advantages and disadvantages of this approach?
Training requirements	What degree of expertise is required for valid and reliable measurements to occur?

related measures of *sensitivity, specificity, positive predictive value*, and *negative predictive value* (defined in Table 7.1) can provide estimates of a diagnostic rating scale's validity, especially in comparison to "gold standard" tests.

Certain rating scales are freely available, whereas others may be obtained only from the author or publisher at a cost. Briefer instruments require less time to administer, which can be essential if large numbers of patients must be screened, but they may be less sensitive or specific than longer instruments and lead to more diagnostic errors. Some rating scales may be self-administered by the patient, reducing the possibility of observer bias; however, such ratings can be compromised in patients with significant behavioral or cognitive impairments. Alternatively, clinician-administered rating scales tend to be more valid and reliable than self-rated scales, but they also tend to require more time and, in some cases, specialized training for the rater. A final consideration is the cultural and linguistic background of the patient (and the rater): culture-specific conceptions of psychiatric illness can profoundly influence the report and interpretation of specific symptoms as well as the assignment of a diagnosis; moreover, rating scales are not available in all languages. When appropriate, a patient's reading level must also be considered. The relative importance of these factors depends on the specific clinical or research milieu, and each factor must be weighed carefully to guide the selection of an optimal rating instrument.[2]

GENERAL DIAGNOSTIC INSTRUMENTS

The general psychiatric diagnostic instruments, described in this section, can provide a standardized measure of psychopathology across diagnostic categories. These instruments are frequently used in research studies to assess baseline mental health and ensure the clinical homogeneity of both patients and healthy control subjects.

One of the most frequently used general instruments is the Structured Clinical Interview for the *Diagnostic and Statistical Manual of Mental Disorders, Fifth Edition (DSM-5)* Axis I Diagnosis (SCID-5).[3] The SCID-5 is a lengthy, semi-structured survey of psychiatric illness across multiple domains (including sections for an Overview, Mood episodes, Psychotic disorders, Bipolar disorders (BPDs), Substance use disorders (SUDs), Anxiety disorders, OCDs, Eating disorders, Externalizing disorders, and Trauma disorders). An introductory segment uses open-ended questions to assess demographics, as well as medical, psychiatric, and medication use histories. The subsequent modules ask specific questions about diagnostic criteria, taken from the DSM-5, in nine different realms of psychopathology. Within these modules, responses are generally rated as "present," "absent (or subthreshold)," or "inadequate information;" and scores are tallied to determine likely diagnoses. The SCID-5 can take several hours to administer, although, in some instances, raters use only portions of the SCID that are relevant to clinical or research areas of interest. Different versions of the SCID-5 can be used for clinical or research settings, including a version focused on personality disorders.

While the SCID-5 is generally considered user-friendly, its length and associated cost precludes its routine clinical use. A shorter and faster-to-administer (15–30 minutes) general rating instrument is the Mini-International Neuropsychiatric Interview (MINI),[4] another semi-structured interview based on DSM-5 criteria. Questions tend to be more limited with this measure than with the SCID-5 and are answered in a "yes/no" format; however, unlike the SCID-5, the MINI includes a module on antisocial personality disorder and has questions that focus on suicidality.

A third general interview, the Schedules for Clinical Assessment in Neuropsychiatry (SCAN),[5] focuses less on DSM-5 categories and provides a broader assessment of psychosocial function. This instrument includes three sections: (I) Present State Examination (Part I: Demographic information; medical history; somatoform, dissociative, anxiety, mood, eating, alcohol, and substance abuse disorders; Part II: Psychotic and cognitive disorders, insight, functional impairment); (II) Item Group Checklist (Signs and symptoms derived from case records, other providers, and other collateral sources); (III) Clinical History Schedule (Education, personality disorders, social impairment). Like the SCID-5, the SCAN can be time-consuming, and administration requires familiarity with its format. It also does not lend itself to making a DSM-5 diagnosis as linear as the SCID-5 and the MINI.

Two additional general diagnostic scales may be used to track changes in global function over time and in response to treatment. Both are clinician-rated and require only a few moments to complete. The Global Assessment of Functioning Scale[3] consists of a 100-point single-item rating scale, which is included in Axis V of the DSM-5 diagnosis. Higher scores indicate better overall psychosocial function. Ratings can be made for the current function and the highest function in the past year. The Clinical Global Impressions (CGI) Scale[6] consists of two scores, one for the severity of illness (CGI-S), and the other for the degree of improvement following treatment (CGI-I). For the CGI-S, scores range from 1 (normal) to 7 (severe illness); for the CGI-I, they range from 1 (very much improved) to 7 (very much worse). A related score, the CGI Efficacy Index, reflects a composite index of both the therapeutic and adverse effects of treatment. Here,

scores range from 0 (marked improvement and no side effects) to 4 (unchanged or worse and side effects outweigh therapeutic effects).

General diagnostic instruments can be useful screening tools for both patients and research subjects. However, they do not permit detailed investigations of affective, behavioral, or cognitive symptoms, and often do not provide diagnostic clarification for individuals with atypical or complex presentations. Diagnostic rating scales that focus on specific domains (such as mood, psychotic, or anxiety symptoms) can be of greater value in these situations. The following section discusses rating scales that are tailored to explore specific clusters of psychiatric illness and medication-related side effects.

SCALES FOR MOOD DISORDERS

The cardinal features of major depressive disorder (MDD) can mimic several distinct neuropsychiatric illnesses, including (but not limited to) dysthymia, anxiety, bipolar-spectrum disorders, substance abuse, personality disorders, dementia, and movement disorders. Moreover, most antidepressant medications and psychotherapies take effect gradually, which makes daily or even weekly progress difficult to gauge subjectively. Diagnostic rating scales can therefore be invaluable in the clarification of the diagnosis and the objective measurement of incremental progress during treatment.

The Hamilton Rating Scale for Depression (HAM-D)[7] is a reliable and valid clinician-administered instrument that is widely used in both clinical and research settings. Its questions focus on the severity of symptoms in the preceding week; as such, the HAM-D is a useful tool for tracking patient progress after the initiation of treatment. The scale exists in several versions, ranging from 6 to 31 items; longer versions include questions about symptoms of atypical depression, psychosis, obsessive-compulsive disorder (OCD), and somatic concerns. Patient answers are scored by the rater from 0 to 2 or 0 to 4 and are tallied to obtain an overall score. Scoring for the 17-item HAM-D-17, which is used frequently in research studies, is summarized in Table 7.2. A decrease of 50% or more in the HAM-D score suggests a positive response to treatment.

The Montgomery-Asberg Depression Rating Scale (MADRS),[8] another clinician-administered instrument, also measures depressive severity, and correlates well with the HAM-D. The MADRS contains 10 items, each reflecting symptom severity from 0 to 6, with a maximum possible score of 60. The MADRS generally has symptoms similar to those of the HAM-D-17 but may be more sensitive to antidepressant-related changes than the HAM-D Scale. It is not as well suited for assessing atypical depression, since it does not examine increased appetite or sleep (see Table 7.2).

The most frequently used self-administered depression rating scale is the Beck Depression Inventory, Second edition (BDI-II).[9] The BDI is a 21-item scale in which patients must rate their symptoms on a scale from 0 to 3; the total score is tallied and interpreted by the clinician (Table 7.2). Like the HAM-D, the BDI may be used as a repeated measure to follow progress during a treatment trial. Although easy to administer, the BDI tends to focus more on cognitive symptoms of depression, and it excludes atypical symptoms (such as weight gain and hypersomnia). The BDI-II replaced four BDI items (weight loss, body image change, somatic preoccupation, and work difficulty) with four new items (agitation, worthlessness, concentration difficulty, and loss of energy). An alternative rating scale, the Inventory of Depressive Symptomatology (IDS),[10] provides more thorough coverage of atypical depression and symptoms of dysthymia. The IDS is available in clinician-rated and self-administered versions and contains 28 or 30 items. Suggested interpretation guidelines are provided in Table 7.2.

The Quick Inventory of Depressive Symptomatology-Self-Report (QIDS-SR)[11] is a 16-item self-rated instrument derived from the IDS, for measuring self-reported changes in symptom severity during antidepressant clinical trials. Each question is rated on a scale of 0 to 3 and the total score is obtained by summing the scores on most of the individual items and by summing the highest scores of three categories (sleep, appetite/weight, and psychomotor activity). The highest possible total score is 27 (see Table 7.2).

Two other self-administered scales, the Zung Self-Rating Depression Scale (Zung SDS)[12] and the Harvard Department of Psychiatry National Depression Screening Day Scale (HANDS),[1] are frequently employed in primary care settings and other screening sessions due to their simplicity and ease of use. The Zung SDS contains 20 items, with 10 items keyed positively and 10 keyed negatively; subjects score each item as present from 1 (or "a little of the time") to 4 (or "most of the time"). To obtain the total score, positively keyed items are reversed and then all the items are summed (Table 7.2). The HANDS has 10 questions about depression symptoms, and it is scored based on the experience of symptoms from 0 (or "none

TABLE 7.2					
Various Depression Scales					
	Not (or Minimally) Depressed	**Mildly Depressed**	**Moderately Depressed**	**Severely Depressed**	**Very Severely Depressed**
17-Item Hamilton Rating Scale for Depression (HAM-D-17)	0–7	8–13	14–18	19–22	≥23
Montgomery-Asberg Depression Rating Scale (MADRS)	0–6	7–19	20–34	≥35	
Beck Depression Inventory (BDI-II)	0–9	10–16	17–29	≥30	
Inventory of Depressive Symptomology (IDS)	0–13	14–25	26–38	39–48	≥49
Quick Inventory of Depressive Symptomatology-Self-Report (QIDS-SR)	0–5	6–10	11–15	16–20	21–27
Zung Self-Rating Depression Scale (Zung SDS)	0–49	50–59	60–69	≥70	
Harvard Department of Psychiatry National Depression Screening Day Scale (HANDS)	0–8 (unlikely)	9–16 (likely)	≥17 (very likely)		

of the time") to 3 (or "all of the time") (Table 7.2). Although the Zung SDS and HANDS take only a few minutes to administer, they are less sensitive to change than the HAM-D and the BDI; like these other scales, the Zung SDS lacks coverage for atypical symptoms of depression.

For assessing the severity of manic symptoms, two clinician-administered scales, the Manic State Rating Scale (MSRS)[13] and the Young Mania Rating Scale (Y-MRS),[14] have both been used extensively on inpatient units; the Y-MRS also correlates well with the length of hospital stay. The MSRS contains 26 items and is rated on a 0 to 5 scale, based on the frequency and intensity of symptoms. Weight is emphasized for symptoms related to elation-grandiosity and paranoia-destructiveness. The Y-MRS consists of 11 items and is scored following a clinical interview. Four items are given extra emphasis and are scored on a 0 to 8 scale (irritability, speech, thought content, and aggressive behavior); the remaining items are scored on a 0 to 4 scale.

SCALES FOR PSYCHOTIC DISORDERS

During interviews with thought-disordered patients, it can be challenging to cover the spectrum of psychotic symptoms—not only because of their heterogeneity but also because they can be difficult to elicit in impaired or uncooperative individuals. Moreover, antipsychotic medications can predispose patients to movement disorders that are elusive to diagnose; for example, the overlap between negative symptoms and neuroleptic-induced akinesia can be difficult to disentangle during the diagnostic interview. Several diagnostic rating scales have been developed to aid clinicians in categorizing and monitoring psychotic symptoms, as well as movement disorders. Each psychotic symptom scale is administered by a clinician.

The Positive and Negative Syndrome Scale (PANSS)[15] is a 30-item instrument that emphasizes three clusters of symptoms: seven positive symptoms (e.g., hallucinations, delusions, disorganization), seven negative symptoms (e.g., apathy, blunted affect, social withdrawal), and 16 general psychopathology items (including a variety of symptoms, e.g., somatic concerns, anxiety, impulse dyscontrol, psychomotor retardation, mannerisms, posturing). Separate scores are tallied for each of these clusters, and a total PANSS score is calculated by adding the scores of the three subscales. Each item is rated on a scale from 1 (least severe) to 7 (most severe) following a semi-structured interview (the Structured Clinical Interview for Positive and Negative Syndrome Scale, SCI-PANSS). Total positive and negative symptoms scores range from 7 to 49 (50th percentile score ~20), and for general psychopathology from 16 to 112 (50th percentile score ~40).[16] Designed to organize data from a broad range of psychopathology, the PANSS provides an ideal scale for monitoring baseline symptoms and response to antipsychotic medications. However, it can take 30 to 40 minutes to administer and score the PANSS, and examiners must have familiarity with each of the PANSS items.

Several additional instruments are available to assess global psychopathology and positive and negative symptom severity in psychotic patients. The 18-item Brief Psychiatric Rating Scale (BPRS)[17] evaluates a range of positive and negative symptoms, as well as other categories (such as depressive mood, mannerisms and posturing, hostility, and tension). Each item is rated on a 7-point scale following a clinical interview. The BPRS has been used to assess psychotic symptoms in patients with both primary psychotic disorders and secondary psychoses, such as depression with psychotic symptoms. More detailed inventories of positive and negative symptoms are possible with the 30-item Scale for the Assessment of Positive Symptoms (SAPS)[18] and the 20-item Scale for the Assessment of Negative Symptoms (SANS).[19] For each of these instruments, items are rated on a scale of 0 to 5 following a semi-structured clinical interview, such as the Comprehensive Assessment of Symptoms and History. Correlations between SAPS and SANS scores with their counterpart subscales in the PANSS are quite high.[16]

An additional consideration in evaluating negative symptoms is whether they occur as a primary component of the disorder, or because of co-morbid processes, such as depression, drug effects, or positive symptoms. The Schedule for the Deficit Syndrome (SDS)[20] uses four criteria to establish whether negative symptoms are present, enduring, and unrelated to secondary causes. Each of the four criteria must be satisfied for a patient to qualify for the deficit syndrome, as defined by Carpenter and colleagues.[21] These criteria include (1) the presence of at least two out of six negative symptoms; (2) at least two of these symptoms must have been present for at least 12 months; (3) symptoms must be unrelated to secondary causes; and (4) patients must meet DSM criteria for schizophrenia.

Patients who take antipsychotic medications are at increased risk for motor disorders due to chronic dopamine blockade. Several rating scales have been designed to evaluate these motoric side effects, which can include extrapyramidal symptoms (EPS), akathisia, and tardive dyskinesia. Each scale is readily administered at baseline and then at follow-up intervals to track drug-induced movement disorders. The Abnormal Involuntary Movement Scale[22] consists of 10 items that evaluate orofacial movements, limb-truncal dyskinesias, and global severity of motor symptoms on a 5-point scale; additional items rule out contributions of dental problems or dentures. Specific instructions are provided with the scale for asking the patient certain questions or having him or her perform motor maneuvers. Both objective measures of akathisia and subjective distress related to restlessness are assessed by the Barnes Akathisia Rating Scale,[23] which also comes with brief instructions for proper rating. Of note, this scale can also be of use for patients taking serotonin reuptake inhibitors, as such patients may also be at risk for akathisia. Finally, the Simpson-Angus Extrapyramidal Side Effects Scale (EPS)[24] contains 10 items for rating Parkinsonian and related motor symptoms. Each item is rated from 0 to 4; the score is summed and divided by 10. A score of 0.3 was cited by the authors as the upper limit of normal.

SCALES FOR ANXIETY DISORDERS

Because many patients have anxiety symptoms that do not meet the DSM-5 threshold for any formal diagnosis, rating scales can also help characterize and follow anxiety symptoms in these individuals.

The Hamilton Anxiety Rating Scale (HAM-A)[25] is the most used instrument for the evaluation of anxiety symptoms. The clinician-implemented HAM-A contains 14 items, with specific symptoms rated on a scale from 0 (no symptoms) to 4 (severe, grossly disabling symptoms). Covered areas include somatic complaints (cardiovascular, respiratory, gastrointestinal [GI],

genitourinary, and muscular), cognitive symptoms, fear, insomnia, anxious mood, and behavior during the interview. Administration typically requires 15 to 30 minutes. Clinically significant anxiety is associated with total scores of 14 or greater.

A frequently used self-rated anxiety scale is the Beck Anxiety Inventory (BAI).[26] In this 21-item questionnaire, patients rate somatic and affective symptoms of anxiety on a four-point Likert scale (0 = "not at all," 3 = "severely: I could barely stand it"). Guidelines for interpreting the total severity score are as follows: normal (0–9), mild to moderate (10–18), moderate to severe (19–29), and severe (>29). The BAI is brief and easy to administer, but like the HAM-A, it does not identify specific anxiety diagnoses or distinguish primary anxiety from co-morbid psychiatric conditions.

Other anxiety rating scales are geared toward specific clinical syndromes. For example, the Yale-Brown Obsessive-Compulsive Scale[27,28] is a clinician-administered semi-structured interview designed to measure the severity of obsessive-compulsive symptoms. The interview is preceded by an optional checklist of 64 specific obsessive and compulsive symptoms. Following the interview, the examiner rates both obsessive and compulsive subscales, with a score of 0 corresponding to no symptoms and 4 corresponding to extreme symptoms in the following five domains: (1) amount of time occupied by symptoms, (2) interference with normal function, (3) subjective distress caused by symptoms, (4) degree that the patient resists symptoms, and (5) degree to which the patient can control symptoms. Total scores average 25 in patients with OCD, compared with less than 8 in healthy individuals.

The Brief Social Phobia Scale (BSPS)[29] consists of clinician-administered ratings in 11 domains related to social phobia covering two general categories: (1) Avoidance and Fear (public speaking, talking to authority figures, talking to strangers, being embarrassed or humiliated, being criticized, social gatherings, and doing something while watched) and (2) Physiological Symptoms (blushing, trembling, palpitations, and sweating). The severity of each symptom is rated from 0 (none) to 4 (extreme), generating three subscale scores: Fear (BSPS-F), Avoidance (BSPS-A), and Physiological (BSPS-P). Total Avoidance and Fear scores range from 0 to 28. Physiological scores range from 0 to 16. These scores are summed in the

Total Score (BSPS-T). A total score greater than 20 is considered clinically significant. Post-traumatic stress–associated symptoms can be measured with the Clinician Administered PTSD Scale (CAPS),[30] which is closely matched to DSM-5 criteria. The CAPS contains 17 items assessed by the clinician during a diagnostic interview; each item is rated for frequency, from 0 (never experienced) to 4 (experienced daily), and for intensity, from 0 (none) to 4 (extreme). The items follow each of the four DSM-5 diagnostic criteria for post-traumatic stress disorder (PTSD), as well as several extra items related to frequently encountered co-morbid symptoms (such as survivor guilt and depression). Scores are tallied within all DSM-5 diagnostic criteria to determine whether the patient qualifies for a PTSD diagnosis.

SCALES FOR SUBSTANCE USE DISORDERS

SUDs are highly co-morbid with other Axis I conditions and can seriously complicate the identification, clinical course, and treatment of other psychiatric disorders. Effective screening for substance abuse or dependence in all settings in which psychiatric patients are encountered, be it the emergency department, a primary care clinic, an inpatient ward, or a non-clinical setting (such as a screening day event), can be a critical initial step in the treatment of these individuals. Diagnostic rating scales can offer a rapid and effective screen for SUDs, as well as assist with treatment planning and follow-up.

The CAGE questionnaire[31] is used ubiquitously to screen for alcohol abuse and dependence. Consisting of four "yes/no" questions (organized by a mnemonic acronym) about alcohol consumption patterns and their psychosocial consequences, the CAGE takes only a few moments to administer and includes four questions: C: Have you ever felt you should *cut down* on your drinking? A: Have people *annoyed* you by criticizing your drinking? G: Have you ever felt bad or *guilty* about your drinking? E: Have you ever had a drink first thing in the morning ("*eye-opener*") to steady your nerves or to get rid of a hangover? Positive answers to at least two questions signify a positive screen and the necessity of a more extended work-up; sensitivity of a positive screen has been measured at 0.78 to 0.81, and specificity at 0.76 to 0.96.[32] Further, the psychometric measures for the CAGE are significantly better than are single questions (e.g., "How much do you drink?)" or laboratory values (such as Breathalyzer or LFTs).

A slightly longer, self-administered instrument called the Michigan Alcoholism Screening Test (MAST)[33] contains 25 "yes/no" items concerning alcohol use. The MAST also includes questions about tolerance and withdrawal, and thus it can point out longer-term problems associated with chronic alcohol abuse. While "no" answers are scored as 0, "yes" answers are weighted from 1 to 5 based on the severity of the queried symptom. Interpretation of the total MAST score is as follows: no alcoholism (0–2), possible alcoholism (3–5), and probable alcoholism (≥6).

A readily administered screen for drug abuse or dependence, the Drug Abuse Screening Test (DAST)[34] is a self-rated survey of 28 "yes/no" questions. As with the MAST, the DAST includes questions about tolerance and withdrawal and can therefore identify chronic drug-use problems. A briefer, 20-item version of the DAST is also available and has psychometric properties that are nearly identical to the longer version; however, each takes only a few minutes to administer and score. A total score on the 28-item DAST of ≥5 is consistent with a probable SUD.

Smoking among psychiatric patients represents a concern not only because it places them at substantially higher risk for developing life-threatening medical problems but also because it can interact with hepatic enzymes and significantly alter the metabolism of psychotropic drugs. The Fagerstrom Test for Nicotine Dependence (FTND)[35] is a six-item, self-rated scale that provides an overview of smoking habits and the likelihood of nicotine dependence. The FTND asks about the number of cigarettes smoked per day, whether the patient smokes more in the morning, how early they have their first cigarette of the day, which cigarette is the hardest to give up, whether it is difficult to refrain from smoking in forbidden places, and whether the patient smokes when very ill. Questions are scored from 0 to 3 or from 0 to 1, with higher scores indicating greater severity. Although there is no recommended cutoff score for dependence, the average score in randomly selected smokers is 4 to 4.5.[32]

SCALES FOR COGNITIVE DISORDERS

Diagnostic rating scales can help identify primary cognitive disorders (e.g., dementia) and screen out medical or neurological causes of psychiatric symptoms (e.g., stroke-related depression). A positive screen on the cognitive tests described in this section often indicates the need for a more extensive work-up, which may include laboratory tests, brain imaging, or formal neurocognitive testing. As with formal cognitive batteries (which are described in detail in Chapter 6), it is important to keep in mind that the level of intellectual functioning, years of education, native language, and literacy can greatly influence performance on screening tests that assess cognition, and these factors should be carefully considered when interpreting the results.

Useful as both a baseline screening tool and an instrument to track changes in cognition over time, the clinician-administered Mini-Mental State Exam (MMSE)[36] is one of the most widely used rating scales in psychiatry. The MMSE provides information on function across several domains: orientation to place and time, registration and recall, attention, concentration, language, and visual construction. It consists of 11 tasks, each of which is rated and summed to determine the total MMSE score (Table 7.3). A score of 24 (of a possible 30) or lower is widely considered to be indicative of possible dementia; however, in early Alzheimer disease (AD), patients can still perform comparably to unaffected individuals. A second limitation of the MMSE is that it does not include a test of executive function, and thus might fail to detect frontal lobe pathology in an individual with otherwise intact brain function.

The Montreal Cognitive Assessment (MoCA)[37] is a rapid screening instrument for mild cognitive dysfunction. It assesses several cognitive domains: attention and concentration, executive function, memory, language, visuo-constructional skills, conceptual thinking, calculations, and orientation. It can be administered in about 10 minutes (Table 7.3). The Clock-Drawing Test[38] found in the MoCA provides an excellent screen of executive function and can be a useful adjunct to the MMSE. In the test, patients are asked to draw a clock, including placing the numbers and drawing the hands to show a specified time. Fig. 7.1 illustrates the clock drawn by a patient with a frontal lobe lesion; the patient was asked to indicate the time "10 to 2." Note how the numbers are drawn outside the circle (which was provided by the examiner in this case) and are clustered rather than evenly spaced, indicating poor planning. The hands are joined near the top of the clock, near the numbers 10 and 2, instead of at the center, indicating that the patient was stimulus-bound to these numbers. The Clock-Drawing Test can also detect neglect syndromes in patients with parietal lobe lesions; in these individuals, all the numbers may be clustered together on the right side of the circle, with the left side neglected.

The clinician-administered Mattis Dementia Rating Scale (DRS)[39] is a longer, but often more prognostically valid instrument, for dementia screening and follow-up. The DRS covers five cognitive domains (listed in Table 7.3), taking 30 to 40 minutes to complete. Within each domain, the most difficult items are presented first. If individuals successfully perform the difficult items, many of the remaining items in the section are skipped and scored as correct, leading to a briefer administration time. A cutoff score of 129 or 130 (of 143 points) has been associated with 97% sensitivity and 99% specificity in diagnosing AD in a large cohort of patients with dementia and healthy control subjects. Repeated measures of the DRS have been able to predict the rate of cognitive decline in AD; further, performance deficits in specific domains have been significantly correlated with localized brain pathology. The DRS may also have some utility in differentiating AD from other causes of dementia, including Parkinson disease, progressive supranuclear palsy, and Huntington disease.

The Massachusetts General Hospital Cognitive and Physical Functioning Questionnaire[40] is a self-administered instrument with 7 items covering various cognitive symptoms (motivation, wakefulness, energy, focus, memory, word-finding, and mental acuity). Items are graded on an ordinal scale (1 = greater than normal, 2 = normal, 3 = minimally diminished, 4 = moderately diminished, 5 = markedly diminished, and 6 = totally absent). Clinicians can use the total score as an overall measure of severity. There are not yet validated cutoff points for total severity scores, as there are for some of the other instruments reviewed, but this is currently under development. Suggested

TABLE 7.3
Mini-Mental State Exam (MMSE), Montreal Cognitive Assessment (MoCA), and Dementia Rating Scale (DRS)

MMSE	MoCA	DRS
Orientation to state, country, town, building, floor (maximum 5 points)	Alternating trail making	Attention: forward and backward digit span, one- and two-step commands, visual search, word list, matching designs; score range 0–37
Orientation to year, season, month, day of week, date (maximum 5 points)	Visuo-constructional skills (cube)	Initiation and perseveration: verbal fluency, repetition, alternating movements, drawing alternating designs; score range 0–37
Registration of three words (maximum 3 points)	Visuo-constructional skills (clock)	Construction: copying simple geometric figures; score range 0–6
Recall of three words after 5 minutes (maximum 3 points)	Naming: identifying animals in figures	Conceptualization: identifying conceptual and physical similarities among items, simple inductive reasoning, creating a sentence; score range 0–39
Serial 7's or spelling "world" backward (maximum 5 points)	Memory: recall of 5 words	Memory: delayed recall of sentences, orientation, remote memory, immediate recognition of words and figures; score range 0–25
Naming two items (maximum 2 points)	Attention: forward and backward digit span, vigilance, serial 7's	
Understanding a sentence (maximum 1 point)	Sentence repetition	
Writing a sentence (maximum 1 point)	Verbal fluency: give words starting with a particular letter of the alphabet	
Repeating a phrase ("No ifs, ands, or buts") (maximum 1 point)	Abstraction: explain what two particular words have in common	
Following a three-step command (maximum 3 points)	Delayed recall: repeat the 5 previous words from the recall test	
Copying a design (maximum 1 point)	Orientation: year, month, exact date, and day of the week; place and city	
Scoring: range 0 to 30.	Scoring: sum all subscores. Add one point for an individual who has 12 years or fewer of formal education, for a possible maximum of 30 points. A final total score of 26 and above is considered normal.	Scoring: range 0–144

interpretations of total function scores are as follows: greater than normal (7), normal (8–14), minimally diminished (15–21), moderately diminished (22–28), markedly diminished (29–35), and absent (36–32). This instrument is used primarily in research settings.

Conclusion

In this chapter, the importance of global and disorder-specific diagnostic rating scales in psychiatry has been described. The indications, format, and utility of some commonly used diagnostic instruments

were presented, and some practical considerations surrounding their use were discussed. No diagnostic rating scale can replace a thorough interview, a carefully considered differential diagnosis, and an individualized treatment plan in psychiatry. However, rating scales can fine-tune each of these components by providing focused information in a time- and cost-efficient manner, by revealing subtle elements of psychopathology that have important treatment implications, and by supplying an objective and often sensitive means of tracking clinical changes over time. Diagnostic rating

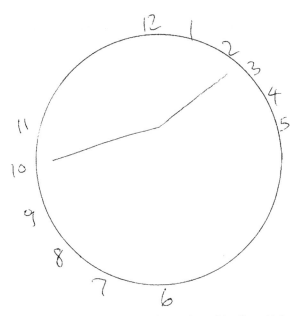

Fig. 7.1 ■ Clock-Drawing Test in a patient with a frontal lobe lesion. Draw "10 to 2."

scales also provide standardized measures that ensure the integrity and homogeneity of subject cohorts in clinical investigations, improving the reliability and validity of psychiatric research studies. Thus, regardless of the setting in which they are used, diagnostic rating scales can enhance the precision of psychiatric assessment.

LABORATORY TESTS

Although primary diagnoses in psychiatry are based on clinical phenomenology, physical examination, and laboratory studies are often important adjuncts in working through a thorough differential diagnosis for psychiatric symptoms.[41,42] Consideration should be given to dysfunction in multiple organ systems, toxins, malnutrition, infections, vascular abnormalities, neoplasm, and other intracranial problems (Table 7.4 organizes many of these using the mnemonic VICTIMS DIE). Certain presentations are especially suggestive of a non-psychiatric cause, including onset after the age of 40 years, history of chronic medical illness, or a precipitous course. Laboratory tests are also important for following serum levels of certain psychiatric medications and for surveillance for treatment-related side

TABLE 7.4	
Organic Causes for Psychiatric Symptoms, Recalled by the Mnemonic "VICTIMS DIE"	
Vascular	Multi-infarct dementia
	Other stroke syndromes
	Hypertensive encephalopathy
	Vasculitis
Infectious	Urinary tract infection and urosepsis
	Acquired immunodeficiency syndrome
	Brain abscess
	Meningitis
	Encephalitis
	Neurosyphilis
	Tuberculosis
	Prion disease
Cancer	Central nervous system tumors (primary or metastatic)
	Endocrine tumors
	Pancreatic cancer
	Paraneoplastic syndromes
Trauma	Intracranial hemorrhage
	Traumatic brain injury
Intoxication/ withdrawal	Alcohol or other drugs
	Environmental toxins
	Psychiatric or other medications (side effects or toxic levels)
Metabolic/ nutritional	Hypoxemia
	Hyper/hyponatremia
	Hypoglycemia
	Ketoacidosis
	Uremic encephalopathy
	Hyper/hypothyroidism
	Parathyroid dysfunction
	Adrenal hypoplasia (Cushing syndrome)
	Hepatic failure
	Wilson disease
	Acute intermittent porphyria
	Pheochromocytoma
	Vitamin B_{12} deficiency
	Thiamine deficiency (Wernicke-Korsakoff syndrome)
	Niacin deficiency (pellagra)
Structural	Normal pressure hydrocephalus
Degenerative	Alzheimer disease
	Parkinson disease
	Huntington disease
	Pick disease
Immune (autoimmune)	Systemic lupus erythematosus
	Rheumatoid arthritis
	Sjögren syndrome
Epilepsy	Partial complex seizures/temporal lobe epilepsy
	Postictal or interictal states

effects. The following sections describe routine screening tests as well as specific serum, urine, cerebrospinal fluid (CSF), and other studies that are considered in the determination of the differential diagnosis and treatment monitoring. The use of electroencephalograms (EEGs) and neuroimaging studies is also described later in this chapter vis-à-vis diagnosis of neuropsychiatric conditions.

Routine Screening

The decision to order a screening test should account for its ease of administration, the likelihood of an abnormal result, and the clinical implications of abnormal results (including management). Although no clear consensus exists about which tests to order in a routine screening battery for new-onset psychiatric symptoms, in practice routine screening tests include the complete blood cell count (CBC); serum chemistries including electrolytes, glucose, calcium, magnesium, phosphate, and tests of renal function; erythrocyte sedimentation rate; and levels of vitamin B_{12}, folate, thyroid-stimulating hormone, and rapid plasma reagin (RPR). Often urine and serum toxicology screens, liver function tests (LFTs), human immunodeficiency virus, and urinalysis are also added.

Psychosis and Delirium

Evaluation of new-onset psychosis or delirium must include a full medical and neurologic work-up; potential causes for mental status changes include infections (both systemic and in the central nervous system [CNS]), CNS lesions (e.g., stroke, traumatic bleed, or tumors), metabolic abnormalities, medication effects, intoxication or states of withdrawal, states of low perfusion or low oxygenation, seizures, and autoimmune illnesses. Given the potential morbidity (if not mortality) associated with many of these conditions, prompt diagnosis is essential (Table 7.5 organizes the life-threatening causes of delirium, using the mnemonic WWHHHHIMPS).[43] If an organic causal agent is not established by virtue of the history, physical examination, and screening studies listed previously, additional testing should include an EEG and neuroimaging. Blood or urine cultures should be sent if there is suspicion of a systemic infectious process. A lumbar puncture is indicated (once an intracranial lesion and elevated intracranial pressure have been ruled out) if

TABLE 7.5
Life-Threatening Causes of Delirium, Recalled by the Mnemonic "WWHHHHIMPS"

Wernicke encephalopathy
Withdrawal
Hypertensive crisis
Hypoperfusion/hypoxia of the brain
Hypoglycemia
Hyper/hypothermia
Intracranial process/infection
Metabolic/meningitis
Poisons
Status epilepticus

patients present with fever, headache, photophobia, or meningeal symptoms; in addition to sending routine CSF studies (e.g., opening pressure, appearance, Gram stain, culture, cell counts, and levels of protein and glucose), depending on the clinical circumstances, consideration should also be given to specialized markers (e.g., antigens for *Cryptococcus*, herpes simplex virus, Lyme disease, and other rare forms of encephalitis, including paraneoplastic syndromes, autoimmune encephalitides (see below), and prion diseases; acid-fast staining; and cytological examination for leptomeningeal metastases). With appropriate clinical suspicion, other blood tests include those for heavy metals (e.g., lead, mercury, aluminum, arsenic, copper), ceruloplasmin (which is decreased in Wilson disease), and bromides.

Autoimmune encephalitis is a severe inflammatory neurologic disorder that results in encephalopathy and significant neuropsychiatric symptoms and merits special mention here due to its increasing prevalence. The diagnosis should be suspected in cases with a subacute onset (less than 3 months) of neuropsychiatric symptoms, especially when paired with new neurologic findings or seizures. Work-up should include CSF studies (pleocytosis is consistent with the diagnosis) as well as magnetic resonance imaging (MRI) of the brain (a typical finding would be bilateral brain abnormalities restricted to the medial temporal lobes) and an EEG. Autoimmune encephalitis can occur without detectable auto-antibodies, however, CSF auto-antibody measurements should nevertheless be obtained to identify co-morbidities, tumor association, and prognosis by immunological subgroup.[44]

Patients receiving antipsychotic medications should have a baseline electrocardiogram (ECG) as well as periodic follow-ups to monitor for QTc prolongation. The atypical antipsychotic clozapine causes agranulocytosis in 1% to 2% of patients taking the medication, necessitating weekly CBC testing for the first 6 months. At the initiation of treatment, a patient must have a white blood cell (WBC) count of >3500 cells/mm^3 and an absolute neutrophil count (ANC) >2000 cells/mm^3. If treatment proceeds without interruption (i.e., with laboratory values remaining above these thresholds), CBC testing can be spaced to biweekly testing after 6 months and to monthly after 1 year of treatment. If the WBC or ANC drops significantly (by more than 3000 or 1500 cells/mm^3, respectively), or in the case of mild leukopenia (with a WBC count of 3000–3500 cells/mm^3) or granulocytopenia (with an ANC of 1500–2000 cells/mm^3), the patient should be monitored closely and have biweekly CBCs checked. In the case of moderate leukopenia (with a WBC count of 2000–3000 cells/mm^3) or granulocytopenia (with an ANC of 1000–1500 cells/mm^3), treatment should be interrupted, CBCs checked daily until abnormalities resolve, and the patient may be re-challenged with clozapine. If the WBC count drops below 2000 cells/mm^3 or the ANC drops below 1000 cells/mm^3, clozapine should be permanently discontinued (i.e., patients should not be re-challenged). In this case, the patient may need inpatient medical hospitalization with daily CBC counts. Physicians and pharmacists who dispense clozapine must report laboratory values through national registries. As an aside, if a patient on clozapine develops signs of myocarditis, treaters should immediately check the WBC count, troponin levels, and an ECG; interrupt treatment with clozapine; and refer the patient for medical evaluation.

Other adverse neuropsychiatric side effects of antipsychotic medications include the risk of seizures, increased prolactin levels, and the onset of neuroleptic malignant syndrome (NMS). A baseline EEG can be helpful in patients taking more than 600 mg/day of clozapine because of an increased incidence of seizures at higher doses. Patients taking typical antipsychotics and risperidone should have prolactin levels checked if they develop galactorrhea, menstrual irregularities, or sexual dysfunction. NMS should be suspected in patients who develop a high fever, delirium, muscle rigidity, and elevated serum creatine phosphokinase levels while taking an antipsychotic medication.

Finally, antipsychotic medications, particularly second-generation antipsychotics, are associated with weight gain and the development of metabolic syndrome. This is particularly concerning in patients with schizophrenia, who are more likely to be overweight or obese than those in the general population. Consensus guidelines recommend baseline and routine monitoring of weight, body mass index, waist circumference, blood pressure, and fasting glucose and lipid profiles.[45]

Mood Disorders and Affective Symptoms

Although depressive symptoms often reflect a primary mood disorder, they may also be associated with numerous medical conditions, including thyroid dysfunction, folate deficiency, Addison disease, rheumatoid arthritis, systemic lupus erythematosus, pancreatic cancer, Parkinson disease, and other neurodegenerative disorders. Clinical suspicion for any of these disorders should drive further laboratory testing, in addition to the routine screening battery listed previously. First-break manic symptoms warrant especially careful medical and neurologic evaluations, and patients who present with these symptoms often receive a laboratory work-up analogous to that described previously for a new-onset psychosis.

Patients who receive pharmacotherapy for mood disorders often require serum levels of the drug being prescribed (and its metabolite) to be checked periodically, as well as baseline and follow-up screening for treatment-induced organ damage. Tricyclic antidepressants (TCAs) can cause cardiac conduction abnormalities, including prolongation of the PR, QRS, or QT intervals; patients taking TCAs should have a baseline ECG to assess for conduction delays, especially if they have a history of pathologic cardiac conditions. TCA levels are useful in several clinical situations, including when the patient reports side effects at low doses, in geriatric or medically ill patients, when there is a question of adherence, or in an urgent clinical situation that requires the rapid achievement of therapeutic levels (e.g., in a severely suicidal patient). Steady-state levels are usually not achieved for 5 days after starting the medication or changing the dose; TCA trough levels should be obtained 9 to 12 hours after the last dose.

No guidelines support routine checking of blood levels once a stable maintenance dose has been achieved, except in the noted circumstances or with changes in the clinical picture.

The selective serotonin reuptake inhibitors (SSRIs), while considered very safe, require precautions in the cases of citalopram and escitalopram, since doses higher than 40 mg/day of citalopram and 20 mg of escitalopram have been associated with QT prolongation.[46] Patients who require high doses of these agents should have a baseline ECG and periodic monitoring to ensure that QT interval prolongation has not developed.

Lithium, a remarkably effective drug for BPD, has a bevy of adverse effects spanning numerous organ systems. Lithium can induce adverse effects on the thyroid gland, the kidney, and the heart, as well as cause a benign elevation of the WBC count; accordingly, baseline and follow-up measures of the CBC with a differential, serum electrolytes, blood urea nitrogen, creatinine, thyroid function tests (TFTs), urinalysis, and ECG should be obtained. Pregnancy tests should also be obtained in females of childbearing years given the risk of teratogenic effects (e.g., Ebstein anomaly) that are associated with use in the first trimester. There is a consensus that therapeutic lithium levels range from 0.4 to 1.2 mEq/L, although certain patients may have idiosyncratic responses outside of this range. Elderly patients with slower rates of drug metabolism and lower volumes of distribution, for example, may experience side effects within this typical range and may require maintenance at lower serum levels with a narrower therapeutic window. Steady-state levels can be checked after 4 to 5 days. Lithium levels can change dramatically during or immediately after pregnancy or if patients are taking thiazide diuretics, non-steroidal anti-inflammatory drugs, angiotensin-converting enzyme inhibitors, angiotensin receptor blockers, or in those who have deteriorating renal function or are dehydrated. Patients on a stable maintenance dose of lithium should have levels checked no less than once every 6 months, along with routine renal and thyroid function testing.

Patients taking carbamazepine or valproic acid for BPD should have baseline and follow-up CBCs, electrolytes, and LFTs, in addition to routine level monitoring, typically every 6 months. In the case of carbamazepine, which can cause agranulocytosis, the CBC should be checked every 2 weeks for the first 2 months of treatment, and then at least once every 3 months thereafter. Given teratogenic effects, these medications are often avoided in females of childbearing age—pregnancy testing should be part of a treatment plan when the risk-benefit analysis results in using these medications.

Anxiety

The medical differential for new-onset anxiety is broad; it includes drug effects, thyroid or parathyroid dysfunction, hypoglycemia, cardiac disease (including myocardial infarction and mitral valve prolapse), respiratory compromise (including asthma, chronic obstructive pulmonary disease, and pulmonary embolism), and alcohol or benzodiazepine withdrawal. Rare causes, such as pheochromocytoma, porphyria, and seizure disorder, should be investigated if suggested by other associated clinical features. Based on this broad differential diagnosis, laboratory work-up may include TFTs, serum glucose or glucose tolerance testing, a chest x-ray examination, pulmonary function tests, a cardiac work-up, porphyrin levels, and an EEG.

Care of the Geriatric Population

Given the increased likelihood of medical conditions that cause psychiatric symptoms in older adults, special attention should be given to non-psychiatric etiologies. Especially common are mental status changes that result from urinary tract infections, anemia, thyroid disease, dementia, and iatrogenic effects from medications. Although the National Institutes of Health Consensus Development Conference identified the history and physical examination as the most important diagnostic tests in elderly psychiatric patients, they also specifically recommended checking a CBC, serum chemistries, TFTs, CBC, vitamin B_{12}, and folate levels. If indicated clinically, additional testing should include neuroimaging, an EEG, and a lumbar puncture. With suspected early dementia, in addition to the DRS (see Rating Scales, discussed earlier), positron emission tomography (PET) may be useful diagnostically.[47]

Substance Abuse

Substance abuse and withdrawal should always be considered in patients with mental status changes.

TABLE 7.6
Serum and Urine Toxicology Screens

Substance	Serum Detection	Urine Detection
Alcohol	1–2 days	1 day
Amphetamine	Variable	1–2 days
Barbiturates	Variable	3 days to 3 weeks
Benzodiazepines	Variable	2–3 days
Cocaine	Hours to 1 day	2–3 days
Codeine, morphine, heroin	Variable	1–2 days
Delta-9-tetrahydrocann abinol (THC)	N/A	~30 days, longer if chronic use
Methadone	15–29 h	2–3 days
Phencyclidine	N/A	8 days
Propoxyphene	8–34 h	1–2 days

N/A, Not applicable.

Substances available for testing in serum and urine are summarized in Table 7.6. Alcohol levels can be quickly assessed using breath analysis (breathalyzer). It is important to remember that serum levels of alcohol do not necessarily correlate with the timing of withdrawal symptoms, especially in patients with chronically high alcohol levels (e.g., withdrawal starts well before the serum alcohol level reaches zero). Patients who present with a history of alcohol abuse should have LFTs and a CBC checked; if macrocytic anemia is present, vitamin B_{12} and folate levels should also be assessed. Chronic liver damage can lead to coagulopathy (as manifested by an elevated prothrombin time [PT] or international normalized ratio) and other manifestations of synthetic failure (e.g., a low albumin level). In the case of cocaine abuse, there should be a low threshold for obtaining an ECG with any cardiac symptom.

Eating Disorders

As part of their medical evaluation, patients presenting with a severe eating disorder should have routine laboratory studies to evaluate electrolyte status and nutritional measures (e.g., an albumin level). Patients who are actively purging can present with metabolic alkalosis (manifested by an elevated bicarbonate level), hypochloremia, and hypokalemia. Serum aldolase levels can be increased in those who abuse ipecac; chronic emesis can also lead to elevated amylase levels. Cholecystokinin levels can be blunted in bulimic patients, relative to controls, following ingestion of a meal. Finally, patients who abuse laxatives chronically may present with hypocalcemia.

Pharmacogenomic Testing

In recent years, research has greatly expanded knowledge of individual genetic variability, particularly as it applies to the metabolism of, and response to, psychotropic medications. A major focus has been on the cytochrome P450 (CYP) system, responsible for the metabolism of many psychotropic agents (summarized in Table 7.7). Commercially available tests, including one US Food and Drug Administration–approved test, permit examination of an individual's CYP polymorphisms through gene chip technology, suggesting patients who may be slow or rapid metabolizers of the substrate drugs.[48] For example, the advent of Deplin (5-methyltetrahydrofolate [5-MTHF]), a prescription form of folate, has stimulated interest in testing for a methylene tetrahydrofolate reductase (MTHFR) polymorphism found in about 10% to 12% of the population. Individuals with the C→T MTHFR polymorphism, particularly in the homozygotic form, cannot convert folic acid normally and may develop deficiencies that could contribute to depression.[49] Because 5-MTHF can cross the blood-brain barrier directly without undergoing the various chemical conversions of the folic acid pathway, individuals with the MTHFR polymorphism could benefit from the addition of 5-MTHF to their medication regimen, both from the standpoint of general health as well as alleviation of depression.[50]

In theory, knowledge gained from these kinds of tests might help clinicians make dosing decisions for patients, potentially facilitating treatment with certain medications with a narrow therapeutic window. Recent guidelines, however, have not supported the clinical use of such tests in treating non-psychotic major depression with SSRIs, for example, because of the relatively high cost and lack of available evidence for clinical benefit.[51] Other pharmacogenomic tests work to predict the clinical response to clozapine, development of agranulocytosis from clozapine, and development of antipsychotic-induced metabolic syndrome, though none is in routine clinical use at this time. Genotype testing for serotonin receptor and

TABLE 7.7

Cytochrome P450 Isoenzymes Active in Metabolizing Commonly Prescribed Psychotropic Medications

CYP1A2	CYP2C9	CYP2C19	CYP2D6	CYP3A3/4/5
Amitriptyline	Fluoxetine	Amitriptyline	Amitriptyline	Alprazolam
Clomipramine	Moclobemide	Citalopram	Amphetamines	Amitriptyline
Clozapine	Ramelteon	Clomipramine	Aripiprazole	Aripiprazole
Duloxetine	Tetrahydrocanna binol (THC)	Clozapine	Atomoxetine	Buspirone
Fluvoxamine		Diazepam	Clozapine	Carbamazepine
Haloperidol		Imipramine	Codeine	Clozapine
Imipramine		Moclobemide	Desipramine	Haloperidol
Methadone		Ramelteon	Dextromethorphan	Imipramine
Mirtazapine		Sertraline	Duloxetine	Lamotrigine
Olanzapine			Fluoxetine	Methadone
Ramelteon			Haloperidol	Midazolam
Tacrine			Hydrocodone	Nefazodone
			Methadone	Oxcarbazepine
			meta-Chlorophenylpiperazine (m-CPP)	Pimozide
			Mianserin	Quetiapine
			Nortriptyline	Risperidone
			Olanzapine	Trazodone
			Oxycodone	Triazolam
			Paliperidone	Zaleplon
			Paroxetine	Zolpidem
			Phenothiazines	Ziprasidone
			Risperidone	
			Sertraline	
			Thioridazine	
			Tricyclics (tricyclic antidepressants)	
			Venlafaxine	

transporter variations is available but not yet clinically proven. Current research focuses heavily on the pharmacogenetics of antidepressants, and the use of peripheral blood-based biomarkers as predictors of clinical response,[52] but no tests for clinical response are yet available outside of the research setting. The concept of personalized prescriptions, or tailoring drugs to an individual's genetic makeup, remains a future goal and research interest for psychiatry, but pharmacogenomic tests have not yet reached routine clinical practice.

Case 1

Mr. B, a 30-year-old molecular biologist, was diagnosed with MDD two years earlier. He had tried several antidepressants, with only a partial response at best. He was currently taking paroxetine (40 mg daily) when he presented to his psychiatrist's office for a regular follow-up visit. At the time, Mr. B was endorsing mildly depressed mood, anhedonia, mild fatigue, diminished concentration, and poor appetite. He was reluctant to have his paroxetine dose increased, because he felt it was already contributing to his daytime fatigue.

During the visit, Mr. B reported that he had recently gone to a commercial lab where they tested people for various enzymatic polymorphisms. Mr. B's profile, which he gave to the psychiatrist, showed that he had a heterozygous C-to-T mutation in the gene for methylene tetrahydrofolate reductase

(MTHFR), an enzyme involved in the interconversion of folate. Mr. B wondered whether he might be deficient in folate and if this could be contributing to his depression.

The psychiatrist ordered a test for folate levels and instructed the patient to return in two weeks. The test results showed folate levels in the low-to-normal range, which is often seen in individuals with this polymorphism. Because folate metabolism is important to many vital cellular functions, the psychiatrist prescribed Deplin (5-MTHF) 15 mg/day as an adjunct to the paroxetine, since a study had shown the benefit of 5-MTHF augmentation in depressed individuals. One month later, Mr. B reported that his depression was considerably improved with the addition of 5-MTHF.

THE ELECTROENCEPHALOGRAM

The EEG employs surface (and sometimes nasopharyngeal) electrodes to measure the low-voltage electric activity of the brain. Used primarily in the evaluation of epilepsy and other neurologic disorders, the EEG is often useful in evaluating organic causes of psychiatric symptoms.

EEG signals are presumed to reflect primarily cortical activity, especially from neurons in the most superficial cortical cell layers. The frequencies of electric activity have been divided into four bands: delta (0–4 Hz), theta (4–8 Hz), alpha (8–12 Hz), and beta (>12 Hz). The awake state is characterized by an alpha predominance. Beta waves emerge during stage 1 sleep (drowsiness); during stage 2, vertex sharp theta and delta waves are observed. Delta waves are seen in stages 3 and 4 of sleep. During rapid eye movement sleep, the EEG will record low-voltage fast waves with ocular movement artifacts. Sleep deprivation, hyperventilation, and photic stimulation can sometimes activate seizure foci. For patients with non-epileptiform EEGs but a residual high suspicion for seizure activity, serial studies, sleep-deprived studies, or long-term monitoring can produce a higher yield. Long-term video monitoring can often help link infrequent clinical events with associated electrical patterns.

EEG patterns associated with neuropsychiatric conditions are summarized in Table 7.8. EEG findings in

TABLE 7.8
EEG Findings Associated With Neuropsychiatric Conditions

Seizure	
■ Generalized	■ Bilateral, symmetric, synchronous, paroxysmal spikes; sharp waves followed by slow waves
■ Absence	■ 3-Hz spike-wave complexes
■ Complex partial	■ Temporal lobe spikes, polyspikes, and waves
■ Psychogenic non-epileptic seizure (PNES)	■ Normal EEG
Delirium	■ Generalized theta and delta activity
■ Hepatic or uremic encephalopathy	■ Triphasic waves
Dementia	
■ Alzheimer and vascular	■ Alpha slowing of the background
■ Subacute sclerosing panencephalitis and Creutzfeldt-Jakob disease	■ Periodic complexes accompanying myoclonic jerks
Locked-in syndrome	■ Normal EEG
Persistent vegetative state	■ Slow and disorganized EEG
Death	■ Electrocerebral silence
Medications	
■ Benzodiazepines and barbiturates	■ Beta activity
■ Neuroleptics and antidepressants	■ Non-specific changes
Focal lesion	■ Focal delta slowing
Increased intracranial pressure	■ FIRDA

EEG, Electroencephalogram; FIRDA, frontal, intermittent, rhythmic delta activity; PNES, psychogenic non-epileptic seizure.

generalized, absence, and partial complex seizure disorders are well characterized and are diagnostic. When interpreted within the context of the clinical presentation, abnormal EEG data can help support several other broad diagnostic categories, including delirium, dementia, medication-induced mental status changes, and focal lesions. Normal data can provide support for diagnoses of non-epileptiform seizures and locked-in syndrome, but they are not able to rule out a variety of ictal states because of limitations on the placement of surface electrodes. Although an increased number

Indications for Neuroimaging in Patients With Psychiatric Symptoms

New-onset psychosis[a]
New-onset delirium[a]
New-onset dementia
Onset of any psychiatric problem in a patient > 50 years old[a]
An abnormal neurologic examination
A history of head trauma
During an initial work-up for electroconvulsive therapy

[a]When initial history, physical examination, and laboratory studies are not definitive.

of EEG abnormalities has been described in a variety of primary psychiatric disorders, at present the EEG is not clinically useful to definitively rule in any primary psychiatric diagnosis.

NEUROIMAGING

Neuroimaging has emerged as a powerful tool in both neuropsychiatric research and in the clinical investigation of organic etiologies for psychiatric presentations; however, rarely do neuroimaging studies establish a primary psychiatric diagnosis. Although less invasive than other diagnostic tests, imaging studies come with their own risks to the patient, and they remain costly.[53] Following a thorough initial evaluation, the decision to use neuroimaging should be made on a case-by-case basis; at present, the major objective of neuroimaging studies in patients with psychiatric symptoms is to prevent missing a treatable brain lesion. A suggested list of indications for brain imaging in psychiatric patients is given in Table 7.9. The following sections describe the major neuroimaging techniques currently available, as well as their clinical utility.

Computed Tomography

Computed tomography (CT) scans use multiple x-rays to provide cross-sectional images of the brain. On CT films, areas of increased beam attenuation (e.g., of the skull) appear white, whereas those of low attenuation (e.g., gas) appear black, and those of intermediate attenuation (e.g., soft tissues) appear in shades of gray. Contrast material may be used to visualize areas where the blood-brain barrier has been compromised, for example, by tumors, bleeding, inflammation, and

abscesses; however, up to 5% of patients can develop idiosyncratic reactions to contrast media, manifested by hypotension, nausea, flushing, urticaria, and anaphylaxis. CT scans can be obtained rapidly and are the imaging modality of choice in identifying acute hemorrhage and trauma and in situations in which MRI is contraindicated. CT scans are generally better tolerated by patients with anxiety or claustrophobia. Although useful in examining gross pathological conditions, CT lacks the resolution to detect subtle white matter lesions or changes in smaller structures, such as the hippocampi and basal ganglia. Because CT scans use ionizing radiation, they are contraindicated in pregnancy.

Although CT scans have a well-established role in the identification of structural abnormalities responsible for psychiatric symptoms in patients with organic lesions, they cannot be used to diagnose primary psychiatric illness. However, there are non-specific structural changes visible on CT that have been consistently identified in the brains of psychiatric patients. Since Weinberger and co-workers[54] first described increased ventricular-to-brain ratios in patients with schizophrenia, several investigators have observed enlarged ventricles in those with eating disorders, alcoholism, BPD, dementia, and depression.

Magnetic Resonance Imaging

MRI, which provides detailed images of the brain in axial, sagittal, and coronal planes, takes advantage of the interaction between protons and an external magnetic field. In the magnetic field of the MRI scanner, hydrogen protons in the water molecules of the brain become aligned as dipoles with, or against, the field. A radiofrequency pulse is applied, shifting the spin on the protons to a higher energy level; when the signal is turned off, the spin returns to the ground state and the proton releases energy. The frequency of energy release (or relaxation) depends on the chemical environment surrounding the proton. A coil that detects the energy emission generates signals that are processed by the scanner to create images. Adjusting the relaxation time parameters (known as T1 and T2) can result in images that are "weighted" differently; whereas T1-weighted images provide anatomic detail and gray-white matter differentiation, T2-weighted images highlight areas of pathologic conditions.

MRI is considered superior to CT for differentiation of white and gray matter, identification of white matter lesions (e.g., in multiple sclerosis, vasculitis, and leukoencephalitis), and visualization of the posterior fossa. As with CT, a contrast medium may be used to identify lesions where the blood-brain barrier has been compromised. MRI is contraindicated in patients with metallic implants (including pacemakers) and is often less tolerable to patients because of the longer length of the study, the enclosed space, and the noise.

MRI may be used clinically to rule out structural brain lesions in patients with psychiatric symptoms, including acute psychosis or delirium, severe mood disorder, and abrupt personality changes. In addition to the structural changes that CT scans are capable of detecting, MRI appears to be more sensitive to detecting atrophic changes in dementia, inflammation-induced edema, and white matter lesions. Compared with CT, MRI can detect acute strokes earlier, using a method called diffusion-weighted imaging.

Functional MRI (fMRI) uses a process of acquisition sequences to approximate cerebral blood flow; accordingly, one can infer regions of brain activation and deactivation at rest, as well as during the execution of sensory, motor, or cognitive tasks. Certain patterns of activation have emerged consistently in dementia, major depression, schizophrenia, and OCD. Although fMRI is used in research to provide enhanced knowledge about psychiatric illnesses and psychotropic medications, it will likely help guide research, drug development, and clinical practice in the future.

A related imaging modality, magnetic resonance spectroscopy (MRS), permits in vivo measurements of certain markers of brain tissue metabolism and biochemistry. For example, using proton-based MRS, one can measure local concentrations of N-acetyl aspartate (a putative marker of neuronal integrity), choline (a marker of membrane turnover), creatine (a marker of intracellular energy metabolism), glutamine, glutamate, and gamma-aminobutyric acid. Localized reductions in N-acetyl aspartate have been implicated in multiple neuropsychiatric disorders, including schizophrenia, temporal lobe epilepsy, AD, acquired immune deficiency syndrome dementia, and Huntington disease. In the future, the combined use of fMRI and MRS holds great promise for delineating

abnormal structure-function relationships underlying psychopathologic conditions.[55]

Positron Emission Tomography/Single Photon Emission Computed Tomography

PET employs radioactive markers to visualize directly cortical and subcortical brain functioning. Some examples of these markers include F^{18} fluorodeoxyglucose (which provides a picture of brain glucose metabolism), oxygen[15] (a surrogate for regional cerebral blood flow), and receptor-specific radioligands (which indicate activity at neurotransmitter receptors). Studies can be performed only where an on-site cyclotron is present to prepare the emitter tracers. Single photon emission computed tomography (SPECT) uses photon-emitting nucleotides measured by gamma detectors to localize brain activation or pharmacologic activity; commonly used tracers include xenon[133] and technetium Tc-99m hexamethylpropyleneamine (which measure cerebral blood flow) and, as in PET, radioligands with specific receptor activity. Although PET scans provide greater spatial and temporal resolution, signal-to-noise ratio, and variety of ligands, SPECT is more readily available, better tolerated, and less expensive.

PET and SPECT may be used in concert with the EEG to determine seizure foci, especially in patients with partial complex seizures; during a seizure, scans can demonstrate areas of increased metabolism, whereas interictally the focus will be hypometabolic and hypoperfused. Moreover, in both AD and multi-infarct dementia, abnormal patterns of cortical metabolism and receptor function as evidenced by PET and SPECT appear to predate structural changes visible on MRI. With the continued development of receptor-specific ligands and other functional markers, these imaging modalities may continue to find a more prominent role in clinical diagnosis and management.

CONCLUSION

Although diagnosis in psychiatry continues to rely primarily on the interview and other clinical phenomenology, diagnostic rating scales and laboratory testing serve important roles in eliminating organic etiologies from the differential diagnosis, monitoring the effects of treatment, and guiding further management decisions. Neuroimaging has provided a non-invasive means to detect subtle neurophysiological dysfunction in psychiatric patients and has begun to find meaningful clinical and research applications. These quantitative measures will assume increasing prominence and importance in 21st-century psychiatry.

REFERENCES

Access the reference list online at https://expertconsult.inkling.com/.

MOOD DISORDERS: DEPRESSION AND BIPOLAR DISORDER

MAURIZIO FAVA, MD ■ ROY H. PERLIS, MD, MSC ■ DAVID MISCHOULON, MD, PHD ■ ALEXANDRA K. GOLD, PHD ■ PAOLO CASSANO, MD, PHD ■ MICHAEL J. OSTACHER, MD, MPH, MMSC ■ GEORGE I. PAPAKOSTAS, MD ■ MASOUD KAMALI, MD ■ SHARMIN GHAZNAVI, MD, PHD ■ AMY T. PETERS, PHD ■ ANDREW A. NIERENBERG, MD ■ LOUISA G. SYLVIA, PHD ■ THEODORE A. STERN, MD

DEPRESSION

INTRODUCTION

Depressive disorders, especially major depressive disorder (MDD), are prevalent conditions associated with significant suffering, psychosocial impairment, and increased mortality. Despite numerous effective treatments, these disorders remain under-recognized and under-treated; this is due largely to the stigma of depression itself and the relative lack of systematic ascertainment of depressive symptoms by healthcare professionals. The public health significance of depression is noteworthy; apart from the direct psychosocial burden, these disorders also heighten the risk of developing other medical diseases and increase their associated morbidity and mortality.

According to the World Health Organization (WHO), MDD ranks among the leading causes of global burdens of disease.[1] An episode of MDD serious enough to warrant professional care affects approximately 16% of the general population during their lifetime.[1] Both the Epidemiological Catchment Area (ECA) study and the National Co-morbidity Survey study have found that MDD is prevalent, with cross-sectional rates of up to 6.6%.[2] Although this condition ranks first among reasons for psychiatric hospitalization (23.3% of total hospitalizations), an estimated 80% of all persons suffering from it are either treated by non-psychiatric personnel or go untreated.[3]

Depression is second only to hypertension as the most common chronic condition encountered in general medical practice.[4] Only 57% of depressed patients actively seek help for their depression, and most of them consult a primary care physician (PCP).[5] Four risk factors (female sex, stressful life events, adverse childhood experiences, and certain personality traits) have consistently been associated with MDD, and the level of evidence suggests that at least some of the association is causal. In the National Co-morbidity Study, the lifetime prevalence of MDD in the United States was estimated to be 21% in women and 13% in males.[6] A wide range of adversities (such as job loss, marital difficulties, major health problems, and loss of close personal relationships) are associated with a substantial increase in the risk for MDD.[7] A range of difficulties in childhood (e.g., physical and sexual abuse, poor parent-child relationships, parental discord, and divorce) increase the risk for MDD later in life.[8] A family history of depression is another risk factor: first-degree relatives of those with MDD have a three-fold increased risk of being affected by MDD themselves.[8] It is widely accepted that MDD is a heritable disorder, but the genes that convey susceptibility have not been well characterized.[9]

Depression is thought to rival virtually every medical illness regarding its burden of disease morbidity.[10] MDD has also been characterized by increased mortality.[11,12] In the general population, suicide accounts for about 0.9% of all deaths, and depression is the most important risk factor for suicide.

Depressed patients often have co-morbid medical conditions. Similarly, the presence of one or more chronic medical problems raises the recent (6-month) and lifetime prevalence of mood disorders. Patients affected by chronic and disabling physical illnesses are at a higher risk of developing depressive disorders, typically at a rate >20%. Among patients hospitalized for coronary artery disease (CAD), 30% have some degree of depression.[13] Patients with diabetes mellitus (DM) also have a two-fold increased prevalence of depression, with rates of 20% and 32% in uncontrolled and controlled studies, respectively.[14,15] Depression is also highly co-morbid with obesity.[16]

At the Massachusetts General Hospital (MGH), psychiatric consultants make a diagnosis of MDD in approximately 20% of medical inpatients, making MDD among the most common problems for which assistance with diagnosis and treatment is requested. The prevalence of a chronic medical condition in depressed patients ranges from 65% to 71%.[17] Depression dramatically influences the course of concurrent medical diseases; in general, the more severe the illness, the more likely depression is to complicate it.[18] Some degree of depression in patients hospitalized for CAD is associated with an increased risk of mortality and an ongoing depression seen during at least the first year following hospitalization.[13] Undergoing cardiac surgery while suffering from MDD, for example, is known to increase the chance of a fatal outcome.[19] Depression in the first 24 hours after myocardial infarction (MI) has been associated with a significantly increased risk of early death, re-infarction, or cardiac arrest.[20] Even among depressed outpatients, the risk of mortality, chiefly due to cardiovascular disease, is more than doubled.[21] The increased risk of cardiac mortality has also been confirmed in a large community cohort of those with cardiac disease who presented with either MDD or minor depression.[18] Those individuals without cardiac disease but with depression also had an increased risk (from 1.5- to 3.9-fold higher) of cardiac mortality.[22]

In patients with DM (type 1 or 2), depression has been associated with a significantly higher risk of DM-specific complications (e.g., retinopathy, nephropathy, neuropathy, macrovascular complications, and

sexual dysfunction).[23] Death rates in an elderly Hispanic population were substantially higher when multiple depressive symptoms were co-morbid with DM (odds ratio, OR 3.84).[24] Depression symptom severity has also been associated with a poor diet and poor medication adherence, functional impairment, and higher healthcare costs in primary care patients with DM.[25]

In acutely ill elderly inpatients, those with more depressive symptoms were more likely to worsen and were less likely to improve medically during and after hospitalization.[26] Under-recognition and under-treatment of depression in the elderly have been associated in primary care settings with increased medical care utilization.[27] Among those aged ≥65 years, depression and the risk of recurrent falls have been linked, with an OR of 3.9 when ≥4 depressive symptoms were present. Patients with cancer and co-morbid depression were at higher risk for mortality[28] and for longer hospital stays. Unfortunately, despite the impact of depression on overall morbidity, functional impairment, and mortality, close to half of those with depression (43%) fail to seek treatment for their depressive symptoms.[29]

Failure to treat depression leaves patients at risk for further complications and death. Any seriously ill individual with neurovegetative symptoms, and who wishes to be dead, is likely to do worse than if he or she had hope and motivation.

Prompt and effective treatment of co-morbid medical conditions is equally important for the outcome of depression. In a study of patients with DM, the severity of depression during follow-up was related to the presence of neuropathy at study entry, and to incomplete remission during the initial treatment trial.[30] By the 10th year of having insulin-dependent DM, nearly half (roughly 48%) of young individuals developed at least one psychiatric disorder, with MDD being the most prevalent (28%).[31] In addition to DM, other medical and neurologic conditions have been associated with an increased risk of developing MDD. For example, Fava and colleagues'[32] review showed that MDD is a life-threatening complication of Cushing syndrome, Addison disease, hyperthyroidism, hypothyroidism, and hyperprolactinemic amenorrhea, and that treatment that primarily addresses the physical condition may be more effective than antidepressant drugs for such organic affective syndromes. A study of computerized medical records at a large staff-model health maintenance organization showed that patients with depression had significantly higher annual healthcare costs and higher costs for every category of care (e.g., primary care, medical specialty care, medical inpatient care, and pharmacy and laboratory costs) than patients without depression.[33] Depressive disorders are associated with more disability than most other chronic diseases (e.g., osteoarthritis, DM), with a possible exception of MI.[34]

MAKING THE DIAGNOSIS OF MAJOR DEPRESSIVE DISORDER (MDD)

Depression is a term often used to describe even minor and transient mood fluctuations. The criteria for MDD according to the *Diagnostic and Statistical Manual of Mental Disorders, 5th edition* (DSM-5)[35] should be applied to the those with medical illnesses in the same way as they are applied to those without a co-morbid medical condition. The DSM-5 has a category for mood disorders "due to" another medical condition. Our recommendation is to diagnose a mood disorder using the DSM-5 criteria. A depressive disorder that does not meet full criteria (due to an insufficient duration or too few symptoms), causing clinically significant distress or impairment, can now be diagnosed as an "Other Specified Depressive Disorder" according to the DSM-5 (a condition that is often referred to as minor depression in the medically ill).

Diagnosis is crucial to treatment. Three questions face the psychiatrist at the outset: (1) Does the patient manifest depression? (2) If so, is there a medical/neurological cause, such as the use of a medication that can be eliminated, treated, or reversed? (3) Does it arise from a medical condition (e.g., Cushing disease), and treatment of that condition will alleviate it, or must it be treated in a fashion like other depressive disorders (e.g., post-stroke depression [PSD])?

Depressed mood is ubiquitous and is often thought to be normal; therefore, it is likely to be dismissed even when it is serious. For example, if a man has terminal cancer and meets the criteria for MDD, this mood state is regarded by some as "understandable" or "appropriate," that is, that anyone with that condition would be depressed. However, MDD is not always triggered by

sadness or despondency. Most patients with terminally ill cancer do not develop MDD no matter how despondent they become. Depression is a dreaded complication of medical illnesses that requires swift diagnosis and treatment.

Patients who suffer from unipolar depressive disorders typically present with a constellation of psychological and cognitive, behavioral, and somatic symptoms. Because far less epidemiologic information is available on depression in the medically ill, the requirement that dysphoria be present for ≥2 weeks should be regarded as an approximation in the medically ill. According to the DSM-5,[35] five or more of the following nine symptoms should be present most of the day, nearly every day, and they should include either depressed mood or the loss of interest or pleasure:

1. Depressed mood (subjective or observed)
2. A markedly diminished level of interest or pleasure in all, or almost all activities (anhedonia), including a reduced libido (with or without decreased arousal or difficulty climaxing)
3. A decrease or an increase in appetite, with significant (more than 5% of body weight per month) weight loss or gain
4. Insomnia or hypersomnia
5. Psychomotor agitation or retardation (that is observable by others)
6. Fatigue or loss of energy
7. Feelings of worthlessness or excessive or inappropriate guilt (which may be delusional), not merely about being sick
8. A diminished ability to think or concentrate, or indecisiveness
9. Recurrent thoughts of death (not just a fear of dying), recurrent thoughts of suicide without a plan, or a suicide attempt or a specific plan for taking one's life.

These symptoms are recalled by using the SIG:E CAPS mnemonic: sleep disturbance (insomnia/hypersomnia) (S), interests/pleasure diminished (I), guilt or feelings of worthlessness (G), reduced energy or fatigue (E), concentration ability reduced (C), appetite/weight disturbance (increased or decreased [A]), psychomotor agitation/retardation (P), and thoughts of suicide or an actual suicide attempt/plan (S).

Other associated psychological/cognitive symptoms may include apathy, irritability, anxiety/nervousness/worrying, indecisiveness, hypersensitivity to criticism or rejection, reward dependency, perfectionism, obsessiveness, ruminations, pessimism, hopelessness/helplessness, cognitive distortions, hypochondriacal concerns, and thoughts of hurting others. Behavioral symptoms may include crying spells, interpersonal friction or confrontation, anger attacks or outbursts, avoidance of anxiety-provoking situations, social withdrawal, avoidance of emotional and sexual intimacy, reduced leisure-time activities, development of rituals or compulsions, compulsive eating, compulsive use of the internet or video games, workaholic behaviors, substance use or abuse, intensification of personality traits or pathologic behaviors, excessive reliance or dependence on others, excessive self-sacrifice or victimization, reduced productivity, self-cutting or mutilation, suicide attempts or gestures, and violent or assaultive behaviors. Associated physical/somatic symptoms may include leaden feelings in the arms or legs, aches and pains, back pain, musculoskeletal complaints, chest pain, headaches, muscle tension, gastrointestinal (GI) upset, palpitations, burning or tingling sensations, and paresthesias.

On first inspection, the DSM-5 criteria for MDD may appear invalid in the medically ill. If a patient has advanced cancer, one might wonder how anorexia or fatigue could be attributed to something other than the malignancy? Four of the nine diagnostic symptoms could be viewed as impossible to ascribe exclusively to depression in a medically ill patient: sleep difficulty, anorexia, fatigue or energy loss, and difficulty concentrating.

The first help comes from the discovery of symptoms that are more clearly the result of MDD, such as the presence of self-reproach ("I feel worthless"), the wish to be dead, or psychomotor retardation (few medical illnesses in and of themselves produce psychomotor retardation; hypothyroidism and Parkinson disease are two of them). Insomnia or hypersomnia can also help to make the diagnosis, although a patient may have so much pain, dyspnea, or frequent clinical crises that sleep is impaired by these events. In addition, the ability to think or concentrate, as with the other symptoms, needs to be asked about in every case.

Functional impairment is also helpful for distinguishing MDD and other depressive disorders from normal mood variability. Responses to a significant loss (e.g., death of a loved one, financial ruin, and other misfortunes) may include intense sadness, rumination about the loss, insomnia, poor appetite, and weight loss often resembling symptoms of a depressive episode. Although such symptoms may be understandable and appropriate to the loss, the presence of a major depressive episode (MDE) in addition to the normal grief response should be considered. This decision inevitably requires that clinical judgment be based on the individual's history and the cultural norms for the expression of distress in the context of loss.

Physicians should always inquire about thoughts of suicide since suicide is one of the most serious complications of depressive disorders. Typically, generic questions such as "Have you been thinking that life is not worth living?" are appropriate to introduce the subject, which can be followed by, "Have you also been thinking that you would be better off dead?" and, finally, "Have you considered taking your own life recently?" and "Have you tried to hurt or kill yourself?" Of course, should a patient report suicidal thoughts/intent, referral to a specialist or to a local psychiatric emergency facility (when appropriate) is strongly recommended. History of mania (e.g., with elevated mood, increased energy, and impulsivity), that is frequently suggested by a history of uncharacteristic behaviors, buying sprees, and excessive risk-taking behavior, is often reported by family members, should lead to referral of depressed patients to a psychiatric specialist for the evaluation of a bipolar disorder (see "Bipolar Disorder" section of this chapter). Referral is also indicated in cases of treatment-resistant depression, psychotic depression, and when there is a danger that the patient will harm someone else.

Case 1

Mr. H, a 24-year-old graduate student without a psychiatric history, reported unusual aches during his annual physical. Medical work-up revealed that his hemoglobin A_{1C} and fasting blood sugar levels were elevated, and he was thought to have type 2 DM. His physician provided instructions to manage his newly diagnosed condition (including how to eat healthily, exercise, and monitor his serum glucose), and scheduled a follow-up visit in 3 months.

At his follow-up visit, Mr. H reported being unable to follow the doctor's instructions, and indeed his blood sugar levels remained elevated. Mr. H also described being shocked by the news and feeling as though there was no hope. He also reported feeling tired all the time, sleeping poorly, and concentrating poorly in classes. Due to these new symptoms, his physician requested a consultation to assess whether Mr. H was also struggling with depression, which might have been adversely impacting his adherence to instructions.

The consulting psychiatrist interviewed Mr. H and reviewed his medical records and medications. He ruled out that his mood change was due to medications. Although aware of normative reactions to a new diagnosis, the psychiatrist considered whether Mr. H's presenting concerns were a result of DM or co-occurring MDD (given problems with sleep, concentration, and energy). On further questioning, Mr. H also described considerable guilt over his present condition, as well as feelings of hopelessness and pessimism. He also reported spending more time watching television alone and socializing less, and that the doctor's exercise and diet plan was too hard.

The psychiatrist determined that Mr. H met the criteria for MDD, based on having five of nine MDD symptoms present most of the day, nearly every day. These also represented a change after his diagnosis of DM and significant functional impairment. While some symptoms may be ascribed to DM, these symptoms would have also presented prior to his diagnosis. In addition, the presence of low self-esteem, guilt, hopelessness, and apathy were more clearly a result of MDD. The psychiatrist conveyed these results to Mr. H's PCP and recommended starting adjunctive treatment for MDD.

If the history reveals five or more of nine symptoms, the psychiatrist may not be certain that some of them have anything to do with depression but may just as likely stem from a co-morbid medical illness. For example, if a patient were found to be hypothyroid, the treatment of choice would not be antidepressants but judicious thyroid replacement. In most medical settings, however, everything is usually being done to alleviate the patient's symptoms of the primary illness. If this appears to be the case, our recommendation is to make the diagnosis of MDD and proceed with treatment.

SUBTYPES OF MAJOR DEPRESSIVE DISORDER

MDD is a heterogeneous clinical entity.[36] Therefore, to allow clinicians and researchers to differentiate individuals with distinct clinical presentations, several subtypes have been defined.[2]

Anxious Depression

When patients with depression experience some symptoms (such as restlessness, tension, excessive worry, or a fear of panicking), it is referred to as "anxious depression." Among the depressed patients participating in the multi-center Sequenced Treatment Alternatives to Relieve Depression (STAR*D) project, the prevalence of anxious depression was approximately 45%.[37] Patients with anxious depression tend to have a slower response to treatment and are less likely to respond to antidepressants than those without anxious depression.[38]

Depression with Anger Attacks

In about 30% to 40% of outpatients with MDD, intermittent outbursts of anger (termed anger attacks) are observed.[39] These individuals may be predominantly irritable when depressed, rather than sad, and these anger episodes are generally not typical of their personality when they are euthymic.

Mixed Depression

Patients who, in addition to meeting criteria for depression, also display symptoms of elevated mood, grandiosity, pressured speech, racing thoughts, increased energy, risk taking, and a decreased need for sleep (without meeting the full criteria for hypomania or mania) should be assigned the diagnosis of "mixed depression." These patients are at increased risk of developing bipolar I or bipolar II disorder.

Melancholic Depression

Those with "melancholic depression" are severely depressed individuals who are unable to experience pleasure (anhedonia) or who lose normal emotional responsiveness to positive experiences. Afflicted patients also exhibit a distinct quality of depressed mood (despondency, despair, moroseness, or empty mood), a worsening of mood in the morning, excessive/inappropriate guilt, early morning awakening, reduced appetite/weight loss, and psychomotor retardation/agitation.

Atypical Depression

Atypical depression is characterized by mood reactivity (defined by an ability to temporarily respond to positive experiences) accompanied by rejection sensitivity, hypersomnia, hyperphagia, and prominent physical fatigue (leaden paralysis, with feelings of heaviness in the arms and legs).

Psychotic Depression

Patients with psychotic depression suffer from delusions and/or hallucinations in addition to depression. The content of their psychotic symptoms is typically mood congruent (i.e., consistent with the depressive themes of guilt, nihilism, and deserved punishment), but may also be mood incongruent (e.g., persecutory or self-referential delusions and hallucinations without an affective component). Psychotic depression is typically accompanied by significant cognitive dysfunction, and it has shown distinctive responsivity to treatment with electroconvulsive therapy (ECT) and to the combination of antidepressants and antipsychotics (being superior to either drug alone).[40]

Catatonic Depression

Catatonia is defined by abnormalities of movement and behavior that arise secondary to a disturbed mental state. Catatonic features include stupor (with a lack of motion/motion response to the environment), posturing (maintenance of a posture held against gravity), negativism (motiveless resistance to all instructions), stereotypy (repetitive purposeless movements), mannerisms (odd/peculiar/circumstantial caricatures of normal movements/actions), echolalia (mimicking another person's speech), and echopraxia (mimicking another person's actions).

Peri-partum Depression

Peri-partum depression is characterized by its onset during pregnancy or within 4 weeks of delivering a child. The symptomatology does not, in general, differ from that seen in non-peri-partum depressive episodes; however, psychotic features (such as delusions involving the newborn infant) are relatively common. Other common symptoms involve mood fluctuations, severe anxiety, panic attacks, thoughts of suicide, spontaneous crying, insomnia, and a general disinterest in the infant.

Seasonal Depression (Seasonal Affective Disorder)

In this subtype of recurrent depression, the onset occurs at a particular time of the year, most often in the fall or winter. Remissions also display a seasonal pattern, that is, a patient with recurrent depressions during the fall, which often remits in the spring. Seasonal depression is more prevalent at higher latitudes; a lack of daylight is believed to be an important etiological factor.

OTHER DEPRESSIVE DISORDERS

Additional categories of depressive disorders listed in the DSM-5 are disruptive mood dysregulation disorder, premenstrual dysphoric disorder, substance/medication-induced depressive disorder, depressive disorder due to another medical condition, other specified depressive disorders, and unspecified depressive disorder.[35]

Persistent Depressive Disorder (i.e., Dysthymic Disorder)

The DSM-5 consolidated chronic MDD and dysthymic disorder into persistent depressive disorder. For the diagnosis of persistent depressive disorder, DSM-5 specifies a state of depression lasting more than 2 years. To qualify, the patient must have a depressed mood for most of the day, on more days than not, and have two or more of the following six symptoms: (1) poor appetite or overeating, (2) insomnia or hypersomnia, (3) low energy or fatigue, (4) low self-esteem, (5) poor concentration or difficulty making decisions, and (6) feelings of hopelessness.

More than 70% of patients with dysthymic disorder develop MDD and have recurrent MDEs superimposed on their dysthymic disorder (i.e., double depression). As in MDD, most individuals with dysthymia have co-morbid medical or psychiatric disorders. Although milder than MDD, dysthymic disorder may have profound effects on one's quality of life and function in multiple life roles; this degree of morbidity is more reflective of the duration of dysthymic disorder than the number of symptoms experienced.

Adjustment Disorder with Depressed Mood

Adjustment disorder with depressed mood (code 309.00) is probably the most over-used diagnosis by consultation psychiatrists. It should not be applied to a medical patient unless the depressive reaction is maladaptive, either in intensity of feeling (an over-reaction) or in function (e.g., when a despondent patient interacts minimally with caregivers and family).

Bereavement

Bereavement (code V62.82) refers to the death of a loved one. In a medically ill patient, it is the self that is mourned after a narcissistic injury (e.g., an MI). DSM-5 cautions clinicians to consider the normative response to loss versus a depressive episode. Distinguishing features of grief are feelings of emptiness and loss, whereas, in an MDE, they are feelings of a persistent depressed mood and the inability to anticipate happiness or pleasure.[35] In acute grief, MDD can be difficult to distinguish, but, when present, it requires treatment (perhaps even more than when it occurs in the absence of acute grief). The dysphoria associated with grief is likely to decrease in intensity over days to weeks and often occurs in waves associated with thoughts of, or reminders of, the deceased. The depressed mood in MDEs is more persistent and not tied to specific thoughts or preoccupations.

Clues helpful to establish a diagnosis of MDD include (1) guilt about things other than actions taken around the time of the death of the loved one, (2) thoughts of death (other than wanting to be with the lost person) or feeling one would be better off dead—suicidal ideation should count in favor of MDD, (3) morbid preoccupation with worthlessness, (4) marked psychomotor retardation, (5) prolonged and marked functional impairment, and (6) hallucinations other than seeing, hearing, or being touched by the deceased person. The principal symptoms of complicated grief are yearning for, and preoccupation with, thoughts of the deceased, crying, searching for the deceased, disbelief about the death, being stunned by the death, and inability to accept the death.

States Commonly Mislabeled as Depression

Up to one-third of patients referred for depression have neither MDD nor minor depression. By far the most common diagnosis found among these mislabeled referrals at the MGH has been an organic brain syndrome. A quietly confused patient may look depressed. The patient with dementia or with a frontal lobe syndrome caused by a brain injury can lack spontaneity and appear depressed. Fortunately, the physical and mental status examinations frequently reveal tell-tale abnormalities. Another unrecognized state, sometimes called "depression" by the consultee and easier for the psychiatrist to recognize, is anger. The patient's physician, realizing that the patient has been through a long and difficult illness, may perceive a patient's reduction in speech or smiling as a manifestation of depression. The patient may thoroughly resent the illness, be irritated by therapeutic routines, and be fed up with the hospital environment but may remain reluctant to express their wrath to the physician or nurses.

Excluding Organic Causes of Depression

In addition to obtaining information regarding the duration and course of all physical and psychological symptoms of a depressed patient, a thorough physical examination should be performed, as well as a mental status examination with close attention paid to thoughts of self-harm or hurting others, and whether psychotic symptoms are present. Practitioners should be aware of the societal stigma of depression and, thus, the reluctance of some patients to report psychological distress.

Routine laboratory tests (e.g., complete blood count, thyroid [and parathyroid] function tests, liver enzymes, blood sugar, lipids, C-reactive protein, and levels of sodium, potassium, creatinine, calcium, folate, vitamin D, and vitamin B_{12}) are also important for ruling out metabolic disorders, infections, and anemia that may cause depressive symptoms. A full report of previous/co-morbid psychiatric disorders must also be obtained, including a systematic evaluation of drug or alcohol abuse/dependence. The clinician must then review the medical history and the use of concomitant medications, since those may also alter mood.

Regarding suspected depression secondary to medication side effects, one should try to establish a relationship between the onset of depressive symptoms and either the start of, or a change in, a medication. If such a connection can be established, the simplest course is to discontinue the agent and monitor the patient for improvement. When the patient requires continued treatment, as for hypertension, the presumed offending agent can be changed, with the hope that the change to another antihypertensive will be followed by the resolution of depressive symptoms. When this fails or when clinical judgment warrants no change in medication, it may be necessary to start an antidepressant along with the antihypertensive drug. The literature linking drugs to depression is inconclusive at best. Clinicians have seen depression following the use of reserpine and steroids[10] and from withdrawal from cocaine, amphetamine, and alcohol. Despite anecdotal reports, beta-blockers do not appear to cause depression.[41] The most common central nervous system (CNS) side effect of drugs is confusion or delirium, and this is commonly mislabeled as depression because a mental status examination has not been conducted.

Several medical conditions must be considered in the differential diagnosis of MDD since careful studies have found a high incidence of MDD in hospitalized medical patients.[22] The diagnosis of a depressive disorder may be complicated by the fact that a patient with certain medical conditions (e.g., cancer, as well as endocrine, cardiovascular or neurological diseases) may present with physical symptoms that resemble those of depression (e.g., fatigue, weight loss, sleep disturbances). For example, carcinoma of the pancreas has been associated with psychiatric symptoms, especially depression, which in some cases seems to be the first manifestation of the disease.[42] Two carefully controlled studies have shown these patients have significantly more psychiatric symptoms and MDD than patients with other malignancies of GI origin, leading some to suspect that depression in this case is a manifestation of a paraneoplastic syndrome.[42,43]

Although MDD is frequently associated with medical illnesses, the DSM-5 specifies that "the depressive episode is not attributable to the physiological effects of a substance or to another medical condition."[35] Therefore, the medical history along with the physical examination and laboratory tests should guide any further diagnostic work-up to discover and treat non-psychiatric medical conditions, which may account for depressive symptoms that "mimic" MDD. However, many patients suffer from concomitant non-psychiatric medical conditions and MDD and should receive treatment for both problems.

Other mental disorders should be included in the differential diagnosis when evaluating MDD and other depressive disorders. As specified in the DSM-5 criteria for MDD, "The occurrence of the major depressive episode is not better explained by schizoaffective disorder, schizophrenia, schizophreniform disorder, delusional disorder, or other specified and unspecified schizophrenia spectrum and other psychotic disorders."[35] Consequently, these disorders represent other diagnoses that can produce symptoms of MDD and a patient who meets full diagnostic criteria for a psychotic disorder should be diagnosed as such, despite meeting the criteria for MDD or other depressive disorders. Similarly, a patient with a history of a manic/hypomanic episode should be diagnosed with bipolar disorder if they meet the criteria for MDD (bipolar depression). These two examples emphasize the need for a thorough assessment of depressed patients, as depressive syndrome may be a consequence of a "primary" psychotic disorder or a depressive episode during bipolar disorder. Distinguishing among psychotic disorders, bipolar disorder, and MDD/other depressive disorders is essential for optimal treatment.

Many mental/behavioral disorders may be co-morbid with depression. These conditions include anxiety disorders, obsessive-compulsive disorder (OCD), trauma- and stressor-related disorders, eating disorders, substance-related and addictive disorders, personality disorders, and neurodevelopmental disorders (e.g., autism, attention-deficit/hyperactivity disorder [ADHD]).[35]

Mood Disorders Secondary to Medical Conditions

Stroke

Direct injury to the brain can produce changes in affect that progress to MDD. Morris and co-workers[44] have intensively studied mood disorders that result from strokes. Left-hemisphere lesions involving the pre-frontal cortex or basal ganglia are the most likely to be associated with post-stroke depression (PSD) and to meet the criteria for MDD or dysthymia.[44] Depressive symptoms appear in the immediate post-stroke period in about two-thirds of patients, with the rest manifesting depression by the sixth month. Additional risk factors for developing MDD were a prior stroke, pre-existing subcortical atrophy, and a family or personal history of an affective disorder. Aphasia did not appear to cause depression, but non-fluent aphasia was associated with depression; both seemed to result from lesions of the left frontal lobe. Although the severity of functional impairment at the time of acute injury did not correlate with the severity of depression, depression appeared to impede recovery. Among patients with left-hemispheric damage, those who were depressed showed significantly worse cognitive performance, which was seen in tasks that assessed temporal orientation, frontal lobe function, and executive motor function. Successful treatment of PSD has been demonstrated by double-blinded studies with nortriptyline[45] and trazodone[46] and has been reported with ECT[47] and the use of psychostimulants.[48] In fact, one study has shown that nortriptyline was more effective than fluoxetine in treating depressive symptoms in patients with PSD.[49] Early and aggressive treatment of PSD is required to minimize the cognitive and performance deficits that this mood disorder inflicts on patients during their recovery.

Right-hemispheric lesions deserve special attention. When the lesion was in the right anterior location, the mood disorder tended to manifest by an apathetic state associated with "inappropriate cheerfulness." However, such patients seldom look cheerful and may complain of a loss of interest, or of worry. This disorder was found in 6 of 20 patients with solitary right-hemisphere strokes (and in none of 28 patients with a single left-hemisphere lesion).

Prosody is also a problem for those with a right-hemisphere injury. Ross and Rush[50] focused on the presentation of aprosodia (with a lack of prosody or inflection, rhythm, and intensity of expression) when the right hemisphere is damaged. A patient with such a lesion might appear quite depressed and be labeled as having depression by staff and family; however, they simply lack the neuronal capacity to express or recognize emotion. If one stations oneself out of the patient's view, selects a neutral sentence (e.g., "The book is red"), asks the patient to identify the mood as mad, sad, frightened, or elated, and then speaks the sentence with the emotion to be tested, one should be able to identify those patients with a receptive aprosodia. Next, the patient is asked to deliver the same sentence with a series of different emotional tones to test for the presence of an expressive aprosodia. Stroke patients can suffer from both aprosodia and depression, but separate diagnostic criteria and clinical examinations exist for each one.

Dementia

Primary dementia increases the likelihood of the patient suffering from MDD, even though the incidence with Alzheimer disease (AD) is not as high as it is with multi-infarct (or vascular) dementia. The careful post-mortem studies of Zubenko and colleagues[51] supported the hypothesis that the pathophysiology of secondary depression is consistent with theories of etiology for primary depression. Comparing dementia patients with and without depression, the ones with MDD showed a 10- to 20-fold reduction in cortical norepinephrine levels.

Since multi-infarct dementia commonly includes depression as a symptom, Hachinski and associates[52] included it in the Ischemia Scale. Cummings and co-workers[53] compared 15 patients with multi-infarct dementia with 30 patients with AD and found that depressive symptoms (60% vs. 17%) and episodes of MDD (4/15 vs. 0/30) were more frequent in patients with the former.

Subcortical Dementias

Patients with Parkinson disease and Huntington disease commonly manifest MDD. Huntington disease may even present as MDD before the onset of either chorea or dementia.[54] Some have noted that as depression in those with Parkinson disease is treated, parkinsonian symptoms also improve, even before the depressive symptoms have subsided. This is especially striking when ECT is used,[55] although the same improvement has been reported after the use of tricyclic antidepressants (TCAs). Treatment of MDD in either disease may increase patient comfort and is always worth trying. Because individuals with Huntington disease may be sensitive to the anticholinergic side effects of TCAs, anticholinergics should be tried first.

Because HIV-1 is neurotropic, even asymptomatic HIV-seropositive individuals when compared with seronegative controls, demonstrate a high incidence of electroencephalographic abnormalities (67% vs. 10%) and more abnormalities on neuropsychological testing.[56] The unusually high lifetime and current rates of mood disorders in HIV-seronegative individuals at risk for AIDS[57] demand an exceedingly high vigilance for their appearance in HIV-positive persons. Depression, mania, or psychosis can appear with acquired immunodeficiency syndrome (AIDS) encephalopathy, but the early, subtler signs (e.g., impaired concentration, complaints of poor memory, blunting of interests, lethargy) may respond dramatically to antidepressants, such as psychostimulants.[58] The selective serotonin reuptake inhibitors (SSRIs) (such as sertraline, fluoxetine, and paroxetine) have also been effective in the treatment of depression in HIV-positive patients.[59] A small open trial also supports the use of bupropion in these patients.[60]

CHOICE OF AN APPROPRIATE TREATMENT FOR DEPRESSION

Whenever MDD is diagnosed, the effort to alleviate symptoms almost always includes the use of psychotherapy (particularly cognitive-behavioral therapy [CBT] and interpersonal therapy), antidepressants, rapid transcranial magnetic stimulation, and in more severe cases, somatic therapies, such as ECT (the single most effective treatment for depression). Newer therapies such as ketamine have gained prominence over the past decade, although insurance coverage remains limited, at least for intravenous infusions. Intranasal esketamine is more widely covered by insurance. Difficulties in finding access to therapists make the use of antidepressants easier. The consulting psychiatrist who understands the interactions among antidepressants, illnesses, and non-psychotropic drugs is best prepared to prescribe these agents effectively.

Prescribing Antidepressants for the Medically Ill

Ever since sudden death in cardiac patients was first associated with amitriptyline,[61] physicians have tended to fear the use of TCAs when cardiac disease is present. However, depression itself is a life-threatening disease and should be treated. Fortunately, the advent of newer antidepressants, such as SSRIs, that are safer and better tolerated than TCAs, has broadened options for the psychiatrist who must select the proper treatment (see Table 8.1).

All cyclic antidepressants, SSRIs, and monoamine oxidase inhibitors (MAOIs) usually correct sleep disturbances (insomnia or hypersomnia) when these are symptoms of depression. Insomnia is a common complaint that often leads to psychiatric consultation in the medical setting. In patients with certain medical illnesses, the choice of an antidepressant must be made on a case-by-case basis, accounting for the side effect profile (risk), the anticipated benefits, and the potential drug-drug interactions. With respect to insomnia, the sedative potency of antidepressants can generally be predicted by their in vitro affinity for the histamine H_1 receptor (antihistaminic property). One exception is trazodone, which has a low affinity for the H_1 receptor but is nonetheless a sedating agent.

This same property can also be used to predict how much weight gain may be associated with the use of the antidepressant. For the most part, the SSRIs, bupropion, nefazodone, trazodone, and venlafaxine have negligible antihistaminic potency and often have a limited effect on weight. The MAOIs, in general, have a low sedative potency, although phenelzine can produce drowsiness. Mirtazapine, a powerful antagonist of the H_1 receptor, is quite sedating and is associated with significant weight gain, particularly at lower doses. Doxepin, possibly the most potent antihistamine in clinical medicine, may also be used when sedation is desired; however, weight should be monitored.

There are three additional categories of side effects that are relevant for the treatment of depression in acute medical settings: orthostatic hypotension (OH), anticholinergic effects, and cardiac conduction effects. We will discuss side effects specific to each antidepressant class, and side effects associated with abrupt discontinuation of antidepressant treatment. When these side effects are understood, safe clinical prescription of antidepressant drugs is far more likely.

TABLE 8.1

Characteristics of Antidepressant Drugs

	Elimination Half-life (hr)	Sedative Potency	Anticholinergic Potency	Orthostatic Hypotension	Cardiac Arrhythmia Potential	Target Dosage (mg/d)	Dosage Range (mg/d)
Tricyclics/Tetracyclics							
Doxepin	17	High	Moderate	High	Yes	200	75–400
Amitriptyline	21	High	Highest	High	Yes	150	75–300
Imipramine	28	Moderate	Moderate	High	Yes	200	75–400
Trimipramine	13	High	Moderate	High	Yes	150	75–300
Clomipramine	23	High	High	High	Yes	150	75–300
Protriptyline	78	Low	High	Moderate	Yes	30	15–60
Nortriptyline	36	Moderate	Moderate	Moderate	Yes	100	40–150
Desipramine	21	Low	Moderate	Moderate	Yes	150	75–300
Maprotiline	43	High	Moderate	Moderate	Yes	150	75–300
SSRIs							
Citalopram	33	Low	Low	Low	Low	20	20–80
Escitalopram	22	Low	Low	Low	Low	10	10–20
Fluoxetine	87	Low	Low	Lowest	Low	20	40–80
Sertraline	26	Low	Low	Lowest	Low	50	50–200
Paroxetine	21	Low	Low-moderate	Lowest	Low	20	20–60
Fluvoxamine	19	Low	Low	Low	Low	200	50–300
Vilazodone	25	Low	Low	Low	Low	40–80	20–160
Vortioxetine	66	Low	Low	Low	Low	10–20	5–40
SNRIs							
Venlafaxine	3.6	Low	Low	Low	Low	300	75–375
Desvenlafaxine	10	Low	Low	Low	Low	50	50–400
Duloxetine	12	Low	Low	Low	Low	40	40–120
Levomilnacipran	12	Low	Low	Low	Low	40–120	20–240
Others							
Bupropion	15	Low	Low	Lowest	Low	200	75–300
Trazodone	3.5	High	Lowest	Moderate	Yes	150	50–600
Nefazodone	3	Moderate	Low	Low	Low	300	300–600
Mirtazapine	30	High	Low	Low	Low	15	15–45
Selegiline (transdermal)	18	Low	Low	Moderate	Low	6	6–12
Monoamine oxidase inhibitors	–	Low	Low	High	Low	–	–
Brexanolone	9	High	Low	Low	Low	IV: Infusion over 2.5 days Hours (Hr) 0–4: 30 mcg/kg/hr Hr 4–24: 60 mg/kg/hr Hr 24–52: 90 mg/kg/hr Hr 52–56: 60 mg/kg/hr Hr 56–60: 30 mg/kg/hr	30–90 mcg/kg/hr as noted under target dosage
Esketamine	7–12	High	Low	Low	Low	Intranasal: Administered in a physician's office with a 2-hr observation period following administration Induction phase (weeks 1–4): 56 mg twice weekly (may increase to 84 mg after first dose) Maintenance phase (weeks 5–8): 56 mg or 84 mg weekly; thereafter (week 9 onward) 56 mg or 84 mg weekly or biweekly	As noted under target dosage

IV, Intravenous; SNRIs, serotonin-norepinephrine reuptake inhibitor; SSRIs, selective serotonin reuptake inhibitors.

Orthostatic Hypotension

OH is not directly related to each drug's in vitro affinity for the α_1-noradrenergic receptor. In general, among the TCAs, tertiary amine agents are more likely to cause an orthostatic fall in blood pressure (BP) compared to secondary amines. For reasons that are not entirely clear, imipramine, amitriptyline, and desipramine are the TCAs most commonly associated with clinical mishaps, such as falls and fractures. The orthostatic effect appears earlier than the therapeutic effect for imipramine and is objectively verifiable at less than half the therapeutic plasma level. Hence, the drug may need to be discontinued long before a therapeutic plasma level is reached. Once postural symptoms develop, increasing the dosage of the antidepressant may not worsen the symptoms.

Paradoxically, a pre-treatment fall of more than 10 mm Hg in orthostatic BP predicts a good response to antidepressant medication in older adult depressed patients.[62] Naturally, younger patients may tolerate a fall in BP more easily than older patients, so an orthostatic fall in BP may not produce symptoms serious enough to require discontinuation of the drug. The presence of cardiovascular disease increases the likelihood of OH. When patients without cardiac disease take imipramine, the incidence of significant OH is 7%. With conduction system disease, such as a bundle-branch block (BBB), the incidence rises to 33%, and with congestive heart failure (CHF), it reaches 50%.[63] Of the TCAs, nortriptyline is the least likely to cause OH, an extremely valuable factor when depression in cardiac or older adult patients requires treatment.[64] MAOIs cause significant OH with roughly the same frequency as imipramine (i.e., often). Moreover, the patient starting a MAOI usually does not experience OH until the medication is having a significant therapeutic effect, roughly 2 to 4 weeks after its initiation.

Among other agents, trazodone and mirtazapine are associated with OH moderately often. Fluoxetine, sertraline, paroxetine, citalopram, fluvoxamine, bupropion, venlafaxine, and psychostimulants are essentially free of this side effect. Bupropion, psychostimulants, and venlafaxine may raise systolic BP slightly. Some have noted that even though the objective fall in standing BP continues for several months, some patients with initial symptoms accommodate and no longer complain of the side effects.

Anticholinergic Effects

The anticholinergic effects of TCAs are a nuisance for many patients. Urinary retention, constipation, dry mouth, confusion, and tachycardia are the most common. The higher heart rate is usually a sinus tachycardia that results from a muscarinic blockade of vagal tone on the heart. Amitriptyline is the most anticholinergic of the antidepressants, with protriptyline a close second. These agents regularly induce tachycardia, and one should monitor the heart rate as the dosage is increased. If significant tachycardia results, another agent may need to be used. Many inpatients, particularly those with ischemic heart disease, are already being treated with β-blockers, such as propranolol. When this is the case, the β-blocker usually protects the patient from developing a significant tachycardia.

Trazodone is almost devoid of activity at the muscarinic receptor, and it is a reasonable choice when another agent has caused unwanted anticholinergic side effects.

Fluoxetine, bupropion, venlafaxine, and the MAOIs exert minimal activity at the acetylcholine muscarinic receptor; hence, they can also be useful alternatives when these side effects impair a patient's access to an antidepressant. Laboratory evidence, supplemented by anecdotal clinical reports, reveals that paroxetine is more anticholinergic, close in its in vitro potency to imipramine. Similar but mild effects, such as dry mouth, accompany the use of mirtazapine. The effects of fluvoxamine and nefazodone are generally mild.

Cardiac Conduction Effects

All TCAs prolong ventricular depolarization. This tends to produce a lengthening of the PR and QRS intervals as well as of the QT interval corrected for heart rate (QTc) on the electrocardiogram (ECG). The His-ventricular portion of the conduction system is preferentially prolonged. That is, these drugs, which are sodium-channel blockers, tend to slow the electric impulse as it passes through the specialized conduction tissue known as the His-Purkinje system. Depressed cardiac patients with premature ventricular contractions (PVCs), when started on an antidepressant, such as imipramine, are likely to have less ventricular irritability, even if the abnormality is as serious as inducible ventricular tachycardia. Both imipramine and nortriptyline have been efficacious as antiarrhythmics and share the advantage of a half-life long enough to permit twice-daily doses.

Ordinarily, this property does not pose a problem for cardiac patients who do not already have conduction system disease. First-degree heart block is the mildest pathologic form and it should not pose a problem when using antidepressant treatment. When the patient's abnormality exceeds this (e.g., right BBB, left BBB, bifasicular block, BBB with a prolonged PR interval, alternating BBB, or second- or third-degree atrioventricular [AV] block), extreme caution is necessary when treating their depression. Cardiology is almost always involved in the care of these patients. Electrolyte abnormalities, particularly hypokalemia or hypomagnesemia, increase the danger, and patients with these abnormalities require careful monitoring.

Occasionally, the question arises whether one of the cyclic agents is less likely than another to prolong conduction, particularly when the patient already shows some intraventricular conduction delay. Maprotiline should be viewed like the TCAs regarding its cardiac conduction effects. Amoxapine has been touted as having fewer cardiac side effects, based on patients who had taken an overdose on this drug; however, atrial flutter and fibrillation have been reported in patients taking amoxapine. Trazodone does not prolong conduction in the His-Purkinje system, but aggravation of the pre-existing ventricular irritability has been reported. Hence, clinical caution should not be abandoned.

MAOIs are remarkably free of arrhythmogenic effects, although there are several case reports of atrial flutter or fibrillation, or both, with the use of tranylcypromine. Consultees tend to dread MAOIs, however, fearing drug and food interactions.

How, then, should the consulting psychiatrist approach the depressed patient with conduction disease? Depression can itself be life threatening and be more damaging to cardiac function than a drug. In the case of a depressed patient with cardiac conduction problems, one can begin with an SSRI, bupropion, venlafaxine, nefazodone, or mirtazapine. Should the depression not remit, reasonable options include augmentation with a psychostimulant or switching to a psychostimulant. Should the patient improve, the stimulant can be continued for as long as it is helpful. By starting with a low dosage (2.5 mg of either

dextroamphetamine or methylphenidate), one is reasonably assured that toxicity will not result. The fragile patient can have heart rate and BP monitored hourly for 4 hours after receiving the drug. If no beneficial response is noted, the next day the dosage should be raised to 5 mg (our usual starting dosage), then to 10, 15, and 20 mg on successive days, if necessary. Some response to the stimulant should be seen, even a negative one (e.g., feeling tenser, "wired," or agitated). Of course, an elevation of heart rate or BP may be a reason to stop the trial. The degree of clinical vigilance must match the clinical precariousness of the patient. Discussion of the type and intensity of monitoring takes place with the consultee.

The adage, "start low, go slow," used in the treatment of older adult patients, is also a good rule for medically unstable patients.

If the depression has left the patient dangerously ill, suicidal, or catatonic, ECT is the treatment of choice. When an antidepressant can be used, monitoring must account for both the development of a steady state (which typically takes about five half-lives of the drug) and the rate at which the dosage is being increased. When the patient requires a daily dosage increase, a daily rhythm strip may be necessary as well as another one, five half-lives after reaching the level thought to represent the therapeutic dosage. Plasma levels are especially useful when a 4- to 8-week drug trial is judged worthwhile. Reliable levels have been established only for nortriptyline hydrochloride (50–150 ng/mL), desipramine hydrochloride (>125 ng/mL), and imipramine hydrochloride (>200 ng/mL).

Myocardial Depression

Antidepressants have not been shown to impair left ventricular function significantly in depressed or non-depressed patients with either normal or impaired myocardial contractility. Even following a TCA overdose, impairment of left ventricular function is generally mild.[65] Hence, CHF is not an absolute contraindication to antidepressant therapy.[65] The patient with heart failure is far more vulnerable to OH; hence, the SSRIs, bupropion, venlafaxine, and nortriptyline, are the preferred agents.

A severely depressed patient could suffer an acute MI. Both conditions are a threat to survival, and the MI is not an absolute contraindication to antidepressant treatment. ECT or drugs may be mandatory. Using the previously mentioned principles, psychiatrists and cardiologists should combine their efforts to restore the patient's health.

Other Side Effects

Other common side effects of bupropion include anxiety and nervousness, agitation, insomnia, headache, nausea, constipation, and tremor. Bupropion is contraindicated in the treatment of patients with a seizure disorder or bulimia, because the incidence of seizures is approximately 0.4% at dosages up to 450 mg/day and it increases almost 10-fold at higher dosages.

Common side effects of venlafaxine include nausea, lack of appetite, weight loss, excessive sweating, nervousness, insomnia, sexual dysfunction, sedation, fatigue, headache, and dizziness.

Mirtazapine's side effects include dry mouth, constipation, weight gain, and dizziness. The relative lack of significant drug-drug interactions with other antidepressants makes mirtazapine a good candidate for combination strategies (i.e., combining two antidepressants together at full dosages).

Trazodone's most common side effects are drowsiness, dizziness, headache, and nausea, with priapism being an extremely rare but potentially serious side effect in males.

Antidepressant Discontinuation Syndrome

Several reports have described discontinuation-emergent adverse events with abrupt cessation of SSRIs and venlafaxine, including dizziness, insomnia, nervousness, nausea, and agitation. The likelihood of developing these symptoms is inversely related to the half-life of the SSRI used because these symptoms are more likely to develop after abrupt discontinuation of paroxetine and to a lesser degree with sertraline, with few symptoms seen with fluoxetine discontinuation.

Hepatic Metabolism

Essentially all antidepressants are metabolized by the hepatic P450 microsomal enzyme system. The interactions produced by the competition of multiple drugs for these metabolic pathways are complex. For example, mirtazapine is a substrate for, but not an inhibitor of, the 2D6, 1A2, and 3A4 isoenzymes.

How long antidepressants need to be maintained in patients with MDD associated with medical illness is not known. Even though patients with primary affective disorder should be maintained on their antidepressant for more than 6 months, the same requirement is not clear for patients with MDD in medical settings. In patients with PSD, and possibly in other instances in which primary brain disease or injury appears to cause depression, antidepressants should be continued for 6 months or longer.

BIPOLAR DISORDER

Overview

Bipolar disorder (BPD) lies on a spectrum; it is characterized by periods of depressed or elevated/irritable mood that last for weeks to years. Sometimes referred to as manic-depressive illness or manic-depressive disorder, it is traditionally considered a recurrent illness, although a growing body of evidence suggests that symptoms are chronic in many patients. The defining features of BPD are manic or hypomanic episodes; however, depressive symptoms contribute to most of the disabilities associated with this illness.

Epidemiology and Risk Factors

The National Co-morbidity Survey—Replication (NCS-R) study estimated a lifetime prevalence of 1% for bipolar I disorder and 1.1% for bipolar II disorder.[66] A previous population-based survey estimated the prevalence of BPD at 3.4% to 3.7%.[67] In the NCS-R, the prevalence of "sub-threshold" BPD—that is, two or more core features of hypomania, without meeting criteria for BPD—was estimated at 2.4%. With this broader definition, the prevalence of all "bipolar spectrum" disorders has reached 4.4%.

The prevalence of BPD is similar for males and females [68] although sex differences may exist in illness features. The risk for BPD also appears to be similar across racial groups and geographical regions. The NCS-R survey found no differences in the prevalence of BPD by race/ethnicity or by socioeconomic status (defined by family income).[66]

The strongest established risk factor for BPD is a family history of BPD. Individuals with a first-degree relative (a parent or sibling) with BPD have a risk of approximately 7 to 10 times that of those in the general population. Importantly, however, their risk for MDD is also increased more than twofold; given the greater prevalence of MDD, this means that family members of individuals with BPD are at greater risk for MDD than BPD, although many people diagnosed with MDD simply have unrecognized BPD.

Several putative environmental risks have been described for BPD[69]; these include pregnancy and obstetrical complications, season of birth (winter or spring birth, perhaps indicating maternal exposure to infection), stressful life events, traumatic brain injuries (TBIs), and multiple sclerosis (MS). In MS, for example, the prevalence of BPD is roughly doubled; this increase does not appear to result from adverse effects of pharmacotherapy. The prevalence may also be increased among individuals with certain neurological disorders, including epilepsy.

Clinical Features and Phenomenology

BPD is characterized by the presence of mood episodes—periods of change in mood and energy with associated symptoms. These episodes are described as depressive, hypomanic, manic, or mixed depending on the predominant mood and the nature of associated symptoms. Criteria for each mood state are included in the DSM-5.[35] The key feature for the diagnosis of BPD is the presence of at least one period of mood elevation or significant irritability meeting criteria for a manic, mixed, or hypomanic episode. These episodes typically recur over time.

A manic episode is identified when an individual experiences an elevated or irritable mood for at least 1 week, along with at least three associated symptoms (i.e., increased self-esteem or grandiosity, a decreased need for sleep, talking more than usual or feeling pressure to keep talking, racing thoughts, distractibility, an increase in goal-directed activity or psychomotor agitation, and engaging in more pleasurable activities that are associated with a high possibility for undesired consequences).

An important change in the DSM-5 requires the presence of increased activity or energy as a core criterion, to improve diagnostic specificity. If the predominant affect is irritable, four rather than three associated symptoms are required. If the symptoms

result in hospitalization at any point, the 1-week criterion is not required—for example, a patient hospitalized after 3 days of manic symptoms is still considered to have experienced a manic episode. As with episodes of MDD, DSM-5 criteria also require that symptoms markedly impair occupational or social function or be associated with psychotic symptoms.

The reliability of a bipolar I diagnosis was modest in DSM-5 field trials, with a kappa of 0.56. Hypomanic symptoms are generally like those of mania, but less severe and impairing. DSM-5 criteria require at least 4 days of mood elevation or irritability, along with associated symptoms; as with mania, required core symptoms now include an increase in energy or activity.

Three important, but often overlooked, aspects of these criteria bear highlighting. First, symptoms must be observed by others—that is, a purely subjective report of hypomania is not enough for a diagnosis. Second, symptoms represent a change from the individual's baseline; those who are "always" cheerful, impulsive, and talkative are not considered chronically hypomanic. Third, symptoms do not cause significant functional impairment—hypomanic-like symptoms that lead to the loss of a job, for example, could be considered mania.

An MDE in the context of bipolar illness is defined exactly as it is in MDD. DSM-5 also includes a modifier—"with mixed features"—recognizing the common co-occurrence of manic and depressive features, setting a lower threshold than the full criteria for each episode type.

Having identified the presence and type of current and past mood episodes, the clinician may then categorize the type of mood disorder and make a diagnosis as follows: (1) Individuals with at least one manic or mixed episode (with or without a prior depressive episode) are considered to have bipolar I disorder; (2) Individuals with at least one hypomanic and one depressive episode, but never a manic episode, are considered to have bipolar II disorder. In practice, the prevalence of hypomania without a single depressive episode is quite rare.

Individuals with persistent mood instability who never meet the full criteria for BPD or MDD are considered to have *cyclothymia*, a heterogeneous diagnosis whose relationship to other diagnostic categories is poorly understood. Specific criteria include at least 2 years marked by periods with hypomanic symptoms that do not meet the criteria for a hypomanic episode, as well as periods of depressed mood that do not meet the criteria for an MDE and no more than 2 months without symptoms. Other specified bipolar and related disorders may be diagnosed in individuals with features of BPD (including mood elevation or depression) who do not meet the criteria for another bipolar diagnosis (for example, where too few symptoms of hypomania are present).

ASSOCIATED ILLNESS FEATURES

Bipolar I versus II

The distinction between bipolar I and II disorder was initially described in 1976, based on apparent stable differences in the illness course. Indeed, modern studies suggest that the transition from bipolar II to bipolar I among adult patients is rare.[70] Some studies suggest that bipolar II patients experience more frequent episodes and have a greater risk for rapid cycling,[71] as well as a greater burden of depressive symptoms.[72] These differences belie the common misconception that bipolar II is less disabling than bipolar I.

Psychosis

Psychosis is not represented in the diagnostic features of BPD. However, psychotic symptoms are common during both manic/mixed and depressive episodes. A recent meta-analytic review suggests that the pooled lifetime prevalence of psychotic symptoms is 63% in those with bipolar I disorder.[73] So-called "mood-congruent" psychotic symptoms are often seen—for example, grandiose delusions during mania or delusions of decay and doom during depression. Psychosis among patients with BPD should resolve along with mood symptoms.

Suicide

Thoughts of suicide and suicide attempts are also not required for diagnosing BPD, although they are among the criteria for a depressive episode. In one large cohort of patients with bipolar I and II, between 25% and 50% reported at least one lifetime suicide attempt.[74] In population-based studies, the risk of death from suicide among patients with BPD is estimated at between 10 and 25 times that of the general population, like that observed in MDD.[75]

Cognitive Symptoms

BPD is often characterized by cognitive deficits that frequently persist after remission, with up to 60% of remitted patients demonstrating reduced performance in at least one cognitive domain relative to healthy comparisons.[76] The most pronounced difficulties are typically with attention, processing speed, and executive functioning, and more variably, the strategic aspects of learning and memory skills, which also involve engaging attention and executive functioning. Cognitive deficits can have a negative impact on functioning in daily life, but there are no approved treatments specifically for cognitive symptoms in BPD. In addition, many commonly used pharmacotherapies for BPD (e.g., anticonvulsants, antipsychotics) can have cognitive side effects, whereas lithium was recently observed to be beneficial for cognitive functioning.[77]

FEATURES OF LONGITUDINAL COURSE

Age at Onset and Prodrome

In a large cohort study of adults with BPD, nearly one-third of individuals reported the onset of symptoms before age 13, and another third became symptomatic between the ages of 13 and 18 years.[74] In this study, earlier onset was associated with a more chronic and recurrent course, greater functional impairment, and greater Axis I co-morbidity. Unfortunately, most such studies rely on retrospective reporting and have frequently failed to distinguish between the onset of mood symptoms and the onset of a syndromal mood episode. In the NCS-R survey, the mean age at onset for bipolar I disorder was 18.2 years, and for bipolar II disorder, it was 20.3 years.[66] However, one systematic review suggested that the age of onset did not reliably differentiate between bipolar I and bipolar II disorder, and that this variable should be considered in the context of other clinical features.[78]

Mood Episodes and Chronicity

For many patients, BPD symptoms may be chronic and persist beyond discrete episodes. In general, while hypomania and mania are considered the defining features of BPD, patients spend a far greater amount of time ill—around two-thirds of the time—with depressive symptoms. In general, the persistence of sub-syndromal symptoms appears common, which may explain in part the persistence of functional impairment as well.

Up to 40% of patients with bipolar I disorder experience a mixed state at some point in their disease course.[79] Recently, the concept of sub-threshold mixed states has received increasing attention: patients who do not meet the stringent criteria for a mixed state (who do not meet criteria for both a manic and a depressive episode simultaneously), but nonetheless have some degree of both types of symptoms. Depressive symptoms are common during manic or hypomanic episodes, underscoring the importance of inquiring about both poles. Conversely, during depressive episodes, patients may experience some degree of hypomanic symptoms, such as racing thoughts. The change in DSM-5 to incorporate mixed symptoms as modifiers of a manic or depressive episode rather than distinct states is an effort to better capture such symptoms.

Rapid Cycling

DSM-5 criteria describe rapid cycling as a specifier in BPD—that is, an illness feature that may be present at times, but it is not necessarily present throughout the course of the illness. Specifically, individuals with at least four mood episodes (major depressive, manic, or hypomanic) within a single year, separated by full recovery or a switch to the opposite pole, are considered to experience rapid cycling. According to a systematic review, the lifetime prevalence of rapid cycling among patients with BPD ranges from 25.8% to 43% and is likely related to a poorer illness course.[80]

Antidepressant-Induced Mania/Hypomania

Some patients with depression experience the onset of mania or hypomania after the initiation of an antidepressant. This presents two separate questions for the clinician. Does the individual have BPD triggered by the antidepressant, or is the mood change only due to the antidepressant and will it resolve with its discontinuation? DSM-5 considers those who develop a full manic episode following antidepressant treatment as BPD. However, many patients do not experience the

full spectrum of symptoms and the symptoms resolve when the antidepressant is stopped. The true prevalence and time course of this phenomenon are difficult to estimate, particularly for a switch to hypomania, because in clinical practice and randomized controlled trials (RCTs), such symptoms of elevated mood may not be investigated aggressively. Most short-term randomized trials of antidepressants report very low rates of mood conversion, but a large meta-analysis of reports of mood switches while on antidepressants, found a switch rate of over 8%, with the highest risk being in the first 2 years.[81] Adding an antidepressant for a patient with BPD on a mood stabilizer or antipsychotic was not associated with an increase in the rate of emerging mania or hypomania in the acute phase of treatment, but the risk significantly increased over the course of a year.[82] Transitions, even in patients taking antidepressants, may also represent part of the natural history of BPD.

Importantly, the switch must be discriminated from the resolution of depressive symptoms; manic/hypomanic symptoms must be present. Again, close longitudinal follow-up may be required to clarify the diagnosis. Even among patients with BPD, induction of a switch with one antidepressant does not necessarily imply that there will be an induction with a switch to another agent. Still, in general, patients with an antidepressant-induced mood elevation that does not resolve shortly after discontinuation of the antidepressant require close monitoring and potential treatment with mood-stabilizing or antipsychotic medications.

EVALUATION, TESTING, AND LABORATORY WORK-UP

Diagnosis of Bipolar Disorder

The diagnosis of BPD relies on a careful clinical assessment to identify current or past manic, hypomanic, mixed, or MDEs. Several tools have been developed to facilitate diagnosis, but none is a substitute for detailed questioning about the mood and associated symptoms for each episode type.

A crucial and often overlooked aspect of diagnosis in BPD is the importance of longitudinal assessment. Despite careful history taking, in the setting of an acute episode, it may be difficult to arrive at a definitive diagnosis. For example, a depressed patient may report "always" being depressed and fail to recall periods of mood elevation consistent with hypomania.

In assessing symptoms of BPD, it is essential to take a detailed history that assesses not only current episodes of depression and hypomania but also potential historical episodes of depression and hypomania. One common error in clinical practice is to establish a diagnosis that is based solely on current symptoms, as it is possible for someone to meet the criteria for BPD based on past episodes of mania and hypomania.

Differential Diagnosis

The following sections review specific diagnoses to be considered in the differential diagnosis for BPD, but several principles apply broadly. First, diagnosis requires the identification of mood episodes, not simply isolated symptoms of mania or depression. Second, longitudinal follow-up is often the key to clarifying the diagnosis. While difficult to implement in practice, a willingness by the clinician to make a provisional diagnosis, and to re-visit it once additional data have been gathered, eliminates some of the misplaced pressure to make an immediate diagnosis with inadequate data.

Schizophrenia and Schizoaffective Disorder

While psychosis is common among patients with BPD, the key feature that distinguishes schizophrenia and BPD is the presence of psychotic symptoms outside of mood episodes, which is not seen in BPD. In acutely psychotic and agitated patients, it may be difficult to distinguish a psychotic episode associated with schizophrenia from a bipolar mixed state. In such cases, longitudinal follow-up is required to clarify the diagnosis: in a patient with BPD, psychotic symptoms should resolve along with mood symptoms.

Patients with schizoaffective disorder, like patients with BPD, may experience both depressive and manic episodes. However, psychotic symptoms (e.g., delusions or hallucinations) that occur in the absence of prominent mood symptoms (i.e., depressive or hypomanic symptoms) for 2 weeks or longer would be consistent with schizoaffective disorder rather than with BPD.

Major Depressive Disorder

The primary distinguishing feature between MDD and BPD is the presence of a current or past manic or hypomanic episode. As such, to distinguish MDD from BPD, it is important to assess for both current and past episodes of mood elevation (mania or hypomania) as well as for mixed episodes.

Some symptoms may be common among people with BPD but are also present in MDD and thus are not diagnostic. For instance, the symptom of irritability should prompt further questioning for mixed/manic symptoms (given the potential presence of irritability during manic or hypomanic episodes), but the high prevalence of irritability during depressive episodes again mandates that this symptom not be relied on to make a diagnosis. Psychotic features may be more commonly seen in BPD than in MDD, although here too they are not diagnostic, as symptoms of psychosis may also occur in MDD.

Among other risk factors, perhaps the best characterized is a family history of BPD. Thus, all evaluations should inquire about a psychiatric family history. Another well-investigated risk factor is an early age of illness onset. In general, the median age of onset for MDD is later than for BPD. Therefore, those with an earlier onset of mood symptoms—particularly with an onset in childhood or adolescence—must be followed closely for BPD.

Anxiety and Related Disorders

Anxiety and related disorders—including panic disorder, generalized anxiety disorder, social anxiety disorder, post-traumatic stress disorder (PTSD), specific phobia, OCD, and agoraphobia—are among the most common psychiatric co-morbidities in BPD, with one recent meta-analytic review finding the lifetime prevalence of any anxiety disorder in BPD to be 42.7%.[83] As a caveat, patients with severe anxiety may report symptoms suggestive of mania or hypomania—particularly racing thoughts or psychomotor restlessness. These symptoms in patients without BPD are often intermittent and do not coincide with periods of mood elevation.

Substance Use Disorders

Substance use disorders (SUDs) are highly prevalent among individuals with BPD and the causal directionality of symptoms is not always clear. Determining that a patient has a SUD does not end the need for screening for BPD, and vice versa. SUDs associated with the highest prevalence rates in treatment-seeking patients with BPD are related to the use of alcohol (42%), cannabis (20%), and other illicit drugs (17%).[84] A factor that complicates the recognition of BPD is that abused substances may cause symptoms that mimic depression, mania, and mixed states. For example, cocaine binges not only represent risk-seeking behavior but are also associated with a decreased need for sleep, pressured speech, increased social behavior, and increased impulsivity in other domains. Likewise, impulsivity during a period of mood elevation may increase the likelihood of substance misuse.

Traditional teaching holds that BPD may be recognized among patients with SUDs by identifying mood episodes during periods of sobriety—if sobriety can be attained long enough to detect a "pure" mood episode, which is not always the case. However, mood symptoms among individuals without BPD are typically confined to and change in parallel with, periods of substance intoxication or withdrawal: a patient might be agitated and euphoric during a cocaine binge, but these symptoms would be unlikely to persist for days after the last cocaine use. In practice, definitively identifying BPD in a patient with frequent and severe substance use can be difficult. Substance use should always be addressed simultaneously with BPD as it leads to an overall worse outcome.

Borderline Personality Disorder

Many symptoms overlap between the DSM-5 definitions of BPD and borderline personality disorder. Notable features in common include irritability, lability, impulsivity, and suicidality. These features may be particularly difficult to distinguish in a patient believed to have current rapid cycling, with rapid fluctuations in mood state. However, several aspects of the presentation bear consideration. First, symptoms of personality disorders are typically more pervasive and less episodic; while they may wax and wane, they would typically not "remit" in the way a mood episode would. Second, while patients with a borderline personality may satisfy multiple manic or depressive criteria, they would be unlikely to meet the full criteria for a hypomanic or manic episode. However, borderline personality disorder and BPD are highly co-morbid; according to one review, 20% of participants across 70 studies met the criteria for co-morbid BPD and borderline personality disorder.[85]

Secondary Mania

In 1978 a group of clinicians described a small cohort of patients who developed manic symptoms in the context of medical illness, particularly after exposure to certain medications, such as corticosteroids. Typically, in such cases, there are other clues that the culprit is not BPD per se: late onset in a patient with no prior mood symptoms, close temporal correlation with a previously implicated medication, or presence of other neurological or systemic symptoms. Further medical work-up is often warranted when such features are present.

CONSEQUENCES OF MISDIAGNOSIS

Some pharmacotherapies for BPD may be effective for other disorders, but a patient incorrectly diagnosed with BPD is likely to receive sub-optimal treatment. Moreover, these pharmacotherapies all carry some degree of potential toxicity, to which these patients may be unnecessarily exposed. On the other hand, a patient whose diagnosis of BPD is missed is also likely to receive sub-optimal treatment because it is less likely that they will be started on a gold standard treatment regimen for BPD. Overall, the risks of misdiagnosis highlight the importance of careful screening and assessment for BPD.

TREATMENT STRATEGIES

Treatment strategies are typically divided into two stages: an acute phase (focused on eliminating or managing acute symptoms) and a maintenance phase (focused on prevention of recurrence and maximization of function). To some extent, this dichotomy is false: acute treatments are often selected with an eye toward future use in maintenance, while maintenance treatments often require adjustment to manage residual or sub-threshold symptoms. Still, it provides a useful framework for consideration of treatment options and helps patients better understand the duration and course of treatment, particularly for those early in the course of their illness.

Multiple guidelines or algorithms have been developed to aid clinicians in the evidence-based treatment of BPD. Using a chronic disease management model, most guidelines emphasize the value of psychoeducation of patients and families about the illness, recognizing and systematically monitoring symptoms, and making sure that patients understand and adhere to treatment. Regarding pharmacotherapy, recommendations are remarkably consistent. The guidelines generally take a step-by-step algorithmic approach, summarize the available data, and assign a level of certainty to their recommendations.

Traditional discussions of bipolar pharmacotherapy rely on the concept of a mood stabilizer, typically short-hand for lithium, valproate, and in some cases carbamazepine. With the broadening of the bipolar pharmacopoeia, particularly the growth of atypical antipsychotics with indications for treatment of mania, depression, or maintenance therapy, the term "mood stabilizer" is more difficult to define. Evidence-based interventions will be discussed in terms of their efficacy in achieving specific treatment goals: acute treatment versus prevention of recurrence, and alleviation of depression versus mania.

Approach to Manic and Mixed States

As with any acute episode, the first element of managing mania is to ensure the safety of patients and those around them; this may require hospitalization. Medical contributors (including drugs of abuse) to mania should be ruled out. Antidepressants or stimulants, which may precipitate or exacerbate mania, should be discontinued.

Multiple first-line agents have been established for mania. Those with the greatest evidence of efficacy include lithium, valproate, and several second-generation antipsychotics (SGAs). Among the SGAs, CANMAT guidelines place quetiapine, asenapine, aripiprazole, paliperidone, risperidone, and cariprazine as first-line interventions. Carbamazepine, olanzapine, ziprasidone, and the first-generation antipsychotic (FGA), haloperidol, are considered second-line options, as well as brexpiprazole, lurasidone, and lumateperone. The choice reflects tolerability since there is little evidence that various antipsychotics have different efficacy. Whether the antipsychotics are used alone or in combination with lithium or valproate typically depends on the severity of illnesses—combination therapy may have modestly greater efficacy. If a single pharmacotherapy does not achieve improvement within a short period, a second one may be added, or the patient may be switched to an alternative first line agent. ECT or clozapine are reserved for cases who do not respond to these options and generally gabapentin, topiramate, and lamotrigine are not efficacious in acute treatment. Benzodiazepines are sometimes used as adjunctive treatments for manic patients, specifically to reduce agitation and promote sleep; they have shown greater efficacy than placebo in RCTs for agitation.

A question of substantial clinical interest has been whether combining multiple anti-manic agents achieves a better response than monotherapy. Meta-analyses suggest a modest advantage in efficacy for combination therapy, although this must be weighed against an increase in adverse effects.[86] In general, monotherapy is preferred for less ill patients, whereas combination therapy is used for those who are more ill (e.g., hospitalized).

The approach to mixed states generally follows that of mania. While one study suggested that lithium might be less effective in these patients than in those with euphoric mania, this is by no means a consistent finding.

Approach to Depression

Efficacy for lithium, valproate, and carbamazepine has been suggested, but not definitively established, in RCTs. Multiple SGAs, including quetiapine and olanzapine (the latter in combination with fluoxetine), as well as lurasidone, cariprazine, and lumateperone were more effective than placebo.[87–89] The anticonvulsant lamotrigine has also been extensively studied in bipolar depression and found to have modest benefits for acute depression.[90]

Most guidelines agree that antidepressant monotherapy is not recommended, particularly for patients with bipolar I disorder. However, in a meta-analysis that included 1383 patients, adding a second-generation antidepressant to a mood stabilizer or an antipsychotic was associated with a small but statistically significant improvement in clinician-rated depressive symptom scores when compared to placebo, but no difference in response and remission rates. The risk of a switch to mania was not increased during the acute phase of treatment but it did increase by 52 weeks.[91] This indicates that some patients with BPD may benefit from adding an antidepressant to their mood stabilizer or SGA. If possible, the antidepressant should be discontinued once the episode has resolved to avoid future mood instability.

Approach to Maintenance Treatment

The goals during maintenance are preventing the recurrence of symptoms and improving functioning. Critical to this is adherence to the treatment regimen. Stopping medications is the main reason for symptom recurrence. Clinicians should avoid using judgmental or critical language when inquiring about treatment adherence. Understanding reasons for non-adherence, such as side effects, is also very important. If symptoms recur, clinicians should evaluate for co-morbidities, such as SUDs or anxiety disorders. Pharmacologically, most studies of lithium and valproate suggest that they are effective in the prevention of recurrence of mood episodes. The optimum therapeutic dose of each, and their relative benefit for prevention of manic versus depressive recurrence, is debated. Two RCTs also found efficacy for lamotrigine in the prevention of depressive recurrence.[92] Evidence of benefit in preventing manic recurrence was much more modest. Numerous SGAs have also been shown to prevent the recurrence of mood episodes. Despite the efficacy of these interventions, BPD remains highly recurrent for many patients, with residual mood symptoms as one of the primary risk factors.

As in acute treatment, the role of antidepressants in maintenance is not established. As noted previously, antidepressants may contribute to an increase in mood episode frequency. On the other hand, one study suggested that discontinuing antidepressants among patients who achieved remission was associated with a greater risk of recurrence. In practice, most guidelines suggest avoiding antidepressants in long-term treatment, when possible. Long-term benzodiazepine treatment has also been suggested to increase recurrence risk.[93]

Use of Psychosocial Interventions

Several trials have evaluated psychosocial interventions alongside pharmacotherapy for improving acute mood episodes and reducing mood episode recurrences. A recent meta-analytic review evaluating 39 RCTs suggested that skills-based psychological interventions can improve outcomes among individuals with BPD when administered alongside pharmacotherapy.[94] Specifically, there is strong support for an adjunctive group or family-based psychoeducation (compared to individual psychoeducation) involving the active practice of illness management tools in reducing mood episode recurrences. There is also strong support for CBT (compared to treatment-as-usual) for stabilizing depressive symptoms.[94]

SPECIAL CONSIDERATIONS IN TREATMENT

Psychotic Symptoms

Psychotic symptoms are common during both manic and depressive episodes. Typical management involves the use of an antipsychotic, with or without a mood stabilizer. Historically, FGAs would be tapered following the acute psychotic episode. However, several SGAs show efficacy for the maintenance phase of illness, either as monotherapy or with a mood stabilizer. Psychotic symptoms that remain after mood symptoms have resolved are indicative of a diagnosis of schizoaffective disorder, rather than BPD.

Bipolar II

Most RCTs in BPD have focused on patients with bipolar I disorder. Treatment recommendations therefore suggest the same approach to both bipolar I and II. Some treatment guidelines include antidepressant monotherapy as an option (not as first-line care) for depressive episodes in bipolar II disorder, given that the risk of mood switching is lower. They suggest caution in escalating the dose and monitoring for worsening symptoms while avoiding it in patients with mixed features or rapid cycling.[95] Some of the newer atypical antipsychotics have shown effectiveness in bipolar II depression.[89]

Pregnancy

Most studies find that, on average, recurrence risk neither increases nor decreases during pregnancy. The post-partum period, however, is a period of dramatically increased risk for recurrence, and patients with BPD are at particular risk for post-partum psychosis. Whether this is a result of hormonal changes or other factors (such as sleep disruption) during the post-partum period has not been well studied. Treatment of BPD during pregnancy is beyond the scope of this chapter. In general, all pharmacological treatment strategies carry some risk to the fetus, although data from the Massachusetts General Hospital national pregnancy registry for atypical antipsychotics, agents that are commonly used in BPD, indicate that the SGAs as a class are unlikely to have a major teratogenic effect.[96] Any risk of treatment must be balanced against the substantial consequences of recurrence during or after pregnancy.

Childhood, Adolescence, and Geriatric Patients

Retrospective studies in adults make it clear that many individuals with BPD were symptomatic before age 18. Lithium and many of the SGAs (e.g., aripiprazole, asenapine, lurasidone, olanzapine, quetiapine, risperidone) have Food and Drug Administration (FDA) approval for use in youth for mania. Options for depression remain more limited (lurasidone).

In geriatric populations, standard treatment approaches are generally adopted but with more attention paid to potential toxicities. Lithium, for example, maybe used at lower target levels, recognizing that brain levels may correspond poorly to plasma levels in this group. Notably, pharmacovigilance studies suggest that atypical antipsychotics may increase the risk of death among older patients, particularly those with dementia,[97] so use of SGAs requires more caution here.

PROGNOSIS

By comparison with other chronic and recurrent medical illnesses, remarkably few data exist to guide clinicians in the estimation of prognosis. Some factors associated with worse outcomes in BPD include the presence of sub-syndromal depressive symptoms, longer duration of illness, a history of psychosis, and co-morbid substance use or personality disorders.

An open question is whether interventions targeting those prognostic factors that may be modifiable might improve outcomes. For example, more aggressive treatment of residual mood symptoms to target remission, as has been emphasized in MDD, might reduce recurrence risk, though this has not been formally studied.

MEDICAL CO-MORBIDITY AMONG PATIENTS WITH BPD

A persistent concern is the observation that patients with BPD are at elevated risk of morbidity and mortality from multiple causes, not only suicide. For example, they show elevated incidences of cardiovascular risk factors (including obesity, hyperlipidemia, and diabetes), with risk compounded by greater rates of tobacco use compared to the general population. Several explanations have been suggested for this co-morbidity: it may be another feature of the disorder itself or a consequence of poorer health maintenance arising from chronic illness. Moreover, many first-line treatments for BPD can precipitate or exacerbate these risk factors.

CONCLUSIONS

The recognition, diagnosis, and treatment of MDD and bipolar disorder has tremendous public health significance. These are prevalent, serious conditions associated with significant suffering and disability. The main challenges in the recognition and diagnosis of these disorders are that these conditions are manifest by a constellation of psychological, behavioral, and physical symptoms and, at the same time, they often co-occur with other psychiatric and non-psychiatric medical disorders. Finally, it is important to remember that the continuum of mood disorders from mild, short-lasting, syndromes toward severe, chronic/recurrent and disabling disorders has been repeatedly stressed.[98,99]

REFERENCES

1. Ferrari AJ, Santomauro DF, Herrera AM, et al. Global, regional, and national burden of 12 mental disorders in 204 countries and territories, 1990–2019: a systematic analysis for the Global Burden of Disease Study 2019. *Lancet Psychiatry*. 2022;9:137–150.
2. Kessler RC, Berglund P, Demler O, et al. The epidemiology of major depressive disorder: results from the National Comorbidity Survey Replication (NCS-R). *JAMA*. 2003;289:3095–3105.
3. Regier DA, Goldberg ID, Taube CA. The de facto U.S. Mental Health Services systems. *Arch Gen Psychiatry*. 1978;35:685–693.
4. Wells KB, Sturm R, Sherbourne CD, et al. *Caring for Depression*. Harvard University Press; 1996.
5. Lepine JP, Gastpar M, Mendlewicz J, et al. Depression in the community: the first pan-European study DEPRES [Depression Research in European Society]. *Int Clin Psychopharmacol*. 1997;12:19–29.

6. Wells KB, Stewart A, Hays RD, et al. The functioning and well-being of depressed patients. Results from the Medical Outcomes Study. *JAMA*. 1989;262:914–919.

7. Charney DS, Manji HK. Life stress, genes, and depression: multiple pathways lead to increased risk and new opportunities for intervention. *Sci STKE*. 2004 16:re5.

8. Fava M, Kendler K. Major depressive disorder. *Neuron*. 2000;28:335–341.

9. Major Depressive Disorder Working Group of the Psychiatric GWAS Consortium A mega-analysis of genome-wide association studies for major depressive disorder. *Mol Psychiatry*. 2013;18: 497–511.

10. Greden JF. The burden of recurrent depression: causes, consequences, and future prospects. *J Clin Psychiatry*. 2001;62(suppl 22): 5–9.

11. Zheng D, Macera CA, Croft JB, et al. Major depression and all-cause mortality among white adults in the United States. *Ann Epidemiol*. 1997;7:213–218.

12. Penninx BW, Geerlings SW, Deeg DJ, et al. Minor and major depression and the risk of death in older persons. *Arch Gen Psychiatry*. 1999;56:889–895.

13. Frasure-Smith N, Lesperance F. Recent evidence linking coronary heart disease and depression. *Can J Psychiatry*. 2006;51:730–737.

14. Anderson RJ, Freedland KE, Clouse RE, et al. The prevalence of comorbid depression in adults with diabetes: a meta-analysis. *Diabetes Care*. 2001;24:1069–1078.

15. Gavard JA, Lustman PJ, Clouse RE. Prevalence of depression in adults with diabetes: an epidemiological evaluation. *Diabetes Care*. 1993;16:1167–1178.

16. Wyatt SB, Winters KP, Dubbert PM. Overweight and obesity: prevalence, consequences, and causes of a growing public health problem. *Am J Med Sci*. 2006;331:166–174.

17. Wells KB, Rogers W, Burnam A, et al. How the medical comorbidity of depressed patients differs across health care settings: results from the Medical Outcomes Study. *Am J Psychiatry*. 1991;148:1688–1696.

18. Cassem EH. Depression and anxiety secondary to medical illness. *Psychiatr Clin North Am*. 1990;13:597–612.

19. Tufo HM, Ostfeld AM, Shekelle R. Central nervous system dysfunction following open-heart surgery. *JAMA*. 1970;212:1333.

20. Silverstone PH. Depression and outcome in acute myocardial infarction. *BMJ*. 1987;294:219–220.

21. Rabins PV, Harvis K, Koven S. High fatality rates of late-life depression associated with cardiovascular disease. *J Affect Disord*. 1985;9:165–167.

22. Pennix BW, Beekman AT, Honig AT, et al. Depression and cardiac mortality: results from a community-based longitudinal study. *Arch Gen Psychiatry*. 2001;58:221–227.

23. De Groot M, Anderson R, Freedland KE, et al. Association of depression and diabetes complications: a meta-analysis. *Psychosom Med*. 2001;63:619–630.

24. Black SA, Markides KS. Depressive symptoms and mortality in older Mexican Americans. *Ann Epidemiol*. 1999;9:45–52.

25. Ciechanowski PS, Katon WJ, Russo JE. Depression and diabetes: impact of depressive symptoms on adherence, function, and costs. *Arch Intern Med*. 2000;160:3278–3285.

26. Covinsky KE, Fortinsky RH, Palmer PM, et al. Relation between symptoms of depression and health status outcomes in acutely ill hospitalized older persons. *Ann Intern Med*. 1997;126: 417–425.

27. Reynolds CF, Alexopoulos GS, Katz IR, et al. Chronic depression in the elderly: approaches for prevention. *Drugs Aging*. 2001;18: 507–514.

28. Prieto JM, Atala J, Blanch J, et al. Role of depression as a predictor of mortality among cancer patients after stem-cell transplantation. *J Clin Oncol*. 2005;23:6063–6071.

29. Lepine JP, Gastpar M, Mendlewicz J, et al. Depression in the community: the first pan-European study DEPRES [Depression Research in European Society. *Int Clin Psychopharmacol*. 1997;12:19–29.

30. Lustman PJ, Griffith LS, Freedland KE, et al. The course of major depression in diabetes. *Gen Hosp Psychiatry*. 1997;19:138–143.

31. Kovacs M, Goldston D, Obrosky DS, et al. Psychiatric disorders in youths with IDDM: rates and risk factors. *Diabetes Care*. 1997;20:36–44.

32. Fava GA, Sonino N, Morphy MA. Major depression associated with endocrine disease. *Psychiatr Dev*. 1987;5:321–348.

33. Simon GE, Vonkorff M, Barlow W. Health care costs of primary care patients with recognized depression. *Arch Gen Psychiatry*. 1995;52:850–856.

34. Hays RD, Wells KB, Sherbourne CD, et al. Functioning and well-being outcomes of patients with depression compared with chronic general medical illnesses. *Arch Gen Psychiatry*. 1995;52:11–19.

35. American Psychiatric Association. *Diagnostic and Statistical Manual of Mental Disorders*. 5th ed. American Psychiatric Association; 2013.

36. Ostergaard SD, Jensen SO, Bech P. The heterogeneity of the depressive syndrome: when numbers get serious. *Acta Psychiatr Scand*. 2011;124:495–496.

37. Fava M, Rush AJ, Alpert JE, et al. What clinical and symptom features and comorbid disorders characterize outpatients with anxious major depressive disorder: a replication and extension. *Can J Psychiatry*. 2006;51:823–835.

38. Papakostas GI, Fan H, Tedeschini E, et al. Severe and anxious depression: combining definitions of clinical sub-types to identify patients differentially responsive to selective serotonin reuptake inhibitors. *Eur Neuropsychopharmacol*. 2012;22:347–355.

39. Fava M, Rosenbaum JF. Anger attacks in patients with depression. *J Clin Psychiatry*. 1999;60(Suppl. 15):21–24.

40. Kruizinga J, Liemburg E, Burger H, et al. Pharmacological treatment for psychotic depression. *Cochrane Database Syst Rev*. 2021(12): Art. No.: CD004044.

41. Long TD, Kathol RG. Critical review of data supporting affective disorder caused by nonpsychotropic medication. *Ann Clin Psychiatry*. 1993;5:259–270.

42. Joffe RT, Rubinow DR, Denicoff KD, et al. Depression and carcinoma of the pancreas. *Gen Hosp Psychiatry*. 1986;8: 241–245.

43. Holland JC, Korzun AH, Tross S, et al. Comparative psychological disturbance in patients with pancreatic and gastric cancer. *Am J Psychiatry*. 1986;143:982–986.

44. Morris PL, Robinson RG, Raphael B, et al. Lesion location and poststroke depression. *J Neuropsychiatry Clin Neurosci.* 1996;8:399–403.

45. Lipsey JR, Robinson RG, Pearlson GD, et al. Nortriptyline treatment of post-stroke depression: a double-blind study. *Lancet.* 1984;1:297–300.

46. Reding MJ, Orto LS, Winter SW, et al. Antidepressant therapy after stroke: a double-blind trial. *Arch Neurol.* 1986;43:763–765.

47. Murray GB, Shea V, Conn DK. Electroconvulsive therapy for poststroke depression. *J Clin Psychiatry.* 1987;47:258–260.

48. Masand P, Murray GB, Pickett P. Psychostimulants in post-stroke depression. *J Neuropsychiatry.* 1991;3:23–27.

49. Robinson RG, Schultz SK, Castillo C, et al. Nortriptyline versus fluoxetine in the treatment of depression and in short-term recovery after stroke: a placebo-controlled double-blind study. *Am J Psychiatry.* 2000;157:351–359.

50. Ross ED, Rush AJ. Diagnosis and neuroanatomical correlates of depression in brain-damaged patients. *Arch Gen Psychiatry.* 1981;38:1344–1354.

51. Zubenko GS, Moossy J, Kopp U. Neurochemical correlates of major depression in primary dementia. *Arch Neurol.* 1990;47:209–214.

52. Hachinski VC, Iliff LD, Zilhka E, et al. Cerebral blood flow in dementia. *Arch Neurol.* 1975;32:632–637.

53. Cummings JL, Miller B, Hill M, et al. Neuropsychiatric aspects of multi-infarct dementia and dementia of the Alzheimer type. *Arch Neurol.* 1987;44:389–393.

54. Folstein SE, Abbott MH, Chase GA, et al. The association of affective disorder with Huntington's disease in a case series and in families. *Psychol Med.* 1983;13:537–542.

55. Asnis G. Parkinson's disease, depression, and ECT: a review and case study. *Am J Psychiatry.* 1977;134:191–195.

56. Koralnick IJ, Beaumanoir A, Hausler R, et al. A controlled study of early neurologic abnormalities in men with asymptomatic human immunodeficiency virus infection. *N Engl J Med.* 1990;323:864–870.

57. Perry S, Jacobsberg LB, Fishman B, et al. Psychiatric diagnosis before serological testing for human immunodeficiency virus. *Am J Psychiatry.* 1990;147:89–93.

58. Fernandez F, Adams F, Levy JK, et al. Cognitive impairment due to AIDS-related complex and its response to psychostimulants. *Psychosomatics.* 1988;29:38–46.

59. Rabkin JG, Wagner GJ, Rabkin R. Fluoxetine treatment for depression in patients with HIV and AIDS: a randomized, placebo-controlled trial. *Am J Psychiatry.* 1999;156:101–107.

60. Currier MB, Molina G, Kato M. A prospective trial of sustained-release bupropion for depression in HIV-seropositive and AIDS patients. *Psychosomatics.* 2003;44:120–125.

61. Robinson DS, Barker E. Tricyclic antidepressant cardiotoxicity. *JAMA.* 1976;236:1089–1090.

62. Stack JA, Reynolds CF, Perel JM, et al. Pretreatment systolic orthostatic blood pressure (PSOP) and treatment response in elderly depressed inpatients. *J Clin Psychopharmacol.* 1988;8:116–120.

63. Roose SP, Glassman AH. Cardiovascular effects of tricyclic antidepressants in depressed patients with and without heart disease. *J Clin Psychiatry Monogr.* 1989;7:1–18.

64. Roose SP, Glassman AH, Siris S, et al. Comparison of imipramine and nortriptyline-induced orthostatic hypotension: a meaningful difference. *J Clin Psychopharmacol.* 1981;1:316–319.

65. Glassman AH, Johnson LL, Giardina E-GV, et al. The use of imipramine in depressed patients with congestive heart failure. *JAMA.* 1983;250:1997–2001.

66. Merikangas KR, Akiskal HS, Angst J, et al. Lifetime and 12-month prevalence of bipolar spectrum disorder in the National Comorbidity Survey replication. *Arch Gen Psychiatry.* 2007;64:543–552.

67. Hirschfeld RM, Calabrese JR, Weissman MM, et al. Screening for bipolar disorder in the community. *J Clin Psychiatry.* 2003;64:53–59.

68. Weissman MM, Bland RC, Canino GJ, et al. Cross-national epidemiology of major depression and bipolar disorder. *JAMA.* 1996;276:293–299.

69. Tsuchiya KJ, Byrne M, Mortensen PB. Risk factors in relation to an emergence of bipolar disorder: a systematic review. *Bipolar Disord.* 2003;5:231–242.

70. Coryell W, Endicott J, Maser JD, et al. Long-term stability of polarity distinctions in the affective disorders. *Am J Psychiatry.* 1995;152:385–390.

71. Baldessarini RJ, Tondo L, Floris G, et al. Effects of rapid cycling on response to lithium maintenance treatment in 360 bipolar I and II disorder patients. *J Affect Disord.* 2000;61:13–22.

72. Judd LL, Akiskal HS, Schettler PJ, et al. A prospective investigation of the natural history of the long-term weekly symptomatic status of bipolar II disorder. *Arch Gen Psychiatry.* 2003;60:261–269.

73. Aminoff SR, Onyeka IN, Ødegaard M, et al. Lifetime and point prevalence of psychotic symptoms in adults with bipolar disorders: a systematic review and meta-analysis. *Psychol Med.* 2022;52(13):1.

74. Perlis RH, Miyahara S, Marangell LB, et al. Long-term implications of early onset in bipolar disorder: data from the first 1000 participants in the systematic treatment enhancement program for bipolar disorder (STEP-BD). *Biol Psychiatry.* 2004;55:875–881.

75. Ösby U, Brandt L, Correia N, et al. Excess mortality in bipolar and unipolar disorder in Sweden. *Arch Gen Psychiatry.* 2001;58:844–850.

76. Van Rheenen TE, Lewandowski KE, Tan EJ, et al. Characterizing cognitive heterogeneity on the schizophrenia-bipolar disorder spectrum. *Psychol Med.* 2017;47:1848–1864.

77. Burdick KE, Millett CE, Russo M, et al. The association between lithium use and neurocognitive performance in patients with bipolar disorder. *Neuropsychopharmacology.* 2020;45:1743–1749.

78. Dell'Osso B, Grancini B, Vismara M, et al. Age at onset in patients with bipolar I and II disorder: a comparison of large sample studies. *J Affect Disord.* 2016;201:57–63.

79. Swann AC. Mixed or dysphoric manic states: psychopathology and treatment. *J Clin Psychiatry.* 1995

80. Carvalho AF, Dimellis D, Gonda X, et al. Rapid cycling in bipolar disorder: a systematic review. *J Clin Psychiatry.* 2014;75:e578–586.

81. Baldessarini RJ, Faedda GL, Offidani E, et al. Antidepressant-associated mood-switching and transition from unipolar

major depression to bipolar disorder: A review. *J Affect Disord.* 2013;148:129–135.

82. McGirr A, Vohringer PA, Ghaemi SN, et al. Safety and efficacy of adjunctive second-generation antidepressant therapy with a mood stabiliser or an atypical antipsychotic in acute bipolar depression: a systematic review and meta-analysis of randomised placebo-controlled trials. *Lancet Psychiatry.* 2016;3:1138–1146.

83. Nabavi B, Mitchell AJ, Nutt D. A lifetime prevalence of comorbidity between bipolar affective disorder and anxiety disorders: a meta-analysis of 52 interview-based studies of psychiatric population. *EBioMedicine.* 2015;2:1405–1419.

84. Hunt GE, Malhi GS, Cleary M, et al. Prevalence of comorbid bipolar and substance use disorders in clinical settings, 1990–2015: Systematic review and meta-analysis. *J Affect Disord.* 2016;206:331–349.

85. Frías Á, Baltasar I, Birmaher B. Comorbidity between bipolar disorder and borderline personality disorder: prevalence, explanatory theories, and clinical impact. *J Affect Disord.* 2016;202:210–219.

86. Perlis RH, Welge JA, Vornik LA, et al. Atypical antipsychotics in the treatment of mania: a meta-analysis of randomized, placebo-controlled trials. *J Clin Psychiatry.* 2006;67:509–516.

87. Loebel A, Cucchiaro J, Silva R, et al. Lurasidone monotherapy in the treatment of bipolar I depression: a randomized, double-blind, placebo-controlled study. *Am J Psychiatry.* 2014;171:160–168.

88. Durgam S, Earley W, Lipschitz A, et al. An 8-week randomized, double-blind, placebo-controlled evaluation of the safety and efficacy of cariprazine in patients with bipolar I depression. *Am J Psychiatry.* 2016;173:271–281.

89. Calabrese JR, Durgam S, Satlin A, et al. fficacy and safety of lumateperone for major depressive episodes associated with bipolar I or bipolar II disorder: a phase 3 randomized placebo-controlled trial. *Am J Psychiatry.* 2021;178:1098–1106.

90. Geddes JR, Calabrese JR, Goodwin GM. Lamotrigine for treatment of bipolar depression: independent meta-analysis and meta-regression of individual patient data from five randomised trials. *Br J Psychiatry.* 2009;194:4–9.

91. McGirr A, Vöhringer PA, Ghaemi SN, et al. Safety and efficacy of adjunctive second-generation antidepressant therapy with a mood stabiliser or an atypical antipsychotic in acute bipolar depression: a systematic review and meta-analysis of randomised placebo-controlled trials. *Lancet Psychiatry.* 2016;3:1138–1146.

92. Goodwin GM, Bowden CL, Calabrese JR, et al. A pooled analysis of 2 placebo-controlled 18-month trials of lamotrigine and lithium maintenance in bipolar I disorder. *J Clin Psychiatry.* 2004;65:432–441.

93. Perlis RH, Ostacher MJ, Miklowitz DJ, et al. Benzodiazepine use and risk of recurrence in bipolar disorder: a STEP-BD report. *J Clin Psychiatry.* 2010;71:194–200.

94. Miklowitz DJ, Efthimiou O, Furukawa TA, et al. Adjunctive psychotherapy for bipolar disorder: a systematic review and component network meta-analysis. *JAMA Psychiatry.* 2021;78:141–150.

95. Yatham LN, Kennedy SH, Parikh SV, et al. Canadian Network for Mood and Anxiety Treatments (CANMAT) and International Society for Bipolar Disorders (ISBD) 2018 guidelines for the management of patients with bipolar disorder. *Bipolar Disord.* 2018;20:97–170.

96. Viguera AC, Freeman MP, Góez-Mogollón L, et al. Reproductive safety of second-generation antipsychotics: updated data From the Massachusetts General Hospital National Pregnancy Registry for Atypical Antipsychotics. *J Clin Psychiatry.* 2021;82

97. Maust DT, Kim HM, Seyfried LS, et al. Antipsychotics, other psychotropics, and the risk of death in patients with dementia: number needed to harm. *JAMA Psychiatry.* 2015;72:438–445.

98. Kendler KS, Gardner CO. Boundaries of major depression: an evaluation of DSM-IV criteria. *Am J Psychiatry.* 1998;155:172–177.

99. Judd LL, Akiskal HS. Delineating the longitudinal structure of depressive illness: beyond clinical subtypes and duration thresholds. *Pharmacopsychiatry.* 2000;33:3–7.

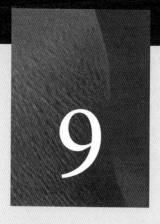

9 DELIRIUM

JASON P. CAPLAN, MD ■ THOMAS H. McCOY, JR., MD ■ NOOR
BECKWITH, MD ■ THEODORE A. STERN, MD

■ ■

OVERVIEW

Delirium may be considered something of a diagnostic chameleon, as its varied presentations can result in misdiagnoses that span almost every major category of mental illness. A syndrome caused by an underlying physiologic disturbance and marked by a fluctuating course of impairments in consciousness, attention, and perception, delirium is often mistaken for depression (when the patient has a withdrawn or flat affect); mania (when the patient has agitation and confusion); psychosis (when the patient has hallucinations and paranoia); anxiety (when the patient has restlessness and hypervigilance); dementia (when the patient has cognitive impairments); and substance abuse (when the patient has impairment in consciousness). With such a diverse array of symptoms, delirium assumes a position of diagnostic privilege in the *Diagnostic and Statistical Manual of Mental Disorders, 5th Edition, Text Revision* (DSM-5-TR),[1] in that almost no other diagnosis can be made de novo in its presence.

Sometimes, delirium is referred to as an acute confusional state, a toxic-metabolic encephalopathy, or acute brain failure; unquestionably, it is the most common cause of agitation and one of the most common triggers for psychiatric consultation in the general hospital. Clinically, delirium is a signifier of consequential somatic illness.[2] Delirium has been associated with a longer length of stay in hospitals[3] and higher costs for care.[4,5] One meta-analysis reported a delirium prevalence of 23% among all medical inpatients.[6] Among intensive care unit (ICU) patients, meta-analyses have noted that delirium occurs in 31.8% of all admissions[7]; when intubation and mechanical ventilation are required, the incidence soars to 81.7%.[2]

Case 1

Mr. J, a 67-year-old man, was admitted to the hospital for elective lumbar spine surgery in the context of chronic back pain. His medical history was significant only for hypertension and hypercholesterolemia treated with losartan and simvastatin, respectively. He had no history of psychiatric illness. His hospital course was complicated by the dehiscence of his surgical wound that required a protracted hospitalization and total bed rest.

Psychiatry was consulted on hospital day 15 to assess for depression. In speaking with the nurse practitioner from the neurosurgery service, the consultant learned that over the prior several days, Mr. J had stopped speaking with staff and family, was not allowing his vital signs to be checked, and was now refusing oral medications. The consultant spoke with the bedside nurse who confirmed these behaviors and further noted "he's just given up!"

The consultant introduced himself to Mr. J, whose response was to raise an eyebrow and turn his head away. The consultant then further explained the purpose of his visit, noting that staff and family were concerned that he may be depressed. Mr. J remained non-verbal. The consultant stated "Sometimes I speak to folks who have had the sort of surgery you have had and are on all the medications you're on and they tell me that sometimes they worry that they see things or hear things that other people don't seem to see or hear. Has anything like that happened to you?" Mr. J then turned his head back to the consultant and nodded his head in the affirmative. The consultant went on to discuss the phenomenon of delirium; that it is due to a medical illness, is not representative of a primary psychiatric illness, and the symptoms can be effectively managed. Mr. J then engaged in the interview, revealing that he had been seeing animals running through his hospital room and was worried that he was "losing my marbles." Cognitive examination revealed prominent deficits in attention and short-term memory.

A battery of laboratory studies revealed a previously undiagnosed urinary tract infection (UTI); therefore antibiotic treatment was initiated. After reviewing an electrocardiogram (ECG) to check Mr. J's QTc, haloperidol 1 mg intravenously (IV) every 6 hours was initiated with resultant resolution of Mr. J's hallucinations and improvement in his attention and memory. This regimen was tapered over the subsequent several days without re-emergence of symptoms of delirium.

DIAGNOSIS

The essential features of delirium, according to the DSM-5-TR,[1] are a disturbance of attention and awareness accompanied by cognitive deficits that develop over a short period and tend to wax and wane over the course of the day in the setting of evidence that these deficits are the direct physiologic consequences of a physiologic condition (including medical illness, substance intoxication or withdrawal, and toxin exposure). The International Classification of Diseases (ICD)-11 also includes disturbances in behavior (e.g., agitation, restlessness, impulsivity), perception (e.g., illusions, hallucinations, delusions), sleep, and emotion (e.g., anxiety, depressed mood, fear, anger, euphoria, apathy) in its diagnostic guidelines.[8] Disturbance of the sleep-wake cycle is also common, sometimes with nocturnal worsening (sundowning) or even complete reversal of the night-day cycle, although, despite previous postulation and ongoing hospital folklore, sleep disturbance alone does not cause delirium.[9] Similarly, the term *ICU psychosis* persists in the medical lexicon; this is an unfortunate and lazy misnomer because it assigns the environment of the ICU as the cause of delirium, effectively allowing the clinician to shrug off any burden of having to explore this syndrome further, and it inaccurately limits the symptomatology of delirium to psychosis.[9]

Despite wide variation in the presentation of the delirious patient, the hallmarks of delirium (although perhaps less immediately apparent) remain similar from case to case. Inattention is the *sine qua non* of delirium in that it serves to differentiate the syndrome from any other psychiatric diagnosis. This inattention (along with an acute onset, a waxing and waning course, and an overall disturbance of consciousness) forms the core of delirium, while other related symptoms (e.g., withdrawn affect, agitation, hallucinations, paranoia) serve as a "frame" that can sometimes be so prominent as to distract from the picture itself.

Psychotic symptoms (such as visual or auditory hallucinations and delusions) are common among patients with delirium.[10] Sometimes the psychiatric symptoms are so bizarre or so offensive (e.g., an enraged and paranoid patient shouts that pornographic movies are being made in the ICU) that diagnostic efforts are distracted. The delirium-inducing hypoglycemia of a man with diabetes can be missed in the emergency department if the accompanying behavior is threatening, uncooperative, and resembling that of an intoxicated person.

While agitation may distract practitioners from making an accurate diagnosis of delirium, disruptive behavior alone will almost certainly garner some attention. The DSM-5-TR includes motoric subtypes for the diagnosis of delirium (i.e., hyperactive, hypoactive, or mixed). The "hypoactive" presentation of delirium is more insidious since the patient is often thought to be depressed or anxious because of his or her medical illness. Studies of quietly delirious patients show the experience to be equally as disturbing as the agitated variant[11]; quiet delirium is still a harbinger of serious illness.[12,13] In addition to motoric specifiers, the DSM-5-TR also allows for differentiation based on chronicity with the "acute" form lasting for hours to days and the "chronic" form lasting weeks or months.

The core similarities found in cases of delirium have led to the postulation of a final common neurologic pathway for its symptoms, although none has yet been clearly proven. Multiple hypotheses, including disturbances of supplies of oxygen and glucose that result in increased oxidative stress, activation of various inflammatory pathways, and neurochemical disturbances that interrupt neural network connectivity, have all been proposed along with theories of neurotransmitter imbalance. Symptoms of delirium have long been attributed to a state of relative hyperdopaminergia and hypocholinergia.[14] The ascending reticular activating system (RAS) and its bilateral thalamic projections regulate alertness, with neocortical and limbic inputs to this system controlling attention. Because acetylcholine is the primary neurotransmitter of the RAS, medications with anticholinergic activity can interfere with its function, resulting in deficits in alertness and attention, which are the heralds of delirium. Similarly, loss of cholinergic neuronal activity in the elderly (e.g., resulting from microvascular disease or atrophy) could be the basis for their heightened risk of delirium. The release of endogenous dopamine due to oxidative stress is thought to be responsible for the perceptual disturbances and paranoia that so often lead to the mislabeling of the delirious patient as "psychotic." Moreover, dopamine could exacerbate agitation by potentiating the neuroexcitatory action of glutamate. Both cholinergic agents (e.g., physostigmine) and dopamine blockers (e.g., haloperidol) have evidence of efficacy in delirium symptom management.

Early detection of cognitive changes can be key to timely identification and treatment of delirium (and perhaps of a heretofore undiagnosed somatic illness responsible for the delirium). Unfortunately, studies have revealed that non-psychiatric physicians are quite unreliable in their ability to identify delirium accurately, and most patients referred to psychiatric consultation services with purported depression are ultimately found to have delirium.[15]

Several screening instruments can be administered by nursing staff at the bedside on a recurring basis to facilitate early identification of delirium. Of these, the Confusion Assessment Method—ICU (CAM-ICU) is probably the most broadly validated and used (and is available online at www.icudelirium.org), although many other options exist (e.g., Stanford Proxy Test for Delirium or Nursing Delirium Screening Scale).[16,17] These screening instruments can serve as a trigger to initiate psychiatric consultation and timely verification of the diagnosis and search for an underlying etiology. In addition to bedside screening, health record–driven risk stratification for delirium is possible[18,19] although

model performance varies widely with specificity between 0.50 and 0.97 and sensitivity between 0.45 and 0.96 reported in a systematic review of the topic.[20,21]

These ranges present a challenge given that age as a univariate predictor has produced an area under the receiver operator characteristic curve of 0.65, and models using only age and dementia history have produced acceptable calibration.[22]

DIFFERENTIAL DIAGNOSIS

As useful as screening protocols may be, treatment relies on a careful diagnostic evaluation; there is no substitute for a systematic search for the specific cause of delirium. The temporal relationship to clinical events often gives the best clues to potential causes. Nursing notes, or documentation of structured screening instruments, should be studied to help discern the first indication of an abnormality (e.g., restlessness, mild confusion, anxiety). Laboratory values should be scanned for abnormalities that could be related to an encephalopathic state. Initiation or discontinuation of a drug, the onset of fever or hypotension, or the acute worsening of renal function, if they are in proximity to the time of mental status changes, become likely culprits.

Without a convincing temporal connection, causes of delirium should be investigated based on their likelihood in the patient's unique clinical situation. In critical care settings, several (life-threatening) should be considered by clinicians. These are states in which an intervention needs to be especially prompt because failure to make the diagnosis may result in permanent central nervous system (CNS) damage. These conditions are Wernicke disease, hypoxia, hypoglycemia, hypertensive encephalopathy, hyper- or hypothermia, intracerebral hemorrhage, meningitis or encephalitis, poisoning (exogenous or iatrogenic), and status epilepticus (i.e., seizures). These conditions are usefully recalled by the mnemonic device "WHHHHIMPS." Other less urgent but still acute conditions that require intervention include intracranial bleeds, sepsis, hepatic or renal failure, thyrotoxicosis or myxedema, delirium tremens, and complex partial seizures. If not already ruled out, when present, they are easy to verify. A broad review of conditions commonly associated with delirium is provided by the mnemonic "I WATCH DEATH" (Table 9.1).

TABLE 9.1

Conditions Commonly Associated With Delirium: "I WATCH DEATH"

Category	Conditions
Infectious	Encephalitis, meningitis, syphilis, pneumonia, urinary tract infection
Withdrawal	From alcohol or sedative-hypnotics
Acute metabolic	Acidosis, alkalosis, electrolyte disturbances, liver or kidney failure
Trauma	Heatstroke, burns, following surgery
CNS pathology	Abscesses, hemorrhage, seizure, stroke, tumor, vasculitis, or normal-pressure hydrocephalus
Hypoxia	Anemia, carbon monoxide poisoning, hypotension, pulmonary embolus, lung or heart failure
Deficiencies	Of vitamin B_{12}, niacin, or thiamine
Endocrinopathies	Hyper- or hypoglycemia, hyper- or hypo-adrenocorticism, hyper- or hypothyroidism, hyper- or hypoparathyroidism
Acute vascular	Hypertensive encephalopathy or shock
Toxins or drugs	Medications, pesticides, or solvents
Heavy metals	Lead, manganese, or mercury

In the elderly, regardless of the setting, the onset of confusion should trigger concern about infection, with UTIs or pneumonia as likely candidates. In one study of elderly females with a UTI, almost half (44.8%) were found to be delirious or to have experienced symptoms of delirium in the prior month.[23] Once a consultant has eliminated these common conditions as possible causes of a patient's disturbed brain function, there is time for an exhaustive approach to the differential diagnosis based on disturbances in each organ system. While the long-used medical admonition to think of horses when one hears hoofbeats remains true, once the consultant has ruled out "horses" (i.e., common diagnoses), attention should turn to "zebras" (i.e., uncommon diagnoses) and potentially to "unicorns" (i.e., diagnoses read about in textbooks but not usually seen in practice). Indeed, the potential causes of oxidative stress (and thus potential causes of delirium) span the entirety of medical practice (Table 9.2). The spectrum of medical pathology is constantly expanding, requiring the psychiatric consultant to maintain an updated awareness of novel diagnoses. A prominent example of this requirement is the phenomenon

TABLE 9.2

Differential Diagnosis of Delirium

General Cause	Specific Cause
Vascular	Hypertensive encephalopathy
	Cerebral arteriosclerosis
	Intracranial hemorrhage or thrombosis
	Emboli from atrial fibrillation, patent foramen ovale, or endocarditic valve
	Circulatory collapse (shock)
	Systemic lupus erythematosus
	Polyarteritis nodosa
	Thrombotic thrombocytopenic purpura
	Hyperviscosity syndrome
	Sarcoid
	Posterior reversible encephalopathy syndrome (PRES)
	Cerebral aneurysm
Infectious	Encephalitis
	Bacterial or viral meningitis, fungal meningitis (*cryptococcal, coccidioidal, Histoplasma*)
	Sepsis
	General paresis
	Brain, epidural, or subdural abscess
	Malaria
	Human immunodeficiency virus
	Lyme disease
	Typhoid fever
	Parasitic (*toxoplasma, trichinosis, cysticercosis, echinococcosis*)
	Behçet syndrome
	Mumps

(Continued)

TABLE 9.2	
Differential Diagnosis of Delirium—cont'd	
General Cause	**Specific Cause**
Neoplastic	Space-occupying lesions, such as gliomas, meningiomas, abscesses
	Paraneoplastic syndromes
	Carcinomatous meningitis
Degenerative	Dementias
	Huntington disease
	Creutzfeldt-Jakob disease
	Wilson disease
Intoxication	Chronic intoxication or withdrawal effects of drugs, including sedative-hypnotics, opiates, tranquilizers, anticholinergics, dissociative anesthetics, anticonvulsants
Neurophysiologic	Epilepsy
	Postictal states
	Complex partial status epilepticus
Traumatic	Intracranial bleeds
	Postoperative trauma
	Heatstroke
	Fat emboli syndrome
Intraventricular	Normal-pressure hydrocephalus
Vitamin deficiency	Thiamine (Wernicke-Korsakoff syndrome)
	Niacin (pellagra)
	B_{12} (pernicious anemia)
Endocrine/metabolic	Diabetic coma and shock
	Uremia
	Myxedema
	Hyperthyroidism
	Parathyroid dysfunction
	Hypoglycemia
	Hepatic or renal failure
	Porphyria
	Severe electrolyte or acid/base disturbances
	Cushing or Addison syndrome
	Sleep apnea
	Carcinoid
	Whipple disease
Autoimmune	Autoimmune encephalitides
	Steroid-responsive encephalopathy associated with thyroiditis (SREAT)/Hashimoto encephalopathy
	Systemic lupus erythematosus
	Multiple sclerosis
Poisoning	Heavy metals (lead, manganese, mercury)
	Carbon monoxide
	Anticholinergics
	Other toxins
Anoxia	Hypoxia and anoxia secondary to pulmonary or cardiac failure, anesthesia, anemia
Psychiatric	Depressive pseudodementia, catatonia, Bell mania

of autoimmune encephalitis which, over the course of two decades, has rapidly changed from its status as a unicorn, to that of a zebra, to that of a horse as awareness and diagnostic capabilities have expanded.

Autoimmune encephalitis may become an even more common cause of delirium as the use of immune checkpoint inhibitors (which increase autoimmunity) expands as the treatment of choice for a variety of cancers.[24] Prior medical records, no matter how lengthy, cannot be overlooked without risk. Some patients have had psychiatric consultations for similar difficulties on prior admissions. Others, in the absence of psychiatric consultations, have caused considerable trouble for their caregivers. Examination of current and past medications is essential because pharmacologic agents (in therapeutic doses, in overdose, or with withdrawal) can produce psychiatric symptoms. These medications must be reviewed routinely, especially in patients whose drugs have been stopped because of surgery or hospitalization or whose drug orders have not been reconciled during transfer between services or institutions. Drug-drug interactions (especially those involving the addition of a CYP 450 inhibitor or discontinuation of a CYP 450 inducer) that can raise blood levels and induce toxicity should be considered. Of all causes of an altered mental status, the use of and withdrawal from drugs is probably the most common. Some agents are commonly known to have neuropsychiatric effects (e.g., corticosteroids), while others are less well-known as precipitants of delirium (e.g., fluoroquinolone antibiotics); thus it may be advisable to review the current literature with an eye to the patient's entire medication list given the possibility of additive or less frequently reported effects. Table 9.3 lists some drugs used in clinical practice that have been associated with delirium.

The list of directly or indirectly acting deliriogenic drugs (e.g., because of drug interactions) is extensive. Fortunately, there is an array of resources (including websites and smartphone applications) that easily allow for the identification of these issues.[25] Once identified, the usual treatment is to stop the offending drug or to reduce the dosage; however, at times this is not possible. Elderly patients, those with impairments of metabolism (e.g., hepatic or renal failure), and those with neurodevelopmental disorders or a history of a significant head injury are more susceptible to the toxic effects of many of these drugs.

THE EXAMINATION OF THE PATIENT

Appearance, level of consciousness, thought, speech, orientation, memory, mood, judgment, and behavior should all be assessed. In the formal mental status examination (MSE), one begins with the examination of consciousness. If the patient does not speak, a handy common-sense test is to ask oneself, "Do the eyes look back at me?" (i.e., does the patient regard and track in a meaningful manner?) One could formally rate consciousness by using the Glasgow Coma Scale (Table 9.4), a measure that is readily understood by consultees in other specialties.[26]

Delirious patients are occasionally unwilling to participate in a psychiatric examination, often because they fear that they are "going crazy," and the presence of a psychiatric consultant at the bedside magnifies these concerns. Indeed, patients may be reluctant to report subjective experiences, such as hallucinations or paranoia, because they do not want hospital staff or family to think that they have "lost it." Leading the interview with an explanation that such symptoms are relatively normal in the setting of illness, do not represent a primary psychiatric illness, and can be effectively managed may serve to establish rapport with these reluctant interviewees.

If the patient cooperates with an examination, attention should be examined first because if this is disturbed, other parts of the examination may be invalid. Forward digit span is a pure test of attention, and most non-delirious elderly patients should be able to recall a list of at least four digits. Verbal vigilance testing is another useful test of attention: one can ask the patient to repeat the letters of the alphabet that rhyme with "tree." (If the patient is intubated, ask that a hand or finger be raised whenever the letter of the recited alphabet rhymes with "tree.") Then the rest of the MSE can be performed. The Folstein Mini-Mental State Examination (MMSE),[27] is usually included. Specific defects are more important than the total score. Other functions, such as writing, are often abnormal in delirium. Perhaps the most dramatic (though difficult to score objectively) test of cognition is the clock drawing test, which can provide a broad survey of the patient's cognitive state (Fig. 9.1).[28] A more recently developed and validated bedside test, the Montreal Cognitive Assessment (MoCA),[29] usefully incorporates some aspects of the MMSE (i.e., tests of memory, attention, and orientation) with tests of more complex visuospatial and executive function (including clock drawing and an adaptation of the Trail Making B task). Although not specifically

TABLE 9.3
Drugs Commonly Used in Clinical Practice That Have Been Associated With Delirium

Antiarrhythmics	Tricyclic Antidepressants	Dopamine Agonists (Central)	Monoamine Oxidase Inhibitors
Disopyramide	Amitriptyline	Amantadine	Tranylcypromine
Lidocaine	Clomipramine	Bromocriptine	Phenelzine
Mexiletine	Desipramine	Levodopa	Procarbazine
Procainamide	Imipramine	Selegiline	**Narcotic Analgesics**
Propafenone	Nortriptyline	Ergotamine	Meperidine (normeperidine)
Quinidine	Protriptyline	**GABA Agonists**	Pentazocine
Tocainide	Trimipramine	Baclofen	Podophyllin (topical)
Antibiotics	**Anticonvulsants**	Benzodiazepines	**Non-steroidal Anti-**
Aminoglycosides	Phenytoin	Eszopiclone	**inflammatory Drugs**
Amodiaquine	Levetiracetam	Zaleplon	Ibuprofen
Amphotericin	**Antihypertensives**	Zolpidem	Indometacin
Cephalosporins	Captopril	**Immunosuppressives**	Naproxen
Chloramphenicol	Clonidine	Aminoglutethimide	Sulindac
Gentamicin	Methyldopa	Azacitidine	**Other Medications**
Isoniazid	Reserpine	Chlorambucil	Cimetidine
Metronidazole	**Antiviral Agents**	Cytosine arabinoside	Clozaril
Rifampin	Acyclovir	(high dose)	Cyclobenzaprine
Sulfonamides	Interferon	Dacarbazine	Digitalis preparations
Tetracyclines	Ganciclovir	FK-506	Disulfiram
Ticarcillin	Nevirapine	5-Fluorouracil	Ketamine
Vancomycin	**Barbiturates**	Hexamethylmelamine	Lithium
Anticholinergics	**β-Blockers**	Ifosfamide	Mefloquine
Atropine	Propranolol	Interleukin-2 (high dose)	Ranitidine
Benztropine	Timolol	L-Asparaginase	Sildenafil
Diphenhydramine	**Diuretics**	Methotrexate (high dose)	Trazodone
Eye and nose drops	Acetazolamide	Procarbazine	**Steroids**
Scopolamine		Tamoxifen	**Sympathomimetics**
Thioridazine		Vinblastine	Aminophylline
Trihexyphenidyl		Vincristine	Amphetamine
		Immune Checkpoint Inhibitors	Cocaine
		Atezolizumab	Ephedrine
		Avelumab	Phenylephrine
		Cemiplimab	Phenylpropanolamine
		Durvalumab	Ranitidine
		Pembrolizumab	Theophylline
		Nivolumab	

GABA, Gamma aminobutyric acid.
Adapted from Cassem NH, Lake CR, Boyer WF. Psychopharmacology in the ICU. In: Chernow B, ed. *The Pharmacologic Approach to the Critically Ill Patient*. Williams & Wilkins; 1995:651–665; Drugs that may cause psychiatric symptoms. *Med Letter Drugs Ther*. 2002;44:59–62.

validated for detecting delirium, the MoCA (available at www.mocacognition.com in a variety of languages) has been consistently shown to have greater sensitivity than the MMSE for mild cognitive impairment in a variety of conditions and typically requires less than 10 minutes to administer. Note that poor performance on the MMSE or MoCA, demonstrated in the setting of suspected delirium, does not imply that the patient

necessarily has a chronic neurocognitive disorder or will be incapable of performing better following recovery from delirium.

The patient's problem can involve serious neurologic syndromes as well; however, the clinical presentation of the patient should direct the examination. In general, the less responsive and more impaired the patient is, the more one should look for neurological *hard signs.* A directed search for an abnormality of the eyes and pupils, rigidity (nuchal or otherwise), hyper-reflexia, "hung-up" reflexes with delayed recovery (as in myxedema), one-sided weakness or asymmetry, gait (as in normal-pressure hydrocephalus), Babinski

reflexes, *gegenhalten, mitgehen,* absent vibratory and position senses, hyperventilation (as in acidosis, hypoxia, or pontine disease), or other specific clues can help verify or reject hypotheses about causality that are stimulated by the abnormalities in the examination.

Frontal lobe function deserves specific attention. Grasp, snout, palmomental, suck, and glabellar responses are helpful when present. Hand movements thought to be related to the premotor area (Brodmann's area 8) can identify subtle deficiencies. The patient is asked to imitate, with each hand separately, specific movements. The hand is held upright, a circle formed by the thumb and first finger ("okay" sign), and then the fist is closed and lowered to the surface on which the elbow rests. In the Luria sequence, one hand is brought down on a surface (e.g., a table or one's own leg) in three successive positions: perpendicular to the surface, extended with all five digits parallel ("cut" or "chop"); then as a fist ("punch"); and then flat on the surface ("slap"). Finally, both hands are placed on a flat surface in front of the patient, one flat on the surface and the other resting as a fist. Then the positions are alternated between right and left hands, and the patient is instructed to do the same; and/or the patient may be instructed to repeat the sequence until directed to stop, during which time errors in inhibition, sequencing, and error detection may become apparent.

For verbally responsive patients, their response to the "Frank Jones story" can be gauged ("I have a

TABLE 9.4
Glasgow Coma Scale

Criterion	Score
Eye Opening (E)	
Spontaneous	4
To verbal command	3
To pain	2
No response	1
Motor (M)	
Obeys verbal command	6
Localizes pain	5
Flexion withdrawal	4
Abnormal flexion (decortication)	3
Extension (decerebration)	2
No response	1
Verbal (V)	
Oriented and converses	5
Disoriented and converses	4
Inappropriate words	3
Incomprehensible sound	2
No response	1
Coma Score = (E + M + V)	Range 3–15

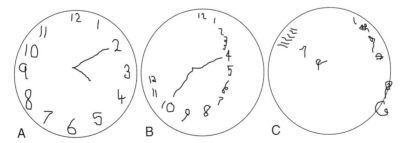

Fig. 9.1 ■ The clock drawing test. The patient is provided with a circular outline and asked to draw the numbers as they appear on the face of a clock. Once the numbering is complete, the patient is asked to set the hands to a particular time (often "ten past" the hour to test if the patient can suppress the impulse to include the number 10). (A) This drawing demonstrates good planning and use of space. (B) This drawing features some impulsiveness because the numbers are drawn out without regard for the actual location, and the time "ten past four" is represented by hands pointing to the digits 10 and 4. Note the perseveration indicated by the extra loops on the digits 3 and 6. Impulsiveness and perseveration indicate frontal lobe dysfunction. (C) This drawing demonstrates gross disorganization, although the patient took several minutes to draw the clock and believed it to be a good representation.

friend, Frank Jones, whose feet are so big he has to put his pants on over his head. How does that strike you?"). Three general responses are given. Type 1 is normal: the patient sees the incongruity and smiles (a limbic response) and can explain (a neocortical function) why it cannot be done. Type 2 is abnormal: the patient smiles at the incongruity (a limbic connection) but cannot explain why it cannot be done. Type 3 is abnormal: the patient neither gets the incongruity nor can explain its impossibility. Even in patients unable to respond verbally, attempts to elicit a limbic response through humor or absurd incongruity can help gauge their level of impairment.

Laboratory studies should be carefully reviewed, with special attention paid to indicators of infection or metabolic disturbance. Toxicology screens are also helpful in allowing the inclusion or exclusion of substance intoxication or withdrawal from the differential diagnosis. Neuroimaging can prove useful in the detection of intracranial processes that can result in altered mental status. Of all the diagnostic studies available, the electroencephalogram (EEG) may be the most useful tool in the diagnosis of delirium. Engel and Romano[30] reported in 1959 their (now classic) findings on the EEG in delirium, namely, generalized/diffuse slowing to the theta-delta range in the delirious patient, the consistency of this finding despite wide-ranging underlying conditions, and resolution of this slowing with effective treatment of the delirium. EEG findings might even clarify the etiology of delirium because delirium tremens is associated with low-voltage fast activity superimposed on slow waves, sedative-hypnotic toxicity produces fast beta activity (>12 Hz), and hepatic encephalopathy is classically associated with triphasic waves.[31] When faced with a consultee who insists that a patient's delirium is actually a primary psychiatric illness requiring admission to a psychiatric unit (i.e., transfer off their service), an abnormal EEG can provide incontrovertible evidence to the contrary.

SPECIFIC MANAGEMENT STRATEGIES FOR DELIRIUM

Psychosocial or environmental measures are alone and rarely effective in the treatment of a *bona fide* delirium of uncertain or unknown cause. Nevertheless, it is commendable to have hospital rooms with windows,

calendars, clocks, and a few mementos from home on the walls; soft and low lighting at night; and, when available, a loving family in attendance to reassure and reorient the patient. Indeed, these measures have been codified into several delirium-prevention protocols. However, once the proverbial genie is out of the bottle, it is unlikely that management of environmental factors will resolve the syndrome. The psychiatric consultant is often summoned because psychosocial measures have failed to prevent or treat the patient's delirium. Mechanical restraints (e.g., geriatric chairs, "vests," helmets, padded mitts, locked leather restraints) are available and quite useful to protect patients from inflicting harm on themselves or staff. One or several of these are often in place when the consultant arrives. One hoped-for outcome of the consultation is that the use of these devices can be reduced or eliminated.

When the cause of the delirium seems straightforward, the treatment revolves around the resolution or reversal of the underlying cause. A discovered deficiency can be replaced (e.g., of blood, oxygen, thiamine, vitamin B_{12}, or glucose). Pathologic conditions can be treated (e.g., volume replacement for hypotension, diuretics for pulmonary edema, antibiotics for infection, calcium for hypocalcemia, or dialysis for acute lithium toxicity). Implicated drugs can be stopped or reduced.

The antiepileptic medication levetiracetam has been associated with several neuropsychiatric adverse effects, including delirium.[32] In these cases, this medication can usually be switched to an alternate antiepileptic, but problems are seldom so simple. Often the drugs (such as corticosteroids) that induce delirium cannot be changed without causing harm to the patient. Alternatively, pain can cause agitation in a delirious patient. Opioids can relieve pain and unfortunately lead to intoxication and decrease in blood pressure and respiratory rate; among opioids, rational selection of agents with relatively less propensity to cause delirium (such as hydromorphone and oxycodone; as opposed to meperidine, tramadol, and morphine) may be beneficial.

Specific antidotes can reverse delirium that is caused by some drugs. Flumazenil and naloxone can reverse the effects of benzodiazepines and opioid analgesics, respectively. However, caution is required because flumazenil can precipitate seizures in a benzodiazepine-dependent patient, and naloxone can precipitate opioid withdrawal in an opioid-dependent patient.

Anticholinergic delirium can be reversed by administration of IV physostigmine in doses starting at 0.5 to 2 mg. Caution is essential with the use of this agent because the autonomic nervous system of the medically ill is generally less stable than it is in a healthy patient who has developed an anticholinergic delirium as a result of a voluntary or accidental overdose. Moreover, if there is a reasonably high amount of an anticholinergic drug on board that is clearing from the system slowly, the therapeutic effect of physostigmine, although sometimes quite dramatic, is usually short lived. The cholinergic reaction to intravenously administered physostigmine can cause profound bradycardia and hypotension, thereby multiplying the complications.[33,34] A continuous IV infusion of physostigmine has been successfully used to manage a case of anticholinergic poisoning.[35] Because of the diagnostic value of physostigmine, one might wish to use it even though its effects will be short lived. If one uses a 1 mg IV injection of physostigmine, protection against excessive cholinergic reaction can be provided by preceding this injection with an IV injection of 0.2 mg of glycopyrrolate. This anticholinergic agent does not cross the blood-brain barrier and should protect the patient from the peripheral cholinergic actions of physostigmine.

While theory, anecdote, and small studies have suggested there could be benefits from the use of oral cholinesterase inhibitors in delirious patients, a randomized, multi-center, double-blind, placebo-controlled trial of rivastigmine in delirium had to be abruptly halted due to significantly increased mortality in the group receiving the cholinesterase inhibitor.[36] The mechanism for this increased mortality remains obscure. Based on the data obtained before the trial was halted, rivastigmine did not decrease the duration of delirium. In the absence of evidence of any clinical utility and with the suggestion that they may increase mortality, these agents are not recommended for use in delirium.

DRUG MANAGEMENT

Definitive treatment of delirium requires identification and treatment of the underlying somatic etiology, but all too often, the cause of delirium is not readily identified or treated. Even when the cause has been identified, effective treatment can still take considerable time. These situations call for the management of the symptoms of delirium.

Benzodiazepines (e.g., lorazepam) are often effective for mild agitation in the setting of withdrawal from drugs that work at the chloride channel (including alcohol, benzodiazepines, and barbiturates). Morphine is also often used because it calms agitation and is easily reversed if hypotension or respiratory depression ensues. These agents should be used with caution since they themselves can cause, or exacerbate, confusion. This occurs much less often with the use of neuroleptics.

Neuroleptics are the agent of choice for delirium. Haloperidol is probably the agent most commonly used to treat agitated delirium in the critical care setting; its effects on blood pressure, pulmonary artery pressure, heart rate, and respiration are milder than those of benzodiazepines, making it an excellent agent for delirious patients with impaired cardiorespiratory status.[37]

Although haloperidol can be administered orally, acute delirium with extreme agitation typically requires the use of parenteral medication. IV administration is preferable to intramuscular (IM) administration for several reasons. First, because drug absorption may be poor in distal muscles if delirium is associated with circulatory compromise or shock, the deltoid is probably a better IM injection site than the gluteus muscle, but neither is as reliable as the IV route. Second, because the agitated patient is commonly paranoid, repeated painful IM injections can increase the patient's sense of being attacked or harmed. Third, IM injections can complicate interpretations of muscle enzyme studies if enzyme fractionation is not readily available. Fourth, and most importantly, haloperidol is less likely to produce extrapyramidal symptoms (EPS) when given IV than when given IM or by mouth (PO), at least for patients without a prior serious psychiatric disorder.[38]

In contrast to the immediately observable sedation produced by IV benzodiazepines, IV haloperidol has a mean distribution time of 11 minutes in normal volunteers[39]; this may be even longer in critically ill patients. The mean half-life of IV haloperidol's subsequent, slower phase is 14 hours. This is still a more rapid metabolic rate than the overall mean half-lives of

21 and 24 hours for IM and PO doses. The PO dose has about half the potency of the parenteral dose, so 10 mg of PO haloperidol corresponds to 5 mg given IV or IM.

Haloperidol has not been approved by the US Food and Drug Administration (FDA) for IV administration, and since it has been off-patent since the 1980s, there is no pharmaceutical company that will fund the studies required to gain such approval. IV haloperidol is, however, the standard of care for the management of delirium in hospitals around the world.

Over decades of clinical use in medically ill patients, IV haloperidol has been associated with few side effects on blood pressure, heart rate, respiratory rate, or urinary output, and it has been linked with few EPS. The reason for the latter is unknown. Studies of the use of IV haloperidol in psychiatric patients have not shown that these side effects were fewer, perhaps because patients with psychiatric disorders are more susceptible to EPS.

Before administering IV haloperidol, the IV line should be flushed with 2 mL of normal saline. Occasionally, haloperidol precipitates with heparin, and because many lines in critical care units are heparinized, the 2-mL flush is advised. Phenytoin precipitates with haloperidol; therefore mixing the two in the same line must be avoided. The initial bolus dose of haloperidol usually varies from 0.5 to 20 mg; usually 0.5 mg (for an elderly person) to 2 mg is used for mild agitation, 5 mg is used for moderate agitation, and 10 mg for severe agitation. A higher initial dose should be used only when the patient has already been unsuccessfully treated with reasonable doses of haloperidol. To adjust for haloperidol's lag time, doses are usually staggered by at least a 30-minute interval. If one dose (e.g., a 5-mg dose) fails to calm an agitated patient after 30 minutes, the next higher dose, 10 mg, should be administered. Calm is the desired outcome. Partial control of agitation is usually inadequate; moreover, settling for this only prolongs the delirium or guarantees that excessively high doses of haloperidol will be used after the delirium is controlled.

Haloperidol can be combined every 30 minutes with simultaneous parenteral lorazepam doses (starting with 1–2 mg). Because the effects of lorazepam are noticeable within 5 to 10 minutes, each dose can precede the haloperidol dose, be observed for its impact on agitation, and be increased if it is more effective.

Some believe that the combination leads to a lower overall dose of each drug.[40]

After calm is achieved, agitation should be the sign for a repeat dose. Ideally the total dose of haloperidol on the second day should be a fraction of that used on day 1. After complete lucidity has been achieved, the patient needs to be protected from delirium only at night by small doses of haloperidol (1–3 mg), which can be given orally. As in the treatment of delirium tremens, the consultant is advised to stop the agitation quickly and completely at the outset rather than barely keep up with it over several days. The maximum total dose of IV haloperidol to be used as an upper limit has not been established, although IV administration of single bolus doses of 200 mg has been used,[41] and more than 2000 mg has been used in a 24-hour period. The highest requirements have been seen with delirious patients on the intra-aortic balloon pump.[42] A continuous infusion of haloperidol has also been used to treat severe, refractory delirium.[43] It has previously been argued that (despite strong empirical clinical evidence) high-dose haloperidol made little pharmacologic sense, given the high rates of dopamine receptor blockade at relatively low doses. In vitro and animal model research has revealed that the butyrophenone class of neuroleptics (haloperidol and droperidol) protects neurons from oxidative stress via their effects on the sigma receptor.[44,45] This mechanism of action may provide the physiologic basis for the clinical benefits of high-dose haloperidol.[46]

When delirium does not respond and agitation is unabated, one might wonder if the neuroleptic (e.g., haloperidol) is producing akathisia. The best indication as to whether the treatment is causing agitation is the patient's description of an irresistible urge to move—usually the limbs, lower more often than upper. If dialogue is possible, even nodding yes or no (provided that the patient understands the question) can confirm or exclude this symptom. If the patient cannot communicate, limited options remain: decreasing or increasing the dose and judging by the response. In our experience, it is far more common for the patient to receive more haloperidol and to improve.

Hypotensive episodes following the administration of IV haloperidol are rare and almost invariably result from hypovolemia. Local caustic effects on veins do not arise. IV haloperidol is generally safe for patients with epilepsy and for patients following head trauma, unless psychotropic drugs are contraindicated because the patient needs careful neurologic monitoring. Although IV haloperidol may be used without mishap in patients receiving epinephrine drips, after large doses of haloperidol a pressor other than epinephrine (e.g., norepinephrine) should be used to avoid unopposed β-adrenergic activity. IV haloperidol does not block a dopamine-mediated increase in renal blood flow. It also appears to be the safest agent for patients with chronic obstructive pulmonary disease.

As with all neuroleptic agents, IV haloperidol has been associated with the development of torsades de pointes (TDP).[47-51] Particular caution is urged when levels of potassium and magnesium are low (because these deficiencies independently predict TDP), when a baseline prolonged QT interval is noted, when hepatic compromise is present, or when a specific cardiac abnormality (e.g., mitral valve prolapse or a dilated ventricle) exists. Delirious patients who are candidates for IV haloperidol require careful screening. Serum potassium and magnesium should be within the normal range, and a baseline ECG should be checked for the pre-treatment QT interval corrected for heart rate (QTc). If necessary, potassium and magnesium should be repleted, and the QTc and levels of potassium and magnesium should be monitored regularly for the duration of neuroleptic treatment. QT interval prolongation occurs in some patients with alcoholic liver disease; this finding is associated with adverse outcomes (e.g., sudden cardiac death).[52] A multitude of other commonly used medications also carry the potential for QTc prolongation (some of the usual offenders are summarized in Table 9.5). Medication lists should be reviewed closely for other agents that could be discontinued or therapeutically exchanged if QTc prolongation becomes a concern. Administration of haloperidol is based (as are all decisions in medicine) on a risk-benefit calculus. Thus there may be circumstances where the administration of haloperidol is reasonable even in the face of a prolonged QTc.

Other available parenteral first-generation antipsychotics for the treatment of agitation are perphenazine, thiothixene, trifluoperazine, fluphenazine, and chlorpromazine. Perphenazine is approved for IV use as an antiemetic. Chlorpromazine is extremely effective, but its potent α-blocking properties can be dangerous for

TABLE 9.5
Non-neuroleptic Medications Associated With Prolongation of the QT Interval

Antiarrhythmics	Anti-infectious	Other
Amiodarone	Atazanavir	Alfuzosin
Disopyramide	Azithromycin	Amantadine
Dofetilide	Chloroquine	Arsenic trioxide
Flecainide	Ciprofloxacin	Bepridil
Ibutilide	Clarithromycin	Chloral hydrate
Procainamide	Erythromycin	Cisapride
Quinidine	Foscarnet	Citalopram
Sotalol	Gatifloxacin	Dolasetron
	Gemifloxacin	Escitalopram
	Halofantrine	Felbamate
	Levofloxacin	Granisetron
	Moxifloxacin	Indapamide
	Ofloxacin	Isradipine
	Pentamidine	Lapatinib
	Sparfloxacin	Levomethadyl
	Telithromycin	Lithium
	Voriconazole	carbonate
		Methadone
		Nicardipine
		Octreotide
		Ondansetron
		Oxytocin
		Probucol
		Ranolazine
		Sunitinib
		Tacrolimus
		Tizanidine
		Vardenafil
		Venlafaxine

critically ill patients. When administered IV or IM, it can abruptly decrease total peripheral resistance and cause a precipitous fall in cardiac output. Nevertheless, using IV in small doses (10 mg) can be safe and effective in the treatment of delirium.

The commonplace use of second-generation antipsychotics (SGAs) in general psychiatric practice and the availability of injectable formulations of olanzapine and ziprasidone have prompted the investigation of these agents in managing delirium.[53] Risperidone has the most data available supporting its use, and multiple studies show it to be efficacious and safe for treating delirium symptoms[54-56]; one small randomized double-blind comparative study found no significant difference in efficacy compared with oral haloperidol.[57] Randomized controlled trials (RCTs) of olanzapine and quetiapine have shown some benefit in ameliorating the severity of delirium.[58-62] Studies that have attempted to compare SGAs with haloperidol have, to date, been limited by two key confounders. First, they employ the oral formulation of haloperidol to allow for successful blinding (since none of the SGAs are available intravenously). Second, IV haloperidol is often used as the "bailout" medication for episodes of uncontrolled agitation in the study subjects. Thus subjects in the SGA arms of these studies still receive IV haloperidol (sometimes more frequently than those receiving oral haloperidol). All drugs in this class feature an FDA "black box warning" indicating an increased risk of death when used to treat behavioral problems in elderly patients with dementia. Similar warnings regarding a potential increased risk of cerebrovascular events are reported for risperidone, olanzapine, and aripiprazole. With decades of clinical experience in the use of haloperidol, and a relative dearth of available data on these newer agents, haloperidol remains the agent of choice for treating delirium.

RCTs of medications for delirium prevention have shown that perioperative administration of olanzapine, risperidone, and IV (but not oral) haloperidol may reduce the incidence of delirium.[63-66] A meta-analysis of five such trials supported the prophylactic use of neuroleptics to ward off delirium.[67] Additional RCTs have demonstrated that regularly scheduled doses of ramelteon and ondansetron can also reduce the incidence of delirium.[68,69] There is some limited evidence suggesting that the pro-cholinergic action of cholinesterase inhibitors provides some protection against the development of delirium,[70,71] although multiple trials have failed to demonstrate any efficacy of these agents in the treatment of active delirium. For patients undergoing surgery, one study has demonstrated a 20% to 30% reduction in the use of intraoperative anesthetic agents and a 35% decrease in postoperative delirium when operative anesthesia is measured by bi-spectral index (BIS) monitoring as compared with treatment as usual.[72]

DELIRIUM IN SPECIFIC DISEASES

Critically ill patients with human immunodeficiency virus infection may be more susceptible to the EPS of haloperidol and to neuroleptic malignant syndrome,[73-75] leading an experienced group

to recommend the use of molindone.[76] Molindone is associated with fewer such effects; it is available only as an oral agent, and it can be prescribed from 5 to 25 mg at appropriate intervals or, in a more acute situation, 25 mg every hour until calm is achieved. Risperidone (0.5–1 mg per dose) is another recommended oral agent. If parenteral medication is required, 10 mg of chlorpromazine has been effective. Perphenazine is readily available for parenteral use as well, and 2-mg doses can be used effectively.

Delirious patients with Parkinson disease pose a special problem because dopamine blockade aggravates their condition. If oral treatment of delirium or psychosis is possible, clozapine, starting with a small dose of 6.25 or 12.5 mg, is probably the most effective agent available that does not exacerbate the disease. With the risk of agranulocytosis attendant to the use of clozapine, quetiapine can play a valuable role in this population because of its very low affinity for dopamine receptors is less likely to exacerbate this disorder.[77]

Adding medications to the regimen of a patient with hepatic compromise is always fraught with the risk of toxicity from that agent or from extant drugs whose metabolism is upset by the disturbance of an already over-burdened cytochrome system. In this population, paliperidone is a useful option since it does not require significant hepatic metabolism.[78]

Benzodiazepines (especially diazepam, chlordiazepoxide, and lorazepam) are routinely used to treat agitated states, particularly delirium tremens, and alcohol withdrawal.[79] Neuroleptics have also been used as adjunctive agents successfully, and both have been combined with clonidine. Trials of barbiturates may be successful as well. When all else fails, IV alcohol is also extremely effective in treating alcohol withdrawal states. The inherent disadvantage is that alcohol is toxic to the liver and brain, although its use can be quite safe if these organs do not show already extensive damage, and it is sometimes quite safe even when they do. Nonetheless, the use of IV alcohol should be reserved for extreme cases of alcohol withdrawal when other, less-toxic measures have failed. A 5% solution of alcohol mixed with 5% dextrose in water run at 1 mL per minute often achieves calm quickly. Treatment pathways have been developed to provide non-psychiatric clinicians with guidance on the management of alcohol withdrawal,[80] although care must always be taken to ensure that benzodiazepines are not inappropriately administered because they almost certainly exacerbate a delirium that results from any other cause.[81]

Propofol is commonly used to sedate critically ill patients and can also be extremely effective in managing agitation. It has moderate respiratory depressant and vasodilator effects, although hypotension can be minimized by avoiding boluses of the drug. The impaired hepatic function does not slow metabolic clearance, but clearance does decline with age, and its half-life is significantly longer in the elderly. This drug's rapid onset and short duration make it especially useful for treating short periods of stress. When rapid return to alertness from sedation for an uncompromised neurologic examination is indicated, propofol is a nearly ideal agent[82]; however, its use in treating a prolonged delirious state has specific disadvantages.[83] Delivered as a fat emulsion containing 0.1 g of fat per milliliter, propofol requires a dedicated IV line, and drug accumulation can lead to a fat-overload syndrome that has been associated with overfeeding, and significant CO_2 production, hypertriglyceridemia, ketoacidosis, seizure activity 6 days after discontinuation, and even fatal respiratory failure.[84,85] Obese patients provide a high volume of distribution, and their doses should be calculated using estimated lean, rather than actual, body mass. If the patient is receiving fat by parenteral feeding, this must be accounted for or eliminated, and adequate glucose infusion must be provided to prevent ketoacidosis. Although no clear association has been demonstrated with addiction, tolerance, or withdrawal, doses seem to require escalation after 4 to 7 days' infusion. Seizures seen after withdrawal or muscular rigidity during administration are poorly understood. The drug is costly, especially when used for prolonged infusions.

Dexmedetomidine is a selective α_2-adrenergic agonist used for sedation and analgesia in the ICU setting. Its action on receptors in the locus ceruleus results in anxiolysis and sedation, and agonism of spinal cord receptors provides analgesia. This unique mechanism of action allows effective management in agitation without the risks of respiratory depression, dependence, and delirium associated with benzodiazepines that are traditionally employed in the ICU.[86] Its relative lack of amnestic effect might further limit its use as monotherapy in the treatment of the delirious patient owing to an increased likelihood of distressing recollections persisting from the period of sedation.[87] In current practice, dexmedetomidine can serve as a useful (but costly) adjunct agent to quell agitation when more traditional approaches have met with limited success.

CONCLUSION

Of all psychiatric diagnoses, delirium demands the most immediate attention because a delay in its identification and treatment might allow the progression of serious and irreversible pathophysiologic changes. Unfortunately, delirium is all too often underemphasized, misdiagnosed, or altogether missed in the general hospital setting.[88-90] Indeed, it was not until their most recent editions that major medical and surgical texts corrected chapters indicating that delirium was the result of anxiety, depression, or the hospital milieu, rather than an underlying somatic cause that required prompt investigation. In the face of this tradition of misinformation, it often falls to the psychiatric consultant to identify and manage delirium while alerting and educating others about its significance.

REFERENCES

1. American Psychiatric Association. *Diagnostic and Statistical Manual of Mental Disorders, ed 5, Text Revision.* American Psychiatric Association; 2022.
2. Ely EW, Shintani A, Truman B, et al. Delirium as a predictor of mortality in mechanically ventilated patients in the intensive care unit. *JAMA.* 2004;291:1753–1762.
3. Thomason JW, Shintani A, Peterson JF, et al. Intensive care unit delirium is an independent predictor of longer hospital stay: a prospective analysis of 261 non-ventilated patients. *Crit Care.* 2005;9:R375–R381.
4. Milbrandt EB, Deppen S, Harrison PL, et al. Costs associated with delirium in mechanically ventilated patients. *Crit Care Med.* 2004;32:955–962.
5. Franco K, Litaker D, Locala J, et al. The cost of delirium in the surgical patient. *Psychosomatics.* 2001;42:68–73.
6. Gibb K, Seeley A, Quinn T, et al. The consistent burden in published estimates of delirium occurrence in medical inpatients over four decades: a systematic review and meta-analysis study. *Age Ageing.* 2020;49:352–360.
7. Krewulak KD, Stelfox HT, Leigh JP, et al. Incidence and prevalence of delirium subtypes in an adult ICU: a systematic review and meta-analysis. *Crit Care Med.* 2018;46:2029–2035.

8. World Health Organization. *International Statistical Classification of Diseases and Related Health Problems*. 11th ed. World Health Organization; 2019.

9. McGuire BE, Basten CJ, Ryan CJ, et al. Intensive care unit syndrome: a dangerous misnomer. *Arch Intern Med*. 2000;160:906–909.

10. Webster R, Holroyd S. Prevalence of psychotic symptoms in delirium. *Psychosomatics*. 2000;41:519–522.

11. Breitbart W, Gibson C, Tremblay A. The delirium experience: delirium recall and delirium-related distress in hospitalized patients with cancer, their spouses/caregivers, and their nurses. *Psychosomatics*. 2002;43:183–194.

12. Stagno D, Gibson C, Breitbart W. The delirium subtypes: a review of prevalence, phenomenology, pathophysiology, and treatment response. *Palliat Support Care*. 2004;2(2):171–179.

13. Peterson JF, Pun BT, Dittus RS, et al. Delirium and its motoric subtypes: a study of 614 critically ill patients. *J Am Geriatr Soc*. 2006;54(3):479–484.

14. Trzepacz PT. Is there a final common neural pathway in delirium? Focus on acetylcholine and dopamine. *Semin Clin Neuropsychiatry*. 2000;5(2):132–148.

15. Swigart SE, Kishi Y, Thurber S, et al. Misdiagnosed delirium in patient referrals to a university-based hospital psychiatry department. *Psychosomatics*. 2008;49:104–108.

16. Ely EW, Margolin R, Francis J, et al. Evaluation of delirium in critically ill patients: validation of the Confusion Assessment Method for the Intensive Care Unit (CAM-ICU). *Crit Care Med*. 2001;29(7):1370–1379.

17. Gusmao-Flores D, Figueira Salluh JI, Chalhub RA, et al. The confusion assessment method for the intensive care unit (CAM-ICU) and intensive care delirium screening checklist (ICDSC) for the diagnosis of delirium: a systematic review and meta-analysis of clinical studies. *Crit Care*. 2012;16(4):R115.

18. Wassenaar A, van den Boogaard M, van Achterberg T, et al. Multinational development and validation of an early prediction model for delirium in ICU patients. *Intensive Care Med*. 2015;41:1048–1056.

19. Bhattacharyya A, Sheikhalishahi S, Torbic H, et al. Delirium prediction in the ICU: designing a screening tool for preventive interventions. *JAMIA Open*. 2022;5(2): ooac048.

20. Lindroth H, Bratzke L, Purvis S, et al. Systematic review of prediction models for delirium in the older adult inpatient. *BMJ Open*. 2018;8:e019223.

21. Ruppert MM, Lipori J, Patel S, et al. ICU delirium-prediction models: a systematic review. *Critical Care Explorations*. 2020;2(12):e0296.

22. Castro VM, Sacks CA, Perlis RH, et al. Development and external validation of a delirium prediction model for hospitalized patients with coronavirus disease 2019. *J Acad Consult Liaison Psych*. 2021;62(3):298–308.

23. Eriksson I, Gustafson Y, Fagerström L, et al. Urinary tract infection in very old women is associated with delirium. *Int Psychogeriatr*. 2011;23(3):496–502.

24. Yordduangjun N, Dishion E, McKnight CA, et al. Immune checkpoint inhibitor-associated autoimmune encephalitis. *J Acad Consult Liaison Psychiatry*. 2021;62(1):115–118.

25. Haffey F, Brady RRW, Maxwell S. Smartphone apps to support hospital prescribing and pharmacology education: a review of current provision. *Br J Clin Pharmacol*. 2014;77:31–38.

26. Bastos PG, Sun X, Wagner DP, et al. Glasgow Coma Scale score in the evaluation of outcome in the intensive care unit: findings from the Acute Physiology and Chronic Health Evaluation III study. *Crit Care Med*. 1993;21:1459–1465.

27. Folstein MF, Folstein SE, McHugh PR. "Mini-Mental State," a practical method for grading the cognitive state of patients for the clinician. *J Psychiatr Res*. 1975;12:189–198.

28. Freedman M, Leach L, Kaplan E, et al. *Clock Drawing: A Neuropsychological Analysis*. Oxford University Press; 1994.

29. Nasreddine ZS, Phillips NA, Bédirian V, et al. The Montreal Cognitive Assessment (MoCA): a brief screening tool for mild cognitive impairment. *J Am Geriatr Soc*. 2005;53:695–699.

30. Engel GL, Romano J. Delirium, a syndrome of cerebral insufficiency. *J Chronic Dis*. 1959;9:260–277.

31. Jacobson S, Jerrier H. EEG in delirium. *Semin Clin Neuropsychiatry*. 2000;5:86–92.

32. Hwang ES, Siemianowski LA, Sen S, et al. Levetiracetam: an unusual cause of delirium. *Am J Ther*. 2014;21:e225–e228.

33. Pentel P, Peterson CD. Asystole complicating physostigmine treatment of tricyclic antidepressant overdose. *Ann Emerg Med*. 1980;9:588–590.

34. Boon J, Prideaux PR. Cardiac arrest following physostigmine. *Anaesth Intensive Care*. 1980;8:92–93.

35. Stern TA. Continuous infusion of physostigmine in anticholinergic delirium: case report. *J Clin Psychiatry*. 1983;44:463–464.

36. van Eijk MM, Roes KC, Honing ML, et al. Effect of rivastigmine as an adjunct to usual care with haloperidol on duration of delirium and mortality in critically ill patients: a multicentre, double-blind, placebo-controlled randomised trial. *Lancet*. 2010;376(9755):1829–1837.

37. Sos J, Cassem NH. The intravenous use of haloperidol for acute delirium in intensive care settings. In: Speidel H, Rodewald G, eds. *Psychic and Neurological Dysfunctions After Open Heart Surgery*. Thieme; 1980:196–199.

38. Menza MA, Murray GB, Holmes VF, et al. Decreased extrapyramidal symptoms with intravenous haloperidol. *J Clin Psychiatry*. 1987;48:278–280.

39. Forsman A, Ohman R. Pharmacokinetic studies on haloperidol in man. *Curr Therap Res*. 1976;10:319.

40. Adams F, Fernandez F, Andersson BS. Emergency pharmacotherapy of delirium in the critically ill cancer patient: intravenous combination drug approach. *Psychosomatics*. 1986;27(suppl 1):33–37.

41. Tesar GE, Murray GB, Cassem NH. Use of high-dose intravenous haloperidol in the treatment of agitated cardiac patients. *J Clin Psychopharmacol*. 1985;5:344–347.

42. Sanders KM, Stern TA, O'Gara PT, et al. Delirium after intra-aortic balloon pump therapy. *Psychosomatics*. 1992;33:35–41.

43. Fernandez F, Holmes VF, Adams F, et al. Treatment of severe, refractory agitation with a haloperidol drip. *J Clin Psychiatry*. 1988;49:239–241.

44. Schetz JA, Perez E, Liu R, et al. A prototypical sigma-1 receptor antagonist protects against brain ischemia. *Brain Res*. 2007;1181:1–9.

45. Lee IT, Chen S, Schetz JA. An unambiguous assay for the cloned human sigma-1 receptor reveals high affinity interactions with dopamine D$_4$ receptor selective compounds and a distinct structure–affinity relationship for butyrophenones. *Eur J Pharmacol.* 2008;578:123–136.

46. Fricchione GL, Nejad SH, Esses JA, et al. Postoperative delirium. *Am J Psychiatry.* 2008;165:803–812.

47. Metzger E, Friedman R. Prolongation of the corrected QT and torsades de pointes cardiac arrhythmia associated with intravenous haloperidol in the medically ill. *J Clin Psychopharmacol.* 1993;13:128–132.

48. Wilt JL, Minnema AM, Johnson RF, et al. Torsades de pointes associated with the use of intravenous haloperidol. *Ann Intern Med.* 1993;119:391–394.

49. Hunt N, Stern TA. The association between intravenous haloperidol and torsades de pointes: three cases and a literature review. *Psychosomatics.* 1995;36:541–549.

50. Di Salvo TG, O'Gara PT. Torsades de pointes caused by high-dose intravenous haloperidol in cardiac patients. *Clin Cardiol.* 1995;18:285–290.

51. Zeifman CWE, Friedman B. Torsades de pointes: potential consequence of intravenous haloperidol in the intensive care unit. *Intensive Care World.* 1994;11:109–112.

52. Day CP, James OFW, Butler TJ, et al. QT prolongation and sudden cardiac death in patients with alcoholic liver disease. *Lancet.* 1993;341:1423–1428.

53. Schwartz TL, Masand PS. The role of atypical antipsychotics in the treatment of delirium. *Psychosomatics.* 2002;43:171–174.

54. Horikawa N, Yamazaki T, Miyamoto K, et al. Treatment for delirium with risperidone: results of a prospective open trial with 10 patients. *Gen Hosp Psychiatry.* 2003;25:289–292.

55. Parellada E, Baeza I, de Pablo J, et al. Risperidone in the treatment of patients with delirium. *J Clin Psychiatry.* 2004;65:348–353.

56. Mittal D, Jimerson NA, Neely EP, et al. Risperidone in the treatment of delirium: results from a prospective open-label trial. *J Clin Psychiatry.* 2004;65:662–667.

57. Han CS, Kim YK. A double-blind trial of risperidone and haloperidol for the treatment of delirium. *Psychosomatics.* 2004;45:297–301.

58. Skrobik YK, Bergeron N, Dumont M, et al. Olanzapine vs haloperidol: treatment of delirium in the critical care setting. *Intensive Care Med.* 2004;30:444–449.

59. Devlin JW, Roberts RJ, Fong JJ, et al. Efficacy and safety of quetiapine in critically ill patients with delirium: a prospective, multicenter, randomized, double-blind, placebo-controlled pilot study. *Crit Care Med.* 2010;38:419–427.

60. Maneeton B, Manneton N, Srisurapanont M, et al. Quetiapine versus haloperidol in the treatment of delirium: a double-blind, randomized, controlled trial. *Drug Des Devel Ther.* 2014;24: 657–667.

61. Grover S, Kumar V, Chakrabati S. Comparative efficacy study of haloperidol, olanzapine, and risperidone in delirium. *J Psychosom Res.* 2011;71:277–281.

62. Kim SW, Yoo JA, Lee SY, et al. Risperidone versus olanzapine for the treatment of delirium. *Hum Psychopharmacol.* 2010;25: 298–302.

63. Kalisvaart KJ, de Jonghe JF, Bogaards MJ, et al. Haloperidol prophylaxis for elderly hip-surgery patients at risk for delirium: a randomized placebo-controlled study. *J Am Geriatr Soc.* 2005;53:1658–1666.

64. Larsen KA, Kelly SE, Stern TA, et al. Administration of olanzapine to prevent postoperative delirium in elderly joint replacement patients: a randomized controlled trial. *Psychosomatics.* 2010;51: 409–418.

65. Prakanrattana U, Prapaitrakool S. Efficacy of risperidone for prevention of postoperative delirium in cardiac surgery. *Anaesth Intensive Care.* 2007;35:714–719.

66. Wang W, Li HL, Wang DX, et al. Haloperidol prophylaxis decreases delirium incidence in elderly patients after noncardiac surgery: a randomized controlled trial. *Crit Care Med.* 2012;40: 731–739.

67. Teslyar P, Stock VM, Wilk CM, et al. Prophylaxis with antipsychotic medication reduces the risk of post-operative delirium in elderly patients: a meta-analysis. *Psychosomatics.* 2013;54:124–131.

68. Hatta K, Kishi Y, Wada K, et al. Preventive effects of ramelteon on delirium: a randomized placebo-controlled trial. *JAMA Psychiatry.* 2014;71:397–403.

69. Papadopoulos G, Pouangare M, Papathanakos G, et al. The effect of ondansetron on postoperative delirium and cognitive function in aged orthopedic patients. *Minerva Anestesiol.* 2014;80:444–451.

70. Dautzenberg PL, Wouters CJ, Oudejans I, et al. Rivastigmine in prevention of delirium in a 65 year old man with Parkinson's disease. *Int J Geriatr Psychiatry.* 2003;18(6):555–556.

71. Dautzenberg PL, Mulder LJ, Olde Rikkert MG, et al. Delirium in elderly hospitalized patients: protective effects of chronic rivastigmine usage. *Int J Geriatr Psychiatry.* 2004;19(7):641–644.

72. Chan MTV, Cheng BC, Lee TM, et al. BIS-guided anesthesia decreases postoperative delirium and cognitive decline. *J Neurosurg Anesthesiol.* 2013;25:33–42.

73. Fernandez F, Levy JK, Mansell PWA. Management of delirium in terminally ill AIDS patients. *Int J Psychiatry Med.* 1989;19: 165–172.

74. Breitbart W, Marotta RF, Call P. AIDS and neuroleptic malignant syndrome. *Lancet.* 1988;2:1488–1489.

75. Caroff SN, Rosenberg H, Mann SC, et al. Neuroleptic malignant syndrome in the critical care unit. *Crit Care Med.* 2002;30:2609.

76. Fernandez F, Levy JK. The use of molindone in the treatment of psychotic and delirious patients infected with the human immunodeficiency virus: case reports. *Gen Hosp Psychiatry.* 1993;15:31–35.

77. Lauterbach EC. The neuropsychiatry of Parkinson's disease and related disorders. *Psychiatr Clin North Am.* 2004;27:801–825.

78. Yoon HK, Kim YK, Han C, et al. Paliperidone in the treatment of delirium: results of a prospective open-label trial. *Acta Neuropsychiatr.* 2011;23:179–183.

79. Olmedo R, Hoffman RS. Withdrawal syndromes. *Emerg Med Clin North Am.* 2000;18:273–288.

80. Repper-DeLisi J, Stern TA, Mitchell M, et al. Successful implementation of an alcohol-withdrawal pathway in a general hospital. *Psychosomatics.* 2008;49:292–299.

81. Hecksel KA, Bostwick JM, Jaeger TW, et al. Inappropriate use of symptom-triggered therapy for alcohol withdrawal in the general hospital. *Mayo Clin Proc.* 2008;83:274–279.

82. Mirski MA, Muffelman B, Ulatowski JA, et al. Sedation for the critically ill neurologic patient. *Crit Care Med.* 1995;23: 2038–2053.

83. Valenti JF, Anderson GL, Branson RD, et al. Disadvantages of prolonged propofol sedation in the critical care unit. *Crit Care Med.* 1994;22:710–712.

84. Mirenda J. Prolonged propofol sedation in the critical care unit. *Crit Care Med.* 1995;23:1304–1305.

85. El-Ebiary M, Torres A, Ramirez J, et al. Lipid deposition during the long-term infusion of propofol. *Crit Care Med.* 1995;23: 1928–1930.

86. Maldonado JR, Wysong A, van der Starre PJA, et al. Dexmedetomidine and the reduction of postoperative delirium after cardiac surgery. *Psychosomatics.* 2009;50(3):206–217.

87. Gertler R, Brown HC, Mitchell DH, et al. Dexmedetomidine: a novel sedative–analgesic agent. *Proc (Bayl Univ Med Cent).* 2001;14:13–21.

88. Farrell KR, Ganzini L. Misdiagnosing delirium as depression in medically ill elderly patients. *Arch Intern Med.* 1995;155: 2459–2464.

89. Boland RJ, Diaz S, Lamdan RM, et al. Overdiagnosis of depression in the general hospital. *Gen Hosp Psychiatry.* 1996;18:28–35.

90. Ely EW, Siegel MD Inouye SK. Delirium in the intensive care unit: an under-recognized syndrome of organ dysfunction. *Semin Respir Crit Care Med.* 2001;22:115–126.

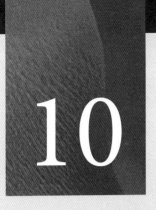

10

PATIENTS WITH NEUROCOGNITIVE DISORDERS

MARC S. WEINBERG, MD, PHD ▪ FRANKLIN KING IV, MD ▪ ILSE R. WIECHERS, MD, MPP, MHS ▪ JENNIFER R. GATCHEL, MD, PHD

As life expectancy extends and the baby boomer generation begins to reach geriatric age, we will confront an epidemic of neurocognitive disorders (NCDs) in general hospitals. The incidence of Alzheimer disease (AD), the most common cause of NCD, is roughly one in nine individuals, or over 6.5 million Americans >65 years, possibly increasing to 12.7 million by 2050.[1] Worldwide estimates of dementia (57 million individuals in 2019) may nearly triple to >152 million by 2050, which is largely attributable to the growth and aging of the population.[2] Unfortunately, most NCDs (used interchangeably in this chapter with the term "dementia"), including AD, are incurable. However, progression can be slowed when the condition is identified and managed appropriately; only a few neurocognitive conditions are reversible. Given that a major task for consultation psychiatrists is to assist in the diagnosis and treatment of NCDs, this chapter provides an overview of these disorders and an approach to their diagnosis and management (Fig. 10.1).

Often, the request to see a medical or surgical inpatient is for a behavioral disturbance thought to be associated with delirium, not for cognitive difficulties alone. Nonetheless, the risk of developing delirium is between two to five times higher in patients with an NCD, and an episode of delirium may unmask a previously undiagnosed NCD. Conversely, delirium is a risk factor for the development of an NCD.[3] Thus, the presence of delirium in an elderly patient should lead the consultant to conduct a thorough evaluation in search of a potentially co-existing NCD. Moreover, behavioral disturbances may be related to an underlying NCD (i.e., behavioral and psychological symptoms of dementia, a.k.a. neuropsychiatric symptoms [NPS]), even in the absence of delirium.

Indeed, another common consultation request is for the evaluation of NPS associated with an NCD. Depression, apathy, and anxiety are among the most common NPS early in the course of many NCDs, although many manifestations (e.g., irritability, impulsivity/disinhibition, psychosis, sleep disturbances, agitation, or aggression) span multiple domains. It is often challenging to determine whether dysregulated mood or other NPS symptoms are causing, co-existing with, or resulting from neurocognitive difficulties.[4] Determining the sometimes subtle differences in the history and presentation of delirium, depression, and AD, can help in the diagnosis of these disorders (Table 10.1).

Other presenting problems should alert the physician to an underlying undiagnosed, misdiagnosed, and/or un-documented NCD. These include poor medication adherence and injuries that could be accounted for by memory impairment. For example, many elderly individuals sustain burns as a result of dangerous cooking methods, or present in the context of other medical conditions that are related to an inability to independently carry out instrumental activities of daily living (IADLs) or even more basic activities of daily living (ADLs) (e.g., bathing, dressing, toileting). Another reason for referral may be the patient's difficulty in coping with care on an inpatient unit, which could signify the earlier stages of an NCD (mild NCD, which will be used interchangeably with mild cognitive impairment [MCI]). Despite a gradual cognitive decline, the patient may have functioned adequately in his or her home setting; however, in the unfamiliar hospital environment,

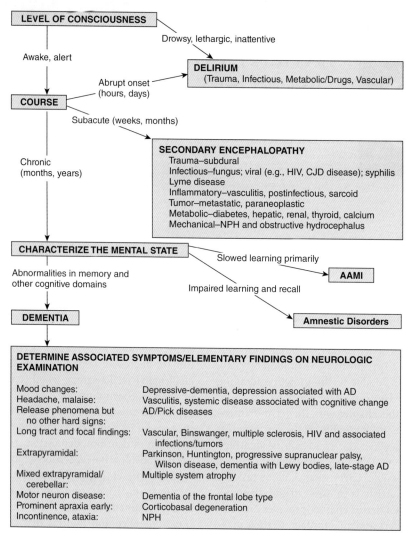

Fig. 10.1 ■ An algorithm for dementia diagnosis. *AAMI*, Age-associated memory impairment; *CJD*, Creutzfeldt-Jakob disease; *AD*, Alzheimer disease; *HIV*, human immunodeficiency virus; *NPH*, normal-pressure hydrocephalus. (Adapted from Schmahmann JD. Neurobehavioral manifestations of focal cerebral lesions. In: *Geriatric Psychiatry. Harvard Medical School and Massachusetts General Hospital Continuing Medical Education Course Syllabus.* 1995.)

care is provided on a different schedule and in a new and complex place. As a result, trusted coping mechanisms may fail and anxiety, dysphoria, agitation, or paranoia can arise or be unmasked.

Case 1

Mr. G, a 74-year-old retired chef with no known psychiatric history and a medical history significant for hypertension, was admitted for treatment of gout after 2 days of worsening foot and knee pain. Colchicine therapy was initiated. His first 24 hours passed uneventfully but on the second night in the hospital, he abruptly yelled at his nurse and showed "aggressive posturing" while she was attempting to take his vital signs. Psychiatry was consulted for the evaluation and management of this behavior.

During the interview, Mr. G was alert and agitated; however, he was oriented only to his name and

TABLE 10.1

Clinical Features of Delirium, Depression, and Alzheimer Disease

	Delirium	Depression	Alzheimer Disease
Onset of initial symptoms	Abrupt	Relatively discrete, maybe insidious	Insidious
	Difficulty with attention and disturbed consciousness	Dysphoric mood or lack of pleasure	Memory deficits—verbal and/or spatial
Course	Fluctuating—over days to weeks	Persistent—usually lasting months if untreated	Gradually progressive, over years
Family history	Not contributory	May be positive for depression	May be positive for AD
Memory	Poor registration	Patchy/inconsistent	Recent > remote
Memory complaints	Absent	Present; may be preoccupied with somatic concerns including memory complaints	Variable—usually absent
Language deficits	Dysgraphia	Increased speech latency	Confrontation naming difficulties
Affect	Labile	Depressed/irritable	Variable—may be neutral, non-tearful

"a hospital" and could not state why he had been admitted. He told the consultant, "The nurses stole my clothes and my wallet! I'm going home! Where's my wife?" The consultant calmly listened to Mr. G's concerns and offered reassurance that his belongings had been stored for safekeeping while he was in the hospital. Mr. G remained suspicious; however, he calmed down after the consultant requested that the staff retrieve his belongings and bring them to Mr. G.

When Mr. G's wife arrived during evening visitation hours, the consultant organized a discussion with her, the nurse, and the night-float resident, whereby the reason for Mr. G's hospitalization was revisited with him. An interview conducted with Mr. G's wife alone revealed that Mr. G had gotten lost several times recently and that she had taken over paying their bills due to errors he had made over the past year. He had also become "confused" during a family trip the previous summer.

For the duration of his stay, Mr. G's personal effects were placed around him to create an atmosphere of familiarity, and the team worked to ensure that he was frequently re-oriented to the date, location, and purpose of the admission. He was discharged without further incident, and outpatient neuropsychology and behavioral neurology appointments were arranged to further evaluate for delirium, NCD, or both.

EPIDEMIOLOGY

Improvements in public health, nutrition, and medical care for the elderly have led to a dramatic increase in the US population over the age of 65. Further, those who live beyond the age of 90, the so-called oldest old, comprise the fastest-growing segment of the US population.[5] This is noteworthy, as aging is a risk factor for dementia. Although the results of epidemiologic studies vary depending on the subjects sampled and the method employed, dementia occurs in approximately 14% of those older than 71 years, and this figure rises to 37% in those over the age of 90, and 50% in older non-agenarians.[6,7] The global prevalence of dementia has been estimated at 57 million individuals in 2019[2]; AD, the most common type of dementia, is the sixth leading cause of death for adults in the USA. In 2022, the direct costs of caring for those with AD in the USA were estimated at $321 billion (in 2021 dollars).[1] Unfortunately, there is a significant racial and ethnic disparity in AD burden.[8] The prevalence and incidence of AD and related dementias in Black and Hispanic populations in the USA is approximately 35% higher than that of White or Asian individuals,[9] based on meta-analyses from the literature and claims data. Interventional AD trials intending to benefit broad swathes of society recruit many fewer individuals from minority backgrounds.[10] Female sex carries an increased risk of AD, even when accounting for differences in longevity; notably, some sex differences in AD risk are related to higher rates of vascular dementia in men.[11]

Approximately 50% to 70% of cases of dementia are due to AD. Vascular dementia (which can have several etiologies) is the second most common type of dementia and it can exist independently, but frequently co-occurs with other dementias, especially AD. Lewy body dementia (LBD) is the next most common type, followed by the less common forms of dementia, such as frontotemporal dementia (FTD), dementias associated with Parkinson disease, and Creutzfeldt-Jakob disease (CJD).

DIAGNOSIS

In an effort to define disorders characterized by cognitive dysfunction, the *Diagnostic and Statistical Manual of Mental Disorders*, 5th edition (DSM-5) has replaced the term "dementia" with "major neurocognitive disorder."[12] The diagnosis of major NCD has also changed; having memory impairment is no longer necessary, but instead, there must be a significant decline from the previous level of functioning in at least one cognitive domain (e.g., memory, executive function, language, or social cognition).

Features of various NCDs may include aphasia (difficulty with any aspect of language), apraxia (the impaired ability to perform motor tasks despite intact motor function), agnosia (an impairment in object recognition despite intact sensory function), or a disturbance of executive function (including the ability to think abstractly, as well as to plan, initiate, sequence, monitor, and stop complex behavior). Associated features include impaired judgment, poor insight, personality change, and psychiatric symptoms (e.g., persecutory delusions and hallucinations—particularly visual). Motor disturbances (e.g., falls, ataxia, parkinsonism, and extrapyramidal symptoms [EPS]) and dysarthria (slurred speech) may be associated with certain NCDs.

Additional essential elements for a diagnosis of a major NCD include a significant impact on independent functioning and the occurrence of impairment outside of the exclusive context of delirium. These final criteria are necessary to rule out age-associated memory impairment, congenital intellectual disability, and life-threatening acute confusional disorders. A comparison of delirium, depression, or AD, the most common form of major NCD, is presented in Table 10.1. Should the differential diagnosis suggest against an acute confusional or depressive disorder, a bevy of specific disorders can cause cognitive impairment (Table 10.2). The consultant may not have in-depth knowledge of these alternative diagnoses but may employ pattern recognition to identify common and unusual presentations.

Many elderly individuals complain of memory difficulties, often involving learning new information or names or finding the right words. In most circumstances, such lapses are normal. The term *mild cognitive impairment (MCI)* was coined to label an intermediate category between the normal cognitive losses that are associated with aging and those linked with dementia and corresponds in the *DSM-5* to the diagnosis of mild NCD. MCI is characterized by a notable decline in memory or other cognitive functions compared with age-matched controls, without significant impairment in independent functioning. MCI is common among the elderly, although estimates vary widely depending on the diagnostic criteria and assessment methods employed. A meta-analysis examining the rate of progression from MCI to AD found that 6.7% progressed to AD each year, and overall, one-third of those with MCI developed AD during their lifetime.[13] Risk factors for progression from MCI to AD include carrier status of the E4 allele of the apolipoprotein E (*APOE*) gene (a major risk factor for AD), clinical severity, brain atrophy, specific patterns of cerebrospinal fluid (CSF) biomarkers and cerebral glucose metabolism, and amyloid-β deposition (Aβ, a pathological finding also AD-related, discussed below). Further work to identify and refine factors that place people at risk for progression of cognitive decline is an area of active research.[14]

Neurocognitive Disorder Due to Alzheimer Disease

Alzheimer disease (AD) is a progressive, irreversible, and fatal brain disease that affects memory, thinking, and behavior. The classic brain lesions of AD include neurofibrillary tangles (composed of hyperphosphorylated tau protein) and neuritic plaques (composed of

TABLE 10.2
Causes of Cognitive Impairment: Diagnoses by Categories with Representative Examples

Degenerative
Alzheimer disease
Frontotemporal dementias
Dementia with Lewy bodies
Corticobasal degeneration
Huntington disease
Wilson disease
Parkinson disease
Multiple system atrophy
Progressive supranuclear palsy

Psychiatric
Depression
Bipolar disorder
Schizophrenia

Vascular
Vascular dementia
Binswanger encephalopathy
Cerebral amyloid angiopathy
Diffuse hypoxic/ischemic injury

Obstructive
Normal-pressure hydrocephalus
Obstructive hydrocephalus

Traumatic
Chronic subdural hematoma
Chronic traumatic encephalopathy
Post-concussion syndrome

Neoplastic
Tumor: malignant—primary and secondary
Tumor: benign (e.g., frontal meningioma)
Paraneoplastic limbic encephalitis

Infections
Chronic meningitis
COVID-19
Post-herpes encephalitis
Focal cerebritis/abscesses
Human immunodeficiency virus (HIV) dementia

HIV-associated infection
Syphilis
Lyme encephalopathy
Subacute sclerosing panencephalitis
Creutzfeldt-Jakob disease
Progressive multifocal leukoencephalopathy
Parenchymal sarcoidosis
Chronic systemic infection
Urinary tract infection

Demyelinatin g
Multiple sclerosis
Adrenoleukodystrophy
Metachromatic leukodystrophy

Autoimmune
Systemic lupus erythematosus
Polyarteritis nodosa

Drugs/Toxins
Medications
Anticholinergics
Antihistamines
Anticonvulsants
β-Blockers
Sedative-hypnotics

Substance Abuse
Alcohol
Inhalants
Phenylcyclidine
Cannabis

Toxins
Arsenic
Bromide
Carbon monoxide
Lead
Mercury
Organophosphates

amyloid β peptides). Although a definitive diagnosis of AD relies on post-mortem findings of these lesions, detailed clinical assessments (by psychiatrists, neurologists, and neuropsychologists), in combination with the use of structural and functional neuroimaging and certain biomarkers, have a high concordance rate with autopsy-proven disease.[15]

Progressive memory loss is the hallmark of AD. Other common cognitive clinical features include impairment of language, visual-spatial ability, and executive function. Patients may be unaware of their cognitive deficits, but this is not uniformly the case. There may be evidence of forgetting conversations, having difficulty with household finances, being disoriented to time and place, and misplacing items regularly. At least two domains of cognitive impairment, including progressive memory decline (that affects functional ability), are required to make a clinical diagnosis of AD.[16] In addition to its cognitive features, AD is associated with several neuropsychiatric symptoms, even in its mildest phases. In particular, irritability, apathy, and depression are common early in the course of the disease, whereas psychosis (including delusions and hallucinations) tends to occur later.[17]

Vascular Neurocognitive Disorder

Vascular neurocognitive disorder, commonly called vascular dementia, refers to a variety of vascular-related causes of dementia, including multi-infarct dementia and small-vessel disease. The pathophysiology of vascular dementia can be related to recurrent or localized embolic strokes, smaller subcortical strokes (e.g., lacunar infarcts), or cerebral hemorrhages. It is important to keep in mind that cerebral hemorrhages (resulting from hypertension or amyloid angiopathy) require a different type of clinical management than does typical vascular occlusive disease, and that dementia develops in 15% to 30% of patients after a stroke.[18]

The clinical features of vascular dementia depend on the lesion location; both the type of cognitive deficits and the time course of the cognitive changes vary. Embolic or large-vessel stroke-related dementia often progresses in a step-wise pattern, with intervening periods of stability punctuated by abrupt declines in cognitive function. Although this might be considered the classic presentation, it is not the most common.[19] Presentations that involve relatively isolated psychotic symptoms in the setting of preserved memory should also raise the possibility of vascular dementia. Similarly, apathy, executive dysfunction, and a relatively intact memory are suggestive of a small-vessel ischemic process.

The main difficulty that arises in the diagnosis of vascular dementia is distinguishing it from AD. Classically, vascular dementia has been distinguished from AD by an abrupt onset and a step-wise course, although with small-vessel, subcortical disease, acute changes may not be appreciated. In addition, prominent executive dysfunction and preserved recognition memory are also suggestive of vascular dementia.

However, the symptoms of vascular dementia frequently overlap with those of AD; in fact, evidence of both is often found at autopsy.

Neurocognitive Disorder with Lewy Bodies

Neurocognitive disorder with Lewy bodies, or Lewy body dementia (LBD), shares clinical features of both AD and Parkinson disease dementia (PDD); therefore making an accurate diagnosis can be challenging. The main pathologic features of LBD are protein deposits called *Lewy bodies*, composed of α-synuclein in the cortex and brainstem.[20] Features that suggest LBD include parkinsonism, visual hallucinations (which occur early, in contrast to the pattern seen in AD), a fluctuating course, an extreme sensitivity to neuroleptic medications, autonomic dysfunction (with falls), and executive and visual-spatial dysfunction (with relatively spared language and memory function). Rapid eye movement sleep-behavior disorder may precede the onset of other symptoms by several years. As in Parkinson disease (PD), depression is common. LBD differs from PDD in that in the former, motor symptoms occur within 1 year of the onset of cognitive problems; in contrast, motor symptoms in PDD typically precede cognitive problems by several years. Although these clinical features are helpful in the identification of the disease, clinical-pathologic concordance remains poor, and post-mortem pathologic findings of Lewy bodies in the cerebral cortex, amygdala, and brainstem are necessary to confirm the diagnosis.[21]

Frontotemporal Neurocognitive Disorder

Frontotemporal neurocognitive disorders, or frontotemporal dementias (FTDs), are a heterogeneous group of disorders that involve the degeneration of different regions of the frontal and temporal lobes, resulting in myriad clinical presentations. Currently included under the category of FTDs are three clinical variants: behavioral-variant frontotemporal dementia (bv-FTD, which accounts for 50% to 70% of FTD in the United States), and primary progressive aphasias (PPAs), which are subdivided into a semantic variant PPA and a non-fluent variant PPA.[22] FTDs tend to manifest at younger ages than typical AD, with most cases occurring in people younger than 65 years of age.

The classic hallmarks of FTD, particularly bv-FTD, are behavioral features, usually out of proportion to, or preceding cognitive impairment. In general, there is a subtle onset and a progression of symptoms (with loss of judgment, disinhibition, impulsivity, loss of empathy and social tact, and interpersonal withdrawal). Other common symptoms involve stereotypies, excessive oral-manual exploration, selective eating habits, wanderlust, excessive joviality, displays of sexually provocative behaviors, and use of inappropriate words or actions. In later stages, parkinsonism is common.

In some cases, language is initially or primarily affected, and can remain as a relatively isolated deficit for years. In these cases, there is often primarily left hemisphere pathology selectively involving the frontal or temporal lobes or the peri-Sylvian cortex. PPA refers to symptomatic involvement of the frontal (or other peri-Sylvian) language areas leading to changes in both expressive and receptive language function. Depending on the localization of left hemisphere pathology, patients may exhibit different degrees of impairment of word-finding, object-naming, syntax, or word-comprehension abilities. Semantic variant PPA is characterized by significant loss of word meaning (i.e., semantic losses) with relatively preserved fluency, which results from left anterior temporal lobe involvement. In contrast, progressive non-fluent aphasia (PNFA) results in difficulty in the production of language. This can manifest as changes in the manner of speech, for example speaking more slowly, with grammatical errors, or with omitted or improperly ordered words. The definitions of these syndromes have been in flux, and in more recent years, PPA syndromes have been further divided into three patterns: semantic variant PPA and PNFA (as above); and logopenic progressive aphasia (LPA) also referred to as the logopenic/phonological variant of PPA. LPA is characterized by impaired naming and single-word retrieval in the absence of motor speech abnormalities and generally preserved object knowledge and comprehension of single words and simple sentences.

Clinical presentations of FTD vary depending on the relative involvement of the hemisphere (right or left) or lobe (frontal or temporal) affected.[23] Patients may initially have more involvement of the right temporal lobe than the left and exhibit primarily a behavioral syndrome with emotional distancing, irritability, and disruption of sleep, appetite, and libido. With initially greater left than right temporal lobe involvement, patients tend to exhibit more language-related problems, including anomia, word-finding difficulties, repetitive speech, and loss of semantic information (i.e., semantic variant PPA).[24] In some cases of FTD, the frontal lobes may be involved more than the temporal lobes. In these instances, patients exhibit symptoms of elation, disinhibition, apathy, or aberrant motor behavior. Depending on the combination of regions involved, patients with FTD exhibit specific cognitive and NPS. As the disease progresses to involve greater expanses of the frontotemporal cortex, the clinical features become similar. The presumption is that the atrophy and underlying pathology that accompanies FTD is regionally specific, but it becomes more generalized as the disease progresses.

Neurocognitive Disorder Due to Another Medical Condition

NCDs caused by other medical conditions include a broad range of disorders that are causally associated with cognitive impairment: structural lesions; trauma; infections; endocrine, nutritional, and metabolic disorders; and autoimmune diseases. Two notable examples include NCDs caused by normal-pressure hydrocephalus (NPH) and CJD.

NPH is recognized by the classic clinical features of gait disturbance, frontal systems dysfunction, and urinary incontinence.[25] Intermittent pressure increases are thought to cause ventricular expansion over time, with damage to the adjacent white matter tracts that connect the frontal lobes. Evaluation usually includes structural brain imaging (magnetic resonance imaging [MRI] and computed tomography [CT]) that demonstrates ventricular enlargement that is out of proportion to the atrophy present.

CJD is a rare disorder that causes a characteristic triad of dementia, myoclonus, and distinctive periodic electroencephalographic complexes. CJD is caused by prions, novel proteinaceous infective agents that induce changes in the cerebral cortex and lead to the distinctive microscopic, vacuolar appearance of spongiform encephalopathy. The CSF in almost 90% of CJD cases contains traces of prion proteins obtained by performing a routine lumbar puncture. Treatment of afflicted individuals is supportive, insofar as the condition follows a characteristic course, with death arriving after an average of 6 months.[26]

Substance/Medication-Induced Neurocognitive Disorder

To establish the diagnosis of substance/medication-induced NCD, there must be evidence from the history, physical examination, or laboratory data that cognitive deficits consistent with dementia are probably caused by exposure to a substance or medication. The diagnosis cannot be made during a period of acute intoxication or drug withdrawal. The most common cause of this type of disorder is chronic alcohol use,[27] but toxins, poisons, inhalants, sedative-hypnotics, and other medications are also causes.

Neurocognitive Disorders Due to Multiple Etiologies

In the diagnostic section of the DSM-5, the phrase "neurocognitive disorder due to multiple etiologies" serves to emphasize that a patient can have more than one cause for cognitive decline. Although many combinations can occur, perhaps the most common is the co-existence of AD and vascular disease. Some authorities refute this assertion, suggesting that diffuse LBD is the second most common primary neurocognitive disorder and that its combination with AD is not sufficiently recognized.[28] AD can also co-exist with reversible causes of dementia (e.g., vitamin B_{12} deficiency, hypothyroidism), further emphasizing the importance of a thorough medical and neurologic work-up to address co-occurring reversible causes.

EVALUATION OF NEUROCOGNITIVE DISORDERS

Evidence of cognitive compromise deserves at least as careful an assessment as evidence of the failure of any other organ. Only through a thoughtful evaluation can potential remediation of the cognitive decline be possible. Although in most cases the goal of treatment is not a cure, there is still much that can be done to help affected patients and their families. The evaluation requires a reliable history (cognitive, psychiatric, medical, and family), complete medical and neurologic examinations, appropriate laboratory testing, and assessments of mental status and cognitive function.

History

A meticulous cognitive history is an extremely sensitive diagnostic tool. Onset, course, and associated symptoms must be elicited carefully because these details of history often provide critical diagnostic clues. Because of time constraints, consultants may be inclined to limit their history-taking to the patient alone. Although some mildly impaired patients may have sufficient capacity to provide an accurate account of their deficits, many (owing to their amnesia, agnosia, or loss of insight) do not. To rely solely on the patient's report will yield a limited history; it may be inaccurate, and it will be incomplete. Additional history is best obtained from people who spend time with the patient, such as family members, close friends, or even healthcare providers who are familiar with the patient. It is important to interview informants away from the patient because informants may be uncomfortable discussing evidence of cognitive decline in the presence of the patient. Even a phone call to a family member or a friend can be helpful, as can a review of old medical records, when available.

A good cognitive history must establish the time at which cognitive changes first became apparent. This information provides important clues regarding the nature of the disorder because some diseases (e.g., CJD) are well known for causing a rapid rate of decline. If the time of onset of the disorder is known, the rate of decline can be estimated by seeing how long it has taken the patient to reach the current level of dysfunction. The rate of progression can only be approximated; however, it is helpful for patients and family members to have such estimates to facilitate planning.

Next, it is important to determine the nature of the behavioral changes that were evident when the disease began. This information can also be helpful in the diagnostic process. For example, an early symptom of FTD is personality change, as manifested by inappropriate behavior, whereas the early symptoms of AD may involve increased passivity or apathy and a gradual, progressive decline in the ability to learn new information. Several years after the onset of the disease, when most patients are diagnosed, the cognitive symptoms of the two disorders may be quite similar, so information about the initial symptoms may be critical.

It is also important to determine whether the initial symptoms developed gradually or abruptly. If the onset of illness was insidious, as in AD, the family may realize only in retrospect that a decline has occurred. In contrast, a series of small strokes may produce symptoms of sudden onset, even if lesions were not evident on CT or an MRI scan of the head. Delirium generally has an acute onset as well. However, if it results from a condition, such as a gradually developing drug toxicity, its onset may be subacute or insidious.

The way symptoms have progressed also provides important diagnostic information. Step-wise deterioration characterized by sudden exacerbation of symptoms is typical of vascular dementia. A physical illness (e.g., pneumonia, a hip fracture) in a patient with AD, however, can also cause a sudden decline in cognitive function. Thus careful questioning is necessary to determine the underlying cause of a step-wise decline in function.

Accurate histories of cognitive function are difficult to obtain because most patients and family members are not attuned to subtle behavioral changes. Important aspects of the medical history may go unrecognized. For example, the family may state that the first symptoms of the disease were the patient's anxiety and depression about work. NPS, such as depression and anxiety, may be among the earliest behavioral changes that occur in the prodrome of a cognitive disorder, as manifestations of underlying disease biology that are closely related to cognitive changes. Indeed, after further inquiry family members may remember several episodes that preceded the onset of work-related anxiety in which the patient could not remember how to deal with a complex situation or learn how to use new equipment.

Family members may also have difficulty understanding why certain subtle distinctions are important for diagnosis. For example, they may report that the patient's first symptom was forgetfulness, but when asked to provide instances of this forgetfulness, they may explain that the patient had difficulty installing a new knob in the kitchen or had trouble finding a familiar location. Both features would suggest spatial difficulty more than memory difficulty. In addition, it may also be difficult for family members to accept and acknowledge that impairments exist, thus limiting the accuracy of the information that they provide.

Finally, it may be more challenging to obtain accurate information from family and caregivers about the early stages of subtle decline. Although a history of a gradual, progressive decline is essential to the diagnosis of AD, informants frequently state that the disorder came on suddenly at the point at which they suddenly became aware that something was wrong. This realization by the family often coincides with external events (e.g., a trip to an unfamiliar place prevented the patient from employing over-learned habits and routines and thus exposed the cognitive decline). The hospital is obviously one such setting; it is not uncommon for family members to state, "He was fine until he got here!" When this happens, it is necessary to attempt to identify when subtle symptoms of cognitive change first occur. Usually, family members can recall episodes that they had overlooked that in hindsight suggested an earlier change in cognitive function. Annual family gatherings or holiday events are useful occasions about which to inquire.

It is also important to determine the patient's current functional status. This information is best obtained informally by asking about the patient's typical day and any changes in his or her home activities and hobbies. Alternatively, the use of scales, such as the activities of daily living (ADL) and the instrumental activities of daily living (IADL) scales (Table 10.3), have been developed for this purpose. The ADL scale surveys six basic areas of function and determines whether the individual can perform these tasks independently or with assistance.[29] The IADL scale provides a sense of a patient's executive functions.[30] A substantial discrepancy between the functional and cognitive status of the patient generally suggests the presence of a psychiatric illness. For purposes of comfort, safety, rehabilitation, and determination of appropriate level of care, ADL and IADL results should be evaluated carefully.

The psychiatric history, with attention paid to reports of past mood or psychotic disorders, may assist in the differentiation of cognitive changes observed in depression from those of a primary NCD. Although cognitive changes can be seen in depression, the history and mental status examination usually allows the physician to separate depression from an NCD or suggest that both are present. Neurovegetative symptoms of depression may be difficult to link specifically to mood or cognitive disorders because anergia, sleep disturbance, and appetite changes can be seen in

TABLE 10.3
Assessment of Functional Status

Activities of Daily Living (ADL)	Instrumental Activities of Daily Living (IADL)
Bathing	Ability to use telephone
Dressing	Shopping
Toileting	Food preparation
Transferring	Housekeeping
Continence	Laundry
Feeding	Mode of transportation
	Responsibility for own medications
	Ability to handle finances

Adapted from Katz S, Downs TD, Cash HR, et al. Progress in the development of the index of ADL. *Gerontologist* 1970;10:20–30; Lawton MP, Brody EM. Assessment of older people: self-maintaining and instrumental activities of daily living. *Gerontologist* 1969;9:179–186.

both depression and NCDs. Thus, it is important to modify the questions asked to encompass the possibility of cognitive impairment. For example, if the tasks are simplified and within the capabilities of a non-depressed, demented patient, the patient is typically able to carry them out. Similarly, if food is presented in a manner that the patient can manage, such as meat cut into bite-size pieces, the patient may show a new-found gusto in his or her appetite.

In reviewing the medical history, the physician should consider whether surgical procedures (e.g., gastrectomy predisposing to vitamin B_{12} deficiency) or medical illnesses (e.g., hypertension, systemic lupus erythematosus) contribute to the symptoms of cognitive dysfunction. It is crucial to determine whether the patient was exposed to toxins (e.g., lead or other heavy metals, carbon monoxide), or has a history of head trauma. Careful questioning should cover alcohol and drug usage (not just current patterns), including a history of abuse or overuse. Many non-psychotropic agents, including those sold over-the-counter, can have negative effects on cognition. For example, antihistamines and antispasmodic drugs can cause cognitive difficulties. Valuable historical data include information regarding impairments in hearing or vision, incontinence, falls, and gait disturbances.

The family history is also helpful. Certain NCDs (e.g., Huntington disease) have definite genetic modes of transmission (e.g., autosomal dominant), whereas for others (e.g., certain vascular dementias) the specific mode of transmission may be unclear, but their

prevalence is much higher in affected families than in the population at large. Familial heritability of AD is also high, leading to the hypothesis that AD risk factors are genetically transmitted.[31] AD is genetically complex, with less than 5% of AD caused by single gene mutations, and the remainder of inheritance is considered polygenic, involving multiple genomic variants and non-genetic contributions.

Early-onset AD is almost always linked to a family history of dementia and it is highly genetically linked (estimated to have 90%–100% heritability[32]), commonly involving autosomal dominant mutations in the *APP*, *PSEN1*, or *PSEN2* genes.[33] Amyloid precursor protein (*APP*) on chromosome 21 was the first identified early-onset AD-linked gene. Presenilin 1 and 2 (*PSEN1* and *PSEN2*) are the other major genes identified as autosomally dominant, also contributing significantly to early-onset AD (as early as in one's 40s[34]).

Late-onset AD (with no universally appreciated age cut-off but commonly construed as >65 years) involves a complex combination of genetic and non-genetic risk factors.

The most well-known AD risk–related gene is apolipoprotein E (*APOE*). Unlike the autosomal dominant genes listed above, *APOE* is a *susceptibility* gene that increases the risk for AD without causing the disease and contributes to 40% to 60% of cases. *APOE* has three alleles: 2, 3, and 4, which have a complex relationship to risk for both AD and cardiovascular disease, with the 2 allele decreasing the risk of both disorders and increasing longevity, and the 4 allele increasing risk and decreasing longevity. The effect of *ApoE4* varies with age; it is most marked in the sixties and it falls substantially beyond the age of 80 or 90 years.

FTD is the most common form of dementia with an onset of <60 years, with most cases presenting between 45 and 64 years of age.[35] In contrast, FTD diagnoses account for only 2.7% of dementia diagnoses for patients >65 years old. FTD sometimes runs in families, and autosomal dominant inheritance is frequently observed. Many of these families are found to harbor a mutation in *MATP*, the gene encoding the tau protein, which is found in NFTs. In addition, FTD can sometimes be associated with mutations in *GRN*, *VCP*, *TARDBP PSEN1*, and *CHMP2B*,[35,36] along with a recently identified C9ORF72 hexanucleotide repeat expansion.[37]

Medical and Neurologic Examination

The consultant should review the results of recent examinations in the medical record to assess their adequacy and accuracy. The cognitive portion of prior examinations may indicate only that the patient was alert and oriented. Additionally, if notes report "disorientation," it is often unclear from the chart whether the patient could not remember the day of the week or whether he or she was confused or psychotic. Consequently, the psychiatric consultant should look for medical and neurologic findings that are associated with NCDs. For example, focal areas of muscle weakness and pyramidal signs may suggest vascular dementia. The presence of extrapyramidal movements may point to one of the NCDs that principally affects subcortical motor areas. Mild to moderate AD, however, may also be associated with EPS and other neurologic signs.[38] A comprehensive neurologic examination should include careful assessment of ocular function, gait, and praxis, as well as the presence of any frontal release signs.

Laboratory Examination

Table 10.4 lists laboratory and other tests that are typically ordered as part of a dementia evaluation. Whenever possible and appropriate, results of prior testing in other settings should be obtained. For example, a chest x-ray examination or CT scan should not be re-ordered if one was recently done unless an acute change has occurred. Additional tests (e.g., serum copper and ceruloplasmin for Wilson disease, antibodies for Lyme disease or autoimmune panels, or serum and urine porphyrins for acute intermittent porphyria) should be requested when the history and examination suggest a specific disorder. Additional work-up, generally reserved for the outpatient setting unless strongly indicated based on clinical evaluation, includes a lumbar puncture, which may be indicated when cancer, infection of the central nervous system (CNS), hydrocephalus, or vasculitis is suspected. Testing of AD biomarkers through CSF (e.g., an AD panel) is beneficial for aiding in diagnostic accuracy. Checking for *ApoE4* status is becoming routine, although it warrants parallel genetic counseling. Testing for the human immunodeficiency virus (HIV) infection is

---

TABLE 10.4
Recommended Laboratory Studies in a Dementia Work-Up

Blood Studies

Complete blood cell count

Vitamin B_{12}

Folate

Liver function tests

Thyroid-stimulating hormone

Syphilis serology

HIV testing

Other Studies

Urinalysis

Sleep study; evaluation for sleep apnea

Electrocardiogram

CT of MRI brain

Representative Additional Studies Based on History and Physical Findings

Chest x-ray examination

Electroencephalogram

Non-invasive carotid studies

Rheumatoid factor, antinuclear antibody, and other autoimmune disorder screens

Lumbar puncture ± Alzheimer biomarker panel

FDG-PET brain

DaT scan

Drug levels

Heavy metal screening

CT, Computed tomography; *DaT*, dopamine transporter; *FDG-PET*, 18F-fluorodeoxyglucose positron emission tomography; *HIV*, human immunodeficiency virus; *MRI*, magnetic resonance imaging.

---

indicated when a patient has relevant risk factors because up to 20% of patients with HIV infection develop dementia. However, dementia is uncommon as an initial sign.

Mental Status Examination

The bedside psychiatric examination covers considerable territory, but it focuses on assessments of affective symptoms and signs of psychosis. The physician should probe for mood symptoms, irritability, disinhibition, tearfulness, and nihilistic or suicidal thinking. Depressed elderly patients may, among their somatic complaints, describe decrements in memory. Depressed patients, as opposed to patients with AD, however, may perform better on more difficult memory tasks than on simple ones. Depressed patients are also more likely to show poor effort on testing (e.g., providing abundant "I don't know" answers) compared with patients with AD, who are more likely to confabulate when they do not know an answer.

Positive psychotic symptoms can be present in primary psychiatric disorders, such as psychotic depression or schizophrenia, but they can also be suggestive of delirium or dementia. The prevalence of psychosis in moderate to severe AD is estimated at approximately 40%, with delusions predominating over hallucinations.[39] Usually, delusions in patients with AD are of a paranoid nature, often involving the mistaken belief that misplaced items have been stolen. With the progression of the disease, *delusional misidentification syndromes* can develop, with the patient believing that loved ones are imposters (i.e., Capgras syndrome).[40] Illusions and hallucinations, usually visual, tend to occur with advanced AD. For example, some patients describe seeing "little people" entering their home. Despite their unusual nature, not all hallucinations or delusions are troublesome to the patient. Mood and psychotic symptoms can occur as part of the clinical picture of many NCDs. Generally, they are non-specific. However, taken together with other elements of the assessment, such symptoms can provide clues as to whether a psychiatric disorder or an NCD is present.

Bedside Neurocognitive Assessment

Domains of cognitive function that require rapid and accurate bedside assessment can be remembered with the mnemonic "A CALM VISAGE" (the face the consultant would put forward when confronted with a patient who is difficult to diagnose). These domains include the following: Attention, Conceptualization, Appearance/behavior, Language, Memory, Visual-spatial, Agnosia and apraxia, General intelligence, and Executive function.

Attention is important to consider because simple attentional abilities must be preserved if any other cognitive task is to be performed adequately. If the patient has difficulty concentrating on a task for even a few minutes, the assessment of other domains will likely be inaccurate. For this reason, attention is evaluated first. Auditory and visual attention can be assessed easily by means of digit span and letter cancellation tests. For the digit span test, the patient is asked to repeat a

series of numbers spaced 1 second apart. The examiner provides gradually increasing spans; unimpaired individuals can repeat five to seven numbers. For the letter cancellation test, the patient is asked to cross off a specific letter each time he or she observes it in any series of letters. A gross assessment can be inferred from how well the patient responds to questions during an interview. The physician should note whether the level of arousal fluctuates or the patient seems easily distracted during the interview.

Tasks that examine conceptualization include tests of concept formation, abstraction, set shifting, and set maintenance. Similarities and proverbs are useful in this regard.

Observation of appearance and behavior is helpful in determining whether patients can care adequately for themselves. Detecting that a patient's buttons are misaligned, for example, may suggest that he or she has spatial difficulties or apraxia.

Language testing for aphasia should include evaluation of comprehension, repetition, reading, writing, and naming. If aphasia has been ruled out or is not suspected, confrontation naming (e.g., of objects and their parts, such as jacket and lapel or watch and strap) should be included in an assessment of the older individual because impairments in naming ability (anomia) occur with age but are prominent in several disorders, including AD. In addition, alterations in verbal fluency (tested by having the patient name as many animals or words as they can in a minute that begins with a certain letter) are seen in many neurocognitive diseases.[41]

The presence of memory dysfunction, despite no longer being essential in the *DSM* criteria, remains common and important in the diagnosis of an NCD. The nature and severity of the memory impairment can serve as a guide to diagnosis, but the assessment of memory is complicated by the fact that changes in memory normally occur with aging. In general, normal elders require more time to retain new information. Therefore careful testing is important to differentiate normal from pathologic memory performance. Testing should include not only short-term memory but also memory of personal events (e.g., details of marriage, names of children) and significant historical dates (e.g., John F. Kennedy's assassination, September 11).

Assessment of visual-spatial abilities may be more difficult in older than in younger individuals because of the frequency of visual-sensory deficits in the elderly. It is difficult to enlarge certain test stimuli to evaluate this domain; therefore figure copying (e.g., of intersecting pentagons or a cube) is the most useful method of assessment.

When agnosia or apraxia is evident, the patient's disease is usually quite advanced. *Agnosia* is diagnosed when a patient fails to recognize a familiar object, despite intact sensory function. With *apraxia*, the patient's ability to carry out motor tasks is impaired, despite intact motor systems and an understanding of the tasks. For example, the patient is unable to mimic the use of common objects (e.g., the use of a toothbrush) or to carry out well-learned motor behaviors (e.g., pretending to blow out a candle). A subtle finding is "organification of praxis" in which the subject, for example, uses a finger as the toothbrush.

In addition to the areas of assessment previously mentioned, examiners should estimate general intelligence to determine whether the patient has access to previously acquired knowledge. A rough approximation can be inferred from the patient's highest level of education. Alternatively, the vocabulary subtest of *The Wechsler Adult Intelligence Scale—Revised* can be used to estimate one's level of intelligence.[42]

A simple, yet often revealing measure of executive functioning is the clock-drawing test, in which the patient is asked to draw a clock face with the hands set at a specific time, such as "ten past eleven" or "ten to two" that involves placing the hands in both hemispheres of the clock face.

Standardized Cognitive Testing

Non-standard testing developed by the clinician can be used to evaluate the cognitive domains noted previously, but a variety of standardized, brief mental status tests can be useful as well. However, although screening tests may identify cognitive difficulties, they are not sufficient to establish a diagnosis of dementia.

Commonly used screening tests are the Mini-Mental State Examination (MMSE)[41] and the Blessed Dementia Scale.[43] Both have high test-retest reliability, and are relatively brief, taking 5 to 15 minutes to administer. Historically, the MMSE has been the most frequently used in clinical settings because it assesses a broad range of cognitive abilities (i.e., attention, concentration, memory, language, spatial ability, and set

shifting) in a simple, straightforward manner. Scores on the MMSE range from 0 to 30, with scores above 26 generally indicating normal cognitive function. Mildly impaired patients typically obtain MMSE scores of 20 to 26; moderate impairment is reflected in scores of 11 to 20; and severe impairment is indicated by scores of 10 or lower. A cut-off score of 23 is generally recommended as suggestive of cognitive dysfunction; however, the application of this cut-off score must be interpreted in the context of the patient's education level. For example, an extremely bright, well-educated person may score 29 or 30, despite having significant impairment.

The MMSE is a useful screening tool in the assessment of patients with mild to moderate cognitive impairments, but it is less helpful in the evaluation of severely impaired patients. The quantification of cognitive abilities in severely impaired patients can serve a variety of needs, including the ability to follow patients throughout an intervention trial, the assessment of spared abilities (which can be used in the development of management strategies), and the examination of the relationship among post-mortem neurochemical and neuropathologic findings and cognitive status shortly before death. The Test for Severe Impairment (TSI) is a useful scale for severely impaired patients and the test can contribute to improved patient management.[44] It minimizes the need for the patient to use language skills because severely impaired patients often have minimally intact verbal skills. Nonetheless, the TSI can evaluate motor performance, language comprehension, language production, immediate and delayed memory, general knowledge, and conceptualization.

Patients with MCI (mild NCD) often score within the normal range on the dementia screening tools discussed previously. The Montreal Cognitive Assessment (MoCA) (Fig. 10.2) was created as a 10-minute screening tool to assist in the detection of MCI.[45] It assesses many cognitive domains, and although somewhat more challenging than the MMSE, it assesses executive and abstract functions in a superior manner. Components of the visual-spatial and executive function testing include a brief "Trails B," copying a cube, and drawing a clock. As the MoCA covers additional cognitive domains and may be more sensitive than the MMSE in detecting MCI, it is increasingly used as the initial measurement of choice at some institutions.[46]

MONTREAL COGNITIVE ASSESSMENT (MoCA)

NAME :
Education :   Date of birth :
Sex :   DATE :

VISUOSPATIAL / EXECUTIVE			POINTS

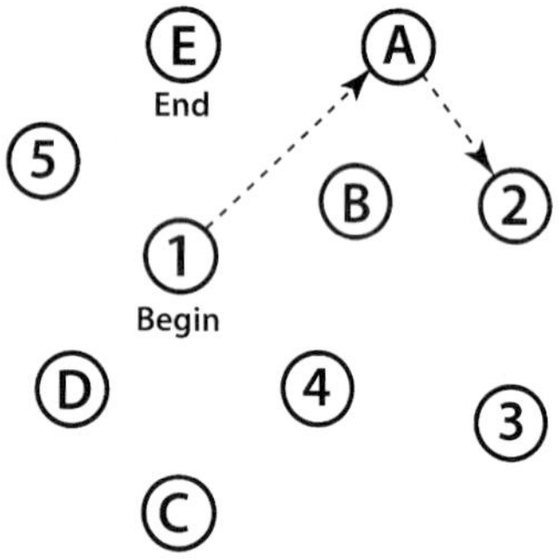

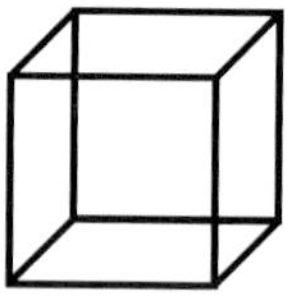

Copy cube

Draw CLOCK (Ten past eleven) (3 points)

[ ]   [ ]

[ ]   [ ]   [ ]
Contour   Numbers   Hands

___/5

NAMING

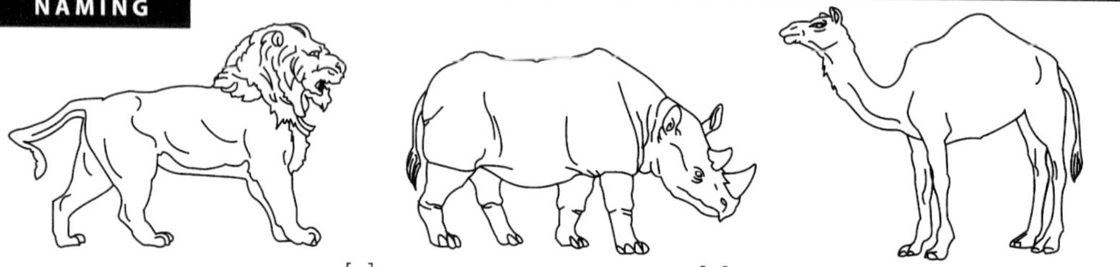

[ ]   [ ]   [ ]   ___/3

MEMORY	Read list of words, subject must repeat them. Do 2 trials, even if 1st trial is successful. Do a recall after 5 minutes.		FACE	VELVET	CHURCH	DAISY	RED	No points
		1st trial						
		2nd trial						

ATTENTION	Read list of digits (1 digit/ sec.).	Subject has to repeat them in the forward order [ ] 2 1 8 5 4	
		Subject has to repeat them in the backward order [ ] 7 4 2	___/2

Read list of letters. The subject must tap with his hand at each letter A. No points if ≥ 2 errors

[ ] F B A C M N A A J K L B A F A K D E A A A J A M O F A A B   ___/1

Serial 7 subtraction starting at 100   [ ] 93   [ ] 86   [ ] 79   [ ] 72   [ ] 65

4 or 5 correct subtractions: **3 pts**, 2 or 3 correct: **2 pts**, 1 correct: **1 pt**, 0 correct: **0 pt**   ___/3

LANGUAGE	Repeat : I only know that John is the one to help today. [ ]	
	The cat always hid under the couch when dogs were in the room. [ ]	___/2

Fluency / Name maximum number of words in one minute that begin with the letter F   [ ] _____ (N ≥ 11 words)   ___/1

ABSTRACTION	Similarity between e.g. banana - orange = fruit [ ] train – bicycle [ ] watch - ruler	___/2

DELAYED RECALL	Has to recall words	FACE	VELVET	CHURCH	DAISY	RED	Points for UNCUED recall only	___/5
	WITH NO CUE	[ ]	[ ]	[ ]	[ ]	[ ]		
Optional	Category cue							
	Multiple choice cue							

ORIENTATION	[ ] Date [ ] Month [ ] Year [ ] Day [ ] Place [ ] City	___/6

© Z.Nasreddine MD   Version 7.1   **www.mocatest.org**   Normal ≥ 26 / 30

Administered by: _____

TOTAL   ___/30

Add 1 point if ≤ 12 yr edu

Fig. 10.2 ■ The Montreal Cognitive Assessment (MoCA). (Copyright Z. Nasreddine, MD. The test and instructions may be accessed at www.mocatest.org)

The MoCA test was previously available online for no cost. However, because of concerns about variability in test administration and to ensure the validity and reliability of the test, a training requirement for the administration of the MoCA went into effect on September 1, 2019, and became a prerequisite for online access. After September 1, 2020, access to the test has been limited to trained and certified users (for a one-time fee of $125), while the paper version of the test remains readily available. Some clinicians, based on their specialty training (neuropsychologists, geriatric psychiatrists), may be exempt from the certification requirement, as are students, residents, and fellows who are supervised by trained senior clinicians.

With all structured tests, the examiner must not simply look at the total score but rather assess the qualitative areas of low and high function. The pattern of deficits may confirm a diagnostic opinion. Conversely, determining that areas of function have been preserved assists the clinician in making recommendations to the patient and the family for adaptive coping with dementia.

TREATMENT CONSIDERATIONS

The approach to treatment of an NCD depends on the specific diagnosis established, as well as on the troublesome symptoms and signs that must be managed. Treatment is divided into three broad categories: medical and surgical interventions, behavioral interventions, and pharmacotherapy. Pharmacotherapy can be divided into treatments for cognitive symptoms and neuropsychiatric symptoms (a.k.a. behavioral and psychological symptoms) of dementia.

Medical and Surgical Interventions

Some NCDs can be helped dramatically by surgical interventions. For example, the treatment for NPH is the removal of CSF via a lumbar puncture or ventriculoperitoneal shunting. It is important to perform cognitive and motor testing before and after the removal of a large volume of CSF.[47] Similarly, draining of frontal subdural hematomas can improve patients' cognition and behavior.

Other reversible medical disorders that contribute to dementia should also be corrected. For example, thyroid hormone repletion in the myxedematous patient improves cognitive function. In many conditions, however, damage has already been done, and repletion may offer only marginal improvement. For example, a patient who had deteriorated over several years was found to have an extremely low vitamin B_{12} level. Her dementia was profound, and it did not respond to intramuscular injections of vitamin B_{12}. Further deterioration of her cognition and other nervous system functions, however, may have been prevented by the treatment.

Sometimes the reduction or elimination of drugs can be beneficial. For example, the elimination of highly anticholinergic (e.g., diphenhydramine, oxybutynin) or sedative-hypnotic medications (e.g., diazepam) can lead to improvement in drug-induced memory impairment. Care must be taken, however, to avoid inducing a withdrawal syndrome caused by too abrupt a taper, especially with benzodiazepines and barbiturates.

Searching for treatable contributors to cognitive decline is important, even when the primary diagnosis is AD. Identification of co-existing medical conditions that have a deleterious effect on the patient's cognition is critical. For example, the aggressive treatment of a urinary tract infection improves not only physical comfort but also intellectual function (because infection in the setting of AD usually causes delirium). Recognition and management of sleep apnea can make a significant difference as well, as disruptions of the sleep-wake cycle can worsen cognition and cause neuropsychiatric symptoms and may even potentiate AD pathophysiological processes, such as CNS Aβ clearance. Pain may also have a negative effect on cognition and it is often overlooked in patients with dementia who are admitted to a general hospital.[48] A patient whose AD was manageable at home became severely aggressive and more confused owing to the discomfort of an impacted bowel. Another patient with presumed vascular dementia showed some improvement in cognition after treatment for congestive heart failure.

Behavioral Interventions

Once drug effects and contributing medical conditions have been identified and managed, acute behavioral symptoms associated with dementia may subside. The environmental strangeness of the hospital, however, may be enough to trigger new psychiatric and behavioral problems, such as paranoid ideation and agitation.

Often, behavioral management alone reduces certain symptoms. Non-pharmacologic interventions are considered first-line treatments because there is evidence to support their efficacy and minimal potential for adverse events; therefore they should be used in every case.[49,50] The basic approaches are well known but are worth repeating (Table 10.5). When considering behavioral interventions, the ABCs of behavioral analysis should be recalled: antecedent, behavior, and consequences. For example, a patient is easily upset and confused when she cannot remember her nurse; as a result, she yells and sometimes throws things at the nurse when she comes into the room, putting both the patient and nurse in danger (e.g., from inadvertent removal of intravenous lines or the nurse being struck by thrown objects). When tailoring behavioral interventions, clinicians should consider each aspect of the behavioral analysis. Possible solutions to the previously mentioned case include posting the names of providers in the patient's room, removing potentially

dangerous objects from within reach of the patient's bed, and reassuring and re-directing the patient.

The way staff members communicate with the patient is also important. Speaking loudly enough (but not too loudly) is a critical first step. Decreased hearing acuity affects all elders, but this does not mean that shouting is necessary. The content of what is said should be simple and to the point. If the patient has considerable expressive language difficulties, questions should be framed so that a yes-or-no response is adequate. Reassurance and distraction are preferred responses to patients who are paranoid or easily distressed.[51] Healthcare staff may initially feel compelled to correct or directly disagree with a patient who endorses a delusional belief. This may result in increased agitation as compared to an approach of gentle redirection, reassurance of core principles of safety and support, and/or distraction.

TABLE 10.5
Examples of Behavioral Management for Patients With Dementia

Re-orient to the environment (e.g., clock, calendar); post names of care providers

Simplify communication (e.g., yes/no questions)

Reassure, distract, and re-direct (e.g., familiar pictures from home)

Use eyeglasses and hearing aids appropriately

Encourage activity and exercise

Offer soothing therapies (e.g., music therapy or aromatherapy)

Provide one-on-one supervision

Avoid direct contradiction in favor of gentle redirection, reassurance, or distraction.

Pharmacotherapy

Cognitive Symptoms

Pharmacotherapies in dementia target both cognitive decline and the NPS of dementia. Because AD is associated with cholinergic dysfunction, cholinesterase inhibitors (ChE-Is) have been developed and are now widely used in treatment (Table 10.6). The commonly used ChE-Is in the United States include donepezil, rivastigmine, and galantamine. A fourth agent, tacrine, was discontinued in 2013 because of its association with hepatotoxicity. The ChE-Is differ in their pharmacologic properties, administration regimens, drug interactions, and effect on hepatic enzymes. The most common side effects include nausea, vomiting,

---

TABLE 10.6
Characteristics of Cholinesterase Inhibitors

Drug	Chemical Class	Total Daily Dose	Regimen	Adverse Events
Donepezil	Piperidine	5–10mg	Daily	GI, headaches, weakness
Rivastigmine	Carbamate	6–12mg (oral), 4.6–9.5mg (transdermal)	Twice daily (oral) or daily (transdermal)	GI, headaches, dizziness
Galantamine	Tertiary alkaloid	16–24mg	Once daily (extended release) or twice daily (immediate release)	GI, insomnia

Adapted from Daly EJ, Falk WE, Brown, P. Cholinesterase inhibitors for behavioral disturbance in dementia. *Curr Psychiatry Rep.* 2001;3:251–258.
GI, gastrointestinal.

and diarrhea; other bothersome adverse effects include insomnia or vivid dreams, fatigue, muscle cramps, incontinence, bradycardia, and syncope. As a result, these drugs may be contraindicated in the setting of bradycardia or sick sinus syndrome; severe asthma and peptic ulcer disease may also be relative contraindications. A patch is now available for rivastigmine, which appears to decrease its gastrointestinal (GI) side effects.

In patients with AD, all of the ChE-Is have been shown to slow the progression of cognitive and functional decline, as well as to potentially improve NPS (see below).[52,53] Treatment with these agents should begin as early as possible in patients with AD.[54] Evidence suggests use of ChE-Is is also warranted in dementia related to vascular disease.[55] Meta-analyses also support the use of ChE-Is in PDD[56] and LBD.[57]

The goals of therapy with ChE-Is include a delay in cognitive decline, a delay of functional decline, and treatment or prevention (or both) of the development of behavioral symptoms. It is important to note that the downhill slope of the illness will continue. ChE-Is also have a small beneficial effect on the burden and active time use among caregivers of persons with AD.[58]

Memantine, an N-methyl-D-aspartate antagonist, is approved by the US Food and Drug Administration (FDA) for the treatment of moderate to severe AD. Memantine normalizes levels of glutamate, a neurotransmitter involved in learning and memory, which in excessive quantities is thought to contribute to neurodegeneration. Common side effects include dizziness, agitation, headache, and confusion. Evidence indicates that adding memantine to the regimen of patients with moderate to severe AD (who were already receiving stable doses of donepezil) results in better outcomes on measures of cognition, ADLs, and behavior.[59,60]

Initiating pharmacotherapy for cognitive symptoms is not usually in the domain of the psychiatric consultant in the general hospital; this is typically the work of outpatient treaters. However, one reason to consider starting these medications in an inpatient medical setting might be to monitor for side effects and tolerability in patients with significant co-morbid medical illnesses. Initiation of ChE-Is may also be considered in this setting for the treatment of NPS, as described later. The consultant may be asked to consider reasons to stop ChE-Is, such as side effects, new medical

contraindications, poor compliance, or rapid decline in the patient's illness. Any benefits of treatment are rapidly lost on discontinuation.

Anti-Aβ Monoclonal Antibodies

Brain Aβ deposition is a hallmark pathological finding in AD pathology,[61] and clearance of this peptide has been shown in preclinical and several recent clinical trials to slow AD progression. As of the second quarter of 2023, there are currently two FDA-approved monoclonal antibody (mAb)–based therapies aimed at targeting Aβ deposits in the brains with MCI or early AD. Aducanumab (Aduhelm), is a human immunoglobulin that targets aggregated amyloid-β (Aβ) in the brain. Aduhelm was FDA-approved in June 2021 through their Accelerated Approval pathway.[62] Aduhelm's approval was controversial due to mixed clinical efficacy findings.[62,63] A decision by the US Centers for Medicare and Medicaid Services (CMS) to restrict coverage of Aduhelm to clinical trials has restricted the commercialization of this first-in-class FDA-approved mAb treatment for AD.

The other monoclonal antibody with current FDA approval is lecanemab (Leqembi), a mAb that binds to soluble Aβ protofibril forms. In an 18-month, double-blinded phase III trial among patients with MCI (with evidence of cerebral amyloid accumulation) or early AD, lecanemab treatment resulted in lower levels of amyloid in the brain and a 27% reduction in the rate of cognitive decline compared to those in the placebo group.[64] Subgroup analyses of cognitive endpoints found that men benefited from the treatment more than women. Leqembi was approved by the FDA in January 2023, through their Accelerated Approval pathway (like Aduhelm). Prescribing information for Leqembi includes indications for initiating treatment for individuals with MCI and early AD. A subcutaneous form of lecanemab is under investigation, and CMS has yet to determine coverage for this medication. Finally, in May 2023, Eli Lilly shared top-line results of their monoclonal antibody treatment, donanemab, which found similar efficacy in slowing cognitive and functional decline to lecanemab[65]; a peer-reviewed complete report is anticipated later this year.

As with ChE-Is, initiating pharmacotherapy with an anti-Aβ monoclonal antibody is not typically in the domain of the psychiatric consultant in the general hospital. However, the consultant will likely evaluate patients who have received or are receiving these medications as outpatients, and thus it is important to have familiarity with their efficacy, side effect profile, overall tolerability, and safety.

Safety of Anti-amyloid Monoclonal Antibodies

Using anti-amyloid mAbs can result in vasogenic cerebral edema and cerebral microhemorrhage. This phenomenon is called amyloid-related imaging abnormalities (ARIA). It was first identified through brain MRI scans of subjects receiving bapineuzumab, one of the first studied amyloid-targeting mAbs for AD.[66] Interestingly, MRI scan abnormalities do not necessarily correlate with symptoms. In clinical trials, the propensity for ARIA has been higher in subjects with homozygous *ApoE ε4* genotype (individuals with the *ApoE ε4* genotype show higher rates of AD and amyloid accumulation, including in cerebral vessels, predisposing them to cerebral amyloid angiopathy—a likely partial link between anti-amyloid mAb treatment and ARIA phenomenology). Risk reduction through patient selection and safety monitoring will be essential as this new class of medications enters widespread use.

Neuropsychiatric Symptoms

Behavioral interventions remain the first-line treatment for managing the NPS of NCDs.[67] However, particularly in the acute hospital setting, pharmacotherapy may also be useful, although certain symptoms are poorly responsive to drug therapies. For example, the motor restlessness and wandering seen in patients with AD are typically unresponsive to medications; in addition, some treatments (e.g., neuroleptics that cause akathisia) may actually aggravate the problem.[68] When other symptoms, such as visual hallucinations or delusions, cause no distress to the patient and are not dangerous, medication is not required. When treatment is necessary, the golden rule of geriatric pharmacotherapy is, "Start low and go slowly." This maxim applies whether target symptoms include apathy, depression, psychosis, agitation, or some combination of these domains.

Apathy is the most common behavioral change in AD.[69] It is defined as a lack of motivation relative to the previous level of function, with a decrease in goal-directed behaviors, goal-directed cognition, and emotional responsiveness.[70] The lack of motivation must not be attributable to intellectual impairment, emotional distress, or a diminished level of consciousness. It is important to distinguish apathy from depression in patients with dementia because the treatments differ (Table 10.7). Treatments for apathy include the use of psychostimulants,[71] dopamine agonists (e.g., bupropion, amantadine),[72] and ChE-Is.[73]

The depressive component of any dementia should be assessed and treated aggressively. If the degree to which affective symptoms are contributing to cognitive dysfunction is unclear, a therapeutic trial of an antidepressant should be employed. The choice of an agent is based principally on the side effects it produces; other considerations include drug-drug interactions and cost. The selective serotonin reuptake inhibitors (SSRIs), for example, citalopram and sertraline, as well as bupropion and mirtazapine have favorable side effect profiles and should be considered. However, there is a paucity of literature to support their use in depression associated with dementia, given somewhat mixed findings on efficacy in recent meta-analyses.[74,75] In addition, a large, multi-center trial developed by a consensus panel assembled by the National Institute of Mental Health found no difference between the administration of 100 mg of sertraline to the placebo-treated group.[76] Care should be taken to avoid those drugs with greater anticholinergic side effects (e.g., paroxetine). Nortriptyline has been used effectively in depression following strokes and is generally well tolerated. Tertiary amine tricyclic antidepressants (TCAs) that are highly anticholinergic (e.g., amitriptyline, imipramine) should be avoided.

TABLE 10.7

Apathy Versus Depression in Alzheimer Disease

	Apathy	Depression
Mood	Blunted	Dysphoric
Attitude	Indifferent	Pessimistic, hopeless
Self-concept	Bland, neutral	Self-critical, nihilistic
Thoughts/ actions	Decreased initiative and persistence	Guilty, suicidal

Hallucinations (particularly visual), delusions (e.g., paranoid, persecutory, somatic), and agitation (which can take the form of motor restlessness, verbal outbursts, or physical aggression) are common in patients with dementia.[77] Before any medication is instituted, reversible causes (e.g., infection, pain, drug effects) should be investigated. If the symptoms are causing significant distress and placing the patient or caregiver at risk, and if non-pharmacologic interventions have failed, the first-line treatment is an antipsychotic medication.

First-generation or typical antipsychotics (e.g., haloperidol, trifluoperazine, perphenazine, thiothixene) have been well studied and show modest improvement in target symptoms.[78] However, elderly patients may be particularly sensitive to the side effects of these agents (e.g., sedation, postural hypotension, EPS) and are at particularly increased risk for developing tardive dyskinesia (TD).[79] Second-generation or atypical antipsychotics (e.g., risperidone) have also been well studied in patients with dementia and are generally better tolerated. Direct comparison of atypical antipsychotics in the CATIE-AD trial (which randomized patients to olanzapine, quetiapine, risperidone, or placebo) found no differences among treatments in the main outcome, time to all-cause discontinuation.[80] Meta-analyses of randomized controlled trials (RCTs) of atypical antipsychotics have found small but statistically significant improvements in NPS of dementia[81]; however, in other studies, trials were limited by high drop-out rates, side effects, and worsening of cognition.[80] While antipsychotics are commonly used off-label for NPS of dementia, in 2023, brexpiprazole (Rexulti) became the first atypical antipsychotic to be FDA approved for agitation in AD[82] based on positive findings in two phase 3 RCTs showing statistically significant and meaningful improvements in caregiver-reported agitation symptoms compared to placebo.

Unfortunately, along with the potential for substantial benefits of atypical antipsychotic use for NPS of dementia, there is also an increased risk of cerebrovascular adverse events in patients with dementia taking atypical antipsychotics.[80] The risk of death in patients taking typical antipsychotics is comparable to, or higher than, the rates in patients taking atypical antipsychotics.[83–85] More recent data have found that the use of both typical and atypical antipsychotic drugs

carries a similar, dose-related increased risk of sudden cardiac death.[86]

Thus, the clinician facing the challenge of treating a person with dementia having psychosis or agitation must weigh the risk of not treating NPS against the risks of the treatment previously discussed. This requires consideration of the evidence that supports the efficacy of a given agent, the morbidity and risk associated with the target symptoms, the patient's medical conditions, and the risks and benefits of the proposed antipsychotic being considered. If an individual lacks the capacity to consent to treatment, it is essential that clinicians obtain informed consent from the patient's healthcare decision-maker before starting an antipsychotic medication. In general, dosing of atypical antipsychotics is lower in elderly patients than those in other populations. In addition to oral forms, some agents may be administered intramuscularly, when required.[87] Usage should be reassessed periodically, particularly because target symptoms may subside with disease progression, and adverse events, such as TD, occur frequently in this population and typically do not resolve spontaneously.[88]

Treatment of psychosis and agitation associated with PDD or LBD requires special mention. High-potency neuroleptics may aggravate tremors and bradykinesia and should be avoided. Clozapine has been found to be useful in controlling psychotic symptoms in patients with PD and LBD[89,90]; however, careful consideration of risk is necessary, given that a recent study found that the use of antipsychotics is associated with an increased mortality risk in patients with PD.[91] In 2016 the FDA-approved pimavanserin, the first drug to be given an indication for the treatment of hallucinations and delusions specifically associated with PD.

Several additional medications can be used off-label in addition to antipsychotics in agitated patients. The short-acting lorazepam (in an oral dosage of 0.25–1 mg) may be helpful when administered before an uncomfortable or potentially frightening procedure, such as a lumbar puncture or an MRI scan. However, due to the many risks associated with the use of benzodiazepines in the elderly (e.g., falls, hip fractures, sedation, worsening cognition), protracted use of benzodiazepines, especially long-acting agents or those with active metabolites (e.g., diazepam, clonazepam), is discouraged.[92–94] The use of buspirone for the treatment of agitation has been reported, but at least several weeks is necessary to achieve a modest benefit with this agent.[95]

Among the antidepressants, a Cochrane review found that sertraline and citalopram were beneficial in reducing agitation. The SSRIs and trazodone were generally well tolerated when compared to antipsychotics.[96] More recently, an RCT showed that citalopram was beneficial in reducing agitation in those with AD, although patients in the citalopram arm experienced worsening of cognition and QTc interval prolongation.[97] Trazodone has been the subject of many case reports demonstrating behavioral improvement in agitated, demented patients,[98] and has been effective for decreasing irritability, agitation, depressive symptoms, and eating disorders in a small, RCT of patients with FTD.[99]

Trazodone has also been effective for the treatment of sleep disturbances in patients with AD, with sedative effects usually achieved rapidly at a dose of 50 mg.[100] Although generally well tolerated, trazodone may induce postural hypotension and priapism. Evidence also supports the use of melatonin to treat sleep disturbance in dementia, showing improvement in sleep efficacy and total sleep time, with no reports of severe adverse events.[101]

Mood stabilizers and other anticonvulsants have also been used off-label to treat agitation associated with dementia. While valproic acid has shown some promise in case reports and open-label studies, results of meta-analyses of fully blinded, RCTs have not supported its routine use for treating agitation in demented patients.[102,103] Pooled data for carbamazepine have been mixed, although two RCTs found efficacy supporting its use.[103] In these studies, both valproate and carbamazepine were better tolerated than atypical antipsychotics, and efficacy was achieved in many cases at subtherapeutic dose ranges. However, drug-drug interactions need to be closely monitored when using these agents. The use of gabapentin and lamotrigine has been shown to be modestly effective in case series, although no RCTs have been published.[104] Of note, gabapentin may worsen NPS in LBD.[105] Lithium is not routinely used unless there is a pre-existing history of bipolar disorder, while oxcarbazepine has not been helpful.[106]

There is also growing evidence that ChE-Is and memantine have modest benefits for NPS in AD and possibly other related dementias with cholinergic deficits.[52,59] Evidence suggests that apathy, depression, or aberrant motor behavior are most likely to improve with the use of ChE-Is; however, they have not been effective in the treatment of either agitation or aggression.[107] Mood symptoms and apathy have most commonly responded to ChE-Is, whereas memantine has been associated with a reduction in irritability and agitation.[73] However, a recent RCT specifically examined the efficacy of memantine in agitation in those with dementia and found no benefit over placebo.[108] Thus, using ChE-Is or memantine for NPS offers an alternative to antipsychotic medications in patients with dementia, although the effects of these drugs appear modest and often provide only temporary improvement.

CONCLUSION

As the population ages, the number of people with NCDs is increasing dramatically; most have AD or vascular dementia. The role of the psychiatric consultant in the diagnosis and treatment of NCDs is important, particularly in the identification of treatable psychiatric and behavioral symptoms.

Family members are the hidden victims of progressive dementia. They typically appreciate the consultant's communication about the diagnosis and the expected course of the disorder. They can benefit from advice about how best to relate to the patient, how to re-structure the home environment, and how to seek legal and financial guidance if appropriate, and how to assess the risk to their own physical and mental health through their roles as caregivers. Family members also should be made aware of the assistance available to them through organizations, such as the Alzheimer's Association, as well as other avenues for seeking individual support and respite.

REFERENCES

1. Alzheimer's Association Alzheimer's disease facts and figures. *Alzheimers Dement.* 2022;18(4):700–789. http://www.alz.org/alzheimers_disease_facts_and_figures.asp.
2. Collaborators GBDDF. Estimation of the global prevalence of dementia in 2019 and forecasted prevalence in 2050: an analysis for the Global Burden of Disease Study 2019. *Lancet Public Health.* 2022;7(2):e105–e125. https://doi.org/10.1016/S2468-2667(21)00249-8.

3. Fong TG, Davis D, Growdon ME, et al. The interface between delirium and dementia in elderly adults. *Lancet Neurol.* 2015;14(8):823–832. https://doi.org/10.1016/S1474-4422(15)00101-5.

4. Mulsant BH, Reynolds CF. Update on the dementia spectrum of depression. *Am J Psychiatry.* 1993;150(2):305–317. https://doi.org/10.1176/ajp.150.2.352.

5. Miller LS, Mitchell MB, Woodard JL, et al. Cognitive performance in centenarians and the oldest old: norms from the Georgia Centenarian Study. *Aging, Neuropsychol Cogn.* 2010;17(5):575–590. https://doi.org/10.1080/13825585.2010.481355.

6. Plassman BL, Langa KM, Fisher GG, et al. Prevalence of dementia in the United States: the aging, demographics, and memory study. *Neuroepidemiology.* 2007;29(1-2):125–132. https://doi.org/10.1159/000109998.

7. Yang Z, Slavin MJ, Sachdev PS. Dementia in the oldest old. *Nat Rev Neurol.* 2013;9(7):382–393. https://doi.org/10.1038/nrneurol.2013.105.

8. Matthews KA, Xu W, Gaglioti AH, et al. Racial and ethnic estimates of Alzheimer's disease and related dementias in the United States (2015–2060) in adults aged ≥65 years. *Alzheimer's Dement.* 2019;15(1):17–24. https://doi.org/10.1016/j.jalz.2018.06.3063.

9. Akushevich I, Kravchenko J, Yashkin A, et al. Expanding the scope of health disparities research in Alzheimer's disease and related dementias. *Alzheimer's Dement.* 2023;15(1):12415. https://doi.org/10.1002/dad2.12415.

10. Canevelli M, Bruno G, Grande G, et al. Race reporting and disparities in clinical trials on Alzheimer's disease: a systematic review. *Neurosci Biobehav Rev.* 2019;101:122–128. https://doi.org/10.1016/j.neubiorev.2019.03.020.

11. Mayeux R, Stern Y. Epidemiology of Alzheimer disease. *Cold Spring Harb Perspect Med.* 2012;2(8):137–152. https://doi.org/10.1101/cshperspect.a006239.

12. *Diagnostic and Statistical Manual of Mental Disorders.* 5th ed. American Psychiatric Association Press; 2013 http://encore.llu.edu/iii/encore/record/C__Rb1280248__SDSM-V__P0,2__Orightresult__X3;jsessionid=ABB7428ECBC4BA66625EDD0E0C5AAFA5?lang=eng&suite=cobalt. Accessed 17.03.23.

13. Mitchell AJ, Shiri-Feshki M. Rate of progression of mild cognitive impairment to dementia - meta-analysis of 41 robust inception cohort studies. *Acta Psychiatr Scand.* 2009;119(4):252–265. https://doi.org/10.1111/J.1600-0447.2008.01326.X.

14. Petersen RC, Roberts RO, Knopman DS, et al. Mild cognitive impairment: ten years later. *Arch Neurol.* 2009;66(12):1447–1455. https://doi.org/10.1001/archneurol.2009.266.

15. Nordberg A. Dementia in 2014: towards early diagnosis in Alzheimer disease. *Nat Rev Neurol.* 2015;11(2):69–70. https://doi.org/10.1038/nrneurol.2014.257.

16. McKhann GM, Knopman DS, Chertkow H, et al. The diagnosis of dementia due to Alzheimer's disease: recommendations from the National Institute on Aging-Alzheimer's Association workgroups on diagnostic guidelines for Alzheimer's disease. *Alzheimer's Dement.* 2011;7(3):263–269. https://doi.org/10.1016/j.jalz.2011.03.005.

17. Lyketsos CG, Carrillo MC, Ryan JM. Neuropsychiatric symptoms in Alzheimer's disease. *Alzheimer's Dement.* 2011;7:532–539.

18. Pendlebury ST, Rothwell PM. Prevalence, incidence, and factors associated with pre-stroke and post-stroke dementia: a systematic review and meta-analysis. *Lancet Neurol.* 2009;8:1006–1018.

19. O'Brien JT, Thomas A. Vascular dementia. *Lancet.* 2015;386:1698–1706.

20. Bonanni L, Thomas A, Onofrj M. Diagnosis and management of dementia with Lewy bodies: third report of the DLB Consortium [1]. *Neurology.* 2006;66(9):1455. https://doi.org/10.1212/01.wnl.0000224698.67660.45.

21. McKeith IG. Consensus guidelines for the clinical and pathologic diagnosis of dementia with Lewy bodies (DLB): report of the Consortium on DLB International Workshop. *J Alzheimer's Dis.* 2006;9(suppl 3):417–423. https://doi.org/10.3233/jad-2006-9s347.

22. Trout AT, Mintz A, Bennett P, Oza UD. Frontotemporal dementia. *Diagnostic Imaging Nucl Med.* 2016;386:44–47. https://doi.org/10.1016/B978-0-323-37753-9.50018-9.

23. Liu W, Miller BL, Kramer JH, et al. Behavioral disorders in the frontal and temporal variants of frontotemporal dementia. *Neurology.* 2004;62(5):742–748. https://doi.org/10.1212/01.WNL.0000113729.77161.C9.

24. Seeley WW, Bauer AM, Miller BL, et al. The natural history of temporal variant frontotemporal dementia. *Neurology.* 2005;64(8):1384–1390. https://doi.org/10.1212/01.WNL.0000158425.46019.5C.

25. Nowak DA, Topka HR. Broadening a classic clinical triad: the hypokinetic motor disorder of normal pressure hydrocephalus also affects the hand. *Exp Neurol.* 2006;198(1):81–87. https://doi.org/10.1016/j.expneurol.2005.11.003.

26. Johnson RT, Gibbs CJ. Creutzfeldt-Jakob disease and related transmissible spongiform encephalopathies. *N Engl J Med.* 1998;339:1994–2004.

27. Ridley NJ, Draper B, Withall A. Alcohol-related dementia: an update of the evidence. *Alzheimer's Res Ther.* 2013;5(1). https://doi.org/10.1186/alzrt157.

28. Beck BJ. Neuropsychiatric manifestations of diffuse Lewy body disease. *J Geriatr Psychiatry Neurol.* 1995;8(3):189–196. https://doi.org/10.1177/089198879500800309.

29. Katz S, Downs TD, Cash HR, et al. Progress in development of the index of ADL. *Gerontologist.* 1970;10(1):20–30. https://doi.org/10.1093/geront/10.1_Part_1.20.

30. Lawton MP, Brody EM. Assessment of older people: self-maintaining and instrumental activities of daily living. *Gerontologist.* 1969;9(3):179–186. https://doi.org/10.1093/geront/9.3_Part_1.179.

31. Heston LL, Mastri AR, Anderson VE, et al. Dementia of the Alzheimer type: clinical genetics, natural history, and associated conditions. *Arch Gen Psychiatry.* 1981;38(10):1085–1090. https://doi.org/10.1001/archpsyc.1981.01780350019001.

32. Wingo TS, Lah JJ, Levey AI, et al. Autosomal recessive causes likely in early-onset Alzheimer disease. *Arch Neurol.* 2012;69(1):59–64. https://doi.org/10.1001/archneurol.2011.221.

33. Karch CM, Goate AM. Alzheimer's disease risk genes and mechanisms of disease pathogenesis. *Biol Psychiatry.* 2015;77(1):43–51. https://doi.org/10.1016/j.biopsych.2014.05.006.

34. Sirkis DW, Bonham LW, Johnson TP, et al. Dissecting the clinical heterogeneity of early-onset Alzheimer's disease. *Mol Psychiatry.* 2022;27(6):2674–2688.   https://doi.org/10.1038/s41380-022-01531-9.

35. Seltman RE, Matthews BR. Frontotemporal lobar degeneration: epidemiology, pathology, diagnosis and management. *CNS Drugs.* 2012;26(10):841–870. https://doi.org/10.2165/11640070-000000000-00000.

36. Forman MS, Farmer J, Johnson JK. Frontotemporal dementia: clinicopathological correlations. *Ann Neurol.* 2006;59:952–962.

37. Van Blitterswijk M, Dejesus-Hernandez M, Rademakers R. How do C9ORF72 repeat expansions cause amyotrophic lateral sclerosis and frontotemporal dementia: can we learn from other noncoding repeat expansion disorders. *Curr Opin Neurol.* 2012;25(6):689–700. https://doi.org/10.1097/WCO.0b013e32835a3efb.

38. Funkenstein HH, Albert MS, Pilgrim D, et al. Extrapyramidal signs and other neurologic findings in clinically diagnosed Alzheimer's disease: a community-based study. *Arch Neurol.* 1993;50(1):51–56. https://doi.org/10.1001/archneur.1993.00540010045016.

39. Ropacki SA, Jeste DV. Epidemiology of and risk factors for psychosis of Alzheimer's disease: a review of 55 studies published from 1990 to 2003. *Am J Psychiatry.* 2005;162(11):2022–2030. https://doi.org/10.1176/appi.ajp.162.11.2022.

40. Devinsky O. Delusional misidentifications and duplications: right brain lesions, left brain delusions. *Neurology.* 2009;72(1):80–87. https://doi.org/10.1212/01.wnl.0000338625.47892.74.

41. Folstein MF, Folstein SE, McHugh PR. "Mini-mental state". A practical method for grading the cognitive state of patients for the clinician. *J Psychiatr Res.* 1975;12(3):189–198. https://doi.org/10.1016/0022-3956(75)90026-6.

42. Franzen MD. *The Wechsler Adult Intelligence Scale-Revised and Wechsler Adult Intelligence Scale-III.* Psychological Corporation; 2000. https://doi.org/10.1007/978-1-4757-3224-5_6.

43. Blessed G, Tomlinson BE, Roth M. The association between quantitative measures of dementia and of senile change in the cerebral grey matter of elderly subjects. *Br J Psychiatry.* 1968;114(512):797–811. https://doi.org/10.1192/bjp.114.512.797.

44. Albert M, Cohen C. The Test for Severe Impairment: an instrument for the assessment of patients with severe cognitive dysfunction. *J Am Geriatr Soc.* 1992;40(5):449–453. https://doi.org/10.1111/j.1532-5415.1992.tb02009.x.

45. Nasreddine ZS, Phillips NA, Bedirian V, et al. The Montreal Cognitive Assessment, MoCA: a brief screening tool for mild cognitive impairment. *J Am Geriatr Soc.* 2005;53:695–699. https://doi.org/10.1111/j.1532-5415.2005.53221.x.

46. Trzepacz PT, Hochstetler H, Wang S, et al. Relationship between the Montreal Cognitive Assessment and Mini-mental State Examination for assessment of mild cognitive impairment in older adults. *BMC Geriatr.* 2015;15(1). https://doi.org/10.1186/s12877-015-0103-3.

47. Devito EE, Pickard JD, Salmond CH, et al. The neuropsychology of normal pressure hydrocephalus (NPH). *Br J Neurosurg.* 2005;19(3):217–224. https://doi.org/10.1080/02688690500201838.

48. Sampson EL, White N, Lord K, et al. Pain, agitation, and behavioural problems in people with dementia admitted to general hospital wards: a longitudinal cohort study. *Pain.* 2015;156(4):675–683. https://doi.org/10.1097/j.pain.0000000000000095.

49. Kales HC, Gitlin LN, Lyketsos CG. Management of neuropsychiatric symptoms of dementia in clinical settings: recommendations from a multidisciplinary expert panel. *J Am Geriatr Soc.* 2014;62(4):762–769. https://doi.org/10.1111/jgs.12730.

50. Brodaty H, Arasaratnam C. Meta-analysis of nonpharmacological interventions for neuropsychiatric symptoms of dementia. *Am J Psychiatry.* 2012;169(9):946–953. https://doi.org/10.1176/appi.ajp.2012.11101529.

51. Marchello V, Boczko F, Shelkey M. Progressive dementia: strategies to manage new problem behaviors. *Geriatrics.* 1995;50(3):40–43.

52. Trinh NH, Hoblyn J, Mohanty S, et al. Efficacy of cholinesterase inhibitors in the treatment of neuropsychiatric symptoms and functional impairment in Alzheimer disease: a meta-analysis. *J Am Med Assoc.* 2003;289(2):210–216. https://doi.org/10.1001/jama.289.2.210.

53. Birks J. Cholinesterase inhibitors for Alzheimer's disease. *Cochrane Database Syst Rev.* 2006;(1): CD00559.

54. Cummings JL. Use of cholinesterase inhibitors in clinical practice: evidence based recommendations. *Am J Geriatr Psychiatry.* 2003;11(2):131–145. https://doi.org/10.1097/00019442-200303000-00004.

55. Malouf R, Birks J. Donepezil for vascular cognitive impairment. *Cochrane Database Syst Rev.* 2004;2010(1). https://doi.org/10.1002/14651858.CD004395.pub2.

56. Rolinski M, Fox C, Maidment I, et al. Cholinesterase inhibitors for dementia with Lewy bodies, Parkinson's disease dementia and cognitive impairment in Parkinson's disease. *Cochrane Database Syst Rev.* 2012;2012(3). https://doi.org/10.1002/14651858.CD006504.pub2.

57. Stinton C, McKeith I, Taylor JP, et al. Pharmacological management of Lewy body dementia: a systematic review and meta-analysis. *Am J Psychiatry.* 2015;172(8):731–742. https://doi.org/10.1176/appi.ajp.2015.14121582.

58. Lingler JH, Martire LM, Schulz R. Caregiver-specific outcomes in antidementia clinical drug trials: a systematic review and meta-analysis. *J Am Geriatr Soc.* 2005;53(6):983–990. https://doi.org/10.1111/j.1532-5415.2005.53313.x.

59. Tariot PN, Farlow MR, Grossberg GT, et al. Memantine treatment in patients with moderate to severe Alzheimer disease already receiving donepezil: a randomized controlled trial. *JAMA.* 2004;291(3):317–324. https://doi.org/10.1001/jama.291.3.317.

60. Van Dyck CH, Schmitt FA, Olin JT. A responder analysis of memantine treatment in patients with Alzheimer disease maintained on donepezil. *Am J Geriatr Psychiatry.* 2006;14(5):428–437. https://doi.org/10.1097/01.JGP.0000203151.17311.38.

61. Murphy MP, Levine H. Alzheimer's disease and the amyloid-beta peptide. *J Alzheimers Dis.* 2010;19(1):311–323. https://doi.org/10.3233/JAD-2010-1221.

62. Shi M, Chu F, Zhu F, et al. Impact of anti-amyloid-beta monoclonal antibodies on the pathology and clinical profile of Alzheimer's disease: a focus on aducanumab and lecanemab. *Front Aging Neurosci.* 2022;14:870517. https://doi.org/10.3389/fnagi.2022.870517.

63. Alexander GC, Knopman DS, Emerson SS, et al. Revisiting FDA approval of aducanumab. *N Engl J Med*. 2021;385(9):769–771. https://doi.org/10.1056/nejmp2110468.

64. van Dyck CH, Swanson CJ, Aisen P, et al. Lecanemab in early Alzheimer's disease. *N Engl J Med*. 2023;388(1):9–21. https://doi.org/10.1056/NEJMoa2212948.

65. Lilly's donanemab significantly slowed cognitive and functional decline in phase 3 study of early Alzheimer's disease | Eli Lilly and Company. Available at: https://investor.lilly.com/news-releases/news-release-details/lillys-donanemab-significantly-slowed-cognitive-and-functional; 2023. Accessed 05.07.23.

66. Lacorte E, Ancidoni A, Zaccaria V, et al. Safety and efficacy of monoclonal antibodies for Alzheimer's disease: a systematic review and meta-analysis of published and unpublished clinical trials. *J Alzheimers Dis*. 2022;87(1):101–129. https://doi.org/10.3233/JAD-220046.

67. Kales HC, Gitlin LN, Lyketsos CG. Education state of the art review. Assessment and management of behavioral and psychological symptoms of dementia. *Br Med J*. 2015;350(8003):h369-5. https://doi.org/10.1136/bmj.h369%5Cnhttp://0-search.ebscohost.com.library.ucc.ie/login.aspx?direct=true&db=a9h&AN=102654524&site=ehost-live.

68. Dubovsky SL. Geriatric neuropsychopharmacology. In: Coffey CE, Cummings JL, eds. *Psychopharmacology Bulletin*. Vol 17. American Psychiatric Association; 1981:141–142.

69. Landes AM, Sperry SD, Straus ME. Apathy in Alzheimer's disease. *J Am Geriatr Soc*. 2001;49:1700–1707.

70. Marin RS. Differential diagnosis and classification of apathy. *Am J Psychiatry*. 1990;147(1):22–30. https://doi.org/10.1176/ajp.147.1.22.

71. Watanabe MD, Martin EM, DeLeon OA, et al. Successful methylphenidate treatment of apathy after subcortical infarcts. *J Neuropsychiatry Clin Neurosci*. 1995;7(4):502–504. https://doi.org/10.1176/jnp.7.4.502.

72. Marin RS, Fogel BS, Hawkins J, et al. Apathy: A treatable syndrome. *J Neuropsychiatry Clin Neurosci*. 1995;7(1):23–30. https://doi.org/10.1176/jnp.7.1.23.

73. Cummings JL, Mackell J, Kaufer D. Behavioral effects of current Alzheimer's disease treatments: a descriptive review. *Alzheimer's Dement*. 2008;4(1):49–60. https://doi.org/10.1016/j.jalz.2007.10.011.

74. Thompson S, Herrmann N, Rapoport MJ, et al. Efficacy and safety of antidepressants for treatment of depression in alzheimer's disease: a meta-analysis. *Can J Psychiatry*. 2007;52(4):248–255. https://doi.org/10.1177/070674370705200407.

75. Nelson JC, Devanand DP. A systematic review and meta-analysis of placebo-controlled antidepressant studies in people with depression and dementia. *J Am Geriatr Soc*. 2011;59(4):577–585. https://doi.org/10.1111/j.1532-5415.2011.03355.x.

76. Weintraub D, Rosenberg PB, Drye LT, et al. Sertraline for the treatment of depression in alzheimer disease: Week-24 outcomes. *Am J Geriatr Psychiatry*. 2010;18(4):332–340. https://doi.org/10.1097/JGP.0b013e3181cc0333.

77. Lyketsos CG, Lopez O, Jones B, et al. Prevalence of neuropsychiatric symptoms in dementia and mild cognitive impairment: results from the cardiovascular health study. *JAMA*. 2002;288(12):1475–1483. https://doi.org/10.1001/jama.288.12.1475.

78. Lanctôt KL, Best TS, Mittmann N, et al. Efficacy and safety of neuroleptics in behavioral disorders associated with dementia. *J Clin Psychiatry*. 1998;59(10):550–561. https://doi.org/10.4088/JCP.v59n1010.

79. Caligiuri MP, Jeste DV, Lacro JP. Antipsychotic-induced movement disorders in the elderly. *Drugs Aging*. 2000;17(5):363–384. https://doi.org/10.2165/00002512-200017050-00004.

80. Schneider LS, Dagerman K, Insel PS. Efficacy and adverse effects of atypical antipsychotics for dementia: meta-analysis of randomized, placebo-controlled trials. *Am J Geriatr Psychiatry*. 2006;14(3):191–210. https://doi.org/10.1097/01.JGP.0000200589.01396.6d.

81. Maher AR, Maglione M, Bagley S, et al. Efficacy and comparative effectiveness of atypical antipsychotic medications for off-label uses in adults: a systematic review and meta-analysis. *JAMA*. 2011;306(12):1359–1369. https://doi.org/10.1001/jama.2011.1360.

82. Harris E. FDA greenlights first drug for agitation related to Alzheimer disease. *JAMA*. Published online 2023. https://jamanetwork.com/journals/jama/article-abstract/2805536.

83. Wang PS, Schneeweiss S, Avorn J, et al. Risk of death in elderly users of conventional vs. atypical antipsychotic medications. *N Engl J Med*. 2005;353(22):2335–2341. https://doi.org/10.1056/nejmoa052827.

84. Gill SS, Bronskill SE, Normand SLT, et al. Antipsychotic drug use and mortality in older adults with dementia. *Ann Intern Med*. 2007;146(11):775–786. https://doi.org/10.7326/0003-4819-146-11-200706050-00006.

85. Schneeweiss S, Setoguchi S, Brookhart A, et al. Risk of death associated with the use of conventional versus atypical antipsychotic drugs among elderly patients. *Can Med Assoc J*. 2007;176(5):627–632. https://doi.org/10.1503/cmaj.061250.

86. Ray WA, Chung CP, Murray KT, et al. Atypical antipsychotic drugs and the risk of sudden cardiac death. *N Engl J Med*. 2009;360:225–235. https://doi.org/10.1097/01.sa.0000360612.83083.3e.

87. Meehan KM, Wang H, David SR, et al. Comparison of rapidly acting intramuscular olanzapine, lorazepam, and placebo: a double-blind, randomized study in acutely agitated patients with dementia. *Neuropsychopharmacology*. 2002;26(4):494–504. https://doi.org/10.1016/S0893-133X(01)00365-7.

88. Steinberg M, Lyketsos CG. Atypical antipsychotic use in patients with dementia: managing safety concerns. *Am J Psychiatry*. 2012;169(9):900–906. https://doi.org/10.1176/appi.ajp.2012.12030342.

89. Friedman JH, Lannon MC. Clozapine in the treatment of psychosis in parkinson's disease. *Neurology*. 1989;39(9):1219–1221. https://doi.org/10.1212/wnl.39.9.1219.

90. Chacko RC, Hurley RA, Jankovic J. Clozapine use in diffuse Lewy body disease. *J Neuropsychiatry Clin Neurosci*. 1993;5(2):206–208. https://doi.org/10.1176/jnp.5.2.206.

91. Weintraub D, Chiang C, Kim HM, et al. Association of antipsychotic use with mortality risk in patients with Parkinson disease. *JAMA Neurol*. 2016;73(5):535–541. https://doi.org/10.1001/jamaneurol.2016.0031.

92. Glass J, Lanctôt KL, Herrmann N, et al. Sedative hypnotics in older people with insomnia: meta-analysis of risks and benefits. *Br Med J.* 2005;331(7526):1169–1173. https://doi.org/10.1136/bmj.38623.768588.47.

93. Chang CM, Wu ECH, Chang IS, et al. Benzodiazepine and risk of hip fractures in older people: a nested case-control study in Taiwan. *Am J Geriatr Psychiatry.* 2008;16(8):686–692. https://doi.org/10.1097/JGP.0b013e31817c6a99.

94. Billioti S, Gage D, Bégaud B, et al. Benzodiazepine use and risk of dementia : prospective. *Br Med J.* 2012;6231(September):1–12.

95. Sakauye KM, Camp CJ, Ford PA. Effects of buspirone on agitation associated with dementia. *Am J Geriatr Psychiatry.* 1993;1(1):82–84. https://doi.org/10.1097/00019442-199300110-00011.

96. Bui Q. Antidepressants for agitation and psychosis in patients with dementia. *Am Fam Physician.* 2012;85(1):20–22.

97. Porsteinsson AP, Drye LT, Pollock BG, et al. Effect of citalopram on agitation in Alzheimer disease: the CitAD randomized clinical trial. *JAMA.* 2014;311(7):682–691. https://doi.org/10.1001/jama.2014.93.

98. Aisen PS, Johannessen DJ, Marin DB. Trazodone for behavioral disturbance in Alzheimer's disease. *Am J Geriatr Psychiatry.* 1993;1(4):349–350. https://doi.org/10.1097/00019442-199300140-00012.

99. Lebert F, Stekke W, Hasenbroekx C, et al. Frontotemporal dementia: a randomised, controlled trial with trazodone. *Dement Geriatr Cogn Disord.* 2004;17(4):355–359. https://doi.org/10.1159/000077171.

100. Camargos EF, Louzada LL, Quintas JL, et al. Trazodone improves sleep parameters in Alzheimer disease patients: a randomized, double-blind, and placebo-controlled study. *Am J Geriatr Psychiatry.* 2014;22(12):1565–1574. https://doi.org/10.1016/j.jagp.2013.12.174.

101. Xu J, Wang LL, Dammer EB, et al. Melatonin for sleep disorders and cognition in dementia: a meta-analysis of randomized controlled trials. *Am J Alzheimers Dis Other Demen.* 2015;30(5):439–447. https://doi.org/10.1177/1533317514568005.

102. Baillon SF, Narayana U, Luxenberg JS, et al. Valproate preparations for agitation in dementia. *Cochrane Database Syst Rev.* 2018;2018(10). https://doi.org/10.1002/14651858.CD003945.pub4.

103. Konovalov S, Muralee S, Tampi RR. Anticonvulsants for the treatment of behavioral and psychological symptoms of dementia: a literature review. *Int Psychogeriatrics.* 2008;20(2):293–308. https://doi.org/10.1017/S1041610207006540.

104. Yeh YC, Ouyang WC. Mood stabilizers for the treatment of behavioral and psychological symptoms of dementia: an update review. *Kaohsiung J Med Sci.* 2012;28(4):185–193. https://doi.org/10.1016/j.kjms.2011.10.025.

105. Rossi P, Serrao M, Pozzessere G. Gabapentin-induced worsening of neuropsychiatric symptoms in dementia with lewy bodies: case reports. *Eur Neurol.* 2002;47(1):56–57. https://doi.org/10.1159/000047948.

106. Sommer OH, Aga O, Cvancarova M, et al. Effect of oxcarbazepine in the treatment of agitation and aggression in severe dementia. *Dement Geriatr Cogn Disord.* 2009;27(2):155–163. https://doi.org/10.1159/000199236.

107. Gauthier S, Cummings J, Ballard C, et al. Management of behavioral problems in Alzheimer's disease. *Int Psychogeriatrics.* 2010;22(3):346–372. https://doi.org/10.1017/S1041610209991505.

108. Fox C, Crugel M, Maidment I, et al. Efficacy of memantine for agitation in Alzheimer's dementia: a randomised double-blind placebo controlled trial. *PLoS One.* 2012;7(5). https://doi.org/10.1371/journal.pone.0035185.

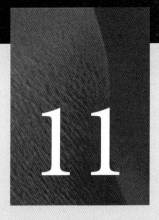

11

PATIENTS WITH PSYCHOSIS

CAROL LIM, MD, MPH ■ ABIGAIL L. DONOVAN, MD
■ OLIVER FREUDENREICH, MD

OVERVIEW

Psychosis, broadly defined, is a gross impairment of reality testing. Psychosis can result from a wide range of psychiatric and medical disturbances, and its presentations vary widely (e.g., an elderly female who lies quietly in bed listening to Satan whispering bears little resemblance to a wildly agitated young man who accuses the nursing staff of trying to poison him). Hallucinations and delusions are the two prototypical symptoms of psychosis. Hallucinations, sensory perceptions in the absence of an external source, occur in any sensory modality and may take the form of voices, visions, odors, or tactile perceptions that may be complex (e.g., electric shocks, the sensation that one is being fondled). Delusions are firmly held beliefs that other members of the patient's societal group judge to be false. Delusions range from plausible, albeit unlikely, beliefs (e.g., an average citizen being monitored by the National Security Agency), to bizarre convictions (e.g., one's internal organs have been replaced with empty beer cans). Delusional individuals cling to their beliefs with unfaltering conviction even in the face of overwhelming evidence to the contrary. While hallucinations and delusions are examples of disordered thought content, the form or organization of thoughts may also be problematic, as occurs in a formal thought disorder such as schizophrenia. Patients with a formal thought disorder may have such disorganized thoughts that their speech is an incoherent word salad, and they may have difficulty making any sense of reality.

When asked to consult on a patient with psychosis, the psychiatric consultant can be of immediate help by ensuring that the patient and staff are safe, and they can demystify this often-frightening condition by approaching psychosis as a disorder of brain function that must be addressed with a thoughtful differential diagnosis, leading to effective treatment.

Case 1

Mr. A, a 45-year-old man who lived in a group home for patients with serious mental illness (SMI), had been receiving his psychiatric care at a community mental health center. He had long-standing schizophrenia that had been well controlled with clozapine for 10 years. Mr. A was brought to the emergency department (ED) for abdominal pain. He was admitted to the surgical service for an acute abdomen and found to have a toxic megacolon that required a hemicolectomy.

Psychiatry was consulted to help manage Mr. A's medications and perioperative agitation. Clozapine was withheld and haloperidol was used to manage his agitation. Even though his clozapine treatment contributed to the development of a toxic megacolon (because of clozapine's anticholinergic and serotonin-blocking properties), Mr. A and his family considered clozapine an essential medication, as it had stabilized his illness after a decade of failed treatments with other antipsychotics. Clozapine was therefore re-started (at a low dose) and carefully titrated to his previous dose during his hospitalization. He was started on a bowel regimen to prevent and manage constipation.

The hospitalization was also used to address two other concerns: Mr. A's basic medical care and his nicotine use. Like many individuals with schizophrenia, Mr. A had not seen his primary care doctor in many years, and he had been smoking cigarettes since high school, currently smoking two packs per day. Thus, the psychiatric consultant requested basic screening laboratory tests (i.e., hemoglobin A_{1c} and a lipid profile) to assess for metabolic side effects that are associated with long-term clozapine treatment. His hemoglobin A_{1c} was elevated, but pre-diabetic. His lipid panel revealed mildly elevated triglycerides and low-density lipoproteins. In addition, Mr. A received nicotine patches during his hospitalization to manage nicotine withdrawal; the psychiatric consultant used motivational interviewing to engage Mr. A around smoking cessation as a critical health goal to reduce his risk of cardiovascular mortality. A follow-up with a primary care doctor was arranged to address diabetes prevention, as part of his hospital discharge plan. Mr. A also agreed to join a smoking cessation group at his community mental health center and discuss pharmacotherapy for smoking cessation (e.g., varenicline) with his outpatient psychiatrist. Last, the group home received a note from the psychiatry consultation-liaison (C-L) service about the prevention of constipation in clozapine patients. As a result of this hospital admission, Mr. A became more engaged in managing his own medical health and better linked to healthcare services.

DIAGNOSTIC EVALUATION

The presence of psychotic symptoms does not mean that a primary psychotic disorder, like schizophrenia, is present; in fact, the differential diagnosis for psychotic symptoms is broad and includes both medical and psychiatric causes. Therefore the assessment of a patient with psychosis begins with a thorough consideration of medical conditions that can present with psychosis (Table 11.1),[1] as well as the drugs and medications that can cause psychosis (Table 11.2). In addition, the diagnostic assessment needs to be informed by a medical history, a review of systems, a family history, and a physical examination. A bedside examination of cognitive function should also be performed. The Mini-Mental State Examination can be supplemented by the clock-drawing test or the Montreal

Cognitive Assessment; this will usually suffice as an initial cognitive screen. Serious deficits in attention, orientation, and memory should suggest delirium or dementia rather than a primary psychotic illness. However, only more comprehensive neurocognitive testing will uncover more subtle, yet functionally relevant, cognitive difficulties with processing speed, working memory, verbal memory, and executive function that almost all patients with schizophrenia, including first-episode psychosis, experience to some degree. Those deficits may not be apparent in a clinical interview alone.

All patients with new-onset psychotic symptoms or a clear change in their chronic psychotic symptoms require a thorough medical evaluation. Laboratory testing should include a complete blood cell count, serum electrolytes, levels of calcium, glucose, creatinine, and blood urea nitrogen, liver function tests, urinalysis, and a urine toxicology screen. In addition, thyroid function tests, vitamin B_{12} and folate levels, erythrocyte sedimentation rate, antinuclear antibodies, and syphilis serology (specific, such as the fluorescent treponemal antibody absorption test), are appropriate. Human immunodeficiency virus (HIV) testing should also be recommended. An extended work-up may include karyotyping for chromosomal abnormalities or urine testing for metabolic disorders. The diagnostic yield from neuroimaging of the brain (magnetic resonance imaging or computed tomography) is low in the absence of localized neurologic findings. Neuroimaging should be obtained, however, in cases with atypical or treatment-resistant psychotic symptoms and should be strongly considered even in cases with new-onset typical psychotic features, because the long-term costs and morbidity of this disorder are quite high in relation to the expense of diagnostic testing. An electroencephalogram (EEG) can be useful when evaluating a confused patient where delirium is suspected, if there is history of serious head trauma, or if symptoms suggestive of a seizure disorder are present. An EEG is rarely helpful if it is employed as a routine screening procedure. Similarly, a lumbar puncture (LP) is not necessary for a routine work-up, but it can be lifesaving if a treatable central nervous system (CNS) infection is suspected. Autoimmune encephalitis is another medical cause of psychosis. Anti-*N*-methyl-d-aspartate (NMDA)

TABLE 11.1
Selected Medical Conditions Associated With Psychosis

Epilepsy

Traumatic brain injury

Dementias
  Alzheimer disease
  Pick disease
  Lewy body dementia

Stroke

Space-occupying lesions and structural brain abnormalities
  Primary brain tumors
  Secondary brain metastases
  Brain abscesses and cysts
  Tuberous sclerosis
  Midline abnormalities (e.g., corpus callosum agenesis, cavum septi pellucidi)
  Cerebrovascular malformations (e.g., involving the temporal lobe)

Hydrocephalus

Demyelinating diseases
  Multiple sclerosis
  Leukodystrophies (metachromatic leukodystrophy, X-linked adrenoleukodystrophy, Marchiafava-Bignami disease)
  Schilder disease

Neuropsychiatric disorders
  Huntington disease
  Wilson disease
  Parkinson disease
  Friedreich ataxia

Autoimmune disorders
  Systemic lupus erythematosus
  Rheumatic fever (history of)
  Paraneoplastic syndromes
  Myasthenia gravis
  Anti-NMDA receptor encephalitis

Infections
  Viral encephalitis (e.g., herpes simplex, measles including SSPE, cytomegalovirus, rubella, Epstein-Barr, varicella)
  Neurosyphilis

Neuroborreliosis (Lyme disease)

HIV infection

CNS-invasive parasitic infections (e.g., cerebral malaria, toxoplasmosis, neurocysticercosis)

Tuberculosis

Sarcoidosis

Cryptococcus infection

Prion diseases (e.g., Creutzfeldt-Jakob disease)

Endocrinopathies
  Hypoglycemia
  Addison disease
  Cushing syndrome
  Hyperthyroidism and hypothyroidism
  Hyperparathyroidism and hypoparathyroidism
  Hypopituitarism

Narcolepsy

Nutritional deficiencies
  Magnesium deficiency
  Vitamin A deficiency
  Vitamin D deficiency
  Zinc deficiency
  Niacin deficiency (pellagra)
  Vitamin B_{12} deficiency (pernicious anemia)

Metabolic disorders
  Amino acid metabolism (Hartnup disease, homocystinuria, phenylketonuria)
  Porphyrias (acute intermittent porphyria, porphyria variegata, hereditary coproporphyria)
  GM_2 gangliosidosis
  Fabry disease
  Niemann-Pick type C disease
  Gaucher disease, adult type

Chromosomal abnormalities
  Sex chromosomes (Klinefelter syndrome, XXY syndrome)
  Fragile X syndrome
  VCFS

CNS, Central nervous system; *HIV*, human immunodeficiency virus; *NMDA*, N-methyl-d-aspartate; *SSPE*, subacute sclerosing panencephalitis; *VCFS*, velo-cardio-facial syndrome.

receptor encephalitis, along with other increasingly recognized antibody-mediated autoimmune encephalitides can present solely with behavioral or psychiatric symptoms. A rapid diagnosis is critical to initiate immunotherapy. A serum autoantibody panel may be cost-effective in routine screening for a first episode of psychosis without clinical "red flags" for encephalitis, given that 5% of first-episode patients have serum antibodies associated with autoimmune encephalitis and there are significant costs related to delayed diagnosis and initiation of treatment.[2] Patients with positive serum screening results should undergo further work-up to confirm an autoimmune encephalitis diagnosis. An LP and cerebrospinal fluid (CSF) analysis is required to make a definitive diagnosis of autoimmune encephalitis.

Several other neuropsychiatric disorders should be considered during the diagnostic evaluation.

TABLE 11.2
Substances Associated With Psychosis

Drugs of Abuse

Associated with Intoxication

Alcohol

Amphetamine

Anabolic steroids

Cannabis

Cocaine

Hallucinogens: LSD, MDMA

Kratom

Inhalants: glues and solvents

Opioids (meperidine)

Phencyclidine (PCP), ketamine

Sedative-hypnotics (including withdrawal): barbiturates and benzodiazepines

Designer drugs (wide variety of chemical classes): synthetic cathinones (bath salts/flakkka), synthetic cannabinoids (spice/K2), synthetic opioid (U4/pinky), and synthetic hallucinogens (N-bomb)

Associated with Withdrawal

Alcohol

Sedative-hypnotics

Medications (Broad Classes with Selected Medications)

Anesthetics and analgesics (including NSAIDs)

Anticholinergics and antihistamines

Antiepileptics (with high doses)

Antihypertensive and cardiovascular medications (e.g., digoxin)

Anti-infectious medications (antibiotics, e.g., fluoroquinolones, TMP/SMX; antivirals, e.g., nevirapine; tuberculostatics, e.g., INH; antiparasitics, e.g., metronidazole, mefloquine)

Antiparkinsonian medications (e.g., amantadine, levodopa)

Chemotherapeutic agents (e.g., vincristine)

Corticosteroids (e.g., prednisone, ACTH)

Interferon

Muscle relaxants (e.g., cyclobenzaprine)

Over-the-counter medications (e.g., pseudoephedrine, caffeine in excessive doses)

Toxins

Carbon monoxide

Heavy metals: arsenic, manganese, mercury, thallium

Organophosphates

Key Diagnostic Questions to Determine Causality Between a Substance and Psychosis

Does the patient have a history of psychosis?

Does the patient have a history of illicit drug use?

Did the psychosis start after a medication was started?

Is there evidence of delirium?

ACTH, Adrenocorticotropic hormone; *INH*, isoniazid; *LSD*, d-lysergic acid diethylamide; *MDMA*, methylenedioxymethamphetamine; *NSAIDs*, non-steroidal anti-inflammatory drugs; *TMP/SMX*, trimethoprim/sulfamethoxazole.

Huntington disease is suggested by a family history of Huntington disease, dementia, and choreiform movements; psychotic symptoms may occur before motor and cognitive symptoms become prominent. Parkinson disease also may present with psychosis, along with bradykinesia, tremors, rigidity, and a festinating gait. With disease progression, psychosis is common and can be the result of either illness or use of medications, or both. The diagnosis of Parkinson disease can be complicated by exposure to antipsychotic medications—a review of the time course of neurologic symptoms in relation to the use of antipsychotics should clarify this diagnostic possibility. Wilson disease may also present with psychotic symptoms, as well as tremors, dysarthria, rigidity, and a gait disturbance. Kayser-Fleischer rings, golden-brown copper deposits around the cornea, are pathognomonic for Wilson disease and may be detected by a slit-lamp examination performed early in the illness. Low levels of serum ceruloplasmin and elevated liver enzymes are typically seen, although a definitive diagnosis also requires the determination of a 24-hour urine copper excretion and often a liver biopsy. Finally, acute intermittent porphyria, characterized by episodes of abdominal pain, weakness, and peripheral neuropathy, may be associated with psychosis. Because the illness is autosomal dominant, a family history may raise suspicion for the diagnosis. During acute attacks, δ-aminolevulinic acid and porphobilinogen urine levels are elevated.

It is impractical and ill advised to attempt to rule out all conceivable diseases that could cause psychosis. The more tests that are ordered without clinical concern for a certain disease, the more false-positive test results will occur. A thoughtful approach that combines findings gathered from a clinical history and a physical examination (including a neurologic examination) with selected laboratory tests will usually suffice to exclude treatable medical illnesses and provide a baseline for future reference. Table 11.3 suggests one screening battery that accomplishes these important initial diagnostic goals.

After medical causes of psychosis have been ruled out, the psychiatric differential diagnosis of psychosis flows from the diagnostic criteria contained in the "Schizophrenia Spectrum and Other Psychotic Disorders" section of the *Diagnostic and Statistical Manual of Mental Disorders, 5th Edition, Text Revision*

TABLE 11.3
Medical Work-up for First-Episode Psychosis

Physical Examination With Emphasis on the Neurologic Examination

Vital signs

Weight and height (BMI), waist circumference[a]

Electrocardiogram[a]

Laboratory Tests
Broad Screening and Medical Baseline:

Complete blood count

Electrolytes including calcium

Renal function tests (BUN/creatinine)

Liver function tests

Erythrocyte sedimentation rate

Antinuclear antibody

Fasting glucose

Fasting lipid profile[a]

Hemoglobin A_{1c}[a]

Consider prolactin level[a]

Hepatitis C (if risk factors are present)[a]

Pregnancy test (in people with a uterus of childbearing age)

Urine toxicology screen

Urinalysis

Exclude Specific Treatable Disorders:

Thyroid-stimulating hormone

Fluorescent treponemal antibody absorption test for syphilis (RPR not sufficient)

HIV screening

Ceruloplasmin

Vitamin B_{12} and folate

Neuroimaging

MRI (preferred over CT) to rule out demyelinating disease, brain tumor, or stroke

Ancillary Tests

Expand the etiological search if indicated, accounting for epidemiology: e.g., chest x-ray, electroencephalogram, blood cultures, lumbar puncture to detect autoantibodies (e.g., anti-NMDA receptor antibodies), serum cortisol, medication drug levels and toxin search, karyotype (early-onset schizophrenia), heavy metal testing, Lyme antibodies. Expand medical monitoring if indicated: e.g., eye examination (if risk factors for cataracts are present)

[a]Not for diagnostic purposes but to establish a baseline for longitudinal medical monitoring.

BMI, Body mass index; *BUN*, blood urea nitrogen; *CT*, computed tomography; *HIV*, human immunodeficiency virus; *MRI*, magnetic resonance imaging; *NMDA*, N-methyl-d-aspartate; *RPR*, rapid plasma reagin.

Modified from Freudenreich O. Secondary schizophrenia. *Psychotic Disorders: A Practical Guide.* 2020:49–67.

(DSM-5-TR).[3] It should be emphasized, however, that these criteria are guidelines for diagnosis and serve as a basis for a common language; they are to be used only in conjunction with a full understanding of the clinical manifestations of the syndrome (Table 11.4). The psychiatric differential diagnosis includes both mood disorders with psychotic features and schizophrenia-spectrum disorders.

Careful delineation of the temporal course of psychotic symptoms (e.g., chronic, episodic, or of recent onset), and their relationship to mood symptoms and substance use is of diagnostic importance. In addition, the range and severity of psychotic and negative symptoms, as well as any neurocognitive impairment, must be assessed. Patients with psychosis are often unable to provide an accurate history; therefore collateral information must be collected from as many sources as possible to understand the evolution of the illness over time. Studies have found that interviews alone are an incomplete source of data in detecting psychotic symptoms and determining a correct diagnosis (e.g., most patients with first-episode psychosis do not discuss their symptoms).[4]

Mood disorders, including both major depressive disorder (MDD) and bipolar disorder (BPD), can feature psychotic symptoms. If the patient meets the diagnostic criteria for MDD and has exhibited psychotic symptoms only during episodes of depression, the diagnosis is MDD with psychotic features. Patients who have experienced manic episodes and who have been psychotic only during affective episodes are diagnosed as having BPD with psychotic features. If psychosis is driven by mood states, the psychotic symptoms should resolve in parallel with the resolution of mood symptoms.

Substance-induced psychoses should be considered if the psychosis has an acute onset (without a clear prodrome), is occurring only in the context of substance use, is not occurring in the context of mood symptoms, if there is no family history of psychosis, and particularly if the patient has previously experienced a substance-induced psychosis. A variety of substances can cause psychosis (see Table 11.2); increasingly common causes of psychosis that lead to ED visits include intoxication with stimulants, synthetic cannabinoids, or other designer drugs.[5] A urine toxicology screening test may detect substance use, but it does not rule

---

TABLE 11.4
Psychiatric Disorders That May Present With Psychosis

Continuous Psychosis

Schizophrenia

Schizoaffective disorder, bipolar type (with prominent episodes of mania)

Schizoaffective disorder, depressed type (with prominent depressive episodes)

Delusional disorder (plausible, circumscribed delusions)

Episodic Psychosis

Depression with psychotic features

Bipolar disorder (manic or depressed)

Schizophreniform disorder (<6 months duration)

Brief psychotic disorder (<1 month duration)

Substance-induced psychotic disorder

Key Diagnostic Questions

Has a reversible, secondary cause (medical issue or substance use) been ruled out?

Are cognitive deficits prominent (delirium or dementia)?

Is the psychotic illness continuous or episodic?

Have psychotic symptoms (active phase) been present for at least 4 weeks?

Has evidence of the illness been present for at least 6 months?

Is there evidence of a decline in the level of functioning?

Are negative symptoms present?

Are mood episodes prominent?

Have there been episodes of major depression or mania?

Do psychotic features occur only during affective episodes?

---

demonstrate a decline in function and display, for at least 4 weeks, symptoms of the active phase, which consist of delusions, hallucinations, or disorganized speech. So-called "Schneiderian first-rank symptoms" (e.g., voices conversing or keeping up a running commentary) are characteristic of schizophrenia but are neither pathognomonic nor obligatory. Other active-phase symptoms include grossly disorganized behavior and catatonia, as well as negative symptoms. Negative symptoms of schizophrenia fall into two main clusters: a cluster of reduced affective experience or expression (i.e., blunted affect and alogia) and an amotivation cluster (i.e., avolition, anhedonia, and asociality). It is important to rule out other causes of negative symptoms, such as dementia, depression, or Parkinson disease. The diagnosis of schizophrenia using DSM-5-TR criteria is made only after evidence of the illness has been present for at least 6 months—if symptoms have been present for less than 6 months, a provisional diagnosis of schizophreniform disorder is used. Patients whose psychotic symptoms remit within 4 weeks of their onset are diagnosed as having a brief psychotic disorder if no secondary cause has been identified.

Recognizing varied duration and symptom admixtures, the term schizophrenia-spectrum disorders is sometimes used as an umbrella term encompassing schizophrenia, schizoaffective disorder, brief psychotic disorder, and schizotypal personality disorder.

If a patient experiences both a major mood episode and the symptoms of schizophrenia have occurred for substantial periods when the patient was euthymic, the illness is classified as schizoaffective disorder. If the mood episode was depressive and depressive episodes have been prominent throughout the course of the illness, the diagnosis would be schizoaffective disorder, depressed type. If episodes of depression have been less frequent and played a less prominent role in the overall course of the illness, schizophrenia with superimposed depression may be a more accurate diagnosis. The bipolar type of schizoaffective disorder includes significant periods of mania as a feature of the illness.

If the patient's condition does not meet the diagnostic criteria for schizophreniform disorder, schizophrenia, or schizoaffective disorder, but one or more delusions are present, the diagnosis of delusional disorder can be made, provided that the patient does not exhibit functional impairment outside of the

out substance-induced psychosis if it is negative, nor does a positive toxicology screening test establish causality for the psychosis, because co-morbid substance use is common in psychotic disorders. In addition, many designer drugs that are readily available over the internet require specialized tests that are not usually available. Psychosis due to substance use is potentially reversible if the substance is removed for a while, which may provide additional support for making the diagnosis.

Schizophrenia often begins with a prodrome of non-specific mood or anxiety symptoms that lasts for several months followed by attenuated psychotic symptoms and increasing role failure that eventually gives rise to a first episode of psychosis. To meet the DSM-5-TR criteria for schizophrenia, patients must circumscribed delusional system. Delusions are often quite plausible and may include the belief that one has a physical defect or medical condition, or that one is being followed, poisoned, infected, loved by a famous person, or cheated on by a spouse. Patients who do not meet the active phase criteria for schizophrenia but who present with chronic, bizarre, or idiosyncratic thoughts or behaviors are classified as having schizotypal personality, which may be a less severe form of schizophrenia.

The proper psychiatric diagnosis of a patient who is psychotic on a cross-sectional examination requires an intimate knowledge of the patient's longitudinal course, something that is often unavailable during an ED visit or inpatient admission. As a result, initial diagnostic impressions may need to be revised as more information and longitudinal history become available.

CLINICAL PICTURES AND CORRESPONDING PROBLEMS DURING A MEDICAL HOSPITALIZATION

During a medical or surgical admission, patients with schizophrenia have higher complication rates from infections and post-operative adverse events compared to patients who do not have schizophrenia.[6] Effective consultation and advocacy could thus have real benefits for some patients with schizophrenia. For these patients, the role of the C-L psychiatrist in the general hospital is threefold: conducting conventional consultations with an emphasis on making a correct diagnosis and instituting proper treatment; educating staff about the symptoms and course of schizophrenia to improve their interactions with patients with schizophrenia; serving as an advocate for someone with a SMI so that they can receive appropriate and comprehensive medical care, including performing capacity assessments when necessary. Interestingly, in one survey the single most common reason for a psychiatric consultation in patients with schizophrenia admitted to the medical service of the Massachusetts General Hospital was "schizophrenia" (30%) (but the referral often lacked a specific question).[7] This finding may reflect concerns of the medical team about how to properly manage a patient with schizophrenia, including fears about potential violence. Other referrals revolve around depression (16%), capacity assessment (14%), and help with the prescription of psychotropic medications (10%).

The specific form of illness that a patient with schizophrenia manifests determines the nature of the staff's concerns, as well as the staff's level of comfort. The symptoms of schizophrenia can be clustered into six symptom domains:[8] positive symptoms (separated into disorganization and paranoid-hallucinatory clusters), negative symptoms (e.g., apathy, anhedonia, social withdrawal, alogia, flat affect), cognitive symptoms (e.g., poor attention, executive function, processing speed, working memory), affective symptoms (e.g., depression, suicidality, maniform symptoms), and motor symptoms (e.g., abnormal movements, catatonia). Patients can have varying presentations due to their specific mixtures of symptoms and differing degrees of response to treatment.

In the general hospital, questions may arise as to whether the patient has the capacity (or competence) to make treatment decisions. Competency refers to the ability of an individual to make decisions in a legal sense, including providing consent for all medical treatment. Competency is determined by a judge and not treatment teams; if a patient lacks the capacity to make decisions, a legal guardian will be appointed to make treatment decisions. Capacity refers to a person's ability to make a specific medical decision in a specific situation. The consultant should make it clear that patients with psychosis may have the capacity to make certain decisions, such as weighing the risks and benefits of proceeding with or refusing medical treatment, even when their judgment is impaired in other realms. The idiosyncratic speech manifest by some patients may give an exaggerated impression of cognitive impairment, whereas their capacity to understand aspects of their medical condition may be adequate. With patience and explanations that account for cognitive limitations, many patients with schizophrenia can participate meaningfully in their medical care, despite some cognitive impairment. Put differently: a diagnosis of schizophrenia per se does not indicate a lack of capacity.

The Paranoid or Delusional Patient

Patients with schizophrenia whose symptoms are limited to delusional systems and hallucinations used to be labeled as having "paranoid schizophrenia." In the absence of overt disorganization and negative symptoms, individuals with paranoid schizophrenia may go unnoticed by hospital staff. Although these patients often conceal psychiatric symptoms and fail to exhibit the bizarre appearance, behavior, and speech that attract attention, they may antagonize nursing staff because of their anger, argumentativeness, or patronizing manner. Nursing staff often appreciate learning that these annoying characteristics are common features of the illness. Even with complex and bizarre delusional beliefs, these individuals may do well when admitted to a medical or surgical service, successfully completing the course of treatment without incident, but difficulties may arise when circumstances in the hospital collide with an individual's delusions. The patient who believes that the Mafia is attempting to kill him may refuse all hospital food for fear of being poisoned. Others become convinced that their physicians are members of the conspiracy that is plotting against them or that the surgeons have implanted a microchip intended to control or monitor their thoughts. To assess safety and to predict potential problems with treatment adherence, the psychiatric consultant must understand the full scope of the patient's delusional system and the nature of any hallucinatory experiences.

Because paranoid patients usually are guarded and reluctant to reveal their delusional beliefs, the consultant must proceed carefully and deliberately. A direct interrogation may backfire and convince the patient that the conspirators sent the interviewer. Because delusional individuals are preoccupied and distressed by their delusional beliefs, it is usually sufficient to engage them in a neutral, non-threatening, discussion about their current interests and activities. Comments that seem out of place or inappropriate to the content may provide clues as to the theme of their delusional system, which can be further explored. Questions should never imply a judgment about psychopathology, but instead demonstrate the interviewer's interest and concern. Examples of such questions include, "Are you safe? Have you noticed any strange coincidences? Are you aware of anyone trying to play with your mind? How do you understand what is happening to you? What have you overheard from others about this?" The interviewer should neither agree with the delusion nor attempt to

reality test—impartial interest and concern are usually a welcome relief to a delusional patient. This technique is sometimes called *partial joining of perspectives*.[9] Ideally, the consultant can serve as an intermediary, listening to the concerns of both the patient and the hospital staff and reconciling their misunderstandings.

In addition to persecutory delusions, somatic delusions may pose a unique problem for the patient with schizophrenia admitted to a medical service. In a retrospective survey, somatic delusions were observed in 8% of patients with schizophrenia, in 24% of patients with schizoaffective disorder, and 13% of patients with delusional disorder.[10] The somatic delusions of schizophrenia-spectrum disorders are typically bizarre and impossible (e.g., feeling one's brain shrinking because of exposure to radioactivity) and can usually be recognized immediately as delusional. However, being aware of a patient's somatic delusions, medical staff may then prematurely discount other somatic complaints. A consultant may be needed to help sort out which physical complaints merit further investigation by hospital staff and which concerns are best viewed as delusions. Especially given the high burden of medical co-morbidities in this population, it is critical to help the medical team avoid diagnostic overshadowing (i.e., misattribution of physical symptoms to "psychiatric" etiologies), which may lead to delayed or inadequate treatment of a potentially treatable medical condition.

The Disorganized Patient

The disorganized patient can be problematic in a medical service. Disorganized speech may make communication about medical symptoms difficult and may interfere with discussions about treatment options. If disorganization is subtle, the patient may appear merely stubborn or oppositional and make routine nursing tasks difficult. One major area of concern for disorganized patients is their lack of judgment and behavioral control. These patients may engage in inappropriate behaviors (e.g., masturbating or disrobing in public, stealing food, and smoking in restricted areas). Of even greater concern is the occasional violent or self-injurious behavior of an agitated, disorganized patient. These patients typically require robust pharmacotherapy and may require physical restraints or around-the-clock observers. A review of past aggressive episodes, which can be provided by outpatient caregivers or family, can help the consultant anticipate problems that are likely to arise during a medical or surgical hospitalization.

The Patient With Negative Symptoms or Neurocognitive Deficits

Individuals with schizophrenia who display prominent negative symptoms may encounter unique difficulties when admitted to medical or surgical services. The deficits in motivation and communication associated with negative symptoms are often compounded by cognitive deficits, particularly in the realms of sustained attention, memory, and executive function. Schizophrenia was once known as *dementia praecox* (premature dementia) because of its prominent cognitive impairments. Patients may seem indifferent to their medical problems and unappreciative of their care. Staff can be easily put off by a patient's poor hygiene and soiled clothing. Sustaining empathy and enthusiasm for the care of a withdrawn and unmotivated patient can require unusual efforts by the entire treatment team. This process may be facilitated by the psychiatric consultant, who can explain that poor hygiene, apathy, and deficits in interpersonal skills are the symptoms of illness that are not willful, but instead are suggestive of the need for additional support and encouragement. Often, the consultant's portrayal of the patient before the onset of illness as a vibrant and healthy young adult helps staff empathize with the patient. When ongoing treatment or rehabilitation is required after discharge, a comprehensive treatment plan should be developed to ensure supervision and support for avolitional patients who would otherwise be unlikely to follow through with treatment. Psychosocial treatments with a recovery orientation, including case management and peer support from people with lived experience, have been shown to improve outcomes.[11] The most important interventions with cognitively impaired patients involve taking ample time to explain information and proposed treatments, avoiding the use of complicated medical terminology, and allowing additional time to ask questions and make decisions—practicing "slow medicine."[12]

The Manic Patient

Although psychotic features in patients with schizophrenia are often bizarre and idiosyncratic, patients who are manic are more likely to present with grandiose delusions that can impair judgment and impulse control. These patients may be difficult to manage because of their boundless energy and grandiose misinterpretation of their situation. Staff may at first mistake mania for unusually high energy, gregariousness, and positive self-esteem; however, eventually, they turn to the psychiatric consultant when the patient refuses to stop pacing or talking to other patients late at night, or when the patient is belligerent, insisting that there is no medical problem. Patients with irritable mania may present with persecutory delusions and can be superficially indistinguishable from patients with paranoid schizophrenia. Management of the patient with mania should begin with containment and isolation from distracting stimuli, as well as access to substances and items that could be used as weapons. Short-term behavioral control can be achieved with the use of antipsychotics in combination with benzodiazepines, whereas long-term treatment may require achieving a therapeutic blood level of a mood stabilizer (e.g., lithium carbonate, valproic acid).

The Psychotic Depressed Patient

Delusions of a psychotically depressed patient usually reflect ruminative concerns about guilt, worthlessness, or physical decrepitude. These patients may puzzle their medical or surgical caregivers with exaggerated bodily concerns and illogical descriptions of organ dysfunction. Their overwhelming hopelessness and sense of being responsible for their plight may also interfere with attempts to involve them in treatment decisions—they may seem more interested in euthanasia than treatment. Some psychotically depressed patients withdraw and may become mute and catatonic. Persecutory delusions also occur in psychotic depression, but these beliefs tend to be less bizarre than those encountered in patients with schizophrenia. In fact, it may be quite difficult to discern whether strangers are attempting to break into the patient's house or whether family members are stealing from the patient's savings. Treatment of psychotic depression typically requires the use of an antipsychotic agent, plus an adequate dose of an antidepressant, or a course of electroconvulsive therapy (ECT) if pharmacotherapy is not effective.

The Elderly Patient With Psychosis

Psychotic symptoms are relatively common among the medically ill or disabled elderly, occurring in 10% to 62% of nursing home patients, up to 27% of elderly psychiatric outpatients in the community, and 5% to 15% of psychiatric inpatients.[13] Isolation and sensory impairment likely contribute to the higher incidence of paranoia and agitation in the elderly. Late-onset schizophrenia and very late-onset schizophrenia-like psychosis (informally referred to as late paraphrenia), which occur after the ages of 40 and 60, respectively, usually occur in females and manifest as paranoia. Older individuals are at particular risk for a host of secondary causes of psychosis, especially delirium and dementia. Psychotic symptoms are present in approximately 50% of cases of delirium[11] and 20% to 70% of cases across various types of dementia.[14] Psychotic symptoms are common in patients with Alzheimer disease (AD); approximately one-third of patients with AD develop psychotic symptoms, and approximately one-fourth develop hallucinations.[13]

Management of psychosis in the elderly requires a comprehensive evaluation for secondary causes, supportive measures, and the judicious use of antipsychotics. Supportive measures should be individualized but can include reassurance, re-orientation strategies, visits from family to alleviate isolation, strategies to maintain the sleep-wake cycle, and measures to compensate for sensory or cognitive deficits, such as providing clear and repeated instructions that counteract misinterpretations of reality. When non-pharmacological interventions are insufficient, short-term use of antipsychotics may be considered, but with great caution given that all antipsychotics carry a US Food and Drug Administration (FDA) black box warning for increased morbidity and mortality in elderly individuals with dementia. Clinical guidelines recommend minimizing the use of antipsychotics in the elderly due to the risk of worsening extrapyramidal symptoms (EPS), sedation, falls, worsening cognition, and metabolic problems. If antipsychotics are used off-label as part of a comprehensive treatment plan to manage agitation or psychosis in a patient with dementia, the response to treatment should be monitored and re-assessed with a rating scale, and periodic attempts should be made to taper and discontinue the antipsychotic. A newer antipsychotic, pimavanserin, a serotonin 5-HT$_{2A}$ inverse agonist and antagonist without dopamine receptor involvement, was FDA approved for the treatment of psychosis in Parkinson disease. Pimavanserin has no affinity for dopamine receptors, which confers advantages due to its inability to exacerbate motor symptoms of Parkinsonism. Pimavanserin is gaining support with promising results from clinical trials for the treatment of various types of dementia-related psychosis given its efficacy in reducing the risk of psychotic relapse as compared to placebo.[14] Selective serotonin reuptake inhibitors (SSRIs) have also been studied for this indication, and citalopram and escitalopram demonstrated some evidence of helping to reduce agitation in this population.[15]

MANAGEMENT OF PATIENTS WITH PSYCHOSIS

General Considerations

As emphasized above, the first step in approaching the treatment of a patient with psychosis is to clarify the diagnosis and obtain a history of psychotropic medication use. Delirium, which is characterized by confusion and fluctuations in mental status, must be recognized and the underlying cause addressed. The pharmacologic management of delirium is described in Chapter 9. Specific information about individual antipsychotic agents and drug-drug interactions is provided in Chapter 37.

Target symptoms for antipsychotics fall into three categories: (1) psychotic symptoms (e.g., hallucinations, delusions, disorganization), (2) agitation (e.g., affective lability, tension, increased motor activity), and (3) negative symptoms (e.g., apathy, flat affect, social isolation, poverty of speech). The last category responds best to an antipsychotic if symptoms are the result of active psychosis (e.g., a patient is withdrawn because of preoccupation with hallucinations). The pharmacologic treatment of acute psychosis is like the treatment of infection with antibiotics—the clinician needs to choose the proper medication at a sufficient dose and then await therapeutic results while monitoring for side effects. For agitation, a response to antipsychotics can often be seen after several days or even after a single dose.

Psychotic symptoms and agitation usually improve with antipsychotics, regardless of the etiology. Most types of secondary psychosis, including psychosis from stimulant intoxication (e.g., amphetamines, cocaine), also respond readily to antipsychotics. The decision around the use of an antipsychotic for a secondary psychosis should be informed by weighing the anticipated duration and severity of the psychosis and the potential side effects of the drug. When psychosis is time-limited and transient (i.e., only occurring in the context of a psychoactive substance or delirium), it is critical not to inadvertently continue the antipsychotic after the patient has been discharged from the hospital. This is particularly important when a first-generation antipsychotic (FGA) (also referred to as typical or conventional antipsychotic) is prescribed given the high risk of irreversible tardive dyskinesia (TD).

Drug Selection

Selection of an antipsychotic agent is guided by efficacy considerations, side-effect profiles, and available formulations (i.e., tablet, rapidly dissolving wafer, patch, liquid, intramuscular [IM], intravenous [IV], or depot preparation). The FGAs act by blocking dopamine D_2 receptors; they all have similar efficacy and differ primarily in their potency (i.e., the dose required for their clinical effect) and in their side effects. Second-generation antipsychotics (SGAs), also referred to as atypical antipsychotics, were developed based on the observation that clozapine while preserving efficacy, did not cause EPS. However, several large, seminal, randomized treatment trials (known by their acronyms, CATIE [Clinical Antipsychotic Trials of Intervention Effectiveness], CAFÉ [Comparison of Atypicals for First Episode], and EUFEST [European First Episode Schizophrenia Trial]) did not establish superior efficacy of SGAs over FGAs. It has, however, also become clear that not all SGAs are alike; each drug needs to be considered individually. Clozapine remains the "gold standard" with regard to efficacy, and it is also preferred for patients who are exquisitely sensitive to dopamine blockade, like patients with Parkinson disease; of the other SGAs, olanzapine has the strongest evidence for enhanced efficacy.[16] Newer medications are no longer full-dopamine antagonists and are sometimes grouped together as third-generation antipsychotics (TGAs).

In the outpatient setting, adherence to antipsychotics is a major treatment goal to reduce relapse. Up to 55% of patients with schizophrenia do not take their medications as prescribed,[17] in part because of ongoing substance use, medication side effects, or lack of insight, but also because of a poor response to treatment. Many but not all antipsychotics are available as long-acting injectable antipsychotics (LAIs) to assist in improving adherence in the maintenance phase of schizophrenia. Patients who are managed with LAIs as outpatients can usually be maintained on their injection schedule if they are admitted to a medical unit. It is important to remember that it takes several months for LAIs to be fully eliminated from the body after stopping them, which can be problematic for patients who develop neuroleptic malignant syndrome (NMS).

If a patient has been taking an antipsychotic with good results, it is often best to maintain the treatment and not to make changes in the regimen unless medical problems or potential drug interactions necessitate a switch, lest the patient be destabilized. Exacerbations in otherwise stable patients, particularly if related to stress and accompanied by depressive symptoms, may improve without altering the medication or raising the dosage. Benzodiazepines can be used temporarily, if needed, to manage worsening of symptoms.

First-Generation Antipsychotics

Low-potency FGAs, such as chlorpromazine (CPZ), should be prescribed in dosages of 300 to 600 CPZ mg-equivalents/day; they are associated with orthostatic hypotension, anticholinergic side effects, sedation, and weight gain, and some are less readily or safely administered parenterally. High-potency agents, such as haloperidol, are more likely to produce EPS, including acute dystonia, parkinsonism, and akathisia. Haloperidol can also be administered parenterally. In the setting of serious medical illness, particularly if other medications with anticholinergic or hypotensive side effects are being administered, haloperidol is typically the antipsychotic of choice. It is important to minimize the risk of Torsades de pointes (TdP) from haloperidol by reducing compounding risk factors (e.g., hypokalemia, hypomagnesemia) and by tracking the QTc.[18] Although considerable inter-individual variability exists, daily oral doses of haloperidol between 5 and 15 mg are adequate for most patients; increasing the dose beyond this range may only aggravate side effects without improving antipsychotic efficacy. IM and IV administration tend to require roughly half that dose. In the elderly, 0.5 to 2 mg of haloperidol at bedtime may be sufficient. If a patient has not previously received an antipsychotic, it is best to start with a low dose (e.g., haloperidol 2–5 mg orally) before increasing it to a usual therapeutic dose.

Second-Generation Antipsychotics

SGAs as a class produce fewer neurologic side effects (e.g., dystonia, akathisia, parkinsonism) than FGAs; they are also associated with less TD. In this class, risperidone is most likely to induce EPS, particularly at dosages higher than 6 mg/day. Lurasidone can also cause EPS at higher doses. It is important to appreciate that SGAs differ substantially from each other regarding other side effects. Risperidone and its active and marketed metabolite, 9-hydroxyrisperidone (paliperidone), are unique among the SGAs because of their propensity to produce hyperprolactinemia. Clozapine, olanzapine, and iloperidone have been associated with substantial weight gain that can be a major obstacle to adherence. Risperidone and quetiapine are associated with intermediate weight gain, and ziprasidone and lurasidone appear to produce less weight gain. Considerable research over the past decade has focused on the effects of SGAs on glucose metabolism and lipids. The observed insulin resistance and dyslipidemia are explained only in part by weight gain, and some antipsychotics seem to affect metabolism differently. Antipsychotics should be carefully monitored for metabolic problems, with close attention paid to pro-active medical management of patients at higher risk (e.g., those with a family history of diabetes, those taking clozapine or olanzapine, or those who already have pre-diabetes or other risk factors). Metformin can be used to mitigate these metabolic side effects. Newer agents used to manage antipsychotic-related weight gain include samidorphan (recently made available as a combination drug co-formulated with olanzapine) and glucagon-like peptide-1 receptor agonists.

Clozapine, risperidone, quetiapine, iloperidone, and ziprasidone have alpha-adrenergic effects that necessitate dose titration to avoid orthostatic hypotension; paliperidone can be given without titration. Of those, clozapine produces the most hypotension and tachycardia. Lurasidone and aripiprazole have minimal effect on QT prolongation.[18] Olanzapine has less risk compared to clozapine, but still confers mild

to moderate risk for QT prolongation. Ziprasidone and iloperidone appear to prolong the QT interval more than other SGAs, but less than thioridazine. For those taking antipsychotics other than thioridazine, ziprasidone, and iloperidone, routine monitoring of the electrocardiogram is generally not necessary unless the patient has other risk factors for QT prolongation.[18] QT prolongation and TdP are more likely when other risk factors (such as pre-existing cardiac rhythm abnormalities or co-administration of agents that delay antipsychotic metabolism by affecting the P450 isoenzyme system) are present.[19] Even in patients treated with ziprasidone, serious cardiac events have been rare (not differing from placebo in registration trials), and overdoses of this agent have been benign. The large observational ZODIAC study of ziprasidone patients found no increase in mortality when compared with olanzapine-treated patients. However, ziprasidone's effect on cardiac repolarization may be problematic in the presence of an underlying heart disease or when it is added to other agents with similar effects. Potential cardiac toxicity remains a clinical concern with all antipsychotics. A large retrospective cohort study did not find a difference between FGAs and SGAs in the risk for sudden death.[20] Instead, both classes produced a dose-related increase in the risk for sudden death.

Clozapine, although clearly possessing superior antipsychotic efficacy, can produce many bothersome and even potentially lethal side effects (Table 11.5). Clozapine carries five black box warnings: agranulocytosis, myocarditis, seizures, orthostatic hypotension with syncope and cardiorespiratory arrest, and increased mortality in elderly patients with dementia-related psychosis. Agranulocytosis and myocarditis are rare (0.8% and 3%, respectively) but serious when they occur, typically within the earlier stages of treatment (within the first 6 months and 2 months, respectively). Seizures are dose dependent with an overall seizure rate of 2.8%, often initially manifesting as myoclonus before progressing to generalized tonic-clonic seizures. Common side effects include orthostatic hypotension, sedation, tachycardia, constipation, weight gain, and sialorrhea. In elderly patients, or in those with cognitive impairment who may not report or recognize symptoms, pro-active management of side effects by a psychiatrist

TABLE 11.5
Side Effects of Clozapine

Five FDA Black Box Warnings
- Agranulocytosis
- Myocarditis
- Seizures
- Orthostatic hypotension with syncope and cardiorespiratory arrest
- Increased mortality in elderly patients with dementia-related psychosis (class warning for all antipsychotics)

Rare but serious side effects
Early side effects
- Agranulocytosis (0.8%)
  - Usually within the first 6 months of clozapine treatment
- Myocarditis (3%)
  - Usually within the first 2 months of clozapine treatment
  - Can be minimized by slow titration

Dose dependent
- Seizures (overall rate 2.8%), initially manifest as myoclonus
  - <300 mg/day—1.0%
  - 300–600 mg/day—2.7%
  - >600 mg/day—4.4%

Common side effects
Early side effects that can be minimized by slow titration
- Orthostatic hypotension
- Sedation
- Tachycardia

Dose-dependent side effects with a potential to become lethal when left untreated
- Constipation
  - Can lead to fecal impaction, paralytic ileus, intestinal obstruction, bowel perforation, toxic megacolon
- Sialorrhea
  - Can lead to aspiration pneumonia

Metabolic side effects that require regular monitoring
- Weight gain
- Diabetes
- Hyperlipidemia

Rare side effects
- Urinary incontinence

Very rare side effects
- Cardiomyopathy
- Pancreatitis
- Pulmonary embolism
- EPS and NMS

EPS, Extrapyramidal symptoms; *FDA,* US Food and Drug Administration; *NMS,* neuroleptic malignant syndrome.

is critical in preventing medical complications and death. Untreated constipation may lead to fecal impaction, paralytic ileus, intestinal obstruction, and/or bowel perforation, highlighting the importance of using laxatives regularly. Sialorrhea is a treatable condition that responds well to glycopyrrolate or atropine drops, but when left untreated it can lead to aspiration pneumonia, which is an alarming condition with an in-hospital mortality rate of approximately 30% in the elderly.[21] Urinary incontinence occurs in 1% of patients taking clozapine, although this statistic is likely under-reported due to stigma and embarrassment. Metabolic side effects need to be monitored routinely as clozapine can lead to metabolic syndromes, including weight gain, diabetes, and lipid abnormalities. Some rare, but not unprecedented, side effects include cardiomyopathy, pancreatitis, pulmonary embolism, TD, and NMS. Despite the list of potentially serious medical complications, clozapine decreased mortality rates more than other antipsychotic agents[22]; this net positive effect on mortality rates probably reflects the magnitude of its protective effect against suicide in contrast to its relatively low frequency of serious adverse effects, coupled with the old adage that there is no physical health without mental health (a psychiatrically ill patient is unlikely to manage his medical problems well). However, any potential protection from death due to suicide must be weighed against the possibility of a premature death from cardiovascular disease in an individual patient.

If a patient is to be started or re-started on clozapine, a provider with experience in the use of this agent should be consulted to determine how frequently to monitor neutrophil counts and to outline strategies for the initiation and optimization of the dosage of this unique agent. Clozapine treatment should not be unnecessarily interrupted when patients are admitted to a medical or surgical service because abrupt discontinuation has been associated with acute worsening of psychosis and with cholinergic rebound.[23] If clozapine has been discontinued for more than 2 days, clozapine should be re-introduced at a low dose and titrated upward toward the patient's previous optimal dose. A cautious approach is necessary to avoid hypotension, bradycardia, or syncope. It is ill advised to start clozapine de novo in a patient during a complicated medical admission.

Third-Generation Agents and the Newest Antipsychotics

Aripiprazole was the first FDA-approved dopamine partial agonist, followed by cariprazine and brexpiprazole. These medications have favorable side-effect profiles regarding metabolic symptoms and cardiac conduction. Aripiprazole is unique in that it can lower prolactin levels and is associated with the least QT prolongation.[18] Lumateperone has a more complex receptor profile, including pre-synaptic dopamine agonism and post-synaptic dopamine antagonism. It causes minimal EPS and metabolic side effects, and it does not require any dose titration. Pimavanserin is a selective serotonin 5-HT$_{2A}$ inverse agonist without dopamine blockade that has an FDA indication for psychosis in Parkinson disease but not for schizophrenia. New antipsychotics under development are non-dopamine-receptor binding medications for schizophrenia, such as a trace amine-associated receptor 1 (TAAR1) agonist called ulotaront and an M1 and M4 muscarinic receptor agonist called xanomeline, which is co-formulated with a peripheral anticholinergic called trospium.

Treating Psychiatric Agitation

Antipsychotics can be used successfully to treat acute agitation associated with psychosis. Given the high risk of EPS with haloperidol, current expert consensus guidelines recommend that SGAs are preferred over FGAs.[24] A sublingual dexmedetomidine preparation (film) has become available to treat acute agitation in schizophrenia and mania. Benzodiazepines can also effectively enhance the tranquilizing effect of antipsychotics or be used alone for the treatment of agitation due to causes other than psychosis. Lorazepam can be combined (in the same syringe) with haloperidol for acute behavioral control—usually 2 mg of lorazepam is given with 5 mg of IM haloperidol. Once agitation is controlled, the patient can be started on a standing dose of an antipsychotic, with a benzodiazepine (e.g., lorazepam 1–2 mg) given as needed, or as a standing order two to three times daily, for as long as is needed. Typically, as psychotic symptoms improve with the use of an antipsychotic, benzodiazepines often become unnecessary. The management of acute agitation in other populations is discussed fully in Chapter 43.

Extrapyramidal Side Effects and Tardive Dyskinesia

Younger patients (i.e., those younger than 40 years of age) started on high-potency FGAs are especially vulnerable to developing acute dystonic reactions during the first week of treatment. Dystonia, the sudden constriction of muscles, is a frightening and uncomfortable experience; when manifested as a laryngeal spasm, it can be life threatening. The occurrence of dystonia early in treatment jeopardizes future compliance with antipsychotics; therefore it is important to anticipate and treat this side effect aggressively. Prophylaxis with an anticholinergic agent, such as benztropine (1–2 mg twice daily), substantially reduces the likelihood of a dystonic reaction even in a high-risk patient. Dystonia is less common with the use of SGAs and TGAs than with high-potency FGAs; moreover, it probably does not occur with either quetiapine or clozapine.

Akathisia is an extremely unpleasant sensation of motor restlessness that is primarily experienced in the lower extremities. For the patient with psychosis hospitalized on a medical service, akathisia can make bedrest unbearable. Akathisia substantially increases the risk that a patient will leave the hospital against medical advice, and it has been associated with self-injurious behaviors as well as with a worsening of agitation.[25] Untrained staff frequently mistake akathisia for psychotic agitation, which leads to unfortunate escalations of antipsychotic doses. For patients in acute distress, diazepam (10 mg) can provide immediate relief. For long-term management, dose reduction may improve akathisia; if relief is not obtained, propranolol (10–20 mg two to four times daily) is often helpful. An even more effective intervention is to switch to an SGA or to a newer antipsychotic, which usually resolves the problem. Akathisia may, however, still occur with the dopamine D$_2$ partial agonists (e.g., aripiprazole) and may take several weeks to resolve spontaneously.

Antipsychotic-induced parkinsonism can easily be mistaken for depression or the negative symptoms of schizophrenia. The presence of tremor and rigidity distinguishes this side effect in more severe cases; subtle cases can easily be missed. Parkinsonian side effects commonly improve with a reduction of the antipsychotic dosage or with the addition of an antiparkinsonian agent (e.g., benztropine 1–2 mg twice daily or preferably amantadine 100 mg two or three times daily given its lack of anticholinergic properties). Because anticholinergic agents impair attention and memory and can produce a vast array of troublesome side effects in the elderly, long-term use of anticholinergics should be avoided. If unsuccessful, switching to either clozapine or quetiapine, which are essentially free of EPS, should be considered.

TD generally appears after more than 6 months of treatment with an antipsychotic; once present, TD may be irreversible. TD usually takes the form of involuntary, choreiform, movements of the mouth, tongue, or upper extremities, although a dystonic form has also been described. Studies suggest that the risk for developing TD with antipsychotic treatment is approximately 3% to 5% per year of exposure, with the prevalence of TD in antipsychotic-treated patients as high as 20% to 30%.[26] The incidence and prevalence of TD are much higher in the elderly (15%–30% per year and 50%–60%, respectively), although some of these cases may represent spontaneously occurring dyskinesias. As part of informed consent, patients requiring prolonged antipsychotic treatment, particularly with FGAs given their higher risk for TD, should be educated about the risk of developing TD as soon as possible after their acute psychosis has been treated. Preliminary evidence that indicated α-tocopherol (vitamin E), at dosages of 400 to 1200 IU daily, improved symptoms of TD was not supported by a much larger controlled trial; thus the best treatment for TD is prevention. Clozapine has generally not been linked to TD; switching a patient from another antipsychotic to clozapine increases the likelihood of improvement in TD. Lowering the dose of an FGA or switching to another antipsychotic can occasionally produce a "withdrawal dyskinesia," which either resolves within 6 weeks or unmasks an underlying dyskinesia that was previously suppressed by the antipsychotic. Tetrabenazine, a vesicular monoamine transporter (VMAT)-2 inhibitor approved to treat chorea in Huntington disease, can be helpful for TD but it has significant side effects, such as drowsiness, parkinsonism, and depression. Newer VMAT-2 inhibitors, such as valbenazine and deutetrabenazine (derivatives of tetrabenazine), are FDA-approved, first-line treatments for TD given their improved tolerability and less frequent dosing.

Neuroleptic Malignant Syndrome

Neuroleptic malignant syndrome (NMS) is a rare, potentially lethal, complication of antipsychotic treatment characterized by hyperthermia (>100.4 °F or >38.0 °C on at least two occasions, measured orally), muscle rigidity, confusion, diaphoresis, autonomic instability, elevated creatine phosphokinase (CPK), and leukocytosis.[27] Although the first symptoms of NMS may involve mental status changes, the syndrome may evolve gradually and culminate in fever and an elevated CPK. Recent studies showed a prevalence of NMS of 0.02% to 0.03% in patients who receive dopamine antagonists,[28] although sub-syndromal cases may be more common. Although parallels have been drawn between NMS and malignant hyperthermia (which results from general anesthesia) largely based on common clinical characteristics, patients with a history of either NMS or malignant hyperthermia do not appear to be at increased risk for developing the other condition. Moreover, analysis of muscle biopsy specimens has not consistently demonstrated physiological overlap between the two conditions. Another overlapping clinical presentation is lethal catatonia, which is a spontaneously occurring syndrome that may be indistinguishable from NMS and that can occur in the absence of antipsychotic treatment.[28] In addition, antipsychotic agents may impair temperature regulation and thus produce low-grade fever in the absence of other symptoms of NMS. The clinician's immediate response to NMS should be to discontinue dopamine-blocking antipsychotics and anticholinergics and hospitalize the patient to allow for IV fluids, cooling, and close monitoring. Because NMS is typically self-limiting, there is limited consensus beyond supportive medical care. The use of benzodiazepines, dopamine agonists (e.g., bromocriptine), dantrolene, and ECT has produced some evidence for efficacy, but it remains a subject of debate.[28]

Re-institution of antipsychotics should be delayed until at least 2 weeks after the episode of NMS has resolved. Studies have suggested a 30% risk of recurrence for antipsychotic re-challenge in those recovering from NMS. NMS has been associated with all antipsychotics, including clozapine, although newer antipsychotics may result in "atypical" presentations, such as the absence of, or less severe symptoms, of rigidity or hyperthermia.[28]

Drug Interactions With Antipsychotic Agents

Antipsychotic drugs interact with other medications because of alterations in hepatic metabolism and the combined use of drugs with additive side effects (such as anticholinergic effects or impairments of cardiac conduction). Most FGAs are extensively metabolized by the 2D6 isoenzyme of the hepatic P450 enzyme system, whereas SGAs generally have more variable hepatic metabolism, typically involving isoenzymes 3A4, 1A2, and 2D6. Fortunately, the therapeutic index (safety/risk ratio) of antipsychotic drugs is quite large, and interactions with agents that inhibit hepatic metabolism are unlikely to be life threatening but may increase side effects. Clozapine produces the most serious adverse effects when blood levels are dramatically elevated; obtundation and cardiovascular effects have been associated with inhibition of clozapine metabolism by fluvoxamine or erythromycin. Fluvoxamine, an SSRI, has been shown to cause a 5- to 10-fold increase in clozapine plasma concentrations by inhibiting the cytochrome P450 1A2 enzyme system. Conversely, cigarette smoking induces the CYP 1A2 enzyme. Thus, smoking cessation leads to a doubling of clozapine blood levels along with increased sedation and worsening of other side effects. Severe systemic inflammation, including severe respiratory illnesses such as COVID-19, can also lead to increased clozapine levels via inhibition of CYP 1A2. The addition of 2D6 inhibitors (e.g., SSRIs) to FGAs would be expected to increase EPS, but in some studies, this increase was not clinically significant, despite substantial increases in blood levels of antipsychotics.[29] Drugs that pan-induce hepatic metabolism, such as certain anticonvulsants (e.g., carbamazepine, phenobarbital, phenytoin), may lower blood concentrations of most antipsychotics substantially and cause a loss of therapeutic efficacy.

Considerable inter-individual variability exists for the metabolism of antipsychotic drugs, even without the complication of drug interactions. Therapeutic drug monitoring (TDM), i.e., the measurement of antipsychotic levels in blood, has become available for most antipsychotics. Application of TDM may be beneficial in challenging clinical situations, such as with a poor therapeutic response, questionable drug adherence, relapse, or adverse effects of antipsychotic treatment, especially in vulnerable patient subgroups, to guide dosing decisions.[30] TDM is recommended with a high level of clinical evidence for clozapine, haloperidol, olanzapine, and perphenazine given the favorable clinical outcomes associated with therapeutic blood levels.[30] For clozapine, an initial target serum level of 350 ng/mL is sufficient, although in patients with a poor response to clozapine, a level of at least 450 ng/mL should be targeted.[31] For maintenance treatment, serum concentrations of between 200 and 300 ng/mL seem adequate. The risk of toxicity, particularly seizures, increases significantly at levels around 1000 ng/mL for the active moiety (clozapine plus norclozapine) although individual vulnerability (due to numerous factors, such as brain damage or chronic substance use) plays a role.

Great care must be taken if low-potency agents (such as chlorpromazine or clozapine) are combined with other highly anticholinergic drugs, because the additive anticholinergic activity may produce and exacerbate confusion, urinary retention, and constipation. In addition, low-potency antipsychotics can depress cardiac function and can significantly impair cardiac conduction when added to class I antiarrhythmic agents (such as quinidine and procainamide). Ziprasidone and iloperidone also affect cardiac conduction in a significant fashion and should not be combined with low-potency phenothiazines or with antiarrhythmic agents.

WORKING TOGETHER WITH THE PATIENT, THE FAMILY, AND THE BROADER CARE TEAM

Patients with schizophrenia may be unable to express their fears or concerns directly; instead, they may exhibit anxiety or insomnia and may become increasingly delusional when stressed. Efforts to anticipate and answer a patient's unspoken fears about his or her medical status can greatly alleviate other symptoms, although this process may need to be repeated daily. Patients with schizophrenia may also lack the capacity to "filter" extraneous stimuli in their world and may become easily overwhelmed or overly stimulated in chaotic environments, like hospitals. Placing a patient with schizophrenia in a quiet and uncluttered room can assist the patient in retaining a sense of control and fostering reality testing. The patient's need for privacy should be respected, and nursing staff should be advised that some patients with schizophrenia do not respond to overly nurturing or what they perceived as intrusive attention.

Families and the broader outpatient care team (e.g., case manager, group home staff, peer support, visiting nurse) of patients with schizophrenia can be invaluable sources of information in any setting. They can help to establish the diagnosis and identify potential triggers for escalation. They might have an idea if poor medication adherence or illicit drug use is contributing to the current psychiatric symptoms. Patients are poor judges of their own cognitive challenges and functional limitations, whereas family members and the care team can often provide a more accurate picture of these domains. Working with families is always important. It is arguably most important when the patient experiences or is recovering from his or her first psychotic episode. Education about the illness, a discussion about the use of medication, and identification of the early signs of relapse can start in the hospital and help with the transition to outpatient care. Families need to know about the risk of suicide in schizophrenia because they could be the first ones to recognize that a patient is becoming hopeless or disillusioned after discharge. It has been well demonstrated that educating families about the illness and helping them develop reasonable expectations for their loved ones with schizophrenia significantly improves the course of the illness.[11] Furthermore, it is important to coordinate and communicate with the broader outpatient care team to ensure continued support and assistance with changes or follow-up recommendations that were initiated in the inpatient setting.

ADDITIONAL CHALLENGES IN THE CARE OF PATIENTS WITH PSYCHOSIS

Assessment of Violence Risk

The relationship between mental illness and violence is complex; having a mental illness per se does not predict violence. Clinicians should assess well-established predictors of violence, the most significant of which is a history of violence. Other risk factors include substance use, cognitive challenges, brain injuries, antisocial personality disorder, and prior exposure to

violence. These risk factors should be assessed both by self-report and by gathering collateral information and reviewing available medical records. A recent review estimated the absolute rate of violence to be 6% to 10% in patients with schizophrenia-spectrum disorders.[32] Furthermore, people with schizophrenia are more likely to become victims of violence than they are to perpetrate violence.[33] Nevertheless, psychiatric treatment of psychosis is a critical violence-prevention task for psychiatrists. While engaging in any treatment may decrease the risk of violence, there is a specific protective effect of clozapine on violence that may not be shared by other antipsychotics. In fact, the American Psychiatric Association Guideline for Schizophrenia strongly recommends the use of clozapine for aggressive behavior in patients with schizophrenia.

Violent or aggressive acts may take different forms depending on the symptom profile of the patient. Paranoid psychosis or manic irritability can result in acts of violence driven by fear or anger. Disorganized patients may act aggressively as a result of impaired self-control, whereas patients with persecutory or religious delusions can plan or enact complex behaviors in alignment with their beliefs (i.e., when they are convinced that they have no alternative but to act violently—either to defend themselves or their family, or to obey God's command). Command hallucinations appear to increase the risk of violence when the individual interprets the voices within a delusional system in such a way that the voices cannot be disobeyed[34]; for example, a patient may believe that it is God's voice giving orders to attack someone believed to be possessed by Satan. Although the potential for violence is a cause for concern, homicides by patients with schizophrenia are rare and are frequently closely related to substance use and social risk factors (e.g., low socioeconomic status).[35] In many cases, family members become victims of violence, rather than innocent by-standers.

Violence against oneself is usually a greater concern in patients with schizophrenia. Suicide is a main cause of premature death in patients with schizophrenia; 5% of patients with schizophrenia commit suicide and as many as 28% attempt suicide.[36] In addition to delusions and hallucinations, depression and substance use are important risk factors for suicide. The consultant must explore carefully these risk factors as well as any history of suicide attempts and self-injurious behaviors.[36] In patients at high risk for suicide, the anti-psychotic clozapine should be considered. Clozapine has an FDA-approved indication for suicidality in schizophrenia-spectrum disorders.

Regardless of its cause, when patients are at high risk of violence or self-harm in the hospital, they should be monitored continuously. The least restrictive methods of preserving safety should be employed, such as the use of a trained observer, the creation of a safe environment, and the limitation of access to sharp objects. However, if the least restrictive measures fail, physical or chemical restraints may be needed to protect the patient, other hospital patients, and staff. Restraints must be used safely, by well-trained staff, and in accordance with hospital and government regulations. Inappropriate use of restraint is not only unjust, but restraints carry morbidity and mortality risks, such as deep vein thrombosis and death from pulmonary embolism.

Pain Insensitivity and Under-Reporting of Physical Symptoms in Schizophrenia

Despite substantially poorer physical health with a higher burden of medical co-morbidities, older studies suggested that patients with schizophrenia may have elevated pain thresholds, which can obscure serious medical problems.[37] In one study, 21% of patients with schizophrenia failed to report pain associated with a perforated peptic ulcer, and 37% felt no pain during acute appendicitis, while it has been estimated that more than 95% of the general public experienced excruciating pain with either condition.[38] In addition, 83% of patients with psychosis undergoing myocardial infarction did not endorse pain.[38] The mechanism underlying this often dramatically elevated pain threshold remains unclear. It had been presumed to involve a different neurobiological response to a painful stimulus, independent of antipsychotic treatment. However, recent studies suggest there may be little or no physiological evidence that supports endogenous analgesia. Instead, patients with schizophrenia might simply be under-recognizing or under-reporting their symptoms, in part due to negative symptoms that impede pain communication.[37] Under- or late-recognition of serious medical conditions could be contributing to this population's premature mortality. Because self-reporting of pain is reduced in schizophrenia,

psychiatric consultants should make medical colleagues aware of this patient characteristics and help them become more sensitive to pain communication. The goal is to assess pain thoroughly using non-verbal behavioral measures and collateral information so that the existence of serious pathologic processes is not dismissed because of an absence of typical manifestations of pain.[37]

Psychogenic Polydipsia (Water Intoxication)

Psychogenic polydipsia is defined as chronic or intermittent ingestion of large volumes of water; it is reported to occur in 15% to 25% of chronically ill patients with SMI.[39] Polydipsia is most frequently observed in patients with schizophrenia, in whom it generally appears 5 to 15 years after the onset of illness. While historically associated with institutionalized patients, 15% of outpatients show excessive water intake.[40] Polydipsia may lead to several complications, including bladder dilatation, enuresis, incontinence, hydronephrosis, renal failure, and congestive heart failure. Approximately 25% to 50% of patients with polydipsia develop hyponatremia within the first 10 years of this condition. Often referred to as *water intoxication*, symptoms of polydipsia with hyponatremia include nausea, vomiting, blurred vision, tremors, cramps, ataxia, confusion, lethargy, seizures, coma, and death. Polydipsia with hyponatremia should be considered a serious complication of psychotic illness that requires careful evaluation and management. Acute care includes supportive treatment, fluid restriction, normal saline, and, in severe cases, the use of hypertonic saline. Fluid restriction can be difficult to implement in patients who have no clear understanding of their contribution to the problem. Rapid correction of an abnormal serum sodium level is unwise because it can lead to congestive heart failure and central pontine myelinolysis. A medical admission is often necessary until the serum sodium normalizes. Long-term management includes frequent monitoring of serum sodium concentrations and restriction of fluid intake when possible. *Vaptans* are a new class of medicines to manage hyponatremia. While clinicians might try them to treat hyponatremia due to psychogenic polydipsia, they are probably prohibitively expensive in most settings, particularly for chronic use. Switching from conventional antipsychotics to clozapine may significantly improve polydipsia and hyponatremia in some patients.

Medical Co-morbidities

As a group, patients with schizophrenia have a reduced life expectancy of up to 20 years and carry a high burden of medical illnesses, including, among others, obesity, diabetes, cardiovascular diseases, pulmonary diseases, and infectious diseases, such as HIV and hepatitis.[22,41] Cardiovascular disease is the primary contributor to an average reduction in life expectancy of two decades or more, a gap that has worsened in recent decades. Studies have shown a 1.4- to 2-fold increased risk across all cardiovascular and metabolic diseases in patients with schizophrenia.[41] Unfortunately, part of the excess mortality related to these medical illnesses is iatrogenic, because antipsychotics, regardless of class, can contribute to cardiac deaths directly (i.e., from sudden death), and indirectly via the development of cardiac disease (due to weight gain, diabetes, and dyslipidemia). Studies have also suggested that patients with schizophrenia are at greater risk of physical multi-morbidity from the onset of diagnosis, even among young people with schizophrenia.[41] Appropriate attention to the medical care of patients with psychotic illnesses has emerged as an important mandate for psychiatrists. A medical hospital admission provides an excellent opportunity to review the adequacy of medical treatment for these patients, with an emphasis placed on screening for the highly prevalent metabolic syndrome (about 40% in the CATIE sample), cardiovascular risk factors, and antipsychotic-related problems. Patients who do not have a primary care provider (PCP) can be identified and linked with community providers.

Cancer (particularly lung cancer) is an important medical cause of death in patients with schizophrenia as they age, just like for other patients. However, cancer detection and treatment are sub-standard for this patient group. In a nationwide Danish register study,[42] the likelihood of having been diagnosed with cancer prior to dying from cancer was markedly reduced in those with schizophrenia compared to controls, suggesting a grave reality that patients with schizophrenia are less likely to be diagnosed with cancer and receive effective treatment.[43]

In selected patients, screening for hepatitis B, hepatitis C, and HIV infection can be accomplished during hospitalization, particularly if it is unlikely to occur otherwise. Studies have suggested that the average incidence of hepatitis B and hepatitis C in patients with schizophrenia in the United States was approximately 20%; the prevalence of HIV among patients with schizophrenia in the United States is almost four times greater than in the general population.[41] Moreover, respiratory conditions, in particular chronic obstructive pulmonary disease and pneumonia, are among the leading causes of death in patients with schizophrenia, accounting for about 20% of all deaths.[44] A recent systemic review and meta-analysis showed that pneumonia confers the highest risk of mortality among natural causes in individuals with schizophrenia.[22] During the COVID-19 pandemic, schizophrenia was the second leading risk factor for COVID-19 mortality after age.[45] Thus, heightened mortality from vaccine-preventable illnesses highlights the importance of vaccinations as preventive care in this population. Psychiatric providers can increase their patients' vaccination rates by proactively providing vaccine education and resolving vaccine hesitancy through motivational interviewing.[46]

Cigarette Smoking and Nicotine Use

While cigarette smoking declined substantially in the general population, the rate of daily smoking and nicotine use among patients with schizophrenia continues to remain higher than the general population level. Individuals with schizophrenia are more likely to smoke tobacco heavily and have more severe dependence.[47] For those patients who use nicotine, quitting should be one of the most important health goals, particularly in light of the high burden of cardiovascular disease in this population. Most patients with schizophrenia want to quit smoking, and with the right support, they can quit. Studies suggest that smoking cessation interventions are particularly effective when initiated in the inpatient setting, which provides a window of opportunity to increase motivation for smoking cessation, particularly if the admission was related in some way to smoking.[48] Clinicians should adopt a pro active "opt-out" approach (using presumptive language assuming that patients want to quit smoking), essentially moving away from the idea that people need to be "ready to quit" prior to being offered smoking cessation interventions. All nicotine users should be offered the most effective pharmacotherapeutic treatments, especially varenicline, and behavioral support and counseling to quit immediately.[49]

While bupropion and nicotine replacement therapy (NRT) alone or in combination are good medication choices to help some patients with schizophrenia quit smoking, varenicline is the most effective medication to help patients quit and remain abstinent. Compared with other populations, where short-term pharmacotherapy is sufficient to assist in quitting and maintaining long-term abstinence, many patients with schizophrenia benefit from maintenance treatment to prevent relapse. Varenicline has been found to be safe in the Evaluating Adverse Events in a Global Smoking Cessation Study (EAGLES) trial, with neuropsychiatric side-effect rates being similar to those who received a placebo.[47]

It is important to note that cigarette smoking reduces the plasma drug concentration levels of most antipsychotic drugs, particularly for drugs that are metabolized by the cytochrome P450 1A2 enzyme system (e.g., olanzapine, clozapine). Therefore, during a lengthy hospital stay when patients are forced to quit smoking, plasma drug levels rise, potentially leading to drug toxicities and increased side effects (e.g., EPS). This effect is not mediated by nicotine, but by tar products, and hence not reversed by NRT, such as patches or gums. Thus, smoking cessation treatment needs to include antipsychotic therapeutic drug monitoring followed by dosage adjustment.

Medication Adherence and Insight Into Illness

One hallmark of schizophrenia is an often-striking lack of insight into the illness: its symptoms, consequences, and need for treatment (also referred to as anosognosia). A patient with psychosis who has just been involuntarily committed to a psychiatric hospital after fighting with police might report that the reason for the admission was that he came for coffee. Thankfully, this example is extreme, and many patients have at least some understanding of the role of psychiatric treatment and can participate meaningfully in decisions regarding the use of antipsychotics. Studies have demonstrated that adherence to antipsychotics, especially LAIs and clozapine, significantly improves morbidity and mortality in this population in part by increasing adherence to medical treatments

(such as antidiabetics, statins, antihypertensives, and beta-blockers).[22] Clinicians should determine the specific reason for poor antipsychotic adherence so that specific remedies can be sought given the protective effect of antipsychotics. Unintentional non-adherence due to individual barriers or structural factors should be considered (e.g., cognitive impairments that make it difficult to access medication and regularly take medication, for which LAIs can be beneficial). In some patients, supervision makes a difference (such as in a group home where medication is administered by staff), whereas in others, one of the assisted treatment options (e.g., assertive community treatment) may be necessary.[11] There is little doubt that for most patients, maintenance antipsychotics must play a pivotal role in preventing psychotic relapse. This is true for patients who have been ill for many years and for patients who are recovering from their first psychotic episode. In a systemic review of patients with first-episode psychosis who discontinued maintenance antipsychotics, 77% and over 90% of patients, experienced another psychotic episode within 1 and 2 years, respectively.[50] The prevention of further psychotic episodes is paramount because psychotic episodes come at a high cost to the patient: work, family, and social lives are interrupted; there is a stigma associated with psychiatric hospitalization; there is a decline in function after each episode in early illness; there is a risk of subsequent progression to treatment-resistant schizophrenia; and there is always the danger of violence, accidental or intentional injury, and death. On the other hand, medical hospital staff can be reassured that antipsychotics can usually be withheld for a brief medical procedure, *if necessary*, because psychotic relapse is typically measured in weeks or months, not days, for remitted patients. For most patients with stable schizophrenia who require medical admission, long-term adherence issues are less relevant, and the treatment team can simply continue the psychiatric outpatient regimen. Patients unwilling to take psychiatric medications usually have no problems taking medical medications.

CONCLUSION

C-L psychiatrists can play several critical roles in the care of patients with schizophrenia who are medically hospitalized. They can assist in making accurate diagnoses of psychotic disorders, based on a thorough medical and psychiatric evaluation, and instituting appropriate treatment regimens. They can help treatment teams understand the nature of psychotic symptoms, resolve their fears and misunderstandings, and facilitate stronger relationships between the patient and the treatment team. They can advocate for appropriate screening, timely detection, and comprehensive treatment of medical illnesses, particularly when patients are unable to advocate for themselves. C-L psychiatrists can assist the medical team with the objective evaluation of patients' symptoms with behavioral assessments and familial input especially when self-reported pain is unreliable or unattainable. C-L psychiatrists can also encourage the medical team to offer preventive care opportunities (such as vaccinations, cancer screenings, and smoking cessation resources), and collect routine blood work to monitor metabolic syndrome can be extremely beneficial for this vulnerable population. Taken together, C-L psychiatrists are well positioned to recognize structural barriers to care for patients with schizophrenia and bridge the disconnect between inpatient and outpatient care settings, which can help address inequities among patients with schizophrenia and improve patient outcomes.

REFERENCES

1. Lim C, Paudel S, Holt DJ. Psychosis and schizophrenia. In: Stern TA, Wilens TE, Fava M, eds. *Comprehensive Clinical Psychiatry*. 3rd ed. Elsevier; 2024.
2. Ross EL, Becker JE, Linnoila JJ, et al. Cost-effectiveness of routine screening for autoimmune encephalitis in patients with first-episode psychosis in the United States. *J Clin Psychiatry*. 2020;82(1).
3. American Psychiatric Association. *Diagnostic and Statistical Manual of Mental Disorders: DSM-5 Text Revision*. 5th ed. American Psychiatric Association; 2022.
4. Kvig EI, Nilssen S. Does method matter? Assessing the validity and clinical utility of structured diagnostic interviews among a clinical sample of first-admitted patients with psychosis: a replication study. *Front Psychiatry*. 2023;14:1076299.
5. Brown HE, Kaneko Y, Donovan AL. Substance-induced psychosis and co-occurring psychotic disorders. In: Donovan AL, Bird S, eds. *Substance Use and the Acute Psychiatric Patient: Emergency Management*. Humana Press; 2019:111–124. Current Clinical Psychiatry.
6. Paredes AZ, Hyer JM, Diaz A, et al. The impact of mental illness on postoperative outcomes among Medicare beneficiaries: a missed opportunity to help surgical patients? *Ann Surg*. 2020;272(3):419–425.
7. Freudenreich O, Stern TA. Clinical experience with the management of schizophrenia in the general hospital. *Psychosomatics*. 2003;44(1):12–23.
8. Freudenreich O. *Diagnostic assessment of schizophrenia* Rosenbaum JF,. *Psychotic Disorders: A Practical Guide*. 2nd ed. Humana Press; 2020:101–113 Current Clinical Psychiatry.
9. Havens L, Sabo A. *Forming effective relationships*. Sabo AN, Havens L, *The Real World Guide to Psychotherapy Practice*. 2000;17–33 eBook.
10. Picardi A, Fonzi L, Pallagrosi M, et al. Delusional themes across affective and non-affective psychoses. *Front Psychiatry*. 2018;9:132.
11. Freudenreich O, Cather C, Stern TA, *Facing Serious Mental Illness: A Guide for Patients and Their Families*. Massachusetts General Hospital Psychiatry Academy; 2021.
12. Sweet V. *Slow Medicine: The Way to Healing*. Penguin; 2017.
13. Reinhardt MM, Cohen CI. Late-life psychosis: diagnosis and treatment. *Curr Psychiatry Rep*. 2015;17:1–13.
14. Tariot PN, Cummings JL, Soto-Martin ME, et al. Trial of pimavanserin in dementia-related psychosis. *N Engl J Med*. 2021;385(4):309–319.
15. Aga VM. When and how to treat agitation in Alzheimer's disease dementia with citalopram and escitalopram. *Am J Geriatr Psychiatry*. 2019;27(10):1099–1107.
16. Huhn M, Nikolakopoulou A, Schneider-Thoma J, et al. Comparative efficacy and tolerability of 32 oral antipsychotics for the acute treatment of adults with multi-episode schizophrenia: a systematic review and network meta-analysis. *Lancet*. 2019;394(10202):939–951.
17. Curto M, Fazio F, Ulivieri M, et al. Improving adherence to pharmacological treatment for schizophrenia: a systematic assessment. *Expert Opin Pharmacother*. 2021;22(9):1143–1155.
18. Beach SR, Celano CM, Sugrue AM, et al. QT prolongation, torsades de pointes, and psychotropic medications: a 5-year update. *Psychosomatics*. 2018;59(2):105–122.
19. Donovan AL, Vyas CM, Petriceks A, et al. Agitation and an altered mental status in the emergency department: differential diagnosis, evaluation, and treatment. *Prim Care Companion CNS Disord*. 2022;24(6):44509.
20. Ray WA, Chung CP, Murray KT, et al. Atypical antipsychotic drugs and the risk of sudden cardiac death. *N Engl J Med*. 2009;360(3):225–235.
21. Shin D, Lebovic G, Lin RJ. In-hospital mortality for aspiration pneumonia in a tertiary teaching hospital: a retrospective cohort review from 2008 to 2018. *J Otolaryngol Head Neck Surg*. 2023;52(1):23.
22. Correll CU, Solmi M, Croatto G, et al. Mortality in people with schizophrenia: a systematic review and meta-analysis of relative risk and aggravating or attenuating factors. *World Psychiatry*. 2022;21(2):248–271.
23. Blackman G, Oloyede E, Horowitz M, et al. Reducing the risk of withdrawal symptoms and relapse following clozapine discontinuation—is it feasible to develop evidence-based guidelines? *Schizophr Bull*. 2022;48(1):176–189.
24. Wilson MP, Pepper D, Currier GW, et al. The psychopharmacology of agitation: consensus statement of the American Association

for Emergency Psychiatry project Beta psychopharmacology workgroup. *West J Emerg Med.* 2012;13(1):26.

25. Bjarke J, Gjerde HN, Jørgensen HA, et al. Akathisia and atypical antipsychotics: relation to suicidality, agitation and depression in a clinical trial. *Acta Neuropsychiatrica.* 2022;34(5):282–288.

26. Caroff SN. A new era in the diagnosis and treatment of tardive dyskinesia. *CNS Spectr.* 2022:4–14.

27. Caroff SN, Mann SC, Sullivan KA, et al. Neuroleptic malignant syndrome. Movement disorder emergencies: diagnosis and treatment. *Nature.* 2022:95–113.

28. Rogers JP, Oldham MA, Fricchione G, et al. Evidence-based consensus guidelines for the management of catatonia: recommendations from the British Association for psychopharmacology. *J Psychopharmacol.* 2023. 02698811231158232.

29. Nguyen T, Liu X, Abuhashem W, et al. Quality of evidence supporting major psychotropic drug-drug interaction warnings: a systematic literature review. *Pharmacotherapy.* 2020;40(5):455–468.

30. Schoretsanitis G, Kane JM, Correll CU, et al. Blood levels to optimize antipsychotic treatment in clinical practice: a joint consensus statement of the American Society of Clinical Psychopharmacology and the Therapeutic Drug Monitoring Task Force of the Arbeitsgemeinschaft für Neuropsychopharmakologie und Pharmakopsychiatrie. *J Clin Psychiatry.* 2020;81(3):3649.

31. Freudenreich O, Schnitzer K. How to use clozapine: a primer for clinicians. *Dir Psychiatry.* 2021;41(1):15–30.

32. Whiting D, Lichtenstein P, Fazel S. Violence and mental disorders: a structured review of associations by individual diagnoses, risk factors, and risk assessment. *Lancet Psychiatry.* 2021;8(2):150–161.

33. Wehring HJ, Carpenter WT. Violence and schizophrenia. *Schizophr Bull.* 2011 Sep;37(5):877–878.

34. Dugré JR, West ML. Disentangling compliance with command hallucinations: heterogeneity of voice intents and their clinical correlates. *Schizophr Res.* 2019;212:33–39.

35. Baird A, Webb RT, Hunt IM, et al. Homicide by men diagnosed with schizophrenia: national case–control study. *BJPsych Open.* 2020;6(6):e143.

36. Donovan AL, Browne J, Freudenreich O, et al. Suicide in schizophrenia spectrum disorders. *Psychiatr Ann.* 2020;50(4):146–151.

37. Onwumere J, Stubbs B, Stirling M, et al. Pain management in people with severe mental illness: an agenda for progress. *Pain.* 2022;163(9):1653–1660.

38. Marchand WE, Sarota B, Marble HC, et al. Occurrence of painless acute surgical disorders in psychotic patients. *N Engl J Med.* 1959;260(12):580–585.

39. Havens TH, Innamorato G, Nemec IIEC. Non-antipsychotic pharmacotherapy of psychogenic polydipsia: a systematic review. *J Psychosom Res.* 2022;152:110674.

40. Iftene F, Bowie C, Milev R, et al. Identification of primary polydipsia in a severe and persistent mental illness outpatient population: a prospective observational study. *Psychiatry Res.* 2013;210(3):679–683.

41. Firth J, Siddiqi N, Koyanagi A, et al. The Lancet Psychiatry Commission: a blueprint for protecting physical health in people with mental illness. *Lancet Psychiatry.* 2019;6(8):675–712.

42. Brink M, Green A, Bojesen AB, et al. Excess medical comorbidity and mortality across the lifespan in schizophrenia: a nationwide Danish register study. *Schizophr Res.* 2019;206:347–354.

43. Irwin KE, Park ER, Fields LE, et al. Bridge: person-centered collaborative care for patients with serious mental illness and cancer. *Oncologist.* 2019;24(7):901–910.

44. Suetani S, Honarparvar F, Siskind D, et al. Increased rates of respiratory disease in schizophrenia: a systematic review and meta-analysis including 619,214 individuals with schizophrenia and 52,159,551 controls. *Schizophr Res.* 2021;237:131–140.

45. Nemani K, Li C, Olfson M, et al. Association of psychiatric disorders with mortality among patients with COVID-19. *JAMA Psychiatry.* 2021;78(4):380–386.

46. Lim C, Van Alphen MU, Maclaurin S, et al. Increasing COVID-19 vaccination rates among patients with serious mental illness: a pilot intervention study. *Psychiatr Serv.* 2022;73(11):1274–1277.

47. Evins AE, West R, Benowitz NL, et al. Efficacy and safety of pharmacotherapeutic smoking cessation AIDS in schizophrenia spectrum disorders: subgroup analysis of eagles. *Psychiatr Serv.* 2021;72(1):7–15.

48. Carson-Chahhoud KV, Smith BJ, Peters MJ, et al. Two-year efficacy of varenicline tartrate and counselling for inpatient smoking cessation (STOP study): a randomized controlled clinical trial. *PLoS One.* 2020;15(4):e0231095.

49. Evins AE, Cather C, Daumit GL. Smoking cessation in people with serious mental illness. *Lancet Psychiatry.* 2019;6(7):563–564.

50. Zipursky RB, Menezes NM, Streiner DL. Risk of symptom recurrence with medication discontinuation in first-episode psychosis: a systematic review. *Schizophr Res.* 2014;152(2-3):408–414.

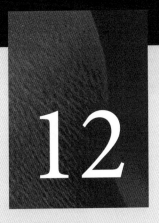

PHARMACOTHERAPY OF ANXIETY DISORDERS

ERIC BUI, MD, PHD ■ AMANDA WATERS BAKER, PHD ■
THEODORE A. STERN, MD

OVERVIEW

Anxiety disorders are associated with significant distress and dysfunction. In this chapter, we will review the treatment of panic disorder (with or without co-morbid agoraphobia), generalized anxiety disorder (GAD), and social anxiety disorder (SAD). Tables 12.1, 12.2, and 12.3 provide dosing information and common side effects associated with the pharmacological agents that are commonly used for the treatment of anxiety.

First-Line Pharmacotherapy for Anxiety Disorders: Selective Serotonin Reuptake Inhibitors and Serotonin-Norepinephrine Reuptake Inhibitors

The selective serotonin reuptake inhibitors (SSRIs) and serotonin-norepinephrine reuptake inhibitors (SNRIs) are first-line agents for the treatment of panic disorder, SAD, and GAD because of their broad spectrum of efficacy (including benefits for disorders that are commonly co-morbid such as major depressive disorder), favorable side-effect profile, and paucity of cardiotoxicity. A meta-analyses of anxiety disorder treatments (with a pooled sample of over 37,000 patients) reported large effect sizes for SNRIs and SSRIs that were greater than those of psychosocial and controlled interventions and comparable to those of tricyclic antidepressants (TCAs) and benzodiazepines, which have less favorable side effects and safety profiles.[1]

Because the SSRIs/SNRIs can cause initial restlessness, insomnia, and increased anxiety, and because patients with anxiety disorders are often sensitive to somatic sensations, the starting doses of these agents should be low, typically half (or less) of the usual starting dose (e.g., fluoxetine 5–10 mg/day, sertraline 25 mg/day, paroxetine 10 mg/day [or 12.5 mg/day of the controlled-release formulation], controlled-release venlafaxine 37.5 mg/day) to minimize the early anxiogenic effect (see Table 12.1). Doses are typically increased after about 1 week of acclimation, to achieve usual therapeutic levels, with further dose titration based on the clinical response and side effects, although an even slower upward titration is sometimes necessary for those who are especially sensitive to side effects or who are somatically focused. Doses for anxiety disorders lie in the typical antidepressant range or are sometimes higher, for example, fluoxetine 20 to 40 mg/day, paroxetine 20 to 60 mg/day (25–72.5 mg/day of the controlled-release formulation), sertraline 100 to 200 mg/day, citalopram 20 to 40 mg/day, escitalopram 10 to 20 mg/day, fluvoxamine 150 to 250 mg/day, and controlled-release venlafaxine 75 to 225 mg/day (although some patients respond at lower doses). In some cases of refractory anxiety disorders, even higher doses may be needed.

Administration of SSRIs and SNRIs has been associated with adverse effects that include sexual dysfunction, sleep disturbances, weight gain, headache, dose-dependent increases in blood pressure (with venlafaxine), gastrointestinal disturbances, the risk of bleeding (with anticoagulants, aspirin, or non-steroidal anti-inflammatory drugs), and provocation of increased anxiety that may make their administration problematic. SSRIs/SNRIs are usually administered in

TABLE 12.1
Selective Serotonin Reuptake Inhibitors (SSRIs) and Serotonin-Norepinephrine Reuptake Inhibitors (SNRIs)

Agent	Initial Dose (mg/d)	Typical Dose Range (mg/d)	Limitations/ Primary Side Effects
Citalopram (Celexa)	10	20–40	Initial jitteriness, GI distress, sedation or insomnia, hypertension (venlafaxine), sexual dysfunction, urinary hesitation (duloxetine), discontinuation syndrome
Duloxetine (Cymbalta)	30	60–90	
Escitalopram (Lexapro)	5–10	10–20	
Fluoxetine (Prozac)	10	20–80	
Fluvoxamine (Luvox)	50	150–300	
Paroxetine (Paxil)	10	20–60	
Paroxetine controlled release (Paxil-CR)	12.5	25–75	
Sertraline (Zoloft)	25	50–200	
Venlafaxine extended release (Effexor-XR)	37.5	75–225	

GI, Gastrointestinal.

TABLE 12.2
Dosing of Tricyclic Antidepressants (TCAs) and Monoamine Oxidase Inhibitors (MAOIs)

Agent	Initial Dose (mg/d)	Typical Dose Range (mg/d)	Limitations/ Primary Side Effects
TCAs			
Imipramine (e.g., Tofranil)	10–25	100–300	Jitteriness, sedation, dry mouth, weight gain, cardiac conduction effects, orthostasis, variably anticholinergic
Clomipramine (Anafranil)	25	25–250	
Monoamine Oxidase Inhibitors (MAOIs)			
Phenelzine (e.g., Nardil)	15–30	45–90	Diet restrictions, hypertensive reactions, serotonin syndrome
Tranylcypromine (e.g., Parnate)	10	30–60	
Benzodiazepines			
Alprazolam (Xanax)	0.25 QID	2–8	Sedation, discontinuation difficulties, potential for abuse, psychomotor and memory impairment, inter-dose rebound anxiety (for shorter-acting agents)
Clonazepam (Klonopin)	0.25 at bedtime	1–5	
Lorazepam (Ativan)	0.5 TID	3–12	
Oxazepam (Serax)	15	30–60	

QID, Four times a day; TID, three times a day.

the morning (although for some individuals, paroxetine and other agents may be sedating and be better tolerated with bedtime dosing); sleep disruption due to these agents can usually be managed by the addition of a hypnotic agent. The typical 2- to 3-week lag in therapeutic efficacy for SSRIs/SNRIs can be problematic for those who are acutely distressed, with some data suggesting that it may take up to 22 weeks for patients to respond.[2] There is also a US Food and Drug Administration (FDA) class warning for the risk of thoughts of suicide and suicide attempts that is based on short-term studies that suggest the need for close monitoring of individuals 24 years or younger, with their use balancing the risk of these adverse effects and clinical need. In addition, data on the dose-dependent QTc prolongation with citalopram in those aged 60 and above have led to recommendations to limit the dose to 20 mg/day and to monitor the electrocardiogram in some populations.

There is no clear evidence of a differential efficacy between the SSRIs and SNRIs to guide selection. On the other hand, differences in their side-effect profiles (e.g., the potential for weight gain and discontinuation-related symptomatology), differences in their drug interactions, and the availability of generic formulations may be clinically relevant.[3–5]

First-Line Therapy for Anxiety Disorders: Cognitive-Behavioral Therapy

Cognitive-behavioral formulations of anxiety disorders focus on the information processing and

TABLE 12.3
Antiepileptic Drugs, Antipsychotics, Beta-Blockers, and Other Agents

Agent	Initial Dose (mg/d)	Typical Dose Range (mg/d)	Limitations/Primary Side Effects
Anticonvulsants			
Gabapentin (Neurontin)	300	600–6000	Light-headedness, sedation
Pregabalin (Lyrica)	200	300–600	Light-headedness, sedation
Lamotrigine (Lamictal)	25	50–500	GI distress, rash (rare Stevens-Johnson)
Valproic acid (Valproate)	250	500–2000	GI distress, sedation, weight gain (rare polycystic ovary disease, hepatotoxicity, pancreatitis)
Antipsychotics			
Aripiprazole (Abilify)	15	15–45	Extrapyramidal symptoms, metabolic syndrome, weight gain, sedation, akathisia, prolonged QTc, blood pressure changes, neuroleptic malignant syndrome
Olanzapine (Zyprexa)	2.5	5–15	
Quetiapine (Seroquel)	25	50–500	
Risperidone (Risperdal)	0.25	0.5–3	
Trifluoroperazine (Stelazine)	2.5	2.5–40	
Ziprasidone (Geodon)	20	40–160	
Beta-blockers			
Atenolol (Tenormin)	25	50–100	Bradycardia, depression, hypotension, light-headedness, sedation; monotherapy efficacy limited to performance anxiety
Propranolol (Inderal)	10–20	10–160	
Other Agents			
Buspirone (BuSpar)	5 TID	15–60	Dysphoria; limited efficacy

GI, Gastrointestinal; *TID*, three times daily.

behavioral reactions believed to be responsible for the maintenance of fear while acknowledging the importance of biologically based sensitivities. In brief, cognitive-behavioral therapy (CBT) is an effective, gold-standard treatment for anxiety disorders. CBT uses specific techniques to target unhelpful thoughts, feelings, and behaviors shown to generate and maintain anxiety. CBT can be used as a stand-alone treatment or combined with anti-anxiety medications (e.g., SSRIs). There is a robust research literature examining the efficacy of CBT for anxiety disorders, and the beneficial effects are considered well established with meta-analyses of randomized controlled trials (RCTs) of CBT for anxiety suggesting that CBT is more efficacious than no treatment and more efficacious than pill or psychotherapy placebos.[6] Out of the many disorder-specific CBT protocols that have been studied across diagnostic categories, anxiety disorder protocols produce some of the strongest results.

PHARMACOTHERAPY OF PANIC DISORDER AND AGORAPHOBIA

The pharmacotherapy of panic disorder targets the prevention of panic attacks, diminishing anticipatory and generalized anxiety, reversing phobic avoidance, improving overall function and quality of life, and treating co-morbid conditions (such as depression). As for all anxiety disorders, the goal of pharmacotherapy is to reduce both the patient's distress and impairment to the point of remission and/or to facilitate their participation, if necessary, in other forms of treatment (such as CBT).

Currently, paroxetine, both the immediate (Paxil) and controlled-release formulations (Paxil-CR), sertraline (Zoloft), fluoxetine (Prozac), and extended-release venlafaxine (Effexor-XR) are FDA approved for the treatment of a panic disorder, although other SSRIs including citalopram (Celexa), escitalopram (Lexapro), and fluvoxamine (Luvox) have also demonstrated anti-panic efficacy.

Should patients fail to respond to several trials of SSRIs and SNRIs, other pharmacological compounds may be considered, including benzodiazepines and TCAs.

Benzodiazepines

Despite guidelines[7] for the use of antidepressants as first-line anti-panic agents, benzodiazepines are still commonly prescribed for the treatment of panic disorder.[8,9] Several high-potency benzodiazepines, including alprazolam (immediate and extended-release forms) and clonazepam, are FDA approved for panic disorder; however, other benzodiazepines of varying potency, such as diazepam and lorazepam,[10] at roughly equipotent doses have demonstrated anti-panic efficacy in RCTs. Benzodiazepines remain widely used for panic (and other anxiety disorders), likely due to their efficacy, tolerability, rapid onset of action, and ability to be used on an "as-needed" basis for situational anxiety. It should be noted, however, that "as-needed" dosing for the monotherapy of panic disorder is rarely appropriate, as this strategy generally exposes patients to the risks associated with benzodiazepine use without the benefit of adequate and sustained dosing to achieve and maintain comprehensive efficacy. Further, "as-needed" dosing engenders dependency on the medication as a safety cue and interferes with exposure to, and mastery of, avoided situations, especially during CBT.

Side effects of benzodiazepines include sedation, ataxia, and memory impairment (which can be particularly problematic in the elderly and in those with prior cognitive impairment).[11] Despite concerns that ongoing benzodiazepine administration results in the development of therapeutic tolerance (i.e., loss of therapeutic efficacy or dose escalation), studies of their long-term use have suggested that benzodiazepines remain effective for panic disorder[12,13] and do not lead to significant dose escalation.[13] However, even after a relatively brief period (i.e., weeks) of regular dosing, rapid discontinuation of benzodiazepines may result in withdrawal symptoms (including increased anxiety and agitation). Discontinuation of longer-acting agents (such as clonazepam) may lead to fewer and less intense withdrawal symptoms with an abrupt taper. Patients who are sensitive to somatic sensations may find withdrawal-related symptoms particularly distressing, and a slow taper as well as the addition of

CBT[14] during discontinuation may help to reduce the distress associated with benzodiazepine discontinuation. A gradual taper is recommended for all patients treated with daily benzodiazepines for more than several weeks to reduce the likelihood of withdrawal symptoms (and, rarely, seizures). Although individuals predisposed to substance use disorders (SUDs) are at risk for benzodiazepine abuse, those without this diathesis do not appear to share this risk.[15] However, benzodiazepines and alcohol may act synergistically in combination, and the use of benzodiazepines in those with a current alcohol use disorder (AUD) can be problematic (thus further supporting the use of antidepressants as first-line anti-panic agents in those with an SUD).

Although co-administration of a benzodiazepine improves the rapidity of response when co-initiated with antidepressants, ongoing use may not be necessary after the initial weeks of antidepressant pharmacotherapy.

Tricyclic Antidepressants

Imipramine (Tofranil) was the first pharmacological agent shown to be efficacious for panic disorder, and TCAs were typically the first-line, gold-standard pharmacological agents for panic disorder until they were supplanted by the SSRIs, SNRIs, and benzodiazepines. Clomipramine may have superior anti-panic properties when compared to other TCAs, possibly related to its greater potency for serotonergic uptake. The efficacy of the TCAs is comparable to that of the newer agents for panic disorder, but they are now used less frequently due to their greater side-effect burden, including associated anticholinergic effects, orthostasis, weight gain, cardiac conduction delays, and greater lethality in overdose. The side-effect profile of the TCAs has also been associated with a high drop-out rate (30%–70%).

Like the recommendations for the use of the SSRIs/SNRIs, treatment with the TCAs should be started at lower doses (e.g., 10 mg/day for imipramine) to minimize the "activation syndrome" (involving restlessness, jitteriness, palpitations, and increased anxiety) that is seen at the onset of treatment (see Table 12.2). Typical antidepressant doses (e.g., 100–300 mg/day for imipramine) may ultimately be used to control symptoms of panic. In cases with a poor response to, or an intolerability to treatment with, standard doses, use of TCA plasma levels, especially for imipramine, nortriptyline (Pamelor), and desipramine (Norpramin), may be informative.

Monoamine Oxidase Inhibitors

Despite their reputation for being efficacious, monoamine oxidase inhibitors (MAOIs) have not been systematically studied in panic disorder as defined by current nomenclature. Reversible inhibitors of monoamine oxidase$_A$ (RIMAs) typically have a more benign side-effect profile and a lower risk of hypertensive reactions than irreversible MAOIs (such as phenelzine).

PHARMACOTHERAPY OF GENERALIZED ANXIETY DISORDER

The pharmacotherapy of GAD is aimed at reducing or eliminating excessive and uncontrollable worry, somatic and cognitive symptoms associated with motor tension and autonomic arousal (e.g., muscle tension, restlessness, difficulty concentrating, disturbed sleep, fatigue, and irritability), and common co-morbidities (including depression) that comprise the syndrome. The anxiety associated with GAD is typically persistent and pervasive, rather than episodic and situational. GAD severity, however, may worsen in response to situational stressors. Thus while the pharmacotherapy of GAD is generally chronic, adjustments may be required in response to worsening during protracted stress.

Like other anxiety disorders, SSRIs and SNRIs are generally considered first-line agents for the treatment of GAD because of their favorable side-effect profile compared to older antidepressants (e.g., TCAs), minimal risk of abuse or dependency compared to benzodiazepines, and a broad spectrum of efficacy for common co-morbidities, such as depression. Currently, the SSRIs, paroxetine and escitalopram, and the SNRIs (including the extended-release formulation of venlafaxine [Effexor-XR] and duloxetine [Cymbalta]) have received FDA approval for GAD; however, all agents in these classes, including sertraline, are likely to be effective for GAD, but with some differences in their side-effect profiles.[16] Long-term trials with SSRIs and SNRIs have demonstrated that treatment for 6 months or longer is associated with significantly lower rates of relapse relative to those who discontinued the drug following acute treatment; further, ongoing treatment appears associated with ongoing gains in the quality of improvement as evidenced by a greater proportion of individuals reaching remission.[17,18]

Benzodiazepines

Benzodiazepines have been widely used for the treatment of generalized anxiety for close to half a century. Although guidelines[19] have emphasized the use of antidepressants for anxiety states including GAD, particularly when co-morbid depression is present, benzodiazepines remain broadly prescribed, either as co-therapy or monotherapy for GAD, because of their ease of use, rapid and generally reliable anxiolytic effect, and relatively favorable side-effect profile.

Given their apparently equivalent efficacy, the selection of a benzodiazepine should be made by matching the pharmacokinetic properties of the agent with the situational parameters and the patient's clinical profile. Agents that are slowly metabolized and have multiple metabolites (such as diazepam and chlordiazepoxide) and those with long half-lives (such as clonazepam) may be easier to taper and are generally associated with fewer symptoms of inter-dose breakthrough compared to shorter-acting and more rapidly metabolized agents (such as oxazepam or lorazepam); the latter agents may be better suited for brief intermittent anxiolysis or for individuals likely to be slower metabolizers (e.g., the elderly or those with hepatic disease). The regular use of benzodiazepines for more than 2 or 3 weeks may be associated with physiological dependence and the potential for withdrawal symptoms with rapid discontinuation or a dramatic dose decrease. Discontinuation of benzodiazepines is best done with a gradual taper to minimize withdrawal symptoms. For some patients switching from a short-acting to a longer-acting agent (e.g., alprazolam to clonazepam) may facilitate discontinuation. The addition of CBT during the tapering process may also facilitate benzodiazepine discontinuation by giving the patient skills to manage recurrent anxiety and withdrawal and addressing concerns about their ability to function without benzodiazepines. Moreover, the abuse liability of benzodiazepines may be problematic in individuals predisposed to SUD, although it is less likely to be a concern for most individuals taking benzodiazepines. Pharmacodynamic interactions due to the co-administration of benzodiazepines and alcohol or other sedating agents may be problematic because of the additive potential for central nervous system (CNS) depression.

Buspirone

Buspirone is a $5-HT_{1A}$ partial agonist belonging to the azapirone class; it is FDA approved for use in generalized anxiety. Although it has demonstrated inconsistent efficacy in clinical practice, it may be useful as an adjunct to standard therapies for refractory anxiety disorders[20]; it may also have weak antidepressant effects when used at higher doses.[21] In general, buspirone has a favorable side-effect profile, although it has a gradual onset of effect; the average therapeutic dose is in the range of 30 to 60 mg/day that is typically administered with twice-a-day dosing.

Anticonvulsants

The alpha-$_2$ delta calcium channel antagonist, pregabalin, has demonstrated efficacy in large RCTs, including several that showed its efficacy for co-morbid depressive symptoms.[22-24] The typical therapeutic dose range for pregabalin is 300 to 600 mg/day, with the most common adverse events being somnolence and dizziness. Data suggest that while low doses of pregabalin are efficacious, there is additional benefit gained by increasing the dose to 450 mg/day, but that beyond 450 mg, reduction in anxiety symptoms does not continue to improve. Of note, pregabalin is approved in Europe for the treatment of GAD.

The selective gamma-aminobutyric acid (GABA) reuptake inhibitor, tiagabine, demonstrated efficacy for the treatment of GAD in one randomized, placebo-controlled trial at doses of 4 to 16 mg/day,[25] although a subsequent series of RCTs failed to confirm this initial observation and do not support the routine use of tiagabine as an anxiolytic.[26]

Tricyclic Antidepressants

Several studies have demonstrated the efficacy of the prototypical TCA, imipramine, for the treatment of GAD, with RCTs showing comparable efficacy but a slower rapidity of onset relative to a benzodiazepine comparator and a greater side-effect burden relative to an SSRI comparator.[26] Again, the unfavorable

side-effect profile and risk for cardiotoxicity account for its second-tier treatment status for GAD.

Antipsychotics

Conventional antipsychotics have long been used in clinical practice for the treatment of anxiety; in fact, based on a large RCT of trifluoperazine (2–6 mg/day),[27] the agent received an FDA indication for the short-term treatment of non-psychotic anxiety. However, concerns regarding the development of extrapyramidal symptoms and tardive dyskinesia (TD) limited the use of typical antipsychotics for the treatment of anxiety. Several second-generation antipsychotics (SGAs), including olanzapine,[28] risperidone,[29] aripiprazole, and ziprasidone,[30] have demonstrated efficacy in RCTs, as well as in case series and case reports for the treatment of GAD, although typically not used exclusively as augmentation in individuals who are refractory to standard interventions. In addition, several RCTs have provided strong support for the efficacy of quetiapine (50–300 mg) monotherapy in the treatment of GAD.[31-33] In addition, the efficacy of the SGAs as mood stabilizers for bipolar disorder,[34] their potential efficacy for use in refractory depression, and their lack of abuse potential suggest they may be useful for those with co-morbid anxiety, mood, and SUDs, particularly those refractory to more standard interventions. Decisions regarding the use of SGAs should consider their potential for serious adverse effects as well as sedation, weight gain, and metabolic syndrome.

Vilazodone and Vortioxetine

A meta-analysis of several RCTs found that vilazodone, a serotonergic antidepressant acting as a 5-HT reuptake inhibitor and a $5-HT_{1A}$ partial agonist, was efficacious (vs. placebo) though the effect size was smaller than SSRI/SNRI or pregabalin. Similarly, a meta-analysis of four RCTs found that vortioxetine, a 5-HT reuptake inhibitor, $5-HT_{3R}$ antagonist, and $5-HT_{1R}$ agonist, was efficacious (vs. placebo) though the effect size was small.

Riluzole

The efficacy of riluzole, an anti-glutamatergic agent, often used in the treatment of amyotrophic lateral sclerosis was examined in individuals with GAD, in an 8-week, open-label, fixed-dose study of 100 mg/day.[35]

Riluzole appeared to be effective and generally well tolerated; although its expense makes it unlikely that its use will be widely adopted, the report suggested that there might be a role for anti-glutamatergic agents in the treatment of anxiety.

PHARMACOTHERAPY OF SOCIAL ANXIETY DISORDER

The pharmacotherapy of SAD is aimed at reducing the patient's anticipatory anxiety prior to, and distress during, social interactions and performance situations, reducing avoidance of social and performance situations, and improving associated impairments in quality of life and function. Of note, individuals with SAD are at increased risk for AUD and SUDs, which may in some cases reflect an attempt to "self-medicate" their anxiety in social situations.

SSRIs and SNRIs have become first-line pharmacotherapy for the treatment of SAD because of their efficacy for this condition, broad-spectrum effects for other anxiety disorders, efficacy for co-morbid depression (in contrast to the benzodiazepines), better tolerability than the TCAs, a more favorable safety profile than the MAOIs, and lack of abuse potential. Currently the SSRIs paroxetine and sertraline, as well as the SNRI venlafaxine (extended release), are FDA approved for SAD, although available evidence suggests that other agents from these classes, including fluvoxamine,[36] citalopram,[37] and escitalopram,[38] are efficacious. Finally, some data suggest that the SNRI, duloxetine, is efficacious for SAD as well.[39] A meta-analysis of the efficacy of second-generation antidepressants in SAD[40] suggested that escitalopram, paroxetine, sertraline, and venlafaxine produced significantly more responders than placebo and that there were no differences in efficacy among them.

Treatment with SSRIs and SNRIs for SAD is typically started at low doses (e.g., paroxetine 10 mg/day, sertraline 25 mg/day, venlafaxine extended release 37.5 mg/day) and titrated against a therapeutic response and tolerability (e.g., paroxetine 20–60 mg/day, sertraline 50–200 mg/day, and venlafaxine 75–225 mg/day). There is usually a therapeutic lag in efficacy of 2 to 3 weeks following initiation of SSRI/SNRI therapy for SAD, although a full response can occur after weeks to months, particularly when social anxiety–related

avoidance develops, and a return to avoided situations should be encouraged alongside pharmacotherapy to both assess and optimize outcomes.

Beta-blockers

Beta-blockers, including propranolol (Inderal) and atenolol (Tenormin), are effective for the treatment of non-generalized social anxiety (i.e., "performance anxiety") about public speaking or other performance situations. Beta-blockers blunt the symptoms of physiological arousal associated with anxiety or fear, such as tachycardia and tremors, which are often the focus of an individual's apprehension in performance situations and lead to an escalating cycle of arousal, agitation, and further elevations in social anxiety. Beta-blockers are effective for performance anxiety, at least in part by blocking these physiological symptoms of arousal, interrupting the escalating fear cycle, and mitigating the individual's escalating concern and focus on their anxiety.

Although effective for physiological symptoms of arousal, beta-blockers are not as effective at reducing the emotional and cognitive aspects of social anxiety, and thus they are not first-line agents for SAD.

Beta-blockers (e.g., propranolol [10–80 mg/day] or atenolol [50–150 mg/day]) are typically administered "as needed" 1 to 2 hours before a performance situation. Beta-blockers have been associated with orthostatic hypotension, light-headedness, bradycardia, sedation, and nausea. Atenolol is less lipophilic[41] and thus less centrally active than propranolol, and, therefore, it may be less sedating. In practice, it is best to administer a "test dose" of the beta-blocker before its use in an actual performance-related event to establish the tolerability of an effective dose and to minimize disruptive side effects during a performance that could further increase anxiety.

Monoamine Oxidase Inhibitors

Before they were supplanted by the SSRIs and SNRIs, the MAOIs were the gold-standard pharmacological treatment for SAD. Interest in their use in SAD grew in part from initial observations of their efficacy for the atypical subtype of depression characterized in part by a marked sensitivity to rejection, and they subsequently demonstrated effectiveness in RCTs in SAD.[42]

Although clearly effective, MAOIs are associated with concerning side effects, including orthostatic hypotension, paresthesias, weight gain, and sexual dysfunction, as well as the need for careful attention to diet and use of concomitant medication because of the risk of potentially fatal hypertensive reactions and serotonin syndrome if the proscriptions are violated. Concerns about the use of MAOIs may have contributed in part to the under-recognition and treatment of SAD that existed until the efficacy of the generally safer and easier-to-use SSRIs and SNRIs was shown. Among the MAOIs, phenelzine has been the best studied for SAD, although tranylcypromine has also been effective.

Phenelzine is typically initiated at 15 mg PO BID and is less likely than reuptake inhibitors (such as TCAs, SSRIs, or SNRIs) to exacerbate anxiety during the initiation of treatment. The usual therapeutic dose range of phenelzine is 60 to 90 mg/day, with some refractory patients responding to higher doses. Careful attention to adherence to a diet free of tyramine-containing foods and avoidance of sympathomimetic and other serotonergic drugs is important to avoid hypertensive or serotonergic crises, and assessment of a patient's ability to maintain these restrictions is a critical component of the risk-benefit analysis of MAOI usage. Because of the need for careful dietary monitoring (including proscriptions against tyramine-containing foods and ingestion of sympathomimetic and other agents) to reduce the risks of hypertensive crises and serotonin syndrome, MAOIs are often used after a lack of response to safer and better-tolerated agents.

Interest in the reversible inhibitors of MAO$_A$ (RIMAs) was stimulated by the significant safety concerns attendant to the administration of irreversible MAOIs. Because they can be displaced from MAO when a substrate (such as tyramine) is presented, the RIMAs do not require strict dietary prohibitions (and the risk of hypertensive crisis and serotonin syndrome associated with the irreversible MAOIs). There are no systematic data available to date regarding the efficacy of the selegiline transdermal patch for the treatment of SAD (or any other anxiety disorder).

Benzodiazepines

Benzodiazepines are efficacious for SAD, with a response noted as early as 2 weeks in non-depressed individuals with SAD.[43]

Benzodiazepines have the advantage of a relatively rapid onset of action, a favorable side-effect profile, and efficacy on an as-needed basis for situational anxiety. The use of benzodiazepines, however, may be associated with adverse effects (including sedation, ataxia, and cognitive and psychomotor impairment), as well as the development of physiological dependence with regular use. Further, they are generally not effective for depression that is often co-morbid with SAD, and they may worsen it. Their potential for abuse in those with a diathesis or a history of an AUD or an SUD, and their potential negative interaction with concurrent alcohol use, is relevant given the increased rates of alcohol and substance use among those with social phobias. Benzodiazepines are started at low doses (e.g., clonazepam 0.25–0.5 mg qhs) to minimize adverse effects (such as sedation) and then titrated as tolerated to therapeutic doses (e.g., clonazepam 1–4 mg/day or its equivalent).

For maintenance treatment, to optimize a continuous anxiolytic effect, longer-acting benzodiazepines (such as clonazepam) are associated with less interdose rebound anxiety than shorter-acting agents and are generally preferred, whereas a shorter-acting agent with a more rapid onset of effect (such as alprazolam or lorazepam) may be more appropriate if used on an as-needed basis for performance situations. Monotherapy with as-needed dosing of benzodiazepines alone is not, however, recommended for non-"performance only" SAD, and as-needed benzodiazepine use may interfere with the reduction of social anxiety and related avoidance with cognitive-behavioral treatments.

CONCLUSIONS AND FUTURE DIRECTIONS

The increased recognition of the prevalence, early onset, chronicity, and morbid impact of anxiety disorders has spurred development efforts to find more effective and better-tolerated pharmacotherapies for this condition. Although SSRIs/SNRIs and benzodiazepines have demonstrated efficacy and favorable tolerability compared to older classes of agents, many patients remain symptomatic despite standard treatment; only a minority remit. In addition to creative uses of available agents alone and in combination, a variety of other pharmacological agents with novel mechanisms of action, including fatty acid amide hydrolase inhibitors, corticotropin-releasing factor antagonists, neurokinin-substance P antagonists, metabotropic glutamate receptor agonists, GABA-ergic agents, and receptor modulators, and compounds with a variety of effects on serotonin, noradrenergic, and dopaminergic receptors and their subtypes, are in various stages of development. In addition, specific agents targeting ways to enhance outcomes with CBT for anxiety disorders, such as the N-methyl-D-aspartate receptor antagonist D-cycloserine, remain an active area of translational research. These efforts may provide more effective and better-tolerated agents for the treatment of anxiety.

REFERENCES

1. Bandelow B, Reitt M, Rover C, et al. Efficacy of treatments for anxiety disorders: a meta-analysis. *Int Clinical Psychopharmacol.* 2015;30(4):183–192.
2. Pollack MH, Van Ameringen M, Simon NM, et al. A double-blind randomized controlled trial of augmentation and switch strategies for refractory social anxiety disorder. *Am J Psychiatry.* 2014;171(1):44–53.
3. Andrisano C, Chiesa A, Serretti A. Newer antidepressants and panic disorder: a meta-analysis. *Int Clin Psychopharmacol.* 2013;28(1):33–45.
4. Fava M, Judge R, Hoog SL, et al. Fluoxetine versus sertraline and paroxetine in major depressive disorder: changes in weight with long-term treatment. *J Clin Psychiatry.* 2000;61(11):863–867.
5. Fava M. Prospective studies of adverse events related to antidepressant discontinuation. *J Clin Psychiatry.* 2006;67(Suppl. 4): 14–21.
6. Carpenter JK, Andrews LA, Witcraft SM, et al. Cognitive behavioral therapy for anxiety and related disorders: a meta-analysis of randomized placebo-controlled trials. *Depress Anxiety.* 2018;35(6):502–514.
7. Work Group on Panic Disorder. American Psychiatric Association Practice guideline for the treatment of patients with panic disorder. *Am J Psychiatry.* 1998;155(5 suppl):1–34.
8. Bruce SE, Vasile RG, Goisman RM, et al. Are benzodiazepines still the medication of choice for patients with panic disorder with or without agoraphobia? *Am J Psychiatry.* 2003;160(8):1432–1438.
9. Noyes R Jr, Burrows GD, Reich JH, et al. Diazepam versus alprazolam for the treatment of panic disorder. *J Clin Psychiatry.* 1996;57(8):349–355.
10. Schweizer E, Pohl R, Balon R, et al. Lorazepam vs. alprazolam in the treatment of panic disorder. *Pharmacopsychiatry.* 1990;23(2):90–93.
11. Stewart SA. The effects of benzodiazepines on cognition. *J Clin Psychiatry.* 2005;66(suppl. 2):9–13.
12. Pollack MH, Otto MW, Tesar GE, et al. Long-term outcome after acute treatment with alprazolam or clonazepam for panic disorder. *J Clin Psychopharmacol.* 1993;13(4):257–263.
13. Soumerai SB, Simoni-Wastila L, Singer C, et al. Lack of relationship between long-term use of benzodiazepines and escalation to high dosages. *Psychiatr Serv.* 2003;54(7): 1006–1011.
14. Otto MW, Pollack MH, Sachs GS, et al. Discontinuation of benzodiazepine treatment: efficacy of cognitive-behavioral therapy for patients with panic disorder. *Am J Psychiatry.* 1993;150(10):1485–1490.
15. Kan CC, Hilberink SR, Breteler MH. Determination of the main risk factors for benzodiazepine dependence using a multivariate and multidimensional approach. *Compr Psychiatry.* 2004;45(2):88–94.
16. Bielski RJ, Bose A, Chang CC. A double-blind comparison of escitalopram and paroxetine in the long-term treatment of generalized anxiety disorder. *Ann Clin Psychiatry.* 2005;17(2): 65–69.
17. Montgomery SA, Sheehan DV, Meoni P, et al. Characterization of the longitudinal course of improvement in generalized anxiety disorder during long-term treatment with venlafaxine XR. *J Psychiatr Res.* 2002;36(4):209–217.
18. Stocchi F, Nordera G, Jokinen RH, et al. Efficacy and tolerability of paroxetine for the long-term treatment of generalized anxiety disorder. *J Clin Psychiatry.* 2003;64(3):250–258.
19. Allgulander C, Bandelow B, Hollander E, et al. WCA recommendations for the long-term treatment of generalized anxiety disorder. *CNS Spectr.* 2003;8(8 suppl 1):53–61.
20. Appelberg BG, Syvalahti EK, Koskinen TE, et al. Patients with severe depression may benefit from buspirone augmentation of selective serotonin reuptake inhibitors: results from a placebo-controlled, randomized, double-blind, placebo wash-in study. *J Clin Psychiatry.* 2001;62(6):448–452.
21. Chessick CA, Allen MH, Thase M, et al. Azapirones for generalized anxiety disorder. *Cochrane Database Syst Rev.* 2006(3):CD006115.
22. Boschen MJ. A meta-analysis of the efficacy of pregabalin in the treatment of generalized anxiety disorder. *Can J Psychiatry.* 2011;56(9):558–566.
23. Stein DJ, Baldwin DS, Baldinetti F, et al. Efficacy of pregabalin in depressive symptoms associated with generalized anxiety disorder: a pooled analysis of 6 studies. *Eur Neuropsychopharmacol.* 2008;18(6):422–430.
24. Kasper S, Herman B, Nivoli G, et al. Efficacy of pregabalin and venlafaxine-XR in generalized anxiety disorder: results of a double-blind, placebo-controlled 8-week trial. *Int Clin Psychopharmacol.* 2009;24(2):87–96.
25. Pollack MH, Roy-Byrne PP, Van Ameringen M, et al. The selective GABA reuptake inhibitor tiagabine for the treatment of generalized anxiety disorder: results of a placebo-controlled study. *J Clin Psychiatry.* 2005;66(11):1401–1408.
26. Pollack MH, Tiller J, Xie F, et al. Tiagabine in adult patients with generalized anxiety disorder: results from 3 randomized, double-blind, placebo-controlled, parallel-group studies. *J Clin Psychopharmacol.* 2008;28(3):308–316.

27. Mendels J, Krajewski TF, Huffer V, et al. Effective short-term treatment of generalized anxiety disorder with trifluoperazine. *J Clin Psychiatry*. 1986;47(4):170–174.

28. Pollack MH, Simon NM, Zalta AK, et al. Olanzapine augmentation of fluoxetine for refractory generalized anxiety disorder: a placebo-controlled study. *Biol Psychiatry*. 2006;59(3):211–215.

29. Brawman-Mintzer O, Knapp RG, Nietert PJ. Adjunctive risperidone in generalized anxiety disorder: a double-blind, placebo-controlled study. *J Clin Psychiatry*. 2005;66(10):1321–1325.

30. Snyderman SH, Rynn MA, Rickels K. Open-label pilot study of ziprasidone for refractory generalized anxiety disorder. *J Clin Psychopharmacol*. 2005;25(5):497–499.

31. Bandelow B, Chouinard G, Bobes J, et al. Extended-release quetiapine fumarate (quetiapine XR): a once-daily monotherapy effective in generalized anxiety disorder. Data from a randomized, double-blind, placebo- and active-controlled study. *Int J Neuropsychopharmacol*. 2010;13(3):305–320.

32. Katzman MA, Brawman-Mintzer O, Reyes EB, et al. Extended release quetiapine fumarate (quetiapine XR) monotherapy as maintenance treatment for generalized anxiety disorder: a long-term, randomized, placebo-controlled trial. *Int Clin Psychopharmacol*. 2011;26(1):11–24.

33. Khan A, Joyce M, Atkinson S, et al. A randomized, double-blind study of once-daily extended release quetiapine fumarate (quetiapine XR) monotherapy in patients with generalized anxiety disorder. *J Clin Psychopharmacol*. 2011;31(4):418–428.

34. Ketter TA, Nasrallah HA, Fagiolini A. Mood stabilizers and atypical antipsychotics: bimodal treatments for bipolar disorder. *Psychopharmacol Bull*. 2006;39(1):120–146.

35. Mathew SJ, Amiel JM, Coplan JD, et al. Open-label trial of riluzole in generalized anxiety disorder. *Am J Psychiatry*. 2005;162(12):2379–2381.

36. Asakura S, Tajima O, Koyama T. Fluvoxamine treatment of generalized social anxiety disorder in Japan: a randomized double-blind, placebo-controlled study. *Int J Neuropsychopharmacol*. 2007;10(2):263–274.

37. Furmark T, Appel L, Michelgard A, et al. Cerebral blood flow changes after treatment of social phobia with the neurokinin-1 antagonist GR205171, citalopram, or placebo. *Biol Psychiatry*. 2005;58(2):132–142.

38. Kasper S, Stein DJ, Loft H, et al. Escitalopram in the treatment of social anxiety disorder: randomised, placebo-controlled, flexible-dosage study. *Br J Psychiatry*. 2005;186:222–226.

39. Simon NM, Worthington JJ, Moshier SJ, et al. Duloxetine for the treatment of generalized social anxiety disorder: a preliminary randomized trial of increased dose to optimize response. *CNS Spectr*. 2010;15(7):367–373.

40. Hansen RA, Gaynes BN, Gartlehner G, et al. Efficacy and tolerability of second-generation antidepressants in social anxiety disorder. *Int Clin Psychopharmacol*. 2008;23(3):170–179.

41. Conant J, Engler R, Janowsky D, et al. Central nervous system side effects of beta-adrenergic blocking agents with high and low lipid solubility. *J Cardiovasc Pharmacol*. 1989;13(4):656–661.

42. Liebowitz MR, Gorman JM, Fyer AJ, et al. Social phobia. Review of a neglected anxiety disorder. *Arch Gen Psychiatry*. 1985;42(7):729–736.

43. Davidson JR, Potts N, Richichi E, et al. Treatment of social phobia with clonazepam and placebo. *J Clin Psychopharmacol*. 1993;13(6):423–428.

SUBSTANCE USE DISORDERS

MLADEN NISAVIC, MD ■ ASHIKA BAINS, MD

OVERVIEW

Substance use disorders (SUDs) present one of the gravest difficulties facing the United States healthcare system. Since the 1990s, the number of patients treated for substance use-related problems in the United States has grown steadily, reaching epidemic proportions in the last decade alone. In 2020 the National Survey on Drug Use and Health found that 162.5 million Americans aged 12 or older (which accounts for 58.7% of the population) used tobacco, alcohol, or an illicit drug in the past month. This number included 138.5 million individuals (50% of the population) who drank alcohol and 37.3 million (13.5%) who used illicit drugs.[1] Of the 138.5 million active alcohol users, 61.6 million engaged in binge drinking and 17.7 million were heavy drinkers. Cannabis was the most commonly used illicit substance (with 49.6 million people reporting use in the past year). Past-year stimulant use was endorsed by 10.3 million individuals; roughly one-third of this cohort used only cocaine, another third reported misusing prescription stimulant medications, and roughly one-sixth (15%) endorsed using methamphetamine. Opioid (e.g., heroin, prescription pain medications) use was reported by 3.4% (9.5 million people), with most admitting to prescription pain reliever misuse (9.3 million people).[1]

The increase in drug use has also led to an increased utilization of healthcare services. The Drug Abuse Warning Network (DAWN) and the Substance Abuse and Mental Health Service Administration have estimated that the top five drugs involved in drug-related emergency department (ED) visits in 2021 were alcohol (41.7%), opioids (14.8%), methamphetamine (11.3%), marijuana (11.12%), and cocaine (4.8%).[2] Fentanyl-related ED visits rose throughout 2021, peaking in the fourth quarter, which reflected the increasing availability of fentanyl in the communities at risk.

Disruption of the brain's endogenous reward systems is a common feature of SUDs; in fact, most addictive drugs act as functional dopamine analogs in the nucleus accumbens/ventral tegmental area reward circuit. Whether through the direct effect of the drug (e.g., cocaine, amphetamines), or indirectly (e.g., opioids, alcohol), a common sequela of acute intoxication is an increase in synaptic availability of dopamine within circuits that mediate motivation and drive, conditioned learning, and inhibitory controls. With chronic drug use, long-lasting compensatory changes (e.g., reduced dopamine availability and receptor density) in the reward circuits, the orbitofrontal cortex (salience attribution), the cingulate gyrus (inhibitory control and mood regulation), the amygdala (fear processing), and the hippocampus (memory) occur. As a result, with chronic use, addiction becomes less about "seeking a high" and more about attempting to retrieve a state of relative normalcy. Compensatory changes related to chronic drug use are related to the emergence of drug tolerance and often physiologically unpleasant reactions on drug discontinuation (related to dependence and withdrawal). Furthermore, chronic changes to dopamine reward circuits may result in a diminished response to other rewarding cues (e.g., food, sex, physical exercise) while changes to the prefrontal circuits may adversely impact a patient's ability to prioritize rational and safe behaviors. Context-based priming of the hippocampus and the amygdala may contribute to the emergence of cravings once the individual is exposed to heightened emotional states, locations, or sensory cues previously associated with drug use.

The chronic relapsing nature of substance use is erroneously thought to imply that treatment for these disorders is futile or even unhelpful and commonly results in clinicians overlooking opportunities to intervene in the disease process. Most clinicians fail to appreciate that the relapse rate of other common chronic medical disorders (e.g., diabetes, hypertension, asthma) exceeds that for SUDs, and that when compared to other chronic conditions, response rates with treatment are comparable to, if not superior to, those of chronic medical conditions.[3] Notably, medical and surgical hospitalizations often provide patients with an extended period of separation from chronic patterns of substance use, and thus present an invaluable opportunity to engage the patient in conversation, and eventually treatment, of their SUDs. Taken together, clinicians should approach patients with SUDs with comparable therapeutic diligence as is offered for those with chronic medical disorders.

Furthermore, substance use is highly co-morbid with other psychiatric conditions, with nearly half of patients with SUDs having at least one co-occurring psychiatric disorder.[1] Accordingly, it is essential for psychiatrists to be knowledgeable about safe and evidence-driven treatment strategies for SUDs. Successful treatment of this expanding group of patients requires that clinicians improve their management of SUDs and their sequelae. This involves providing a timely and accurate diagnosis of the substance use problem, recognizing key symptoms associated with intoxication or acute discontinuation/withdrawal, and initiating evidence-backed SUD treatment. The latter involves a myriad of clinical tools (including the use of motivational enhancement techniques to assess readiness for recovery, identification of outpatient addiction resources, and use of medications to reduce cravings and maintain recovery).

Alcohol Use Disorder

Alcohol remains one of the most prevalent and clinically relevant substances, with an estimated 75 million people worldwide meeting the criteria for an alcohol use disorder (AUD).[4] In the United States, nearly two-thirds of all adults consume alcoholic beverages, while an estimated 8 million Americans meet the criteria for a severe AUD. Furthermore, approximately 500,000 individuals each year experience acute alcohol withdrawal severe enough to require pharmacologic management.[5] The annual healthcare costs related to alcohol use have been estimated to exceed US$250 billion, while the estimated alcohol-associated annual mortality rate is 85,000 to 100,000 individuals in the United States alone.[6,7] In fact, alcohol accounts for roughly one-tenth of all deaths among working-age US adults.[8] Given the prevalence of problematic drinking and AUD, it is no surprise that alcohol is responsible for more neuropsychiatric problems in general hospitals than for all other substances combined. Studies estimate that 25% to 50% of all individuals hospitalized for injuries were intoxicated at the time of their trauma and that the prevalence of alcohol-related problems in medical inpatients ranges from 12.5% to 30%.[8,9] Furthermore, alcohol use is an important risk factor for the development of cancers of the esophagus and liver, heart disease, cirrhosis, and end-stage liver disease. Alcohol is also strongly associated with violent behavior/aggression, homicide, falls/trauma, and motor vehicle accidents.[10]

Given the prevalence of alcohol use in our society and the potential for significant medical, psychiatric, and psychosocial complications associated with chronic alcohol use and alcohol withdrawal, all psychiatrists who work in general hospitals should be skilled in the recognition and treatment of AUDs. Prompt identification of patients with AUD and initiation of acute inpatient treatment have been associated with improved clinical outcomes.[11–13]

Screening for Alcohol Use Disorder

Alcohol use is widespread; roughly 50% of the adult US population reports using alcohol within the past 30 days, although there is considerable variation in the pattern and severity of use. The National Institute on Alcohol Abuse and Alcoholism defines two categories of problematic drinking:

- Use of >14 drinks per week or >4 drinks on any day for males under the age of 65 years
- Use of >7 drinks per week or >3 drinks on any day for females and/or any adult 65 years and older.[14]

TABLE 13.1
AUDIT-C Questionnaire for Alcohol Problems Screening

1. How often did you have a drink containing alcohol in the past year?
   - Never (0 points)
   - Monthly or less (1 point)
   - 2–4 times per month (2 points)
   - 2–3 times per week (3 points)
   - 4 times per week (4 points)
2. In the past year, how many drinks did you have on a typical day when you were drinking?
   - 1–2 (0 points)
   - 3–4 (1 point)
   - 5–6 (2 points)
   - 7–9 (3 points)
   - 10 (4 points)
3. How often did you have six or more drinks on one occasion in the past year?
   - Never (0 points)
   - Less than monthly (1 point)
   - Monthly (2 points)
   - Weekly (3 points)
   - More than once a week, or daily (4 points)

TABLE 13.2
CAGE Questionnaire for Alcohol Problems Screening

C Have you felt the need to **C**ut down on your drinking?
A Have people **A**nnoyed you by criticizing your drinking?
G Have you ever felt bad or **G**uilty about your drinking?
E Have you had a drink first thing in the morning to steady your nerves or to get rid of a hangover (i.e., an "**E**ye opener")?

Nearly one-third (30%) of all US adults who use alcohol do so in a potentially unhealthy manner, including 15% who exceed the recommended daily limit, 10% who exceed both daily and weekly limits, and 2% who exceed the weekly limit alone.[14] The highest rates of risky alcohol use occur in younger adults (18–29 years old), males, and Native Americans.[15]

Many tools are available to providers to help identify risky alcohol use. These include a variety of questionnaires that can be administered to inpatients or outpatients. Laboratory testing can be useful (especially if there is a concern for minimization of reported use), although such tests are not routinely recommended for screening purposes. The most commonly encountered screening tools include the Alcohol Use Disorders Identification Test-Concise (AUDIT-C) screening test (Table 13.1) and the CAGE questionnaire (Table 13.2). The AUDIT-C asks three questions and is considered positive when scores are >4 in males or >3 in females with a 90% sensitivity and an 80% specificity rate. The CAGE asks four questions and >2 positive responses

convey a sensitivity of 77% and a specificity of 79% for the detection of an AUD.[16] If the CAGE is used for screening, even a single response should be considered as screening positive.

Acute Intoxication and the Psychiatric Sequelae of Alcohol Use

Ethanol, the primary active component of alcoholic beverages, is a water-soluble alcohol compound primarily absorbed via the gastrointestinal (GI) mucosa of the small intestine (80%) and the stomach (20%).[17] The compound undergoes hepatic metabolism via alcohol dehydrogenase. In fact, a smaller distribution volume and reduced expression of this enzyme in females are believed to account for their increased susceptibility to alcohol intoxication. In most individuals, peak serum alcohol levels are reached 30 to 90 minutes following alcohol ingestion. Resolution of the acute toxidrome follows steady-state kinetics so that a 70-kg male is expected to metabolize approximately 10 mL of absolute ethanol or 1.5 to 2 drink equivalents (1.5 oz whiskey = 5 oz wine = 12 oz beer) per hour.[18]

The effect of alcohol on the central nervous system (CNS) is complex and involves changes across multiple neurotransmitter systems. The primary mechanism of action is achieved through gamma aminobutyric acid (GABA) agonism, which accounts for the CNS depressant effects of alcohol as well as for the behavioral disinhibition seen with the use of the compound. With chronic exposure, further CNS changes occur, primarily in response to exogenously increased GABA tone, including a decrease in GABA receptors, decreased GABA production, and decreased binding affinity to the receptor complex.[19] More importantly, these changes also lead to an increase in endogenous glutaminergic tone (an attempt to maintain homeostasis) and the development of complicated alcohol withdrawal symptoms.[20–22]

Signs and symptoms associated with acute alcohol intoxication are undoubtedly familiar to virtually all clinicians (see Table 13.3). Mild intoxication can present with impulsivity, elation, slight slurring of speech, and gait impairment. As the blood alcohol content increases, these findings become more pronounced and include marked disinhibition, irritation, or even frankly aggressive behavior. The neurologic examination is notable for nystagmus, impaired coordination (ataxia), and an unsteady gait. Attention and memory consolidation are commonly impaired, resulting in reduced recall of the intoxication, or even full "blackouts" in more severe cases. With severe alcohol poisoning, CNS depression becomes prominent, leading to stupor and coma.

The clinical effect is dose dependent, although much variability exists based on the patient's gender, genetics, amount/rate of intake, co-ingestion of other drugs, and overall duration of alcohol use. While the blood alcohol level (BAL) can reliably predict clinical effects in patients who only use alcohol socially, habituation and tolerance are common with chronic use and, in these individuals, little clinical evidence of intoxication may be seen despite an extremely elevated BAL.[23] In patients who use alcohol intermittently, a BAL <100 mg/dL will produce euphoria, problems with coordination, and impaired attention. Higher levels (e.g., a BAL of 100–200 mg/dL) are associated with a worsening of motor deficits, impaired judgment, and an increased chance of assaultive/aggressive behavior.

As the BAL exceeds 300 mg/dL, encephalopathy and CNS depression become prominent, and coma (and even death) can occur at a BAL of 400 to 500 mg/dL.

The initial work-up for acute alcohol intoxication should involve checking basic chemistry studies (as electrolyte imbalance is common), a serum glucose level, hepatic function, and a BAL. If co-ingestion is suspected, screening for other drugs is recommended, although it may not always be necessary with isolated alcohol intoxication. Treatment depends largely on the degree of intoxication observed:

- Mild-to-moderate intoxication can be managed supportively, and patients may require little more than observation and serial assessments. Intravenous (IV) fluids may be warranted if there is evidence of volume depletion (e.g., persistent tachycardia). Agitation, if present, may respond to reduced stimulation/isolation, and in more severe cases, use of dopamine antagonists, such as IV haloperidol (e.g., 2–5 mg), as it does not exacerbate sedation and can be administered easily. In patients with a preference for the non-parenteral route, various atypical agents (e.g., olanzapine, quetiapine) should be considered. Benzodiazepines are also commonly used in this setting, although using them as sole agents for the management of agitation may exacerbate acute intoxication and therefore result in worsening agitation, over-sedation, and respiratory depression. Once an individual is no longer intoxicated, they can usually be discharged home, although it is prudent to engage a patient in a conversation

TABLE 13.3
Alcohol Withdrawal Syndrome Symptom Clusters, Receptors, and Recommended Treatment Options

Symptom Clusters	Common Symptoms	Neurotransmitters Affected	Recommended Treatment
A	Anxiety, restlessness, general malaise, nausea/emesis; *fine* tremor	Decreased GABA activity	GABA agonists
B	*Coarse* tremor, hypertension, tachycardia, fever, diaphoresis	Increased glutamate and norepinephrine activity	Beta-blockers, alpha-agonists
C	Confusion, encephalopathy, hallucinations, paranoid ideation, agitation	Increased glutamate and dopamine activity	Dopamine antagonists

GABA, Gamma aminobutyric acid.

regarding the extent of use and discussion of potential aftercare resources.

- Severe intoxication may require intensive supportive measures, including frequent assessments of physiologic parameters. With severe obtundation, patients may not be able to protect their airway and may require intubation. Hemodynamic changes (including tachycardia and hypotension) may be seen, and patients may require IV hydration.

Alcohol Withdrawal Syndrome: Identification and Management

Symptoms of alcohol withdrawal are heterogeneous, ranging from mild discomfort to potentially life-threatening complications, including seizures, alcohol withdrawal delirium (AWD) (delirium tremens), and multi-organ failure requiring intensive care. Withdrawal also involves multiple neurotransmitter systems, including not only GABA and glutamate but also monoaminergic neurotransmitters (e.g., serotonin, dopamine, norepinephrine). Variability in withdrawal symptoms reflects a series of changes in CNS receptor expression and function associated with chronic alcohol use. As previously discussed, alcohol enhances GABA activity and inhibits glutamate activity, leading to a CNS depressant effect. In the setting of chronic alcohol use, the GABA system habituates, which leads to a decrease in the number of GABA receptors, changes in the configuration of the receptor subunits, and reduced rates of GABA synthesis. The result is decreased *endogenous* GABA tone. Similarly, chronic exposure to alcohol leads to changes in the glutamate neurotransmitter system, namely with an increase in the number of glutamate receptors. The overall effect is that of increased *endogenous* excitatory tone, representing an attempt to restore homeostasis and balance the increase in *exogenous* GABA tone caused by alcohol use. With abrupt cessation of alcohol use, this tenuous balance becomes disturbed quickly, and a state marked by over-expression of excitatory neurotransmitters (glutamate, norepinephrine, dopamine) and reduced GABA tone develops. The specific types of neurotransmitters affected, and the severity of the aberration seen determine the clinical symptoms and the severity of the alcohol withdrawal syndrome observed.[20-22]

Given the range of neurotransmitters involved, treatment of alcohol withdrawal should be tailored to the specific symptom cluster observed, including the use of GABAergic agents (e.g., benzodiazepines, barbiturates) for active withdrawal management, case-dependent use of beta-blockers or alpha-adrenergic agents to treat refractory tachycardia/hypertension, and use of dopamine antagonists for management of hallucinations, agitation, and paranoid delusions.

Types of Alcohol Withdrawal Syndromes

Clinical hallmarks of the four major alcohol withdrawal syndromes are outlined below:

Early/uncomplicated withdrawal syndrome generally reflects CNS hyperactivity in the setting of alcohol discontinuation and includes subjective sensations of anxiety and restlessness, insomnia, fine tremors, changes in appetite/GI upset, diaphoresis, and headaches. These symptoms generally develop within the first 6 to 12 hours after cessation of use and may even be observed in those with elevated BALs (a reflection of chronic use and habituation). Unless the patient progresses to a complicated withdrawal state, an early withdrawal syndrome is self-limited and will remit spontaneously within 24 to 48 hours. Most patients who experience alcohol withdrawal present with minor withdrawal symptoms and respond well to treatment with benzodiazepines.

Alcohol withdrawal seizures (AWS) occur within 12 to 48 hours after the last drink, although they have been described as occurring as early as 1 to 2 hours after the last use. Despite significant concerns in the hospital setting, AWS are uncommon events that are seen in only 1% of unmedicated patients who undergo alcohol withdrawal. Moreover, the risk for AWS is increased in patients with a pre-existing seizure disorder, prior head trauma, or a history of seizures related to alcohol discontinuation.[24] Classically, most AWS are singular, self-limited, tonic-clonic convulsions; reports of multiple, prolonged seizures and/or progression to status epilepticus should raise concerns for alternative etiologies and prompt further diagnostic assessment. Although most patients do not require head imaging, computed tomography and/or magnetic resonance imaging (MRI) scans can help exclude other causes of ictal activity and should be strongly considered in patients with acute head trauma, new focal neurologic findings, or an acutely altered sensorium not solely attributable to alcohol intoxication. Multiple prior detoxifications increase the risk of withdrawal seizures more than the quantity or duration of drinking; this implies a kindling phenomenon with chronic alcohol use, similar to that observed in patients with epilepsy. Most AWS are treated with benzodiazepines (e.g., IV/ oral lorazepam) or longer-acting barbiturates (e.g., phenobarbital). There are limited data to support the use of other anti-epileptic drugs (AEDs) over benzodiazepines, unless the patient has a co-morbid seizure disorder, in which case concurrent use of benzodiazepines (acutely) in conjunction with home AEDs is appropriate.

Alcoholic hallucinosis is a rare syndrome that reflects increased dopaminergic activity; it is commonly confounded by AWD. The onset of symptoms is typically within the first 12 to 24 hours after the last drink. Without treatment, most symptoms remit within 48 hours after the last drink (the earliest time point associated with AWD).[22] Those who experience alcoholic hallucinosis classically describe vivid visual hallucinations that may occur in the context of an otherwise clear sensorium. Olfactory and tactile hallucinations are also noted with alcoholic hallucinosis, along with paranoid delusions. Unlike AWD, patients with alcoholic hallucinosis do not exhibit significant attention deficits, tremors, or autonomic dysregulation (the combination of these symptoms essentially comprises the diagnosis of AWD). While alcoholic hallucinosis will invariably (and eventually) remit even without treatment, most patients will benefit from a brief course of dopamine antagonists. As with other types of acute psychosis, attention should be paid to patient safety and all patients with alcoholic hallucinosis should be assessed for self-harm and harm to others.

Alcohol withdrawal delirium (delirium tremens) is a clinical syndrome characterized by autonomic hyperactivity (e.g., tachycardia, hypertension, hyperthermia), confusion/disorientation, hallucinations, and not uncommonly agitation. Visual hallucinations, including those of animals (e.g., "white mice" and "pink elephants") are common, although hallucinations involving other sensory modalities have also been described. Delusional thinking and paranoia may exacerbate a patient's distress and lead to agitation or frank

aggression. Most patients will develop AWD within 48 to 72 hours of discontinuing alcohol, although a later onset has also been described. Untreated, the condition typically persists for 3 to 4 days, although it may persist longer; it is associated with a significant risk for morbidity and mortality. While only 5% of patients with AUD will develop AWD, the risk appears to be greater in the following populations:

- Patients with a history of AWD (strongest predictor)
- Patients with a history of chronic sustained daily drinking
- Older individuals (age >40)
- Patients with significant concurrent medical/ surgical illnesses, including long bone fractures, burns, and head trauma
- Patients who develop withdrawal symptoms in the context of an elevated BAL
- Patients admitted >2 days since their last drink.[25-27]

While AWD was associated with a 37% mortality rate at the beginning of the last century, more recently, improved survival rates are undoubtedly a reflection of improved diagnosis, and management, particularly with advances in critical care. Most AWD-associated morbidity and mortality occurs in the setting of cardiopulmonary failure (e.g., arrhythmias, ischemic events, aspiration), infectious concerns (e.g., aspiration pneumonia), metabolic derangements (e.g., acute hepatitis, pancreatitis, electrolyte abnormalities), and CNS injury (e.g., due to falls/head trauma).

Treatment of Alcohol Withdrawal

Treatment of AWS relies on the early recognition of patients at risk for developing the syndrome and on prompt withdrawal of treatment once initial symptoms have been observed. Although it can be challenging to predict which patients may develop AWS, a history of withdrawal or associated complications (e.g., seizures, AWD) is most strongly associated with the risk for recurrent AWS.

Given the heterogeneity of the syndrome, rigid adherence to a single protocol for all cases of alcohol withdrawal is unrealistic. This noted, most patients with AWS should respond well to a symptom-triggered benzodiazepine-based withdrawal protocol, in which benzodiazepine dosage/timing is individualized based on symptom severity/clinical need and only administered once the withdrawal symptoms have been observed. Assessment of the severity of withdrawal is best accomplished with the use of standardized scales, such as the Clinical Institute Withdrawal Assessment for Alcohol—Revised (CIWA-AR).[28] Although it is more involved than standard taper protocols, and may require education of clinical staff (physicians and nurses) before it is used, the benefits of symptom-triggered treatment are considerable, as it ensures that patients receive treatment only when they need it *and* receive as much as they need. This has significant clinical implications (e.g., reducing the overall use of benzodiazepines by a factor of four, shortening the length of treatment, and reducing symptom duration by a factor of six).[29-31] Chlordiazepoxide, diazepam, or lorazepam are the three most commonly used benzodiazepines for the management of alcohol withdrawal, with the first two often utilized in outpatient detoxification or psychiatric hospital settings, while lorazepam is a preferred agent in medical inpatients. Lorazepam, temazepam, and oxazepam each have low rates of hepatic metabolism and thus may be the preferred agents in those with significant liver disease. In patients unable/unwilling to take medications orally, lorazepam can be administered intravenously or intramuscularly (which adds to its versatility in hospital settings).

As previously reviewed, we typically recommend against using standing benzodiazepine tapers or continuous infusions, given a higher risk for complications and overall inferior treatment outcomes when compared to symptom-triggered treatment. This noted, in a small subset of patients, symptom-triggered treatment may prove challenging (e.g., medical confounders that resemble signs of withdrawal or deception by the patient)—in these cases, considering alternatives to benzodiazepines or a structured taper may prove beneficial.

Over the past decade, phenobarbital (a long-acting barbiturate) has increasingly been recognized as a viable and safe alternative to conventional benzodiazepine treatment. A prospective, randomized, double-blind, placebo-controlled study with 102 patients, half of whom received either a single dose of IV phenobarbital (10 mg/kg in 100 mL of normal saline) or placebo (100 mL of normal saline) in addition to a symptom-guided lorazepam-based alcoholwithdrawalprotocol, found that patients who received phenobarbital had fewer intensive care unit (ICU) admissions (8% vs. 25%), and there were no differences in adverse events.[32] Similarly, recent large retrospective work from our institution showed that a phenobarbital-driven protocol was comparable in efficacy and safety to conventional benzodiazepine treatment and was a potentially superior choice in patients with benzodiazepine tolerance and in surgical trauma patients where symptom-triggered treatment may be difficult to institute due to substrate limitations.[33,34]

Although AEDs have generally been shown to be inferior to benzodiazepines for AWS management, there is growing interest in benzodiazepine-sparing protocols, especially for cases of mild alcohol withdrawal.[35] Accordingly, there is some evidence that gabapentin co-administered with clonidine may prove effective in managing most symptoms of mild/moderate AWS.[36]

In addition to active pharmacologic management of alcohol withdrawal, supportive care is key to minimizing the risk of potential complications. In hospitalized patients, this includes consideration of fall and aspiration precautions, and frequent re-direction/orientation if the patient is delirious. As noted, benzodiazepines/barbiturates are essential in the treatment of alcohol withdrawal, yet these agents should not be used solely for agitation management as there is a risk of over-medicating the patient and through this potentiating acute intoxication, disinhibition, agitation, and impulsivity. Neuroleptics, including quetiapine/olanzapine, are commonly used in conjunction with GABAergic agents in hospital settings (when a patient can take medications orally) and haloperidol (when IV medications are required).

Historically, ethanol has been used to mitigate the risk of emergent AWS, especially in patients who report that they intend to resume drinking immediately on discharge.[37] Although the notion of administering "a drink with dinner" in the hospital may appear novel and exciting, several practical complications arise that make other agents preferred alternatives in nearly all cases: ethanol is difficult to titrate, it has many adverse metabolic effects, and it is unsafe in the general medical setting when considering active medical illness and the potential for drug-drug interactions.

Lastly, in the ICU, dexmedetomidine and propofol have each been used as viable alternatives to benzodiazepines/phenobarbital for the treatment of alcohol withdrawal.[38,39]

The risk of respiratory compromise and sedation with propofol, along with bradycardia and hypotension associated with dexmedetomidine, limits the use of these otherwise-helpful agents in the ICU setting.

In addition, to the medications described, all patients treated for alcohol withdrawal should receive thiamine given their increased risk for Wernicke encephalopathy and Korsakoff psychosis. Daily doses (200 mg) are recommended for the prevention of the syndrome and carry no safety risk to the patient, while higher doses are recommended if an actual thiamine deficiency is suspected.

Wernicke-Korsakoff Syndrome

Victor and associates in their classic monograph *The Wernicke-Korsakoff syndrome* stated that "Wernicke encephalopathy and Korsakoff syndrome in the alcoholic, nutritionally deprived patient may be regarded as two facets of the same disease."[40] Although uncommon (by some estimates <5% of patients with chronic alcohol use) the diagnosis is often missed and should be considered in all patients who present with heavy alcohol use, especially if they may have other reasons for malnutrition (e.g., homelessness, head/neck cancer, cognitive impairment).

Wernicke Encephalopathy

Wernicke encephalopathy arises acutely and is classically characterized by a triad of ophthalmoplegia, ataxia, and mental status disturbance, although less than 20% of cases display all three signs.[40] The ocular disturbance, which is necessary for the diagnosis, consists of paresis or paralysis of the lateral rectus muscles, nystagmus, and a disturbance in conjugate gaze. A global confusional state consists of disorientation, unresponsiveness, and derangement of perception and memory. Exhaustion, apathy, and profound lethargy are also part of the picture.

Once thiamine treatment has been initiated for Wernicke encephalopathy, improvement in the ocular findings is often evident within hours, while full recovery occurs after days or weeks. Classically, approximately one-third of patients recover from the state of global confusion within 6 days of treatment, another third recover within 1 month, and the remainder improve within 2 months. The global confusional state is almost always reversible, in marked contrast to the memory impairment of Korsakoff psychosis.

Korsakoff Psychosis

Korsakoff psychosis, also referred to as *confabulatory psychosis* and *alcohol-induced persisting amnestic disorder*, is characterized by impaired memory in an otherwise alert and responsive person. Hallucinations are rarely encountered. Curiously, confabulation, long regarded as the hallmark of Korsakoff psychosis, is not seen in most cases, and its absence should not preclude this diagnosis. The memory loss is generally bipartite. The retrograde component involves an inability to recall the past, and the anterograde component involves the lack of capacity for the retention of new information. In the acute stage of Korsakoff psychosis, the memory gap may be so blatant that the patient cannot recall simple items (such as the examiner's first name, the day, or the time) after a few minutes, even though the patient is provided with this information several times. As memory improves, usually within weeks to months, simple problems can be solved, limited always by the patient's span of recall.

The electroencephalogram may be unremarkable or might show diffuse slowing, while an MRI scan might demonstrate changes in the periaqueductal gray area, hippocampal formations, and the medial dorsal nucleus of the thalamus.[23]

Although often regarded as irreversible, a significant number of patients with Korsakoff psychosis show some improvement over time. Classically, one expects 20% of the patients to recover more or less completely; however, 25% showed no recovery, and the rest recovered partially.

Treatment

Administration of the B vitamin, thiamine, through an IV or intramuscular (IM) injection, should be considered a routine component of early treatment for all intoxicated patients, preferably while still in the ED or immediately on admission, whichever comes earlier.[41] Because subclinical cognitive impairment can occur even in apparently well-nourished patients, we recommend routine treatment with IV thiamine (as prophylaxis) for all intoxicated patients, as this prevents advancement of the disease and reverses at least a portion of the lesions that affect CNS territories.

For preventive measures, we often recommend using >100 mg of IV thiamine immediately, followed by 200 mg of thiamine (orally) while the patient remains in the hospital. If Wernicke/Korsakoff is suspected, treatment should consist of high-dose thiamine (500 mg IV three times per day for at least 3 days) followed by 500 mg IV/IM daily while symptoms persist. Because GI absorption of thiamine may be erratic, IV/IM formulations are much preferred to oral formulations. Lastly, thiamine should be administered before giving glucose, as the latter may precipitate or even exacerbate Wernicke encephalopathy.[41,42]

Pharmacotherapy for Alcohol Use Disorder

Most of the treatments for AUD revolve around modifying the reinforcing effects that the compound has on the cortico-mesolimbic dopamine reward pathways. Thus medications used for the treatment of AUD will work on a variety of receptor systems (e.g., endogenous opioids, GABA, glutamate, and serotonin). Treatment should be initiated while the patient is hospitalized, and patients should remain on the medication for at least 6 months after attaining sobriety. Treatment courses longer than 6 months have not been well studied.

First-line treatment for AUD involves naltrexone and acamprosate. The two are briefly summarized below:

- Naltrexone, available in oral and IM depot form, exerts its pharmacologic effect through mu (μ)-opioid receptor blockade, which reduces the reinforcing effects of alcohol consumption. In animal studies, naltrexone has been found to reduce alcohol self-administration.[43] In humans, naltrexone has reduced the rate and severity of alcohol consumption compared with placebo.[44,45] Oral naltrexone is commonly used at doses of 50 to 100 mg/day, while the IM formulation (Vivitrol) is used at doses of 380 mg every 4 weeks. Patients who require opioid agents (e.g., for pain management) should not be started on naltrexone; otherwise, the drug is well-tolerated with its most common side effects, including nausea, fatigue, and low appetite. Rare cases of interstitial pneumonia and eosinophilic pneumonia have been reported with the use of naltrexone.

- Acamprosate works through modulation of glutamate CNS transmission and has been shown to reduce rates of alcohol consumption compared to placebo in patients with severe AUD, as well as to increase the duration of abstinence by an average of 11%.[44,46] The drug is safe and is generally well tolerated, although dose adjustments may be needed in patients with renal failure (owing to primarily renal metabolism). The primary barrier to treatment may be reduced adherence in the setting of three times daily (TID) dosing.

In addition to these agents, a variety of other compounds have been used for the pharmacologic management of AUD. Some of the most common are summarized below:

- Topiramate has reduced alcohol use in patients with severe AUD, but it does not carry US Food and Drug Administration approval for this indication. It is believed to work by antagonizing kainate glutamate receptors and by interacting with GABA receptors.[47,48] Compared with other drugs listed here, topiramate initiation may require a gradual titration and tapering (to both initiate and discontinue the medication) and it is associated with more frequent side effects, including cognitive dulling, weight loss, mood changes, and depression. As with many AEDs, topiramate use should be avoided by pregnant females.

- Gabapentin, at doses of 600 mg TID, has offered benefits (in a placebo-controlled randomized trial) regarding rates of abstinence, reduction in the extent of drinking, and improved mood/sleep/cravings in the treatment group.[49]

- Baclofen, selective serotonin reuptake inhibitors, and ondansetron have each been studied as potential options for the treatment of AUD, although the data for most of these compounds have not been consistent/encouraging.

- Disulfiram discourages drinking through negative reinforcement, as it precipitates an unpleasant physical reaction when an individual consumes alcohol while on this medication. The compound works by inhibiting aldehyde dehydrogenase, thus preventing the metabolism of acetaldehyde (the primary hepatic metabolite of alcohol breakdown). Accumulation of acetaldehyde leads to flushing, sweating, headache, palpitations, nausea, and vomiting. The efficacy of the compound is limited, and it often requires strong motivation or supervised conditions. With unsupervised treatment, disulfiram is less effective, as most patients will self-discontinue the medication before they resume drinking. Disulfiram should be avoided in patients with severe cardiovascular disease, pregnant females, and patients with psychosis. In general, the use of this medication has waned, given the alternatives.

Psychosocial Treatment of Alcohol Use Disorder

Brief substance use intervention in the general medical setting is well-developed and effective.[50] Even brief contact with an addiction consultant has led to improvement in 30% to 50% of patients several months after their hospitalization. This effect is even more pronounced in those with no history of a psychiatric illness and with good social function and resources.[51] Addiction consultation services to hospital physicians should assist with diagnosis, intervention, pharmacologic management, and post-acute care referral.

AUD causes diverse disruptions in people's self-awareness, communication skills, capacity for relationships, sense of purpose, and spirituality. Alcoholics Anonymous (AA), Self-Management and Recovery Training recovery, and other peer-driven recovery services, have a record of success and benefit greatly from their accessibility and low cost. If already established within AA, patients may benefit from visits from their sponsor or from other group members while hospitalized. Alternatively, some hospitals have established AA meetings on-campus, and (if able and interested) patients should be encouraged to attend these while hospitalized. Recovery coaches offer an excellent alternative to the classic addiction clinician's approach and may be able to engage patients on a deeply personal level through shared experiences. Working with individuals in recovery may motivate patients to engage with the team and be more trusting of the treatment options offered.

Motivational interviewing (MI) is a directed, patient-centered counseling technique for eliciting behavioral change by helping to explore and resolve ambivalence to change.[52] With this approach, the provider assesses the patient's losses and risks, helps the patient to recognize the underlying cause as substance abuse, and uncovers ambivalence about the potential value of treatment. By avoiding a threatening style of confrontation about denial, MI has been found to enhance the motivation for recovery.[52]

To be successful, any attempt at treating AUD in the inpatient setting should focus on much more than diagnosing the disorder and managing withdrawal symptoms. Patients should be assessed for their understanding of the problem and their readiness to engage with addiction work. Pharmacologic treatments should be initiated while in the hospital, and patients should engage with substance use specialists to review outpatient resources and services to facilitate recovery. Issues that may impede recovery, such as inadequate housing and legal problems, should be acknowledged and addressed whenever possible.

STIMULANTS

Cocaine

Cocaine is a tropane alkaloid naturally found in leaves of the *Erythroxylum coca* plant, a bush native to the Andes Mountains region of South America. To this day, leaves of the plant continue to be used by the indigenous people (typically chewed), for their anesthetic, stimulant, and hunger-suppressant effects. Over the past two centuries, the discovery of methods to reliably isolate the alkaloid combined with the ever-increasing demand for the compound has led to cocaine becoming one of the most commonly abused drugs worldwide. An estimated 17 million people (about 0.4% of the world population) have used cocaine, a number only surpassed by cannabis and alcohol.[53] The widespread use of the drug, combined with its potent stimulant effects, has led to cocaine being one of the leading drugs of abuse (in terms of the frequency of ED contacts, general hospital admissions, violence, and other social problems). The DAWN ED data for 2011 reported 505,224 ED visits related to cocaine, compared with 455,668 ED visits for marijuana, and 258,482 ED visits related to heroin use—a staggering 40% of all ED visits related to illicit drug use.[54] Traditionally, the coca leaf is chewed to release the cocaine alkaloid, yet isolated cocaine is rarely ingested (commonly with a highly alkaline compound to prevent neutralization by the acidic milieu of the stomach). More commonly, cocaine is injected, insufflated, or inhaled (as "crack") as the latter methods greatly increase the bioavailability of the drug.

Pharmacology and Mechanism of Action

Cocaine increases the monoamine neurotransmitter activity in the CNS by blocking the pre-synaptic reuptake transporters for dopamine, norepinephrine, and serotonin. Given the potent effects of cocaine on dopamine's availability within the CNS, much of the drug's stimulant and addictive effects have been ascribed to its effects on the cortico-mesolimbic dopamine reward circuits.[55,56] In addition to these effects, cocaine also acts by blocking voltage-gated sodium ion channels, an action that accounts for its effect as a local anesthetic and contributes to its cardiac toxicity.

The route of administration greatly influences the bioavailability of the drug, including its onset and duration of effect. Smoking (i.e., inhalation) and IV use generally lead to near instantaneous (seconds to minutes) effects, and most patients note that the drug's effects wear off within 30 minutes. Intranasal administration results in a slower onset of symptoms (within 30 minutes) and the effects of the drug are similarly extended to up to 1 hour.

Cocaine is commonly co-administered with alcohol, which leads to the formation of cocaethylene, a compound with stimulant effects like those of cocaine, albeit with a longer half-life. This compound has also been noted to convey greater cardiotoxicity compared with cocaine alone.

Cocaine is extensively metabolized by the liver and its metabolites are eliminated in the urine, most commonly as benzoylecgonine. This metabolite (rather than the parent compound) is detected by urine drug tests for cocaine; it can be detected as early as 4 hours after intake and may remain detectable for up to 1 week after cocaine is used. There are no common false positives on urine cocaine screening.

Cocaine intoxication is associated with potent stimulant effects, including an increase in energy and alertness, bright (to frankly euphoric) affect, insomnia, as well as anorexia. Like other stimulants, cocaine is associated with an intensely pleasurable state and is commonly used to potentiate sexual activity. With higher doses, the unintended effects of cocaine may become apparent, including anxiety and panic attacks, restlessness, agitation, and violent behavior, as well as psychosis (manifesting as paranoid ideation, hallucinations, or delusional thinking). Signs of adrenergic hyperactivity (e.g., hyperreflexia, tachycardia, diaphoresis, mydriasis) may also be seen. More severe symptoms (e.g., hyperpyrexia, hypertension, cocaine-induced vasospastic events, such as stroke or myocardial infarction) are relatively rare among recreational users but are seen more commonly in patients who present to the ED for cocaine-related issues. Patients may manifest motor signs of CNS excitability, including tremor, myoclonus, and stereotyped movements of the mouth, face, or extremities (e.g., skin picking, "crack dancing," "boca torcida"). Infrequently, seizures may occur, even with first-time use of the drug—most commonly these are manifest as generalized tonic-clinic seizures within the first 90 minutes after the drug is used.

Given its potent effects on the central and peripheral monoamine neurotransmitter systems, it is not surprising that cocaine has significant effects on most organ systems. In addition to its stimulant and pro-ictal effects described previously, cocaine has been associated with increased rates of hemorrhagic and ischemic stroke, an effect postulated to be due to increased heart rate and blood pressure (due to sympathetic nervous system activation), cerebral vasoconstriction, and vasospasm. Cocaine similarly increases the risk for cardiac ischemia, and chest pain is one of the most frequent complaints among cocaine users who seek medical attention. Cocaine-associated increased heart rate and blood pressure (via increased peripheral adrenergic activity), as well as vasoconstriction, lead to reduced cardiac oxygen availability and an increased risk for cardiac complications, including myocardial infarction. Furthermore, cocaine's action as a sodium channel blocker leads to an increased risk of cardiac arrhythmias and even sudden death.

Use of intranasal cocaine has been associated with rhinitis, sinusitis, and in severe cases, perforation of the nasal septum. Inhalation of cocaine commonly leads to respiratory symptoms, including shortness of breath, wheezing, and cough, but it may also cause bronchitis, pulmonary edema, hemorrhage, and even pneumothorax. While cocaine has not been shown to be a significant source of hepatotoxicity in humans, it can contribute to renal damage through direct (vasoconstriction of renal arteries) and indirect effects (cocaine-induced rhabdomyolysis).

Cocaine discontinuation leads to an unpleasant, though rarely medically concerning, withdrawal syndrome. Nonetheless, DAWN data indicate that up to one-fourth of all drug-related detoxification-related ED visits were attributable to cocaine withdrawal.[54] Patients commonly present with symptoms (including depression, fatigue, anhedonia, difficulties concentrating, as well as increased sleep and appetite) opposite to those seen with cocaine intoxication. Patients may also exhibit drug cravings. In some cases, depression and psychomotor retardation that are observed with cocaine withdrawal may be so severe as to be accompanied by prominent hopelessness and suicidal ideation. In comparison with its behavioral effects, the physical signs of cocaine withdrawal are usually mild and clinically unremarkable.

Psychiatric Sequelae of Cocaine Use

Cocaine use has been associated with the development of cocaine use disorder in up to one-sixth of all individuals exposed to the drug. Although euphoria is an intended effect of the drug, patients who are acutely intoxicated by cocaine may present with symptoms that resemble acute mania, a primary anxiety disorder, or a primary depressive disorder. The most serious psychiatric finding associated with cocaine intoxication is cocaine-induced psychosis, which frequently manifests as visual and auditory hallucinations, paranoid delusions, and (in severe cases) violence. Some studies estimate its prevalence at 80% of all individuals with a cocaine use disorder. While these symptoms resemble those of a primary psychotic process, cocaine-induced psychosis may be differentiated by its transient nature, the relative absence of negative symptoms, as well as more prominent visual and tactile hallucinations (e.g., "coke bugs").

Management

Cocaine intoxication can lead to significant medical and psychiatric sequelae, and acute management should take both domains into consideration. As with all acute toxidromes, the ABCs (airway, breathing, circulation) of stabilization are essential to initial patient management. Given the stimulant effects of cocaine outlined above, monitoring for tachycardia, hypertension, and associated end-organ damage (e.g., coronary ischemia, stroke) is also essential with acute intoxication. Mild-to-moderate tachycardia and hypertension may respond to the use of IV benzodiazepines. For refractory or severe hypertension, alpha-adrenergic agents (e.g., phentolamine) are commonly used. The use of beta-blockers in acute cocaine intoxication remains controversial, but this class of medications has been traditionally avoided for concerns of unopposed alpha-adrenergic stimulation and associated increased chances for vasospasm and cardiac ischemia.

Acute psychomotor agitation and anxiety can similarly be managed with benzodiazepines, while antipsychotics may be administered in cases of severe psychosis. In our experience, co-administration of IV lorazepam and IV haloperidol is often beneficial in these situations, with rapid resolution of agitation.

Sub-acute management of cocaine use may involve a brief course of benzodiazepines (for refractory anxiety and insomnia), as well as dopamine antagonists (for residual psychosis). The former should be used judiciously to avoid complications related to benzodiazepine misuse (e.g., dependence, diversion).

Longitudinally, cocaine use disorder is primarily managed by the use of behavioral interventions, such as therapy and involvement with a peer support group. Most medications (including antidepressants, e.g., citalopram, dopamine antagonists; most anticonvulsants, e.g., carbamazepine, gabapentin; and certain dopamine agonists) have not shown consistent efficacy in the treatment of cocaine dependence. Disulfiram, varenicline, and naltrexone have also been used, again with mixed results. Agonist substitution therapy with long-acting oral stimulants (e.g., amphetamine) alone, or in combination with topiramate, has shown some promise; however, considerable risks exist regarding diversion, and cardiac safety often presents barriers to treatment.[57] A randomized clinical trial of topiramate for the treatment of cocaine addiction showed greater efficacy than placebo at increasing the mean weekly proportion of cocaine non-use days and associated measures of clinical improvement among cocaine-dependent individuals.[58] Various therapeutic approaches have also been utilized to manage cocaine use disorder, including supportive, cognitive-behavioral, and motivational therapies, as well as peer support groups (such as Cocaine Anonymous), with mixed results. The behavioral intervention with the best evidence-based outcomes for the treatment of cocaine is the Matrix Model. This model provides a framework for engaging patients (as they learn about issues critical to addiction and relapse, receive direction and support from a trained therapist, and become familiar with self-help programs). Patients are also monitored closely for drug use through urine testing. Treatment includes elements of relapse prevention, family and group therapies, drug education, and self-help participation. Detailed treatment manuals contain worksheets for individual sessions; other components include family education groups, early recovery skills groups, relapse prevention groups, combined sessions, urine tests, 12-step programs, relapse analysis, and social support groups. Several studies have demonstrated that participants treated using the Matrix Model show statistically significant reductions in drug and alcohol use, improvements in psychological indicators, and reduced high-risk behaviors associated with human immunodeficiency virus (HIV) transmission.[59]

Amphetamines and Other CNS Stimulants

Amphetamines encompass a diverse class of CNS stimulants that have been used since antiquity for medicinal, as well as recreational purposes. The practice of chewing Khat leaves in Ethiopia and Yemen, as well as the use of the *Ephedra sinica* plant in ancient China offer some of the earliest examples of amphetamine use. Amphetamine was initially synthesized in 1887, but it was not until the 1930s that these drugs became widely used for the treatment of colds and congestion and to promote alertness in battle-fatigued troops during World War II. In the 1950s, stimulants re-gained popularity as weight-loss aides and soon thereafter became widely used as drugs of abuse. Despite increasing efforts to regulate the production and distribution of stimulants, the number of synthetic amphetamine compounds has risen in recent decades and now includes not only the traditional amphetamines, but also methamphetamine (crystal meth), MDMA (ecstasy), and synthetic cathinone ("bath salts").

The ongoing popularity of CNS stimulants is reflected in epidemiologic data. According to data from DAWN, the number of ED visits related to non-medical use of CNS stimulants among adults aged 18 to 34 increased from 5,605 in 2005 to 22,949 in 2011. As stimulants can mask the sedating effects of alcohol, the two compounds are commonly used in conjunction, and about 30% of all ED visits related to non-medical CNS stimulant use also involve alcohol.[54] As the number of various amphetamines is considerable and no toxicology tests will reliably screen for all amphetamine compounds, it is essential that consulting physicians be familiar with the pharmacology of these drugs so as to be prepared to recognize the drug-related toxidrome and to provide appropriate management.

Pharmacology and Mechanism of Action

Like cocaine, most amphetamines exert their effect through stimulation of CNS alpha- and beta-adrenergic receptors, leading to a toxidrome marked by increased alertness, euphoria (or in severe cases, anxiety and agitation), tachycardia, hypertension, and mydriasis. The specific mechanism of action is often drug-dependent, but most CNS stimulants propagate the release of amine neurotransmitters, including dopamine, serotonin, and norepinephrine, although some may also act through reuptake inhibition. The propensity of a specific amphetamine drug for a specific set of neurotransmitters may differ from related amphetamine products, and this may in part be reflected by significant variability in clinical findings observed with these compounds. As an example, methamphetamine exerts its effect by increasing dopamine availability in the synaptic cleft by promoting the release of the neurotransmitter, blocking its reuptake and degradation, and increasing the activity of enzymes necessary in dopamine synthesis.[60]

Acute intoxication from amphetamine compounds closely resembles that of cocaine and is marked by central and peripheral hyperactivity, including physiologic changes (tachycardia, hypertension, hyperthermia, diaphoresis, and mydriasis) and mental status changes (euphoria as the intended effect; anxiety, agitation, and violent behavior as unintended effects). Cardiac problems (including chest pain, ischemia, and arrhythmias) are rarely seen, but when present they can lead to serious complications. Signs of CNS hyperexcitability, including seizures, tremors, and myoclonus, may occur with acute intoxication. Electrolyte abnormalities, related to dehydration due to reduced intake and insensible losses through hyperthermia, can lead to significant complications (including arrhythmias and renal failure). In particular, the use of ecstasy (MDMA) has been linked with severe hyponatremia (in the setting of free-water losses), leading to obtundation and potentially fatal cerebral edema.

Psychiatric Sequelae of Amphetamine Use

Acute intoxication with amphetamines may present in a fashion like that of several primary psychiatric conditions, including panic attacks, mania, and/or psychosis. Acute onset of symptoms without a prodrome characteristic for a primary psychiatric disorder, presence of visual and tactile hallucinations, a positive toxicology screen, and a history of drug use may all provide clues towards stimulants as a cause of new-onset mania/psychosis. Amphetamine-associated psychosis can persist beyond the initial drug use and even recur during periods of abstinence from the drug. Findings on the physical examination consistent with stimulant use include pupillary dilatation, poor dentition ("meth teeth" due to a chronically dry mouth), and excoriations (due to skin picking).

It is estimated that up to 40% of all patients with amphetamine use have a co-morbid primary psychiatric disorder, including psychosis (28.6%), a mood disorder (32.3%), an anxiety disorder (26.5%), or ADHD (30%–40%).[61]

As with cocaine, depressive symptoms are common with amphetamine discontinuation and may be severe enough to meet the diagnostic criteria for major depressive disorder. While amphetamine discontinuation can produce a life-threatening physiologic syndrome, in some patients the extent of depression can be so severe that psychiatric hospitalization and suicide precautions are warranted.

Persistent amphetamine use has been associated with CNS neurotoxicity and associated deficits in episodic memory, executive functioning, and language and motor skills; the long-term clinical relevance of these findings remains uncertain.

Management

Acute amphetamine intoxication and withdrawal are managed like that of cocaine (outlined previously in this chapter).

No medications have shown consistent efficacy for the long-term management of stimulant use disorder. Bupropion and mirtazapine have shown some promise, especially in milder cases, or when they can be used in conjunction with therapy. In particular, the data (albeit limited) appear to favor mirtazapine—a 12-week trial of mirtazapine versus placebo in methamphetamine-dependent men who have sex with men showed that the mirtazapine-treated patients were less likely to submit positive urine drug screens compared with the group receiving placebo.[62] The Matrix Model has shown some promise as a therapeutic approach to long-term behavioral management of patients with stimulant use disorders.

HALLUCINOGENS

Hallucinogens comprise a broad and diverse class of drugs, the unifying effect of which is their intended mode of action—to produce alterations in thinking, sensations, and reality perceptions. Widely used across many cultures, this group includes natural (e.g., hallucinogenic mushrooms, peyote, *Salvia divinorum*) as well as synthetic compounds (e.g., lysergic acid diethylamine [LSD]). While these compounds have traditionally been used to heighten spiritual/religious experiences, most modern hallucinogen use is recreational, with the desired intent to produce perceptual alterations, including hallucinations or illusions, or to enhance emotional states. Commonly, the term "tripping" is used to describe acute intoxication with a hallucinogen, with the term "bad trip" used to describe acute intoxication marked by unintended sequelae (including anxiety, agitation, and paranoia).

LSD, synthesized in 1938 by Albert Hofmann, was the first synthetic hallucinogen and one of the best-studied drugs in this class. Initially marketed as an anesthetic and adjunct for psychotherapy, the drug became popular as a psychedelic drug in the 1960s, and was listed as a drug of abuse by 1966. Over the past two decades, the use of LSD has diminished, as more users turn to alternative (and more readily available) compounds, including synthetic cannabinoids, phencyclidine (PCP), ketamine, and naturally-occurring hallucinogenic compounds.

Hallucinogen use is often sporadic, and relatively uncommon when compared with opioids and stimulants. Approximately 4.2 million individuals in the United States used hallucinogens in 2014, and these drugs accounted for only 7% of all US ED visits related to illicit drugs.[54]

Pharmacology and Mechanism of Action

Given the sheer number and diversity of compounds characterized as hallucinogens, a detailed account of the specific biochemical properties of each is beyond the scope of this chapter. Nonetheless, most of these compounds exert their effect through the modulation of serotonin, dopamine, and glutamate—especially through binding of the 5-HT_{2A} receptors in the neocortical pyramidal cells.[63] Sympathomimetic effects, including pupillary constriction, tachycardia, hypertension, and hyperthermia are seen, though commonly they are not as severe as with stimulants and cocaine. A brief overview of the most commonly used hallucinogenic compounds is presented below:

- *Lysergic acid diethylamide (LSD):* LSD is commonly used as a pill or in liquid form (e.g., added to blotter paper). Its intended effect is to produce visual illusions, often characterized by intense colors and distortions, as well as emotional changes marked by euphoria and depersonalization. Time perception may also be distorted, with users often describing experience of reality as if in "slow motion." Most recreational users will maintain awareness that their experiences are drug-induced. Unintended effects are commonly seen with the ingestion of higher doses of LSD and may include intense dysphoria, anxiety, or agitation. Panic, overwhelming fear, and even paranoia, are classically described, and patients may lack the awareness that their bad trip is drug induced. This, in turn, may cause impaired judgment and lead to unintentional injuries or even death.
- *Dextromethorphan (DXM):* DXM is a sigma opioid agonist and *N*-methyl-ᴅ-aspartate (NMDA) receptor antagonist, commonly available in various cough remedies. DXM misuse is most commonly seen in the adolescent population ("robo tripping") with the intended effect of producing a trance-like dissociative state. Overuse may lead to paranoia, hallucinations, and, in severe cases,

coma. As DXM is commonly sold mixed with other compounds (e.g., diphenhydramine and acetaminophen), all cases of suspected DXM intoxication should be monitored for potential additional toxicity related to these compounds.

- *Mescaline:* Mescaline is the active ingredient found in the peyote cactus (*Lophophora williamsii*), a plant native to the south-west United States. It is ingested as a tea prepared from the plant or as dried "buttons." Its effects are like those of LSD, though generally milder. While mescaline can be legally used by members of the Native American Church, reflecting its traditional use in religious ceremonies, all other use of the compound is considered illegal.
- *Psilocybin:* This hallucinogen compound is found in several species of mushrooms that are native to the Pacific Northwest and the southern United States, commonly known by their street names of "magic mushrooms" or "shrooms." The mushrooms are commonly dried (to aid with storage/transport) and consumed with food. The intended effect is like that of LSD, although milder, and may be preceded by significant GI symptoms (e.g., nausea, vomiting) immediately on consuming the compound. Accidental ingestion of otherwise toxic mushrooms can occur, as can unintended ingestion of other hallucinogens (e.g., lacing edible mushrooms with LSD).
- *Salvinorin A:* This compound is a kappa opioid agonist found in the leaves of the *Salvia divinorum* plant. It can be freely obtained through the Internet, and it is not a federally controlled substance in the United States; this further contributes to its rising popularity. Much like other hallucinogens, it can produce sensory distortions, although most users primarily reflect on emotional changes, including elevated mood, euphoria, as well as introspection. It has a relatively short duration of action (generally 1–2 hours), especially when compared with other hallucinogenic compounds.
- *Phencyclidine (PCP, Angel dust):* PCP is a noncompetitive antagonist at NMDA receptors, initially developed as an anesthetic agent. The drug can be insufflated, smoked, ingested, or used intravenously. At low doses, PCP produces

a sense of detachment from one's surroundings and may lead to dissociation as well as amnesia. At higher doses, PCP intoxication may present with markedly bizarre (and often severely violent) behavior, hallucinations, and even catatonia. Physical examination may elicit nystagmus (vertical and horizontal), as well as signs of sympathomimetic toxicity (including mydriasis). Severe agitation is often a presenting problem for PCP-intoxicated patients and appropriate measures to ensure the safety of healthcare staff must be considered when dealing with this toxidrome.

▪ *Ketamine (Special K):* Structurally similar to PCP, ketamine exerts its effect chiefly through NMDA receptor antagonism. Depending on the dosage used, ketamine can produce a wide array of CNS effects, ranging from euphoria and dissociation to agitation, hallucinations, and coma. When used in the hospital setting, ketamine is a safe anesthetic, leading to conscious sedation and anesthesia. As a drug of abuse, ketamine is utilized to alter sensory perceptions, diminish alertness, and induce mild sedation. With overdose, patients may present with obtundation or even coma, while emergence from sedation may be marked by dissociation, confusion, and agitation. Respiratory and cardiovascular support is thus an essential component of acute management of ketamine intoxication. While ketamine overdose can be fatal, most complications have been described in patients co-ingesting drugs (e.g., stimulants or other sedatives). Physical examination may show nystagmus (though it is less common than with PCP), increased muscle tone, and pupillary dilatation. Chronic ketamine use can cause ketamine-induced ulcerative cystitis, which presents as incontinence, hematuria, and decreased bladder compliance/volume.

Psychiatric Sequelae and Management

Acute intoxication with hallucinogens may present similarly to mania (euphoria, overwhelming sense of well-being) as well as psychosis (given sensory misperceptions). Prominent visual phenomena, the patient's awareness that the symptoms are drug-induced, dissociative experiences, and a distorted sense of time may all point towards acute intoxication. Severe vital sign changes are uncommon with these drugs, and if seen they should raise concerns for a co-ingestion. Containment and safety may be the only interventions warranted with milder cases of intoxication, although IV benzodiazepines co-administered with dopamine antagonists have been used to manage the agitated delirium observed in severe cases.

While hallucinogens are not known to induce primary psychosis, they may unmask a latent psychotic illness, as well as lead to brief psychotic episodes (commonly lasting up to a week). Psychiatric containment may be warranted in these cases. Patients may also describe "flashback" experiences like those that develop with acute intoxication; it often arises weeks to months after the discontinuation of the drug.

Serotonin syndrome has been described with several hallucinogens, including LSD, and may occur in those who take hallucinogens while taking serotonergic agents, including SSRIs, MAOIs, or lithium.

CANNABIS AND SYNTHETIC CANNABINOIDS

Cannabis remains the most commonly used drug of abuse worldwide, with an estimated 2.5% of the world population (147 million people) having used the drug in 2014.[64] Cannabis use is particularly common in adolescents and young adults across the United States. While cannabis remains illegal on the federal level, a growing number of states have passed legislation that legalizes the possession and medical use of marijuana. The long-term effects of the liberalization of marijuana use on the prevalence and severity of cannabis use disorder remain to be seen.

Besides cannabis, there has been a steady increase in the availability and use of synthetic cannabinoids over the last two decades. Commonly sold as "herbal remedies" and "natural products" these compounds go by a variety of street names, the most common of which are "K2" and "Spice." While synthetic cannabinoid intoxication resembles a marijuana "high," these drugs can be incrementally more potent and are often associated with pronounced psychiatric and neurologic pathology. As the number of synthetic cannabinoids available far exceeds the detection ability of most drug assays, familiarity with this drug class and its effects remains essential.

Pharmacology and Mechanism of Action

Recreationally, cannabis is used in a variety of modes, including its most common routes, through inhalation and ingestion. The drug exerts its CNS effects primarily through the cannabinoid receptor (CB-1) found in the basal ganglia, substantia nigra, cerebellum, hippocampus, and cerebral cortex. CB-1 activation is associated with inhibition of the release of several neurotransmitters (including acetylcholine, glutamate, GABA, norepinephrine, and dopamine). Synthetic cannabinoids act on the same receptors as cannabis but may differ in their potency (up to 800 times greater) and thus differ in their clinical effects due to differences in their binding strength and affinity. Some of the synthetic cannabinoids interact with other receptors, including the NMDA and serotonin receptors.

Psychiatric Sequelae of Cannabis Use

Recreational cannabis use is seldom associated with medically significant side effects. Most cases of mild intoxication present with CNS depression (e.g., somnolence), while severe cases are often accompanied by unintended behavioral changes (including anxiety, dysphoria, or even agitation). Physical examination is classically notable for a dry mouth, conjunctival injection, increased appetite ("munchies"), slurring of speech, and ataxia/nystagmus. Hyperemesis may be observed, often with chronic cannabis use, and it may indicate cannabis hyperemesis syndrome. Classically, patients will report a pattern of chronic cannabis use, cyclical episodes of nausea/vomiting, and symptomatic relief with hot showers.

Synthetic cannabinoids may present with more pronounced symptoms than cannabis, including delirium, psychosis, severe psychomotor agitation, and (rarely) seizures. These drugs have also been associated with higher rates of cardiovascular and CNS toxicity.

Management

Most cases of marijuana intoxication are mild and self-limited; they typically respond to supportive measures that target reduction of the level of stimulation and reassurance. Severe or persisting cases should raise concerns about exposure to synthetic cannabinoids or alternative psychoactive compounds. As with stimulants, the use of short-acting benzodiazepines may reduce symptoms of anxiety that are often seen with the acute toxidrome. Synthetic cannabinoids may present with severe agitation, and thus may require considerably higher doses of benzodiazepines to achieve sedation. Monitoring (including assessment of electrolyte abnormalities related to insensible fluid losses and rhabdomyolysis, hyperthermia, and seizures) and treatment are crucial. In most severe cases, patients will warrant inpatient medical or psychiatric admission for assistance with symptom management.

OPIOIDS

Opioids are some of the most important medicinal compounds, widely used for their ability to provide effective analgesia. They also constitute one of the most commonly encountered classes of drugs of abuse. With their use stretching back over millennia (opium was originally extracted from the poppy plant *Papaver somniferum*), opiates have played a significant role in religion, culture, and medicine. Over the past three decades, there has been a persistent and dramatic increase in opioid use in the United States, with an estimated 9.5 million people reporting past-year misuse of heroin or prescription pain relievers in 2020. Most of those who have used opioids—9.3 million—used prescription opioids (e.g., fentanyl, oxycodone), reflecting an increased availability and distribution of these drugs.[1] This is more than twice the number of people who used opioids just a decade ago, and starkly emphasizes the ongoing impact of the opioid epidemic in the United States. Nearly one-third (31%) of individuals with acquired immunodeficiency syndrome in the United States are related to injection drug use.[65] An estimated 70% to 80% of new hepatitis C infections that occur in the United States each year are among IV drug users. Other public health problems that have emerged over the last decade include an increased number of ED visits and deaths due to opioid overdoses. Specifically, prescription methadone, oxycodone, and hydrocodone-related ED visits quadrupled between 2004 and 2008.[66] Use of heroin, once the most commonly misused opioid agent, is steadily dropping as the more potent and easily manufactured synthetic alternatives (namely, fentanyl) become increasingly more available.

Clinicians across all disciplines have considerable responsibility to prevent and reverse the epidemic of opioid-related morbidity and mortality. Judicious prescribing of opioids for pain relief remains an essential step in reducing the availability of these drugs. Prompt recognition of the symptoms associated with opioid intoxication and withdrawal, including familiarity with medications used to manage the sequelae of both, is an essential skill of acute inpatient management. Lastly, efforts should be made to ensure that all patients receive appropriate longitudinal assistance with their drug use, including maintenance opioid treatment strategies, medication-assisted strategies for abstinence, expanded access to naloxone, and behavioral treatment resources.

Pharmacology and Mechanism of Action

All opioids exert their effect through an interaction with one of three opioid receptor classes (mu, kappa, delta). Structurally, all opioid receptors are coupled to G proteins, which in turn activate second-messenger pathways in the target cell, including cAMP and calcium-mediated pathways. Although opioid receptors are abundant throughout the central and peripheral nervous system, the distribution of specific receptor subtypes, the type of second-messenger pathway, and the downstream effect on neurotransmitter release are highly variable from site to site and account for the wide range of clinical effects observed following opiate use. Activation of CNS mu receptors is associated with euphoria and reward pathway activation (via dopamine increase in the mesolimbic system), anxiolysis (via noradrenergic neurons in locus ceruleus), and analgesia (via inhibition of nociceptive information). Central mu receptor activation is also responsible for respiratory depression and sedation, while the stimulation of peripheral mu receptors results in cough suppression and GI dysmotility. Miosis, a classic sign of opioid intoxication, is mediated through kappa receptor activation.[67]

Management of Opioid Intoxication and Withdrawal

Acute intoxication with opioids presents with a clinical syndrome characterized by CNS depression (sedation), interpersonal withdrawal to elated mood, and slurred speech. Physical examination is notable for miosis, reduced respiratory rate, decreased bowel sounds, and common dermatologic findings consistent with repeated IV drug use (e.g., track-marks, injection sites). Patients who inject subcutaneously ("skin popping") may also present with multiple abscesses at the injection sites. Beyond changes in respiratory rate and levels of oxygenation (linked with severe intoxication), other vital sign changes are uncommon; hypothermia may reflect prolonged environmental exposure, while hyperthermia may indicate an acute infection related to IV drug use (e.g., aspiration pneumonia, abscesses, bacteremia, or endocarditis).

Acute opioid overdose is a medical emergency and close attention should be paid to the patient's alertness and respiratory status. In severe cases, coma and respiratory arrest may ensue and require ICU-level care. Naloxone, a short-acting opioid antagonist, should be administered in all cases of suspected opioid overdose. It is available in a variety of formulations, including IV, IM, and nasal, and it is generally safe, as it lacks acute toxicity or significant drug-drug interactions. While initial doses of 0.05 mg can be used in patients with spontaneous ventilation, higher doses (up to 2 mg) should be given to patients who are apneic or in cardiopulmonary arrest. Naloxone should be administered to secure adequate ventilation rather than an intact level of consciousness, and the patient may require multiple doses of naloxone (e.g., up to 8), especially if an overdose with high-potency agents (fentanyl) is suspected. If opioid withdrawal is accidentally precipitated, it should be managed through supportive measures; further opioid administration is not recommended. Once stabilized, the patient should be monitored for re-emergence of opioid toxicity, as the half-life of naloxone is relatively short when compared to most opioid agents; thus multiple administrations of the medication may be required to maintain adequate respiration and to prevent re-emergence of respiratory compromise.

Urine toxicology is not necessary for the management of most cases of acute opioid overdose, but we recommend routine checking to potentially differentiate various types of opioids ingested and to assess for the presence of any other substances. Initial laboratory testing following an acute overdose should also include levels of serum glucose, electrolytes, liver enzymes, and creatine kinase (later to assess for rhabdomyolysis). An electrocardiogram should be considered in all cases where a methadone overdose is suspected to monitor for QTc prolongation. Chest imaging may be helpful to rule out aspiration, and an additional infectious work-up should be considered in all febrile patients given their heightened risk for bacteremia, endocarditis, and septic arthritis due to IV drug use. Once stabilized, patients may benefit from infectious disease screening (including HIV, hepatitis, and syphilis).

The classic signs of opioid withdrawal usually begin 8 to 12 hours after the last opioid dosing. These include sweating, yawning, lacrimation, tremors, rhinorrhea, marked irritability, dilated pupils, and an increased respiratory rate. More severe signs of withdrawal (e.g., nausea, vomiting, insomnia, abdominal cramps) occur 24 to 36 hours after the last dose. Untreated, the syndrome subsides in 5 to 10 days, and while uncomfortable, it is not life-threatening. Due to its longer half-life, patients withdrawing from methadone or buprenorphine/naloxone may not show symptoms of withdrawal until 3 days or more after the last dose, and, once present, the symptoms may persist for 2 to 4 weeks.

As the available data clearly show superior treatment outcomes in patients managed with opioid agonist therapy, acute detoxification alone is generally not recommended. However, in settings in which agonist therapy may not be available, or if a patient declines treatment with an agonist agent, acute detoxification can be attempted with a variety of methods, outlined below:

- *Supportive care:* Milder cases of opioid withdrawal can be managed by administering medications that counter some of the most challenging withdrawal symptoms. This includes acetaminophen for muscle aches, clonidine for autonomic symptoms, dicyclomine for GI cramps and diarrhea, and trazodone or quetiapine for insomnia and anxiety. Despite its historic name, "comfort measures," this approach is generally perceived as uncomfortable by the patient and is associated with lower completion rates when compared with withdrawal management via the use of opioid replacement therapy.
- *Methadone:* Methadone is available in a variety of formulations (oral, IV, and IM), and its long half-life makes it particularly suitable for the management of opioid withdrawal. Specific starting doses may be challenging to determine and will depend on the patient's pattern of use; most patients note improvement in withdrawal symptoms with doses between 30 and 40 mg/day. Methadone can be administered as a single daily dose or divided into three doses. The latter approach is favored whenever uncertainty arises regarding the pattern of use or the patient's last exposure to street opioids, as it minimizes the risk of over-sedation. When starting methadone or increasing it, the QTc should be monitored, although prolongation is uncommon in doses less than 60 to 80 mg/day. Once the patient reaches a stable methadone dose that leads to the resolution of most withdrawal symptoms, the medication can be tapered by 10% to 25% per day until it is discontinued.
- *Buprenorphine:* Buprenorphine is an efficacious alternative to methadone for short-term inpatient opioid detoxification. Patients are monitored for signs of opioid withdrawal and treated with sublingual doses of buprenorphine 2 to 4 mg. Once symptoms of acute withdrawal have been stabilized, buprenorphine can be tapered over the next 3 to 5 days. Patients typically report that buprenorphine detoxification is more comfortable than detoxification with either methadone or clonidine.

Although techniques that permit a safe, rapid, and medically effective detoxification from opiates seem highly attractive in an era of managed care, clinicians must understand that detoxification alone is rarely successful as a treatment for any addiction. Unless the patients are started on appropriate maintenance treatment (either with opioid agonists or naltrexone) and given access to appropriate long-term addiction resources, relapse rates following acute detoxification are extremely high. The resulting costs to the patient, to society, and to the healthcare system far outweigh any savings realized from a rapid and supposedly cost-effective detoxification protocol.

Pharmacotherapy for Opioid Use Disorder

Once the patient has completed detoxification, long-term treatment for opioid use disorder (OUD) should be pursued through maintenance pharmacotherapy and/or behavioral interventions. Considerable data support the pharmacologic approach to opioid maintenance treatment over non-pharmacologic options, and inpatient medical/surgical hospitalization commonly presents an excellent opportunity to initiate OUD pharmacologic treatment and identify appropriate community support resources for the patient.

Opioid Agonist Treatment

Opioid agonist treatment involves the use of either methadone or buprenorphine/naloxone to block the acute effects of other opiates, reduce drug cravings, and minimize behavioral consequences of chronic OUD. While the patient remains physiologically dependent on an opiate, maintenance therapy with either drug has not been associated with psychosocial problems associated with illicit drug use. Both methadone and buprenorphine/naloxone have been shown to reduce mortality related to OUD.[68]

Methadone is a long-acting opioid agonist and a schedule II drug in the United States. Although methadone can be prescribed for pain management by any physician, only licensed treatment programs can initiate methadone for OUD.

Compared with placebo, methadone maintenance treatment has been associated with reduced rates of opioid-positive drug treatment, longer treatment duration, and greater retention rates. Methadone treatment has also been associated with a reduced rate of HIV infection, and with reduced mortality rates related to opioid use.[69]

Patients who are about to begin long-term treatment with methadone should be informed about the risks associated with QTc prolongation, although in most cases, this risk is minimal compared with the risks presented by ongoing opioid use. Patients should also be counseled about the possibility of overdose. As a full opioid agonist, methadone has greater potential for overdose compared with buprenorphine, and these effects may be potentiated in patients who are still actively using opioids while on methadone maintenance, or with polypharmacy.

Methadone is generally administered as a single daily dose, although split-dosing can be used in situations when methadone is prescribed for pain or in patients shown to be rapid metabolizers of the drug. Most patients with an OUD will initiate treatment at 30 mg on their first day, with an additional 10 mg given if the patient exhibits significant withdrawal symptoms 1 hour after the 30 mg dose. The dose is titrated in 5 to 10 mg increments every 1 to 2 days until a therapeutic dose is reached (generally, 60–80 mg of methadone/day). Most patients stabilize on methadone doses between 80 and 120 mg/day, although higher doses are not uncommon, including in pregnant patients.

Buprenorphine is a partial μ-opioid agonist that has been shown to be a viable alternative to methadone in the management of OUD. When dispensed as a sublingual tablet in combination with naloxone, it has minimal potential for IV misuse and has demonstrated efficacy for OUD treatment.[70] Buprenorphine is classified as a schedule III controlled substance; historically, only specially certified clinicians could prescribe the medication for the treatment of OUD, though there has recently been increased recognition that these requirements only limit access to what is generally safe, yet highly effective, treatment. As with methadone, buprenorphine treatment has been associated with fewer positive urine toxicology screens and greater treatment retention when compared with patients managed with non-pharmacologic measures alone.[71,72] Patients with OUD who are started on buprenorphine during a hospitalization show increased rates of sobriety and are more likely to follow up with addiction resources post-discharge when compared with patients treated through detoxification alone.[73]

Buprenorphine is largely safe and appears to have a lower potential for lethal overdose compared with methadone (given its partial agonist effect). Most buprenorphine-related fatalities occur in patients who are using the drug with other sedatives (e.g., benzodiazepines, alcohol). Buprenorphine is typically administered in conjunction with naloxone as a sublingual tablet or strip. As naloxone has poor GI absorption, it is inactive when ingested and will not precipitate withdrawal. If the drug is crushed/dissolved and used intravenously, naloxone becomes active and will precipitate acute withdrawal—this effectively deters patients from using buprenorphine-naloxone intravenously.

As buprenorphine is a partial opioid agonist, it can displace full agonist opioids from the receptor and precipitate withdrawal. When initiating the medication, it is thus essential that patients have been abstinent from other opioids and show symptoms consistent with moderate opioid withdrawal (with a short-acting opioid [e.g., heroin] most patients will start buprenorphine within 10–12 hours after last use, although the wait can be considerably longer if the patient is using a long-acting agent [e.g., methadone]). Most patients are started on buprenorphine 4 mg and monitored for resolution of withdrawal. Additional 2 to 4 mg doses are administered if the withdrawal symptoms persist, with most patients needing 8 to 12 mg during the first day of treatment. On the following day, the patient is given a single dose consisting of the total doses received on the first day, and an additional 2 to 4 mg may be given for any residual withdrawal symptoms. Most patients will stabilize on doses of 8 to 16 mg/day, though some may require up to 32 mg/day.

More recently, there has been a growing recognition of the potential benefits of buprenorphine microdosing in the inpatient hospital setting, especially if patients require ongoing treatment with an opioid (e.g., for acute pain control). Specifically, progressively increasing doses of buprenorphine are offered over 7 days, while the patient continues to take the full dose of opioid agonist (including methadone). Patients are usually started on 0.5 mg of buprenorphine per day, and the dose is doubled every 24 hours until the patient reaches a therapeutic dose of 16 mg/day. At this point, patients can be safely tapered off methadone or any other opioid agonist without significant withdrawal or discomfort.

Opioid Antagonist Treatment

Opioid antagonists are used to prevent the user from experiencing opioid intoxication, and thus reinforce abstinence. This form of treatment is particularly effective in patients who are highly motivated or in patients who cannot be placed on opioid agonist treatment for personal/professional reasons, although is otherwise considerably less effective than treatment with methadone or buprenorphine/naloxone. Naltrexone is used as a long-acting injectable administered every 4 weeks (set dose of 380 mg per injection). Compared to placebo, long-acting IM naltrexone reinforces abstinence and increases patient retention better. Oral naltrexone, while available, is generally not recommended for the treatment of OUD, due to its limited compliance rates.

BENZODIAZEPINES AND OTHER SEDATIVE HYPNOTICS

Benzodiazepines are a class of sedative-hypnotic agents with a wide variety of therapeutic roles, including the management of anxiety disorders, seizures, insomnia, and GABA-mediated withdrawal states. Discovered accidentally in 1954 by Leo Sternbach, chlordiazepoxide (Librium) was the first benzodiazepine to be synthesized, followed by diazepam (Valium) in 1963, and some 50 other benzodiazepine compounds since. Nowadays, benzodiazepines are one of the staples of modern medicine and psychiatry— a versatile drug class commonly used in inpatient and outpatient settings, and frequently prescribed by specialists (e.g., psychiatrists) as well as primary care physicians. While immensely useful in the appropriate clinical setting, benzodiazepines have the potential for misuse and dependence, and a withdrawal state produced by discontinuation of the drug may be life-threatening.

Pharmacology and Mechanism of Action

All benzodiazepines exert their effect via modulation of the $GABA_A$ receptor. Unlike many other drugs discussed in this chapter, benzodiazepines do not change the expression or synaptic availability of GABA, but act to increase the binding of the neurotransmitter to the $GABA_A$ receptor by modulating the receptor structure. The resulting effect is that of hyper-polarization of the target neuron and decreased ability to initiate an action potential. While different benzodiazepines generally share a similar molecular structure, the presence of various side chains accounts for the considerable variability observed in the metabolism pharmacodynamics and pharmacokinetics within the drug class.

It is clinically useful to categorize benzodiazepines based on their kinetics (e.g., onset of action, half-life), as well as the primary site of metabolism. These characteristics often determine how a particular drug is used clinically and may also play an important role in its abuse potential. A detailed account of the pharmacokinetics of common benzodiazepines is beyond the scope of this chapter. However, some of the key points are outlined below:

- *Onset of action:* Benzodiazepines with a relatively quick onset of action (e.g., midazolam) have an important role in procedural sedation and management of acute anxiety states (e.g., clonazepam, alprazolam). Clinical experience suggests that the benzodiazepines with a more rapid onset of action (e.g., alprazolam, clonazepam) appear to be more likely sought after by those who abuse benzodiazepines as they produce an acute "high," unlike drugs with a slower onset of action (e.g., oxazepam).[74]
- *Half-life:* Benzodiazepines can be divided into three groups based on their half-life. Benzodiazepines with a short half-life (<12 hours) include oxazepam and midazolam. Generally, these drugs have few active metabolites and are metabolized in a manner unaffected by liver disease. Midazolam is used as an anesthetic, given its rapid onset of action and quick clearance, while oxazepam is used for withdrawal management in patients with known hepatic disease. Intermediate-acting benzodiazepines include lorazepam and temazepam (with a half-life between 12 and 24 hours). Long-acting benzodiazepines (with a half-life >24 hours) include most other benzodiazepine compounds, including diazepam and chlordiazepoxide. Most of these drugs demonstrate significant hepatic metabolism, may have active metabolites, and tend to accumulate in tissues. Their long half-lives make these drugs a preferred choice for the management of withdrawal states.[74]
- *Metabolism:* Most benzodiazepines are metabolized through the P450 system, namely the CYP 3A4 and CYP 2C19 enzymes. Drugs that inhibit the CYP 3A4 enzyme (e.g., grapefruit juice, macrolide antibiotics, HIV protease inhibitors) may reduce benzodiazepine metabolism, and thus potentiate the drug's effect and potential toxicity. The inducers of CYP 3A4 (e.g., phenobarbital, phenytoin, carbamazepine) will increase benzodiazepine metabolism and clearance. Lower benzodiazepine doses should be used in patients with known hepatic dysfunction. Lorazepam, oxazepam, and temazepam (easily remembered by the brief mnemonic "OTL," which stands for "outside the liver") avoid first-pass hepatic metabolism. These drugs are less susceptible to CYP interactions and are safer in patients with known hepatic disease.[74]

Psychiatric Sequelae of Benzodiazepine Use

The intended effect of benzodiazepine use is to reduce anxiety, facilitate sleep, or induce sedation. When taken in excess, benzodiazepines may lead to an overdose characterized by CNS depression like that seen with severe alcohol intoxication. Patients typically present with slurred speech, ataxia, confusion (which may lead to belligerence or agitation), and somnolence. Respiratory depression is uncommon with isolated benzodiazepine overdose, although the risk is increased with co-ingestion of other sedatives, including alcohol, and opioids. Severe intoxication may lead to stupor or coma and patients may require intubation for respiratory support. Commonly, patients will have benign vital signs, despite considerable sedation, which may help rule out other life-threatening causes of CNS depression. Toxicologic screening will help differentiate between the toxicity of benzodiazepines and other sedatives, including alcohol, and may help identify potential co-ingestion.

Flumazenil, a specific benzodiazepine antagonist, reverses the life-threatening effects of a benzodiazepine overdose. An initial IV dose of 0.2 mg can be given over 30 seconds, followed by a second 0.2 mg IV dose if there is no response after 45 seconds. This procedure can be repeated at 1-minute intervals up to a cumulative dose of 5 mg. Although readily available, flumazenil is rarely used in clinical practice as it may precipitate seizures in those who are dependent on benzodiazepines or in those taking tricyclic antidepressants (TCAs). Most cases of benzodiazepine intoxication are thus managed through supportive care.

Benzodiazepine Withdrawal Management

Benzodiazepines can produce a state of physiologic dependence, especially when used in high doses for prolonged periods. Up to 45% of patients who receive stable, long-term doses show physiologic evidence of withdrawal with abrupt drug discontinuation. Withdrawal symptoms resemble those seen with alcohol and other sedative-hypnotics and include a state marked by subjective anxiety, irritability, and insomnia. Patients may show vital sign changes consistent with increased autonomic arousal (tachycardia, hypertension) and commonly present with a tremor ("shakes"). In severe cases, patients may develop delirium tremens or have one or more seizures—as both conditions are potentially life-threatening, prompt recognition and treatment of benzodiazepine withdrawal is a clinical priority.

The simplest approach to benzodiazepine detoxification in an outpatient setting is a gradual reduction in dose that may be extended over several weeks or months. This treatment approach is commonly reserved for highly motivated patients and patients without significant concern for misuse or diversion of the medication. When a more rapid inpatient detoxification is required, several options should be considered (e.g., the use of phenobarbital or a longer-acting benzodiazepine or controlled daily dosage reductions of the benzodiazepine at 15%–25% per day). When phenobarbital is utilized, a target serum level of 15 to 30 µg/mL is utilized, with a controlled taper over the course of at least 7 days.

An alternative approach may involve discontinuing the offending benzodiazepine altogether and starting the patient on a taper of a high-potency, longer-lasting benzodiazepine (e.g., clonazepam or diazepam). This strategy is particularly useful for withdrawal from high-potency, intermediate-acting benzodiazepines (e.g., lorazepam). A clonazepam taper may mitigate acute withdrawal symptoms and adequately manage the anxiety that most patients experience with rapid lorazepam discontinuation. Due to observed decreased sensitivity to other benzodiazepines, for alprazolam detoxification, we recommend either the use of a daily controlled taper of alprazolam at no more than 15% daily or detoxification with the use of phenobarbital, as noted above.

Supplemental medication, such as the use of β-adrenergic blockers (propranolol), α-adrenergic agonists (clonidine), and dopamine antagonists, may offer some relief of the subjective complaints, including anxiety and general malaise. These agents should never be utilized as monotherapy for the detoxification of patients from benzodiazepines.

REFERENCES

1. Substance Abuse and Mental Health Services Administration. *Key Substance Use and Mental Health Indicators in the United States: Results From the 2020 National Survey on Drug Use and Health (HHS Publication No. PEP21-07-01-003, NSDUH Series H-56).* Center for Behavioral Health Statistics and Quality, Substance Abuse and Mental Health Services Administration; 2021. Retrieved from https://www.samhsa.gov/data.
2. Substance Abuse and Mental Health Services Administration. *Drug Abuse Warning Network: Findings From Drug-Related Emergency Department Visits, 2021 (HHS Publication No. PEP22-07-03-002).* Center for Behavioral Health Statistics and Quality, Substance Abuse and Mental Health Services Administration; 2022. Retrieved from https://www.samhsa.gov/data/.
3. O'Brien CP, McLellan AT. Myths about the treatment of addiction. *Lancet.* 1996;347:237–240.
4. World Health Organization (WHO). *WHO Global Status Report on Alcohol 2004.* WHO; 2004.
5. Kosten TR, O'Connor PG. Management of drug and alcohol withdrawal. *N Engl J Med.* 2003;348:1786.
6. Harwood H. *Updating Estimates of the Economic Costs of Alcohol Abuse in the United States: Estimates, Update Methods, and Data, NIH Publication no. 00-1583.* National Institute on Alcohol Abuse and Alcoholism; 2000.
7. Sacks JJ, Gonzales KR, Bouchery EE, et al. 2010 National and state costs of excessive alcohol consumption. *Am J Prev Med.* 2015;49(5):e73–e79.
8. Stahre M, Roeber J, Kanny D, et al. Contribution of excessive alcohol consumption to deaths and years of potential life lost in the United States. *Prev Chronic Dis.* 2014;11:E109.
9. Blondell RD, Looney SW, Hottman LW, et al. Characteristics of intoxicated trauma patients. *J Addict Dis.* 2002;21(4):1–12.
10. World Health Organization (WHO). *Global Status Report on Alcohol and Health.* WHO; 2011.
11. Langenbucher J. Rx for health care costs: resolving addictions in the general medical setting. *Alcohol Clin Exp Res.* 1994;18(5):1033–1036.
12. Alaja R, Seppa K. Six-month outcomes of hospital-based psychiatric substance use consultations. *Gen Hosp Psychiatry.* 2003;25(2):103–107.
13. Hillman A, McCann B, Walker NP. Specialist alcohol liaison services in general hospitals improve engagement in alcohol rehabilitation and treatment outcome. *Health Bull (Edinb).* 2001;59(6):420–423.
14. National Institute on Alcohol Abuse and Alcoholism. *Helping Patients Who Drink Too Much: A Clinician's Guide, NIH Publication no. 05-3769.* National Institute on Alcohol Abuse and Alcoholism; 2005.
15. Hasin DS, Stinson FS, Ogburn E, et al. Prevalence, correlates, disability, and comorbidity of DSM-IV alcohol abuse and dependence in the United States: results from the National Epidemiologic Survey on Alcohol and Related Conditions. *Arch Gen Psychiatry.* 2007;64(7):830–842.
16. Maisto SA, Saitz R. Alcohol use disorders: screening and diagnosis. *Am J Addict.* 2003;12(suppl 1):S12–S15.
17. Norberg A, Jones AW, Hahn RG, et al. Role of variability in explaining ethanol pharmacokinetics: research and forensic applications. *Clin Pharmacokinet.* 2003;42(1):1–31.
18. Barnes EW, Cooke NJ, King AJ, et al. Observations on the metabolism of alcohol in man. *Br J Nutr.* 1965;19(4):485–489.

19. Morrow AL, Suzdak PD, Karanian JW, et al. Chronic ethanol administration alters gamma aminobutyric acid, pentobarbital and ethanol-mediated 36Cl-uptake in cerebral cortical synaptoneurosomes. *J Pharmacol Exp Ther.* 1988;246(1):158–164.

20. Hoffman PL, Grant KA, Snell LD, et al. NMDA receptors: role in ethanol withdrawal seizures. *Ann N Y Acad Sci.* 1992;654:52–60.

21. Tsai G, Gastfriend DR, Coyle JT. The glutamatergic basis of human alcoholism. *Am J Psychiatry.* 1995;152(3):332–340.

22. Victor M, Adams RD. The effect of alcohol on the nervous system. *Res Publ Assoc Res Nerv Ment Dis.* 1953;32:526–573.

23. Brust JCM. *Neurological Aspects of Substance Abuse.* Butterworth-Heinemann; 1993.

24. Essardas H, Daryanani FJ, Santolaria E, et al. Alcoholic withdrawal syndrome and seizures. *Alcohol Alcohol.* 1994;29(3):323–328.

25. Ferguson JA, Suelzer CJ, Eckert GJ, et al. Risk factors for delirium tremens development. *J Gen Intern Med.* 1996;11(7):410–414.

26. Cushman P Jr. Delirium tremens: Update on an old disorder. *Postgrad Med.* 1987;82(5):117–122.

27. Schuckit MA, Tipp JE, Reich T, et al. The histories of withdrawal convulsions and delirium tremens in 1648 alcohol dependent subjects. *Addiction.* 1995;90(10):1335–1347.

28. Sullivan JT, Sykora K, Schneiderman J, et al. Assessment of alcohol withdrawal: the revised clinical institute withdrawal assessment for alcohol scale (CIWA-Ar). *Br J Addict.* 1989;84(11):1353–1357.

29. Daeppen JB, Gache P, Landry U, et al. Symptom-triggered vs fixed-schedule doses of benzodiazepine for alcohol withdrawal: a randomized treatment trial. *Arch Int Med.* 2002;162(10):1117–1121.

30. Jaeger TM, Lohr RH, Pankratz VS. Symptom-triggered therapy for alcohol withdrawal syndrome in medical inpatients. *Mayo Clinic Proceed.* 2001;76(7):695–701.

31. Sellers EM, Naranjo CA, Harrison M, et al. Diazepam loading: simplified treatment of alcohol withdrawal. *Clin Pharmacol Ther.* 1983;34(6):822–826.

32. Rosenson J, Clements C, Simon B, et al. Phenobarbital for acute alcohol withdrawal: a prospective randomized double-blind placebo-controlled study. *J Emerg Med.* 2013;44(3):592–598.

33. Nejad S, Nisavic MD, Larentzakis A, et al. Phenobarbital for acute alcohol withdrawal management in surgical trauma patients—a retrospective comparison study. *Psychosomatics.* 2020;61(4):327–335.

34. Nisavic M, Nejad S, Isenberg B, et al. Use of phenobarbital in alcohol withdrawal management—a retrospective comparison study of phenobarbital and benzodiazepines for acute alcohol withdrawal management in general medical patients. *Psychosomatics.* 2019;60(5):458–467.

35. Minozzi S, Amato L, Vecchi S, et al. Anticonvulsants for alcohol withdrawal. *Cochrane Database Syst Rev.* 2010(3):CD005064.

36. Levine AR, Carrasquillo L, Mueller J, et al. High-dose gabapentin for the treatment of severe alcohol withdrawal syndrome: a retrospective cohort analysis. *Pharmacotherapy.* 2019;39(9):881–888.

37. Hodges B, Mazur JE. Intravenous ethanol for the treatment of alcohol withdrawal syndrome in critically ill patients. *Pharmacotherapy.* 2004;24(11):1578–1585.

38. Rayner SG, Weinert CR, Peng H, et al. Dexmedetomidine as adjunct treatment for severe alcohol withdrawal in the ICU. *Ann Intens Care.* 2012;2(1):12.

39. Coomes TR, Smith SW. Successful use of propofol in refractory delirium tremens. *Ann Emerg Med.* 1997;30(6):825–828. 75.

40. Victor M, Adams R, Collins G, et al. *The Wernicke–Korsakoff Syndrome.* FA Davis; 1971.

41. Thomson AD, Cook CC, Touquet R, et al. The Royal College of Physicians report on alcohol: guidelines for managing Wernicke's encephalopathy in the accident and emergency department. *Alcohol.* 2002;37(6):513–521.

42. Sechi GP, Serra A. Wernicke's encephalopathy: new clinical settings and recent advances in diagnosis and management. *Lancet Neurol.* 2007;6(5):442–455.

43. Roberts AJ, McDonald JS, Heyser CJ, et al. mu-Opioid receptor knockout mice do not self-administer alcohol. *J Pharmacol Exp Ther.* 2000;293(3):1002–1008.

44. Jonas DE, Amick HR, Feltner C, et al. Pharmacotherapy for adults with alcohol use disorders in outpatient settings: a systematic review and meta-analysis. *JAMA.* 2014;311(18):1889–1900.

45. Rösner S, Hackl-Herrwerth A, Leucht S, et al. Opioid antagonists for alcohol dependence. *Cochrane Database Syst Rev.* 2010(12):CD001867.

46. Rösner S, Hackl-Herrwerth A, Leucht S, et al. Acamprosate for alcohol dependence. *Cochrane Database Syst Rev.* 2010(9):CD004332.

47. Skradski S, White HS. Topiramate blocks kainate-evoked cobalt influx into cultured neurons. *Epilepsia.* 2000;41(suppl):S45–S47.

48. White HS, Brown SD, Woodhead JH, et al. Topiramate modulates GABA-evoked currents in murine cortical neurons by a nonbenzodiazepine mechanism. *Epilepsia.* 2000;41(suppl 1):S17–S20.

49. Leggio L, Kenna GA, Swift RM. New developments for the pharmacological treatment of alcohol withdrawal syndrome. A focus on nonbenzodiazepine GABAergic medications. *Prog Neuropsychopharmacol Biol Psychiatry.* 2008;32(5):1106–1117.

50. Fleming MF. Brief interventions and the treatment of alcohol use disorders: current evidence. *Recent Dev Alcohol.* 2002;16:375–390.

51. Alaja R, Seppa K. Six-month outcomes of hospital-based psychiatric substance use consultations. *Gen Hosp Psychiatry.* 2003;25(2):103–107.

52. Miller W, Rollnick S. *Motivational Interviewing: Preparing People to Change Addictive Behavior.* Guilford Press; 2001.

53. United Nations Office on Drugs and Crime. World Drug Report 2015. United Nations Publication Sales No. E.15.XI.6. 2015.

54. U.S. Department of Health and Human Services, Substance Abuse and Mental Health Services Administration, Center for Behavioral Health Statistics and Quality: Drug Abuse Warning Network. National Estimates of Drug-Related Emergency Department Visits. Available at Visits https://www.samhsa.gov/data/sites/default/files/DAWN2k11ED/DAWN2k11ED/DAWN2k11ED.pdf; 2011.

55. Howell LL, Kimmel HL. Monoamine transporters and psychostimulant addiction. *Biochem Pharmacol.* 2008;75(1):196–217.

56. Dackis CA, O'Brien CP. Cocaine dependence: a disease of the brain's reward centers. *J Subst Abuse Treat.* 2001;21(3):111–117.

57. Mariani JJ, Pavlicova M, Bisaga A, et al. Extended-release mixed amphetamine salts and topiramate for cocaine dependence: a randomized controlled trial. *Biol Psychiatry.* 2012;72(11):950–956.

58. Johnson BA, Wang XQ, Penberthy JK, et al. Topiramate for the treatment of cocaine addiction: a randomized clinical trial. *JAMA Psychiatry.* 2013;70(12):1338–1346.

59. Rawson R, Shoptaw SJ, Obert JL, et al. An intensive outpatient approach for cocaine abuse: the matrix model. *J Subst Abuse Treat.* 1995;12(2):117–127.

60. Barr AM, Panenka WJ, MacEwan GW, et al. The need for speed: an update on methamphetamine addiction. *J Psychiatry Neurosci.* 2006;31(5):301–313.

61. Salo R, Flower K, Kielstei A, et al. Psychiatric comorbidity in methamphetamine dependence. *Psychiatry Res.* 2011;186(2,3):356–361.

62. Colfax GN, Santos GM, Das M, et al. Mirtazapine to reduce methamphetamine use: a randomized controlled trial. *Arch Gen Psychiatry.* 2011;68(11):1168–1175.

63. Fantegrossi WE, Murnane KS, Reissig CJ. The behavioral pharmacology of hallucinogens. *Biochem Pharmacol.* 2008;75(1):17–33.

64. World Health Organization. Management of Substance Abuse—Cannabis. Available at: http://www.who.int/substance_abuse/facts/cannabis/en/.

65. Centers for Disease Control and Prevention Reported US AIDS cases by HIV-exposure category—1994. *MMWR.* 1995;44:4.

66. Substance Abuse and Mental Health Services Administration. Center for Behavioral Health Statistics and Quality. *Drug Abuse Warning Network, 2008: National Estimates of Drug-Related Emergency Department Visits, HHS Publication No. SMA 11-4618.* HHS; 2011.

67. Waldhoer M, Bartlett SE, Whistler JL. Opioid receptors. *Annu Rev Biochem.* 2004;73:953–990.

68. Gibson A, Degenhardt L, Mattick RP, et al. Exposure to opioid maintenance treatment reduces long-term mortality. *Addiction.* 2008;103(3):462–468.

69. Mattick RP, Breen C, Kimber J, et al. Methadone maintenance therapy versus no opioid replacement therapy for opioid dependence. *Cochrane Database Syst Rev.* 2009;(3):CD002209.

70. Ling W, Charuvastra C, Collins JF, et al. Buprenorphine maintenance treatment of opiate dependence: a multicenter, randomized clinical trial. *Addiction.* 1998;93(4):475–486.

71. Mattick RP, Breen C, Kimber J, et al. Buprenorphine maintenance versus placebo or methadone maintenance for opioid dependence. *Cochrane Database Syst Rev.* 2014;(2):CD002207.

72. Fudala PJ, Bridge TP, Herbert S, et al. Office-based treatment of opiate addiction with a sublingual-tablet formulation of buprenorphine and naloxone. *N Engl J Med.* 2003;349(10):949–958.

73. Liebschutz JM, Crooks D, Herman D, et al. Buprenorphine treatment for hospitalized, opioid-dependent patients: a randomized clinical trial. *JAMA Intern Med.* 2014;174(8):1369–1376.

74. Greenblatt DJ, Shader RI, Divoll M, et al. Benzodiazepines: a summary of pharmacokinetic properties. *Br J Clin Pharmacol.* 1981;11(suppl 1):11S–16S.

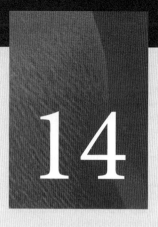

14

SOMATIC SYMPTOM AND RELATED DISORDERS AND FUNCTIONAL SOMATIC SYNDROMES

ALEJANDRA ELIZABETH MORFIN RODRIGUEZ, MD ■ SCOTT R. BEACH, MD ■ NICHOLAS KONTOS, MD ■ FELICIA A. SMITH, MD ■ DONNA B. GREENBERG, MD

OVERVIEW

Somatic symptom and related disorders is one of many terms applied to somatic medical concerns that do not present "as advertised." Other terms that have been utilized over the years include psychosomatic illness, medically unexplained symptoms (MUS), symptoms of unknown origin, and abnormal illness behaviors. Borrowing and extending from Barsky, *symptom amplification* will be used as an umbrella term for this phenomenon.[1] This chapter focuses on somatic symptom and related disorders as well as functional somatic syndromes; deception syndromes are covered in a separate chapter.

Roughly 60% to 80% of the American population experience a somatic symptom in any given week.[2] Many of these individuals do not bring their complaints to the medical system, but those who do present to doctors account for more than half of all ambulatory visits. Only a small minority of them are found to have a clear etiology for their complaints. Among the remainder, only a fraction prove to be diagnostically significant symptom amplifiers. However, given the huge denominator, this fraction accounts for 10% to 24% of outpatient visits and may represent the most frequent form of psychopathology seen by primary care providers (PCPs).[3] Whether this group is better accounted for by primary symptom amplification or by a mood, anxiety disorder, or personality disorder is a matter of debate.[3-5]

The Diagnostic and Statistical Manual of Mental Disorders, Fifth Edition (DSM-5), now updated to the *DSM-5-Text Revision* (DSM-5-TR), changed the classification of these disorders since the existing diagnoses contained redundancies, the prototypical disorder of the previous category (somatization disorder) did not capture many of the patients of concern, and because these patients are most often seen by non-psychiatrists who were generally unfamiliar with the DSM-IV diagnoses.[6] Given the dynamic nature of the field and the ubiquity of somatic symptoms, many other classification systems emerged, each of which was unified by the intent to make the categorization more useful for patients and doctors while maintaining scientific validity.[7] This chapter provides a general overview of the psychosomatic disorders, explores the shared parameters of these diagnoses, and delves deeper into the DSM-5-TR diagnoses of somatic symptom disorder (SSD), illness anxiety disorder (IAD), functional neurological disorder (FND)/conversion disorder, and psychological factors affecting medical illness. This chapter also touches on the most common functional somatic syndromes (e.g., irritable bowel syndrome [IBS], fibromyalgia [FM], and chronic fatigue syndrome [CFS]).

Case 1

A 46-year-old woman with a psychiatric history of generalized anxiety disorder (GAD) and post-traumatic stress disorder and no significant past medical history presented to her PCP with somatic symptoms. She reported intermittent gastrointestinal (GI) symptoms, tingling in her right arm, and headaches that interfered with her day-to-day life. She had been unemployed and received disability benefits due to her persistent physical symptoms. She had presented to the emergency department three times during the last month for shortness of breath, lightheadedness, and tingling in her fingertips. Each time, the work-up was unremarkable, and multiple treatments failed to relieve her symptoms. She was sent home with reassurance and a recommendation to follow up with her PCP. She worried that her symptoms represented a catastrophic medical event. Multiple antidepressant trials were discontinued due to her inability to tolerate even initial doses. She was taking brand name sertraline (12.5 mg), as she reported intolerable nausea, diarrhea, and "zapping" sensations in her neck that resolved immediately after starting the brand name drug. She hoped to see several specialists, including an allergist, pharmacist, and a neurologist, for the work-up of her persistent physical symptoms.

SOMATIC SYMPTOM AND RELATED DISORDERS

In the DSM-5-TR, the term "somatization" is no longer used, in part because many general medical problems (not to mention nearly all psychiatric ones) are poorly understood from an "organic" perspective. Instead, the crux of dysfunction from this condition lies in the *amplification* of the experience or the functional limitations caused by somatic symptoms.[5]

In addition to the DSM-5-TR-acknowledged diagnoses, other common functional somatic syndromes include IBS, FM, and CFS/myalgic encephalitis. These entities share many features with the somatic symptom and related disorders and will be addressed separately below.

SHARED PARAMETERS OF PSYCHOSOMATIC CONDITIONS

In somatic symptom and related disorders (excluding psychological factors affecting medical illness, where

unexplained symptoms are not manifested), functional somatic syndromes, as well as factitious disorder and malingering (see Chapter 15), symptoms are depicted according to how they fall along the parameters discussed below. Each parameter is non-binary, such that most boxes in Fig. 14.1 are, quite literally, "shades of gray." Breaking down these presentations in this manner offers coherence to disparate categories that only share the vague quality of having a somatic focus. The figure and corresponding discussion are not a diagnostic schema but instead a way of thinking about what is going on in these complex conditions.

Manifestations

Diseases are revealed to physicians through symptoms and/or signs. *Symptoms* are "any morbid phenomenon... *experienced by the patient* and indicative of disease." *Signs* are "*discoverable on examination of the patient.*"[8] Both occur together frequently, and the line between the two is not always clear.

Many diseases are discoverable only by their signs. These may be due to the nature of the disease (e.g., early stages of hypertension) or the patient's temperament and culture (e.g., a thigh melanoma evaluated by an allopathic physician once it interfered with walking).[9] SSD, IAD, and the functional somatic symptoms (FSS) all involve amplification or fear of symptoms that are insufficiently associated with signs and diagnostic test results. Patients with FSS also exhibit abnormal illness behavior, although this may represent a self-selected or even iatrogenic majority of those for whom a diagnosis is made or extracted.[5]

Symptoms may be significant in FND (N.B.: the less-preferred name, conversion disorder, remains "officially" allowable), but the diagnosis itself is dependent upon neurologic signs. With sensory manifestations of FND, the distinction between symptoms and signs can be especially blurry. However, these patients do not merely complain of blindness, numbness, or weakness; they are presumed to "have" them. While FND's signs may not come "as advertised" (e.g., they are inconsistent across time or circumstance and lack an anatomically coherent distribution), they should be discernible on examination or observation in the absence of patient commentary.[10]

Most instances of factitious disorder involve self-inflicted disease. As such, factitious disorder is usually

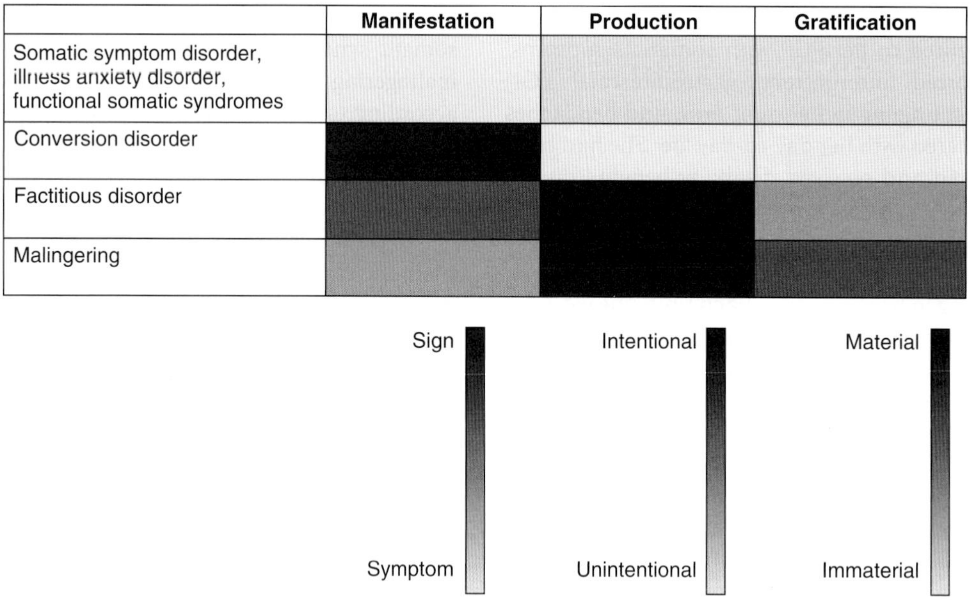

	Manifestation	Production	Gratification
Somatic symptom disorder, illness anxiety disorder, functional somatic syndromes			
Conversion disorder			
Factitious disorder			
Malingering			

Sign — Symptom | Intentional — Unintentional | Material — Immaterial

Fig. 14.1 ■ Three parameters of somatically focused syndromes.

manifested by signs of disease (such as sepsis, hypo-glycemia, and anemia). However, this manner of presentation is likely preceded and/or overlapped by more subtle, undetected phases of elaboration and symptom fabrication without actual physical morbidity.[11] The opposite seems to be the case in malingering, with symptom fabrication being seen more often than sign induction.

Production

The historical influence of psychodynamic theory on psychosomatic medicine leads to terms such as "somatizing" and "conversion" that imply an unconscious transformation of psychological states into physical ones. Cognitive-behavioral models also involve automatic processes that are outside of the patient's awareness. It is more inclusive to describe the manifestations of somatically focused conditions as being on a spectrum of intentionality.

Patients with SSD, IAD, and the FSS are genuine in their identification of the symptoms of which they complain. That these symptoms seem exaggerated might speak to their perceived severity, to the desperation of those who fear that doctors do not take them seriously, or to the intentional exaggeration of distress. The signs of FND are similarly unintentionally produced.

Intentionality and lying are at the heart of the production of signs and symptoms in factitious disorder and malingering. Thus, in the production column they receive the darkest squares in the table. The intentional deception lies in *how* the patient became septic. When symptoms are intentionally falsified, the patient's untrue medical statements are simply called *lying*.

Gratification

Primary and *secondary gain* are sometimes used to describe how the production of symptoms and signs satisfies patients' needs. Secondary gain refers to the gratification derived from tangible items (e.g., for food, shelter, money, illicit substances) or to the items themselves. Primary gain refers to gratification derived from the relief of intrapsychic tension,[12] or to the means used to relieve that tension (sometimes referred to as the "assumption of the sick role").

Privileges of the sick role include blamelessness for the products of sickness, relief from duties that are incompatible with the sickness, and entitlement to care.[13] The psychological benefits of blamelessness, relief, and care for those feeling unworthy, belea-guered, and/or unloved bring some clarity to the nebulous concept of primary gain. Of course, blame-lessness and legal culpability, relief and disability payments, and care and shelter can bleed into one another, reminding us that the distinction between primary and secondary gains, beyond the outer mar-gins, is unsubstantiated.[11]

When it comes to gratification, SSD, IAD, and FSS cluster together, with immaterial sick role privi-leges seeming to dominate. Sick role status depends on social and medical validation of one's sickness. This contingent aspect of sick role privileges may par-tially explain the desperate, sometimes hostile, way that these individuals pursue or cling to the medical legitimacy of their distress. These efforts to legitimize distress can eclipse patients' stated desires for relief, possibly explaining findings such as a diminished pla-cebo response and the powerful negative prognostic effect of support group participation for those with CFS.[14] In the age of social media, this dynamic plays out in the form of followers and likes.

Patients with FSS, SSD, or IAD may eventually bring disability paperwork or other requests to be excused medically to their doctors, but these are secondary pursuits. They straddle the types of gratification delin-eated here. Similarly, depending on one's belief in and "discovery" of a trigger (e.g., an impending divorce hearing, an unacceptable revenge fantasy), it can be difficult to determine the reason behind which type of gratification the signs of conversion disorder are mobilized.

The nature and similarity of the gratifications inherent to SSD, IAD, FSS, and FND can inform treat-ment. Sick role privileges are balanced by a duty to pursue health. Claiming sick role privileges without accepting this duty may be the shared characteristic of "heartsink patients."[15] The idea of bringing a patient's duty into the picture allows for communication and limit setting that embraces, rather than challenges, the patient's sick role status, hinges it on healthier behav-ior, and reins in what patients can expect from physi-cians (and others).

For the deception syndromes, this rationale falls apart, since these patients pursue their sick role status disingenuously. If the difference between immaterial/primary and material/secondary gain is sufficiently blurred, and if this is the main distinguishing char-acteristic between factitious disorder and malinger-ing, then there are two superficial possibilities. One extends the disorder status of factitious disorder to malingering; the other extends the quasi-criminal status of malingering to factitious disorder. Instead, both conditions might be better understood as behav-iors that arise and distract from broader problems. For example, malingering can be part of the broader patterns of non-pathologic criminality, sociopathy, or desperation; factitious disorder can be viewed as mal-adaptive management of attachments in those with borderline or other character disorders.[11]

GENERAL PRINCIPLES IN THE TREATMENT OF SOMATIC SYMPTOM DISORDERS

The first consideration in any medical treatment is making the right diagnosis. Since patients may seek care in different places and physicians may lack access to (due to time or the disinclination to scrutinize) the medical history, the pattern of maladaptive illness behavior may go unrecognized, and the diagnosis can be delayed. Legwork to obtain or review records and to talk with the patient about their past may be necessary to reveal a longitudinal pattern. It is only when physi-cians know the medical data that they can offer clari-fication. The way in which a patient adapts to illness and the way they experience pain or other symptoms often begins early in life, sometimes with a traumatic context.[5]

Whether the symptom is fatigue or pain, it is best to treat co-morbid depression and, anxiety, and to be mindful about how patients use or misuse addictive medications, as such use can adversely affect symp-tom burden. Patients should be told that the goal of treatment is to achieve better functioning rather than to relieve all symptoms. The capacity of the patient to function despite their symptoms and re-engage in physical and social activities is an important dimen-sion. Listening to what a patient believes about their symptoms and what makes them mad, sad, or scared gives them comfort and respect and affords them with a sense of ownership. Power is in the details of knowing what makes them overdo and what makes them avoid activities.[16]

Somatic Symptom Disorder

Somatic symptom disorder (SSD) is the prototypical diagnosis of the category that bears its name. SSD, as defined by the DSM-5-TR, requires only one or more persistent (>6 months) symptoms that form the focus of the patient's excessive thoughts, feelings, and behaviors, regardless of the presence or absence of an explanatory medical diagnosis. The patient with SSD manifests preoccupations, anxiety, and time and energy that is devoted to their symptom(s) that are disproportionate to their severity as determined by providers.[6]

Many theories have attempted to explain the abnormal illness behaviors experienced by these patients, including their mismanagement of the "sick role." A major component of Parsons' sociologic conceptualization of the sick role was that the sick person justly acquires a degree of blamelessness for their symptoms, relief from duties incompatible with their malady, and an entitlement to care; these are balanced by an obligation to pursue health with the help of one's providers. When one considers the plight of the guilt-ridden, over-burdened, and unloved person, sickness can be "one-stop-shopping" from a primary gain point of view. From that same sociologic view, the pathology of SSD is a desperate clinging to the benefits of the sick role without fulfillment of the duty, that, along with sickness, purchases those benefits. This imbalance may be the cause of the variable consternation and desperate indulgence that many providers and family members exhibit toward the patient with SSD.[3,13,17,18]

Theories about SSD exist in proportion to "schools" of psychiatry; they cannot be given full justice here. Psychodynamic theories, originating in conversion hysteria, tend to hinge on defense mechanisms that "convert" unbearable or unacceptable feelings and impulses into bodily sensations. Originally coined by Nemiah, alexithymia is an explanation for why patients who are unable to recognize and describe their own emotions might instead experience them somatically.[19–21] Neural circuit framework studies have sought to explain symptom amplification and identified the associated elements of amplification as a hypervigilance to bodily sensations, the focus given to frequent but weak sensations, and the ability to react to these sensations with affective and cognitive interpretations of danger or alarm. The neural circuit framework

studies have identified neurological correlates for regions in the brain involved in bodily sensation hypervigilance as well as the parallel under-processing of affective information, suggesting a model driven by stress-mediated neuroplastic changes.[20]

In parallel with this theory, a cognitive model developed while studying symptom-amplifying patients is still applicable. Here, the patient is someone who, already having a low threshold for the detection of bodily sensations and variations, applies medical significance to those sensations, and behaves accordingly. This behavior often includes limiting activities and seeking medical validation relentlessly (and usually unsuccessfully) for functionally meaningful relief of their suffering.[1,5,22] This mechanism is borne out by studies of the cognitive biases about health found in symptom-amplifying patients[5,23–25] and overlaps with biological theories as represented by studies of the phenomenon of central sensitization.[26]

Prevalence data regarding SSD remain limited. The prevalence, based on self-reporting, is thought to be between 6.7% and 17.4% in the general population and 35% in general medical patients. In one study, 45.5% of patients with MUS in primary care settings met the criteria for SSD.[18,27] In a population-based study, those with an existing diagnosis of a physical condition scored higher than those in the general population on the Somatic Symptom Disorder B Criteria Scale (SSD-12). In small studies that focus on patients with FM or congestive heart failure, 25.6% and 18.5% of patients, respectively, met the criteria for SSD.[27,28] DSM-5 field trials found that 7% of the general population would meet the criteria for SSD.[29] SSD is more common among females, those with little education, low socio-economic status, older age, unemployment, a recent stressful life event, concurrent psychiatric or medical illnesses, and high neuroticism. Studies have indicated that SSD persists for at least 4 years in nearly one-third of patients.[4,6,30,31]

Treatment of Somatic Symptom Disorder

Approaches to the management of SSD focus on optimizing function, coping with symptoms, and avoiding false dichotomies between the "mind and body."[16] The management of SSD is best carried out by PCPs according to a conservative plan that is based upon being a consistent care provider, preventing unnecessary or dangerous medical procedures, and asking in a supportive manner about the stress in the patient's life. The last occurs during the physical examination, without inferring with or implying that the "real" cause for the patient's somatic complaints is psychosocial stress (which is what most investigators believe). The basic goal is to help the patient cope with the symptoms rather than to eliminate them completely.[16,32]

One strategy includes providing opinions of specialists regarding treatment recommendations in a letter to the PCPs of those with SSD, although this has not improved symptom severity or outcomes.[33] In addition, it is useful to have regularly scheduled appointments (e.g., every 4–6 weeks); a physical examination performed at each visit to look for disease; the avoidance of hospitalization, diagnostic procedures, surgery, and the use of laboratory assessments, unless clearly indicated; and not telling patients, "It's all in your head," with concurrent psychosocial assessments screening for co-morbid psychiatric disorders.[16,32] Some evidence suggests that the longer people go with an untreated somatic disorder, the more pervasive their symptoms are likely to become, and the less likely their symptoms are to remit.[30] Physicians can help their patients work within a treatment model that is at worst considered palliative, and at best considered the same as it is for any other chronic disease. Further, it is important to note that patients with SSD must be worked up appropriately when new symptoms arise, as they are not immune to developing more illnesses; co-morbid medical conditions should be addressed promptly.[5]

Cognitive-behavioral therapy (CBT), delivered in the primary care setting or via the internet, can help to identify and re-structure cognitive distortions, unrealistic dysfunctional beliefs, worries, and behaviors that drive many of these disorders. CBT can reduce symptoms and lower healthcare costs. Short-term psychodynamic psychotherapy has a moderate empirical base to support its use in SSD and multiple studies demonstrate significant and sustained benefits; several studies suggest that treated patients may have fewer physician visits and hospital use. Mindfulness-based therapies and internet-based emotional awareness and expression therapy have also been helpful.[4,30,32,34,35]

There is evidence for antidepressant medications in SSD even when patients do not meet the criteria for a co-morbid psychiatric disorder, especially in patients who present with pain, with a possible role for low-dose atypical antipsychotics in reducing distress. For those who meet the criteria for a psychiatric disorder, medications should be continued for at least a year after remission has been achieved. Repetitive transcranial magnetic stimulation has also improved SSD in patients with co-morbid depression.[27,32,36]

Illness Anxiety Disorder

Whereas patients with SSD are more preoccupied with symptoms than with the meaning of them, those with IAD are preoccupied with the idea of having or contracting a major illness. These patients may not have active symptoms, and instead beset providers with requests for screening tests such as "full-body scans." Alternatively, someone with IAD may avoid the healthcare system altogether, afraid of finding something that they do not wish to know. Thus the DSM-5-TR divides IAD into "care-seeking" and "care-avoidant" types.[6] In addition, repeated health-related internet searches for possible illnesses can be a manifestation of IAD in the age of the internet (i.e., cyberchondria).[37] Overall, those with IAD are thought to account for 2% to 13% of the general population.[22]

Extrapolating from studies of hypochondriasis, patients with IAD hold to a "restrictive concept of good health," as evidenced by their responses on rating scales, such as the Health Norms Sorting Task, which asks if a person could be considered "healthy" while experiencing a variety of different somatic sensations. As with SSD, many schools of thought exist regarding the etiology, including a cognitive model that likens IAD to obsessive-compulsive disorder (OCD). Analogous features include the repeated intrusive nature of the thoughts, the compulsive need to seek care, the performance of health rituals, and the affiliated significant level of health-related distress.[4,22,23]

Although research is limited, IAD typically begins in early to middle adulthood, and it has a fluctuating course. Notably, IAD is highly co-morbid with GAD, panic disorder, OCD, and major depressive disorder (MDD). As with any illness beliefs and behaviors, the patient's cultural and familial upbringing will have had a major influence, and (as with all SSDs) it is worth asking about family illness experiences/models, particularly in childhood.[22] Notably, pediatric clinics are seeing IAD rates rise in children after the COVID-19 pandemic.[38] IAD is a chronic condition, but its prognosis tends to be better in those with a high level of baseline function, a shorter duration of illness, and psychiatric treatment. Factors associated with a chronic course are severe symptoms, functional impairment, childhood physical punishment, a longer duration of illness, and being more harm-avoidant and less cooperative.[22]

Treatment of Illness Anxiety Disorder

IAD can be a chronic and disabling disease. When confronted with IAD, a treater's first step should be to screen for co-morbid affective and anxiety disorders (including OCD). These are likely easier to treat, and their resolution may diminish or bring an end to exaggerated disease fears. Isolated IAD is more difficult to cure.

Three randomized, double-blind, placebo-controlled trials of medication in IAD have demonstrated efficacy for fluoxetine and paroxetine. Sixty percent of patients with IAD no longer met criteria at 8 to 9 years following treatment with selective serotonin reuptake inhibitors (SSRIs), and remission rates have been demonstrated in up to 80%. The combination of SSRIs and CBT has been particularly effective.[22]

Cognitive, behavioral, and educational interventions are also successful. The treatment combination of PCP education and time-limited CBT improves a range of symptoms, with a modest treatment effect. The manualized treatment targets cognitive and perceptual mechanisms of illness, including *hypervigilance* to visceral experience; *beliefs* about symptom etiology; the *context* in which the hypochondriasis occurs; sick role *behaviors*; and *mood*. Randomized controlled trials (RCTs) have shown the benefits of individual, group-based, and internet-based CBT, as well as mindfulness-based interventions.[22]

Patients with IAD tax PCPs. Such patients are difficult to reassure; their care is both time-consuming and expensive and they often provoke strong negative reactions in their frustrated providers. Psychiatrists can be instrumental in easing anxieties and offering management recommendations. The goals of PCPs treating patients with IAD should be threefold: to avoid unnecessary diagnostic tests and obviate overly aggressive medical and surgical intervention; to help a patient tolerate the symptoms rather than strive to eliminate them; and to build a durable doctor-patient relationship based on the physician's interest in the patient as a person and not just in their symptoms. Once a physician views his or her task as palliative, rather than curative, the doctor-patient relationship becomes less contentious and adversarial. Further, patients are more likely to loosen their grip on their concerns when they feel that the physician has acknowledged and accepted their symptoms as "real."[16,22,32]

Several practical measures may be helpful. Physicians can forge a personal connection with their patients by paying attention to their social history and by complimenting the patients on their ability to persevere despite tremendous discomfort. Rather than providing as-needed appointments, physicians can schedule meetings at regular intervals, thereby decoupling professional attention from symptom severity. Patients with IAD tend to develop iatrogenic complications and treatment side effects. This has given rise to the clinical maxim, "Don't just do something, stand there." In other words, the best medical interventions are modest, simple, and benign.

Functional Neurological Disorder (FND)/ Conversion Disorder

FND/conversion disorder involves a loss or change in sensory or motor function that is suggestive of a physical disorder, lacks physical findings consistent with having a known neurological or medical condition, and causes significant functional impairment as well as distress. The diagnosis can be specified by symptom type, persistence (acute and self-limiting versus chronic), and whether it occurs with or without a psychological stressor. The DSM-5-TR accounts for non-neurologic presentations, such as pseudocyesis, separately under the heading "Other Specified Somatic Symptom and Related Disorders."[6]

As with other SSDs, incompatibility between signs and the examination, laboratory tests, or radiologic findings does not necessarily mean the absence of abnormality. The best example of this point is the overrepresentation of psychogenic non-epileptic seizures

(PNES) among patients with electrographic evidence of epileptic seizures. FND can also manifest as a reduced or absent skin sensation, blindness, aphonia, weakness, paralysis, tremors, dystonic movements, gait abnormalities, or abnormal limb posturing.[10]

FND is a "rule in" diagnosis that can only be made after a thorough physical and neurological assessment. The diagnosis considers the full clinical picture with special consideration given to validated signs that have high diagnostic sensitivity for FND. At the center of these physical examination signs is the incompatibility with pathology and the tested function. Some examples of clinical examination findings include Hoover sign (hip weakness that improves with engagement of the contralateral leg), hip abductor sign (abductor weakness that improves with engagement of the contralateral side), tubular visual field for visual impairments, and motor inconsistency (e.g., eliciting physical signs that become positive or negative when tested in a different way). In the case of seizures, or PNES, the following signs are more consistent with non-epileptic seizures: tight eye closure, tearfulness, ictal crying (although this may also indicate dacrystic seizures), pelvic thrusting and dyssynchronous arm movements (though these may be present in certain frontal lobe seizures), and a memory of the seemingly generalized event.

In FND, unintentional production is assumed, and if feigning is suspected strongly enough, the likely diagnosis shifts to factitious disorder or malingering, although the latter is no longer an exclusion for FND.[10]

Outdated presumptions about proximate stressors being causal run counter to the longitudinal course of FND. Often, FND does *not* follow a stressor-conversion-relaxation-resolution pattern. Instead, FND frequently follows a relapsing-remitting or chronic course, which may vary depending on the type of presentation. For example, unilateral sensory and motor signs may persist for several years in most hospitalized neurological patients. The frequency/presence of PNES similarly waxes and wanes in many patients.[39]

Often referred to as "functional" deficits, the signs seen in FND ought to be considered as misunderstood rather than as misleading. The original historic meaning of "functional" in medicine meant hidden or physiologic, as distinguished from visible, anatomic disease. The physiologic underpinnings of conversion disorder remain "hidden," and are difficult to study

given their protean nature (e.g., should FND patients with blindness, hemiparesis, and PNES be grouped together in the same study?). Still, the literature suggests abnormal recruitment and connectivity between brain areas involved in arousal, planning, and execution of movements. Thought to represent disruptions in self-monitoring, attention, emotional processing, and agency, these findings may also reflect the pathophysiologic underpinnings of the association between FND and trauma.[21]

FND is more common in females than in males. The age of onset is variable across most of the life span and across different manifestations of the illness. Its incidence is estimated at 4 to 12 per 100,000, with movement disorders and seizures being the most common manifestations. PNES may peak in the third decade, and motor signs may peak in the fourth decade.[10]

Prognosis and Treatment of FND

The literature supports a mixed outlook for patients with FND. Potential positive prognostic factors include a short duration of symptoms and the absence of psychiatric co-morbidities, whereas co-morbid chronic pain disorders and severe disability are poor prognostic indicators.[10] While 50% of patients may resolve their symptoms during hospitalization, a fraction of these patients develop recurrent conversion symptoms (20%–25% within 1 year). Unilateral functional weakness or sensory disturbance diagnosed in hospitalized neurological patients persisted in more than 80% (of 42 patients over a median of 12.5 years).[40] Patients with one conversion symptom may also develop other forms of somatization.

Treatment begins with education. Guidelines for presenting a diagnosis of FND to patients have been developed. These include naming the condition, emphasizing that it is common, acknowledging disability, reassuring patients that they are not faking, and explaining that symptoms appear to be related to dysfunction of the neurologic system rather than to structural problems. Like any diagnosis, patients may have a broad range of reactions to hearing the news and many may have trouble accepting the diagnosis altogether. In these cases, it is best to avoid confronting or trying to convince the patient, rather than continuing to engage them in treatment planning and education. The historical use of the suggestion that symptoms will gradually improve over time is no longer a cornerstone of the education model.[41]

Physical therapy (PT), occupational therapy (OT), and speech-language pathology therapy have adapted treatment approaches when treating patients with FND with a focus on re-training patients to have volitional control over motor movements while avoiding de-conditioning and helping to identify patterns of symptom exacerbations. Consensus recommendations exist for PT and OT for FND.[42]

Psychotherapy in many of its forms has also been studied for FND. While both psychodynamic psychotherapy and CBT have been used, more research is needed to better understand how to pair a specific psychotherapy modality with a patient's presentation. A meta-analysis suggested that limitations in the literature include a lack of high-quality controlled trials of psychodynamic therapy and a lack of long-term follow-up data in most CBT trials.[35]

Psychotherapy requires significant patient engagement and willingness to discuss not only their symptoms but also the impact of their symptoms on their life and vice versa. When broaching the topic of therapy, it is useful to discuss the role that emotions and recent psychosocial stressors can have on symptom development and progression. An approach acceptable to some individuals has been to say that the body, mysterious in many ways, can be smarter than we are; it may tell us something is wrong before we realize we need help. When the stress in our lives becomes excessive, especially when our nature is to overlook problems or to grit our teeth and prevail, our body, by its symptoms, may blow the "time-out" whistle, forcing us to stop, rest, and get help. This approach invites patients to gain greater insight.

In general, medications are not used to treat FND; however, all co-morbid medical and psychiatric disorders should be treated with medications, as appropriate. Like all other psychosomatic conditions, a designated physician should coordinate care and evaluate all treatment strategies/and the need for additional work-ups.[10]

Psychological Factors Affecting Medical Illness

This diagnosis refers to behaviors that are adversely affecting the course or treatment of a conventionally defined and diagnosed medical condition. Psychological factors affecting medical illness exist in a range of severity from "mild" (i.e., increasing risk) to "extreme" (i.e., causing life-threatening risk), and encompass any psychological state or personality trait (aside from those associated with a distinct psychiatric co-morbidity). It could be said that just about all of us have this condition since almost none of us refrains from all behaviors detrimental to health. Perhaps conspicuously, this "diagnosis" does not end in the word "disorder."[6]

PSYCHIATRIC DIFFERENTIAL DIAGNOSIS

Depressive Disorders

The first consideration in patients with physical symptoms that seem out of proportion to objective findings is depression. MDD has a somatic dimension, and everything hurts more in the setting of depression.

Indeed, 75% of patients seen in primary care with MDD or panic disorder seek treatment exclusively for somatic symptoms (e.g., insomnia, fatigue, anorexia, and weight loss). Depressed patients report more functional somatic symptoms (e.g., aches, pains, constipation, dizziness) than other patients. Among primary care patients, disabling chronic pain was present in 41% of those with MDD compared with 10% of those without MDD.[18,27,31] Those patients with both chronic pain and MDD tended to have more severe affective symptoms and a higher prevalence of panic disorder. Even across cultures, most patients with MDD spontaneously report only somatic symptoms; when pressed, however, 89% also offer psychological symptoms.[32]

When MDD is diagnosed in the context of unexplained bodily complaints, depression should be treated. Both affective and somatic symptoms abate with systematic antidepressant treatment. Of course, MDD (as well as GAD) is also a major co-morbidity of SSDs, seemingly present in most of these patients.[4,5,32] One must also be on guard against the false hope that "if I just treat the depression, the 'somatizing' will disappear." Further, MDD can be difficult to diagnose in patients prone to amplified experiences and somatic symptoms. There is reason to believe they may also be prone to amplify certain psychological "symptoms."[5]

Anxiety Disorders

Anxiety frequently co-occurs with functional somatic symptoms, and anxious patients tend to catastrophize normal physiologic sensations and ailments, commonly overlapping with the aforementioned misinterpretation of body signals as alarming.[22] Many of the symptoms of panic disorder are somatic; they include dyspnea, palpitations, chest pain, choking, dizziness, paresthesia, hot and cold flashes, sweating, faintness, and trembling. As a result, patients during a panic attack may feel that they are unable to breathe or that they are dying. Patients with panic disorder may focus on the most prominent symptom and find the appropriate subspecialist; therefore, patients with MUS and panic disorder present with chest pain to cardiology, nausea or diarrhea to gastroenterology, and dizziness to neurology.[5,23] Anxiety is also one of the most common features of MDD.[6] In addition, given that the thoughts and behaviors in somatic symptom and related disorders can have an intrusive quality as well as involving ritualistic behaviors, OCD must also be considered.[22]

When co-morbid with pain, anxiety can lower the pain threshold. In fact, some patients cannot distinguish anxiety from pain ("No, I am not frightened; I hurt!"). Pleas for pain relief may be related to anxiety rather than addiction or the neediness associated with a personality disorder.

Substance Use Disorders

Physicians should always consider the diagnosis of substance use disorders (SUDs) in a patient with multiple, vague, somatic symptoms. Whether the patient consciously conceals substance use or fails to make the connection, the diagnosis may be elusive. Information from the patient's family may help ("What he calls headache and chest pains, doctor, I call a hangover."). Because substance use systematically disrupts sleep, patients may begin misusing prescribed substances. Insomnia, morning cough, pains in the extremities, dysesthesias, palpitations, headache, GI symptoms, fatigue, bruises—none are strangers to the patient with a SUD.

Psychotic Disorders

Sometimes a somatic complaint has the rigid, stereotyped character of a delusion and is seen in a patient with a psychotic disorder. Here, the key is to consider a psychotic disorder as a possibility with the benefit of a more complete mental status examination and history. Patients with psychotic depression may have nihilistic somatic delusions (such as the conviction that one's abdominal organs are decomposing).

Delusional disorder of the somatic type presents a diagnostic challenge, since the delusions of delusional disorder are, by definition, non-bizarre, at least insofar as they follow the laws of biology and physics. Patients with a delusional disorder of the somatic type tend to be more circumscribed about the nature of their medical complaint, even as its consequences increasingly consume their lives.

In contrast to delusional disorder, the somatic delusions of schizophrenia are generally so bizarre and idiosyncratic (e.g., that foreign bodies are inside an organ or orifice, that body parts are missing or deformed, or that a more mundane somatic issue is being caused by other parties at a distance) as to be easily recognized. But when a patient with schizophrenia complains of a symptom that is not bizarre (e.g., a headache or weakness), the rigid delusional dimension of psychosis may be missed. Making such a diagnosis with a thorough psychiatric history and examination is ordinarily no problem. Patients with schizophrenia can also have functional neurological symptoms (e.g., hemiparesis).

Nonetheless, physical symptoms in a patient with psychotic disorder must be taken seriously. The premature mortality in this population with serious mental illness (SMI) is significant. What component of this is due to symptoms being dismissed by providers distracted or biased by a psychotic disorder diagnosis is not entirely clear, but, either way, a diagnosis of schizophrenia leads to a life foreshortened by an average of 15 years. It may be more common not to hear out a patient with schizophrenia and to miss a straightforward medical complaint. Additionally, baseline neurocognitive dysfunction found in patients with SMI, such as schizophrenia, is thought to be the main contributor to this increased mortality.

Cognitive Impairment

Somatizing cannot be localized to either a specific brain structure or a neurotransmitter system; however, patients with dementia or other structural brain diseases can have functional somatic complaints, and the recognition of cognitive impairment may be the key to better care. Intellectual disability, for example, has been associated with FND.

Personality Disorders

Although included in the differential diagnostic list of Table 14.1, personality disorders do not "cause" functional somatic symptoms. Rather, for the patient with these disturbances, the somatic symptom is a means to an end. For the individual with an antisocial personality disorder, pain may be a means to get narcotics, to get out of work, or to escape trial. For the person with a dependent personality disorder, functional weakness gains the attention and nurturance of others. For the patient with borderline personality traits, somatic symptoms can become the focus for physicians and nurses, who may engage in a sadomasochistic struggle with the patient. The process begins with a helping relationship and ends with the rejection of a disappointed and outraged patient accused of wrongdoing. The "end" for this patient is the emotionally charged (usually hostile) relationship, and the failure to palliate the symptoms means to the patient that the physician simply does not care enough. Sometimes symptoms are reinforced by personality styles. Somatic symptoms are exaggerated by patients with a histrionic personality and may be the object of such intense fixations by those with OCD, paranoid, schizotypal, and schizoid personalities as to make these patients take on a hypochondriacal character.

TABLE 14.1

Differential Diagnosis of Functional Somatic Symptoms

Demonstrable Somatic Illness
- With proportionate vs. disproportionate illness behaviors

Psychiatric Differential Diagnosis
- Depressive disorders
- Anxiety disorders
- Substance use disorders
- Psychotic disorders
- Neurocognitive disorders
- Deception syndromes
  - Malingering
  - Factitious disorders
- Somatic symptom and related disorders
- Personality disorders

Functional Somatic Syndromes

Like somatic symptoms and related disorders, functional somatic syndromes (FSS) are characterized by complaints that seem out of proportion to any abnormalities found, and they lack laboratory confirmation. FSS are seen by many specialties, including rheumatology (FM), GI medicine (IBS), and urology (interstitial cystitis) to name a few. These diagnoses depend on consensus criteria, descriptions of symptoms, and a natural course of illness.

Psychiatrists are unlikely to be called on to make one of these diagnoses. However, given their conceptual similarities to psychopathology, phenomenological similarities to SSD, and significant co-morbidities with affective and anxiety disorders, it behooves one to have some passing familiarity with them. These criteria undergo revisions of their own, much as the DSM does. IBS is found within the numerous functional GI disorders defined by the Rome criteria. FM and myalgic encephalitis/CFS are undergoing re-framing and/or objectification of their criteria.

FSS are characterized by their respective cores of MUS, with associated features, required to "rule in" those that have established diagnostic criteria. Table 14.2 outlines salient features of the better-characterized FSS. Despite this, there is an argument to be made that there are more commonalities than distinguishing features between them, and there is substantial overlap in the phenomenology, epidemiology, and co-occurrence of these various syndromes. Some have gone as far as to suggest that in reality, "there is only one FSS," sometimes conceptualized as bodily distress syndrome.[43] Like SSDs, the FSS carries across-the-board co-morbidity with depressive and anxiety disorders; notably, patients with one FSS, when subjected to diagnostic investigation for another, are found generally to have both illnesses 30% to 70% of the time, with co-morbidities of >70% found in multiple studies.[32]

Those patients who seek medical care for FSS are more distressed, depressed, and under more life stress than community residents who have the same symptoms but who never seek a physician. Indeed, all FSS could be said to have high rates of undiagnosed members of the general population who do not present themselves to the healthcare system or consider themselves markedly disabled, yet nonetheless "meet criteria" for these illnesses.[4] These findings reiterate the hypothesis that important features of FSS may have a low threshold of symptom detection and a tendency to medically interpret somatic cues. Once the patient acquires a functional diagnosis (either by strict research criteria or by looser clinical criteria), that diagnosis is granted greater authority and legitimacy than a co-morbid psychiatric diagnosis and has often been found to form a central part of that person's identity over time. Physicians and patients often collude to focus their attention only on the somatic syndrome.

The fact that a patient has been diagnosed with FSS should not limit aggressive treatment of co-morbid psychiatric diagnoses. The principles of care for all disorders apply here as well. All co-morbid diseases, both psychiatric and non-psychiatric, should be treated.

Knowing the patient, listening with respect for their suffering, setting limits, avoiding unnecessary and costly interventions, and keeping an ear for changes in medical complaints remain pivotal concepts.

Myalgic Encephalomyelitis/Chronic Fatigue Syndrome

Myalgic encephalomyelitis/CFS is defined by three core features: impaired day-to-day functioning compared to pre-morbid baseline because of fatigue that is new and persists for 6 months, post-exertional malaise, and unrefreshing sleep. Patients must also have either cognitive impairment or orthostatic intolerance. The Institute of Medicine recommends a focused physical examination and work-up for other possible medical

TABLE 14.2

Comparison of the Three Major Functional Somatic Syndromes

	Myalgic Encephalomyelitis/ Chronic Fatigue Syndrome[a]	Irritable Bowel Syndrome (IBS)[b]	Fibromyalgia[c]
Exclusion of other somatic/psychiatric cause	Unnecessary	Unnecessary	Required
Duration	Present at least 50% of the time for ≥6 months	≥6 months + symptoms occurring 1 day/week over the last 3 months	≥3 months
Severity criteria	Must be met: must have a substantial reduction in functioning	Unspecified; abdominal pain associated with defecation with changes in stool consistency or bowel habits	Must be met: Symptom Severity Score of 5 or higher
Reproducibility/relief of symptoms	Not relieved by rest, symptoms worsened with exertion	May find relief with defecation, some experience symptom worsening	Assessed via Widespread Pain Index
Ancillary symptoms	Four or more of: ■ Cognitive impairment ■ Sore throat ■ Tender lymph nodes ■ Muscle pain ■ Multi-joint pain ■ New headaches ■ Unrefreshing sleep ■ Post-exertion malaise	Accompanied by ■ Bloating ■ Constipation subtype (IBS-C) ■ Diarrhea subtype (IBS-D) ■ Mixed subtype (IBS-M)	History of: ■ Bilateral pain ■ Somatic pain in any body part ■ Fatigue and cognitive "fog"

[a]Adapted from Committee on the Diagnostic Criteria for Myalgic Encephalomyelitis/Chronic Fatigue, Board on the Health of Select, and Institute of Medicine. The National Academies Collection: Reports Funded by National Institutes of Health. In: *Beyond Myalgic Encephalomyelitis/Chronic Fatigue Syndrome: Redefining an Illness*. US National Academies Press; 2015. Copyright 2015 by the National Academy of Sciences.[44]
[b]Adapted from Mearin F, Lacy BE, Chang L, et al., Bowel disorders. *Gastroenterology*. 2016;150(6):1393–1407.[47]
[c]Adapted from Galvez-Sánchez CM, Montoro CI. Psychoeducation for fibromyalgia syndrome: a systematic review of emotional, clinical and functional related-outcomes. *Behav Sci (Basel)*. 2023;13(5):415.[46]

or psychiatric causes of fatigue, although, unlike prior diagnostic criteria for CFS, no guidelines are given with regards to whether CFS can be diagnosed in the setting of other specific psychiatric disorders.[44]

Although CFS was associated with infection with Epstein-Barr virus, no single virus has been shown to cause persistent, debilitating CFS. Symptoms similar to CFS have been reported as part of the post-acute sequelae of COVID-19.[45] In the primary care setting, patients with post-infectious fatigue after 6 months are more likely to have had fatigue and psychological distress before the infection. A history of dysthymia and more than eight MUS not already listed in CFS criteria may predict prolonged disability in CFS patients.

Suggested screening laboratory tests include a complete blood count, a sedimentation rate, liver and renal function tests, calcium, phosphate, glucose, thyroid-stimulating hormone, and urinalysis. Further tests, such as a magnetic resonance imaging scan of the head to search for multiple sclerosis, should be guided by clinical findings.

There is no specific medical treatment for CFS, and the treatment plans should center on the symptoms that most distress or impair the patient. While antidepressants are not useful for treating CFS specifically, they may improve co-morbid depression. The choice of antidepressants for co-morbid mood disorders depends on their capacity to improve sleep but limit sedation. A 2019 Cochrane review suggested that exercise therapy has a positive effect on fatigue, and noted that there was limited evidence to draw conclusions about the effectiveness of CBT or adaptive pacing for CFS.[44]

Fibromyalgia

Fibromyalgia is a syndrome of generalized muscle pain and tenderness lasting longer than 3 months and without an alternative cause for the pain. It is diagnosed utilizing two self-report scales: the Widespread Pain Index and the Symptom Severity Score. Whereas the prior diagnostic criteria relied on trigger points (both the quantity and physical examination), the 2011 modified criteria eliminated the need for a physical examination and allowed room for more associated symptoms, including fatigue, waking unrefreshed, cognitive symptoms, headaches, pain or cramps in the lower abdomen, and depression. Affective

disorders are common among patients with FM who seek rheumatologists.[46]

Prior to prescribing medication, psychoeducation is critical to ensure that the patient understands their disease, the role of stress and mood disturbances, and the behavioral modifications necessary for symptom management (e.g., exercise, sleep hygiene, and relaxation techniques). A variety of medications have been used for FM, but pregabalin, duloxetine, and milnacipran are the only agents that currently have US Food and Drug Administration approval for the treatment of FM.[46]

Irritable Bowel Syndrome

Symptoms of IBS occur in 15% to 20% of the population and become chronic in two-thirds of cases. Patients with IBS represent 25% to 50% of referrals to gastroenterologists. The disorder affects females more than males and, although its causes are unknown, it appears to have a genetic component. The ROME international criteria for IBS include continuous or recurrent symptoms (at least 1 day per week for the last 3 months) of abdominal pain associated with two or more of the following: associated with defecation, change in stool frequency, or a change in stool consistency. The disorder is subtyped depending on the predominant symptom into diarrhea, constipation, and mixed and un-subtyped types. IBS is not a diagnosis of exclusion and it can be diagnosed without ruling out other causes if clinical criteria are met.[47]

At least half of all patients with IBS have at least one co-morbid psychiatric condition. Those who visit physicians have more severe symptoms and are more likely to have co-morbid psychiatric diagnoses than those who do not. Anxiety disorders are most common, followed by depressive disorders. A history of childhood abuse, high levels of neuroticism, and lower levels of resilience, positive affect, self-efficacy, and emotional regulation are more prevalent among patients than among the general population.[48]

Again, making a diagnosis depends on meeting the criteria, the natural history of illness, and the absence of laboratory confirmation of another diagnosis. In the context of a relationship in which the physician continues to learn about the patient, the physician chooses somatic treatments that target the predominant symptom of pain, constipation, or diarrhea. A tricyclic antidepressant (TCA) has an analgesic effect at low doses but tends to cause constipation and is preferable for patients with recurrent diarrhea. An SSRI seems the better choice for co-morbid panic disorder or OCD, particularly in patients with constipation. Overall, TCAs and SSRIs appear to have similar treatment effects. Fiber, anti-spasmodic agents, and dietary adjustments, including moving to a predominantly plant-based diet, have also been studied.[49]

CBT and interpersonal psychodynamic therapy appear to be effective in improving well-being and quality of life. Exposure therapy may be a promising treatment, according to a 2023 meta-analysis.[50] Relaxation training; stress management techniques; and education about the amplification of visceral symptoms and the vicious circle of anxiety, increased vigilance for symptoms, and resultant increase in symptoms and pain are helpful to both individuals and groups.[25,50]

CONCLUSION

Somatic symptom presentations are a nearly universal experience, and symptom amplification is a problem for a significant subset of patients and the physicians who attempt to understand and treat them. The DSM-5-TR has re-organized many of these presentations within the category of somatic symptoms and related disorders, although other fields of medicine continue to use different classifications for these patients. Ultimately, symptom amplification descriptions and names may be less important than the associated illness behaviors. Addressing abnormal illness behaviors through co-morbidity identification, strategic primary care approaches, psychotherapies, better navigation of the sick role status, and conservative use of medications, consultations, and diagnostic tests, is critical in the management of these patients.

REFERENCES

1. Barsky AJ, Borus JF. Functional somatic syndromes. *Ann Intern Med.* 1999;130(11):910–921.
2. Lipowski ZJ. Somatization: the concept and its clinical application. *Am J Psychiatry.* 1988;145(11):1358–1368.
3. Steinbrecher N, Koerber S, Frieser D, et al. The prevalence of medically unexplained symptoms in primary care. *Psychosomatics.* 2011;52(3):263–271.
4. Frølund Pedersen H, Frostholm L, Søndergaard Jensen J, et al. Neuroticism and maladaptive coping in patients with functional somatic syndromes. *Br J Health Psychol.* 2016;21(4):917–936.
5. Barsky AJ, Silbersweig DA. The amplification of symptoms in the medically ill. *J Gen Int Med.* 2023;38(1):195–202.
6. American Psychiatric Association. *Somatic Symptom Disorder and Related Disorders, Diagnostic and Statistical Manual of Mental Disorders, 5th Edition, Text Revision.* American Psychiatric Association Publishing; 2022.
7. Burton C, Fink P, Henningsenet P, et al. Functional somatic disorders: discussion paper for a new common classification for research and clinical use. *BMC Medicine.* 2020;18(1):34.
8. *Stedmans' Medical Dictionary.* 28th ed. Lippincott Williams and Wilkins; 2006.
9. Benmeir P, Neuman A, Weinberg A, et al. Giant melanoma of the inner thigh: a homeopathic life-threatening negligence. *Ann Plast Surg.* 1991;27(6):583–585.
10. Aybek S, Perez DL. Diagnosis and management of functional neurological disorder. *BMJ.* 2022;376:64.
11. Hamilton J, Feldman M, Cunnien AJ. *Clinical assessment of malingering and deception.* R Rogers, SD Bender. *Factitious Disorder in Medical and Psychiatric Practices.* Guilford Press; 2008:128–144.
12. Taylor MD, Vaidya NA. *Descriptive Psychopathology: The Signs and Symptoms of Behavioral Disorders.* Cambridge University Press; 2009.
13. Parsons T. *The Social System.* The Free Press; 1951.
14. Huibers MJ, Wessely S. The act of diagnosis: pros and cons of labelling chronic fatigue syndrome. *Psychol Med.* 2006;36(7):895–900.
15. O'Dowd TC. Five years of heartsink patients in general practice. *BMJ.* 1988;297(6647):528–530.
16. Hijne K, Van Eck van der Sluijs JF, Van Broeckhuysen-Kloth SM, et al. Individual treatment goals and factors influencing goal attainment in patients with somatic symptom disorder from the perspective of clinicians: a concept mapping study. *J Psychosom Res.* 2022;154:110712.
17. Lehmann M, Pohontsch NJ, Zimmermann T, et al. Diagnostic and treatment barriers to persistent somatic symptoms in primary care - representative survey with physicians. *BMC Fam Pract.* 2021;22(1):60.
18. Lehmann M, Pohontsch NJ, Zimmermann T, et al. Estimated frequency of somatic symptom disorder in general practice: cross-sectional survey with general practitioners. *BMC Psychiatry.* 2022;22(1):632.
19. Nemiah JC. A psychodynamic view of psychosomatic medicine. *Psychosom Med.* 2000;62(3):299–303.
20. Hallett M, Aybek S, Dworetzky BA, et al. Functional neurological disorder: new subtypes and shared mechanisms. *Lancet Neurol.* 2022;21(6):537–550.
21. Drane DL, Fani N, Hallett M, et al. A framework for understanding the pathophysiology of functional neurological disorder. *CNS Spectr.* 2020:1–7.
22. Scarella TM, Boland RJ, Barsky AJ. Illness anxiety disorder: psychopathology, epidemiology, clinical characteristics, and treatment. *Psychosom Med.* 2019;81(5):398–407.

23. Barends H, Dekker J, van Dessel N, et al. Exploring maladaptive cognitions and behaviors as perpetuating factors in patients with persistent somatic symptoms: a longitudinal study. *J Psychosom Res.* 2023;170:111343.

24. Berezowski L, Ludwig L, Martin A, et al. Early psychological interventions for somatic symptom disorder and functional somatic syndromes: a systematic review and meta-analysis. *Psychosom Med.* 2022;84(3):325–338.

25. Blanchard EB, Scharff L. Psychosocial aspects of assessment and treatment of irritable bowel syndrome in adults and recurrent abdominal pain in children. *J Consult Clin Psychol.* 2002;70(3):725–738.

26. Achenbach J, Tran AT, Jaeger B, et al. Quantitative sensory testing in patients with multisomatoform disorder with chronic pain as the leading bodily symptom-a matched case-control study. *Pain Med.* 2020;21(2):e54–e61.

27. Löwe B, Levenson J, Depping M, et al. Somatic symptom disorder: a scoping review on the empirical evidence of a new diagnosis. *Psychol Med.* 2022;52(4):632–648.

28. Axelsson E, Hedman-Lagerlöf E, Lindfors P. Validity and clinical utility of distinguishing between DSM-5 somatic symptom disorder and illness anxiety disorder in pathological health anxiety: should we close the chapter? *J Psychosom Res.* 2023;165:111133.

29. Frances A. The new somatic symptom disorder in DSM-5 risks mislabeling many people as mentally ill. *BMJ.* 2013;346:f1580.

30. Löwe B, Levenson J, Depping M, et al. Somatic symptom disorder: a scoping review on the empirical evidence of a new diagnosis. *Psychol Med.* 2021;52(4):1–17.

31. Behm AC, Hüsing P, Löwe B, et al. Persistence rate of DSM-5 somatic symptom disorder: 4-year follow-up in patients from a psychosomatic outpatient clinic. *Compr Psychiatry.* 2021;110:152265.

32. Henningsen P, Zipfel S, Sattel H, et al. Management of functional somatic syndromes and bodily distress. *Psychother Psychosom.* 2018;87(1):12–31.

33. Hoedeman R, Blankenstein AH, van der Feltz-Cornelis CM, et al. Consultation letters for medically unexplained physical symptoms in primary care. *Cochrane Database Syst Rev.* 2010;12 CD006524.

34. Maroti D, Lumley MA, Schubiner H, et al. Internet-based emotional awareness and expression therapy for somatic symptom disorder: a randomized controlled trial. *J Psychosom Res.* 2022;163:111068.

35. Gutkin M, McLean L, Brown R, et al. Systematic review of psychotherapy for adults with functional neurological disorder. *J Neurol Neurosurg Psychiatry.* 2020. https://doi:10.1136/jnnp-2019-321926

36. Chiu LL, Liu CY, Chen TY. The role of low-frequency repetitive transcranial magnetic stimulation on the right prefrontal cortex in a patient with somatic symptom disorder and comorbid major depressive disorder. *J Acad Consult Liaison Psychiatry.* 2023;64(3):305–306.

37. Stone J, Sharpe M. Internet resources for psychiatry and neuropsychiatry. *J Neurol Neurosurg Psychiatry.* 2003;74(1):10–12.

38. Matsumoto N, Kadowaki T, Takanaga S, et al. Longitudinal impact of the COVID-19 pandemic on the development of mental disorders in preadolescents and adolescents. *BMC Public Health.* 2023;23(1):1308.

39. Pick S, Anderson DG, Asadi-Pooya A, et al. Outcome measurement in functional neurological disorder: a systematic review and recommendations. *J Neurol Neurosurg Psychiatry.* 2020;91(6):638–649.

40. Gelauff J, Stone J, Edwards M, et al. The prognosis of functional (psychogenic) motor symptoms: a systematic review. *J Neurol Neurosurg Psychiatry.* 2014;85(2):220–226.

41. Carson A, Lehn A, Ludwig L, et al. Explaining functional disorders in the neurology clinic: a photo story. *Pract Neurol.* 2016;16(1):56–61.

42. Nielsen G, Stone J, Matthews A, et al. Physiotherapy for functional motor disorders: a consensus recommendation. *J Neurol Neurosurg Psychiatry.* 2015;86(10):1113–1119.

43. Petersen MW, Schröder A, Jørgensen T, et al. The unifying diagnostic construct of bodily distress syndrome (BDS) was confirmed in the general population. *J Psychosom Res.* 2020;128:109868.

44. Committee on the Diagnostic Criteria for Myalgic Encephalomyelitis/Chronic Fatigue, Board on the Health of Select, and Institute of Medicine. The National Academies Collection: reports funded by National Institutes of Health. In: *Beyond Myalgic Encephalomyelitis/Chronic Fatigue Syndrome: Redefining an Illness.* US National Academies Press; 2015. Copyright 2015 by the National Academy of Sciences. All rights reserved.

45. Munipalli B, Seim L, Dawson N, et al. Post-acute sequelae of COVID-19 (PASC): a meta-narrative review of pathophysiology, prevalence, and management. *SN Compr Clin Med.* 2022;4(1):90.

46. Galvez-Sánchez CM, Montoro CI. Psychoeducation for fibromyalgia syndrome: a systematic review of emotional, clinical and functional related-outcomes. *Behav Sci (Basel).* 2023;13(5):415.

47. Mearin F, Lacy BE, Chang L, et al. Bowel disorders. *Gastroenterology.* 2016;150(6):1393–1407.

48. Madva EN, Sadlonova M, Harnedy L, et al. Positive psychological well-being and clinical characteristics in IBS: a systematic review. *Gen Hosp Psychiatry.* 2023;81:1–14.

49. Ford AC, Lacy BE, Harris LA, et al. Effect of antidepressants and psychological therapies in irritable bowel syndrome: an updated systematic review and meta-analysis. *Am J Gastroenterol.* 2019;114(1):21–39.

50. Axelsson E, Kern D, Hedman-Lagerlöf E, et al. Psychological treatments for irritable bowel syndrome: a comprehensive systematic review and meta-analysis. *Cogn Behav Ther.* 2023:1–20.

15

FACTITIOUS DISORDERS AND MALINGERING

FELICIA A. SMITH, MD ■ SCOTT R. BEACH, MD ■ NICHOLAS KONTOS, MD ■ DONNA B. GREENBERG, MD

OVERVIEW

Factitious disorders and malingering both involve voluntary symptom production and deception of medical providers. In this light, Ford has combined these two disorders under the heading of *deception syndromes*.[1] Importantly, not all patients who lie to providers have a deception syndrome. Indeed, most patients may consciously or unconsciously minimize or maximize aspects of their presentation, often for decidedly non-pathologic reasons, including anxiety about the consequences of telling the truth (e.g., will I be locked up if I disclose my suicidal ideation; will I be taken seriously if I tell them that my primary issue is with substance use or abuse?) or a desire to align with, or be liked by, the provider. Even patients who fabricate their symptoms and create signs wholesale often have understandable motives (e.g., an escape or reprieve from an abusive situation through hospitalization) to which their lying and the providers they lie to take a back seat in their minds.

Regardless, medical deception, especially when elaborate, dramatic, protracted, or contested, often angers and confounds providers, making these patients some of the most memorable of our careers. The thought of a patient with an infection that requires multiple diagnostic studies and broad-spectrum antibiotics, only to be seen self-injecting feces into various body parts, seems incredulous to most. The motivation is often difficult to comprehend, but in theory it separates the two diagnoses. In factitious disorder the motivation centers around primary gain and the sick role, while obvious external rewards are absent. Those who malinger, on the other hand, are motivated by a (to them) clear-cut secondary gain, often legal, financial, or pharmaceutical.

In practice, this distinction often breaks down since sick role "gains" associated with blamelessness, excuse from duties, and entitlement to care often blur the lines between so-called primary and secondary gain. If (as in many cases) there is no clear-cut difference between immaterial/primary and material/secondary gain, and if this is held to be the distinguishing characteristic between factitious disorder and malingering, then there are two possibilities. One extends the disorder status of factitious disorder to malingering; the other extends the quasi-criminal status of malingering to factitious disorder. Either way, both conditions might be better understood as behavioral patterns that obscure problems that need to be identified and addressed more adaptively. Malingering might be seen variably as part of broader patterns of non-pathological criminality, sociopathy, or desperation; factitious disorder might be viewed as a manifestation of separation avoidance in those with a borderline personality or another character disorder.[2,3] While this chapter refers largely to the standard primary/secondary gain distinction in deception syndrome diagnosis, the behavioral explanation approach should be kept in mind throughout.

The deceptive nature and the difficulty of confirming these conditions create an investigative challenge; thus prevalence rates are less than reliable. The potential (inter)subjective nature of determining the motivation (that is often murky at best) further complicates matters. It seems clear, however, that the disruption caused by these patients in their own lives, in those of their family members, and to the larger medical system is significant and requires attention.

Case 1

Ms. S, a 25-year-old woman, had a 5-year history of worsening lower back pain that initially occurred only when sitting at a workstation for prolonged periods; it abruptly worsened 2 years later after a seemingly minor "fender bender." A magnetic resonance imaging scan obtained shortly afterward revealed a herniated disc at L3–4. Ms. S had not worked since the accident. She moved back in with her parents shortly afterward and has remained in litigation related to the accident, which she sees as being unfairly drawn out by the other driver's insurance company, especially given her financial situation. Attempts to treat her pain have been reported as ineffective, although she has remained on chronic opioid therapy, as well as on gabapentin and ibuprofen. She has consistently declined referrals for physical therapy and recommendations for exercise, stating that she is too fatigued and in too much pain to tolerate either. Resistant to any inquiry about depressive symptoms, she at one point grudgingly accepted a trial of sertraline and reported severe nausea and diarrhea after two 25-mg doses. Further, the gastrointestinal symptoms failed to resolve after she stopped taking sertraline. Over the next year, she was evaluated by two different gastroenterologists, the second of whom diagnosed her with irritable bowel syndrome. Despite reporting chronic diarrhea and an inability to keep food down, she gained approximately 10 pounds a year since the automobile accident, perhaps relating to a life now dominated by allopathic and homeopathic medical visits and devoid of any recreational activities of note other than watching television from a chair bolstered by memory foam back supports.

Factitious Disorders

Factitious disorders are marked by the conscious production of symptoms and/or signs with the unconscious goal of obtaining the sick role. Patients may fake or exaggerate symptoms and may intentionally worsen or simply create signs. Concealment of the actual causes of their complaints is the frustrating core of this paradoxical condition in which the patient is, by definition, sick (i.e., has factitious disorder), just not in the manifest way, and if they ceased being sick in the manifest way, they would no longer have factitious disorder. This paradox lends further support for the idea of viewing and handling this deception syndrome (and malingering) as a goal-directed behavior more than as a discrete "disorder."

That said, the *Diagnostic and Statistical Manual of Mental Disorders, Fifth Edition* (DSM-5)[4] no longer distinguishes between factitious disorders with physical symptoms and those with psychological features, although clinically this remains a helpful distinction. In a factitious disorder with physical symptoms, the most common presentation is that of a general medical condition. The types of physical symptoms and diseases that have been simulated are limited only by the imaginations of those who feign them.[5-9] Table 15.1 lists some common presentations.[10] Laboratory tests and diagnostic modalities may be particularly useful in distinguishing factitious presentations from their true medical correlates. For example, in the case of suspicious infection, polymicrobial culture results that indicate an uncommon source (e.g., from urine or feces) are highly suggestive. Those who inject insulin to produce hypoglycemia will have a low C-peptide level on laboratory analysis, whereas glyburide can be measured in the urine of those suspected of taking oral hypoglycemics. Laxative abuse to cause ongoing diarrhea is confirmed by testing for phenolphthalein in the stool.[10] Finally, diagnostic studies in cases of suspected thyrotoxicosis (from surreptitious ingestion of thyroid hormone) reveal elevated levels of serum total or free thyroid hormone, undetectable serum thyrotropin levels, low serum thyroglobulin concentration, normal urinary iodine excretion, suppressed thyroidal radioactive iodine uptake, absence of goiter, and absence of circulating antithyroid antibodies.[11]

Detection of other types of physical factitious illness may require more astute physical examinations or observational skills (not to mention catching the patient "in the act"). For example, fever of unknown etiology may be caused by warming thermometers on heat sources. Hematuria may be produced by bloodletting from another body area (commonly from a

TABLE 15.1
Typical Clinical Presentation of Factitious Disorder

Type	Clinical Findings or Symptoms
Acute abdominal type (laparotomaphilia migrans)	Abdominal pain; multiple surgeries may lead to true adhesions and subsequent bowel obstruction
Neurological type (neurologic diabolica)	Headache, loss of consciousness, seizure
Hematological type	Anemia from bloodletting or use of an anticoagulant
Endocrinological type	Hypoglycemia from exogenous insulin; hyperthyroidism from exogenous thyroid hormone
Cardiac type	Chest pain or arrhythmia
Dermatological type (dermatitis autogenica)	Rash; skin eruptions
Febrile type (hyperpyrexia figmentatica)	Thermometer manipulation to produce fever
Infectious type	Wound infected with multiple organisms (often through fecal material)

Adapted from Beach SR, Viguera AC, Stern TA. Factitious disorders. In: Stern TA, Herman JB, Gorrindo T, eds. *Massachusetts General Hospital Psychiatry Update and Board Preparation*. 3rd ed. MGH Psychiatry Academy; 2012:161–164.

finger prick) into the urine sample. With non-healing wounds where self-excoriation or "picking" behavior is suspected, witnessing the act either directly or with the use of video monitoring is diagnostic. Of note, the latter brings up complex ethical and legal considerations. Finally, among the numerous other possible physical expressions of factitious disorder, those that rely on more subjective reports (including joint or muscle pain, headache, renal colic, or abdominal pain) may be present for months or years before a factitious etiology is even considered, much less diagnosed.

Although most published cases of factitious disorder involve physical symptoms, many patients primarily feign psychological symptoms. Psychological complaints encompass a broad spectrum of symptoms (including depression, anxiety, psychosis, bereavement, dissociation, post-traumatic stress, and suicidal and homicidal ideation).[12–16] In the case of factitious bereavement, for example, the patient may report a dramatic or recent loss of a child or other loved one with a display of emotion that invokes significant sympathy from medical treaters. When the truth is discovered, the reported deceased may either be still alive, have died long ago, or perhaps did not really play a major role in the patient's life. Another common feature of factitious disorder with psychological features is pseudohallucination—an absent perceptual disturbance that the patient nonetheless describes consistently with hallucination. Finally, Ganser syndrome, characterized by the provision of approximate answers to questions (as well as by having amnesia, disorientation, and perceptual disturbances), may be related to factitious disorder with psychological symptoms, though the original description that still associates it with deception in incarcerated populations is now joined by its manifestation in dissociative and trauma-spectrum disorders and as a sort of cognitive conversion sign.[17]

Whereas the term *Munchausen syndrome* is often used interchangeably with factitious disorder, the classic Munchausen syndrome is reserved for a subset of patients (approximately 10% of those with factitious disorder) exhibiting the most severe and chronic form, which is marked by the following three components: recurrent hospitalizations, travel (often across long distances and including "prestigious" institutions) from hospital to hospital (peregrination), and *pseudologia fantastica*.[9] Pseudologia fantastica is the production of intricate and colorful stories or fantasies associated with the patient's autobiography, characterized by an overlapping of fact and fiction (with a repetitive quality, grandiosity, or an assumption of the victim role by the storyteller).[1] Impostership, although not a hallmark of Munchausen syndrome, is also a common feature, with patients claiming to be war heroes or former professional athletes. Patients with Munchausen syndrome often make a career out of their illness. Serial hospitalizations render employment or sustained interpersonal relationships impossible. Moreover, patients who produce significant self-trauma or develop untoward complications from medical or surgical interventions become further incapacitated. The prognosis is generally poor in these cases, and patients may die prematurely from complications of their own self-injurious behavior or iatrogenesis. Patients with the Munchausen subtype are more likely to be male, to exhibit antisocial and dependent personality traits, and to display average to above-average intelligence.[1]

Whereas Munchausen syndrome is the most dramatic form of factitious illness, common factitious disorder is, while less easily noticed, more prevalent.[1] As opposed to those with Munchausen syndrome, patients with common factitious disorder do not typically use aliases or travel from hospital to hospital, but rather frequent the same physician. They are well known in their healthcare system because of numerous hospitalizations. Risk factors for common factitious disorder include female sex, a history of abuse, being unmarried, having experience in the healthcare profession, and having borderline personality disorder or masochistic personality traits.

Factitious disorder imposed on another is a subtype of factitious disorder recognized by DSM-5-TR and formerly called "factitious disorder by proxy," in which persons falsify symptoms or induce illness in another person.[18] The perpetrator in this case is most often the biological mother of a young child, although the elderly and those under the medical care of others are also at risk of being victimized. This disorder has two characteristic forms. The classic form involves a parent or caregiver intentionally inflicting injury or inducing illness in a child while deceiving treating clinicians with false or exaggerated information. The other, perhaps more common and potentially insidious, involves a caregiver embellishing or fabricating symptoms to encourage overly aggressive medical evaluations and interventions. In contrast to standard factitious disorder, the motivation here is to satisfy the caregiver's psychological need to care for a chronically or severely ill individual. The former "by proxy" nomenclature could be accurately applied to the caregiver's pursuit of their own sort of sick role by proxy. In a review of 451 cases of factitious disorder imposed on another, Sheridan found that victims are typically 4 years old or younger, with equal percentages of males and females. She further discovered that an average of 21.8 months elapsed between the onset of symptoms and diagnosis, and 6% of the victims died. Perhaps even more alarming, was her finding that 61% of their siblings had illnesses like those of the victims, and 25% of the victims' known siblings had died.[19]

Much like general factitious disorder, the symptoms and signs in factitious disorder imposed on another are more commonly physical than psychological and may involve any symptom within the scope of imagination. The most common presentations seem to be apnea, anorexia, feeding problems, diarrhea, and seizures.[18,19] These may be induced in a variety of ways, from smothering the child to feeding the child laxatives or ipecac. Perpetrators often have some medical training or exposure to the illness that affects the child (e.g., a mother who has a seizure disorder herself). Other clinical indicators or red flags include a patient who does not respond to appropriate treatments, symptoms that improve when the mother does not have access to the child, unexplained illnesses with other children in the family, a mother who becomes anxious when her child improves, or a mother who encourages invasive testing.[20]

In the past two decades, a new variant of factitious disorder has emerged, known as Munchausen by the internet. Although not included in DSM-5-TR, the syndrome has been described in several journal articles.[21,22] Rather than presenting to hospitals with symptoms, sufferers seek attention from other internet users by feigning illness in chat rooms or social media. The expansion of the internet has made it much easier for people to gain a nuanced understanding of certain medical diseases to appear more convincing. Classic behavioral patterns of this variant of the syndrome include verbatim recapitulation of textbook descriptions of illnesses, with a description of recurrent, worsening illness followed by a miraculous recovery, and a reported duration of severe illness that conflicts with the internet user's behavior, such as blogging about being in the intensive care unit with septic shock. Some patients even fake their own deaths in this syndrome as the ultimate ploy for sympathy, often before being reborn with a new identity.

Diagnostic Approach

As previously suggested, making the diagnosis of a factitious illness is often difficult. However, there are several elements of a general strategic approach that may be helpful. Early suspicion is important to avoid colluding with the patient in ordering unnecessary tests and subjecting the patient to further risk of iatrogenic injury. When suspecting factitious illness, one should first obtain information from all pertinent collateral sources. These may include previous or current caregivers, family members, current and old medical records, and laboratory and diagnostic studies.

Technology may be making it easier for clinicians to detect factitious disorders. The expansion and unification of medical records through centralized databases means that many practitioners have access not only to records in their own hospital system but also to records in hospital networks and community health services, and many states have prescription monitoring programs that provide a central database for controlled substance prescriptions. Verification of the "facts" presented by the patient is critical.

Next, one should look for historical elements that are suggestive of factitious disease. Some of these are outlined in the DSM-5-TR.[4] Recognition of typical presentations (including all of those outlined in Table 15.1) may provide further clues. Typical hospitalizations for those who feign medical or psychiatric illness share common characteristics. First, patients often come to emergency departments (EDs) after hours (at night or on the weekend), when staffing is decreased and senior-level staff are likely absent. Patients use medical jargon and generally know which diagnoses or conditions will merit hospitalization. Their histories are often quite dramatic and convincing, and such patients persuade their physicians to provide care by appealing to narcissistic qualities, such as omnipotence. Once hospitalized, treatments are marked by demands for specific interventions (e.g., surgery or certain medications) and by increasing needs for attention. When the demands go unmet, patients become angry. In many cases, the patient correctly predicts worsening of the disease and complains to the staff about mistreatment or misdiagnosis. The patient may play on the clinician's fear of liability to drive further unnecessary testing and treatment. If staff uncovers the deception, strong countertransference feelings of hatred arise. Patients are then rapidly discharged or elope from the hospital only to seek "treatment" at another facility soon thereafter.

When one finds unwarranted or unreasonably explained medical paraphernalia or directly observes the patient intentionally inducing his or her own symptoms, the diagnosis is virtually assured. Of note, searching of rooms and personal belongings without the patient's permission are controversial and, in many cases, considered an illegal invasion of privacy. Before embarking on such an endeavor, it is prudent to consider the potential ramifications carefully and to

seek legal counsel. Sometimes, belongings can be held until discharge if the patient will not allow them to be searched. Knowing one's institutional and regional regulations is important. While something resembling detective work is implied here, one must remember (and sometimes remind others) that we are not, in fact detectives. All kinds of bias can skew an "investigation" and lead to medical vigilantism if we do not work within our skill sets.

True physical disorders (especially rare or unusual diseases with few objective findings) may mimic factitious disorders. It is essential to consider this possibility before prematurely diagnosing a factitious illness. Somatic symptom disorder and conversion disorder (see Chapter 14) may also be mistaken for factitious disorder. These diagnoses, however, are distinguished from factitious illnesses in that their symptoms are not under voluntary control.

As with all factitious illnesses, the diagnosis of factitious disorder imposed on another may prove difficult unless one directly witnesses a perpetrator harming the victim. When the victim is a child or is elderly, legal obligations and privacy rights may differ from those of a typical adult patient. This is particularly pertinent regarding mandated reporting (that varies state by state), as well as when video surveillance is proposed as a mechanism to uncover intentional harm. In general, whenever diagnostic or treatment strategies outside of the standard of care are considered, it is best to consult with medical and legal colleagues before undertaking them.

Malingering

Malingering involves the conscious feigning, induction, or exacerbation of physical or psychological symptoms for conscious gain. This so-called secondary gain is the hallmark of the phenomenon and can include obtaining something desired (such as food, shelter, or medication, especially controlled substances) or avoiding responsibility (such as missing a court date or obtaining time off from work, release from the military, or relief from childcare or elder care obligations). The DSM-5-TR includes malingering under "other conditions that may be a focus of clinical attention."[4] Although the prevalence of malingering is unknown, it may be detected in up to 10% of psychiatric inpatients and up to 40% of patients applying for disability.[23] ED physicians suspect malingering behavior in 13% to 20% of patients.[24,25] Despite the almost-certainly higher prevalence, a study using the National Inpatient Sample of hospital discharges revealed that it is only diagnosed in 0.15% of hospital discharges.[26] It is thought to be more common in males than females and is highly co-morbid with substance use and psychiatric disorders, including antisocial personality disorder, although it has been observed in psychologically normal adults.

Those who malinger most often pick symptoms that are highly subjective and difficult to prove or disprove. Vague pains (such as headache, tooth pain, or back pain) are common. The goal may be to obtain narcotics or to be placed on disability. Psychiatric symptoms are often easier to fake than physical symptoms, and patients may claim that they are suicidal or are suffering from hallucinations or delusions. Along with suicidal ideation, chest pain is a common malingered complaint that can easily lead to hospital admission.

Involvement in the legal system is a risk factor for malingering, particularly among patients who are referred for examination by an attorney. The presence of a lawsuit after a reported injury should also raise suspicion that the patient is malingering. In general, like those with a factitious disorder, individuals who malinger tend to have poor coping skills and use immature defense mechanisms. As a group, they tend to seek medical or psychiatric care frequently, but they vary in terms of their personalities from charming and glib, to dependent and needy, to irritable and demanding.

Another common feature of malingering is a long list of claimed allergies. Malingerers tend to have a list of allergies that precludes the use of whole classes of medications and is structured to guide the physician toward prescribing desired medications, often controlled substances. Because they are desperate to have their needs met, patients who malinger frequently exhibit the "black cloud" phenomenon, in which the number and degree of bad things that have happened to them recently may strike the interviewer as implausible. Finally, perhaps the most consistent telltale sign of malingering is the escalation of symptoms in response to not having demands met.

The presence of clearly identified secondary gain is not absolute evidence of malingering—one must be careful not to miss the diagnosis of a true medical condition in this population. Many patients with true medical or psychiatric illnesses stand to benefit in other ways from treatment. The diagnosis of malingering is ultimately based on a combination of inconsistencies in the history, the presence of secondary gain, a history of suspected deception, and other associated features outlined above. Patients with a history of malingering remain at risk for real medical or psychiatric illness and should be granted a reasonable evaluation at each visit. This evaluation, however, should take prior documentation of malingering into account. Excessive fears of "missing something" can produce unnecessary testing and treatments as easily as feared biases produced by documentation of malingering can impede necessary ones.

When malingering is suspected, certain interview techniques (such as asking repeatedly about details to establish inconsistencies, using gentle assumption to ask about secondary gain [e.g., "When is your next court date?"], and asking about less likely symptoms to highlight exaggeration of distress) can be helpful in building a case for the diagnosis. For example, in patients who malinger psychosis, questions about low-frequency psychotic experiences (such as visual hallucinations of speech bubbles coming from people's mouths) may reveal false symptoms. In some cases, formal psychological testing may also be useful. The Minnesota Multiphasic Personality Inventory-2 may pick up distortions or exaggerations in both physical and psychological symptoms via its embedded scales for faking good and faking bad.[27]

Management of Deception Syndromes

No specific psychiatric treatment has been shown to be effective in the management of deception syndromes. There are, however, a few principles that generally prove helpful. The first is to avoid premature confrontation, which may result in defensiveness, increased elusiveness, or flight from the hospital. Being aware of negative countertransference is also essential if one is to avoid being judgmental or acting on the hostility so often evoked by these patients. Because deception syndromes are often highly treatment resistant, placing an emphasis on management over cure helps to re-frame the treatment goals. Clear and open communication between the psychiatrist and medical and surgical colleagues is essential in this regard.

Direct confrontation of patients manifesting factitious and malingered behaviors tends to be more often reflexively discouraged than productively discussed, but more recently has received more rigorously principled, if not evidence-based, attention.[28,29] A specific framework to guide the permissibility and conduct of confrontation, in general, has been proposed based on reciprocal rights and duties in the physician-patient relationship.[30] Given the complexity of accurately diagnosing a deception syndrome and the need for rigorous documentation, many psychiatrists will offer a "pass" for patients unknown to the system who seem to be engaging in intentional deception, perhaps using gentle confrontation and clearly documenting their suspicions, but without altering the treatment plan. Nonetheless, some established deceivers warrant carefully planned confrontation and security-facilitated discharge from the hospital. The therapeutic parts of this "therapeutic discharge" include discouragement of maladaptive behavioral strategies and minimization of the medical system's role in perpetuating those strategies and/or causing iatrogenic harm. Suggested documentation of such is outlined in Table 15.2.[31,32] Acknowledging one's own anger toward the patient (so as not to base action or inaction on it) is also a key to appropriate treatment. Given that there is often overlap with legal issues for those who engage in malingering or factitious behaviors, consultation with legal experts is frequently advisable.

In the specific case of factitious disorder imposed on another, the first consideration is protecting the victim. In many cases this means placing the child in foster care (at least temporarily). Treatment then addresses both the victim and perpetrator. Although no effective treatment for victims has been established, it is generally thought that therapy to address co-morbid psychiatric diagnoses is a good place to start. Legal interventions are often required. Therapy for perpetrators is generally the mainstay of treatment; however, because many perpetrators never admit to wrongdoing, this often proves difficult.

CONCLUSION

Factitious disorders and malingering share the common feature of the intentional production of symptoms that are either of a physical or psychological nature. The motivation differs from assuming the sick role in the

TABLE 15.2
Suggested Documentation for Deception Syndromes[32]

- Paragraph 1: Summarize the presentation
- Paragraph 2: Document inconsistencies during this encounter and the general attitude toward the interviewer
- Paragraph 3: Document historical inconsistencies, with specific reference to other notes
- Paragraph 4: Document the standard risk assessment using all factors, but then acknowledge any factors about which there may be uncertainty or which may have been manipulated
  - "Of note, although the patient reports a history of four suicide attempts, none of these is documented, and, in fact, the patient has previously denied any history of suicide attempts. The impact of this potential risk factor on assessment is therefore unclear."
  - Highlight future orientation and cite specific examples
  - Remember that a key protective factor is the ability to seek treatment during times of crisis
- Paragraph 5: Document recommendations for the level of care, appropriateness of recommendation, and arguments against recommending a higher level of care, including evidence for prior demonstrated poor use of higher levels of care
- Paragraph 6: If the patient escalated in the face of recommendation, document this occurrence, how it was dealt with, and what it represented
- Paragraph 7: If the patient seems likely to engage in manipulative behavior to exact revenge or spite the physician, consider anticipatory documentation of this future behavior and recommendations for addressing it
- Add deception syndrome to the Problem List

Documentation on deceptive patients is often extensive and time-consuming.

former to obtaining external secondary gain in the latter. *Factitious disorder imposed on another* is further complicated by inflicting harm on someone else (often a young child) to indirectly assume the sick role. Each of these is challenging to diagnose and difficult to treat once the diagnosis is made. Ethical and legal considerations are also pertinent, as are those of avoiding iatrogenesis, which may further harm the patient. The deceptive nature of these illnesses often induces negative countertransference (including anger and hatred toward the patient). Understanding the illnesses (including their clinical presentations, diagnostic approaches, and treatment options) brings clinicians one step closer to providing better care for this difficult population.

REFERENCES

1. Ford CV, Sonnier L, McCullumsmith C. Deception syndromes; factitious disorders and malingering. In: Levenson JL, ed. *The American Psychiatric Publishing Textbook of Psychosomatic Medicine*. 3rd ed. American Psychiatric Publishing; 2019.

2. Gorman WF. Defining malingering. *J Forensic Sci*. 1982;27:401–407.

3. Goldstein AB. Identification and classification of factitious disorders: an analysis of cases reported during a ten-year period. *Int J Psychiatry Med*. 1998;28:221–241.

4. American Psychiatric Association Diagnostic and Statistical Manual of Mental Disorders. 5th ed., text rev. American Psychiatric Association; 2022. https://doi.org/10.1176/appi.books.9780890425787.

5. Sutherland AJ, Rodin GM. Factitious disorders in a general hospital setting: clinical features and a review of the literature. *Psychosomatics*. 1990;31:392–399.

6. Craven DE, Steger KA, La Chapelle R, et al. Factitious HIV infection: the importance of documenting infection. *Ann Intern Med*. 1994;121:763–766.

7. Krahn LE, Li H, O'Connor MK. Patients who strive to be ill: factitious disorder with physical symptoms. *Am J Psychiatry*. 2003;160:1163–1168.

8. Fliege H, Grimm A, Eckhardt-Henn A, et al. Frequency of ICD-10 factitious disorder: survey of senior hospital consultants and physicians in private practice. *Psychosomatics*. 2007;48:60–64.

9. Asher R. Munchausen's syndrome. *Lancet*. 1951;1:339–341.

10. Beach SR, Viguera AC, Stern TA. Factitious disorders. In: Stern TA, Herman JB, Gorrindo T, eds. *Massachusetts General Hospital Psychiatry Update and Board Preparation*. 3rd ed. MGH Psychiatry Academy; 2012:161–164.

11. Bogazzi F, Bartalena L, Scarcello G, et al. The age of patients with thyrotoxicosis factitia in Italy from 1973–1996. *J Endocrinol Invest*. 1999;22:128–133.

12. Thompson CR, Beckson M. A case of factitious homicidal ideation. *J Am Acad Psychiatry Law*. 2004;32:277–281.

13. Mitchell D, Francis JP. A case of factitious disorder presenting as alcohol dependence. *Subst Abus*. 2003;24:187–189.

14. Phillips MR, Ward NG, Ries RK. Factitious mourning: painless patienthood. *Am J Psychiatry*. 1983;140:420–425.

15. Sparr L, Pankratz LD. Factitious posttraumatic stress disorder. *Am J Psychiatry*. 1983;140:1016–1019.

16. Friedl MC, Draijer N. Dissociative disorders in Dutch psychiatric inpatients. *Am J Psychiatry*. 2000;157:1012–1013.

17. Dieguez S. Ganser syndrome. *Front Neural Neurosci*. 2018;42:1–22.

18. Rosenberg DA. Web of deceit: a literature review of Munchausen syndrome by proxy. *Child Abuse Negl*. 1987;11:547–563.

19. Sheridan MS. The deceit continues: an updated literature review of Münchausen syndrome by proxy. *Child Abuse Negl*. 2003;27:431–451.

20. Sadock BJ, Sadock VA. *Factitious disorders. Kaplan and Sadock's Synopsis of Psychiatry*. 9th ed. Lippincott Williams & Wilkins; 2004:668–675.

21. Feldman MD. Munchausen by Internet: detecting factitious illness and crisis on the Internet. *South Med J*. 2000;93:669–672.

22. Feldman MD, Bibby M, Crites SD. 'Virtual' factitious disorders and Munchausen by proxy. *West J Med*. 1998;168:537–539.

23. Rissmiller DJ, Wayslow A, Madison H, et al. Prevalence of malingering in inpatient suicide ideators and attempters. *Crisis*. 1998;19:62–66.

24. Yates BD, Nordquist CR, Schultz-Ross RA. Feigned psychiatric symptoms in the emergency room. *Psychiatr Serv*. 1996 Sep;47(9):998–1000.

25. Rumschik SM, Appel JM. Malingering in the Psychiatric Emergency Department: prevalence, predictors, and outcomes. *Psychiatr Serv*. 2019 Feb 1;70(2):115–122.

26. Punko D, Luccarelli J, Bains A, et al. *The diagnosis of malingering in general hospitals in the United States: a retrospective analysis of the National Inpatient Sample*. November 11, 2022. Academy of Consultation-Liaison Psychiatry Annual Meeting. Brief Oral Paper.

27. Lees-Haley PR, Fox DD. MMPI subtle-obvious scales and malingering: clinical versus simulated scores. *Psychol Rep*. 1990;66(3 Pt 1):907–911.

28. Feldman MD, Yates GP. *Dying to be Ill: True Stories of Medical Deception*. Routledge; 2018.

29. Nisavic M, Flores EJ, Heng M, et al. Case 26-2019: a 27-year-old woman with opioid use disorder and suicidal ideation. *N Engl J Med*. 2019 Aug 22;381(8):763–771.

30. Kontos N, Querques J, Freudenreich O. Fighting the good fight: responsibility and rationale in the confrontation of patients. *Mayo Clin Proc*. 2012;87(1):63–66.

31. Taylor JB, Beach SR, Kontos N. The therapeutic discharge: an approach to dealing with deceptive patients. *Gen Hosp Psychiatry*. 2017;46:74–78.

32. Kontos N, Taylor JB, Beach SR. The therapeutic discharge II: an approach to documentation in the setting of feigned suicidal ideation. *Gen Hosp Psychiatry*. 2018;51:30–35.

16 EATING DISORDERS

YOUNGJUNG RACHEL KIM, MD, PHD ■ KAMRYN T. EDDY, PHD

OVERVIEW

Eating disorders (EDs) are psychiatric illnesses with high rates of morbidity and mortality. They are characterized by abnormal eating patterns that significantly impairs a person's psychosocial functioning. The main EDs described here are anorexia nervosa (AN), bulimia nervosa (BN), binge-eating disorder (BED), avoidant/restrictive food intake disorder (ARFID), and other specified feeding or eating disorder (OSFED).[1] As individuals with EDs can develop serious medical and psychiatric complications; early detection and multi-disciplinary treatment are critical to maximize the chance of recovery.

EPIDEMIOLOGY

EDs affect people of all ages, sexes, races, ethnicities, and socioeconomic statuses. In the USA, it has been estimated that 9% of the population, or over 28 million Americans will develop an ED at some point in their life.[2] The lifetime prevalence rates (with rates for females and males) were estimated at 6.4% for all EDs (8.6%, 4.1%, respectively), 0.6% for AN (0.7%, 0.5%, respectively), 0.8% for BN (1.4%, 0.2%, respectively), 2.2% for BED (2.7%, 1.7%, respectively), and 2.7% for OSFED (3.8%, 1.6%, respectively).[2] Epidemiologic data on ARFID are limited but it is thought to be as common as BED, with comparable rates across sexes.

COURSE OF ILLNESS

The etiology of EDs is multi-faceted. Identified risk factors for developing an ED include biological (e.g., female sex, genetics, metabolic disorders [such as obesity and diabetes]), psychological (e.g., low self-esteem, neuroticism, exposure to sexual abuse or other adversities), and sociocultural (e.g., Westernization, peer influence, and media exposure that affects body dissatisfaction, dieting) factors.

AN typically begins in post-pubertal adolescence, but it can develop during childhood or adulthood. The onset of BN is usually later (i.e., in late adolescence and young adulthood). BED begins even later, often arising in adulthood. ARFID can begin at any age.

A long-term follow-up study of AN and BN has shown that approximately two-thirds of female patients with AN recover by the age of 22 years, whereas two-thirds of patients with BN recover after 9 years, with the remainder following a chronic course.[3] Importantly, for individuals with AN, studies have shown that pathology may shift over time, moving away from restrictive eating towards binge eating and/or purging (with or without changes in body weight), such that individuals cross over from restrictive to binge-eating/purging subtypes (AN-R to AN-BP) or cross over to a different diagnosis, including BN, BED, and OSFED.[4] On the other hand, more than 80% of those with BED achieve remission over a 5-year follow-up, with low rates of relapse, chronicity, or diagnostic crossover.[5]

During the illness, individuals with EDs can develop other medical and psychiatric illnesses, either as a complication of the ED or as a co-morbid condition. This can complicate the management of the ED, affecting treatment response and contributing to high mortality rates and increased morbidity. For instance,

AN has a standardized mortality rate of 5.9—one of the highest among all psychiatric illnesses—and individuals with AN may die from medical complications of starvation (e.g., cardiac arrhythmia), suicide related to severe depression, or a car accident while driving under the influence Although the 2022 US Preventive Services Task Force report found insufficient evidence regarding screening for EDs,[6] because early intervention is associated with better outcomes, it is crucial for clinicians to remain vigilant.

Case 1

Ms. D, a 21-year-old White college student with no psychiatric history, was brought to the clinic by her mother because she was concerned that her daughter was exhibiting abnormal eating habits since returning home for summer break. Her mother described Ms. D as visiting the bathroom with increasing frequency after family meals and she had noticed food disappearing from the fridge and cupboards on several occasions. Her mother was concerned about Ms. D's "secretive" behavior and had witnessed her eating large quantities of chocolates and cookies in her room alone.

During the interview, Ms. D was fully oriented, soft spoken, and avoided eye contact. She presented with depressed and anxious affect without any signs of mania or psychosis. She perceived her weight to be higher than she desired, and she described her low self-esteem; she based her self-worth almost entirely on her shape and weight. She denied having thoughts of suicide, but she acknowledged that she had considered harming herself on several occasions.

Ms. D first engaged in binge eating and purging after a disappointing result on a mid-term examination over the winter. Over the following 5 months, abnormal eating episodes increased to 3 to 4 times per week. Following a binge episode, she described feeling guilty and ashamed. She denied using diuretics or diet pills; however, she reported taking laxatives 5 to 6 times each week. She became increasingly anxious and was afraid to eat around others for fear that her friends might observe her behavior and see her losing control. At home she had begun to store food in her room or binge eat in the kitchen alone during the night.

On examination, her body mass index (BMI) was 20.2 kg/m^2; she had mild parotid swelling and signs of dental erosion. Russell sign was absent, and there was no abdominal bloating or tenderness. Ms. D reported occasional palpitations, generalized fatigue, and regular menstruation. Laboratory tests revealed mild hypokalemia (3.1 mmol/L); her other electrolytes were within normal limits.

Ms. D was diagnosed with BN and depression. She was offered outpatient care and potassium supplementation. The team met with her primary care physician (PCP) who prescribed 60 mg of fluoxetine daily. She was started on a 20-session cognitive-behavioral therapy (CBT) program to interrupt her binge-purge cycle and reduce her over-valuation of her shape and weight.

Within the first 4 weeks of treatment, Ms. D was able to reduce the frequency of her binge eating and purging to once every other week, and by the end of treatment she had no episodes of binge eating or purging in several weeks. Her mood had also improved.

CLINICAL EVALUATION

An accurate diagnostic evaluation of an ED is critical in selecting the optimal treatment strategy. Detection of an ED can be challenging, in part due to the reluctance of many patients to acknowledge or disclose their symptoms, and in part due to the fact that most clinicians neither take the time nor have expertise to detect an ED. Individuals may come to a specialized evaluation for an ED after they have aroused clinical suspicion (e.g., due to unexplained weight changes or after changes in mood or habits are noticed by family members), often after many months or years following symptom onset.

Clinicians should ask sensitive yet direct questions about the patient's weight history, as well as about their eating and exercising habits. Because taking a clinical history does not always elicit accurate or complete information, other data (such as collateral history, physical findings, laboratory studies, and medical records) should be reviewed as part of the comprehensive evaluation.

Medical etiologies of substantial shifts in appetite and weight should be evaluated with a careful history, examination, and diagnostic tests. While an ED diagnosis is not given if symptoms are fully accounted for by another condition (e.g., a malignancy that results in loss of appetite and 35% of pre-morbid body weight), overlapping presentations of co-morbid conditions and an ED (e.g., malignancy in an individual with underlying cognitive distortions of one's body image that results in weight loss related to appetite suppression from the cancer exacerbated by volitional restrictive eating) can occur. Moreover, because the management of one condition can influence the other, practitioners need to assess medical conditions as part of any comprehensive evaluation for an ED to develop an optimal treatment plan. A comprehensive history, review of systems, physical examination, and laboratory testing can often be sufficient, unless suspicion is high for specific conditions (e.g., a strong family history and a known inherited risk variant for early-onset cancer). Conditions to consider include: disorders that affect metabolism (such as hyperthyroidism or cancer), disorders of nutrient absorption (such as celiac disease or malabsorption syndromes following gastrointestinal [GI] surgery), and medical co-morbidities that involve treatments used [or misused] for weight control [insulin]. As such, history taking should include a surgical, medical, and psychiatric history; a family history; a medical and psychiatric review of systems; and a full inventory of current and past use of prescription and over-the-counter (OTC) medications (e.g., supplements, diet pills, stimulants, laxatives, diuretics, enemas, anabolic steroids, insulin, and thyroid replacement hormones). Moreover, because EDs are frequently co-morbid with mood and anxiety disorders, personality disorders, and substance use disorders (SUDs), a complete assessment of the mental status and the psychiatric history should be conducted along with a careful assessment of suicide risk (to facilitate safe discharge planning).

The clinical evaluation for an ED should always include a weight assessment. Determining the weight status is essential to completing a precise diagnostic evaluation and for longitudinal management. Current weight and height should be measured, with the patient in a hospital gown, whenever possible. If gowning is not feasible, the patients should be asked to empty their pockets and take off any jewelry or outer layers of clothing. If water loading is suspected, patients can be asked to void prior to being weighed. Weight and height can be used to calculate the BMI, which is the standard for weight assessment for adults, using the formula BMI = weight in kg/(height in m)^2. For children, patterns during development should be accounted for; the BMI percentiles for age and sex are then used for weight assessments in the context of a growth chart with prior BMI percentiles. Measured weight and height, age, and biological sex data can be used to determine the BMI percentiles through calculators and charts available through the US Centers for Disease Control and Prevention (https://www.cdc.gov).[7]

Aside from assessing the weight status, the rest of the physical examination may not be as high yield, as many ED-associated findings are neither sensitive nor specific, and most do not correlate well with the severity of the medical condition. For instance, a patient with AN may present with hypothermia and a patient with BN may present with Russell sign and/or parotid hypertrophy from recurrent episodes of self-induced emesis, but these can be missing or minimal in many patients. Abnormalities found on the physical examination, including vital signs and mental status changes (e.g., signs of end-organ damage from cardiovascular compromise or hemodynamic instability) can indicate medical acuity and help to determine whether hospitalization is needed.

Laboratory assessment can include a basic metabolic panel, a complete blood count, liver function tests, and a thyroid-stimulating hormone (TSH) level, with free thyroxine levels, as well as a hemoglobin A1c (Hgb A1c) if the fasting blood sugar on the metabolic panel is abnormal. While tests, like TSH and Hgb A1c, may be useful in ruling out thyroid dysfunction and diabetes, laboratory tests are neither sensitive nor specific in detecting any particular ED. Rather, determining the renal, immunologic, and liver function from routine laboratory tests, as well as tests of cardiac function and an electrocardiogram (ECG), can help to rule out a medical cause for weight changes, to assess for co-morbidities, and guide the selection of a psychopharmacologic treatment, if indicated. Nutritional status can be assessed with laboratory tests for vitamin deficiencies, but one should consider the possibility that they may be spuriously normal related to recent patterns of eating and use of supplements, which may downplay the seriousness of the nutritional compromise. Overall, clinicians should refrain from ordering a long list of unnecessary diagnostic tests without direct clinical utility, as this can add to medical costs without adding to clinical care. For instance, while higher levels of endogenous ghrelin have recently been associated with future weight gain in individuals with AN,[8] it is unclear how one might use this information in the clinical setting, such as in stratifying treatment endpoints. Another example is in evaluating a young woman with the clinical picture consistent with AN who reports that her last menstrual period was 5 years ago, in which case the psychiatrist does not need to *see* the abnormal reproductive hormone levels to confirm that there have been impairments in the reproductive axis. On the other hand, if this individual is unable to see the seriousness of her symptoms despite a 5 year history of amenorrhea, it can be helpful for the patient to see the objective medical test results that are clearly "flagged" as abnormal. In general, if a clinician cannot identify the utility of a test, then it may not be necessary to order that test.

A test that is indicated in low-weight patients with AN or ARFID is dual X-ray absorptiometry (DEXA) scan, which is typically ordered in consultation with an endocrinologist or through a PCP, to assess for bone loss associated with low-weight EDs, which can be repeated to monitor for bone health recovery. That said, clinicians may choose to forego certain tests, such as a DEXA scan, if the burden of additional testing becomes a barrier to engaging the patient, and for those who may feel easily overwhelmed and demotivated. In such cases, targeted testing to evaluate and monitor the patient's medical stability, acute medical risks, and immediate treatment plans (i.e., an elevated QTc that precludes the use of an antipsychotic treatment) would need to be identified and prioritized, with a plan to revisit more chronic management aspects, such as a DEXA scan, at a later timepoint in treatment.

Differential Diagnosis

The Diagnostic and Statistical Manual of Mental Disorders, Fifth Edition (DSM-5-TR)[1] characterizes AN by restriction of food intake leading to a significantly low weight, fear of gaining weight or engaging in behaviors that maintain low weight; and body image disturbances or impairment in insight to the seriousness of their low body weight. For adults, low weight is defined as a BMI $<18.5 \, kg/m^2$, and AN severity can be further specified as mild (with a BMI of $17-18.49 \, kg/m^2$), moderate (with a BMI of $16-16.99 \, kg/m^2$), severe (with a BMI of $15-15.99 \, kg/m^2$), or extreme (with a BMI $<15 \, kg/m^2$). For children and adolescents, BMI percentiles for age and sex are used, and although those who fall below the fifth BMI percentile for age and sex are generally considered underweight by the CDC, there is no pre-specified cutoff BMI percentile in the DSM-5 criteria. Instead, clinicians should assess the current weight status relative to one's growth trajectory. Two subtypes of AN include restricting (AN-R) and binge-eating/purging (AN-BP) subtypes, with their subclassification depending on the absence or presence of recurrent binge eating and/or purging over the past 3 months, in addition to the predominantly restrictive pattern of eating that is characteristic of AN.

BN is defined in the DSM-5 as the presence of recurrent episodes of binge eating and inappropriate compensatory purging behaviors at least once per week for 3 months or more, to control one's weight. During a binge eating episode, an individual consumes an objectively large amount of food, coupled with feeling a lack of control. Individuals with BN also overvalue the importance of shape and weight in ascertaining their self-worth. The key difference between AN-BP and BN is weight status; individuals with BN are not underweight and are normal weight or even overweight. Patients may utilize a variety of inappropriate behaviors to compensate for the calories consumed. Self-induced vomiting is a common purging method, although it is an inefficient means of ridding the body of calories; one study found that individuals retain more than half of the calories they consume after vomiting.[9] Individuals who purge may also use laxatives, diuretics, enemas, and other medications. For instance, patients with co-morbid type I diabetes mellitus should be assessed for unexplainable episodes of hyperglycemia from inappropriate purging by withholding their insulin, often called "diabulimia." Poorly controlled blood sugar in patients with type I diabetes is well known to accelerate the development of long-term vascular complications (e.g., blindness, limb amputation), as well as a potentially fatal acute complication of diabetic ketoacidosis. Patients with co-morbid attention-deficit hyperactivity disorder (ADHD) who are prescribed stimulants, such as Adderall, may suddenly report a need for much higher doses relative to their baseline, coupled with attempts to lose weight, which can be dangerous for the patient's well-being and predispose them to develop an SUD. As such, it is important for clinicians outside of the ED field to be aware of ED behaviors. The severity rating for BN is based on the number of *compensatory* episodes per week (mild: 1–3, moderate: 4–7, severe: 8–13, extreme: ≥14).

BED is characterized primarily by recurrent episodes of binge eating, at least once per week over 3 months, without compensatory purging. Binge-eating episodes must be associated with three or more of the following: eating rapidly; eating until uncomfortably full; eating large amounts despite a lack of hunger; eating in solitude to avoid embarrassment; and/or feelings of disgust or guilt following the episode. If an individual who is binge eating is also underweight, with or without purging behaviors, an AN-BP diagnosis is more appropriate. If an individual who is binge eating also has recurrent inappropriate compensatory purging behaviors without being underweight, a BN diagnosis is more appropriate. BED is associated with overweight and obese weight status, but not all individuals who are overweight or obese have BED, and not all individuals who have BED are overweight or obese. Unlike AN and BN, BED criteria do not require an over-valuation of shape and weight. However, this feature is common in BED and those who are preoccupied with this concern have had worse outcomes.[10] The severity rating for BED depends on the number of binge-eating episodes per week (mild: 1–3, moderate: 4–7, severe: 8–13, and extreme: ≥14).

ARFID is characterized by a restrictive eating pattern that results in weight loss or growth failure, nutritional deficiency, dependence on enteral feeding or supplements, and/or other impairments to psychosocial functioning. Individuals with ARFID may demonstrate restriction of food volume or variety, or both, related to: sensory sensitivity (e.g., avoidance of specific foods related to negative sensory experiences), fear of aversive consequences (e.g., avoidance of eating related to a prior episode of choking, vomiting, or an allergic reaction), and/or lack of interest in eating

(e.g., a lack of hunger signals). In addition, symptoms of ARFID may be unrelated to any issues of food insecurity and access, or cultural meaning (e.g., religious fasting or culturally normative avoidance of certain foods). Although certain medical conditions may coexist with ARFID, the symptoms of ARFID would not be fully explained by the medical condition alone. There are no severity ratings for ARFID.

OSFED serves as a diagnosis for individuals who clearly have clinically impairing eating disturbances but do not meet the criteria for a specific ED. OSFED comprises five example presentations, including atypical AN (i.e., AN without low body weight); sub-threshold BN (binge eating and purging behaviors occur less than once per week, or BN criteria met for less than 3 months); sub-threshold BED (binge eating occurs with no purging less than once per week, or BED criteria met for less than 3 months); purging disorder (recurrent purging behavior without binge-eating episodes); and night eating syndrome (recurrent nighttime awakenings coupled with eating, or excessive eating after dinner). Of note, as individuals with AN-BP can have purging behaviors without any binge-eating episodes and vice versa, AN-BP can be differentiated from different OSFED types by both the prominence of restrictive eating and the low-weight criteria. For instance, OSFED-atypical AN would demonstrate predominantly restrictive eating and weight loss with or without binge-eating and/or purging episodes much like AN-R and AN-BP, but *without being clinically underweight*. OSFED-BN would not demonstrate a predominantly restrictive eating pattern or significant weight loss, and the distress from binge-eating and purging episodes would be prominent. OSFED-purging disorder would not have a low body weight or the predominance of restrictive eating (i.e., as the presence of restrictive eating, purging, and low body weight would meet criteria for AN-BP, and the presence of restrictive eating and purging without a low body weight would be OSFED-atypical AN). Lastly, night-eating syndrome can be differentiated from sleep-related eating disorders, manifested by parasomnias related to sleep cycle disturbances or associated with certain medications used to treat insomnia (e.g., Ambien), in which patients *do not recall* the excessive mid-sleep food intake. Individuals with night eating syndrome engage in recurrent excessive eating after awakening from sleep or in the late evening after dinner with full awareness and recall of the night-eating episodes despite being unable to control them.[11]

The DSM-5 also includes a diagnosis called "unspecified feeding or eating disorder" (UFED) for instances in which there is insufficient information to confer a specific ED diagnosis and while the symptoms are clearly causing distress or impairment, for when it may not be possible or appropriate to conduct a comprehensive evaluation to diagnose the ED. For instance, in a busy emergency room, the psychiatrist evaluating an acutely suicidal patient with recent weight loss and distress from recurrent episodes of purging may choose to make note of the presence of an UFED in favor of facilitating the patient's expeditious disposition to an inpatient psychiatric setting while making sure that it is noted as part of the risk assessment and history, to be expanded during inpatient treatment.

TREATMENT PLANNING OVERVIEW

Although acute treatment of medical complications, nutritional compromise, and associated acute psychiatric symptoms can begin in the general hospital setting, treatment will eventually move to specialized outpatient psychiatric care. Therefore, the psychiatrist has a critical role in the evaluation and management of eating-disordered patients in general hospitals, involving: (1) a psychiatric evaluation to establish the presence of an ED and other psychiatric diagnoses together with a general medical evaluation to rule out medical etiologies of ED symptoms, to establish the presence of any medical co-morbidities, and to identify the need for more specialized medical consultations; (2) designing a treatment framework that considers the medical and psychiatric risks, acutely and over the longer-term, to *triage towards an optimal treatment setting* without compromising safety (e.g., from an acutely elevated risk due to suicidality or to hemodynamic instability), and *to build a multi-disciplinary care team* to address the treatment needs with a clearly aligned treatment plan. The treatment plan is best finalized and implemented together with the multi-disciplinary care team, to address the: (1) education of the care team; (2) patient and family engagement and education; (3) nutritional rehabilitation and medical monitoring; (4) a behavioral plan to monitor and deter maladaptive

behaviors and encourage regular eating with reinforcing mechanisms; and (5) pharmacologic treatments for ED or for co-morbid conditions, as appropriate.

Considerations in Treatment Planning

The goals of hospitalization for those with an ED are guided by the severity and duration of the condition as well as its medical complications. Initial goals generally encompass stabilization of medical parameters and behavioral symptoms, safety and containment when appropriate, and a plan for nutritional rehabilitation.

A behavioral protocol can be implemented on an inpatient medical or psychiatric service with sufficient medical monitoring capacity based on staff experience and resources, to promote refeeding or control inappropriate compensatory behaviors. Some services have standardized protocols, while in others, the consulting psychiatrist and staff can develop a plan to meet the needs of individual patients. A description of such protocols is beyond the scope of this chapter, but one such protocol for nutritional rehabilitation of a low-weight patient can include supervised meals to monitor for meal completion and to deter compensatory behaviors (e.g., restrictions on bathroom trips within an hour of meals) and clear goals for weekly weight gain and over the course of treatment (e.g., a gain of 2 pounds per week; a pre-specified final weight goal), together with mechanisms to reward and reinforce desired behaviors (e.g., privileges/passes to leave the unit with supervision) with a readout that may be contingent on meeting a dietary plan and/or weight goals.

Some patients who have been hospitalized on a medical service for complications of an ED may eventually be transitioned to an inpatient psychiatric service or to a residential treatment program to complete their course of specialized ED treatment at a higher level of care, even after the stabilization of acute medical issues. Others may be discharged to an ED-focused lower level of treatment that may be appropriate and available depending on the region (such as being an outpatient, in an intensive outpatient program [IOP], or in a partial hospitalization program [PHP]). During outpatient, IOP, or PHP treatments, patients may develop new signs and symptoms that necessitate another hospitalization. Table 16.1 provides a list of signs and symptoms that may indicate the need for hospitalization of eating-disordered patients.

TABLE 16.1
Possible Indications for Hospitalization of Patients With an ED

Domain	Symptom/Sign[a]	Example
Weight	Substantially low body weight or a rapidly falling weight	<75%–85% of expected body weight
Behavioral	Severity of ED symptoms or a concerning escalation in the frequency of symptomatic episodes	Binge eating and/or vomiting 16 times daily that results in social and occupational functional impairments as well as dangerous levels of electrolyte disturbances
		Acute food or water refusal
Medical	Hemodynamic instability	SyncopeSeizures
	Severe medical complications	Dangerous derangements in electrolytes
		Diabetic ketoacidosis from insulin misuse
		Hematemesis or severe and progressive anemia from gastric perforation following purging episodes
		Altered mental status
Psychiatric	Acutely elevated risk of harm to oneself or others	Thoughts of suicide
		Aggression or impulsivity
	Functional impairments related to the overall psychiatric symptom burden	Exacerbation of a co-morbid substance use disorder during treatment of an ED, related to patients substituting a maladaptive coping behavior with another
		Severe co-morbid depression, even in the absence of an active suicidality, that may result in significant functional impairments and interfere with a patient's ability to engage with ED treatment at a lower level of care
Treatment Related	Lack of objective response despite engagement in treatment	Sustained or persistent inability to eat without supervision or to abstain from intractable purging after food intake
	Necessity of close supervision for symptom control	Reaching a threshold weight at which the patient repeatedly has deteriorated rapidly or not achieving a clinically meaningful weight gain even with reported outpatient adherence to the treatment plan, which may suggest the need for closer monitoring for adherence and for treatment-interfering factors

[a]Weight, vital signs, metabolic, and other parameters for hospitalization are best interpreted in the context of the patient's overall health, medical and psychiatric history, support systems, and engagement in treatment. As such, the indication for hospitalization may be appropriate for one patient but not necessarily for another patient. For instance, the level of care determination may not be identical for the following three patients with AN of extreme severity: a patient who has recently lost weight from a BMI of 20 to 14 kg/m^2 in the past few months with rapid deterioration in the medical stability; a patient who has been at a BMI of 14 kg/m^2 for several years in the community without current evidence of an acutely elevated medical or psychiatric risk and no desire to be hospitalized; and a patient who has been at a BMI of 14 kg/m^2 for several years in the community without any issues who recently developed frequent episodes of hematemesis and seizures.
AN, Anorexia nervosa; BMI, body mass index; ED, emergency department.

In the outpatient setting, there is no single way to build an optimal treatment plan. For instance, a consolidated psychiatric treatment plan may be designed, such that a psychiatrist provides weekly psychotherapy, medication management, and medical monitoring, in discussion with the PCP, which may be preferred if the PCP is unable to provide frequent appointments or if there are certain patient-specific factors for which there is a consolidated approach would be more beneficial. Often an ED treatment plan is designed on a split care model, with a psychologist or social work therapist providing weekly psychotherapy and remaining in communication with a PCP or an ED medical specialist who may or may not be a psychiatrist, to provide close medical monitoring, together with, or without, a psychiatrist for any psychopharmacologic treatments. Certain treatment plans include a dietitian who is familiar with ED care and who consults with the patient directly or the patient's caregivers. When involving multiple care team members, it is useful to have clearly delineated non-overlapping roles and responsibilities (e.g., who will monitor weight on a weekly basis, or who will be responsible for medical monitoring) should be established at the time of treatment planning. An important aspect of effective collaboration about the treatment plan, progress, and concerns, is establishing a clear modality and frequency of communication between team members (e.g., via weekly or monthly Zoom meetings, phone calls, email updates; each clinician conducts chart reviews of visits and contacts only when new concerns or issues arise).

Clinicians should strongly encourage their patients to consent to communicate all clinical information that is relevant to treatment planning among team members and should scrutinize how exceptions will impact treatment. Because splitting and miscommunication are both strong possibilities in such treatment situations, the team should make every effort to reach a consensus about the treatment plan and develop contingency plans that depend on progress or difficulties and should present a unified front to the patient. When evaluating an ongoing treatment or a new treatment plan, clinicians should bear in mind that medical, nutritional, and psychological goals are integral to any treatment plan.

Engaging the Reluctant Patient

For the patient who has difficulty admitting the extent of their symptoms or acknowledging that symptoms are problematic, gentle confrontation is recommended. This may include psychoeducation about worrisome clinical signs, the availability and efficacy of treatment, and the risks of not pursuing treatment.

In addition, collaboratively creating a cognitive-behavioral formulation that highlights the predictable and self-defeating links among eating-disordered behaviors can be illuminating for patients who perceive their symptoms as disparate or uncontrollable. Many patients believe that their symptoms have an important primary gain (i.e., controlling their weight) and unduly base their self-worth on their body shape, weight, and appearance. Sometimes, positive feedback and self-efficacy can be so reinforcing that it induces them to lose weight. Not infrequently, the restrictive eating often gives way to bouts of binge eating, which in turn can segue into purging and other inappropriate

compensatory behaviors. Binge eating can be further complicated by a preoccupation with food—so extreme that many patients report being constantly distracted by the tally of calories they have consumed or that they plan to consume that day. Thus a vicious self-reinforcing cycle ensues.

Engaging a patient in ED treatment can also be challenging because the patient may perceive treatment as a threat to the benefits one has accrued from the symptoms. For instance, many patients experience distraction and emotional numbing as a result of their restrictive, binge eating, and purging behaviors that can be a self-soothing coping strategy for those who cannot access more adaptive defenses. Moreover, patients often believe that they will be happier at a low weight; however, the sad reality is that, even after attaining a low body weight, the maladaptive eating habits coupled with malnourished brain physiology preclude patients from attaining sustained happiness regardless of one's body weight. Yet, their associated cognitive inflexibility limits insight into this aspect, undermines therapeutic engagement, and perpetuates the cycle of illness for eating-disordered patients.

For general hospital inpatients who are reluctant to discuss or to allow treatment of their symptoms, engaging the patient around mutually identified goals and identifying key points of leverage are key strategies. Even if the patient provides a seemingly off-target reply (e.g., a patient with AN who hopes to get her parents "off her back," or a patient with BN who would like to lose weight), the stated rationale can prompt the development of specific goals with which to ally with the patient, such as autonomy or health. In addition to informing the patient and family about medical complications and risks associated with the disorder, concrete evidence about the adverse health impacts of the disorder can be presented as a strategy to motivate treatment engagement.

When appropriate, clinicians should work collaboratively with parents, teachers, coaches, or school administration to identify incentives for patients to meet their therapeutic goals. For example, patients may be required to meet specific clinical benchmarks to be eligible to participate in school or extracurricular activities.

Especially when motivation or treatment adherence is in question or the risk of decompensation is high, a treatment agreement that specifies interim goals and the patient's responsibilities provides clarity to the team and to the patient. For example, a patient may be asked to agree to attend all appointments, to allow weighing and laboratory work at intervals specified by the team, and to consent to communication among all members of the treatment team. In addition, parameters to be used in considering a higher level of care should be specified, so that if a patient's weight is unstable, all team members and the patient can agree about the point at which an increased intensity of care (e.g., adding a group, adding medication, or being admitted to an inpatient unit for eating disorders) is necessary. To be maximally therapeutic, non-negotiable outcomes (e.g., hospitalization for persistence of low body weight from treatment nonresponse) should sound rational, be implemented consistently throughout the treatment, avoid surprises, and provide opportunities for the patient to prevent implementation by altering undesirable behaviors.[11,12] Of course, involuntary hospitalization may be necessary when a patient is at imminent risk for self-harm or is unable to care for themselves (e.g., as evidenced by ongoing untreated serious medical complications).

Medical Management

Medical complications of EDs are common, can affect every organ system, and are potentially severe and even lethal. Complications are associated with behaviors that can occur across the spectrum of body weight and EDs.

Poor nutrition associated with a restrictive diet, binge eating and purging behaviors, and/or low body weight from an ED can result in fluid and electrolyte disturbances that require medical attention. Loss of electrolytes, e.g., sodium, may be coupled with a concomitant loss of water, and signs and symptoms that include dehydration, hypotension, tachycardia, postural dizziness, and syncope. Electrolyte imbalances in those with EDs are often asymptomatic, which may lead some to think that the signs are not serious. However, dangerously low or high levels of electrolytes (such as potassium, phosphate, and magnesium) can be precipitated by restrictive eating and starvation or by recurrent purging behaviors (e.g., vomiting and use of laxatives or diuretics) and can result in serious sequelae including life-threatening cardiac arrhythmias, which warrant timely repletion.

Cardiac complications of EDs are often asymptomatic until they become lethal. Bradycardia, orthostasis, and non-specific arrhythmias are common in patients with AN, and they may lead to a reduced left ventricular mass and impairments in systolic function.[13,14] Both QT dispersion and QT interval prolongation may be common in AN,[15] which increases the risk of ventricular arrhythmias and sudden death. Historically, patients with EDs who purged were also at risk of fatal cardiomyopathies due to the once widespread availability of syrup of ipecac with the US Food and Drug Administration (FDA) approval of the OTC status in 1965 (e.g., see the case of Karen Carpenter[16]), but this has become rare over the past decade. Assessment of vital signs and an ECG should be a routine part of the initial evaluation as well as the treatment plan so that acute cardiac complications of EDs can be recognized and addressed.

While fluid and electrolyte imbalances and cardiac complications can lead to life-threatening complications of ED, osteopenia and osteoporosis are among the most serious long-term complications of chronic low-weight status in AN. Low bone mineral density (BMD) of osteopenia or osteoporosis in patients with AN increases the risk of fractures from falling, which contributes to the high burden of morbidity and mortality.[17,18] While there are no FDA-approved therapies for bone loss in AN, the most effective treatment for improving BMD in AN is weight restoration. Supplementation of vitamin D and calcium either individually or with a daily multivitamin is often utilized. That said, some patients who have recovered from AN have persistently reduced BMD,[18] and treatments, such as estrogen replacement, are under investigation for bone health in AN.[19] DEXA scanning at the initial assessment and every 12 to 24 months can assist in counseling those at high risk for fractures and bone loss.

Gastrointestinal (GI) symptoms in patients with EDs, while more benign than cardiac complications, are more common and symptomatic, and can be a barrier to treatment. They include early satiety, indigestion, bloating, flatulence, constipation, abdominal pain, and nausea. These symptoms typically resolve with treatment and with establishing regular eating. GI symptoms of EDs are non-specific, can be related to weight changes or disordered eating, and maybe a manifestation of a co-morbid primary GI illness; therefore, patients with EDs should be evaluated for GI co-morbidities.

Dental erosion and caries develop in patients who purge by vomiting because of the effects of gastric acid on tooth enamel. Patients who engage in vomiting should be referred for dental care.

TREATMENT OF PATIENTS WITH ANOREXIA NERVOSA

The framework of treatment for patients with AN can be the most complex among the EDs. Treatment plans for patients with AN should address aspects of medical monitoring, nutritional rehabilitation, and psychotherapy, with or without adjunctive psychopharmacology.

Medical Monitoring

Treatment plans for patients with AN should include provisions for regular monitoring of body weight on a pre-determined schedule in a consistent setting. Weight checks may be on a weekly basis in the outpatient setting or three times per week in an inpatient unit, depending on the treatment plan, which may build weight gain-dependent reinforcements such as certain in-unit privileges to encourage behavioral change. Depending on clinician and patient preference, blind or open weights for regular weight checks are used without a clear consensus, but this decision should be guided by, and be consistent with, individualized treatment goals. At the time of weight checks, vital signs and a focused physical examination should also be performed, as indicated by the clinical status and the stage of treatment.

Nutritional Rehabilitation

The most important treatment goal for patients with AN addresses weight restoration, which is required for a full return to health. While protocols have a range of weight goals, a good rule of thumb for weight restoration can be a BMI of 20 to 21 kg/m² for adults with AN. Relapse to low-weight status is common shortly after weight restoration (i.e., occurring in up to half of weight-restored patients), and weight restoration should be followed by a relapse-prevention stage of treatment to maintain the restored weight and achieve long-term recovery. Psychological symptoms often resolve more slowly during the weight maintenance stage.

Patients with AN may begin nutritional rehabilitation at any level of care if there are mechanisms in place to monitor for medical stability as part of the treatment plan. If patients are persistently underweight (e.g., ≤75% of expected body weight), or present with a dangerous medical complication, they may require a higher level of care than outpatient treatment. In the absence of any acute medical or psychiatric risks that necessitate higher levels of care (Table 16.1), there is no rule for determining the optimal level of care for patients with AN; the capacity of the clinical team to provide sufficient monitoring of sustained medical stability without acute issues is the major determinant in maintaining or transitioning the level of care to prioritize patient safety. A hospital setting for nutritional rehabilitation can be helpful in addressing acute medical complications in a timely manner and may allow for more careful monitoring of dietary intake, deterring purging and excessive exercising, and facilitating the implementation of behavioral reinforcements to initiate behavioral change. Extreme malnutrition that is recalcitrant to treatment may lead to nasogastric or parenteral feeding approaches, although these are less common. Patients who require inpatient-level care to gain weight, but who repeatedly relapse after discharge, may be best served by care in a residential care setting for an extended period to achieve and stabilize an adequate weight.

Patients with AN who embark on nutritional rehabilitation require close monitoring of their electrolytes in the first week to mitigate the development of refeeding syndrome. It is thought that rapid refeeding stimulates the release of insulin, which results in intracellular shifts in potassium, magnesium, and phosphorus to meet the demand of metabolizing the increased supply of glucose. Sensing the shift, the kidneys attempt to retain sodium, which results in water retention and edema. If not addressed, this can result in volume overload followed by multi-organ failure and death. Therefore regardless of the level of care, any abnormal potassium, magnesium, and phosphorus values should be repleted, to at least 4.0 mmol/L, 2.0 mg/dL, and 3.0 mg/dL, respectively. After several days without significant laboratory abnormalities or other medical issues while sufficiently escalating daily caloric goals (typically in the first 2 weeks), laboratory tests can be checked less frequently.

Calories should be increased incrementally, but rapidly, to achieve desired weight gains of 1 to 2 pounds weekly for outpatients and 2 to 3 pounds weekly in hospital settings. Caloric requirements vary, but patients may require up to 4000 kcal/day as refeeding progresses. Historically, low-calorie refeeding protocols, such as starting at 1400 kcal/day and increasing the daily calorie goal by 200 kcal every other day, have been utilized to mitigate the risk of an adverse event known as the refeeding syndrome. However, slow weight gain may result in underfeeding, which has been associated with negative outcomes; recent evidence has demonstrated the efficacy and safety of higher-calorie refeeding without an increased risk of refeeding syndrome.[20,21] Higher-calorie protocols often start with refeeding at 2000 kcal/day and increasing the daily calorie goal by 200 kcal/day. Energy needs may be greater in young, growing adolescents; nutritional supplements may be beneficial, as can the use of daily multivitamins and empiric or prophylactic repletion of thiamine, which are critical in metabolizing glucose and other nutrients.

Patients may benefit from nutritional consultation, as they are often overly preoccupied with minor details of nutrition (such as calorie counting or carbohydrate avoidance), and their dietary knowledge may come from unreliable sources, such as fad diet books or websites. Nutritional counseling can also be framed as an activity to assist with judgment and motivation. Especially with underweight patients, establishing a caloric requirement and developing a dietary plan to meet the weight goals that are set is highly useful. At a minimum, this plan includes three meals daily to establish expectations of eating in alignment with social norms and nutritional adequacy, and it generally includes snacks or caloric supplements (or both).

Psychological Therapies

For adolescents with AN who are medically stable, manualized family-based treatment (FBT) has the strongest empirical support (reviewed in Refs. 22 and 23). This three-phase outpatient treatment spans 20 sessions over approximately 1 year and is based on the premise that the patient cannot control his or her symptoms, so the parents must temporarily claim responsibility for re-nourishment.[24] In phase one, parents are asked to correct the patient's malnutrition by providing an energy-dense meal plan as well as empathic but firm encouragement for increased calorie consumption. After steady weight gain, food choices are gradually returned to the patient during phase two, and the family is invited to explore the ways in which the AN has affected the family dynamics. In the final phase, when the patient has reached a stable weight, therapy focuses on orchestrating a smooth return to normal adolescent development. As with many behavioral therapies, early change is critical to FBT success.

There are fewer empirical findings to guide psychological treatments in adults with AN (reviewed in Refs. 23 and 25), and randomized controlled trials (RCTs) in adult outpatients with AN have shown only modest weight gain with many patients remaining symptomatic.

No psychological interventions have demonstrated superiority over treatment-as-usual for weight and psychopathology,[25] across modalities including CBT, Maudsley Model of Anorexia Nervosa Treatment for Adults (MANTRA), interpersonal therapy (IPT), and specialist supportive clinical management (a combination of supportive therapy and case management), and focal psychodynamic therapy.[23,25-27] Given the lack of a single treatment with superior efficacy in adults with AN, clinicians should select a therapeutic modality after considering various patient-specific factors. Novel treatments, such as an exposure-based 20-session CBT that promotes early change rather than the usual 40 sessions of CBT for underweight patients, are being evaluated.

Pharmacologic Management

To date, no RCTs testing pharmacologic agents for primary symptoms of AN have been shown to be efficacious. As such, there are no FDA-approved medications for AN.

Because atypical antipsychotics induce significant weight gain and are efficacious for altered cognition, studies have tested antipsychotics as a treatment for the core symptoms of AN (i.e., low weight and rigid cognitive distortions about body image). Results from a meta-analysis that combined the data from small RCTs have shown a lack of efficacy for AN, including a non-significant increase in BMI, no effects on the drive for thinness or body dissatisfaction, and overall ED symptoms.[28] A recent large multi-site RCT conducted at five sites, found that outpatient treatment of adults with AN with olanzapine (2.5–10 mg/day for 16 weeks) was associated with a modest yet significant benefit regarding body weight, with about 1 pound of additional weight gained every month over placebo.[29] This was not accompanied by any significant benefits for the psychological symptoms of AN and its co-morbidities, such as symptoms of depression and obsessive-compulsive disorder (OCD). Nevertheless, olanzapine may be a reasonable adjunctive agent for the treatment of AN. If it is used, treatment plans should monitor vital signs for any changes to blood pressure, the ECG for QTc interval prolongation, laboratory tests that look for any new or worsening metabolic abnormalities (i.e., with a lipid panel and an Hgb A1c every 6 months), as well as a regular physical examination to assess for any abnormal movements suggestive of extrapyramidal symptoms.

RCTs have tested antidepressants with efficacy for depression, anxiety, and OCD in those with AN. The use of selective serotonin reuptake inhibitors (SSRIs) and tricyclic antidepressants (TCAs), as well as other antidepressants, have not shown efficacy regarding the core symptoms of AN or for depressive symptoms (reviewed in Ref. 30), which may be related to the effects of starvation. Anxiolytics, such as benzodiazepines, have not demonstrated any efficacy for the core symptoms of AN or for anxiety.[31] In practice, many providers prescribe psychotropics in an attempt to address the high burden of depression and anxiety in most individuals with AN, and it may be a reasonable addition to the treatment plan if this psychopharmacologic treatment is desired by the patient. Given the overall lack of efficacy across antidepressant and anxiolytic classes in those with AN, SSRIs can be considered given their favorable side effect profile. Benzodiazepines, given the lack of benefits in this population and given the high risk of misuse and dependency, should be avoided when possible.

Agents that promote weight loss or diminish appetite, such as stimulants, should also be avoided whenever possible. Diversion and misuse of such medications or use of illicit substances, like cocaine, maybe a part of the clinical picture that may not be readily apparent but nevertheless poses a barrier to weight gain, and patients should be screened for drug use, given that the shame and guilt over these behaviors may preclude spontaneous disclosure. Lastly, medications that promote appetite or weight gain can inadvertently trigger binge-eating episodes, and should be used judiciously—and with full transparency to the patient—if indicated for other symptom targets for patients with AN.

TREATMENT OF PATIENTS WITH BULIMIA NERVOSA

Psychotherapy, using CBT along with appropriate medical management, has the strongest evidence; therefore it has been the first-line treatment for BN. More than 60% of those with BN do not achieve full remission with psychotherapy alone,[32] highlighting the need for pharmacological options for BN. The use of antidepressants for BN is increasingly accepted as another first-line treatment, either in combination with or as an alternative to psychotherapy, with studies consistently demonstrating the robust benefits of medications for BN. Importantly, patient-factors (such as cultural barriers and attitudes towards the use of psychiatric medications), as well as access to care issues can be considered in designing a treatment plan.

Psychological Therapies

CBT has the best empirical support as the psychotherapy for BN. More specifically, enhanced CBT (CBT-E) is the first-line psychotherapy modality for patients with BN.

CBT-E is a manualized outpatient therapy for use across ED diagnoses.[12] For individuals who are medically stable and not underweight (e.g., those with BN), CBT is designed to span 20 sessions over four stages. In Stage 1, patients are introduced to the general model of EDs in which shape and weight concerns and strict dietary restraint to lose weight promote binge eating and purging in a self-perpetuating cycle (to develop a personalized formulation for the patient's illness). Patients and therapists co-create a schedule of regular eating (i.e., three meals and two snacks daily), and the patient is asked to self-monitor food intake to identify individualized triggers for binge eating and purging and to use the information from the self-monitoring records to identify alternative pleasurable activities to distract from urges to binge. Stage 2 involves taking stock of progress and identifying maintaining mechanisms that will be addressed in Stage 3. In Stage 3, the therapist assists the patient in reducing factors that maintain the ED psychopathology (e.g., over-valuation of shape and weight in self-evaluation) through behavioral interventions. For instance, the therapist may assist the patient in reducing body-checking and avoidance behaviors that exacerbate body dissatisfaction, by cultivating alternative aspects of self-evaluation other than shape and weight. In Stage 4 the patient develops a relapse-prevention plan (by identifying stressful situations that may trigger symptoms) as well as problem-solving potential solutions. CBT-E for BN has demonstrated consistently good empiric support, e.g., in a waitlist-controlled trial, over half of the patients with BN achieved remission of binge eating and purging along with improvements in BN psychopathology by 1 standard deviation of community norms by the end of 20-session treatment and at a 60-week follow-up.[33]

For adolescents with BN, FBT has demonstrated comparable efficacy to CBT-E, and either therapy modality may be offered.[34] In adults, CBT-E is the "gold standard" therapy modality for BN, but treatment alternatives should be considered for those who do not respond to CBT, do not wish to participate, or do not have access to specialized treatments. For example, self-help versions of CBT using books like *Overcoming Binge Eating*[35] have demonstrated some efficacy for BN. Moreover, self-guided CBT that augments this with a limited number of brief meetings with a therapist has been shown to be more effective than pure self-help.[36,37] Self-help and guided self-help versions of CBT enhance access to care for patients. In addition, studies of CBT-E outcomes have shown that regularizing eating patterns within the first 4 weeks of 20-session CBT predicts better overall treatment response, a 10-session CBT for non-underweight patients, such as those with BN, has been developed with a focus on promoting early behavioral change, with findings that appear to support efficacy of this approach. While IPT may be efficacious for BN it may take longer to achieve results than with CBT, increasing the length of time the patient is suffering from bulimic symptoms. Other therapies that have some empirical support for BN include emerging approaches that incorporate third-wave behavioral therapy techniques, such as those drawn from acceptance and commitment therapy and dialectical behavior therapy.

Pharmacologic Management

Fluoxetine has been FDA approved for BN since 1996. Treatments with high doses of fluoxetine (e.g., 60 mg daily) for 8 weeks have shown efficacy over placebo in reducing the core behavioral symptoms of BN (i.e., binge eating and purging) in adults in a large RCT across 13 sites,[38] together with consistently robust benefits in other RCTs. Fluoxetine is also well tolerated and reduces co-morbid depressive symptoms in patients with BN. Given the observed dose-dependent efficacy, fluoxetine (60 mg daily) is the first-line pharmacotherapy for BN, either starting on this dose as in the studies or with a short titration period. Subsequently, small studies using fluoxetine for BN have also demonstrated efficacy after a limited treatment response to psychological interventions such as CBT or IPT for BN[39] and in maintenance therapy over the course of a year.[40]

Other SSRIs, such as sertraline and citalopram, and other classes of antidepressants, such as TCAs (like imipramine) and monoamine oxidase inhibitors (MAOIs) (like phenelzine) have demonstrated efficacy in reducing BN symptoms, and the norepinephrine-dopamine reuptake inhibitor bupropion is contraindicated in BN due to the increased risk of seizures.[41] Among these options, SSRIs have the best evidence base for efficacy in BN and the most benign side effect profile, which can be trialed bearing in mind that higher doses may be optimal to address the symptoms of BN. Because of this, closer monitoring may be required when trialing citalopram for BN (if considering doses >40 mg daily, given the potential for QTc prolongation).

Other classes of medications also show promise. A 10-week topiramate trial, in doses ranging from 25 to 400 mg (median dose, 100 mg) daily in one study, was found to significantly reduce BN symptoms over placebo in RCTs.[42] However, topiramate can induce side effects that include cognitive issues and paresthesia, as well as weight loss; therefore the potential benefits of topiramate for BN should be weighed against the potential risk of substantial weight loss and cross-over to AN-BP that could add to the morbidity and impair the life of the patient. Other medications that have demonstrated some benefits for BN include naltrexone and ondansetron, however, it is widely accepted that no medications match the robust benefits of high-dose fluoxetine for BN.

In summary, the first-line pharmacotherapy for BN is high-dose fluoxetine, which has the best efficacy and side effect profile. It may also have efficacy for adolescents with BN[43] and if fluoxetine or other SSRIs are used for adolescents and young adults with BN, practitioners should provide close monitoring for treatment-emergent thoughts of suicide,[44] as described in the FDA's black box warning. Regardless of the medication choice, the risk:benefit ratio should be considered for each patient. Lastly, it is essential to ensure that the dosing schedule is arranged with consideration of the pattern of purging throughout the day so that the medication can be sufficiently absorbed to take effect.

TREATMENT OF PATIENTS WITH BINGE EATING DISORDER

Patients with BED are often quite willing to seek and accept treatment. Because BED is frequently co-morbid with obesity, patients often come to treatment motivated to address binge eating that poses a barrier to weight loss attempts. CBT is the first-line treatment for BED, with or without SSRI antidepressants, which also have efficacy for BED.

Psychological Therapies

CBT has the strongest empirical support for BED (reviewed in Ref. 45). Because BN and BED share clinical features and CBT-E is meant to be transdiagnostic, CBT for BED is quite similar to that for BN, featuring psychoeducation, self-monitoring, normalization of eating, reducing the extent to which self-evaluation is based on shape and weight, and relapse prevention. In studies that compared CBT to pharmacotherapy for BED, CBT treatments with or without pharmacotherapy were superior to both pharmacotherapy and placebo alone. And, as with BN, CBT can also be delivered in a guided self-help style or in group formats with promising results for BED.[46,47] IPT is a second-line treatment for patients with BED who do not respond rapidly to CBT. Despite the efficacy of CBT and other psychological treatments for binge

eating in those with BED, treatments for BED are not associated with significant weight loss in patients with BED who are overweight or obese,[46,47] which may be disheartening for patients. If so, concepts from the Health at Every Size may offer some comfort as this philosophy is grounded on how healthy behaviors are more important for one's health than the number on the scale.[48] Alternatively, pharmacologic augmentation can be considered as data supports modest benefits for weight loss for pharmacologic interventions for BED. As such, while psychotherapy remains the first-line treatment for BED, adjunctive pharmacotherapy can be beneficial for some patients.

Pharmacologic Management

Several medications have demonstrated efficacy for BED in RCTs (reviewed in Ref. 49). While antidepressants have efficacy for BED,[50,51] because CBT has been shown to be consistently superior to antidepressants,[52] antidepressants are a second-line option for those who do not respond to CBT or when access to psychotherapy is limited. When patients with BED are overweight or obese, SSRIs are preferred over TCAs and MAOIs given the weight neutrality of SSRIs.

Lisdexamfetamine (LDX; Vyvanse), a stimulant pro-drug used in the treatment of patients with ADHD, remains the only FDA-approved medication for BED. LDX works by enhancing norepinephrine and dopamine levels in the brain. Several large RCTs have found that LDX led to fewer binge episodes per week in those with moderate-to-severe BED, with one large 30-site RCT demonstrating efficacy at 8 weeks with either 50 mg or 70 mg daily doses of LDX over placebo in moderate-to-severe BED.[53] Continuation of LDX therapy for maintenance treatment of BED after initial response was associated with a lower risk of relapse.[54] The safety profile and tolerability of LDX in this population were consistent with previous findings in adults with ADHD.[55] Common side effects include insomnia, irritability, anxiety, and dry mouth, along with elevations in blood pressure and heart rate. As such, medical and psychiatric health and co-morbidities must be evaluated prior to initiating treatment. Given the risks of misuse and diversion and the potential for dependency on stimulant treatments, LDX should be used with caution in individuals with an SUD history.

Although LDX is not FDA approved for obesity, LDX treatment in those with BED can be associated with weight loss.[53,55] As BED is more commonly associated with obesity than other EDs, other treatments that address symptoms of BED and obesity are of interest. FDA-approved medications for obesity are being actively tested for patients with BED and obesity. For instance, a small RCT has demonstrated the efficacy of phentermine-topiramate (Qysmia) with doses of 3.75 to 15 mg and 23 to 92 mg, respectively, which led to a reduction in BED symptoms along with a 6 kg weight loss over 12 weeks.[56] Of the combination regimens, topiramate monotherapy over 14 weeks at 50 to 600 mg (median dose 212 mg) daily[57] or 16 weeks at 25 to 400 mg (median dose 300 mg) daily[57,58] has also been effective for reducing the frequency of binge eating along with a 5-kg weight loss.[57,58] However, patients may not tolerate the high side effect burden, such as impaired cognition, paresthesia, and taste perversion.

In summary, treatment for BED may benefit from pharmacologic augmentation with agents that target depression, ADHD, and obesity, depending on the patient-specific factors together with patients' verbalized goals, such as weight loss.

TREATMENT OF PATIENTS WITH AVOIDANT/RESTRICTIVE FOOD INTAKE DISORDER

Treatments for ARFID are being actively investigated. Proof-of-concept studies have demonstrated the early promise of CBT (CBT-AR),[59,60] FBT,[61] and supportive parenting for anxious childhood emotions (SPACE-ARFID)[62] for children and adolescents with ARFID. Preliminary findings of CBT-AR in adults with ARFID have also been promising.[63]

There are no FDA-approved medications or any large RCTs that support the use of pharmacotherapy for ARFID, and any off-label pharmacologic treatments can be considered as adjunctive if the risk-benefit profile is acceptable.

SUMMARY

EDs may affect individuals of all ages, sexes, races, ethnicities, and socioeconomic status and may be more common than previously thought, affecting about 28 million Americans at some point in their lives. EDs can occur with limited overt clinical signs that may mask the severity of the condition, and treatment planning should always address medical health and psychological symptoms. Optimal management of patients with EDs starts with a comprehensive evaluation that encompasses psychiatric and medical symptoms, signs, and history pertinent to the diagnostic clarification of the ED, which is important in guiding treatment planning. In addition, stratification of psychiatric and medical risk profiles with information from the evaluation is necessary to triage to the appropriate level of care that ensures patient safety. Treatment planning for AN, which has one of the highest mortality rates across psychiatric disorders, should address elements of medical monitoring, nutritional rehabilitation, and psychological treatments to normalize the disordered eating towards weight normalization. While adjunctive use of olanzapine can be considered, no medications have been FDA approved for AN. In contrast, both CBT-E and high-dose fluoxetine are considered first-line interventions to address binge eating and purging in BN. For BED, while CBT-E remains a first-line treatment, LDX has been FDA approved for use in BED, and there may be additional benefits for those who wish to lose weight. For ARFID, cognitive-behavioral approaches that target interruption of restrictive eating behaviors show promise. Overall, the burden of morbidity and mortality remains high for EDs and early intervention may be beneficial. Given the limited treatment options with robust efficacy for AN, ARFID, and OSFED, additional research is needed.

REFERENCES

1. American Psychiatric Association. *Diagnostic and Statistical Manual of Mental Disorders, Text Revision.* 5th ed. American Psychiatric Association; 2022.
2. Harvard T. H. Chan School of Public Health and Boston Children's Hospital. *The Social and Economic Cost of Eating Disorders in the United States of America: A Report for the Strategic Training Initiative for the Prevention of Eating Disorders and the Academy for Eating Disorders.* Available at: https://www.hsph.harvard.edu/striped/report-economic-costs-of-eating-disorders/. June 2020.
3. Eddy KT, Tabri N, Thomas JJ, et al. Recovery from anorexia nervosa and bulimia nervosa at 22-year follow-up. *J Clin Psychiatry.* 2017;78:184–189.

4. Eddy KT, Dorer DJ, Franko DL, et al. Diagnostic crossover in anorexia nervosa and bulimia nervosa: implications for DSM-V. *Am J Psychiatry*. 2008;165:245–250.

5. Fairburn CG, Cooper Z, Doll HA, et al. The natural course of bulimia nervosa and binge eating disorder in young women. *Arch Gen Psychiatry*. 2000;57:659–665.

6. Feltner C, Peat C, Reddy S, et al. Screening for eating disorders in adolescents and adults: evidence report and systematic review for the US Preventive Services Task Force. *JAMA*. 2022;327:1068–1082.

7. Kuczmarski RJ, Ogden CL, Guo SS, et al. 2000 CDC growth charts for the United States: methods and development. *Vital Health Stat*. 2002;11:1–190.

8. Kim YR, Lauze MS, Slattery M, et al. Association between ghrelin and body weight trajectory in individuals with anorexia nervosa. *JAMA Netw Open*. 2023;6:e234625.

9. Kaye WH, Weltzin TE, Hsu LK, et al. Amount of calories retained after binge eating and vomiting. *Am J Psychiatry*. 1993;150:969–971.

10. Grilo CM. Psychological and behavioral treatments for binge-eating disorder. *J Clin Psychiatry*. 2017;78(Suppl 1):20–24.

11. Geller J, Srikameswaran S. Treatment non-negotiables: why we need them and how to make them work. *Eur Eating Disord Rev*. 2006;14:212–217.

12. Fairburn CG. *Cognitive Behavior Therapy and Eating Disorders*. Guilford Press; 2008.

13. Romano C, Chinali M, Pasanisi F, et al. Reduced hemodynamic load and cardiac hypotrophy in patients with anorexia nervosa. *Am J Clin Nutr*. 2003;77:308–312.

14. Olivares JL, Vazquez M, Fleta J, et al. Cardiac findings in adolescents with anorexia nervosa at diagnosis and after weight restoration. *Eur J Pediatr*. 2005;164:383–386.

15. Swenne I, Larsson PT. Heart risk associated with weight loss in anorexia nervosa and eating disorders: risk factors for QTc interval prolongation and dispersion. *Acta Paediatr*. 1999;88:304–309.

16. Schmidt R. Karen Carpenter's tragic story. *The Guardian*. 2010. Available from: https://www.theguardian.com/books/2010/oct/24/karen-carpenter-anorexia-book-extract

17. Schorr M, Miller KK. The endocrine manifestations of anorexia nervosa: mechanisms and management. *Nat Rev Endocrinol*. 2017;13:174–186.

18. Misra M, Golden NH, Katzman DK. State of the art systematic review of bone disease in anorexia nervosa. *Int J Eat Disord*. 2016;49:276–292.

19. Misra M, Katzman D, Miller KK, et al. Physiologic estrogen replacement increases bone density in adolescent girls with anorexia nervosa. *J Bone Miner Res*. 2011;26:2430–2438.

20. Golden NH, Cheng J, Kapphahn CJ, et al. Higher-calorie refeeding in anorexia nervosa: 1-year outcomes from a randomized controlled trial. *Pediatrics*. 2021:147.

21. Garber AK, Cheng J, Accurso EC, et al. Short-term outcomes of the study of refeeding to optimize inpatient gains for patients with anorexia nervosa: a multicenter randomized clinical trial. *JAMA Pediatr*. 2021;175:19–27.

22. Datta N, Matheson BE, Citron K, et al. Evidence based update on psychosocial treatments for eating disorders in children and adolescents. *J Clin Child Adolesc Psychol*. 2022:1–12.

23. *A Guide to Selecting Evidence-Based Psychological Therapies for Eating Disorders*. 1st ed. Academy for Eating Disorders; 2020.

24. Lock J. *Treatment Manual for Anorexia Nervosa: A Family-Based Approach*. Guilford Press; 2001.

25. Solmi M, Wade TD, Byrne S, et al. Comparative efficacy and acceptability of psychological interventions for the treatment of adult outpatients with anorexia nervosa: a systematic review and network meta-analysis. *Lancet Psychiatry*. 2021;8:215–224.

26. McIntosh VV, Jordan J, Carter FA, et al. Three psychotherapies for anorexia nervosa: a randomized, controlled trial. *Am J Psychiatry*. 2005;162:741–747.

27. Fisher CA, Skocic S, Rutherford KA, Hetrick SE. Family therapy approaches for anorexia nervosa. *Cochrane Database Syst Rev*. 2019(5): CD004780.

28. Dold M, Aigner M, Klabunde M, et al. Second-generation antipsychotic drugs in anorexia nervosa: a meta-analysis of randomized controlled trials. *Psychother Psychosom*. 2015;84:110–116.

29. Attia E, Steinglass JE, Walsh BT, et al. Olanzapine versus placebo in adult outpatients with anorexia nervosa: a randomized clinical trial. *Am J Psychiatry*. 2019;176:449–456.

30. Claudino AM, Hay P, Lima MS, et al. Antidepressants for anorexia nervosa. *Cochrane Database Syst Rev*. 2006 CD004365.

31. Steinglass JE, Kaplan SC, Liu Y, et al. The (lack of) effect of alprazolam on eating behavior in anorexia nervosa: a preliminary report. *Int J Eat Disord*. 2014;47:901–904.

32. Linardon J, Wade TD. How many individuals achieve symptom abstinence following psychological treatments for bulimia nervosa? A meta-analytic review. *Int J Eat Disord*. 2018;51:287–294.

33. Fairburn CG, Cooper Z, Doll HA, et al. Transdiagnostic cognitive-behavioral therapy for patients with eating disorders: a two-site trial with 60-week follow-up. *Am J Psychiatry*. 2009;166:311–319.

34. Le Grange D, Lock J, Agras WS, et al. Randomized clinical trial of family-based treatment and cognitive-behavioral therapy for adolescent bulimia nervosa. *J Am Acad Child Adolesc Psychiatry*. 2015;54:886–894. e882.

35. Fairburn CG. *Overcoming Binge Eating: The Proven Program to Learn Why You Binge and How You Can Stop*. 2nd ed. The Guilford Press; 2013.

36. Banasiak SJ, Paxton SJ, Hay P. Guided self-help for bulimia nervosa in primary care: a randomized controlled trial. *Psychol Med*. 2005;35:1283–1294.

37. Wagner G, Penelo E, Wanner C, et al. Internet-delivered cognitive-behavioural therapy v. conventional guided self-help for bulimia nervosa: long-term evaluation of a randomised controlled trial. *Br J Psychiatry*. 2013;202:135–141.

38. Fluoxetine Bulimia Nervosa Collaborative Study Group Fluoxetine in the treatment of bulimia nervosa. A multicenter, placebo-controlled, double-blind trial. *Arch Gen Psychiatry*. 1992;49:139–147.

39. Walsh BT, Agras WS, Devlin MJ, et al. Fluoxetine for bulimia nervosa following poor response to psychotherapy. *Am J Psychiatry*. 2000;157:1332–1334.

40. Romano SJ, Halmi KA, Sarkar NP, et al. A placebo-controlled study of fluoxetine in continued treatment of bulimia nervosa after successful acute fluoxetine treatment. *Am J Psychiatry*. 2002;159:96–102.

41. Horne RL, Ferguson JM, Pope HG Jr, et al. Treatment of bulimia with bupropion: a multicenter controlled trial. *J Clin Psychiatry*. 1988;49:262–266.

42. Hoopes SP, Reimherr FW, Hedges DW, et al. Treatment of bulimia nervosa with topiramate in a randomized, double-blind, placebo-controlled trial, part 1: improvement in binge and purge measures. *J Clin Psychiatry*. 2003;64:1335–1341.

43. Kotler LA, Devlin MJ, Davies M, Walsh BT. An open trial of fluoxetine for adolescents with bulimia nervosa. *J Child Adolesc Psychopharmacol*. 2003;13:329–335.

44. Bridge JA, Iyengar S, Salary CB, et al. Clinical response and risk for reported suicidal ideation and suicide attempts in pediatric antidepressant treatment: a meta-analysis of randomized controlled trials. *JAMA*. 2007;297:1683–1696.

45. Iacovino JM, Gredysa DM, Altman M, Wilfley DE. Psychological treatments for binge eating disorder. *Curr Psychiatry Rep*. 2012;14:432–446.

46. Wilson GT, Wilfley DE, Agras WS, Bryson SW. Psychological treatments of binge eating disorder. *Arch Gen Psychiatry*. 2010;67:94–101.

47. Brownley KA, Berkman ND, Peat CM, et al. Binge-eating disorder in adults: a systematic review and meta-analysis. *Annals Int Med*. 2016;165:409–420.

48. Bacon L. *Health at Every Size: The Surprising Truth About Your Weight*. Rev. & updated ed. BenBella Books; 2010.

49. Heal DJ, Gosden J. What pharmacological interventions are effective in binge-eating disorder? Insights from a critical evaluation of the evidence from clinical trials. *Int J Obes (Lond)*. 2022;46:677–695.

50. Leombruni P, Piero A, Lavagnino L, et al. A randomized, double-blind trial comparing sertraline and fluoxetine 6-month treatment in obese patients with Binge Eating Disorder. *Prog Neuropsychopharmacol Biol Psychiatry*. 2008;32:1599–1605.

51. McElroy SL, Hudson JI, Malhotra S, et al. Citalopram in the treatment of binge-eating disorder: a placebo-controlled trial. *J Clin Psychiatry*. 2003;64:807–813.

52. Devlin MJ, Goldfein JA, Petkova E, et al. Cognitive behavioral therapy and fluoxetine as adjuncts to group behavioral therapy for binge eating disorder. *Obes Res*. 2005;13:1077–1088.

53. McElroy SL, Hudson JI, Mitchell JE, et al. Efficacy and safety of lisdexamfetamine for treatment of adults with moderate to severe binge-eating disorder: a randomized clinical trial. *JAMA Psychiatry*. 2015;72:235–246.

54. Hudson JI, McElroy SL, Ferreira-Cornwell MC, et al. Efficacy of lisdexamfetamine in adults with moderate to severe binge-eating disorder: a randomized clinical trial. *JAMA Psychiatry*. 2017;74:903–910.

55. Gasior M, Hudson J, Quintero J, et al. A phase 3, multicenter, open-label, 12-month extension safety and tolerability trial of lisdexamfetamine dimesylate in adults with binge eating disorder. *J Clin Psychopharmacol*. 2017;37:315–322.

56. Safer DL, Adler S, Dalai SS, et al. A randomized, placebo-controlled crossover trial of phentermine-topiramate ER in patients with binge-eating disorder and bulimia nervosa. *Int J Eat Disord*. 2020;53:266–277.

57. McElroy SL, Arnold LM, Shapira NA, et al. Topiramate in the treatment of binge eating disorder associated with obesity: a randomized, placebo-controlled trial. *Am J Psychiatry*. 2003;160:255–261.

58. McElroy SL, Hudson JI, Capece JA, et al. Topiramate for the treatment of binge eating disorder associated with obesity: a placebo-controlled study. *Biol Psychiatry*. 2007;61:1039–1048.

59. Thomas JJ, Becker KR, Kuhnle MC, et al. Cognitive-behavioral therapy for avoidant/restrictive food intake disorder: feasibility, acceptability, and proof-of-concept for children and adolescents. *Int J Eat Disord*. 2020;53:1636–1646.

60. Thomas JJ, Eddy K. *Cognitive-Behavioral Therapy for Avoidant/Restrictive Food Intake Disorder: Children, Adolescents, and Adults*. Cambridge University Press; 2019.

61. Lock J, Sadeh-Sharvit S, L'Insalata A. Feasibility of conducting a randomized clinical trial using family-based treatment for avoidant/restrictive food intake disorder. *Int J Eat Disord*. 2019;52:746–751.

62. Shimshoni Y, Silverman WK, Lebowitz ER. SPACE-ARFID: a pilot trial of a novel parent-based treatment for avoidant/restrictive food intake disorder. *Int J Eat Disord*. 2020;53: 1623–1635.

63. Thomas JJ, Becker KR, Breithaupt L, et al. Cognitive-behavioral therapy for adults with avoidant/restrictive food intake disorder. *J Behav Cogn Ther*. 2021;31:47–55.

17 PAIN

SHAMIM H. NEJAD, MD, FASAM ■ MENEKSE ALPAY, MD

OVERVIEW

Of all human experiences, pain is the most absorbing; it is the only human experience that generally confers a sense of relief and joy when it comes to an end. Moreover, by its very nature, it is solitary. Despite its intensity and its unequaled power over the mind and body, pain can be difficult to recall once it subsides.[1] The International Association for the Study of Pain (IASP) has re-defined pain as "an unpleasant sensory and emotional experience associated with or resembling that associated with actual or potential tissue damage," and has added six clinical components.

- Pain is always a personal experience that is influenced to varying degrees by biological, psychological, and social factors.
- Pain and nociception are different phenomena. Pain cannot be inferred solely from activity in sensory neurons.
- Through their life experiences individuals learn the concept of pain.
- A person's report of an experience of pain should be respected.
- Although pain usually serves an adaptive role, it may have adverse effects on function and social and psychological well-being.
- Verbal descriptions are only one of several ways to express pain, and the inability to communicate does not negate the possibility that a human or non-human animal experiences pain.[2,3]

This definition recognizes the fact that pain has both an acute nociceptive aspect and an emotional-affective dimension; these factors suggest that psychiatrists may have a significant role in the treatment of patients who suffer from pain. Conceptualizing pain in this manner underscores the fact that pain is an important and complicated sensation.

In this chapter, the pathophysiology of pain along with common pain syndromes and terminology is reviewed. In addition, the role of the psychiatric consultant and psychiatric assessment of the patient with pain is discussed. Furthermore, general principles of pain management, including the use of medications for symptomatic pain management, as well as approaches to the treatment of pain behavior are outlined. The problem of pain being co-morbid with substance use disorders (SUDs) is also discussed.

PATHOPHYSIOLOGY OF PAIN

To understand pain, one needs to know about the pathophysiology of nociception and realize that the threshold, intensity, quality, time course, and perceived location of pain are determined by CNS mechanisms.[3] For example, neurosurgeons have shown that interruption of the specific pain pathways often does not eliminate pain; numbness does not confer analgesia. Peripheral nerve damage may result in changes in the receptive fields and recruitment of neurons at multiple levels of the nervous system (from the dorsal horn to the brainstem and the thalamus and cortex). Somatic therapies directed only at nociceptive input may be ineffective.[4]

Detection of noxious stimuli (i.e., nociception) starts with the activation of peripheral nociceptors (somatic pain) or with the activation of nociceptors in bodily organs (visceral pain). Somatic pain is usually well localized, attributable to certain structures or areas, and described as stabbing, aching, or throbbing. In contrast, visceral pain may be poorly localized, not necessarily attributable to the involved organ (i.e., as is the case with referred pain), and is characteristically described as dull and crampy.

Tissue injury stimulates the nociceptors by the liberation of substances (e.g., prostaglandins, arachidonic acid, histamine, and bradykinin). Subsequently, axons transmit the pain signal to the spinal cord (to cell bodies in the dorsal root ganglia; see Fig. 17.1).

Three different types of axons are involved in the transmission of a painful stimulus from the skin to the dorsal horn. A-β fibers are the largest and most heavily myelinated fibers that transmit awareness of light touch. A-δ fibers and C fibers are the primary nociceptive afferents. A-δ fibers are 2 to 5 μm in diameter and are thinly myelinated. They conduct immediate, rapid, sharp, and brief pain (first pain) with a velocity of 20 m/second. C fibers are 0.2 to 1.5 μm in diameter and are unmyelinated. They conduct prolonged, burning, and unpleasant pain (second pain) at a speed of 0.5 m/second. A-δ and C fibers enter the dorsal root and ascend or descend one to three segments before

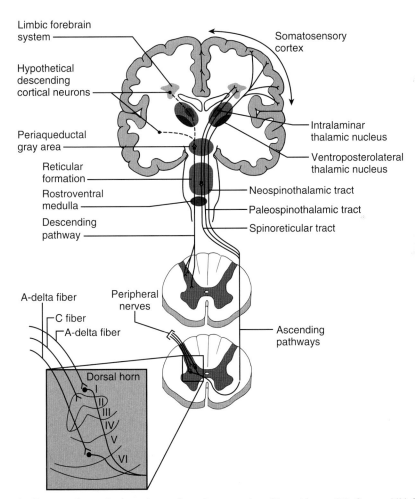

Fig. 17.1 ■ Schematic diagram of neurologic pathways for pain perception. (From Hyman SH, Cassem NH. Pain. In: Rubenstein E, Federman DD, eds. *Scientific American Medicine: Current Topics in Medicine. Subsection II.* Scientific American; 1989.)

synapsing with neurons in the lateral spinothalamic tract (*substantia gelatinosa* in the gray matter).

Substance P, an 11-amino-acid polypeptide, considered to be a major pain neurotransmitter, is released from the fibers at many of these synapses. Capsaicin, which is extracted from red hot peppers, inhibits nociception by inhibiting substance P. Inhibition of nociception in the dorsal horn is functionally quite important. Stimulation of the A-δ fibers not only excites some neurons but also inhibits others. This inhibition of nociception through A-δ fiber stimulation may explain the effects of acupuncture and transcutaneous electrical nerve stimulation (TENS). The lateral spinothalamic tract crosses the midline and ascends toward the thalamus. At the level of the brainstem, more than half of this tract synapses in the reticular activating system (in the *spinoreticular tract*), in the limbic system, and in other brainstem regions (including centers for the autonomic nervous system). Another site of projections at this level is the periaqueductal gray (PAG; see Fig. 17.2), which plays an important role in the brain's endogenous analgesia system. After synapsing in the thalamic nuclei, pain fibers project to the somatosensory cortex, located posterior to the sylvian fissure in the parietal lobe (Brodmann's areas 1, 2, and 3).[5]

Developments in imaging technology have clarified the relationship between pain pathways and cortical and limbic areas. These findings may help explain the relationship among emotions, cognition, and pain modulation that are observed in clinical practice as heightened pain perception in depressed patients and high rates of depression in those with chronic pain. Functional imaging studies utilizing both functional magnetic resonance imaging and positron emission tomography (PET) have shown that acute traumatic nociceptive pain activates the hypothalamus and the PAG as well as the prefrontal cortex, insular cortex, anterior cingulate cortex (ACC), posterior parietal cortex, primary motor/somatosensory areas, supplementary motor area, thalamus, and cerebellum.[6] Additionally, functional imaging studies have helped clinicians understand cognitive and emotional modulation of pain perception. Researchers have shown that with hypnotic suggestion the activity in the ACC is dependent on the intensity of the suggestion (i.e., the same stimulus with the suggestion of "highly

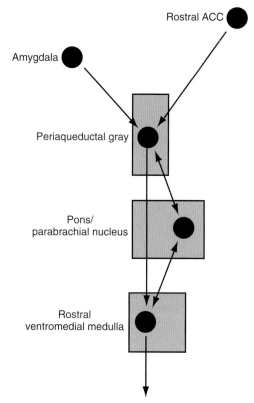

Fig. 17.2 ■ Endogenous opioid systems. *ACC*, Anterior cingulate cortex. (From Petrovic P, Ingvar M. Imaging cognitive modulation of pain processing. *Pain.* 2002;95:1–5.)

unpleasant" induces significantly more ACC activation than when suggestions are less unpleasant).[7,8] In another study, when subjects were distracted during a painful stimulus, pain perception was attenuated in somatosensory regions and the PAG.[9] The short-acting opioid, remifentanil, as well as placebo analgesia, have been shown to activate the ACC, which is rich in opioid receptors.[10] It is of interest that analgesia induced by both opioids and placebos has been reversed with the opioid antagonist naloxone.[11] These findings suggest that cortical areas may exert control over lower brain areas involved in opioid analgesia.[10]

Endogenous analgesic systems involve numerous endogenous peptides with opiate-like activity in the central nervous system (CNS) (e.g., endorphins, enkephalins, dynorphins, nociception/orphanin FQ). Different opiate receptors are involved in different opiate effects.[12]

Mu (μ) receptors are involved in the regulation of analgesia, respiratory depression, constipation, and miosis. Mu receptors (located in the PAG, rostral ventral medulla, medial thalamus, and dorsal horn of the spinal cord) are the receptors that are mainly responsible for supraspinal analgesia.

Kappa (κ) receptors in the dorsal horn (spinal analgesia), deep cortical areas, and other locations are involved in spinal analgesia, sedation, and miosis; pentazocine preferentially acts on these receptors.

Delta (δ) receptors, like κ-receptors, mediate spinal analgesia, hypotension, and miosis. Enkephalins (located in the limbic system, the dorsal horn, and other locations unrelated to pain) have a higher affinity for these receptors than opiates. δ-Receptors also mediate psychotomimetic effects (i.e., psychosis) in the CNS. Their effects are not reversed by naloxone, an opiate antagonist.[5]

In terms of anatomic organization, the centers involved in endogenous analgesia include, in addition to PAG, the rostral ACC, amygdala, parabrachial plexus in the pons, and rostral ventromedial medulla.[10] The descending analgesic pain pathway starts in the PAG (which is rich in endogenous opiates), projects to the rostral ventral medulla, and from there descends through the dorsolateral funiculus of the spinal cord to the dorsal horn. The neurons in the rostral ventral medulla use serotonin to activate endogenous analgesics (enkephalins) in the dorsal horn. This effect inhibits nociception at the level of the dorsal horn since neurons that contain enkephalins synapse with spinothalamic neurons.

In addition, there are noradrenergic neurons that project from the locus coeruleus (the main noradrenergic center in the CNS) to the dorsal horn and inhibit the response of dorsal horn neurons to nociceptive stimuli. The effects of tricyclic antidepressants (TCAs) and other newer antidepressants are thought to be related to an increase in serotonin and norepinephrine that inhibits nociception at the level of the dorsal horn.[5]

PAIN TERMINOLOGY

Acute pain is usually related to an identifiable injury or a disease; it is self-limited and resolves over hours to days or in a time frame that is associated with healing.

Acute pain is usually associated with objective autonomic features (e.g., tachycardia, hypertension, diaphoresis, mydriasis, or pallor).

Chronic pain (i.e., pain that persists beyond the normal time of healing or lasts longer than 6 months) may have a neurologic origin, involving lowered firing thresholds for spinal cord cells that modulate pain (triggering pain more easily); anatomic plasticity and recruitment of a wide range of cells in the spinal cord (so that touch or movement causes pain); convergence of cutaneous, vascular, muscle, and joint inputs (where one tissue refers pain to another); or aberrant connections (electric short circuits between the sympathetic and sensory nerves that produce causalgia). Muscle pains often add to the pain experience. Vascular and other visceral mechanisms share features with neurologic mechanisms; however, these mechanisms involved are not mutually exclusive.[13,14] Table 17.1[15-27] summarizes the clinical implications of the mechanisms of chronic pain. Characteristic features include vague descriptions of pain and an inability to describe the pain's timing and localization. Unlike acute pain, chronic pain lacks signs of heightened sympathetic activity. Depression, anxiety, and premorbid personality problems are common in this patient population. It is usually helpful to determine the presence of a dermatomal pattern (Fig. 17.3), determine the presence of neuropathic pain, and assess pain behavior.

Continuous pain in the terminally ill tends to originate from well-defined tissue damage due to terminal illness (e.g., cancer pain). It is a variant of nociceptive pain. Stress, sleep deprivation, depression, and premorbid personality problems may exacerbate this pain.

Neuropathic pain is caused by an injured or dysfunctional central or peripheral nervous system; it is manifest by spontaneous, sharp, shooting, or burning pain that is usually distributed along dermatomes (Fig. 17.3). Neuropathic pain is often observed in deafferentation pain, complex regional pain syndrome (CRPS), diabetic neuropathy, central pain syndrome, trigeminal neuralgia, or post-herpetic neuralgia.

Terms commonly used to describe neuropathic pain include hyperalgesia (an increased response to stimuli that are normally painful); hyperesthesia (an exaggerated painful stimulus to noxious stimuli, e.g., pressure or heat); allodynia (pain with a stimulus not normally painful, e.g., light touch or cool air); and

TABLE 17.1
Chronic Pain: Nervous System Pathophysiology[15–27]

Neurologic Mechanisms	Physiologic Effects	Clinical Implications
Neuroplasticity[15,16]	Recruitment of cortical and subcortical neurons so wide dynamic range cells can be activated by low-threshold mechanoreceptors Allodynia Allesthesia	Early, concurrent, multi-modal treatment of nociceptive, central, vascular, sympathetic, and psychiatric aspects of the pain Block glutamate, substance P Early use of anti-epileptic drugs, membrane stabilizers, sympatholytics NMDA antagonists
NMDA excess and glutamate-GABA imbalance[17–20] Glutamate up, GABA down	Opioid tolerance Central hyperalgesia Hyperexcitability of peripheral and central pain cells	Normally non-painful light touch, muscle, and joint movements are painful Treatment options: benzodiazepines, baclofen, anti-epileptic drugs, substance P antagonists, or other NMDA antagonists (e.g., ketamine), GABA agents
Neurotoxins[21]	Excitotoxic (e.g., quinolinic acid) Neuropathy	AIDS pain: anti-epileptic drugs, serotoninergic/noradrenergic agents, free radical scavengers
Opioid "off" mechanisms[22,23] Off cells in the medulla Morphine 3 G/morphine up Side effect intolerance	Hyperalgesia as opioids increase (particularly intrathecal) Tolerance as morphine 3 G increases Side effects greater than benefit	Maintaining steady blood levels of opioids, or decreased opioids may increase pain Switching to a different opioid if one does not work Trial off opioids if minimal response
Sympathetic pain[16]	Mechano-allodynia, swelling Dystrophic changes	Sympathetic blockade and/or α-blocking drugs may be useful in CRPS, trauma, facial pain, arthritis
Monoamines (5-HT, NE, dopamine)[24–27]	5-HT increase lessens opioid analgesia 5-HT$_1$ dysregulation leads to vascular pain 5-HT$_1$ involved in affective disorders/suffering of pain	Full dosage, early use of antidepressant drugs, including TCAs, SSRIs, and dopamine agonists, alone or in combination NE reuptake inhibitors (e.g., desipramine, venlafaxine) are useful for pain whether depressed or not Pergolide and methylphenidate are useful adjuvants
Psychiatric illness	Decreased sleep Decreased muscle relaxation Alienation, anxiety	Differential diagnosis of psychiatric conditions and appropriate treatments

5-HT, 5-Hydroxytryptamine; *CRPS*, complex regional pain syndrome; *GABA*, γ-aminobutyric acid; *NE*, norepinephrine; *NMDA*, N-methyl-D-aspartate; *SSRIs*, selective serotonin reuptake inhibitors; *TCAs*, tricyclic antidepressants.

hyperpathia (pain from a painful stimuli with a delay and a persistence that is distributed beyond the area of stimulation).

CRPS is a syndrome of sympathetically maintained pain or pain in an extremity that is mediated by sympathetic overactivity. The syndrome is usually caused by injury; however, the cause is unknown in approximately 10% of cases. Any type of trauma (e.g., a sprain, a fracture, or a contusion) may cause it; iatrogenic causes include amputation, lesion resection, myelography, and intramuscular (IM) injections. CRPS may be disease-related (e.g., due to myocardial infarction, shoulder-hand syndrome,

herpes zoster, cerebrovascular accidents, diabetic neuropathy, disc herniation, degenerative disc disease, neuraxial tumors or metastases, multiple sclerosis, or poliomyelitis). CRPS is divided into two types. In type I CRPS, which typically develops after minor trauma or fracture, no overt nerve lesion is detectable. In type II CRPS, a definable nerve injury is present. Per diagnostic criteria set forth by the IASP, the diagnosis of CRPS can be made if the following criteria are met:[28]

1. Preceding noxious event without (CRPS I) or with obvious nerve lesion (CRPS II).

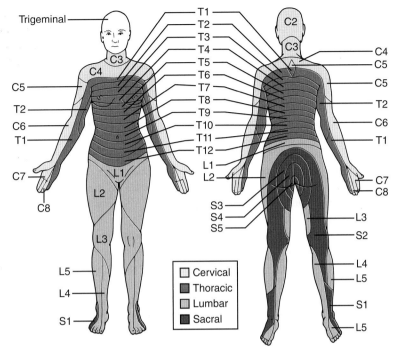

Fig. 17.3 ■ Schematic diagram of segmental neuronal innervation by dermatomes. (From Hyman SH, Cassem NH. Pain. In: Rubenstein E, Federman DD, eds. *Scientific American Medicine: Current Topics in Medicine. Subsection II.* Scientific American; 1989.)

2. Spontaneous pain or hyperalgesia/hyperesthesia is not limited to a single nerve territory and is disproportionate to the inciting event.
3. Edema, skin blood flow (temperature) or sudomotor abnormalities, motor symptoms, or trophic changes are present on the affected limb, especially at distal sites.
4. Other diagnoses have been excluded.

The clinical course (which may last up to 6 months) starts with an acute phase that involves pain, edema, and warm skin. Subsequently, dystrophic changes dominate the picture with cold skin and trophic changes (3–6 months after the onset of the untreated acute phase). Irreversible atrophic changes (atrophy and contractures) eventually occur. There may be symptom improvement with inhibition of sympathetic output; sympathetic blockade may be both diagnostic and therapeutic.[29]

Idiopathic pain, previously referred to as "*psychogenic pain*," is poorly understood. The presence of pain does not imply or exclude a psychological component. Typically, there is no evidence of an associated organic etiology or an anatomical pattern consistent with symptoms. Symptoms are often grossly out of proportion to an identifiable organic pathology.

Jurisigenic pain results from perceived physical or emotional damage related to medical, personal, work, or product injury. Patients with this pain syndrome usually maintain the sick role for as long as possible to maximize financial return. It is important to recognize the existence of a conflict and to educate patients and attorneys; maintenance of a helping and neutral posture is critical.

Phantom limb pain refers to severe and excruciating pain in the body part that is no longer present following amputation. The amputation of a limb is commonly followed by sensations that the deafferented body part is still present. These may include non-painful phantom sensations in specific positions, shapes, or movements, sensations of warmth or cold, itching, tingling, or electric sensations, and other paresthesias.[30] However, pain may also be present, and occurs in 50% to 80% of all those who have undergone an amputation.[31] Although this condition is most common after the amputation of a limb, it can also occur after the surgical removal of other body parts (e.g., the breast, rectum, penis, testicle, eye, tongue, or teeth).[32] The pathophysiology of this pain is poorly understood, however, it is likely secondary to CNS[33–35] and peripheral factors (e.g., nociceptive input from the residual limb),[36] with psychological factors influencing the course and severity of the pain.[37] Consistent with the impact of the "psyche" on pain, one study showed that it is possible to induce pain following an amputation with hypnotic suggestion.[38]

Myofascial pain can arise from one or several of the following problems: hypertonic muscles, myofascial trigger points, arthralgias, and fatigue with muscle weakness. Myofascial pain is generally used to describe muscle and connective tissue sources of pain. Myofascial pain can be a primary diagnosis (e.g., fibromyalgia) or, as more often is the case, a co-morbid diagnosis (e.g., with vascular headache or with a psychiatric diagnosis). Psychiatric symptoms are common in patients with muscle pain; other symptoms often involve decreased energy, impaired sleep, and changes in psychomotor activity. Myofascial pain syndromes may involve muscle trigger points, hypersensitive skin, a subjective sense of swelling and numbness, somatic symptom disorders (SSDs), affective and anxiety disorders, non-restorative sleep, as well as pain of the head and neck. The diagnosis should be considered if there are multiple muscle trigger points in the temporalis, sternocleidomastoid, rhomboids, or trapezius muscles; if the person cannot get at least 5 hours of uninterrupted sleep; and if chronic fatigue is present.[39] Deficient Stage 4 sleep is thought to underlie the lack of deep muscle relaxation, aching muscles, arthralgias, and general malaise.[40–42]

PAIN MEASUREMENT

The experience of pain is always subjective. However, objective measurement of the patient's subjective response is possible. Several sensitive and reliable clinical instruments for pain measurement are available. These include:

1. *The pain drawing.* This involves having the patient draw the anatomic distribution of the pain as it is felt in their body. The patient draws the outline of the body, labels where the pain is, and keeps this document as part of the medical record. The drawing serves as a clue to the anatomy of the problem, the psychological state of the patient, and the patient's level of knowledge.

2. *The visual analog scale.* A 100-mm visual analog scale (with 0 signifying no pain and 100 representing severe pain) is readily understood by most patients. It is also exquisitely sensitive to change; consequently, the patient can mark this scale once a day or even hourly during treatment trials, if desired. Two separate scales can be kept for the least and the greatest pain. Concurrent scales for mood, overall progress, and pain allow for comparison of the relationship of pain to the total clinical picture, thereby rounding out the clinician's understanding of the patient's syndrome.

3. *Categorical rating scales.* Ad hoc categorical rating scales may be devised that comprise three to five categories for the ranking of pain severity.

THE PSYCHIATRY CONSULTANT AS PAIN PHYSICIAN

The common reasons that patients in pain or their treating physicians seek consultation and treatment from psychiatrists include:

- To separate functional from non-functional factors.
- To resolve inconsistencies between symptoms and physical findings.
- To assess the patient for depression, anxiety, or some other co-morbid neuropsychiatric disorder, personality problems, and their relation to the experience of pain.
- To address a patient's or physician's concerns about opioid use (e.g., use of high-dose analgesics, maintenance treatment, or toxicity).
- To determine if the use of psychopharmacologic agents might help to alleviate pain and suffering.

The psychiatrist begins with a clarification of the reason for the consultation, creates some initial hypotheses, and examines the patient. If possible, the psychiatric consultant should be brought into the case early on and introduced as a member of the medical team. The referring physician should take care to ensure that the patient does not interpret the referral as a sign that the patient is not believed, and the physician should state that a psychiatrist is routinely asked to evaluate patients with longstanding pain, and mental health referrals are a part of pain treatment.

Gathering Important Preliminary Information

The psychiatric consultant's job begins by answering five questions: (1) Is the pain intractable because of nociceptive stimuli (e.g., from the skin, bones, muscles, or blood vessels)? (2) Is the pain maintained by non-nociceptive mechanisms (i.e., have the spinal cord, brainstem, limbic system, and cortex been recruited as reverberating pain circuits)? (3) Is the complaint of pain primary, as occurs in disorders such as major depressive disorder (MDD), an anxiety disorder, or a delusional disorder? (4) Is there a more efficacious pharmacologic treatment? (5) Have pain behavior and disability become more important than the pain itself? Table 17.2 provides a useful guideline for organizing the questions, testing hypotheses, and determining the diagnosis.

The Physical Examination

A clinician's physical examination of a patient in pain includes examination of the painful area, muscles, and sensation to pinprick and light touch (Table 17.3). The examination is essential to the psychiatric evaluation for pain and it serves three purposes. First, examination of the patient allows for better history taking, formation of a therapeutic alliance, and integration of data. Second, the psychiatrist can search for signs of different types of pain and distinguish them from symptoms of a somatoform disorder, including functional neurological symptom disorder (FND).

The Psychiatric Examination

Interviewing the patients with chronic pain demands a holistic approach to their presentation; it is helpful to ask the patient to write a detailed account of their pain from its onset to the present. A detailed history of when and how the pain began, inquiring about the various treatments received, and the patient's relationships with other physicians are also important in the evaluation of pain. Throughout history, it is prudent to assess fluctuations in the pain. Why did it improve? Did the medication help, or was it some other factor that proved palliative? In addition, one should explore the patient's past and present mental state and consider the family history and cultural beliefs. Open-ended questions may include: Have you ever suffered like this before? What do you think about in the early morning hours when you cannot sleep? What do others think is the nature of the problem? The psychiatrist also plays an important role in the treatment of pain by their ability to recognize co-morbid psychiatric conditions that may be co-morbid with pain. Non-medical treatments and approaches that may have helped should be included in this inquiry.

Depression

Major depressive disorder (MDD) can be diagnosed in approximately one-fourth of patients who suffer from chronic pain. Recurrent affective illness, a family history of depression, and psychiatric co-morbidity (with anxiety and substance use) are often present. Often, depression pre-dates pain; overall, most patients in pain have co-morbid depressive symptoms. Although some depressive syndromes are secondary to pain (e.g., adjustment disorder with affective symptoms), many patients have MDD that is masked by denial or by medications that promote sleepiness. Denial of affect, particularly anger, is observed in many patients who suffer from chronic pain and who are referred for consultation. Diagnosing an affective illness when an abnormal mood is minimized by the patient may be difficult, but the following tactics can be used to help unearth affective disorders. Depression should not be rationalized as being appropriate in those with a pain disorder and the treatment of the depressed patient in pain is no different than treatment of any other depressed patient. Education of the patient as to the rationale for antidepressant treatment is advised for good treatment adherence; maintenance treatment, for 3 to 6 months, is usually necessary.

It is essential to ask questions about neurovegetative symptoms. Examples of such questions include: How often do you awaken from sleep during the night? How long does it take for you to return to sleep? Do you have an early morning awakening? When was the last time you enjoyed yourself? Does food taste the same as it always has? Do you enjoy eating? What do you do

TABLE 17.2
Questions to Ask When Pain Persists

Pain Syndromes: What Is the Problem?	Selected Diagnostic Considerations	Consider
Is there an ongoing physical disease? (e.g., infection, cancer)	MRI for anatomic pathology Gallium scan for infection ESR for infection, cancer prostate-specific antigen, carcinoembryonic antigen, p24 testing Pelvic, breast, prostate, gastrointestinal examination	Progression of disease Metastatic disease Visceral pain: adhesions, referred pain, central pain
Is there a problem with the use and response to opioids? (e.g., misuse, lack of efficacy)	Central pain Opioids masking a psychiatric problem Opioid dosing error or inconsistency Opioid toxicity	Intravenous agents Antidepressants, anxiolytics, or sleep medications Opioid potency P450 2D6 codeine or oxycodone/SSRI interaction Meperidine toxicity
Is there a psychiatric disorder associated with pain? Depression Anxiety Somatic symptom disorder Psychosis Does CNS pain exist? (e.g., neuropathic pain)	Loss of all pleasure and mid-late insomnia Panic depersonalization, benzodiazepine failure, anxiety not relieved by analgesics Hypochondriasis Increased sensory threshold, decreased pain threshold Non-dermatomal distribution of pain Hyperpathia Allodynia, often opioid-resistant	Depression often masked by opioids or anxiolytics Co-morbid somatoform, mood, or anxiety disorders Pain drawing and explanation helpful for diagnosis Sharp sensation perceived as light touch is common A light touch is painful and sustained and has a delayed crescendo Tuning a fork/moving a hair examination detects allodynia best
Is it a pain behavior syndrome?	Somatic symptom disorder; rule out depression, substance use disorder, physical/sexual abuse, missed physical disorder	Anger and anxiety: denied Counter dependent, demanding style Passive and endearing
Is the patient faking? Malingering Factitious disorder	Malingering for drugs/disability Factitious deception to maintain the sick role	Malingering or factitious disorders with physical symptoms are rare, and much more likely to be something else
Is an unusual problem responsible for pain? Myofascial pain Porphyria Gastrointestinal pain Pelvic-visceral pain Neuropathic pain Sexual pain disorder	Muscle trigger points absent, deep sleep Laxative abuse, anorexia/bulimia Adhesions Hypoesthesia, allodynia Wasting illness, subcortical deficits/AIDS Conversion symptoms, especially pelvic, and gastrointestinal head pain	Myofascial pain is often co-morbid with other pain syndrome Visceral pain is diffuse, non-dermatomal, with sympathetic symptoms, and may mimic psychiatric presentations Physical/sexual abuse antidote pain

AIDS, Acquired immunodeficiency syndrome; *CNS, central nervous system; ESR,* erythrocyte sedimentation rate; *MRI,* magnetic resonance imaging; *SSRI,* selective serotonin reuptake inhibitor.

for fun? Can you still smile? Do you have an interest in people, such as your grandchildren or friends? Do you have difficulty with decision-making? What do you do when you are angry? Do you sometimes feel you would rather be dead?

It is also important to evaluate the person's limbic (i.e., genuine and uncensored) response to emotionally charged stimuli. One should look for denial of any strong emotion, particularly anger or sadness, and note if the patient answers affective questions with an

TABLE 17.3
General Physical Examination of Pain by the Psychiatrist

Physical Finding	Purpose of Examination
Motor deficits	Does the patient give way when checking strength? Does the person try? Is there a pseudoparesis, astasia-abasia, or involuntary movements suggesting a somatoform disorder?
Trigger points in head, neck, shoulder, and back muscles	Are any of the common myofascial trigger points present, suggesting myofascial pain? Presence of evoked pain (such as allodynia, hyperpathia, or anesthesia) suggests neuropathic pain
Evanescent, changeable pain, weakness, and numbness	Does the psychological complaint pre-empt the physical?
Abnormal sensory findings	Detection of lateral anesthesia to pinprick ending sharply at the midline Presence of topographic confusion Presence of non-dermatomal distribution of pain and sensation suggests either a somatoform or CNS pain disorder Presence of abnormal sensation suggests neuropathy or CNS pain
Sympathetic or vascular dysfunction	Detection of swelling, skin discoloration, or changes in sweating or temperature suggests a vascular or sympathetic element to the pain
Uncooperativeness, erratic responses to the physical examination	Detection of an interpersonal aspect to the pain, causing abnormal pain behavior, as in somatoform disease

CNS, Central nervous system.

affective response or only replies with avoidance and denial. Denial, displacement, or suppression of emotions may contribute to pain syndromes. If necessary, neuropsychological testing and assessment of personality styles can be added to the evaluation in difficult-to-diagnose situations.

Anxiety Disorders

When pain exists, denial of fear, worry, or nervousness is a more ominous sign than the mere expression of modulated fear or worry about pain. Given that it is normal to worry about painful threats to the body and the mind, pathologic denial of any affect may suggest psychosis, a FND, an illness anxiety disorder, a factitious illness, or a personality disorder. Questions, such as the following, may help to obtain information: "Does the pain make you panic? Do you feel your heart beating fast, have an overwhelming feeling of dread or doom, or experience a sense of sudden high anxiety?"

Anxiety disorders occur in approximately one-third of patients with intractable pain (usually in the form of generalized anxiety or panic disorder). More than half of patients with anxiety disorders also have a current or a history of MDD or another psychiatric disorder. Alcohol and SUDs are the most common co-morbid diagnoses; consequently, recognition and treatment of co-morbid depression and substance use are critical to long-term treatment outcomes.

A variety of agents, including TCAs, selective serotonin reuptake inhibitors (SSRIs), serotonin-norepinephrine reuptake inhibitors (SNRIs), mirtazapine, and clonazepam, alone or in combination, improve panic, anxiety, and depression as well as neuropathic pain, muscle tension, and sleep. Anxiety that results from disruptions of bodily integrity, a sense of self, or attachment to caregivers occurs in one-third to one-half of patients with chronic pain. Anger is often linked to anxiety, although it can be denied and expressed in terms of somatic symptoms. SSRIs are helpful with anger, anxiety, and mood disorders. Existential anxiety may increase when cancer is first diagnosed, when death nears, or when pain engenders feelings of helplessness. Spending time with the person, telling the truth, accepting the situation, and reconnecting with family members (parents and children) often decreases existential anxiety.

Somatic Symptom Disorders

SSDs occur in 5% to 15% of patients with chronic pain, and somatoform disorders account for approximately one-third of all cases of psychiatric disability, as well as nearly half of all sick-leave occasions.[43]

Among those with a history of somatic complaints, pain in the head or neck, epigastrium, and limbs predominates. Visceral pain from the esophagus, abdomen, and pelvis associated with psychiatric co-morbidity, especially somatoform disorders, can be challenging to diagnose.[44] Missed ovarian cancers, central pain following inflammatory disorders, and referred pain are often overlooked because of the nonspecific presentations of visceral pain. Moreover, in one study, nearly two-thirds of women with chronic pelvic pain reported a history of sexual abuse.[45] Those who experience SSDs often have painful physical complaints and excessive anxiety about their physical illness. Most of their pain complaints do not have a well-defined cause, and a psychiatric diagnosis may be difficult to establish (Table 17.4).

Functional Neurological Symptom Disorder

Functional neurological symptom disorders (FNDs) may manifest as pain syndrome with a significant loss or alteration in physical functioning that mimics a physical disorder. Symptoms may include paresthesia, numbness, dysphonia, dizziness, seizures, globus hystericus, limb weakness, sexual dysfunction, or pain. If pain or sexual symptoms are the sole complaints,

the diagnosis is pain disorder or sexual pain disorder rather than FND. Pain, numbness, and weakness often form a conversion triad in the pain clinic.

Psychological factors are judged to be associated when a temporal relationship between the symptoms and a psychosocial stressor exists—the person must not be intentionally producing their symptom. A mechanism of primary or secondary gain needs to be evident before the diagnosis can be confirmed. *La belle indifference* and histrionic personality traits have little value in making or excluding the diagnosis of FND. A conversion V on the Minnesota Multiphasic Personality Inventory (MMPI) denotes the hypochondriacal traits and relative absence of depression that may accompany FND. Evoked responses, an electromyogram, an electroencephalogram, an MRI, PET scans, and repeated physical examinations are useful for the identification of patients who had been diagnosed erroneously as "hysterical."[46]

Factitious Disorder with Physical Symptoms

Factitious disorder with physical symptoms involves the intentional production or feigning of physical symptoms. Onset is usually in early adulthood with successive hospitalizations forming the life-long pattern.

TABLE 17.4	
Somatoform and Related Disorders	
Disorders	**Diagnostic Tips**
Somatic symptom disorder	Physical symptoms that suggest physical illness or injury—symptoms that cannot be explained fully by a general medical condition, or by the direct effect of a substance, and are not attributable to another mental disorder
	Central and visceral pain, especially pelvic pain, can mimic somatic symptom disorder(s)
	Pain may improve with psychopharmacologic medications or psychological interventions without a clear psychiatric diagnosis
Functional neurological symptom disorder (FND) (conversion disorder)	Identifiable physical illness and FND symptoms often co-occur
	An undiagnosed medical condition may underlie the psychiatric diagnosis
	Deciding if psychological factors are causative or response is often impossible in patients with chronic pain
	Culturally determined stress responses, numbness, total body pain, weakness, astasia-abasia, fainting, voices, and non-epileptiform seizure activity are transient and not included as FND.
Illness anxiety disorder (hypochondriasis)	Transient hypochondriasis is particularly common in the elderly
	Psychosis and depression may be concealed because of the patient's fears
Malingering/factitious disorder	Pseudomalingering with dissociative features (Ganser syndrome) presents with malingering, but also underlies real psychiatric illness. Some classify it as a conversion, dissociative, or factitious disorder

The cause is a psychological need to assume the sick role, and as such, the intentional production of painful symptoms distinguishes factitious disorder from SSDs, in which the intention to produce symptoms is absent. Renal colic, orofacial pain, and abdominal pain are three of the common presenting complaints in factitious disorder; of these, abdominal pain and an abdomen with scars herald the diagnosis most often. Despite the seeming irrationality of the behavior, those with factitious disorder are not psychotic.

Pain may be described as occurring anywhere in the body, and the patient often uses elaborate technical details with *pseudologia fantastica* (to capture the attention of the listener). Opioid medication-seeking behavior, multiple hospitalizations under different names in different cities, inconclusive invasive investigations and surgery, lack of available family, and a truculent manner are characteristic of this disorder. An assiduous inquiry into the exact circumstances of the previous admission and discharge leads to a sudden outraged discharge against medical advice. There is typically no effective treatment. If the patient were willing to receive care, however, psychotherapy would be the treatment of choice, coupled with addiction recovery services if there is an underlying SUD.

Malingering

In malingering, the patient feigns a complaint, although no pain is felt, because of an external incentive, such as obtaining money or drugs or avoiding work. The conscious manipulation by malingering patients precludes much diagnostic help from amytal interviews or hypnosis because of the patient's willful withholding of information. The patient typically refuses psychological tests; this raises suspicion even before a diagnosis is made. Even when agreeable to testing, the MMPI can be skewed to normality by some patients, although differences (>7) between obvious and subtle scale scores and high L, F, and K scale scores (T>70) may be suggestive. A mnemonic for suspicion of the diagnosis is WASTE (*W*ithholding of information; *A*ntisocial personality; *S*omatic examination inconclusive and changeable; *T*reatment erratic with non-adherence and vagueness; *E*xternal incentives exist, such as occur in a medicolegal context). The psychiatrist's familiarity with the neurologic examination is always useful, but it is of critical importance for the diagnosis of malingering when non-anatomic findings arise. Once a non-functional etiology has been excluded, scrutiny of old records and calls to previous physicians may unearth evidence of prior similar behaviors. Like lying, malingering tends to be a character trait used in times of stress from early adolescence. Once revealed, psychotherapy can be offered; unfortunately, non-adherence is typical, and the prognosis is guarded.

Dissociative States

Dissociation is caused by psychological trauma, and it involves a disturbance or alteration in the normally integrative functions of identity, memory, or consciousness. Pelvic pain, sexual pain disorders, headaches, and abdominal pain are the most common pain complaints in developmentally traumatized individuals. Walker and associates[45] reported that in 22 women with chronic pelvic pain, 18 experienced childhood trauma. Of the 21 women selected as controls (i.e., without pelvic pain), 9 had childhood trauma ($P < .0005$). Dissociation, somatic distress, and general disability were more frequent in the group with pain. Denial makes the diagnosis of dissociative disorders in patients with pain a longitudinal process because the truth is shared slowly with the physician only when the patient can tolerate it. Signs of an underlying dissociative disorder are periods of amnesia, nightmares, and panic, as well as anxious intolerance of close personal relationships. These patients can be helped in long-term therapy relationships with special attention paid to their trauma symptoms.

GENERAL PRINCIPLES OF PAIN THERAPY

Pain Is Not Psychological by Default

The patient should not have their pain called "psychological" or "supratentorial" merely because it is not understood or because it is unresponsive to treatment. The physician should assure the patient that there is no question about the degree of suffering involved. Furthermore, psychological factors may play a role, but this by no means diminishes either the quality or the quantity of pain the patient endures. Education about the close relationship of "psyche and soma" in CNS is often useful for establishing an effective doctor-patient relationship.

Longstanding pain is difficult to assess largely because what we learn about pain is based on our concept of acute pain. The patient with acute pain moans, writhes, sweats, begs for help, and gives every appearance of being in great distress. Those nearby someone in acute pain typically feel an urge to help. When pain persists over days and weeks, the individual adapts to it, often without realizing it and the pain behavior diminishes. This may be accounted for by several explanations: the sensation may become intermittent, or the CNS inhibits the pain. The physician must understand the pathophysiology of pain, employ the full range of neurologic, pharmacologic, and psychological therapies, and work with those in chronic pain to help their suffering.

Care Does Not Only Involve Symptom Management

An important principle of pain management is to assure the patient that treatment will continue, even if there is no immediate improvement. The physician should also guard against being affected by the patient's sense of discouragement. One of the fears expressed by many patients who suffer from chronic pain is that of abandonment; they believe that if they do not improve, the physician will no longer treat them. In this case, an endless series of medications, without continuing examination, psychotherapy, or critical thinking, is tantamount to non-involvement or abandonment. Education about relaxation techniques, yoga, acupuncture, TENS, ultrasound, and massage, all have their place in the therapeutic armamentarium. Mind Body Medicine programs are very helpful for patients in pain since they work on stress management and increasing resiliency through teaching the connection between stress and pain. These programs teach relaxation response, appreciation of the role of positive thoughts and beliefs, healthy eating, restorative sleep, and physical activity. The value is not only in soothing the pain but also in helping the person to feel more in control, to suffer less, and to become an active, educated participant while under the physician's care.

Deafferentation Surgery is Usually Not the Answer

An abiding principle in the treatment of chronic pain is to avoid surgery whenever possible. Few surgical procedures on the CNS cure or control pain, and often result in side effects, including pain that is worse than before the operation. In particular, CNS pain is notoriously refractory to surgeries that interrupt afferent pain pathways. The pain is often made worse by procedures, such as a neurectomy, rhizotomy, tractotomy, and cordotomy. Surgery, except for cingulotomy, is not a treatment for depression that manifests as pain. A central procedure, such as cingulotomy, performed stereotactically using radiofrequency lesions, may be useful for intractable pain, especially because it has a low risk of psychiatric and physical morbidity. Personality changes, mental dulling, and memory impairment are rare. Unfortunately, even when pain is reduced with cingulotomy, it can return within 3 to 6 months. To exemplify this multiform plasticity of pain, consider the following account of an extraordinary case.

Case 1

Mr. C, a 28-year-old mechanic, was thrown from his motorcycle *en route* to his wedding. Injury occurred to his brachial plexus and arm, requiring an amputation at the shoulder. He then developed severe phantom limb pain. Six months later, the stump was revised and a neurectomy was performed; the pain, however, remained unaltered. The nerve was then severed further into the stump with a similar result. An unsuccessful rhizotomy was then performed, followed by a chordotomy with the same outcome. He engaged in individual psychotherapy for a year, but there was no improvement. After six sessions of electroconvulsive therapy, the pain only intensified. A higher cervical chordotomy was performed without success, and then a mesencephalic tractotomy; again, there was no relief. He next had both dorsomedial thalamic nuclei ablated using stereotactic electrocautery. He emerged from this procedure with his personality intact but still with his original pain. Then electrolytic lesions were made bilaterally in the inferior mesial quadrant of the frontal lobe in stages; still, the pain remained. Following this, he had a left radiofrequency amygdalotomy followed by a left cingulotomy. Nonetheless, the pain continued. The pain remained for 4 years after the accident, as pristine as it was 2 weeks after the injury.

Talking and Listening

A strategy to evaluate the feelings and behaviors observed in patients with pain is as necessary as the strategy for evaluating the physical aspects of the pain.[47] The skill required is not only a matter of diagnosing the major psychiatric illnesses that can present with pain—these patients often have a maladaptive style of interaction that requires a different kind of interpretive skill—but also a question of the physician's ability to relate to the patient with long-suffering pain who shows poor judgment of surgical risk, denies anger and rapidly alternates between idealizing and denigrating the medical caretaker. The fluctuations of both mood and cooperation frequently encountered in the clinical interview are symptomatic of the patient's damaged self-esteem or their injured sense of self. Patients with chronic pain invariably feel damaged not only in the body part afflicted with discomfort but also in self-image and spirit—a phenomenon known as narcissistic injury.[48] The techniques for interviewing the patient with narcissistically injured pain are designed to establish a diagnostic working relationship. They allow for an accurate medical history to be elicited, mistrust between physician and patient to be avoided, an effective treatment plan to be developed, and the outcomes through compliance and education to be enhanced.

The interviewer should allow the patient to tell their own story. An initial degree of catharsis may help decrease the patient's anxiety and in giving the physician a sense of the patient's character. The physician must actively facilitate an alliance with the patient while still maintaining neutrality and avoiding misplaced sympathy. The patient's underlying feelings of fear, anger, resentment, and mistrust are best uncovered by asking how others view the situation, essentially a counter-projective method. This approach sometimes bares unpleasant affects without the use of intrusive questions from the physician. Labeling overt and covert roles assigned by the patient to the physician is an important early intervention. Specifically, this means that the physician should point out when the patient is attributing unrealistic curative powers to him or her or appears to believe that the physician is indifferent to the patient's suffering. The longer one waits to confront these fantasies, the less effective any intervention will be. Expression of affect should be encouraged, and the physician should help the patient express the feelings he or she is having but does not want to acknowledge. These interventions are most successful with a neutral and kind approach by giving the patient the necessary emotional space to process without denial and difficulties related to the situation.

Optimal care of patients with intractable pain requires processing neurologic and psychiatric data while delineating and responding to the phrase-by-phrase manifestations of suffering and pain behavior. In essence, being able to get patients to talk about what they are angry about is just as important as discussing their insomnia or disc herniation. Progress occurs with needy and angry patients, only when there is clear processing and separation of the reality-based facts of the case from unrealistic expectations. In that way, every clarification of an unrealistic idea can be an introduction to a more realistic alternative. The overall goal is to improve the patient's self-awareness and capacity for insight, thereby gaining control.

MEDICATION FOR PAIN: ANALGESIA AND ADJUVANTS

Judicious and effective use of medicine in patients with chronic pain rests on the concise evaluation of the four main components of the pain complaint: nociceptive pain, CNS mechanisms of pain, suffering, and pain behavior. In its most elemental form, the medical management of these four components employs opioids, anti-epileptic drugs (AEDs), antidepressants, and behavioral treatment. Non-steroidal anti-inflammatory drugs (NSAIDs), aspirin, and nerve blocks are often helpful in the early stages of these conditions.

Non-Steroidal Anti-Inflammatory Drugs

The World Health Organization (WHO) has established a three-step guideline for pain treatment (Fig. 17.4). Step 1 involves the use of NSAIDs, aspirin, or acetaminophen. Step 2 adds codeine to the NSAID, with other adjuvants (e.g., TCAs, antidepressants, AEDs, stimulants). Step 3 employs opioids with adjunctive medication. Conceived for cancer pain, and reporting efficacy in 90% of cancer patients, the three steps are a useful template for many kinds of acute pain, adjusted for the specific pain mechanism being treated. NSAIDs

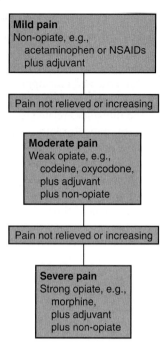

Fig. 17.4 ■ The analgesic ladder. (From Borsook D, Lebel AA, McPeek B. *MGH Handbook of Pain Management*. Little Brown; 1995.)

are useful for acute and chronic pain, such as inflammation, muscle pain, vascular pain, and post-traumatic pain, or when the physician wants to use a potent non-opioid analgesic. NSAIDs are generally equally efficacious and have similar side effects.[49]

Side Effects

Most NSAIDs can cause bronchospasm in aspirin-sensitive patients, induce gastric ulcers, interact with angiotensin-converting enzyme inhibitors (thereby contributing to renal failure), precipitate lithium toxicity, and impair renal function in the long term. NSAIDs can elevate blood pressure in patients treated with β-blockers and diuretics. The exception to this general rule is the non-acetylated (non-aspirin) salicylates that do not inhibit the synthesis of prostaglandins. These include choline magnesium trisalicylate and diflunisal; these agents do not cause bronchospasm in aspirin-sensitive patients, precipitate renal failure, or inhibit platelet aggregation. Certain NSAIDs, however, have features that make some preferable over others

in certain situations. The discovery of the enzyme cyclooxygenase (COX) isoforms (1 and 2) led to the increased use of selective COX-2 inhibitors. COX-2 tends to facilitate the inflammatory response selectively, and it has been argued that the use of new agents (parecoxib, etoricoxib, lumiracoxib, and celecoxib) may increase gastrointestinal (GI) safety.[50]

Based on currently available data, the US Food and Drug Administration (FDA) has concluded that an increased risk of cardio- and cerebrovascular events has been demonstrated for all of the cyclooxygenase-2 (COX-2) selective NSAIDs, including rofecoxib, valdecoxib, and celecoxib.[50] Rofecoxib was voluntarily removed from the market in 2004 following the finding of increased cardiovascular events compared with placebo in a long-term study. Valdecoxib was voluntarily withdrawn from the market in 2005 after the FDA concluded that the overall risk versus benefit profile for the drug was unfavorable. Although an increased risk of cardiovascular events has also been demonstrated with celecoxib, the FDA has found that the benefits of celecoxib outweigh potential risks in properly selected and informed patients.

Special Features

Synergistic combinations of acetaminophen, aspirin, and caffeine are the cornerstone for temporary relief of pain (e.g., headaches and muscle pain) and potentiation of the effects of opioids. They do, however, have a limit on dosing and have only moderate potency; they are also not well tolerated by those who may be medically ill. NSAID variations then need to be considered. Choline magnesium trisalicylate (1000–1500 mg) is safe in aspirin-sensitive patients, and it does not prolong bleeding. Misoprostol can reduce GI erosions in patients on maintenance NSAIDs, but its use can be limited by diarrhea, pain, and flatulence in about one-third of patients. Ibuprofen (800 mg) is a rapid-release agent that produces higher blood levels over the first half hour than the other preparations at equal dosage. Ketorolac (up to 30 mg every 6 hours) intramuscularly followed by oral dosing has a rapid onset and a high potency, enabling it to be substituted for morphine (note: 30 mg of ketorolac is equivalent to 10 mg of morphine). It should be used for no more than 5 days. Extended-release preparations can be useful when long, steady analgesia and simple dose regimens are needed (e.g., nabumetone, oxaprozin, ketoprofen, piroxicam). Naproxen (375–500 mg twice a day with enteric-coated, delayed-release tablets) can be well tolerated over time. Ketoprofen (200 mg) extended-release tablets can be taken once a day, but they are not intended for patients with renal disease or those over 75 years of age. Ibuprofen works well as an opioid adjuvant for bone pain. Naproxen (up to 1500 mg a day), but not flurbiprofen, has also had positive results for bone pain. The newer COX-2 inhibitors may cause fewer GI problems compared with other NSAIDs. Celecoxib does not impair platelet function. Parecoxib, etoricoxib, or lumiracoxib are not currently available in the United States. (For a list of NSAIDs, see Table 17.5.)

Opioids

Opioids help some patients with cancer as well as those with non-cancer-related chronic pain.[51,52] Cancer pain is the most common indication for maintenance use of opioids.[53] Acute, severe, and unremitting pain also requires opioid treatment, as outlined in the WHO analgesic ladder. At times, opioids may be the only effective treatment for chronic, non-malignant pain, such as the pain associated with degenerative disorders, and vascular conditions.[54] Bouckoms and colleagues[55] demonstrated that non-malignant pain treated with long-term oral opioids provides effective pain relief in about two-thirds of those treated. Nociceptive pain, absence of depression, and absence of any substance

TABLE 17.5
Properties of Aspirin and Non-Steroidal Anti-inflammatory Drugs

Drug	Dose (mg)	Dosage Interval (h)	Daily Dose (mg/day)	Peak Effect (h)	Half-life (h)
Aspirin	81–975	4	4500	0.5–1	0.25
Celecoxib	100–200	12	1200	1	11
Diclofenac	25–75	6–8	200	2	1–2
Diflunisal	250–500	12	1500	1	13
Etodolac acid	200–400	6–8	1600	1–2	7
Fenoprofen	200	4–6	3200	1–2	2–3
Flurbiprofen	50–100	6–8	300	1.5–3	3–4
Ibuprofen	200–400	6–8	3200	1–2	2
Indometacin	25–75	6–8	200	0.5–1	2–3
Ketoprofen	25–75	6–8	300	1–2	1.5–2.0
Ketorolac[a]					
Oral	10	6–8	40	0.5–1	6
Parenteral	60 load, then 30	6–8	120	0.5	6
Meclofenamic acid	500 load, then 275	6–8	400	1	2–4
Mefenamic acid	500 load, then 250	6	1250	2–4	3–4
Nabumetone	1000–2000	12–24	2000	3–5	22–30
Naproxen	500 load, then 250	6–8	1250	2–4	12–15
Naproxen sodium	550 load then 275	6–8	1375	1–2	13
Oxaprozin	60–1200	24	1800	2	3–3.5
Phenylbutazone	100	6–8	400	2	50–100
Piroxicam	40 load, then 20	24	20	2–4	36–45
Sulindac	150–200	12	400	1–2	7–18
Tolmetin	200–400	8	1800	4–6	2

Adapted from Borsook D, Lebel AA, McPeek B. *MGH Handbook of Pain Management.* Little Brown Publishers; 1995.
[a]Use no longer than 5 days.

use were all significantly associated with long-term opioid treatment efficacy. Patients with neuropathic pain or MDD fared especially poorly; a bad outcome was four times more likely than a good outcome. Even when patients were carefully selected (i.e., lack of previous addiction or gross personality disorder), one-third of patients developed tolerance or addiction over 3 years. Even so, those patients with SUDs and chronic pain may still benefit from closely monitored physician-prescribed opioids for their physical pain if it stops them from turning to illicit supplies. These patients may require specific non-opioid strategies for their neuropathy and depression if gains are to be made. The use of buprenorphine products may be helpful given its less harmful potential versus opioid medications, coupled with its ability to also provide analgesia.

Opioid Potencies

Codeine is a good opioid for mild-to-moderate pain, but it has limited efficacy for severe pain. Morphine is the medication of choice for acute and chronic pain because of its long history of safety and decreased cost. Beyond these starting points, the basic principles of opioids are outlined in Table 17.6.

Principles of Opioid Administration

Potency and Administration. Potency and administration are consistent with the characteristics of the drug, its half-life, and absorption by different routes; such knowledge helps to ensure that the dosage schedule is consistent with these parameters.

Oral Potency. Oral potency must be high so that parenteral use can be avoided if possible. Methadone is a good first choice because of its oral potency and relatively slow clearance. Morphine and hydromorphone are useful alternatives for initial treatment. Once oral doses have been initiated and titrated to a satisfactory level (e.g., 4-hourly dosing of morphine or methadone), the analgesic effect needs to be sustained by minimizing fluctuations in blood levels and the variable effects of dosing schedules. Controlled-release morphine sulfate (MSC) is ideal for this homeostasis because it is released more slowly than conventional oral morphine. Furthermore, morphine's effect is not significantly affected by minor

hepatic disease. Only 50% of the morphine in its controlled-release formulation reaches the CNS after 1.5 hours, three times longer than it takes conventional oral morphine to reach the CNS. Steady state is reached with MSC in about 1 day. A steady state with MSC at any fixed dose and dosing interval has a lower maximum blood concentration than conventional morphine, thereby reducing fluctuations in blood levels. Note that MSC does not release morphine continuously and evenly, so a dosing schedule of every 12 hours has more peaks and troughs than conventional oral morphine given every 4 hours. It is also important to be aware that chewing or crushing MSC further increases erratic release. MSC should not be given less than every 12 hours.

Avoid As-Needed Dosing. A steady-state opioid blood level requires approximately 4 half-lives to achieve consistency, and a steep dose-response curve makes pain relief erratic (e.g., if one dose is missed, it can take 23 hours to return to therapeutic analgesia). Dosing on an as-needed basis makes steady relief impossible. It may also predispose the patient to medication-respondent conditioning and subsequent behavioral problems.

Toxicity. Morphine and hydromorphone uncommonly cause toxicity and hence are prescriptions of choice. Even so, when the glomerular filtration rate is poor and morphine or hydromorphone doses are high, toxicity may occur, even when equivalent doses of morphine are used without signs of toxicity. Meperidine hydrochloride should be avoided in difficult cases because of its short duration of action (2–4 hours) and because even at normal doses, its principal metabolite (normeperidine) can cause irritability, auditory and visual hallucinations, agitation, confusion, disorientation, hypomania, paranoia, and myoclonus, in addition to partial and generalized seizures.[56,57] This CNS excitement is more likely to occur in patients with malignancy or renal impairment, or when the drug is given intravenously and the dose exceeds 300 mg/day for more than 3 days—all conditions in which there may be significant accumulation of the pro-convulsant normeperidine. Methadone, once initiated, may accumulate in the body given its longer half-life, and care should be taken to ensure there is no excessive

TABLE 17.6
Potencies and Special Features of Opioids

Drug	Parenteral (mg Equivalent)	Oral (mg)	Duration (h)	Special Features
Morphine	10	30	4	Morphine sulfate controlled release has 12-h duration
Codeine	120	200	4	Ceiling effect as dose increases, low lipophilic
Oxycodone	4.5	30	4	Oxycodone controlled release has an 8–12 h of duration (10, 20, 40 slow-release mg)
Hydromorphone	2	8	5	Suppository 6 mg = 10 mg parenteral morphine
Levorphanol	2	4	4	Low nausea and vomiting, low lipophilic
Methadone	5	10	2	Cumulative effect; days 3–5 decrease respiration
Meperidine	100	300	3	κ, pro-convulsant metabolite, peristaltic slowing and sphincter of Oddi dysfunction
Fentanyl	0.1	25 μg SL	1 (patch 72 h)	50 μg patch = 60 mg/day morphine IM/IV
Sufentanil	Not recommended	15 μg SL	1	High potency with low volume of fluid
Propoxyphene	Not available	325	4	High dose leads to psychosis
Buprenorphine	0.3	0.3	4–6	μ-Partial agonism; κ-antagonism; may precipitate withdrawal in patients already on full agonist opioids
Tramadol	Not available	150	4	μ-Agonist, decreased reuptake 5-HT and NE, P450 metabolism
Nalbuphine	10	Not available	3	Agonist-antagonist

5-HT, 5-Hydroxytryptamine; *IM*, intramuscular; *IV*, intravenous; *NE*, norepinephrine; *SL*, sublingual.

sedation or other signs of toxicity. Trouble-shooting checklists for opioids may be required when the basic principles mentioned above have not been successful.[58]

Are Opioids the Drugs of Choice in Our Case?

Unduly long clinical trials and ongoing patient suffering may be avoided by giving the patient 10 mg of IV morphine as a single-blinded test dose. This is a diagnostic procedure designed to determine if opioids will relieve the pain. If there is a positive result with relief of pain, one concludes that morphine works well enough to continue its use. A negative outcome might result in a repeat dose of morphine at 20 mg to ensure that it was not just tolerance that failed to produce a benefit at 10 mg. If there is neuropathic pain, for example, opioids may not produce a good enough response at normal doses. In about 50% of patients with intractable pain, opioids do not have a good enough analgesic effect. In a minority, it is the anxiolytic effect rather than the analgesic effect that is helpful.

Dosing. Prescriber inexperience and resulting fear are the usual reasons that analgesics are given at inadequate dosage and frequency. Appropriate dosing requires knowledge of the potency and half-life of the drug. Common errors that occur at critical moments include failure to adjust the dosage when switching from parenteral to oral use (e.g., not increasing the dose of opioid medication when switching from IM/IV to oral dosing); failure to administer the drug at longer intervals than its half-life (e.g., methadone's analgesic half-life is 4–8 hours; consequently, methadone is usually needed at least three times a day when it is given for pain, not once a day as when it is given for opioid use disorder); and under-dosing when beginning MSC or fentanyl patches because both require at least 24 hours to reach steady-state (supplementary opioids are required for the first 24 hours).

Drug Delivery. An important question to bear in mind is whether the method of administration and type of opioid has been optimized. The most common problem in severe pain is the three-fold to eight-fold variability of IM absorption. This can be decreased by using hydrophilic agents (e.g., morphine and hydromorphone) rather than lipophilic (e.g., fentanyl, methadone, and meperidine). When more lipophilic agents, such as methadone, are used intramuscularly, injections into the deltoid rather than the gluteus muscle are preferable. If an erratic response occurs, it might be due to inconsistent drug delivery. Alternative methods include delivery of the drug intravenously, sublingually, intrathecally, ventricularly, or transdermally. For example, Kunz and co-workers described the innovative use of sublingual sufentanil, 25 mg every 3 minutes (for three doses) for severe but episodic pain.[59] The drug and route were preferable to patient-controlled analgesia (PCA), fentanyl sublingually, or MSC because the volume of fluid was small, the speed of onset was within 1 minute, and the half-life was short (and therefore not sedating the rest of the day); in addition, the cost was comparable with PCA, albeit more expensive than sublingual fentanyl. The patient could get out of bed and remain alert and comfortable with a low-tech intervention that is ideal for hospice or home care.

Tolerance or Excessive Sedation. The age of the patient is an important factor in the efficacy of the drug. The duration of effect may double as age increases; as it does, so does the analgesic effect in a 70-year old versus a 20-year old. Opioid adjuvants (e.g., methylphenidate) may decrease or increase (e.g., with antidepressants) sedation.

Partial Agonists. Buprenorphine is a partial agonist with high binding affinity at μ-opioid receptors, an agonist with low binding affinity at the nociceptin opioid receptor (NOP), and an antagonist with high binding affinity at κ- and δ-opioid receptors. The term "partial agonist" has been utilized due to a partial effect on stimulating the receptor with in vitro assays. This does not necessarily translate to partial analgesic efficacy in vivo or clinical practice, as the analgesic signaling pathway can be sufficiently activated by a partial agonist. Partial agonism at the μ-opioid receptor by buprenorphine yields effective analgesia and a ceiling effect on respiratory depression and euphoria and reduces other adverse events commonly observed with conventional full agonist opioids. As buprenorphine does not occupy all μ-opioid receptors, this allows for the efficacy of concomitant full μ-opioid receptor agonists. Antagonism at the δ- and κ-opioid receptors may limit constipation, respiratory depression, dysphoria, and substance abuse. In addition, kappa-opioid receptor antagonists are currently being considered promising therapeutics for psychiatric conditions (including depression, anxiety, and SUDs). Agonism at NOP contributes to spinal analgesia and may limit the potential for substance misuse and tolerance commonly observed with full μ-opioid receptor agonists.

Buprenorphine is approved by the FDA for acute pain, chronic pain, opioid use disorder (OUD), or opioid dependence, depending on the formulation. Buprenorphine formulations exist as either a combination therapy with naloxone (utilized to minimize IV misuse of buprenorphine) or as stand-alone products.

Clinical safety and efficacy data suggest that buprenorphine may be an alternative with equivalent or superior analgesia to conventional opioids for patients with pain. IV buprenorphine has been the most extensively studied formulation and is FDA approved for acute pain, while the transdermal patch and buccal film are FDA approved for patients with chronic pain. The transdermal patch has demonstrated efficacy for chronic pain with once-weekly dosing, however, clinicians may find that the buprenorphine buccal film formulation has favorable bioavailability, available doses, efficacy, adverse event profile, and benefit-risk assessments for the treatment of chronic pain.

Due to buprenorphine's partial agonist properties, historical concerns have arisen as to preferred strategies for their use in the peri-operative period. While there is no risk of precipitated withdrawal when opioids are utilized in patients already on buprenorphine, there is a risk of inducing precipitated withdrawal in patients receiving full agonist opioids (FAO) and have buprenorphine (BUP) newly introduced. In the case of patients who are already receiving BUP for MOUD and require an FAO for surgery or a significant procedure, continuation and/or reduction in BUP dosing is recommended with the use of FAO as needed for optimal analgesia. BUP is maintained at lower dosing until the increased pain event has passed, FAO is tapered down and BUP is returned toward the patient's baseline dose.

The concept of stopping BUP pre-op with a washout period before introducing FAO has been abandoned and replaced by this blended approach.

Addiction. The risk of opioid addiction in a population of medically ill patients is approximately 0.3%. Therefore, if a patient has a SUD based on difficulties with managing opioids should only be done cautiously. Acute sympathetic symptoms from drug withdrawal or tolerance are more likely to be the problem than SUD *per se.* Rather than addiction, unrecognized depression alone or co-morbidity with anxiety is a more frequent, immediate explanation for the excessive need for opiates.

In recent years, oxycodone has attracted significant attention in the media due to its addictive potential. Clinical practice and research trials show that it is a good medication for pain due to its efficacy, tolerable side effect profile, and short onset of action. In patients who cannot tolerate or respond to other opioids, it remains a good option.[60] More controlled and cautious prescribing, and avoidance of extended-release formulations, which have high misuse potential, has decreased the misuse potential.

Recent data suggest, however, that the risk of prolonged administration of opioid medication can be as high as 3% in patients following major surgery, and thus the use of careful prescribing guidelines, distribution of small, controlled amounts, along informed consent of risk to the patient are advised.[61]

For those patients who require longer-term opioid prescribing for chronic pain, consideration for use of BUP should be considered.

Opioid Adjuvants. Opioid adjuvants are indicated when toxic or pharmacokinetic factors limit further increases in the patient's opioid dosage or when pain remains uncontrolled by opioids in combination with other secondary treatments, such as decompression surgery, nerve blocks, or anxiolytic drugs. The choice of adjuvant should be individualized; one should aim for the simplest and most potent combination of drugs. The selection of the adjuvant depends on the symptoms associated with the pain; the character of the pain; and the physician's knowledge of any special issues, risks, drug interactions, or special mechanisms.

Guidelines for Opioid Maintenance Adjuvants

- Maintenance opioids should be considered only after other methods of pain control have been proven unsuccessful. Alternative methods vary from case to case but typically include NSAIDs; oral, transdermal, IV, intrathecal, or epidural opioids; membrane-stabilizing drugs; AEDs, monoaminergic agents, local nerve blocks; nerve stimulation; and physical therapy.
- Opioids should not be prescribed for those with an OUD unless there is a new major medical illness with severe pain (e.g., cancer or trauma). In such cases, a second opinion from another physician is suggested for all opioids used for longer than 2 months.
- If opioids are prescribed for longer than 3 months, the patient should have a second opinion consultation, ideally with a formal pain specialist, plus a follow-up consultation at least once per year.
- There should be one pharmacy and one prescriber designated.
- Opioid dosage should be defined, as should expectations of what will happen if there are deviations from it. For example, misuse leads to rapid tapering of the drug and a detoxification program, if necessary. There should be no doubt that the physician will stop the medication if there is safety concern.
- Informed consent as to the rationale, risks, benefits, and alternatives should be documented. In addition, the patient should always be instructed to lock up medications, including the risk it may pose to children at home.
- The course of treatment, especially the ongoing indication(s), changes in the disease process, efficacy, the presence of tolerance, or emerging signs of a use disorder should be documented.

Justification for the maintenance of opioids, given the mixed benefits and risks, involves humanitarian and public health principles. If opioids are the only effective treatment for intractable suffering, they should be used for humanitarian reasons. The risk of episodic misuse may be justified in certain patients with high-risk histories or those with chronic pain if the use of medication lessens functional disability and illicit drug use. For example, a patient with a history of an OUD with chronic pain may benefit from a methadone maintenance program, which may also provide some level of pain management; furthermore, it may be an effective public health means of reducing the risk of human immunodeficiency virus (HIV) infection.

Analgesic Adjuvants

Pain may be refractory, despite the most judicious application of traditional anti-nociceptive measures, such as surgery, nerve blocks, and opioids. Stimulants, dopamine antagonists, TCAs, benzodiazepines, AEDs, antihistamines, peptides, and prostaglandin inhibitors, also have roles as non-opioid pain treatment adjuvants[62] (Table 17.7). The type of pain is as important as its cause in guiding the choice of an adjuvant. The pain may be characterized as a constant aching somatic pain, as in a fracture, or as a paroxysmal burning deafferentation sensation, as in phantom limb pain. The primary cause of the pain, however, does not necessarily determine its type or character. For example, the pain of metastatic cancer may be either neuropathic or visceral (and may or may not respond well to NSAIDs). Neuropathic pain is often refractory to opioids, and it covers a diverse group of conditions, which range from herpetic neuralgia to atypical facial pain. Patients suffering from this type of pain may respond to AEDs or TCAs. In the most difficult or ambiguous cases, a valuable technique is to use an IV dose of the drug to gain a rapid and accurate assessment of its effectiveness in the long term. IV morphine, lidocaine, and lorazepam can be used in this way to see whether any of these classes of drugs are worth pursuing.

Antidepressants for Pain

The mechanisms of action of TCAs are multiple and probably co-modulate the pain-relieving effect.[63] First, they have an effect in augmenting the descending periaqueductal spinal inhibitory control of pain mediated by serotonin and norepinephrine. In the spinal cord, the dorsolateral funiculus is a serotonergic inhibitory descending spinal pain pathway that modulates 80% of the spinal analgesic effect of opiates. Second, they potentiate naturally occurring or administered opiates. For example, desipramine, 8-OH-amoxapine, and imipramine are twice as potent as amitriptyline and four times as potent as trazodone and clomipramine at

binding to opiate receptors. Third, antihistamine and α-receptor effects may be important regarding potentiation. Fourth, there may be membrane-stabilizing anesthetic, anti-kindling anti-epileptic effects, which may also give secondary symptom relief of insomnia or anxiety.

The pain relief obtained from antidepressants is often independent of their effects on mood or the alleviation of MDD.[64,65] In fact, the greatest response to antidepressants in patients with pain may occur in those who are not depressed.[66] Antidepressants as analgesics are best thought of as monoaminergic cell stabilizers rather than just antidepressants. Serotonin, norepinephrine, and dopamine all modulate pain via their actions in the periphery of the CNS.

Serotonin presents a paradox because more serotonin is not necessarily better, yet function must be intact for pain to be inhibited. One type of peripheral serotonin receptor, 5-HT$_{1D}$, is found in cerebral blood vessels. Sumatriptan, a selective 5-HT$_{1D}$ antagonist, acts to produce vasoconstriction and migraine headache relief. The raphe and mesolimbic structures are important sites of subcortical serotonin receptors, mainly types 1 A, 2 A, and B. These areas modulate pain and mood—the neurobehavioral sites of action. Despite the important role serotonin plays in pain, there are several exceptions to the simplistic notion of more serotonin, and less pain.[67] For example, buspirone, fluoxetine, and trazodone have all been shown to be ineffective in attenuating certain pain syndromes.[68-70]

Norepinephrine-modulating medications also have value in treating chronic pain. Desipramine (average dose of 200 mg daily) relieved pain in diabetic neuropathy, in both non-depressed and depressed patients,[71] and also relieved post-herpetic neuralgia.[72] Duloxetine, an SNRI, has become the first antidepressant to have a specific pain indication for the treatment of painful diabetic neuropathy.[73] Duloxetine has also been studied in several large studies for the treatment of fibromyalgia and found to be efficacious, not only in pain reduction but also in reduction of tender points and stiffness scores, while also increasing the tender-point pain threshold when compared with placebo.[74] These results have also been reproduced by other SNRIs, with milnacipran and venlafaxine also having been shown to be efficacious for the treatment of pain associated with fibromyalgia.[75,76]

TABLE 17.7
Analgesic Adjuvants

Agent	Dosage	Indications	Special Issues
Prostaglandin Inhibitors	Variable, limited by side effects and medical co-morbidity	Metastatic bone pain Inflammation Vascular pain	NSAID risks: gastrointestinal bleeding, renal impairment
Dopamine Antagonists Phenothiazines Butyrophenones	Antipsychotic D_2 receptor-blocking doses	Post-herpetic pain Cancer pain Diabetic neuropathy Adjunct to TCAs Co-morbid anxiety or delirium	Haloperidol binds to opioid receptors Membrane stabilizing
Stimulants			Stimulants decrease pain and sedation
Methylphenidate Dextroamphetamine Pergolide	5–50 mg/day (t½: 2–7 h)5–20 mg/day (t½: 4–21 h)0.05 mg TID (t½: 6–72 h)	Post-operative pain and pain in pediatric and cancer patients respond well to analgesic-stimulant combinations	Appetite and cognition improve; methylphenidate shows better long-term efficacy than amphetamine
Steroids Prednisone Methylprednisolone	15+ mg/day PO 15 mg/kg IV boluses	Bone metastases Brain swelling Spinal cord compression Anorexia and pain Sickle cell pain	Risks: mood lability, withdrawal, anxiety, insomnia, gastrointestinal upset
Peptides Calcitonin	100–200 IU SC BID nasal 200 IC/day	Paget's, metastatic, and myeloma pain	Intrathecal, nasal, and SC are used
Somatostatin	500 µg	Vascular headaches	Somatostatin inhibits SP
Capsaicin crème	0.075%	Neuralgia, cancer pain Hyperalgesia, post-herpetic neuralgia, cluster headache, CRPS, inflammatory dermatoses, itching secondary to dialysis, psoriasis	Capsaicin effect peaks 4–6 weeks, for diabetic, post-mastectomy, and arthritic pain
Antihistamines Diphenhydramine	150 mg	Opioid adjunct	Decreased inflammation, 5-HT, NE, dopamine, opiate clearance increased opiate binding
Hydroxyzine	100 mg		
Benzodiazepines Clonazepam Lorazepam	1–4 mg/day 2–16 mg/day	Adjuvant tricyclics Allodynia	Not a substitute for a diagnosis of depression or substance abuse
Anti-Epileptic Drugs Phenytoin	300–450 mg/day	Cancer pain	Paroxysmal pain responds best to anti-epileptic drugs
Carbamazepine	400–1600 mg/day	Headaches, neuralgia	
Valproate	500–2000 mg/day	Central pain	
Gabapentin	900–1800 mg/day	Neuropathy	
Lamotrigine	100–300 mg/day	Migraine headaches	
Oxcarbazepine	300–1600 mg/day	Neuropathy	
Pregabalin	600–1200 mg/day	Neuropathy; PHN	
Topiramate	200–400 mg/day	Neuropathy	

(Continued)

	TABLE 17.7		
	Analgesic Adjuvants—Cont'd		
Agent	**Dosage**	**Indications**	**Special Issues**
Tricyclics	25–300 mg/day	Neuropathy	Burning
Desipramine		Post-herpetic neuralgia	Deafferentation pains respond best to tricyclic drugs
Imipramine			Increased side effects with amitriptyline
SSRIs		Diabetic neuropathy	
Paroxetine	20–60 mg/day		
Citalopram	20–60 mg/day		
SNRIs		Diabetic neuropathy	
Duloxetine	60–120 mg/day	Diabetic neuropathy; fibromyalgia	
Venlafaxine	75–375 mg/day	Fibromyalgia	

5-HT, 5-Hydroxytryptamine; BID, two times daily; CRPS, complex regional pain syndrome; IV, intravenous; NE, norepinephrine; NSAID, non-steroidal anti-inflammatory drug; PHN, post-herpetic neuralgia; SC, subcutaneous; SNRIs, serotonin-norepinephrine reuptake inhibitors; SSRIs, selective serotonin reuptake reuptake inhibitors; SP, substance P; TCAs, tricyclic antidepressants.

Reviews of Efficacy

Earlier reports by Lindsay and Wyckoff showed an efficacy of 70% to 80% for antidepressants for the treatment of patients with chronic pain and depression.[77] Stein and associates reported that amitriptyline (150 mg/day) was more effective than acetaminophen 2 g/day in a controlled, double-blind study, with mild depression being one of the predictors of pain relief at the end of the 5-week study.[78] Blumer and Heilbronn showed twice the improvement (60%) in outcome and a halving of the dropout rate (25%) in those patients with pain treated with antidepressants.[79]

Pain syndromes that may be responsive to antidepressants include those associated with cancer, post-herpetic neuralgia, arthritis, vascular and tension headaches, and facial pain. The literature reports a wide range of generally positive but poorly designed studies. Feinmann reviewed the 11 largest and best-designed studies on pain relief from antidepressants when depressive symptoms were present.[80] TCAs (amitriptyline hydrochloride) and MAOIs (phenelzine sulfate) were used, and the results demonstrated that these antidepressant drugs were beneficial in the treatment of chronic pain associated with depression.

A review by Goodkin and co-workers found that 37 of 53 trials (70%) of heterocyclic antidepressant drugs for chronic pain syndromes failed to meet minimum criteria for adequate design.[81] Of the remaining 16 trials that met design and protocol criteria, seven evaluated headache pain and documented positive effects with low-dose regimens. Complicating these findings was that smaller than typical antidepressant doses were used in many studies. In this same review, another non-random series of 17 studies was selected, of which five (29%) met minimum design and protocol criteria (i.e., clear protocol, placebo-controlled, and defined outcome measurements); only two of the five trials showed positive results. One study was for low-dose amitriptyline in mixed pain syndromes, and the other study was for desipramine in post-herpetic neuralgia. Max found that in 13 well-designed, randomized trials, antidepressants reduced pain in diabetic neuropathy and post-herpetic neuralgia, particularly the mixed serotonin and norepinephrine agents (e.g., imipramine, desipramine, and amitriptyline).[82]

Saarto and Wiffen, in a Cochrane-based review, reviewed available randomized clinical trials (RCTs) of antidepressants in neuropathic pain.[26] In total, 61 RCTs were included, and it was found that TCAs were effective, with a number needed to treat (NNT) of 3.6 for the achievement of at least moderate pain relief. Venlafaxine had an NNT of 3.1 and there was limited evidence for the effectiveness of the SSRIs based on current available data.

In a meta-analysis conducted to assess the efficacy of antidepressants in treating back pain in adults, it was found that antidepressants were more effective than placebo in reducing pain severity but not functional status in chronic back pain.[83] TCAs have been shown to be an option for patients with chronic back pain, with SSRIs showing limited effectiveness. To date, SNRIs have not been studied for the treatment of chronic back pain.[27]

When is it worth trying a monoaminergic agent? A trial of an antidepressant medication is useful in any intractable pain condition because analgesic effects are at least partly independent of antidepressant effects. Furthermore, the size of the analgesic effect does not differ significantly in the presence of depression.

There is no clear evidence for the superiority of any one antidepressant over another. Amitriptyline, desipramine, and doxepin hydrochloride have been used most often in clinical studies. Even though sedating and non-sedating properties of drugs have no significant association with analgesic effects, the antihistaminic profile of an antidepressant correlates with the effect.[84] Potent serotonin reuptake blockade is not essential to pain relief; moreover, there is doubt about the efficacy of purely serotonergic drugs for neuropathic pain (e.g., fluoxetine, zimelidine, and trazodone).[85,86] Buspirone does not appear to relieve pain. Except paroxetine, all antidepressants studied in placebo-controlled trials of neuropathic pain have some inhibition of norepinephrine reuptake (i.e., amitriptyline, desipramine, nortriptyline, imipramine, and maprotiline).[71] Venlafaxine has some agonist-antagonist opiate activity as well as norepinephrine, 5-hydroxytryptamine, and dopamine reuptake effects, but it has yet to be rigorously proven as an analgesic.[87]

MAOIs may be particularly helpful in the attenuation of atypical pain associated with atypical depression. Both MAOIs and TCAs, however, may require a trial of at least 6 weeks for the full benefit to be evident.

Dopamine agonists can also augment analgesia. Dopamine has been associated with pain in clinical and experimental trials and has also been shown to co-modulate opioid and substance P effects in the CNS. Psychostimulants can potentiate the effects of opioid analgesics.[88,89] Methylphenidate has been studied as adjuvant therapy for cancer patients receiving opioids. In a randomized, double-blind, placebo-controlled crossover trial of 32 patients with advanced cancer receiving chronic opiate therapy, statistically significant reductions in pain intensity and sedation were seen with the use of methylphenidate.[90] In another study of 50 patients with advanced cancer and opiate-induced sedation, 44 had a decrease in sedation after initiation of methylphenidate.[91] Patients with incident cancer pain (mild or no pain at rest, severe pain during movements) showed better pain control, and they tolerated higher doses of opioids when supplemented with methylphenidate.[92] A placebo-controlled trial demonstrated that the addition of oral methylphenidate resulted in improved cognitive function in 20 patients receiving continuous subcutaneous opioids for cancer pain,[93] and similarly, 5 of 11 adolescent cancer patients receiving opiates exhibited improved interaction with family or decreased somnolence when methylphenidate was added to their medication regimen.[94] While classified as a dopamine reuptake inhibitor, bupropion also has noradrenergic activity. Evidence of an analgesic effect is still very limited, although in one double-blind, placebo-controlled, crossover trial, 73% of 41 subjects with neuropathic pain obtained pain relief with bupropion treatment.

Monoaminergic agents in combination with clonazepam, valproate, or opioids, for cancer pain, are often safe and desirable.

Although some patients may respond to low doses of antidepressants for pain, a complete trial of antidepressants in those with pain requires a full dose of an antidepressant, the same as is used in MDD. The placebo-controlled study of McQuay and colleagues found that low doses of antidepressants (25 mg of amitriptyline) did not have the efficacy of higher doses.[95] The best results in the largest number of people are obtained, however, when the usual antidepressant dosage of the drug is used (e.g., 300 mg/day of imipramine hydrochloride or its equivalent).

Anti-Epileptic Drugs

Anti-epileptic drugs (AEDs) have a long history of effectiveness in the treatment of pain, especially neuropathic in origin, dating back to case reports for the treatment of trigeminal neuralgia with phenytoin in 1942 and carbamazepine in 1962.[96] Blocking abnormally high-frequency and spontaneous firing in afferent neurons in the dorsal horn and thalamus are the putative mechanisms for the efficacy of anticonvulsants with regard to pain. The consequence of blocking the hyperexcitability of low-threshold mechanoreceptive neurons in the brain leads to pain relief.[97] Phenytoin, carbamazepine, valproic acid (VPA), benzodiazepines, along with gabapentin, pregabalin, lamotrigine, topiramate, and oxcarbazepine, are agents used to help manage pain. These drugs have several shared cellular effects, which include antagonism of excitatory amino acids, γ-aminobutyric acid (GABA)-receptor agonism, sodium and calcium pump stabilization, and antagonism of adenosine. Indirectly, they all antagonize the effects of excitatory amino acids, which are believed to kindle the hyperexcitability of CNS neurons.

Phenytoin has been shown to be effective in alleviating pain associated with various neuropathies, particularly trigeminal, diabetic, and post-stroke pain. Sharp, shooting, and lancinating pain has been shown to respond especially well to this drug. It has more behavioral toxicity, however, and is less effective than carbamazepine, thus making it a second choice for analgesia.

Carbamazepine is generally superior to phenytoin for pain. The effect of carbamazepine on pain suppression is likely mediated by central and peripheral mechanisms. The ability of carbamazepine to block ionic conductance appears to be frequency dependent, which enables the drug to suppress the spontaneously active Aδ and C fibers responsible for pain without affecting normal nerve conduction. Since Blom[96] reported the analgesic properties of carbamazepine for patients with trigeminal neuralgia in 1962, carbamazepine has been shown to be effective also for post-herpetic pain, post-sympathetic pain, diabetic neuropathy, multiple sclerosis, and assorted neuralgias.[98] Higher levels (8–12 µg/L) are typically necessary for optimal efficacy.

The first reports of VPA used in neuropathic pain appeared in the early 1980s. VPA prolongs the repolarization of voltage-activated Na^+ channels, and increases the amount of GABA in the brain, enhancing the activity of glutamic acid decarboxylase and inhibiting GABA degradation enzymes. VPA has been shown to decrease post-herpetic neuralgia, episodic and chronic cluster headaches, migraine, and postoperative pain, as well as various neuralgias. It has also been demonstrated that VPA is effective in treating migraine headaches in two double-blind, placebo-controlled trials.[99,100] These demonstrations of efficacy in pain reduction are in addition to the traditional place for VPA in the treatment of psychiatric disorders (bipolar and schizoaffective disorders). VPA sprinkles are well tolerated and can substitute for carbamazepine and lithium in pain states, although no head-to-head comparisons have been completed.

Benzodiazepines have been controversial in the alleviation of pain; however, they may be effective and safe in certain clinical situations.[101] Combinations of benzodiazepines with antidepressants or opiates may be particularly useful clinically. IV lorazepam was superior to morphine, lidocaine, and placebo in a single-blind study of neuropathic pain,[102] however, these results were not reproduced in a randomized, double-blind trial in which lorazepam was less effective than amitriptyline in patients with post-herpetic neuralgia.[103] Orally, clonazepam is the drug of choice. It binds more slowly to central than to peripheral benzodiazepine receptors, and it is synergistic with serotonergic pain mechanisms, a factor that distinguishes it from other benzodiazepines. A useful diagnostic test for benzodiazepine-sensitive pain is to administer lorazepam 2 mg IV in a single-blind manner evaluated by visual analog scale (VAS) monitoring. Positive results (>3 cm decrease in VAS) signify relief of ongoing pain. If positive results are achieved, it is recommended to give sequential IV lorazepam doses to break the pain cycle (in severe cases) or clonazepam (e.g., 2–4 mg orally at bedtime and 1 mg twice a day).

Of the newer AEDs used for the treatment of neuropathic pain, gabapentin is perhaps the best studied so far. Developed as a structural GABA analog, it has no direct GABAergic action. It is believed that gabapentin acts on the α-2-δ type of Ca^{2+} channels. Gabapentin has been shown to relieve pain and associated symptoms in patients with peripheral diabetic neuropathy, post-herpetic neuralgia, HIV-related neuropathy, and cancer-related neuropathic pain.[104-107] The dosages used in these studies typically ranged from 900 to 3600 mg daily in three divided doses. Additional studies are required to evaluate if gabapentin has efficacy in other pain states.

Topiramate works via multiple mechanisms, including prolongation of voltage-sensitive sodium channel inactivation, $GABA_A$ agonism, and non-N-methyl-D aspartate (NMDA) glutamate receptor antagonism. Topiramate has been found to be useful in the treatment of trigeminal neuralgia, along with diabetic neuropathy.

Oxcarbazepine is a keto-analog of carbamazepine, with the analgesic mechanism likely due to inhibition of voltage-dependent Na^+ channels and to a lesser extent, K^+ channels. While studies seem to show mixed results for the use of oxcarbazepine for diabetic neuropathy, it seems to have similar efficacy to carbamazepine in the treatment of trigeminal neuralgia; however, there are limited data regarding the efficacy and safety of this drug in the treatment of other neuropathic pain syndromes.

Pregabalin is a GABA analog believed to exert its analgesic effect by binding to the α_2 delta subunit of voltage-gated calcium channels on primary afferent nerves and reducing the release of neurotransmitters from their central terminals. Evidence seems to show that pregabalin is effective in reducing the intensity of pain associated with diabetic polyneuropathy and post-herpetic neuralgia.[108,109]

Lamotrigine is a direct glutamate antagonist that also inhibits sodium channels. While initial case reports seemed to show some promise for the use of lamotrigine in neuropathic pain states, most randomized, double-blind studies to date have not shown any significant efficacy.[110–114]

Sympathetically Maintained Pain

Sympathetically maintained pain (SMP)—regardless of whether it is due to reflex sympathetic dystrophy, opiate tolerance, hyperalgesia, inflammation, vascular headache, post-herpetic neuralgia, trauma, facial pain, or arthritis—may respond to sympathetic blockade.[115] Sympathetic efferent fibers release norepinephrine, which in turn activates α-adrenergic receptors. Activation of these receptors, either directly or indirectly, excites nociceptors. Activity in the nociceptors then evokes pain and causes further discharge of nociceptors. α-Adrenergic receptor super-sensitivity has been postulated as a likely mechanism for both the hyperalgesia and the autonomic disturbances associated with SMP.[116] The clinician can consider the early use of sympathetic blockade in any chronic pain syndrome with

features of sympathetic dysfunction. SMP is diagnosed and treated using the method of injecting or transdermally applying an α-adrenergic-blocking agent selected from the group consisting of an α-1-adrenergic antagonist, α-2-adrenergic agonist, or other drug that depletes sympathetic norepinephrine. One method to assess for SMP is to infuse 500 mL of one-half normal saline before putting phentolamine into an ischemic regional block, then administer phentolamine 10 mg IV over 10 minutes. A positive test result is marked by relief of evoked pain stimulated by light touch or a tuning fork.[117] α-Blocking drugs (e.g., phentolamine, α-blocking antidepressants) and α_2-agonists, such as clonidine, given with or without opiates, are all potentially useful in patients with chronic pain. Intrathecal, epidural, and systemic administration of clonidine also produce analgesia and clonidine is often useful in patients who have developed tolerance to opiates and who have some types of vascular or neuropathic pain.[118,119] Transdermal clonidine (0–3 mg/day) is sometimes useful in neuropathy, although the results of the treatment are mixed.

The mechanism of action of dexmedetomidine resembles that of clonidine, although its affinity for the α-2-adrenoceptor is approximately eight times that of clonidine,[120] and it has a significantly higher α-2/α-1 selectivity ratio than does clonidine.[121,122] Besides its analgesic effects, its sedative effects are thought to be secondary to action on α-2-adrenoreceptors located in the locus coeruleus. Similar to clonidine, dexmedetomidine decreases the requirement for opioids in patients undergoing a variety of surgical procedures[123] and in a clinical trial where it was administered as a single agent for sedation, it reduced by approximately 60% the number of patients who needed opioids for the control of pain.[124] Dexmedetomidine was approved in the United States in 2000 for up to 24 hours of pain treatment in surgical patients.

β-Blockers are not efficacious in the treatment of sympathetically maintained pain except in their use for alleviating migraine headaches. Guanethidine, bretylium, reserpine, and phentolamine have been used successfully to produce a chemical sympathectomy.[125,126]

TREATMENT OF CENTRAL NEUROPATHIC PAIN STATES

The clinical hallmark of central pain is that it persists without an obvious nociceptive stimulus; the physiologic goal of treatment is to stabilize hyperexcitable neurons. Table 17.8 outlines some clinical approaches to central pain.

Carbamazepine has been shown to be among the most effective agents for some facial neuralgias, which may be associated with severe pain and discomfort. Within 24 hours of attaining a steady state, it is effective in 80% of patients with trigeminal neuralgia, making it clinically superior to phenytoin. Other types of lancinating pain, such as postherpetic neuralgia, post-sympathectomy pain, and post-traumatic pain, may also respond to AEDs. IV trials offer a quick, definitive way of identifying drug responders in complex or pressured situations. For routine CNS pain, clonazepam is well tolerated for pain syndromes, especially when allodynia is present. It facilitates both pre-synaptic and post-synaptic inhibition, increases recurrent inhibition, and decreases the firing rate of normal and epileptic neurons in the brain; it also enhances sleep, relaxes muscles and blood vessels, and treats anxiety

TABLE 17.8
Pain Management and Treatment

Pain Characteristics	What Treatment Is Next?	Comments
Nociceptive element present?	Nerve block for diagnostic and therapeutic reasons Imaging: MRI, looking for lesions	Even in pain that appears central (e.g., trigeminal neuralgia), nociceptive triggers can initiate pain and peripheral deafferentation
Allodynia present? (vibration, cold, or light touch)	Low-dose clonazepam (1–4 mg/day) if the person can tolerate benzodiazepines alone or in combination with desipramine 50 mg at bedtime (up to 300 mg eventually, if necessary) Mexiletine 150–400 mg TID	Allodynia predicts response to clonazepam Clonazepam relaxes muscles, improves sleep and anxiety Membrane stabilizers are useful but cardiotoxicity needs to be checked Peptides useful
Paroxysmal attacks? (lightning like)	Anti-epileptic drugs (AEDs) Carbamazepine 400–1600 mg/day (serum 8–12 g/L) Valproate 500–2000 mg/day Gabapentin 300–1200 mg TID Lamotrigine 100–300 mg/day	Clonazepam should usually be tried first but works well synergistically with the AEDs listed Valproate for vascular headache Gabapentin: few drug interactions
Central pain— Allodynia Paroxysmal attacks Sharp perceived as a light touch Decreased pain threshold Non-dermatomal distribution of pain Hyperpathia	Definitive trial is a single-blind random assignment of IV lorazepam (2–4 mg) vs. lidocaine (100 mg) vs. morphine 10 mg, rated on a VAS pain Amitriptyline 25 mg IV infusion as test dose with VAS pain	Careful physical examination essential Is sharp perceived as a light touch? A light touch is painful, sustained, and has a delayed crescendo Tuning fork/moving a hair examination best for allodynia
Co-morbid central pain? Vascular and myofascial pain	Valproate 250–2000 mg/day Physical therapy Monoaminergic prescription antidepressants Nasal calcitonin 200 IU/day Capsaicin 4-6-week trial Topical preparation	Common in head, neck, and face pain Mixed results with SSRIs Rule out sympathetically maintained pain

(Continued)

TABLE 17.8		
Pain Management and Treatment—Cont'd		
Pain Characteristics	What Treatment Is Next?	Comments
Psychiatric component? Rule out or treat	Co-morbid psychiatric and CNS pain: consider prescription with dual efficacy for pain and psychiatric diagnosis	Rule out depression and anxiety, and consider mimics of central pain, such as somatoform, factitious, or psychotic disorders
	Benzodiazepine for allodynia and anxiety	
	Antidepressants for neuropathy, depression, and anxiety	Pain drawing by the patient is a good tool to uncover psychosis and myofascial pain
	Dopamine antagonists for neuralgia, anxiety, psychosis, and nausea	Rule out akathisia, restless leg syndrome
	AEDs for lancinating pain and mood stabilization	

CNS, Central nervous system; IV, intravenous; MRI, magnetic resonance imaging; SSRIs, selective serotonin reuptake inhibitors; TID, three times daily; VAS, visual analog scale.

symptoms. It is the drug that exemplifies the need to select prescriptions based not only on their efficacy and tolerability but also on their mechanisms of action for disease processes that have multiple pathophysiological causes.

TREATMENT OF CHRONIC PAIN AND THE USE OF MULTI-DISCIPLINARY PAIN CLINICS

Rehabilitative approaches to chronic pain management have been the most widely recommended intervention. These typically focus more on improving function and quality of life through enhancing self-management rather than symptom relief. Typically, these approaches are conducted by a multi-disciplinary team of health professionals who attempt to address identified physical, psychological, and social factors that may contribute to the experience and impact of chronic pain. This requires medical providers who can work in a collaborative, inter-disciplinary manner, with the patient also playing an active role. The disciplines involved typically include physical therapists, clinical psychologists, nurses, and physicians also often comprised of different fields of medicine (e.g., physical medicine and rehabilitation, pain medicine, psychiatry). Not surprisingly, such multi-disciplinary approaches can require significant resources and organizational support for their implementation.[127]

Guidelines

Medicare guidelines offer one set of standards for multi-disciplinary pain management. The pain must be of at least 6 months duration (resulting in significant life disturbance and limited functioning); it must be attributable to a physical cause; and it must be intractable to the usual methods of treatment. Desirable characteristics of pain treatment facilities and standards of care in pain management have now been published (in response to skepticism about cost, quality, control, and diversity of pain treatment facilities).[117] Quality control guidelines developed by the Commission on Accreditation of Rehabilitation Facilities (CARF), under the umbrella of the Joint Commission on Accreditation of Healthcare Organizations (JCAHO), have led to the certification of numerous chronic pain management programs nationwide. It should be noted, that behavioral treatments often employed in this setting, however, are not primarily for pain relief but rather to assist the patient in extinguishing the maladaptive behaviors associated with their pain experience.[128] Furthermore, proof of the cost-effectiveness of inpatient multi-disciplinary treatment remains sparse and consequently somewhat ill defined.

Reasons for Referral to a Multi-disciplinary Pain Clinic

Multi-disciplinary pain clinics should be considered in the following circumstances:

- When consultation with an independent physician who is an expert in the treatment of chronic pain is necessary for further assessment or to confirm that no single modality of outpatient treatment is likely to work.
- When the patient has already obtained maximum benefit from outpatient treatments (such as NSAIDs, nerve blocks, antidepressants, and simple physical and behavioral rehabilitation).
- When intensive daily interventions are required, usually with multiple concurrent types of therapy, such as nerve blocks, physical therapy, and behavior modification.
- When the patient exhibits abnormal pain behavior and agrees to the goals of improved coping, work rehabilitation, and psychologic assessment.
- When medications for pain relief are so complex or compliance management so difficult further supervision or recommendations of medical therapy may be necessary.

Rehabilitation

Rehabilitation of patients who have chronic pain syndromes may require some combination of input from specialists in psychiatry, physical therapy, physical medicine and rehabilitation, behavioral psychology, and neurology. It is important to bear in mind that no special therapy, including exercise therapy, spinal manipulation, bed rest, orthoses, acupuncture, traction therapy, back schools, and epidural steroids, works well. Successful rehabilitation aims to decrease symptoms, increase independence, and allow the patient to return to work. A positive, rapid return to light-normal activities and work is essential if disability is to be minimized. Psychologically, this is the key to coping with acute trauma. Even with patients who experience low back pain, 50% of whom have a recurrence within 3 years of the initial episode, there is no evidence that a return to work adversely affects the course of the pain syndrome.[129]

Hypnosis

The use of hypnosis in chronic pain syndromes is well known. Self-hypnosis is particularly helpful, but only about one in four subjects can achieve a state of concentration of sufficient magnitude for lasting pain control. Hypnosis is a method worth considering,

provided that the physician knows its limitations and how to apply it to the individual patient's needs.

Education

Education is needed for the caregivers as well as the patient. A thorough investigation of patients' past and present history, and the emotional reactions of caregivers and medical staff to the levels of opioid use, and pain versus substance dependence can help the care team to create a safe treatment program. Education of the care team by mental health professionals may decrease significant anxiety and conflicts around the care of patients with pain.

Cognitive and Behavioral Therapies

Cognitive-behavioral therapy (CBT) has been shown to be effective in patients who suffer from either continuous or chronic pain. Negative, or catastrophic, thoughts are often present in patients with pain disorders. Such thoughts are highly correlated to the intensity of pain complaints. CBT focuses on re-structuring this negative cognitive schema into a more realistic appraisal of the patient's current condition. When a realistic perspective regarding the past, present, and future can be gained, patients may be able to deal with their pain more effectively. Relaxation training is often a component of CBT for patients with pain. Progressive muscle relaxation, stretch-based relaxation, deep breathing, and autogenic training are all relaxation techniques that may be learned.[130,131]

Relaxation Response and Mindfulness Therapies

The purpose of relaxation techniques is to decrease the activity of the sympathetic nervous system, by evoking an opposite reaction to the stress response, namely a relaxation response.[131] The use of relaxation techniques is associated with reduced blood pressure, oxygen uptake, respiratory frequency, heart frequency, and muscle tension, and has several detectable physiological effects, including lower cortisol levels and inhibition of inflammatory processes.[132,133]

Several different types of relaxation techniques exist, including mindful meditation, breathing techniques, visualization, autogenic training, and progressive muscle relaxation. One possible explanation of why relaxation techniques relieve chronic pain is that chronic pain may be maintained and increased by psychological stress and physical tensions.[134] It has been estimated that three months of regular practice is necessary to obtain pain reduction with effects likely dependent on individual differences and the type of chronic pain experienced.[135]

Numerous systematic reviews on the effects of mindfulness meditation have been published, and in those that report pain outcomes, several have focused on specific types of pain such as low back pain, fibromyalgia, or somatic symptoms. Several comprehensive reviews have focused on controlled trials of mindfulness interventions for chronic pain including a review that showed improvements in depressive symptoms and coping, and another review on mindfulness for chronic back pain, fibromyalgia, and musculoskeletal pain that showed small positive effects for pain. In addition, reviews on various pain conditions have found improvements in pain, pain acceptance, quality of life, and functional status.[136]

Coping and Psychotherapy

Coping with chronic pain always threatens two fundamentals of survival: attachment behaviors and intrapsychic defenses. To cope means to have people of quality around to fortify one's courage and to have adaptive defense mechanisms to negotiate the thoughts and feelings that arise in one's head. Helping the patient develop evidence-based coping skills is more effective for decreasing pain and psychological disability than education alone.[137] Coping is also context-dependent and most effective when the focus includes the couple or family.[138,139]

The psychodynamic aspects of coping involve conflicts over autonomy and care. Old conflicts about nurturance suggest there may be mixed feelings about recovery. Shame may mimic depression, trigger conservation-withdrawal, and produce counter-dependent behavior. Regression, some of which is normal, can be manifest as non-adherence, help-rejecting behavior, complaining, and behaviors akin to the metaphoric "cutting off your nose to spite your face." The hateful patient and the hateful physician are often compatriots in partnership with chronic pain, and the task of the psychiatrist is to clarify how these problems become played out in the physician-patient relationship. One should understand that the physician may be a protective figure who is the recipient

of both idealized and angry feelings when a cure is not forthcoming. Modern healthcare, with its fragmentation, multiple caregivers, and bureaucracies, guarantees rifts in the physician-patient relationship. To help the patient cope, the psychiatrist must be sensitive to the unconscious feelings of the patient and be prepared to manage denial and employ counseling, relaxation, exercise, physical rehabilitation, and pharmacotherapy, while still functioning as a teacher and physician.

REFERENCES

1. Fleming P. *My Aunt's Rhinoceros and Other Reflections*. Simon and Schuster; 1958.
2. Raja SN, Carr DB, Cohen M, et al. The revised International Association for the Study of Pain definition of pain: concepts, challenges, and compromises. *Pain*. 2020;161(9):1976–1982.
3. Wall PD. The prevention of postoperative pain. *Pain*. 1988;33(3):289–290.
4. Wall PD, McMahon S. The relationship of perceived pain to afferent nerve impulses. *Trends Neurosci*. 1986;9:254–255.
5. Hyman S, Cassem NH. Pain. In: Rubenstein E, Federman DD, eds. *Scientific American Medicine: Current Topics in Medicine. Subsection II*. Scientific American; 1989.
6. Seifert F, Maihofner C. Central mechanisms of experimental and chronic neuropathic pain: findings from functional imaging studies. *Cell Mol Life Sci*. 2009;66(3):375–390.
7. Rainville P, Hofbauer RK, Paus T, et al. Cerebral mechanisms of hypnotic induction and suggestion. *J Cogn Neurosci*. 1999;11(1):110–125.
8. Faymonville ME, Laureys S, Degueldre C, et al. Neural mechanisms of antinociceptive effects of hypnosis. *Anesthesiology*. 2000;92(5):1257–1267.
9. Valet M, Sprenger T, Boecker H, et al. Distraction modulates connectivity of the cingulo-frontal cortex and the midbrain during pain – an fMRI analysis. *Pain*. 2004;109(3):399–408.
10. Petrovic P, Ingvar M. Imaging cognitive modulation of pain processing. *Pain*. 2002;95(1–2):1–5.
11. Levine JD, Gordon NC, Fields HL. The mechanism of placebo analgesia. *Lancet*. 1978;2(8091):654–657.
12. Corder G, Castro DC, Bruchas MR, et al. Endogenous and exogenous opioids in pain. *Annu Rev Neurosci*. 2018 Jul 8;41:453–473.
13. Meller ST, Gebhart GF. Nitric oxide (NO) and nociceptive processing in the spinal cord. *Pain*. 1993;52(2):127–136.
14. Fields HL, Liebeskind JC. *Pharmacological Approaches to the Treatment of Chronic Pain: New Concepts and Critical Issues*. IASP Press; 1994.
15. May A. Chronic pain may change the structure of the brain. *Pain*. 2008;137(1):7–15.
16. Zhuo M. A synaptic model for pain: long-term potentiation in the anterior cingulate cortex. *Mol Cells*. 2007;23(3):259–271.
17. Dickenson AH. *Mechanisms of Central Hypersensitivity: Excitatory Amino Acid Mechanisms and Their Control*. Springer-Verlag; 1997.

18. Bell RF, Dahl JB, Moore RA, et al. Perioperative ketamine for acute postoperative pain. *Cochrane Database Syst Rev.* 2006(1): CD004603.

19. Vaughan CW, Ingram SL, Connor MA, et al. How opioids inhibit GABA-mediated neurotransmission. *Nature.* 1997;390(6660): 611–614.

20. Wu LJ, Xu H, Ren M, et al. Genetic and pharmacological studies of GluR5 modulation of inhibitory synaptic transmission in the anterior cingulate cortex of adult mice. *Dev Neurobiol.* 2007; 67(2):146–157.

21. Heyes MP, Saito K, Crowley JS, et al. Quinolinic acid and kynurenine pathway metabolism in inflammatory and non-inflammatory neurological disease. *Brain.* 1992;115:1249–1273.

22. Holloway M. No pain, no gain? *Science.* 1990;248(4961):1313.

23. Paix A, Coleman A, Lees J, et al. Subcutaneous fentanyl and sufentanil infusion substitution for morphine intolerance in cancer pain management. *Pain.* 1995;63(2):263–269.

24. Benarroch EE. Descending monoaminergic pain modulation: bidirectional control and clinical relevance. *Neurology.* 2008;71(3):217–221.

25. Furst S. Transmitters involved in antinociception in the spinal cord. *Brain Res Bull.* 1999;48(2):129–141.

26. Saarto T, Wiffen PJ. Antidepressants for neuropathic pain. *Cochrane Database Syst Rev.* 2007(4):CD005454.

27. Chou R, Huffman LH. Medications for acute and chronic low back pain: a review of the evidence for an American Pain Society/American College of Physicians clinical practice guideline. *Ann Intern Med.* 2007;147(7):505–514.

28. Harden RN, Bruehl S, Stanton-Hicks M, et al. Proposed new diagnostic criteria for complex regional pain syndrome. *Pain Med.* 2007;8(4):326–331.

29. Albazaz R, Wong YT, Homer-Vanniasinkam S. Complex regional pain syndrome: a review. *Ann Vasc Surg.* 2008;22(2): 297–306.

30. Kooijman CM, Dijkstra PU, Geertzen JH, et al. Phantom pain and phantom sensations in upper limb amputees: an epidemiological study. *Pain.* 2000;87(1):33–41.

31. Jensen T, Nikolajsen L. *Phantom Pain and Other Phenomena After Amputation.* Churchill Livingstone; 1999.

32. Luo Y, Anderson TA. Phantom limb pain: a review. *Int Anesthesiol Clin.* 2016;54(2):121–139.

33. Doubell TP, Mannion R, Woolf CJ. The dorsal horn: state-dependent sensory processing, plasticity and the generation of pain. In: Wall P, ed. *Textbook of Pain.* Churchill Livingstone; 1999.

34. Ramachandran VS, Rogers-Ramachandran D, Stewart M. Perceptual correlates of massive cortical reorganization. *Science.* 1992;258(5085):1159–1160.

35. Finnerup NB, Attal N, Haroutounian S, et al. Pharmacotherapy for neuropathic pain in adults: a systematic review and meta-analysis. *Lancet Neurol.* 2015;14(2):162–173.

36. Wall PD, Gutnick M. Ongoing activity in peripheral nerves: the physiology and pharmacology of impulses originating from a neuroma. *Exp Neurol.* 1974;43(3):580–593.

37. Niraj S, Niraj G. Phantom limb pain and its psychologic management: a critical review. *Pain Manag Nurs.* 2014;15(1): 349–364.

38. Willoch F, Rosen G, Tolle TR, et al. Phantom limb pain in the human brain: unraveling neural circuitries of phantom limb sensations using positron emission tomography. *Ann Neurol.* 2000;48(6):842–849.

39. Travell JG, Simons DG. *Myofascial Pain and Dysfunction: The Trigger Point Manual.* Williams & Wilkins; 1983.

40. Moldofsky H. Sleep and pain. *Sleep Med Rev.* 2001;5(5): 385–396.

41. Drewes AM. Pain and sleep disturbances with special reference to fibromyalgia and rheumatoid arthritis. *Rheumatology (Oxford).* 1999;38(11):1035–1038.

42. Boakye PA, Olechowski C, Rashiq S, et al. A critical review of neurobiological factors involved in the interactions between chronic pain, depression, and sleep disruption. *Clin J Pain.* 2016;32(4):327–336.

43. Sigvardsson S, von Knorring AL, Bohman M, et al. An adoption study of somatoform disorders. I. The relationship of somatization to psychiatric disability. *Arch Gen Psychiatry.* 1984;41(9):853–859.

44. McDonald JS. Management of chronic pelvic pain. *Obstet Gynecol Clin North Am.* 1993;20(4):817–838.

45. Walker EA, Katon WJ, Neraas K, et al. Dissociation in women with chronic pelvic pain. *Am J Psychiatry.* 1992;149(4):534–537.

46. Reed JL. The diagnosis of 'hysteria.' *Psychol Med.* 1975;5(1): 13–17.

47. Evans W, Hoyle C. The comparative value of drugs used in the continuous treatment of angina pectoris. *J Med.* 1933;2: 311–338.

48. Elton NH, Hanna MM, Treasure J. Coping with chronic pain. Some patients suffer more. *Br J Psychiatry.* 1994;165(6): 802–807.

49. Acute Pain Management Guideline Panel. *Acute Pain Management: Operative or Medical Procedures and Trauma–Clinical Practice Guidelines.* Department of Health and Human Services; 1992.

50. Dajani EZ, Islam K. Cardiovascular and gastrointestinal toxicity of selective cyclo-oxygenase-2 inhibitors in man. *J Physiol Pharmacol.* 2008;59(suppl 2):117–133.

51. Arkinstall W, Sandler A, Goughnour B, et al. Efficacy of controlled-release codeine in chronic non-malignant pain: a randomized, placebo-controlled clinical trial. *Pain.* 1995;62(2): 169–178.

52. Ventafridda V, Tamburini M, Caraceni A, et al. A validation study of the WHO method for cancer pain relief. *Cancer.* 1987;59(4):850–856.

53. Portenoy RK, Foley KM. Chronic use of opioid analgesics in non-malignant pain: report of 38 cases. *Pain.* 1986;25(2): 171–186.

54. Gourlay GK. Long-term use of opioids in chronic pain patients with nonterminal disease states. *Pain Rev.* 1994;1(1):62–76.

55. Bouckoms AJ, Masand PS, Murray GM, et al. Non-malignant pain treated with long-term oral narcotics. *Ann Clin Psychiatry.* 1992;4:185–192.

56. Bruera E, Schoeller T, Montejo G. Organic hallucinosis in patients receiving high doses of opiates for cancer pain. *Pain.* 1992;48(3):397–399.

57. Fogarty T, Murray GB. Psychiatric presentation of meperidine toxicity. *J Clin Psychopharmacol.* 1987;7(2):116–117.

58. Hill RG. Pharmacological considerations in the use of opioids in the management of non-terminal disease states. *Pain Rev.* 1994;1(1):47–61.

59. Kunz KM, Theisen JA, Schroeder ME. Severe episodic pain: management with sublingual sufentanil. *J Pain Symptom Manage.* 1993;8(4):189–190.

60. Rischitelli DG, Karbowicz SH. Safety and efficacy of controlled-release oxycodone: a systematic literature review. *Pharmacotherapy.* 2002;22(7):898–904.

61. Clarke H, Soneji N, Ko DT, et al. Rates and risk factors for prolonged opioid use after major surgery: population-based cohort study. *BMJ.* 2014;348:g1251.

62. Lussier D, Huskey AG, Portenoy RK. Adjuvant analgesics in cancer pain management. *Oncologist.* 2004;9(5):571–591.

63. Breitbart W. Psychotropic adjuvant analgesics for pain in cancer and AIDS. *Psychooncology.* 1998;7(4):333–345.

64. Staiger TO, Gaster B, Sullivan MD, et al. Systematic review of antidepressants in the treatment of chronic low back pain. *Spine.* 2003;28(22):2540–2545.

65. Russell IJ, Mease PJ, Smith TR, et al. Efficacy and safety of duloxetine for treatment of fibromyalgia in patients with or without major depressive disorder: results from a 6-month, randomized, double-blind, placebo-controlled, fixed-dose trial. *Pain.* 2008;136(3):432–444.

66. Max MB, Culnane M, Schafer SC, et al. Amitriptyline relieves diabetic neuropathy pain in patients with normal or depressed mood. *Neurology.* 1987;37(4):589–596.

67. Lance JW. 5-Hydroxytryptamine and its role in migraine. *Eur Neurol.* 1991;31(5):279–281.

68. Bragin EO, Korneev AY, Vasilenko GF. Buspirone effect on the development of antinociceptive reactions. *Pain.* 1989;36(2):257–261.

69. Kishore-Kumar R, Schafer SC, Lawlor BA, et al. Single doses of the serotonin agonists buspirone and m-chlorophenylpiperazine do not relieve neuropathic pain. *Pain.* 1989;37(2):223–227.

70. Davidoff G, Guarracini M, Roth E, et al. Trazodone hydrochloride in the treatment of dysesthetic pain in traumatic myelopathy: a randomized, double-blind, placebo-controlled study. *Pain.* 1987;29(2):151–161.

71. Max MB, Lynch SA, Muir J, et al. Effects of desipramine, amitriptyline, and fluoxetine on pain in diabetic neuropathy. *N Engl J Med.* 1992;326(19):1250–1256.

72. Kishore-Kumar R, Max MB, Schafer SC, et al. Desipramine relieves postherpetic neuralgia. *Clin Pharmacol Ther.* 1990;47(3):305–312.

73. Smith TR. Duloxetine in diabetic neuropathy. *Expert Opin Pharmacother.* 2006;7(2):215–223.

74. Arnold LM, Rosen A, Pritchett YL, et al. A randomized, double-blind, placebo-controlled trial of duloxetine in the treatment of women with fibromyalgia with or without major depressive disorder. *Pain.* 2005;119(1–3):5–15.

75. Gendreau RM, Thorn MD, Gendreau JF, et al. Efficacy of milnacipran in patients with fibromyalgia. *J Rheumatol.* 2005;32(10):1975–1985.

76. Sayar K, Aksu G, Ak I, et al. Venlafaxine treatment of fibromyalgia. *Ann Pharmacother.* 2003;37(11):1561–1565.

77. Lindsay PG, Wyckoff M. The depression-pain syndrome and its response to antidepressants. *Psychosomatics.* 1981;22(7):571–573. 576–577.

78. Stein D, Peri T, Edelstein E, et al. The efficacy of amitriptyline and acetaminophen in the management of acute low back pain. *Psychosomatics.* 1996;37(1):63–70.

79. Blumer D, Heilbronn M. Chronic pain as a variant of depressive disease: the pain-prone disorder. *J Nerv Ment Dis.* 1982;170(7):381–406.

80. Feinmann C. Pain relief by antidepressants: possible modes of action. *Pain.* 1985;23(1):1–8.

81. Goodkin K, Vrancken MA, Feaster D. On the putative efficacy of antidepressants in chronic, benign pain syndromes. *Pain Forum.* 1995;4(4):237–247.

82. Max MB. Thirteen consecutive well-designed randomized trials show that antidepressants reduce pain in diabetic neuropathy and post-herpetic neuralgia. *Pain Forum.* 1995;4(4):20–23.

83. Salerno SM, Browning R, Jackson JL. The effect of antidepressant treatment on chronic back pain: a meta-analysis. *Arch Intern Med.* 2002;162(1):19–24.

84. Onghena P, Van Houdenhove B. Antidepressant-induced analgesia in chronic non-malignant pain: a meta-analysis of 39 placebo-controlled studies. *Pain.* 1992;49(2):205–219.

85. Watson CP, Evans RJ. A comparative trial of amitriptyline and zimelidine in post-herpetic neuralgia. *Pain.* 1985;23(4):387–394.

86. Gourlay GK, Cherry DA, Cousins MJ, et al. A controlled study of a serotonin reuptake blocker, zimelidine, in the treatment of chronic pain. *Pain.* 1986;25(1):35–52.

87. Gallagher HC, Gallagher RM, Butler M, et al. Venlafaxine for neuropathic pain in adults. *Cochrane Database Syst Rev.* 2015;(8):CD011091.

88. Dalal S, Melzack R. Psychostimulant drugs potentiate morphine analgesia in the formalin test. *J Pain Symptom Manage.* 1998;16(4):230–239.

89. Dalal S, Melzack R. Potentiation of opioid analgesia by psychostimulant drugs: a review. *J Pain Symptom Manage.* 1998;16(4):245–253.

90. Bruera E, Chadwick S, Brenneis C, et al. Methylphenidate associated with narcotics for the treatment of cancer pain. *Cancer Treat Rep.* 1987;71(1):67–70.

91. Bruera E, Brenneis C, Paterson AH, et al. Use of methylphenidate as an adjuvant to narcotic analgesics in patients with advanced cancer. *J Pain Symptom Manage.* 1989;4(1):3–6.

92. Bruera E, Fainsinger R, MacEachern T, et al. The use of methylphenidate in patients with incident cancer pain receiving regular opiates. A preliminary report. *Pain.* 1992;50(1):75–77.

93. Bruera E, Miller MJ, Macmillan K, et al. Neuropsychological effects of methylphenidate in patients receiving a continuous infusion of narcotics for cancer pain. *Pain.* 1992;48(2):163–166.

94. Yee JD, Berde CB. Dextroamphetamine or methylphenidate as adjuvants to opioid analgesia for adolescents with cancer. *J Pain Symptom Manage.* 1994;9(2):122–125.

95. McQuay HJ, Carroll D, Glynn CJ. Low dose amitriptyline in the treatment of chronic pain. *Anaesthesia*. 1992;47(8):646–652.

96. Blom S. Trigeminal neuralgia: its treatment with a new anticonvulsant drug (G-32883). *Lancet*. 1962;1(7234):839–840.

97. Rogawski MA, Loscher W. The neurobiology of antiepileptic drugs for the treatment of nonepileptic conditions. *Nat Med*. 2004;10(7):685–692.

98. Maciewicz R, Bouckoms AJ, Martin JB. Drug therapy of neuropathic pain. *Clin J Pain*. 1985;1:39–45.

99. Hering R, Kuritzky A. Sodium valproate in the treatment of cluster headache: an open clinical trial. *Cephalalgia*. 1989;9(3):195–198.

100. Freitag FG, Collins SD, Carlson HA, et al. A randomized trial of divalproex sodium extended-release tablets in migraine prophylaxis. *Neurology*. 2002;58(11):1652–1659.

101. Nakamura-Craig M, Follenfant RL. Effect of lamotrigine in the acute and chronic hyperalgesia induced by PGE2 and in the chronic hyperalgesia in rats with streptozotocin-induced diabetes. *Pain*. 1995;63(1):33–37.

102. Bouckoms AJ. *Intravenous lorazepam for pain of intractable neuralgia*. Paper presented at the 5th World Congress of Pain, Hamburg, Germany, 1987.

103. Max MB, Schafer SC, Culnane M, et al. Amitriptyline, but not lorazepam, relieves postherpetic neuralgia. *Neurology*. 1988;38(9):1427–1432.

104. Backonja M, Beydoun A, Edwards KR, et al. Gabapentin for the symptomatic treatment of painful neuropathy in patients with diabetes mellitus: a randomized controlled trial. *JAMA*. 1998;280(21):1831–1836.

105. Rowbotham M, Harden N, Stacey B, et al. Gabapentin for the treatment of postherpetic neuralgia: a randomized controlled trial. *JAMA*. 1998;280(21):1837–1842.

106. Hahn K, Arendt G, Braun JS, et al. A placebo-controlled trial of gabapentin for painful HIV-associated sensory neuropathies. *J Neurol*. 2004;251(10):1260–1266.

107. Caraceni A, Zecca E, Bonezzi C, et al. Gabapentin for neuropathic cancer pain: a randomized controlled trial from the Gabapentin Cancer Pain Study Group. *J Clin Oncol*. 2004;22(14):2909–2917.

108. Lesser H, Sharma U, LaMoreaux L, et al. Pregabalin relieves symptoms of painful diabetic neuropathy: a randomized controlled trial. *Neurology*. 2004;63(11):2104–2110.

109. Sabatowski R, Galvez R, Cherry DA, et al. Pregabalin reduces pain and improves sleep and mood disturbances in patients with post-herpetic neuralgia: results of a randomised, placebo-controlled clinical trial. *Pain*. 2004;109(1–2):26–35.

110. Vinik AI, Tuchman M, Safirstein B, et al. Lamotrigine for treatment of pain associated with diabetic neuropathy: results of two randomized, double-blind, placebo-controlled studies. *Pain*. 2007;128(1–2):169–179.

111. Jose VM, Bhansali A, Hota D, et al. Randomized double-blind study comparing the efficacy and safety of lamotrigine and amitriptyline in painful diabetic neuropathy. *Diabet Med*. 2007;24(4):377–383.

112. Silver M, Blum D, Grainger J, et al. Double-blind, placebo-controlled trial of lamotrigine in combination with other medications for neuropathic pain. *J Pain Symptom Manage*. 2007;34(4):446–454.

113. Rao RD, Flynn PJ, Sloan JA, et al. Efficacy of lamotrigine in the management of chemotherapy-induced peripheral neuropathy: a phase 3 randomized, double-blind, placebo-controlled trial, N01C3. *Cancer*. 2008;112(12):2802–2808.

114. Wiffen PJ, Rees J. Lamotrigine for acute and chronic pain. *Cochrane Database Syst Rev*. 2007(2):CD006044.

115. Gracely RH, Lynch SA, Bennett GJ. Painful neuropathy: altered central processing maintained dynamically by peripheral input. *Pain*. 1992;51(2):175–194.

116. Raja SN. Role of the sympathetic nervous system in acute pain and inflammation. *Ann Med*. 1995;27(2):241–246.

117. Fishbain DA, Rosomoff HL, Steele-Rosomoff R, et al. Pain treatment facilities referral selection criteria. *Clin J Pain*. 1995;11(2):156–157.

118. Coombs DW, Saunders RL, Fratkin JD, et al. Continuous intrathecal hydromorphone and clonidine for intractable cancer pain. *J Neurosurg*. 1986;64(6):890–894.

119. Eisenach JC, DuPen S, Dubois M, et al. Epidural clonidine analgesia for intractable cancer pain. The Epidural Clonidine Study Group. *Pain*. 1995;61(3):391–399.

120. Peden CJ, Prys-Roberts C. Dexmedetomidine – a powerful new adjunct to anaesthesia? *Br J Anaesth*. 1992;68(2):123–125.

121. Aantaa R, Kanto J, Scheinin M, et al. Dxmedetomidine, an alpha 2-adrenoceptor agonist, reduces anesthetic requirements for patients undergoing minor gynecologic surgery. *Anesthesiology*. 1990;73(2):230–235.

122. Jaakola ML, Salonen M, Lehtinen R, et al. The analgesic action of dexmedetomidine – a novel alpha 2-adrenoceptor agonist – in healthy volunteers. *Pain*. 1991;46(3):281–285.

123. Arain SR, Ruehlow RM, Uhrich TD, et al. The efficacy of dexmedetomidine versus morphine for postoperative analgesia after major inpatient surgery. *Anesth Analg*. 2004;98(1):153–158.

124. Alhashemi JA, Kaki AM. Dexmedetomidine in combination with morphine PCA provides superior analgesia for shockwave lithotripsy. *Can J Anaesth*. 2004;51(4):342–347.

125. Bonelli S, Conoscente F, Movilia PG, et al. Regional intravenous guanethidine vs. stellate ganglion block in reflex sympathetic dystrophies: a randomized trial. *Pain*. 1983;16(3):297–307.

126. Hylden JL, Thomas DA, Iadarola MJ, et al. Spinal opioid analgesic effects are enhanced in a model of unilateral inflammation/hyperalgesia: possible involvement of noradrenergic mechanisms. *Eur J Pharmacol*. 1991;194(2–3):135–143.

127. Chowdhury AR, Graham PL, Schofield D, et al. Cost-effectiveness of multidisciplinary interventions for chronic low back pain: a narrative review. *Clin J Pain*. 2021;38(3):197–207.

128. Fordyce WE. *Back Pain in the Workplace: Management of Disability in Non-specific Conditions*. IASP; 1995.

129. Nachemson A. Work for all. For those with low back pain as well. *Clin Orthop Relat Res*. 1983;179:77–85.

130. Williams AC, Fisher E, Hearn L, et al. Psychological therapies for the management of chronic pain (excluding headache) in adults. *Cochrane Database Syst Rev.* 2020(8):CD007407.

131. Benson H. *Relaxation Response.* William Morrow and Company; 2000.

132. Chang BH, Dusek JA, Benson H. Psychobiological changes from relaxation response elicitation: long-term practitioners versus novices. *Psychosomatics.* 2011;52:550–559.

133. Bhasin MK, Dusek JA, Chang BH, et al. Relaxation response induces temporal transcriptome changes in energy metabolism, insulin secretion and inflammatory pathways. *PLoS One.* 2013;8(5).

134. Chen YLE, Francis AJ. Relaxation and imagery for chronic, nonmalignant pain: effects on pain symptoms, quality of life, and mental health. *Pain Manag Nurs.* 2010;11(3):159–168.

135. Payne RA, Donaghy M. *Payne's Handbook of Relaxation Techniques. A Practical Guide for Health Care Professionals.* Churchill Livingstone; 2010.

136. Hilton L, Hempel S, Ewing BA, et al. Mindfulness meditation for chronic pain: systematic review and meta-analysis. *Ann Behav Med.* 2017;51:199–213.

137. Keefe FJ, Williams DA. A comparison of coping strategies in chronic pain patients in different age groups. *J Gerontol.* 1990;45(4):161–165.

138. Manne SL, Zautra AJ. Couples coping with chronic illness: women with rheumatoid arthritis and their healthy husbands. *J Behav Med.* 1990;13(4):327–342.

139. Kopp M, Richter R, Rainer J, et al. Differences in family functioning between patients with chronic headache and patients with chronic low back pain. *Pain.* 1995;63(2):219–224.

18

NEUROPSYCHIATRIC CONDITIONS: SEIZURES, HEADACHES, STROKE SYNDROMES, AND TRAUMATIC BRAIN INJURIES

FELICIA A. SMITH, MD ■ SAMUEL I. KOHRMAN, MD ■
TAHA GHOLIPOUR, MD ■ JEFFERY C. HUFFMAN, MD ■
THEODORE A. STERN, MD

OVERVIEW

The structure and function of the central nervous system (CNS) are altered by many neurologic disorders. Because the CNS controls affect, behavior, and cognition, neurologic disorders may lead to neuropsychiatric symptoms that resemble those found in primary psychiatric conditions. Therefore, the general hospital psychiatrist is frequently called on to assess patients who have classic psychiatric symptoms caused by an underlying neurologic disease. In this chapter, we review the management of patients with neurologic conditions that are commonly associated with neuropsychiatric phenomena, including seizures, headaches, stroke syndromes, and traumatic brain injuries (TBIs).

Case 1

Ms. A, a 23-year-old woman, was admitted to the medical service after she presented to the emergency department with a self-reported "big seizure" a few days earlier at home, and 2 weeks of recurrent brief spells of "panic" and out-of-body experience. A psychiatric consultation was requested given her extensive psychiatric history and suspected psychogenic non-epileptic seizures.

She reported having bipolar disorder, post-traumatic stress disorder (PTSD) (related to childhood abuse by a relative), and being a victim of physical assault as a teenager (involving a skull fracture and a reported seizure). She endorsed smoking marijuana daily to control her anxiety and a history of heavy drinking. She was currently unemployed and struggled with keeping her current living situation. She had stopped her lamotrigine, which she was prescribed as a mood stabilizer, around 1 month ago. On examination, she appeared anxious, but was euthymic. Other than a report of out-of-body (autoscopic) visual hallucinations along with the "panic spells" there were no other positive findings identified on the examination. She denied having thoughts of suicide or violence. A toxicology screen was positive for marijuana, and her alcohol and lamotrigine levels were undetectable. A computerized tomography (CT) scan of her head was reported as unremarkable.

The consultant confirmed the psychiatric history, provided input regarding management during the hospitalization, and expressed concern about the etiology of the spells; a neurology consultation was recommended as well as a video-electroencephalogram (EEG) during the admission. An extended bedside EEG with video recording captured three events during which Ms. A remained conscious but appeared fearful. These were accompanied by slowing of her heart rate that lasted for approximately 10 seconds, after which she reported the event to her nurse.

A review of the EEG showed focal seizures arising from the right posterior temporal region.

The diagnosis of focal seizures with impairment of awareness from the right temporal lobe with presumed occasional secondary generalization and associated ictal bradycardia was made. The history of significant head trauma was considered the most likely etiology. Ms. A was re-started on lamotrigine and levetiracetam was added as a second antiepileptic drug (AED) to protect her from generalized seizures while lamotrigine remained sub-therapeutic. As well as addressing co-morbid psychiatric diagnoses, the treatment team counseled Ms. A about medication adherence, contraception, avoidance of driving, and the risk of mood symptoms, aggression, or suicidal ideation with her new medication, levetiracetam. A neurology follow-up appointment was also made to address her new diagnosis, consider further work-up, and consider stopping the second AED.

MANAGEMENT OF PSYCHIATRIC SYMPTOMS IN PATIENTS WITH SEIZURE DISORDERS

Approximately half of all patients with seizure disorders have co-morbid psychiatric syndromes[1]; therefore, the general hospital psychiatrist should have a working knowledge of seizure disorders and the neuropsychiatric syndromes that are commonly associated with them. Patients with seizures may have psychiatric symptoms that occur during a seizure (*ictal* symptoms), immediately before or after a seizure (*peri-ictal* symptoms), or between seizures (*inter-ictal* symptoms).

By way of definition, a clinical seizure is an abnormal paroxysmal discharge of cerebral neurons sufficient to cause clinically detectable events that are apparent to the patient or an observer.[2] Patients with a chronic course of repeated, unprovoked seizures are said to have epilepsy. Seizures can be *focal* (starting in a particular area of the brain, i.e., the focus) or *generalized* (involving both hemispheres simultaneously). Focal seizures (formerly called "partial seizures") may remain limited to their focus in the same brain hemisphere, or propagate throughout the rest of the cortex, often called *secondary generalization*. Consciousness is often fully or partially preserved if the seizure activity is restricted to only limited parts of the brain. Clinical symptomatology may be variable in this setting, correlating with the involved brain areas. Generalized seizures are associated with loss of consciousness (LOC), ranging from seconds of staring spells in *absence* seizures (formerly called *petit mal*) to *generalized tonic-clonic* convulsions (*grand mal*). Generalized tonic-clonic (GTC) seizures can occur after an immediate or a delayed spread of focal seizure activity to the rest of the brain, or so-called *secondary generalization*. A *primary* generalized seizure occurs in the absence of a suspected focus and in the setting of a genetic/idiopathic epilepsy syndrome, or due to metabolic disarray (such as hypoglycemia, hyponatremia, or toxic exposure). GTCs are characterized by a sudden LOC with a brief tonic phase marked by contraction of skeletal muscles and upward deviation of the eyes. A more prolonged clonic phase (characterized by rhythmic movements and jerking of the extremities) follows.[3] These seizures are almost always followed by a *post-ictal* state with decreased responsiveness and a state similar to deep sleep that lasts minutes to hours. *Absence* seizures are characterized by brief (usually 5–10 seconds) lapses in consciousness and by motionless staring, without loss of muscle tone and without any post-ictal change in consciousness. These seizures occur primarily in children and rarely occur after puberty. *Myoclonic* seizures are characterized by brief and sudden, often bilateral, muscle contractions that may occur singly or repeatedly; these are seen in a variety of epileptic syndromes in children but also occur in adults with advanced neurodegenerative diseases. *Atonic* seizures ("*drop attacks*") are a type of generalized seizure characterized by sudden loss of muscle tone that leads to falls, without clonic activities that are seen in tonic-clonic seizures.

The terminology for focal seizures has changed repeatedly over recent decades which has caused some confusion. Focal seizures are generally described based on how they affect consciousness. Focal seizures with impairment of consciousness or awareness (formerly "complex partial seizures," also known as focal-unaware seizures) deserve special mention, insofar as they are the most common type of seizure in adults and are commonly associated with neuropsychiatric phenomena.[4] Certain types of focal seizures that also have a high prevalence of neuropsychiatric symptoms during and between seizures include *temporal lobe seizures* and *psychomotor seizures*. On the other hand, focal seizures without impairment of consciousness or awareness (formerly "simple partial seizures," also known as focal aware seizures) have symptoms limited to the area of the cortex that is stimulated. Examples of these include simple motor seizures with twitching of corresponding muscle groups, or simple visual seizures with the occurrence of visual experiences in the visual field corresponding to the seizing cortex.

Focal seizures may involve sensory, affective, perceptual, behavioral, or cognitive symptoms. Symptoms may include hallucinations of any sensory modality; they can be olfactory (e.g., a noxious odor, like burning rubber), gustatory (metallic or other tastes), auditory, visual, or tactile hallucinations. The most common affective symptoms are fear and anxiety, although depression may also occur. Rage may also occur but is uncommon. Such affective symptoms usually have a sudden onset and offset.

Behavior during focal seizures with impairment of awareness may also be abnormal; *automatisms* are common and may include oral or buccal movements (e.g., lip smacking or chewing), picking behaviors, or prolonged staring. Cognitive symptoms associated with focal seizures include *déjà vu* (a feeling of familiarity), *jamais vu* (a feeling of unfamiliarity), macropsia, micropsia, and dissociative, or "out-of-body" experiences. Patients with neuropsychiatric symptoms secondary to seizures may be mistakenly diagnosed with a primary psychiatric disorder because the symptoms are often like those of primary psychiatric disorders, and because the inter-ictal (and even ictal) scalp electroencephalogram (EEG) may appear normal due to deep localization of involved cortices. Therefore, the general hospital psychiatrist must be particularly astute in differentiating patients with focal seizures from those with primary psychiatric disorders.

In the following discussion, the phenomenology and treatment of neuropsychiatric symptoms among patients with seizure disorders are outlined. The ictal, peri-ictal, and inter-ictal neuropsychiatric symptoms will be discussed, as will ways to delineate how these symptoms differ from those seen in patients without seizure disorders.

Ictal Neuropsychiatric Phenomena

Ictal psychiatric symptoms are most often associated with focal seizures, although they can also occur with generalized seizures.[1] Anxiety, fear, and psychosis are the most common psychiatric symptoms experienced during a seizure. Up to one-third of patients with focal seizures with impairment of awareness have anxiety or fear as part of their seizures[5,6]; the anxiety is often intense and may last throughout the seizure. It is important to keep in mind that subtle focal seizures, such as stereotyped anxiety, might be described as an "aura" (a term that is no longer recommended to describe these seizures) by patients and by some physicians. Such symptoms may resemble those of panic attacks with autonomic symptoms, nausea, intense anxiety, and depersonalization. Therefore, patients with epilepsy may have both ictal anxiety and inter-ictal panic attacks that are difficult to distinguish. The more circumscribed the symptoms are to the associated seizure phenomena (e.g., automatisms or hallucinations during an episode, or confusion or severe lethargy after the event), the more likely it is that the anxiety is ictal.

Ictal psychosis has also been seen in patients with focal seizures. Ictal psychotic symptoms are most often associated with temporal lobe foci, but nearly one-third of patients have non-temporal lobe foci.[7] Hallucinations during a seizure are much more likely to be olfactory or gustatory; auditory hallucinations (common in primary psychotic disorders) are less common, but simple auditory symptoms, such as echoing, might occur in the setting of a simple focal seizure involving auditory perception cortices. Paranoia is uncommon and is usually short lived. In contrast to patients with a primary psychosis, consciousness is usually impaired during ictal psychosis and affected patients are usually amnestic for the episode.[8]

Ictal depression is uncommon; it occurs as part of the aura in approximately 1% of patients with epilepsy.[9] Such depressive symptoms, as with other ictal symptoms, appear abruptly, in a stereotypic manner, and without obvious psychosocial precipitants. Although depressive symptoms often disappear abruptly, some authors have noted that ictal depressed mood may extend beyond the presence of other ictal or post-ictal symptoms.[9,10] Ictal crying (a so-called *dacrystic seizure*) has been described in seizures with the involvement of limbic structures.

Ictal anger, agitation, and aggression have also been reported, but appear to be exceedingly rare (fewer than 0.5% of patients in one large series[11]). Furthermore, ictal aggression is poorly directed and generally does not involve significant interactive behaviors. Stereotyped shouting and pushing are among the most common manifestations; patients rarely perform intricate, directed acts of violence during a seizure.

Determining whether anxiety, depression, or other psychiatric symptoms are ictal events or part of primary psychiatric conditions can be difficult. Table 18.1 describes some distinguishing characteristics of ictal and non-ictal symptoms. In general, ictal symptoms have an abrupt onset and offset, occur in concert with other stereotyped manifestations of seizures, and are frequently short lived, usually lasting less than 3 minutes.[1] The most convincing evidence for the ictal nature of a symptom is a more or less stereotyped pattern; that is, a patient will not experience fear with one seizure and depressive symptoms with another—the pattern of symptoms will generally be the same.

Prolonged or frequent focal seizures, sometimes qualifying as *status epilepticus*, may result in prolonged ictal psychiatric symptoms that further complicate the diagnosis. Therefore, the EEG remains a key tool for establishing whether symptoms are ictal. Since most focal seizures have an identifiable *focus* (such as an ischemic, neoplastic, or vascular lesion), brain imaging should be considered early if ictal symptoms are suspected. A patient's history (such as a history of systemic malignancy, cerebrovascular risk factors, or suspicion of an inflammatory or infectious process in the brain), should decrease the threshold for brain imaging. Unfortunately, CT scans have low sensitivity and specificity for detecting many etiologies, despite their ready availability and lower cost; a magnetic resonance imaging (MRI) protocoled and reviewed by a radiologist for finding seizure foci, is strongly recommended.

Treatment of ictal psychiatric symptoms requires a careful evaluation. Primary psychiatric symptoms and ictal psychiatric symptoms are similar, frequently co-morbid, and have different treatments. Therefore, working with a neurologist for careful clinical evaluation, EEG monitoring, and when indicated, other diagnostic procedures should be arranged to distinguish these phenomena. Once symptoms have been identified as ictal, treatment of the associated psychiatric symptoms requires treatment of the seizure with

TABLE 18.1
Clinical Characteristics That Help Distinguish Epileptic From Non-Epileptic Events

	Epileptic Seizures	Non-Epileptic Seizures/Events
Onset	Sudden onset and offset	Often gradual
Duration	Often <3 min	Variable
Perception	May experience olfactory, gustatory, visual hallucination; déjà vu; derealization	May experience auditory hallucinations; paranoia
Eyes during event	Open	Closed
Incontinence	Common	Rare
Awareness	Often impaired; can stay aware during some focal seizures	Variable; may be responsive during parts of the event
Recall of event	None or limited (e.g., aura)	Usually intact
Ictal EEG	Almost always abnormal	Unchanged from baseline
Inter-ictal EEG	Normal or abnormal	Often normal
Tongue bite	Lateral tongue	None or tip of the tongue
Injury	May be present	Rarely present (suggestive of serious psychopathology)
Incontinence	May be present	Rare
Post-ictal state	Confusion or drowsiness is common	Rare
Prolactin	Elevated; or normal	Normal; rarely elevated from baseline

EEG, Electroencephalogram.

AEDs. Treatment of ictal psychosis with antipsychotics or ictal anxiety with non-anticonvulsant anxiolytics may be used in the short term until seizures are controlled with an AED, although longer-term treatment with these agents is generally not indicated. Measures to reduce the risk of falls or other injuries are crucial for patients whose seizure disorders remain active.

Peri-ictal Neuropsychiatric Phenomena

Despite the above-mentioned rarer ictal neuropsychiatric phenomena, most neuropsychiatric disturbances are seen in peri-ictal, and mostly post-ictal phases of seizures. They usually occur several hours after a seizure. Pre-ictal symptoms can occur and include psychosis, mood changes, or aggression in the hours or minutes before a seizure and they should not be confused with focal seizures, which are sometimes called *auras*.[5,12] These symptoms tend to increase until the onset of the clinical seizure,[13] and, depending on the time course and nature of the symptoms, may be conceptualized as prodromes separate from the ictus or as ictal events.

Post-ictal neuropsychiatric symptoms are relatively common. Approximately 8% to 10% of patients with seizures have post-ictal behavioral disturbances.[14] These symptoms may occur in the context of a diffuse post-ictal suppression of the cortical activity that involves disinhibited, sub-cortical behavior (e.g., moaning, crying, laughing, cursing, demonstrating sexual behavior, or expressing rage). Autonomic instability may contribute to what is observed as a post-ictal behavior as well. Patients are often amnestic for these events, and during these periods are difficult to control. Neuropsychiatric symptoms may also arise post-ictally, despite the presence of a clear consciousness. Patients may remember parts of events or even try to justify their behavior. Post-ictal symptoms should remit spontaneously and are often short lived, and persistence of symptoms beyond 72 hours should be considered as a possible inter-ictal symptom. However, such symptoms may persist for days or even weeks. Patients with well-defined, prolonged post-ictal neuropsychiatric syndromes may be more likely to develop persistent inter-ictal symptoms.[15]

Psychosis is the most common post-ictal neuropsychiatric symptom, occurring in up to nearly 8% of patients with epilepsy,[16] and it often appears after a non-psychotic post-ictal period. It occurs most commonly in patients with focal-unaware seizures that become secondarily generalized,[9] especially in those with temporal lobe or bilateral foci. Psychotic symptoms vary widely, and affective symptoms (depressive or manic) may also be present. Symptoms can include paranoid or grandiose delusions and hallucinations in a variety of sensory modalities; Schneiderian first-rank symptoms of schizophrenia are rare.[15] Symptoms tend to resolve spontaneously but recur an average of two to three times per year. In a minority of patients, such symptoms become chronic, even in the absence of clear clinical seizures.

Post-ictal depression is also associated with focal-unaware seizures but is less common than is post-ictal psychosis.[17] Patients with post-ictal depression may have flattened affect and anhedonia more often than they would sadness, and post-ictal depression is commonly associated with delirium and with other post-ictal cognitive disturbances. Kanner and Balabanov[17] found that symptoms last an average of 24 hours, although symptoms may be more prolonged. In most cases, post-ictal depressive symptoms do not just represent a reactive response to the stress of having a seizure. Other post-ictal symptoms are less common. Acute post-ictal anxiety is relatively infrequent and is usually associated with post-ictal depression. Post-ictal mania and hypomania occur infrequently. Post-ictal aggression can also occur; however, it is generally associated with delirium, psychotic symptoms, or abnormal mood states.

The management of patients with post-ictal neuropsychiatric symptoms has several tenets. First, enhanced treatment of the seizure disorder is crucial; patients whose seizure disorders are poorly controlled appear to have a greater tendency toward post-ictal affective and psychotic symptoms. In addition to the use of AEDs for seizure prophylaxis, other psychotropic medications may be indicated, especially if symptoms are prolonged, present a risk to the patient or others, or adversely affect the patient's ability to receive appropriate treatment. Such situations occur most commonly with psychosis, and low doses of antipsychotics can reduce agitation and can diminish psychotic symptoms. If such symptoms are limited to the post-ictal period, these medications can be discontinued once symptoms resolve, because the best prophylaxis against recurrence of psychosis is treatment with

AEDs to prevent seizures. Antidepressants are uncommonly indicated for depressive symptoms limited to the post-ictal period.

In addition to medications, behavioral treatments can be instituted to facilitate coping and to maintain the patient's safety. Such interventions may include the use of restraints or observers, frequent re-orientation, or the presence of familiar family members. Finally, it is important to know the patient's post-ictal pattern of symptoms to prepare caregivers and family members for what lies ahead. Seizures and their neuropsychiatric sequelae are commonly stereotyped; that is, patients tend to have the same post-ictal symptomatology from seizure to seizure. If a patient is known to become psychotic or dangerous after a seizure, the treatment team can be prepared with antipsychotic treatments or with other safety-enhancing measures.

Inter-ictal (Chronic) Neuropsychiatric Phenomena

Psychiatric syndromes are also common in the period between seizures; patients with seizure disorders have chronic psychiatric disorders at substantially higher rates than do those in the general population and those with similar quality-of-life burdens from other chronic medical conditions. Depression, anxiety, and psychosis are all common with depressive disorders being the most prevalent. In contrast, inter-ictal hypomanic or manic symptoms are uncommon and often point to a possible primary mood disorder.

Inter-ictal depression is common and can be disabling. Rates of depression and suicide among patients with epilepsy are four to five times greater than those in the general population,[1,18,19] and up to 80% of patients with epilepsy report having some feelings of depression.[20] A constellation of biological and psychosocial factors likely coalesces to result in these elevated rates of depression, but risk factors for depression that are specific to seizure disorders include poor seizure control and focal seizures with impairment of awareness,[21,22] especially with left-sided temporal lobe seizure foci. Suicide may be 25 times more likely among patients with TLE than among those in the general population.[23] A history of depression has also been associated with the onset of seizures, given that a history of depression increases (by three-fold) the risk of developing a seizure disorder.[17,24] Some

have hypothesized that depression and epilepsy share neurotransmitter abnormalities (e.g., reduced noradrenergic, dopaminergic, and serotonergic activity) and that these shared abnormalities may explain the link between the two conditions.

The symptoms of inter-ictal depression are often distinctive. Atypical features are common,[20] and many patients have depressive symptoms that are more consistent with dysthymia than with major depressive disorder (MDD).[25] Blumer and associates[26] have described a clinical syndrome called *inter-ictal dysphoric disorder*, which is characterized by inter-ictal dysthymic symptoms with intermittent irritability, impulsivity, anxiety, and somatic symptoms. Some people with epilepsy and their families may report that the worsening of these behavioral symptoms is predictive of a breakthrough seizure in the upcoming hours to days.

Inter-ictal anxiety disorders vary in their frequency. Anxiety symptoms are more common in patients with epilepsy than they are in the general population, and, of the anxiety disorders, panic disorder appears to be the most common. Inter-ictal panic disorder is present in approximately 20% of patients with epilepsy,[5] with symptoms that differentiate the panic attacks from the feelings of panic that occur during a seizure. The treating neurologist may want to capture some of these events on video-EEG monitoring, preferably in an inpatient epilepsy monitoring study, to ascertain the non-ictal nature of these panic symptoms, especially in epilepsy with a temporal lobe focus. Other anxiety disorders, such as generalized anxiety disorder (GAD) or obsessive compulsive disorder (OCD) are less common.[1] Inter-ictal personality disorder; however, may involve prominent obsessive traits.

Inter-ictal psychosis can be intermittent (with brief, recurrent episodes), but more commonly it is continuous and chronic. Psychotic symptoms are approximately 10 times more likely to occur in patients with epilepsy.[1] Psychosis is also more common in patients with epilepsy with a temporal lobe focus, with multiple seizure types, with a poor response to seizure treatment, or with a history of status epilepticus.[27] Clinically, inter-ictal psychotic symptoms most often consist of paranoid delusions with associated visual or auditory hallucinations. Affective blunting, a lack of motivation, and catatonia are also common.[27] Compared with patients with schizophrenia, patients with inter-ictal psychosis have greater preservation of affect and more visual hallucinations.

An inter-ictal personality change among patients with TLE was described several decades ago and repeatedly reported by practicing epileptologists. The TLE personality syndrome, reported primarily by Gastaut and co-workers[28] and detailed by Geschwind,[4] has features that include moral rigidity, hyper-religiosity, hypergraphia, hyposexuality, and hyperviscosity ("a sticky personality"). However, some authors have questioned the existence of such a syndrome.[29]

The management of inter-ictal psychiatric phenomena is like the treatment of primary psychiatric disorders. However, there are several special considerations in this population. Given that most inter-ictal psychiatric symptoms are more common when seizures are poorly controlled, effective treatment with AEDs is of vital importance. Treatment of psychiatric symptoms associated with epilepsy should also include behavioral and educational interventions that reduce the risk related to their seizure disorder (e.g., having family ensure that depressed patients take their AEDs or keeping manic or psychotic patients from driving when this is unsafe).

One caveat in the treatment of patients with co-existing neuropsychiatric symptoms with AEDs is the potential behavioral side effects of some of these drugs. The US Food and Drug Administration (FDA) has issued a class label change, asking AED manufacturers to warn patients and providers about a possible increased risk of suicidal thoughts and behavior, even when used for indications other than seizure control. This warning was issued in response to a large meta-analysis that showed an association with such outcomes but did not investigate the possible causality from underlying conditions, in patients who are prescribed an AED.[30] Some AEDs are better known to affect a patient's underlying or co-morbid behavioral symptoms in both positive and negative ways. Lamotrigine, valproate, oxcarbazepine, and carbamazepine have long been used as mood stabilizers and are generally favored by neurologists when mood disorders or disturbances are established (or even perceived) in a patient with epilepsy. Phenobarbital may cause increased irritability in children with epilepsy, but not in adults. Topiramate (particularly at higher doses), zonisamide, phenobarbital, and vigabatrin can cause depressed mood. Lamotrigine and felbamate are generally considered stimulating and may produce anxiety or insomnia.[31]

Perampanel is a broad-spectrum AED that targets the central glutamate alpha-amino-3-hydroxy-5-methyl-4-isoxazolepropionic acid (AMPA) receptors. During pivotal clinical trials, an increased risk of psychiatric adverse effects, consisting of alteration of mood and hostility was noted. This led to a "black box warning" for aggression and homicidal ideation. The behavioral side effects seem to be dose dependent and improved in most patients by decreasing the dose.[32,33]

Levetiracetam, one of the most frequently used first-line AEDs has a great medical safety profile but it has become infamous for affecting mood and behavior. Different studies suggest around 10%[34] of patients started on levetiracetam report a change in their mood or behavior in the form of irritability (most common), aggression, depression, or worsening depression, and labile mood, and rarely suicidality. Some patients will need to switch AEDs due to this side effect. There are observational studies that suggest that supplementation of pyridoxine (vitamin B_6) may improve behavioral change in a group of pediatric patients with epilepsy.[35]

Treatment of psychiatric symptoms with psychotropics is frequently indicated, but the effects of these agents on the seizure threshold should be considered. The risk of seizure with most antidepressant drugs is quite small when these agents are used at standard doses.[36] Citalopram,[37] sertraline,[36] venlafaxine,[17] and tricyclic antidepressants (TCAs)[26] have all been used successfully in patients with epilepsy without significantly exacerbating the underlying seizure disorder. Given their relative safety regarding seizure exacerbation and their overall safety and tolerability, selective serotonin reuptake inhibitors (SSRIs) should be considered as first-line treatment for patients with inter-ictal depression. In general, starting with a low dose and increasing the dose gradually should minimize the risk of seizure in these patients. Bupropion and maprotiline are more strongly associated with the development of seizures. Among the TCAs, clomipramine may be associated with a greater risk of seizure and should probably be avoided as well. Monoamine oxidase inhibitors (MAOIs) have not been associated with an elevated risk of seizure, although they have not been studied in patients with seizure disorders.

Finally, electroconvulsive therapy (ECT) can be used to treat patients with epilepsy and severe depression[38]; ECT appears to increase the seizure threshold between treatments,[39] and it has been used safely in patients with epilepsy.[40]

Patients with anxiety disorders can be treated with antidepressants or with benzodiazepines; buspirone, sometimes used for the treatment of GAD, can lower the seizure threshold, and generally is not recommended for this population.[41] Patients on rapid dose escalation of buspirone may present with new-onset or breakthrough seizures, some of them a symptom of underlying epilepsy.

Inter-ictal psychosis can be treated with anti-psychotics. It appears that all antipsychotics may modestly lower the seizure threshold; however, low-potency antipsychotics, such as chlorpromazine, may have greater effects on the seizure threshold than higher-potency agents.[42] Clozapine has been associated with an elevated seizure risk and, in general, it should be avoided if reasonable alternatives are available. Therefore, when needed, recommended agents are atypical antipsychotics, such as risperidone, or high-potency typical antipsychotics. Again, titrating the dosage slowly and using the lowest effective dose should minimize the risk of seizure in this population.

In summary, virtually any psychiatric symptom can occur before, during, or after the seizure. However, anxiety is most common during a seizure, psychosis is most common post-ictally, and depression is the most common chronic symptom between seizures. All behavioral symptoms are more common in patients with focal seizures with impairment awareness (formerly complex partial seizures) than with other types of seizure disorders. Treatment of ictal phenomena involves treatment of the seizure, whereas post-ictal and inter-ictal phenomena may require the use of antipsychotics, anxiolytics, or antidepressants for optimal symptomatic relief. Careful attention to the patient's safety is always an important consideration (whether from seizure or suicidality), and a knowledge of the patient's pattern of symptoms associated with their seizures helps caregivers and family members prepare for sequelae.

NON-EPILEPTIC SEIZURES

Patients who appear to be having epileptic seizures may be having abnormal movements as the result of another medical or neurologic problem or, most often, because of psychological factors (e.g., a conversion reaction or functional neurologic pathology). These events, called *psychogenic non-epileptic seizures (PNESs)*, pose a common and important problem. The terms *pseudoseizure* and *hysterical seizures* have been used in the past and are antiquated, and discouraged to avoid the assumption of these being voluntary events by family and other providers. The incidence of PNES is higher in people with a personal history of seizures as well as in those with a history of knowing or taking care of patients with seizures, such as in family members or among healthcare providers at any level. The prevalence of PNES increases significantly within outpatient and inpatient referral centers for epilepsy.[43] Clarification of the nature of events (epileptic vs non-epileptic, often psychiatric, non-epileptic seizures) is a common reason for admission to an epilepsy monitoring unit or inpatient video-EEG monitoring. Patients with PNES are often significantly disabled by these events. When they have concurrent epileptic seizures, these may be easier to control with AEDs or with surgical procedures.[44]

As with other conversion disorders or functional neurologic disorders, the presence of PNES imposes a high burden on the patient's health, as well as on the healthcare system, and is often hard to diagnose and treat. Even after a diagnosis of PNES has been made, affected patients continue to be disabled by recurrent convulsive events.[43,45]

The general hospital psychiatrist is frequently called on to assess patients suspected of having PNES. Knowledge of the epidemiology, differential diagnosis, clinical features, and relevant diagnostic studies that may suggest the presence of PNES can significantly facilitate making the diagnosis. Once the diagnosis of PNES is suspected, the psychiatrist needs to be able to discuss the diagnosis of PNES with the patient in a way that is validating, reassuring, and supportive.[43,46,47]

PNES is common, occurring in approximately 10% of outpatients with intractable seizure disorders and in approximately 20% of patients with intractable seizures referred to epilepsy monitoring units.[43] About three-fourths of those with PNES are females, and they most often exhibit symptoms when they are between the ages of 15 and 35.[45] A history of sexual abuse is common among patients with PNES, occurring in at least 25% of those with the condition.[48,49] Roughly 25% of patients with PNES also suffer from epileptic seizures.[50] Unfortunately, some patients with either epileptic seizures (or cardiovascular events) are mistakenly diagnosed with PNES without an adequate work-up, sometimes by a provider biased by the pre-existing psychiatric diagnosis or substance use, psychosocial history, and (as discussed earlier in this chapter) undiagnosed ictal or inter-ictal neuropsychiatric phenomena. Other non-epileptic events without a presumed psychiatric nature are less frequently, but occasionally, presented to the consulting psychiatrist, and it is important to recognize them. Syncope and undiagnosed cardiovascular causes with unusual symptoms are probably the most important to recognize. Table 18.2 displays several conditions that can be mistaken for epilepsy. Among PNES semiologies, recurrent unconscious, psychologically mediated hypermotor spells (essentially conversion GTC seizure-like spells) are the most common. Other causes of psychosomatic symptoms such as other functional neurologic pathology, somatic symptomatology, factitious disorder and malingering, are more extensively covered in Chapter 15.

Clinical Considerations

This section addresses the approach to the diagnosis of PNES. Although almost all the features suggestive

---

TABLE 18.2
Differential Diagnosis of Non-epileptic Events

General Medical Conditions
Transient ischemic attack
Complicated migraine
Syncope
Hypoglycemia
Parasomnia (e.g., rapid eye movement, behavior disorder, or night terrors)
Narcolepsy
Myoclonus (from metabolic disturbance)

Psychiatric Causes
Functional Neurologic Disorder
Somatic symptom disorder or illness anxiety disorder
Dissociative disorder
Panic disorder (simulating partial seizures)

Volitional Deception
Factitious disorder (goal is to maintain the sick role)
Malingering (goal is to obtain secondary gain, e.g., disability income)

---

of PNES (discussed later) can also occur in true seizure disorders, certain clinical features of the peri-ictal and convulsive phases can help distinguish these two, although a single clinical feature taken in isolation should not be used to confirm a diagnosis of PNES. It is useful to know the usual characteristics of GTC seizures, and careful observation throughout the seizure can be very useful in the diagnostic assessment. This is why inpatient admission and prolonged video-EEG monitoring to capture the event on video for review is considered the best way of making the diagnosis.

GTC seizures are usually sudden in onset; although there may be an aura before the seizure, there is usually a sudden LOC, followed by a brief tonic period of <30 seconds. A more prolonged period of convulsive, clonic, activity follows. This activity is characterized by bilateral, symmetrical, and rhythmic jerking of the upper and lower extremities; trunk activity and pelvic thrusting are uncommon. Loss of continence, tongue biting, and other injuries may occur. The patient remains unconscious and unresponsive throughout the event and is amnestic for the episode. After the event, the patient may be confused or drowsy or complain of headache; the patient is rarely completely lucid in the immediate post-ictal period. Most GTC seizures are quite brief, lasting less than 3 minutes, and they have a stereotyped pattern in a given individual. On the other hand, Table 18.3 lists the clinical features that suggest PNES. It should be emphasized again that certain types of seizures are marked by symptoms that appear to suggest PNES. For example, focal motor seizures may involve asymmetrical jerking with preserved consciousness. Focal seizures with impairment of awareness can manifest with only behavioral or psychiatric symptoms. Frontal lobe seizures may cause pelvic thrusting and pedaling movements, but characteristically tend to occur in sleep. Automatisms during focal seizures with impairment of awareness may result in acts that appear volitional. However, a combination of atypical features suggests that PNES is the more likely diagnosis.[43,45]

The use of video-EEG monitoring allows one to correlate EEG changes (or the lack thereof) during a convulsive event. If a patient experiences a typical event and the EEG remains normal, this suggests PNES, especially when other clinical features are inconsistent with epilepsy. However, it should be noted that

TABLE 18.3
Features That Suggest Non-Epileptic (Conversion) Seizures

Historical Features

History of sexual abuse

History of other unexplained neurologic symptoms occurring during stress

Seizures despite multiple adequate trials of anticonvulsants at therapeutic levels

Features of Event

Events occur with suggestion/provocation

Gradual onset and offset of symptoms

Responsiveness during event

Weeping, speaking, or yelling during the event

Asymmetrical clonic activity

Head bobbing or pelvic thrusting

Rapid kicking or thrashing

Prolonged duration of symptoms (>3 min)

No EEG abnormalities during the event

Post-event Features

Lucid during immediate post-ictal period

Able to recall event

Lack of incontinence, tongue biting, or physical injury despite numerous events

Post-ictal prolactin is normal

Neuropsychological testing suggestive of conversion symptoms

EEG, Electroencephalogram.

focal seizures may give rise to normal EEGs in 10% to 40% of cases.[51–53] The EEG capture of multiple events reduces the likelihood of such false-negative EEG findings. If the patient reports multiple semiologies, there is always a chance that the unwitnessed etiology is indeed a seizure, even if one other type of spell is determined to be PNES.

In addition to using video-EEG monitoring, the use of suggestion or provocative stimuli may provide evidence for the diagnosis of PNES. The use of provocative stimuli was practiced regularly in the past but has been a topic of ethical controversy as they are considered deceptive; examples include the injection of normal saline or placement of a tuning fork on the head after a suggestion has been given that the procedure will likely cause a seizure. Much discussion has ensued about the ethics of deception under these circumstances; researchers have found that such provocative testing can be approached honestly with the patient with high rates of suggestibility and little adverse effect on the patient-physician alliance.[50] However, these techniques are now generally discouraged, while the use of hyperventilation, photic stimulation, and verbal suggestion without creating explicit misinformation for the patient are commonly used.[54]

In terms of laboratory studies, the usefulness of prolactin levels to distinguish between epileptic and non-epileptic events is questionable, given that in more than 10% of patients with GTC seizures, 30% of patients with temporal lobe seizures, and 60% of patients with frontal lobe seizures, prolactin is not elevated.[55] Other diagnostic laboratory values, such as creatine phosphokinase, may be even less sensitive and specific, especially when taken in isolation.

Neuropsychological testing can be a useful adjunct to clinical and laboratory evaluation. Such testing can provide information about co-morbid psychiatric diagnoses, personality styles, and tendencies toward conversion reactions. Some studies demonstrate that patients with PNES, when compared with patients with epilepsy, exhibit less objective evidence of cognitive impairment and are more likely to show impairments that are a function of poor effort rather than real deficits.[56,57] Also, some studies of patients with PNES using the Minnesota Multi-phasic Personality Inventory report an association with the "conversion V" profile with elevations in scales 1 (Hs, hypochondriasis), 3 (Hy, hysteria), and 2 (D, depression).[55] However, such testing cannot definitively make or exclude a diagnosis of PNES, and there is a significant overlap of results, particularly on cognitive testing, between patients with PNES and those with epilepsy.[58]

TREATMENT

Making a definitive diagnosis of PNES can be difficult. As presented in the clinical vignette at the beginning of this chapter, there are characteristic features of epidemiology, clinical events, laboratory values, and EEG monitoring that may suggest PNES, but for each thought to have PNES, there are others in whom true epilepsy can result in a diagnosis of PNES. However, a thorough evaluation using each of these domains—with EEG-video monitoring being the best diagnostic test—can help the psychiatrist determine whether PNES is more or less likely. Finally, it is important to allow for the possibility that one's diagnosis of PNES may be incorrect; but this should not prevent clinicians from moving forward based upon their clinical findings. It should simply serve as a reminder to maintain an open mind about the diagnosis.

General medical providers often feel that once the diagnosis of PNES has been made, treatment is over. However, treatment is truly just beginning. After the diagnosis is made, patients with PNES continue to have frequent and disabling PNES events; only about 30% will stop having convulsive events.[43,45] However, early diagnosis is associated with a better outcome,[59] and presentation of the diagnosis and a treatment plan in a way that is acceptable to the patient is critical.

Table 18.4 lists the important features of NES diagnosis and the treatment plan for patients with the disorder. First, the diagnosis should be framed positively: it is tremendously reassuring that these events are not due to abnormal electrical discharges in the brain, and there is no need to take anticonvulsant medications and deal with their side effects. If a patient feels as if he or she is being told that there is nothing wrong, it can be useful to emphasize that although there is not a *structural* or *electroencephalographical* abnormality

present, there is an abnormality of *function* of the nervous system that will require integrated treatment. Furthermore, the physician should make it clear that he or she understands that these events are having a significant impact on the patient's life and require ongoing efforts to reduce their negative impact.

Next, the physician should describe the impact of mood, anxiety, and stress on these symptoms and inform the patient that reduction of these symptoms is imperative to help the patient improve his or her function and quality of life. However, rather than simply making a referral to a psychiatrist, the physician should also emphasize that the patient will continue to see his or her neurologist or primary care physician regularly as a crucial part of the treatment. The regularity of this follow-up is important: the patient should have an appointment with the caregiver, regardless of whether he or she is having active symptoms, thus disconnecting the link between symptoms and medical attention.

In one of the few controlled trials conducted to compare treatment options for PNES, LaFrance and colleagues[47] conducted a small, randomized study.

TABLE 18.4

Guidelines for Presenting a Diagnosis of Non-Epileptic Seizures and Developing a Treatment Plan

Presentation of the Diagnosis	Treatment Plan
1. Frame the diagnosis in a positive way: Symptoms are not due to abnormal electrical activity, and risks of anticonvulsants need not be undertaken.	1. The treatment plan should include as much psychiatric care as the patient will allow. Weekly psychotherapy to assess unconscious motivation, to allow psychoeducation, and to provide support is ideal.
2. Explain that symptoms are likely due to a problem with the *function* of the nervous system, rather than electrical or structural abnormalities.	2. Psychotropic medications should be used to treat co-morbid psychiatric symptoms (e.g., associated with major depression).
3. Explain that these symptoms are common and are likely to improve gradually over time. Give specific suggestions regarding how they will improve (e.g., episodes will become less prolonged, then become less frequent, then have fewer symptoms during each episode, and so forth).	3. Regular follow-up from other caregivers is a key component of the treatment plan. Appointments should be scheduled at regular intervals, whether or not the patient is symptomatic, and patients should receive positive reinforcement (and not a decrease in frequency of follow-up) when symptoms subside.
4. Acknowledge the disability that such symptoms have caused and the importance of developing a treatment plan that will improve the function of the nervous system and reduce disability.	4. Physical examinations should be done regularly, but diagnostic studies should be avoided unless clearly indicated.
5. Introduce the idea that anxiety, stress, and mood significantly affect the frequency and severity of these events and that reduction of these symptoms is crucial in the patient's treatment.	5. Despite the diagnosis of non-epileptic seizures, all caregivers should remain vigilant for the possibility that an organic diagnosis has been missed or that non-epileptic seizures and epilepsy are both present.
6. Describe a treatment plan that includes integrated, consistent treatment from providers in psychiatry, neurology, and primary care.	

Patients in this study were fairly motivated and had some insight into their PNES diagnosis, which is not always the case. The study had the following arms: medication (flexible-dose sertraline) only, cognitive-behavioral therapy informed psychotherapy (CBT-ip) only, CBT-ip with medication (sertraline), or treatment as usual. The results showed significant seizure reduction and improved co-morbid depression and anxiety symptoms, as well as global functioning with CBT-ip both without and with sertraline, while medication alone and treatment, as usual, did not show any improvement.[47] This study and similar studies, despite the limitations regarding study population and study size, suggest that there might be more effective treatments for this group of patients.

MANAGEMENT OF PATIENTS WITH HEADACHE

Headache is one of the most common medical complaints; up to 93% of males and 99% of females have experienced headaches.[60] At any point in time, roughly 16% of the world's population has a headache.[61]

Prevalence peaks during the average individual's most productive years, from ages 25 to 55, resulting in a marked reduction in productivity. Although most headaches are not life threatening, they do cause significant impairment. The Global Burden of Disease (GBD) study reveals that headache disorders are a major global public health issue. In the 2019 version (GBD 2019), headaches were the third leading cause of years lost to disability (YLD), and the leading cause of YLD in adults under the age of 50 years.[62] Most people with recurrent and troublesome headaches have tension-type, migraine, cluster headaches, or other trigeminal autonomic cephalalgias. These are referred to as "primary headaches" in the widely used International Classification of Headache Disorders—III; primary headaches include migraine, tension-type headache (TTH), and trigeminal autonomic cephalalgias (e.g., cluster headaches) (Table 18.5).[63] However, it is vitally important that clinicians rule out life-threatening medical conditions that are associated with headaches that can be encountered with a higher index of suspicion in the general hospital setting by consultation psychiatrists.

TABLE 18.5
Primary Headaches

Syndrome	Epidemiology	Symptoms	Acute Treatment	Miscellaneous
Tension type	27% of females 23% of males	Band-like pain, lack of associated symptoms, not usually incapacitating, may be relieved by alcohol	NSAIDs, acetaminophen, relaxation techniques, biofeedback	Not associated with increased muscle tension
Migraine	17% of females 9% of males	Recurrent stereotyped episodes of pain; presentation varies between patients, unilateral pulsating pain in front of the head, often the pain generalizes, may have multiple associated symptoms, 4–24 h	Avoid precipitating factors; NSAIDs, triptans, ergots	70% of patients have family history. 70% of females have a decrease in migraine attacks during pregnancy. Migraine tends to wane as a patient enters the forties
Cluster	Overall <0.2%, most are in males, onset before age 25	Grouping of excruciating, sharp, pain located usually behind one eye occurring several times daily; may occur during sleep; peaks within 5–10 min, <3 h; associated with reddened conjunctiva, sweating, ptosis	Oxygen, triptans	May repeat in spring. Patients often smoke cigarettes and drink alcohol excessively

NSAIDs, non-steroidal anti-inflammatory drugs.

Head Pain Pathophysiology

Although the brain contains no nociceptive fibers, head pain may arise from several areas. The "trigeminocervical complex," a large ipsilateral nuclear group spanning the trigeminal nucleus caudalis (rostrally) to the high cervical dorsal horn cells (caudally), receives distributed cervical and trigeminal nociceptive information. Nociceptive C and A-delta fibers innervate the skin, periosteum, large vessels (arteries, veins, and sinuses), and meninges.[64] Except for the posterior fossa, which is supplied by the high cervical nerve roots, most head pain is mediated through the first division of the trigeminal nerve.[65]

From this "trigeminocervical complex," second-order pathways then cross and terminate in the thalamus; third-order pathways then bring the information to the cortex. Descending endogenous inhibitory pain systems may influence incoming signals at the juncture between the first- and second-order neurons. This simplified schema may mediate most, if not all, head pain. In addition to this peripheral sensitization, there are likely central processes at work during headaches (such as the recruitment of previously non-nociceptive neurons).[64] Allodynia, a term that describes pain caused by an activity that normally does not elicit pain (such as coughing or brushing one's hair) may be an example of this central sensitization.

As to the specific cause of migraine, one theory of migraine generation is dysfunction in brainstem systems, possibly genetically determined. In addition, cortical spreading depression, now thought to be the mechanism of the aura in migraine, may result in local ionic and chemical changes that might sensitize perivascular trigeminal fibers and impair glymphatic flow, causing a cascade of changes to produce the clinical symptomatology of migraine with aura by way of the simplified schema above.[66] Included in this process, trigeminal neural impulses may subsequently "feedback" through various routes to the meninges, leading to local release of neuropeptides (e.g., calcitonin gene-related peptide [CGRP], substance P, and vasoactive intestinal polypeptide) that can amplify and sustain the headache cascade. Migraine is associated with structural changes in the brain, including strokes[67] and white matter hyperintensities on MRI scans that increase with disease progression.[68] Stimulation of nearby brainstem nuclei by this cascade may also explain some of the associated constitutional symptoms that are commonly seen in migraine.

TTH may be a misnomer as recent studies have demonstrated that this type of headache is not reliably associated with increased muscle contractions or physiological tension.[69] The mechanism of TTH may be related to the hyper-excitability of afferent neurons from muscles or impairments in pain inhibitory systems and may share many of the pathophysiological features of migraine. Whether TTH is ultimately viewed as a variation of migraine or as a separate pathological condition remains unsettled.

Recent information suggests a central, possibly hypothalamic, cause for cluster headaches with important peripheral trigeminovascular and autonomic activation as well.

Tension-Type Headaches

TTH is the most common headache disorder; however, since most individuals with TTH experience mild-to-moderate and episodic TTH, the disorder is less often encountered in clinical settings. TTH is more common in females, with nearly one-fourth of people (23.4% of males and 27.1% of females) having an active disorder.[61] In TTH, the high prevalence confounds the detection of a genetic influence; studies of several large populations suggest a complex multi-factorial mode of inheritance in favor of a sporadic condition.

Chronic TTH is rare, but it can be disabling, and it places patients at risk of developing a medication overuse headache (MOH). Pain is the main symptom, usually described as bilateral, band like, steady, and mild to moderate in intensity. An increased tenderness in the muscles of the head and neck can often be demonstrated on palpation, but its absence does not rule out the disorder. Other symptoms (such as nausea, vomiting, photophobia, or phonophobia) do not typically occur.

Non-pharmacologic treatment of TTH includes reassurance (i.e., there is no life-threatening cause). Biofeedback for TTH, as noted in a review of 94 studies, yielded a significant medium-to-large effect compared with waiting-list controls and a significant medium-sized effect compared with placebo.[70] There were also significant improvements in perceived self-efficacy and symptoms of depression and anxiety, as well as less medication use.

Pharmacologically, simple analgesics (such as a non-steroidal anti-inflammatory drug [NSAID]) are used to treat individual headaches. The best evidence of efficacy is for aspirin (in doses of 500–1000 mg).[71] Preventative treatment may be needed when headaches are disabling or frequent. Good evidence supports the use of amitriptyline, a tertiary amine TCA, which is generally effective for headaches (used at doses lower than those needed to treat depression).[72] Tizanidine and mirtazapine have demonstrated some benefit.[72,73] Botulinum toxin (botox) is currently not indicated for TTH; there is mixed evidence for a possible benefit of botox injections into the head and neck.[74] Opioid- and barbiturate-containing medications should be avoided, as tolerance, dependence, or MOH can develop.

Migraine Headaches

Migraines are the most common headache type as they pertain to urgent or emergent headache attacks. Migraine attacks are episodic, usually disabling headaches associated with nausea and photophobia (see Box 18.1 for migraine diagnostic criteria).

Approximately 17% of females suffer from migraine, as opposed to 8.6% of males.[61] In females, migraine attacks often begin at menarche and recur pre-menstrually. Contraceptive medication may worsen migraine in some females, while in others it

BOX 18.1
DIAGNOSTIC CRITERIA FOR MIGRAINE HEADACHES

At least five attacks fulfilling the criteria below:
Headache attacks that last for 4–72 hours (when untreated or unsuccessfully treated)
Headache that has at least two of the following four characteristics:
1. Unilateral location
2. Pulsating quality
3. Moderate or severe pain intensity
4. Aggravation by or causing avoidance of routine physical activity (e.g., walking or climbing stairs)
During the headache, at least one of the following:
1. Nausea and/or vomiting
2. Photophobia and phonophobia
Not better accounted for by another International Classification of Headache Disorders—III diagnosis.

may improve symptoms. Pregnancy offers relief from migraine in nearly three-fourths of females.[69]

The inheritance in migraine is complex, with over 40 gene locations contributing to risk. Heritability estimates range from 34% to 64%. First-degree relatives of those with migraine (but without an aura) are twice as likely to have the condition. However, a first-degree relative of an individual who has migraine with an aura is four times more likely to have that type of migraine.[75] In patients with a rare form of migraine, familial hemiplegic migraine (FHM), the responsible genetic defects result in ion channel dysfunction (channelopathy) that is thought to explain the migraine symptoms in these patients. FHM has been associated with three mutations: CACNA1A gene (coding for a calcium channel) on chromosome 19 in FHM1; ATP1A2 (coding for a K/Na-ATPase) on chromosome 1 in FHM2; and SCN1A gene (coding for a sodium channel) on chromosome 2 in FHM3.[63]

Migraine attacks occur in four phases. The premonitory (prodromal) phase may include emotional/behavioral symptoms (including depressed mood, anxiety, euphoria, talkativeness, restlessness, hyperactivity, and irritability), and neurologic symptoms (e.g., difficulty concentrating, drowsiness, dysphasia, hyperosmia, photophobia, and phonophobia) that may continue into the headache phase. Gastrointestinal (GI) symptoms, anorexia, thirst, urination, stiff neck, and food cravings (that a patient may misconstrue as a migraine trigger) may also occur. The second phase, aura, develops over minutes and lasts up to an hour, although migraine without aura is more common than migraine with aura. Visual auras occur in 99% of patients with an aura, and could include scotomata (blind spots), phosphenes (images of light or color visible with closed eyes), geometric forms, fortification spectra (bright, shimmering, jagged lines spread across the visual field), scintillations (flashing zig-zag lines), or visual distortions. Other aura symptoms include hallucinations (e.g., visual, olfactory, auditory, or gustatory), motor deficits (e.g., weakness, ataxia, hemiparesis or hemiplegia), paresthesia, (e.g., of the lips and hands especially), aphasia or dysarthria, or perceptual impairments (déjà vu, dissociation, disturbed consciousness). In some individuals, an aura may not be followed by a headache, and it can mimic other neurological disorders (e.g., stroke, psychosis, or intoxication). The headache phase is often characterized by unilateral pulsatile pain in the frontotemporal region or around the eye. In half of patients, the pain switches sides of the head during the attack or in different attacks.[69] The pain may become dull and symmetrical, like that of TTH. Photophobia and phonophobia are common features. Autonomic dysfunction arises and includes slowed gastric emptying, nausea, and vomiting, which can cause severe disability. The length of a headache can vary greatly, but it usually lasts from 4 to 74 hours. Patients may attempt to avoid sensory input and movement, and may seek out dark, quiet, spaces. Following cessation of the headache, the post-drome phase may be characterized by asthenia, impaired concentration, fatigue, sadness, and irritability, although others may experience euphoria.

Treatment for migraine headaches begins with avoidance of any identifiable precipitants. To identify potential triggers, patients should record, in a headache diary, their headache episodes and their severity, as well as suspected triggers (e.g., the timing of menses, ingestion of foods, stressors, and response to medication). For migraine prevention, the United States Headache Consortium offers Grade A (from multiple well-designed randomized clinical trials [RCTs] yielding consistent findings) recommendations for several non-pharmacologic interventions (including relaxation training, electromyography biofeedback, and cognitive-behavioral therapy [CBT]).[76] Mindfulness-based cognitive therapy improved migraine disability index scores more than those of a waitlist control group in one study.[77] Clinicians can reduce stigma and patient self-blame by de-emphasizing the role of "avoiding triggers" or medication "overuse" in headache propagation, supporting the patient with messages of empowerment rather than pity, and even using re-framing language when describing the disease.

Abortive pharmacotherapy for mild-to-moderate migraine is like that of TTH. More severe migraine attacks are effectively treated with ergotamine, dihydroergotamine, and the $5-HT_{1B/1D}$ agonists known as triptans (e.g., sumatriptan, naratriptan, zolmitriptan, rizatriptan, almotriptan, eletriptan, and frovatriptan). Triptans are considered first-line abortive treatments for severe migraine attacks. The $5-HT_{1F}$ agonist lasmiditan may be considered an abortive agent in patients for whom the potential vasoconstrictive properties of triptans may be contraindicated. The CGRP antagonists, referred to as "gepants," (rimegepant, ubrogepant, atogepant) may be used for abortive treatment and as a preventive treatment.

In 2006 the FDA issued a warning about the possibility of serotonin syndrome in patients given triptans while taking a serotonergic antidepressant (e.g., an SSRI or serotonin-norepinephrine reuptake inhibitor [SNRI]). However, the American Headache Society contends that insufficient evidence exists to support limiting the use of triptans.[78] From a pathophysiologic perspective, serotonin syndrome is most likely caused by overstimulation at the $5-HT_{2A}$ receptor, with a smaller contribution from the $5-HT_{1A}$ receptor. Triptans have no significant binding activity at these specific serotonin receptor subtypes. A 2018 retrospective review of over 19,000 patients who were co-prescribed a triptan and an antidepressant found a clinical suspicion for serotonin syndrome in only 17 patients, while only seven met the criteria for serotonin syndrome, and only two of the case vignettes appeared credible.[79] In sum, the association of triptans with serotonin syndrome appears to be very rare, and as the potential benefits exceed the risk, triptans should not be contraindicated in patients using other serotonergic medications.

For those with frequent migraine attacks, prophylactic medication (referred to as preventives) may be necessary. Beta-blockers (e.g., propranolol) are one of the most frequently used preventatives. Anticonvulsants (e.g., topiramate, valproic acid) are also effective; lamotrigine, gabapentin, and carbamazepine have less evidence for their efficacy in this population. Amitriptyline, at low doses, is the only TCA with proven efficacy as a preventative, although nortriptyline is used occasionally. The SNRI venlafaxine is probably effective at usual or at high doses, while there is even less evidence for the use of duloxetine and limited evidence for milnacipran. Other preventatives include calcium channel blockers (e.g., verapamil), NSAIDs, angiotensin receptor blockers (candesartan), angiotensin-converting enzyme inhibitors (lisinopril), and serotonin antagonists (e.g., methysergide, cyproheptadine), which have all been effective. Evidence also supports the use of Petasites (Butterbur), riboflavin, co-enzyme Q 10, and magnesium as preventatives. The recently introduced CGRP monoclonal antibodies (eptinezumab, erunumab, remanezumab, galcanezumab) have a longer half-life and are less likely to cause hepatic toxicity than the aforementioned "gepants"; they have demonstrated efficacy as migraine preventives and for chronic migraine. Onabotulinum toxin A (Botox) received FDA approval for headache prevention in adults with chronic migraine; multiple injections into the head and neck are given every 12 weeks.

For those who suffer from status migrainosus (migraines that last longer than 72 hours), first-line treatment typically includes the use of parenteral ketorolac in addition to a parenteral dopamine antagonist (e.g., metoclopramide, prochlorperazine, chlorpromazine, haloperidol, droperidol), and parenteral dihydroergotamine. Parenteral steroids or valproate may also be considered. A continuous infusion of intravenous (IV) lidocaine may be efficacious, yet evidence is still being gathered and such treatment is available in only a few hospital settings.[80]

Cluster Headache and Other Trigeminal Autonomic Cephalalgias

Cluster headache is considered one of the trigeminal autonomic cephalalgias (TACs) in the ICDH-3 classification. Cluster headache is much less common than other primary headaches, with a prevalence of less than 0.2%. The male-to-female ratio with cluster headaches is 4:1.[81] Cluster headaches may be autosomal dominant in about 5% of cases.[2] Recent information suggests a central, possibly hypothalamic, cause for cluster headaches with important peripheral trigeminovascular and autonomic activation as well.

Cluster headache is characterized by severe unilateral pain in the orbital or temporal region lasting 15 to 180 minutes, associated with autonomic symptoms, including injected conjunctiva, profuse facial sweating or flushing, ptosis, or miosis[69] The pain may occur every other day up to eight times daily for several weeks (known as bouts or clusters) followed by periods of remission that may last months or years. Headaches may be triggered by using alcohol or tobacco. Risk factors include smoking and excessive alcohol intake. The onset is usually before age 25 and there may be a cyclical pattern that repeats in the spring. Cluster headaches often occur during REM sleep.

Cluster headaches may be aborted by breathing 100% oxygen for 15 minutes at a flow of at least 7 L/minute. Along with oxygen, injectable or intranasal triptans are considered first-line treatments. Corticosteroids may also provide short-term relief. Prophylactic medications include verapamil and lithium. Successful dosing for lithium is based on blood levels in the therapeutic range for the treatment of bipolar disorder. The response usually takes 3 weeks. Topiramate (at doses of 25–200 mg/day) has also shown some efficacy.[82]

Other TACs include paroxysmal hemicrania (PH), a severe unilateral orbital or temporal pain lasting 2 to 30 minutes multiple times each day, with associated ipsilateral autonomic findings. In contrast, hemicrania continua (HC) is a severe chronic headache with associated ipsilateral autonomic findings that persist for more than 3 months. Both PH and HC respond to indomethacin (at doses of 150–225 mg daily). Short-lasting unilateral neuralgiform headache attacks with conjunctival injection and tearing (SUNCT), and short-lasting unilateral neuralgiform headache attacks with cranial autonomic symptoms (SUNA) are described as having severe unilateral stabbing head pains that last seconds to minutes, with ipsilateral autonomic findings. Lamotrigine may be the preferred initial treatment.

Primary Headache Treatment and Secondary Medication Overuse Headache

Specific treatment of headaches depends on their underlying cause; however, general rules apply. Symptomatic treatment of most headache types begins with an analgesic (such as acetaminophen or an NSAID), and many medications can be used for multiple types of headaches (Table 18.6). The use of opiates is generally discouraged in the treatment of headaches, although for severe post-surgical pain, they may offer short-term relief. In the treatment of chronic daily headaches, opiates have been unsuccessful, with nearly three-fourths of patients either failing to demonstrate marked improvement or showing problematic drug behaviors, such as dose violations.[83]

Frequent and consistent use of medications used for the treatment of pain can lead to a set of secondary headaches (such as chronic daily headaches, e.g., MOH). This pattern of use may disrupt the normal pain pathways that exacerbate headache syndromes. Perturbations in normal vasoconstriction may also

TABLE 18.6

Pharmacological Treatment of Headache

Medication	Dosing	Side Effects	Headache Type
Acetaminophen	1000 mg every 4 h as needed to a maximum of 4000 mg/day	Hepatotoxicity	Tension type
Beta-blockers (e.g., propranolol)	40 mg bid, increase as heart rate tolerates	Dizziness, interferes with asthma treatment	Migraine, sexual, exertional, pheochromocytoma
Botulinum toxin type A	25–260 units injected every 3 months	Muscle weakness, ptosis	Chronic migraine
Calcium channel blockers (e.g., verapamil)	40 mg tid	Hypotension, A-V block	Migraine
Carbamazepine	100 mg bid and increase until relief	Leukopenia, hepatotoxicity, weight gain, somnolence	Trigeminal neuralgia
Combination analgesics (e.g., Fiorinal)	1–2 caplets every 4 h as needed	Somnolence, palpitations (due to caffeine), addiction	Tension type
Dopamine blockers (e.g., prochlorperazine)	10–25 mg as needed	Sedation, dystonia, parkinsonism	Migraine (for nausea)
Ergots (e.g., ergotamine tartrate)	2 mg SL every 30 min (up to 6 mg/day) as needed	Dizziness. Should not be used with triptans or MAOIs	Migraine, cluster
Gabapentin	900–3600 mg daily	Dizziness, somnolence	Migraine, CDH, trigeminal neuralgia
Lithium	600–1200 mg daily (based on therapeutic blood levels)	Renal toxicity, polyuria, polydipsia, edema, weight gain, thyroid disease, nausea, diarrhea	Cluster
NSAIDs (e.g., ibuprofen)	400–800 mg every 6 h	Increased bleeding time, renal toxicity, GI side effects	Migraine, CDH, tension-type, sexual, exertional
Serotonin antagonists (e.g., methysergide)	2–8 mg daily	Retroperitoneal and retropleural fibrosis	Migraine
Serotonin-norepinephrine reuptake inhibitors (e.g., venlafaxine)	150 mg daily	Nausea, sexual dysfunction, hypertension	Migraine
Serotonin reuptake inhibitors (e.g., fluoxetine)	20–60 mg daily	Sexual dysfunction, nausea, somnolence	Migraine, tension-type
Steroids (e.g., methylprednisolone)	24 mg the first day and taper over 6 days	Nausea, vomiting, insomnia, anxiety	Cluster, migraine, IIH, temporal arteritis (higher doses), medication overuse
Tizanidine	8–20 mg daily	Dry mouth, hypotension, bradycardia	Migraine, CDH
Topiramate	25–100 mg bid	Somnolence, weight loss, kidney stones	Migraine, CDH, cluster
Tricyclic antidepressants (e.g., amitriptyline)	10–150 mg at bedtime	Dry mouth, hypotension, constipation, arrhythmia, fatigue	Migraine, tension type, cluster
Triptans (e.g., sumatriptan)	6 mg subcutaneously hourly × 2/daily as needed	Nausea. Interaction with ergots; contraindicated in stroke, coronary artery disease	Migraine, exertional, sexual
Valproic acid	500–2000 mg/day	Nausea, somnolence, weight gain, alopecia; avoid if possible, in pregnancy	Migraine, trigeminal neuralgia

bid, Twice per day; CDH, chronic daily headache; GI, gastrointestinal; IIH, idiopathic intracranial hypertension; qhs, every night; SL, sublingually; tid, three times per day.

contribute. Implicated medications include barbiturates, benzodiazepines, ergots, triptans, opioids, and, NSAIDs.[69] Evidence suggests that patients who overuse triptans experience MOHs faster and with lower doses than patients who use analgesics or ergots.[84] Patients who overuse triptans are more likely to have daily migraine-like symptoms, while those over-using analgesics or ergots typically have daily TTH.[84] Patients' headaches rarely respond to preventive or prophylactic measures if the patient is over-using abortive treatments. If the patient is over-using narcotics, avoidance of opiate withdrawal may play a role in the medication overuse.

Management of MOH due to substances that can cause withdrawal (such as opioids or caffeine) may require tapered detoxification, not just to mitigate withdrawal symptoms, but to minimize rebound headache and thus reduce the psychological reinforcement for the substance. Detoxification for MOH due to a butalbital-containing combination of analgesics requires further research to determine best practices, although some headache centers taper with phenobarbital.[85] A short course of steroids (such as 60 mg of prednisone for 5 days) may also help.[86]

Psychiatric Co-morbidity and Headaches

Headache disorders are not psychiatric conditions. However, the co-morbidity of psychiatric disorders and headaches is high, and the influence is bi-directional, with increasing headache burden causing more psychiatric morbidity, and increasing psychiatric burden worsening headaches. Depression and anxiety have the highest co-morbidity in patients with headache disorders. Compared to those in the general population, the risk of depression is two to four times higher in people with migraine, and three times higher in people with cluster headaches.[87,88] Bipolar disorder is relatively rare compared to MDD; however, about one-third of patients with bipolar disorder also have migraine.[89,90] Depression is associated with an increased risk of transformation of episodic migraines into chronic migraines.[91] Patients with migraine are at increased risk for suicide attempts and severe pain is associated with a higher rate of suicide attempts.[92] Patients may experience anxiety during a headache attack, develop generalized anxiety under conditions of chronic headache, or encounter anticipatory anxiety about the next attack between headaches.

At least 30% of patients with post-traumatic headaches also have post-traumatic stress disorder (PTSD).[93] Attention-deficit/hyperactivity disorder (ADHD) is more common in those with migraines, people with ADHD are at higher risk for concussions, and those with a concussion are more likely to have a prolonged recovery if they have both ADHD and migraine.[94,95] People with MOH have a 40% risk of developing a substance use disorder (SUD).[96]

There is a paucity of evidence to guide the management of psychiatric disorders in patients with headaches, although there are some important caveats. The risk of medication-induced mood exacerbation in patients with bipolar disorder and migraine is likely higher, as patients with migraine and bipolar disorder are more likely to be rapid cyclers, and are more likely to be exposed to TCAs and SNRIs, which carry a higher risk for medication-induced mood exacerbation compared to other antidepressants.[97,98] Headache is often reported following initiation of an antidepressant medication, however, headaches typically dissipate over time and they should not be a reason to defer treatment.[99] Among antidepressants, bupropion and escitalopram carry a significant risk of headaches, while trazodone and vilazodone confer a large but statistically insignificant risk.[100] The latter two agents, which are phenylpiperazine derivative antidepressants, may cause more headaches in those with migraines or with a family history of migraines, possibly due to the migraine-inducing effects of their shared active metabolite, and they might be best avoided in those with migraines.[101,102]

The importance of communication among treaters of headaches and psychiatric disciplines is essential to avoid needless duplication of similar serotonergic medications used for ostensibly different purposes. There is insufficient evidence to show that the addition of low-dose TCA to a second antidepressant is more effective for depression or headache. One study (involving 88 subjects) demonstrated that citalopram plus amitriptyline had better outcomes for depression and headache than either agent used alone.[103]

HEADACHE RED FLAGS

Historical features that may indicate a dangerous underlying cause for headache include the so-called "first and worst" headache or "thunderclap headache":

DIFFERENTIAL DIAGNOSIS FOR THUNDERCLAP HEADACHE

- Intracerebral hemorrhage
- Arterial dissection
- Cerebral venous thrombosis
- Unruptured vascular malformation
- Pituitary hemorrhagic infarct (pituitary apoplexy)
- Central nervous system hypotension
- Acute sinusitis
- Third ventricular colloid cyst
- Hypertensive encephalopathy
- Spontaneous low-pressure headache
- Reversible cerebral vasoconstriction syndrome

BOX 18.3
CLUES TO DANGEROUS HEADACHES

- First time to have this type of headache → investigate with diligence
- Acute onset → SAH, other thunderclap headaches (see Box 19.2)
- Chronic, progressive → rule out brain tumor, chronic SAH
- Fever → meningitis, encephalitis
- Worse when lying down → increased ICP secondary to mass (tumor or hemorrhage)
- Worse when standing up → decreased ICP secondary to LP
- Pain worse after time spent in a particular location → carbon monoxide poisoning
- Associated with N/V → mass
- Associated with localizing signs → mass
- Papilledema or increase in pain with cough or straining → mass, intracranial hypertension
- Scalp tenderness or skull fracture → subdural hematoma
- Orbital or temporal bruit → AVM, sinus thrombosis
- Nuchal pain or rigidity → acute or chronic meningitis or SAH
- Onset after age 50 or chronic and progressive → tumor, SDH

AVM, Arteriovenous malformation; ICP, intracranial pressure; LP, lumbar puncture; N/V, nausea, and vomiting; SAH, subarachnoid hemorrhage.

that is, the sudden onset of a de novo severe headache (that reaches maximal intensity in 1–3 minutes), possibly indicating a subarachnoid hemorrhage (SAH) from an aneurysmal bleed. This pattern has been investigated in some detail, and there is a differential diagnosis beyond SAH, with both primary and secondary types described (Box 18.2). Some of these headaches are benign; however, given the risks associated with missing an aneurysmal bleed, this pattern cannot be assumed to be benign, and it must be evaluated.

Headache associated with fever, chills, and a change in mental status is a matter of concern and one that is not often confused with primary headache syndrome. Similarly, a new-onset headache in an immune-compromised individual (e.g., someone with acquired immunodeficiency syndrome [AIDS]) or someone with a concerning past medical history (e.g., with a history of metastatic cancer) should also prompt concern.

New-onset migraine after the age of 50 is unusual; thus, an evaluation (including an evaluation for temporal arteritis) is warranted, to prevent the often-sudden complication of irreversible visual loss.

DIFFERENTIAL DIAGNOSIS AND CLINICAL APPROACH

While most patients with dangerous headaches are treated in emergency settings, a psychiatrist familiar with the presentation of rare headache syndromes may be a lifesaver. Differentiating among all potential causes of headaches can be daunting. A host of conditions should be considered when an individual complains of a headache. The task can be made less difficult

by ruling out dangerous causes of headaches (Box 18.3). Once this has been done, the clinician can match the headache history to the headache syndrome.

Taking the headache history is the most crucial aspect of the work-up. Elucidation of such features of the pain, as timing (e.g., acute or chronic), onset (e.g., sudden or insidious), duration, severity, location (e.g., unilateral, bilateral, including the neck or eyes), associated symptoms (e.g., visual changes, motor symptoms, nausea, diaphoresis, anxiety), body position (e.g., after standing up or lying down), and setting (e.g., during sleep, at work, or after exercise) is important. The effects of medication, meals (including specific foods [such as chocolate]), substances (such as caffeine and alcohol), sleep (including patterns and changes), and exercise also offer important clues to the diagnosis. A family history of certain types of headaches may also shed light on the etiology. For patients with more than one type of headache, a separate history should be obtained for each type.

Physical examination of a patient with a headache must include a full neurological examination, a funduscopic examination, and an examination of the head.

Vital signs must also be assessed (as either low or high blood pressure may be contributing factors). A fever may point toward a CNS infection. The neurological examination may reveal focal findings that indicate a stroke or multiple sclerosis (MS). The fundoscopic examination will search for signs of raised intracranial pressure (ICP), such as papilledema. Physical examination of the head will search for signs of trauma, and one should palpate for tenderness or masses, and auscultate over the temples and eyes for bruits that may signal the presence of an arteriovenous malformation (AVM). The neck must also be checked for rigidity.

Further testing may be indicated to evaluate etiologies suggested by the history and physical examination (Table 18.7). For a patient with a new-onset severe headache, a CT scan is the preferred imaging modality in the emergency setting. On the other hand, a CT head scan may miss abnormalities within the posterior fossa, venous sinuses, optic nerve, or when signs of low/high cerebrospinal fluid (CSF) pressure, or Chiari malformations are present. For patients with subacute or chronic headaches, the American Headache Society recommends MRI over CT scanning.[104]

TABLE 18.7
Laboratory and Other Tests During Headache Evaluation

Suspected Condition	Order
Acute stroke or bleed	CT
Aneurysm	MRA or CT angiogram
CVT	MRI and MRA or CT and CT angiogram
MS	MRI
Infection	LP
Temporal arteritis	ESR, CRP
Seizures	EEG
Carbon monoxide poisoning	Carboxyhemoglobin
CNS tumor	CT
Pheochromocytoma	24-hour urine metanephrine; abdominal CT

CNS, Central nervous system; CRP, C-reactive protein; CT, computed tomography; CVT, cerebral venous thrombosis; EEG, electroencephalogram; ESR, erythrocyte sedimentation rate; LP, lumbar puncture; MRA, magnetic resonance angiogram; MRI, magnetic resonance imaging; MS, multiple sclerosis.

A lumbar puncture (LP) can help to evaluate for infectious or inflammatory etiologies, SAH, spontaneous intracranial hypotension (SIH), or idiopathic intracranial hypertension (IIH). In an elderly person with a new-onset headache, an elevated erythrocyte sedimentation rate (ESR) suggests a possible giant cell arteritis or temporal arteritis. An EEG and evoked responses have no particular role in primary headache diagnosis but may help sort out causes for several secondary headaches.

SECONDARY HEADACHES: ACUTE AND SUBACUTE

Structural causes should be evaluated if the patient's headache pattern does not follow that of one of the primary headache syndromes, is accompanied by an abnormal neurological examination, is progressive, or is of acute onset. Secondary headaches carry a prevalence related to the underlying condition. The pathogenesis of secondary headaches depends on the etiology of each headache. Discussed below are some of the dangerous causes of headaches.

Post-Traumatic Headache

Headache attributed to a traumatic injury to the head is one of the most common causes of secondary headaches.[63] Nearly half of those who have suffered a concussion have headaches that last for up to 2 months after the injury.[105] Headaches after trauma may be due to several factors, including acceleration and deceleration forces that can cause shear injuries to neurons. Psychological, social, and medicolegal issues may also play a role. Nausea, vomiting, dizziness, vertigo, depression, and anxiety can accompany the headaches. The headaches often begin within 2 weeks of the injury and may resemble migraines or TTHs.

Intracranial Hemorrhage

Cerebral bleeds are usually manifest by the sudden onset of focal neurological deficits that reflect the location and size of the bleed. Larger bleeds can cause an altered mental status, headache, nausea, vomiting, LOC, and hemiplegia. Herniation and death can occur within 24 hours. The most common risk factor for intracranial hemorrhage (ICH) is chronic systemic hypertension, but trauma, anticoagulation therapy, a saccular aneurysm, an AVM, a CNS tumor, clotting disorders, an angiopathy, and vasculitis are also associated with ICH.

Subarachnoid Hemorrhage

A "thunderclap" headache is the classic description of the presentation of SAH, but there are other causes of an excruciating and sudden headache (see Box 18.2). SAH is caused by a rupture of the wall of a cerebral aneurysm or of a cerebrovascular malformation. The fatality rate with SAH is nearly 50%, and half of the survivors develop severe deficits.[63] The most common site of such a rupture is in the circle of Willis. The sudden onset (reaching its peak within a minute) of a severe headache is the most common presentation, and it is often associated with nuchal rigidity. SAH often occurs during exertion (e.g., exercise, sexual intercourse, or straining on the toilet). Initially, there may be fever, nausea, vomiting, seizures, lethargy, and even coma. Focal neurological deficits and retinal hemorrhages point toward SAH. The diagnosis can usually be made upon seeing blood on a non-contrast CT or in the CSF during an LP. Occasionally, SAH may be the result of a vascular leak from a pathological vessel, or a sentinel bleed, and the presentation is not quite as dramatic. At times, no cause can be found to explain a documented SAH; in these patients, the prognosis appears to be benign. Risk factors for SAH include head trauma, thrombocytopenia, use of warfarin or heparin, a clotting factor deficiency, cocaine use, and ingestion of tyramine while taking an MAOI. Treatment of SAH and intracranial bleeds depends on their etiology, location, and symptoms. Neurosurgical consultation is indicated for larger bleeds that may cause compression and herniation. Evacuation of the bleed may be considered. Supportive care includes prevention of increases in ICP that may cause herniation, while avoiding hypotension that could cause ischemia.

Aneurysms

Headache, likely attributed to either a sentinel bleed or local compression, is present in roughly one-fifth of those with an unruptured cerebral aneurysm.[63] This can be an important and potentially life-saving warning, considering the morbidity and mortality rates of SAH. The classic presentation of an enlarging posterior communicating cerebral artery aneurysm is severe posterior orbital pain associated with third nerve palsy and a "blown pupil." Between 2% and 9% of autopsies reveal berry aneurysms; half of them are detected in the circle of Willis.[106]

Intracranial Mass Lesions

Brain tumors and subdural hematomas (SDHs) may cause headaches that may initially be confused with TTHs when the headache is mild, bilateral, and dull. They may worsen as ICP rises while coughing, straining, or bending over, or during REM sleep. Objective evidence of increased ICP (such as papilledema) may not be evident until late in the course. Similarly, localizing findings on the neurological examination may not be apparent, although subtle cognitive and personality changes are usually seen. Chronic SDH can be a cause of a fluctuating headache accompanied by confusion and lethargy. Headache is found in 25% to 100% of those with acute SDHs.[63] SDHs develop more frequently in the elderly, in those who are anticoagulated, and in those with an alcohol use disorder (AUD). Brain tumors are also seen more often in those over the age of 50.

Ischemic Stroke

Up to one-third of patients with an ischemic stroke complain of headache.[63] The presence of focal neurological deficits helps to differentiate the headache from a stroke from a primary headache. The pain is usually mild to moderately severe. The complaint of headache is more often seen with the basilar territory rather than with carotid strokes.

Cerebral Venous Thrombosis

Thrombosis of the cerebral veins and sinuses causes swelling of cerebral veins and reduces absorption of CSF. The increased pressure in the skull leads to infarcts and hemorrhages. The condition can be fatal. Headache is the most common symptom of cerebral venous thrombosis, occurring in over 90% of cases, and it is often the initial complaint.[107] In over 90% of cases additional neurological signs and symptoms (such as seizures, encephalopathy, papilledema, or a focal deficit) develop.[4] Cerebral venous thrombosis is more likely to affect young adults and children. In adults, 75% of the cases occur in females, and are exacerbated by the use of hormonal contraception, head trauma, or ear and sinus infections.[107] Treatment usually involves anticoagulation with heparin in the hospital, followed by oral anticoagulation for an extended period, as an outpatient.

Acute Meningitis

Acute meningitis is manifest in a severe, rapid-onset headache associated with fever, neck stiffness, photophobia, and malaise. This condition often occurs as an epidemic in young adults in areas of relative confinement (such as military barracks or college dormitories). Treatment of meningitis involves treatment of the underlying condition, and use of supportive measures (including IV fluids, antipyretics, anticonvulsants, and bed rest) as needed.

Temporal Arteritis

Temporal arteritis is almost always seen in patients over the age of 55 years with a constant, but dull, headache over one or both temples. Jaw claudication (increasing jaw pain on chewing) is rare, but it was once considered pathognomic for the condition.[69] In advanced cases, the temporal arteries can be red and tender.[66] Often there are systemic signs (such as low-grade fever, malaise, and weight loss) and there may be joint pain or other signs of rheumatoid disease, and visual loss, including amaurosis fugax. Blindness because of ophthalmic artery occlusion and ischemia from cerebral artery occlusion can lead to serious and permanent complications. An ESR above 40 is present in over 90% of cases.[69] A biopsy of the temporal artery that shows focal granulomatous arteritis with giant cells is the definitive test, but it is often unnecessary. Risk factors for temporal arteritis include an age over 55 years and a history of polymyalgia rheumatica. Although the cause is unknown, the condition is associated with inflammation of the temporal and other medium-to-large cerebral and extracerebral arteries. Histologically, a focal granulomatous arteritis with giant cells is seen. Temporal cell arteritis is treated with high-dose steroids to prevent blindness or other stroke syndromes. The patient's symptoms and ESR should be monitored closely for 1 to 2 years.

SECONDARY HEADACHES: SUBACUTE TO CHRONIC

Trigeminal Neuralgia

Patients who suffer from trigeminal neuralgia, also known as tic douloureux, experience sharp pain along one of the three divisions of the trigeminal nerve, most commonly the V2 division. Stimulation of the affected area often triggers pain. This can be by brushing the teeth, eating, touching the affected area, or drinking cold water. The pain is often described as "shocks" of severe pain that last 20 to 30 seconds; shocks do not occur during sleep. The pain begins after age 60, usually the result of a blood vessel pressing against the trigeminal nerve root as it emerges from the brainstem. Tumors of the cerebellopontine angle can also produce tic douloureux. The elderly and those with MS are more likely to suffer from trigeminal neuralgia. Carbamazepine is the "gold standard" for providing at least partial pain relief in 80% to 90% of patients, but many other AEDs (including gabapentin, lamotrigine, phenytoin, and pregabalin) have been effective for trigeminal neuralgia. If a blood vessel is noted to be pressing on the trigeminal nerve, microvascular decompression surgery may be recommended. Injection of an anesthetic at the root of the trigeminal nerve can also stop the pain.

Headaches Attributed to Increased Cerebrospinal Fluid Pressure

A variety of secondary headaches can be attributed to high CSF pressures. IIH, formally known as pseudotumor cerebri, is diagnosed by the presence of intracranial hypertension and elevated CSF pressure. The headache may be accompanied by a "whooshing" noise (pulsatile tinnitus), and in most cases, papilledema is present on fundoscopy. While it often presents in obese females of childbearing age, SIH is also a common misdiagnosis in this population. Other potential causes for increased CSF pressure, including cerebral venous sinus thrombosis, which can have an almost identical presentation, should be excluded. In addition to weight loss, treatment for SIH may include medications with carbonic anhydrase inhibitor activity (e.g., acetazolamide, topiramate, and possibly zonisamide). Surgical intervention (optic nerve sheath fenestration, CSF shunting) is reserved for only the most severely affected patients who are recalcitrant to medical treatment or those with progressive vision loss.

Chronic Meningitis

Chronic meningitis causes a continuous dull headache, accompanied by signs of systemic illness, typically with cognitive decline. Chronic meningitis can irritate and compromise cranial nerve (CN) function (creating, for example, blurred or double vision [CN III, CN IV, and CN VI], facial palsy [CN VII], or hearing impairment [CN VIII]). An LP shows elevated white blood cells, low glucose, and elevated levels of protein. Chronic meningitis is most often caused by *Cryptococcus*, but Lyme disease and fungal infections are also potential culprits. Having a compromised immune system (e.g., having AIDS, being elderly, receiving steroids) is a risk factor for developing chronic meningitis.

COVID-19

Headache is one of the most common symptoms of acute coronavirus disease 2019 (COVID-19) infection, affecting 16% to 40% of patients. Characteristically the headache is an early symptom, lasting 1 to 2 weeks, usually in the frontotemporal or occipital regions. Approximately 18% of patients who develop long-COVID have a prominent headache, which is more common in those with hyposmia; these headaches can take on different phenotypes, such as TTH and migraine headache-like phenotypes.[108] Treatment for long-COVID headaches is based on suggested treatments for the primary headache phenotype. Further elucidation of COVID-19-related headaches will likely develop as clinicians and scientists obtain more data.

MANAGEMENT OF PATIENTS WITH STROKE SYNDROMES

Given that cerebrovascular accidents (CVAs) result in brain areas with reduced or absent function, it is not surprising that abnormalities of affect, behavior, and cognition are common after a CVA. This section discusses the prevalence, diagnosis, and management of patients with psychiatric symptoms after a CVA.

Stroke is a leading cause of morbidity and mortality around the globe. In 2019 there were 12.2 million new strokes and 6.55 million deaths associated with stroke, which constitutes the second-leading cause of death worldwide.[109] In the United States, there were 150,000 new strokes in that same year.[110] Stroke is also a major contributor to disability, leading to 143 million disability-adjusted life years lost around the globe as of 2019.[111] Cognitive impairments and neuropsychiatric syndromes, including depression and apathy, are frequent impairments following stroke,[112,113] and they adversely affect the long-term prognosis (leading to a higher mortality rate and more disability) and the quality of life of stroke survivors.[114,115] Such neuropsychiatric sequelae of strokes have been recognized for decades. More than 50 years ago, both Kraeplin[116] and Bleuler[117] noted an association between cerebrovascular disease and depressive illness. Ironside,[118] in 1956, was the first to describe pathologic crying and laughing associated with cerebral infarction, now a well-described post-stroke syndrome termed *pseudobulbar affect*. Despite the high incidence of these disorders and their frequent description in the literature, acute emotional and behavioral sequelae of stroke go largely unrecognized and untreated.[119]

One way to conceptualize certain neuropsychiatric syndromes caused by stroke is based on the lesion location. Whereas our current understanding of brain circuitry is much more sophisticated than it was from prior models that postulated that certain cortical lobes performed specific cognitive functions, it remains true that lesions in specific cortical areas are more likely to cause characteristic cognitive and neuropsychiatric deficits. For example, strokes in the left frontal lobe are more likely to result in non-fluent aphasia, and strokes affecting the right parietal lobe most frequently cause anosognosia, an unawareness of illness, or neurologic deficits. Table 18.8 provides a list of some correlations between neuropsychiatric deficits and lesion locations.

Neuropsychiatric syndromes caused by strokes can also be categorized by their symptomatology. The following section discusses post-stroke cognitive impairment and delirium, depression, mania, psychosis, anxiety, and other common neuropsychiatric sequelae of stroke.

TABLE 18.8
Correlations Between Cortical Lesion Location and Neuropsychiatric Symptoms

Cortical Area	Potential Neuropsychiatric Symptoms
Frontal lobes	
Orbitofrontal region	Disinhibition, personality change, and irritability
Dorsolateral region	Executive dysfunction: poor planning, organizing, and sequencing
Medial region	Apathy and abulia
Left frontal lobe	Non-fluent (Broca) aphasia, post-stroke depression (possibly)
Right frontal lobe	Motor dysprosody
Temporal lobes	
Either side	Hallucinations (olfactory, gustatory, tactile, visual, or auditory), episodic fear, or mood changes
Left temporal lobe	Short-term memory impairment (to verbal or written stimuli), fluent (Wernicke) aphasia (left temporoparietal region)
Right temporal lobe	Short-term memory impairment (non-verbal stimuli, e.g., music), sensory dysprosody (right temporoparietal region)
Left parietal lobe	Gerstmann syndrome (finger agnosia, right/left disorientation, acalculia, and agraphia)
Right parietal lobe	Anosognosia, constructional apraxia, prosopagnosia, and hemineglect
Occipital lobes	Anton syndrome (cortical blindness with unawareness of visual disturbance)

Case 2

Mrs. B, a 75-year-old widowed executive with a history of GAD, was admitted to the hospital with a left middle cerebral artery CVA. Her presentation was marked by left-sided hemiplegia and a non-fluent aphasia. Because more than 3 hours had elapsed since the onset of her symptoms, she was not eligible for tissue plasminogen activator. Over the course of her hospitalization, she was diagnosed with atrial fibrillation and was placed on an anticoagulant. She worked with physical therapy and made slow gains in terms of motor function. Psychiatry was consulted at the rehabilitation facility 2 weeks after the stroke, to assess her for depression.

On interview, Mrs. B was alert and lucid, sitting upright in her hospital bed. She had prominent broken speech, and she became frustrated quickly with her inability to communicate, slamming her fist on the bedside table. Language comprehension was intact. Discussion with nursing revealed that Mrs. B was sleeping poorly, had a poor appetite, and had a low energy level. The physical therapist added that while Mrs. B had been very motivated to participate in the rehabilitation exercises at the beginning of her stay, her motivation to participate in physical therapy had ebbed over the past few days. The speech therapist noted a similar pattern when working with Mrs. B to improve her speech.

When asked if she felt depressed, Mrs. B nodded her head "yes." She quickly teared up when asked if she felt hopeless, and she appeared quite distressed when asked if she found pleasure in anything. She also endorsed significant loneliness, as she had lost her husband 2 years earlier and her grown children lived out of state. Finally, Mrs. B admitted to feeling more anxious than usual, and was especially fearful about the significant changes in store for her given that she had always been proudly independent and now was having difficulty with her activities of daily living (ADLs) as well as her ability to communicate. Despite feeling depressed, anxious, and hopeless, Mrs. B denied suicidal ideation and was amenable to treatment.

The consultant diagnosed Mrs. B with depressive disorder due to a CVA, with major depressive-like episode (post-stroke depression) in addition to her ongoing GAD. She was re-started on an SSRI, fluoxetine, as it had reduced her anxiety in the past. Mrs. B was also referred for close follow-up with a psychiatrist given her increased risk of poor outcomes both in terms of post-stroke functional improvement and her higher-than-usual suicide risk in the setting of post-stroke depression and anxiety.

Cognitive Impairment and Delirium

Approximately 25% to 40% of patients develop delirium in the first week after a stroke[120,121] with those who suffered a hemorrhagic stroke having a higher risk. Since delirium may be difficult to differentiate from cognitive deficits that result from focal brain lesions, it is essential to assess for waxing and waning symptomatology that is characteristic of delirious states. Risk factors for delirium include older age, impaired vision, impaired swallowing, and a prior history of stroke.[122,123] The presence of delirium post-stroke confers a poorer overall prognosis and is associated with longer lengths of stay in the hospital, an increased risk of dementia, and an increased overall mortality rate.[124]

Cognitive impairment is also common post-stroke and occurs in about one-fourth of patients examined 3 months after the event.[124,125] The term "vascular cognitive impairment (VCI)" includes the full spectrum from mild to severe cognitive impairment, both in people with cerebrovascular disease and those with vascular (post-stroke) dementia.[110] Post-stroke risk factors of VCI include severity of infarct, large legion size, older age, low education level, history of diabetes or atrial fibrillation, and the number of recurrent strokes.[110,126] The first year after stroke confers the highest risk of developing dementia, with an estimated incidence of 20% to 30%.[110,126]

Post-Stroke Depression

Post-stroke depression (PSD) is the prototypical acute psychiatric manifestation of stroke. It is common; approximately 30% of patients meet the criteria for MDD in the first 3 months after stroke, and this often develops into a chronic remitting-relapsing condition.[127,128] Stroke-associated depression may reduce survival and increase the risk of recurrent vascular events and of cognitive impairment.[129-131] Risk factors for PSD include a history of depression, pre-stroke functional impairment, living alone, post-stroke social isolation, and possibly female gender.[132]

Both biological and psychological theories of etiology have been studied. Biological hypotheses include lesion location (e.g., of the left frontal region and left basal ganglia),[133-135] neurotransmitter mechanisms (decreased serotonin and norepinephrine), inflammatory cytokine-mediated (increased interleukins, IL-1β, IL-18, IL-6, and tumor necrosis factor alpha), and gene polymorphism mechanisms (e.g., a short variant of serotonin transporter gene-linked promoter region).[136,137] One study also showed an association between elevated serum levels of neopterin both in the acute post-stroke phase and in those with PSD at

6-month follow-up.[138] Psychological factors, largely related to the various functional and personal losses associated with stroke, also contribute to the development of PSD. The correlation between the stroke location and the likelihood of developing PSD has been controversial; some studies have found positive correlations, and a large meta-analysis of 143 studies by Carson and co-workers[139] found no correlation between lesion location and the risk of PSD.

PSD is associated with significant long-term negative effects on social function, motor abilities, and quality of life.[140] Moreover, the negative effect of depression on functional impairment continues well beyond the period of abnormal mood symptoms.[141] Such extended functional disability may be due to poor initial rehabilitation efforts by patients with PSD that limit the recovery of strength and mobility.

The diagnosis of PSD is straightforward in many cases, although certain situations can make diagnosis quite challenging. Several non-depressive neurologic stroke sequelae may resemble symptoms of depression. Patients with expressive aprosodias have monotonous speech that may make them appear sad or withdrawn, and their affect may appear blunted. The presence of anosognosia (neurologically mediated unawareness of illness usually associated with right parietal lesions) may look like denial associated with depression, and this symptom can itself lead to frustration and anger when others insist that the patient has a problem that he or she simply cannot recognize. Finally, aphasias can make the diagnosis of depression—or any diagnosis—more difficult because of the difficulty of communicating with such patients. By being aware of these potential neurologic sequelae and by carefully using criteria from the *Diagnostic and Statistical Manual of Mental Disorders, Fifth Edition* (DSM-5),[142] with particular attention paid to depressive symptoms that overlap less with concurrent medical and neurologic symptoms (e.g., feelings of guilt, worthlessness, hopelessness, suicidality), in most cases the psychiatrist can verify the presence or absence of PSD.

Despite the significant consequences of PSD (both because of under-diagnosis[119] and of the fear of intolerable side effects from antidepressant medications), it is often under-treated. However, early and effective treatment of depression is perhaps even more crucial in this patient population than it is in other populations, given the need for full mobilization for occupational and physical therapy and other functional re-training early in the course of recovery.

Several placebo-controlled trials have demonstrated that antidepressants are effective in the treatment of PSD. The majority of studies assessed for PSD in the setting of ischemic rather than of hemorrhagic stroke. SSRIs[143-146] and nortriptyline[147] have been shown to relieve symptoms of PSD; another study of nortriptyline found that treatment of depression resulted in improved cognitive outcomes.[148] A study by Robinson and associates[149] found that nortriptyline was more effective than was either fluoxetine or placebo in treating PSD and improving functional outcomes. Studies of PSD have found disruptions of both noradrenergic and serotonergic pathways[145]; the effectiveness of venlafaxine was demonstrated in a case series by Kucukalic and colleagues,[150] and only 2 of 30 patients studied had mild elevations in blood pressure, which would be a side effect of concern with venlafaxine in post-stroke patients. Finally, a 2008 systematic review of 12 pharmacotherapy trials found that antidepressant therapy is modestly beneficial for remission of PSD; however adverse events were more common with antidepressants.[151] More studies are needed to fully assess the risks versus benefits in this regard.

Psychostimulants have also been used in the treatment of PSD. Retrospective studies using psychostimulants (methylphenidate and dextroamphetamine) to treat PSD found these medications to be effective, with response rates of 47% to 80%.[152,153] Response to psychostimulants was rapid (usually within 48 hours), and adverse events were rare. However, unlike SSRIs and TCAs, psychostimulants have not been studied under placebo-controlled, double-blind conditions for the treatment of PSD.

ECT also appears to be an effective treatment for PSD, with high rates of response and low rates of medical complications.[154] ECT is more extensively discussed in Chapter 36. In addition, to the somatic treatments of PSD, there is evidence to suggest that care management programs, which include education, antidepressant treatment guided by algorithm, and close monitoring of therapy may be more effective than somatic treatments alone.[155] In addition to this, group and family psychotherapy have also been reported to safely and effectively treat PSD,[156,157] but there are few randomized and controlled trials of individual psychotherapies for PSD. One study found that problem-solving therapy reduced the incidence of depression and delayed the time to onset, compared with placebo, for post-stroke patients.[158] Although there is some positive evidence for CBT as a treatment of PSD,[151] other studies have found no significant difference between CBT, attention placebo, and standard care.[159] More studies are needed in this area.

Administration of psychiatric medications to at-risk populations to prevent the onset of psychiatric illness is an increasingly popular area of study. In this regard, several studies have evaluated whether antidepressant medication can prevent PSD.[158,160-162] Although initial studies have demonstrated differences in the rates of depression in post-stroke patients who received medication compared to placebo, they were not statistically significant and were under-powered.[160,161] A more methodologically sound study by Robinson and associates[158] evaluated 176 non-depressed patients within 3 months of stroke and randomized them to three groups, a double-blinded escitalopram and placebo group and a non-blinded problem-solving therapy group. Rates of MDD and minor depression were statistically significantly lower for both escitalopram and problem-solving therapy, although escitalopram remained significant only with an intention-to-treat analysis. The potential clinical impact of these studies is impressive, but more studies are needed to definitively guide clinical care.

For most patients with mild-to-moderate PSD, SSRIs are the treatment of choice, given their proven efficacy, favorable side effect profile, and cardiovascular safety. However, TCAs, despite higher rates of side effects than SSRIs, might also be considered first-line agents for PSD because of their potentially superior efficacy. For more severe depression that impairs decision-making capacity, nutritional intake, or ability to participate in rehabilitation, psychostimulants should be considered; methylphenidate or dextroamphetamine can be started at 2.5 to 5 mg in the morning, and a protocol for dosing and patient monitoring can be followed (Table 18.9). ECT can also be considered in patients with incapacitating depression. Prophylactic treatment with antidepressants to prevent depression is supported by preliminary studies and may be prudent in patients with numerous risk factors; careful analysis of risks and benefits for the individual patient is still required.

TABLE 18.9
Guidelines for the Use of Psychostimulants to Treat Depression

1. Consider possible (relative) contraindications to psychostimulant use:

   a. history of ventricular arrhythmia

   b. recent myocardial infarction

   c. congestive heart failure with reduced ejection fraction

   d. poorly controlled hypertension

   e. tachycardia

   f. concurrent treatment with monoamine oxidase inhibitors.

2. Initiate treatment with a morning dose of 5 mg methylphenidate or dextroamphetamine (2.5 mg in frail elderly or medically tenuous patients).

3. Check vital signs and response to treatment in 2–4 h (the period of peak effect).

4. If the initial dose is well tolerated and effective throughout the day, continue with a single daily morning dose.

5. If the initial dose is well tolerated and effective for several hours, with a loss of effect in the afternoon, give the same dose twice per day (in the morning and the early afternoon).

6. If the initial dose is well tolerated but is without significant clinical effect, increase the dose by 5 mg/day until a clinical response is achieved, intolerable side effects arise, or 20 mg dose is ineffective (i.e., a failed trial).

7. Continue treatment throughout the hospitalization; stimulants can usually be discontinued at discharge

Post-Stroke Apathy

Apathy is a disorder of diminished motivation and initiative that is characterized by restricted social engagement, lack of emotional response, and diminished cognitive abilities. In the post-stroke period, apathy has been historically seen as a symptom of other syndromes, such as depression or dementia, but emerging evidence suggests that it might be a distinct entity.[163,164] Post-stroke apathy (PSA) is as frequent as is PSD and is also associated with poor functional recovery and low QoL.[113,129] PSA has been associated with hemorrhagic stroke as well as with right hemispheric subcortical lesions with a particular focus in the basal ganglia and anterior cingulate circuit which is involved in motivation.[165] Although more studies on the treatment of PSA are needed, early work suggests the same treatment as PSD, including SSRIs and particularly psychostimulants.

Other Post-Stroke Psychiatric Phenomena

Other psychiatric syndromes that occur in the post-stroke period include anxiety, mania, and psychosis. Post-stroke anxiety is common, and usually arises in concert with PSD. Approximately one-fourth of patients meet the criteria for GAD (except for duration criteria) in the acute post-stroke period; at least three-fourths of these patients with post-stroke GAD symptoms have co-morbid depression.[166,167] Post-stroke anxiety has a negative impact on the functional recovery of stroke patients and has been associated with impairment of ADLs up to 3 years after the event.[167] The functional impairment of PSD and post-stroke GAD appear to be additive, insofar as patients with both GAD and PSD have greater ADL impairment at follow-up than those with isolated PSD.[168]

Post-stroke mania occurs in fewer than 1% of patients. Symptoms of post-stroke mania are like those of primary mania (with a flight of ideas, pressured speech, a decreased need for sleep, grandiosity, and associated psychotic symptoms). Lesions in the right orbitofrontal cortex, right basal temporal cortices, dorsomedial thalamus, and head of caudate appear to be associated most often with post-stroke mania.[169–174] Stroke in the right hemisphere, compared with the left, has led to increased serotonin binding, and it is hypothesized that this may result in post-stroke mania.[175]

Post-stroke psychosis is also uncommon, occurring at a rate of approximately 1% to 2%.[176] Such patients usually have right temporoparietal lesions and a high rate of associated seizures.[176,177] This suggests that temporal lobe damage that leads to complex partial seizures (CPS) and associated psychosis may account for symptoms in a significant percentage of these patients.

Finally, two other clinical neuropsychiatric syndromes are common in the post-stroke period. The first is termed *catastrophic reaction*, a collection of symptoms involving patient desperation and frustration. This syndrome is relatively common—especially in the acute phase; rates of post-stroke catastrophic reaction are 3% to 20%.[178,179] Catastrophic reactions are strongly associated with PSD, with roughly three-quarters of patients with catastrophic reactions having PSD.[179] Catastrophic reactions are also associated with a personal and family history of psychiatric disorders.[178]

Catastrophic reactions also appear to be associated with anterior sub-cortical lesions and with left cortical lesions.[178-180] Given the strong association of catastrophic reactions and depression, some feel that such a reaction is a behavioral symptom of depression (provoked by anterior sub-cortical damage) rather than a discrete syndrome. Others feel that catastrophic reactions result from damage to areas in the left hemisphere involved in the regulation of emotions related to social communication.[179]

The second of these clinical syndromes is *pseudobulbar affect*, also termed *pseudobulbar palsy*. This syndrome (which consists of frequent and easily provoked spells of laughing or crying) occurs to some degree in approximately 15% of post-stroke patients.[181,182] The pathophysiology is unknown but is thought to involve frontal release of brainstem emotional centers.[183] It is usually seen in a mild form, with brief fits of crying or laughing linked with appropriate changes in mood; however, in more serious cases, it may involve frequent and spontaneous fits of laughing and crying that are inappropriate to the context. It can cause embarrassment, curtailment of social activities, and a decreased quality of life.[184]

Treatment of these post-stroke phenomena generally parallels the treatment of primary psychiatric syndromes. Post-stroke anxiety can be treated like any primary anxiety syndrome. SSRIs are effective in the treatment of a variety of anxiety disorders, including GAD, and, given that most patients with post-stroke anxiety have co-morbid PSD, these agents are often the treatments of choice. Benzodiazepines can also be given for isolated anxiety, but they can lead to ataxia, sedation, and paradoxical disinhibition; therefore they must be used with caution in this population. Furthermore, these agents do not treat co-morbid depression.

Treatment of post-stroke mania follows the same rules as the treatment of primary mania. Mood stabilizers and adjunctive antipsychotic medications or benzodiazepines are used to control symptoms. Treatment studies of post-stroke mania have found that lithium, valproic acid, carbamazepine, neuroleptics, and clonidine are variably efficacious, although none of these treatments has been examined in placebo-controlled, double-blind trials for this condition.[170,175,185-187] Post-stroke psychosis can be treated symptomatically with antipsychotics. However, anticonvulsants (especially valproic acid and carbamazepine) should be used when psychotic symptoms are the result of CPS, because psychotic symptoms should improve with better seizure control.

Finally, pseudobulbar affect and catastrophic reaction may respond well to antidepressants. A few trials of TCAs and SSRIs, some of which were placebo-controlled, have demonstrated efficacy in reducing symptoms of pseudobulbar affect.[188-191] Additionally, the combination of dextromethorphan and quinidine has been shown to reduce laughing and crying spells due to pseudobulbar affect in patients with ALS[192] and may also be of benefit in the post-stroke setting. Symptoms of a catastrophic reaction may also improve with antidepressant treatment of co-morbid PSD.

In short, psychiatric symptoms after stroke are common and have a significant impact on the long-term outcome of post-stroke patients. Awareness of neurologic symptoms that may mimic psychiatric illness (e.g., anosognosia) and careful diagnostic interviews can allow accurate diagnosis and prompt treatment. In general, psychiatric symptoms secondary to stroke are treated in the same way as non-stroke-related psychiatric syndromes with similar symptoms.

MANAGEMENT OF PATIENTS WITH TRAUMATIC BRAIN INJURIES

TBIs are a leading cause of death and disability in the United States, contributing to 30% of injury deaths each year.[193] Recent data from the Centers for Disease Control and Prevention reveals that 1.7 million head injuries occur each year while 223,135 individuals were hospitalized due to TBI in 2019.[194] Of this group, psychosocial and psychological impairments lead to substantial disability and cause significant stress to their families. The consulting psychiatrist plays an important role in evaluating and treating these patients. This section will address the epidemiology and pathophysiology of TBI, followed by a discussion of the clinical features and treatment of the affective, behavioral, and cognitive aspects of TBI.

Epidemiology

Disorders that result from TBI are more common than any other neurologic disease, except for headache. Falls cause the majority: 28% of TBIs, and motor vehicle accidents (20%); assaults (11%); having one's head struck against an object (19%); other trauma (13%); and unknown trauma (9%) account for the remaining TBIs.[193] Among adults, alcohol is a contributing factor in 40% to 56% of cases.[193,195] The highest rates of hospitalization and death after TBI are found in persons older than 75 years.[193] Individuals who have had one brain injury are three times as likely, compared with the general population, to sustain a second, and after a second TBI the risk of another is 10 times higher.[193] It should be noted, however, that even more mild TBIs (i.e., without an associated hospital stay) may result in neuropsychiatric sequelae.

Pathophysiology

TBI can be divided into primary and secondary brain injuries. Primary injury consists of focal and diffuse lesions. Focal TBI generally results from a blow to the head that produces cerebral contusions or hematomas. Epidural hematomas, SDHs, and cerebral contusions are all types of focal lesions. The location, size, and progression of the injury determine the resultant morbidity and mortality.[195] Most injuries occur in the polar temporal lobes and on the inferior surface of the frontal lobes because of contact with the bony prominences along the base of the skull, often a result of a coup-contrecoup mechanism of injury. All are diagnosed by CT scanning or an MRI scan of the brain. An epidural hematoma is usually caused by head trauma that is associated with a lateral skull fracture and with tearing of the middle meningeal artery and vein and therefore is most often located in the temporal or temporoparietal region.[195] There is often LOC followed by a period of lucidity, and then neurologic deterioration. Prompt surgical evacuation of the hematoma is essential. SDH is more common than epidural hematoma and generally results from the tearing of a bridging vein between the cortex and a venous sinus. Much of the force of an impact is often transmitted to the brain, and the underlying brain injury determines the outcome in approximately 80% of cases.[195] Treatment also involves surgical evacuation. Finally, traumatic cerebral contusion is often associated with an initial bout of unconsciousness, generally followed by recovery. Edema may cause fluctuations in the level of consciousness, seizures, or focal neurologic signs. Surgery is rarely undertaken for cerebral contusions.

Diffuse lesions, or *diffuse axonal injury*, are seen more commonly in injuries that involve rapid acceleration, deceleration, or rotational forces.[196] The sites most prone to such injury are the reticular formation, basal ganglia, superior cerebellar peduncles, limbic fornices, hypothalamus, and corpus callosum.[196] Patients who suffer diffuse axonal injury have high rates of morbidity and mortality. The diagnosis, often missed on CT, may be made by the use of diffusion-weighted MRI, which is sensitive to the axonal swelling seen after injury. The lack of radiographic evidence of injury does not translate into an absence of damage. Deficits in arousal, attention, and cognition (i.e., processing speed) often result from diffuse axonal injury.

Whereas primary brain injury (focal and diffuse) results from mechanical injury at the time of the trauma, secondary brain injury is caused by the physiologic responses to the initial injury. This is thought to involve a cascade of events, with edema and hematomas leading to increased ICP, which leads to compression and deformation of surrounding brain tissue and further damage. Neuronal damage is also mediated by the release of neurotoxic substances. Although a full discussion of each of these is beyond the scope of this chapter, each substance must be considered when evaluating the status of a brain-injured individual in the acute care setting.

Clinical Presentation

TBI is often divided into three categories according to the severity and the duration of altered mental status; however, there is no definitive breakdown of specific types of sequelae that may be affiliated with each. Whereas more severe injuries are often thought to have more persistent and pervasive consequences, there are certainly instances of significant morbidity even with mild TBI. The severity of the injury is classified by the Glasgow Coma Scale (GCS; Table 18.10). Mild head injury correlates with a GCS score of 13 to 15, moderate injury with a GCS score of 9 to 12, and severe head injury corresponds to a GCS score of less than 8. Lower scores are associated with more severe injury and poorer recovery outcomes.[194]

Other factors that may increase morbidity include the following: lower intelligence quotient (IQ), a concomitant SUD, older age, and a history of brain injury. Moreover, the DSM-5[142] suggests the following

TABLE 18.10
Glasgow Coma Scale

Eye Opening

Spontaneous	4
To voice	3
To painful stimulus	2
None	1

Verbal Response

Oriented	5
Confused	4
Inappropriate words	3
Unintelligible sounds	2
None	1

Motor Response

Follows commands	6
Localizes pain	5
Withdraws from pain	4
Flexor response	3
Extensor response	2
None	1

criteria to establish the severity of injury significant enough to cause a neurocognitive disorder (NCD) due to TBI (one or more of the following): (1) LOC; (2) post-traumatic amnesia; or (3) disorientation and confusion; (4) neurologic signs (e.g., neuroimaging demonstrating injury; a new onset of seizures; a marked worsening of a pre-existing seizure disorder; visual field cuts; anosmia; hemiparesis). The NCD must present immediately after the TBI or immediately after recovery of consciousness and persist past the acute post-injury period. Diagnostic features of this disorder also include cognitive disturbances as well as fatigue; disordered sleep; headache; vertigo or dizziness; irritability or aggression; anxiety, depression, or affective lability; changes in personality; and apathy or a lack of spontaneity. Of note, this syndrome is known to neurologists and the lay public as post-concussive syndrome.

These features are representative of the three major categories of neuropsychiatric sequelae that may be seen with TBI: cognitive impairment, changes in personality and behavior, and Axis I psychiatric disorders (e.g., mood, anxiety, and psychotic disorders). Each of these is outlined briefly.

Cognitive Impairment

Cognitive difficulties in acute care settings following TBI may be due to the brain injury itself, delirium, or other factors. As recovery progresses, deficits related to the TBI (e.g., attentional impairment, associated with the reticular activating system and prefrontal white matter) become more apparent.[197] Impairments in language and executive function (those skills necessary for independence in the world) as well as memory, often follow TBI.[197] Examples of executive dysfunction include poor planning, impaired abstraction, and difficulties with calculations. Neurocognitive testing is essential to further specify and quantify deficits. Moreover, neuropsychological testing is invaluable in designing an individualized rehabilitation program to meet the specific needs of each patient.

Personality Changes

Personality change due to TBI is a DSM-5[142] diagnosis characterized by a persistent personality disturbance that represents a change from the individual's prior personality; it is a direct consequence of the injury and is not better explained by delirium, dementia, or another Axis I disorder. The disturbance must also cause clinically significant distress or impairment in occupational or social function.[142] The terms *frontal lobe syndrome* and *organic personality syndrome* are often used to describe these personality changes.[198] Personality changes and behavioral manifestations often include labile affect, disinhibition, poor social judgment, apathy, lewdness, loss of social graces, perseveration, aggressive behavior, paranoia, and inattention to personal hygiene. In a 30-year follow-up study of patients with TBI, Koponen and colleagues[199] found that 23% of injured adults manifested an Axis II diagnosis. These changes may be a direct result of the TBI but also may be exacerbated or caused by delirium, seizures, or use of medications or substances. When evaluating personality changes, the physician should note that the patient may have little insight into the change, so including supportive family members in the evaluation and planning of treatment is essential. Additionally, families may need significant support to cope with changes present in their loved ones.

Mood and Anxiety Disorders

As many as 40% of patients with TBI will develop an Axis I disorder, most commonly MDD, an AUD, panic disorder, a specific phobia, or a psychotic disorder.[199] Depression occurs in 26% to 77% of those with mild TBI, whereas higher rates of depression are associated with more severe injuries.[200-203] These individuals have a higher risk because of the neuroanatomic and physiologic changes that occur and because of lost capabilities, changes in roles, and financial and other losses that have occurred.[204] Pre-morbid substance abuse, poor functioning, a lower education level, and an unstable work history predict depression after TBI.[205,206] Because there may be a significant overlap between cognitive impairment and personality changes, the diagnosis must be made with care. MDD is associated with poor outcomes across multiple domains; this makes its early diagnosis and treatment particularly important. Prominent signs and symptoms include fatigue, distractibility, anger, irritability, and rumination. Neuropsychological testing may be helpful in these individuals. Finally, there is an increased risk of suicide after TBI; up to 15% of individuals make a suicide attempt in the 5 years after TBI. In this population, intense despair, hopelessness, worthlessness, and loss of sense of integrity, as well as relationship breakdown and isolation, contribute to the risk of suicide.[204,207] Additionally, prominent insomnia and chronic headaches often exacerbate the situation. The combination of depression and disinhibition associated with frontal lobe injury is also thought to contribute to higher rates of suicide.

Mania has also been shown to occur more often after TBI than it does in the general population.[203] Predisposing factors may include a family history of affective illness, right temporal lobe lesions, and right orbitofrontal cortex injuries; unfortunately, consensus is lacking. Furthermore, seizures seem to be more common in this group;[203] this makes the EEG an important diagnostic tool following TBI. For this reason, AEDs are the preferred mood stabilizers after TBI (see Treatment, below).

Regarding anxiety disorders after TBI, GAD, and PTSD appear to be the most common.[203-209] OCD, specific phobias, and panic disorder have also been reported.[210] GAD is co-morbid with depression in approximately 11% of patients. There is some evidence that early intervention with CBT for acute stress disorder may prevent PTSD after mild TBI.[208] Other investigators have shown a relationship between impaired memory of the traumatic event and lower rates of PTSD;[209] however, more research is needed in this area.

Psychosis

Psychosis due to TBI is thought to be relatively rare. Although some authors doubt that a correlation exists,[203] others argue that psychosis may appear immediately after brain injury or years later (with rates between 0.7% and 9.8%).[211] Frontal and temporal lobe injuries are associated with psychosis, as are post-traumatic seizures.[212] Cognitive impairment and behavioral changes (already described) may mimic the symptoms of schizophrenia. Because individuals with schizophrenia have also been found to have a higher incidence of brain injury than those in the general population,[212] it may be true that head injury predisposes these individuals to schizophrenia. Alternatively, it may be that individuals who are already predisposed to schizophrenia have a higher incidence of brain injury for other reasons.

Treatment

Treatment of neuropsychiatric sequelae of TBI is best accomplished with a comprehensive, multi-disciplinary, rehabilitative approach. This may include psychiatric, neurologic, psychological, behavioral, occupational, and vocational evaluations. Specific brain injury centers are best equipped to undertake this; however, not all communities have such resources. Psychiatric evaluation and consultation generally focus on several areas of intervention: pharmacological, behavioral, cognitive, and social (family support). These are discussed in the following sections.

Pharmacology

In general, medications effective for primary psychiatric disorders in non-TBI patients are similarly effective in patients who have sustained a TBI. Because brain-injured patients are often more sensitive to certain medications and their side effects, several guidelines should be considered. The principle of "start low and go slow" is wise; however, being overly cautious may lead to inadequate medication trials if therapeutic doses are not achieved or medications are not given enough time to work. Slow titration as tolerated by side effects and adequate duration of trials should be the goal.

Although the treatment of depression and anxiety in patients with TBI follows the same principles as those for the treatment of depression and anxiety in the general population, careful attention should be paid to medication side effects. Medications with a high potential for lowering the seizure threshold (such as some dopaminergic agonists and antagonists), causing sedation (typically mediated by antihistamine effects), and inducing anticholinergic side effects and hypotension (usually mediated by peripheral alpha antagonism) should be avoided or used with great care if no better alternative exists. TCAs and bupropion, which both lower the seizure threshold, are generally avoided. SSRIs are usually well tolerated. Several studies (only one of which was an RCT) with citalopram, fluoxetine, and sertraline have demonstrated improvements in mood and aggression.[213–216] Psychostimulants may be employed for depressive symptoms (irritability, apathy, and depressed mood), cognitive symptoms (arousal, processing speed, and attention), and fatigue,[217,218] although paradoxical dysphoria, agitation, and paranoia may be seen in those following a brain injury. Improvements have also been seen in depression, anxiety, irritability, and aggression with buspirone; it has a more favorable side effect profile and less abuse potential than benzodiazepines.[219–221] Propranolol (a β-blocker) has been shown to reduce the intensity of agitation and aggression following TBI.[211] Amantadine hydrochloride is a treatment considered to have potential therapeutic value in this population and has been shown to accelerate recovery in patients with severe TBI.[222] Finally, ECT remains a good option and is often under-utilized. Care should be taken to assess memory and cognitive dysfunction before recommending ECT, given the potential side effects of this treatment.

Mania should be treated using standard agents. However, neurotoxicity from lithium may develop at higher rates in patients with TBI; anticonvulsant mood stabilizers, such as valproic acid or carbamazepine, may be preferable. For patients with co-morbid seizures, AEDs are the treatment of choice.

Neuroleptics are frequently used for agitation and aggression in TBI patients, as well as psychosis. The use of neuroleptics in this population is controversial given research, largely conducted on animals, that indicates they interfere with neural plasticity and are associated with longer post-traumatic amnesia and worse outcomes.[217,223] That said, there is also evidence that antipsychotics may be effective for the management of agitation and aggressive behavior.[224] Because patients following a brain injury are at increased risk for extrapyramidal symptoms (e.g., dystonias, akathisias, and parkinsonian side effects), high-potency agents should be used with care, and atypical antipsychotics are generally preferred over typical (first generation) antipsychotics. Antipsychotics with significant anticholinergic side effects (e.g., clozapine and low-potency typical agents) and antipsychotics that lower the seizure threshold, such as clozapine, should be monitored carefully.

Finally, benzodiazepines and barbiturates should be used sparingly in patients with TBI because of their potential to cause paradoxical disinhibition, sedation, and worsening of cognitive and motor impairments.[217] If rapid sedation is desired in an agitated patient, low doses may be used with caution.

Behavioral, Cognitive, and Social Interventions

Once deficits related to TBI have been delineated, a comprehensive plan of treatment can be instituted. Behavioral treatments are helpful for the management of maladaptive social behaviors (including aggression) and personality disorders. For patients with prominent mood or anxiety symptoms, who are easily agitated, or who have low thresholds to anger and aggression, environmental modification (e.g., increasing structure, simplifying tasks, reducing or increasing stimulation, and removing triggers and irritations) helps reduce symptoms.[225] Specific cognitive rehabilitation programs may be helpful, depending on individual deficits. These deficits are best assessed by the administration of neuropsychiatric testing. Teaching about stress management and coping skills may also be particularly useful. Finally, psychotherapeutic and social interventions, including family education and supportive therapy, may prove useful given the sense of loss and distress often felt by family members and loved ones.

CONCLUSION

TBI is an important cause of neuropsychiatric disability in the United States. A thorough assessment of mood, anxiety, personality change, and cognition should be a routine part of post-injury screening. The consulting psychiatrist plays an important role in the evaluation and treatment of these patients. Prompt diagnosis and treatment, as well as appropriate referral using a multidisciplinary approach, will greatly benefit patients and their families.

REFERENCES

1. Marsh L, Rao V. Psychiatric complications in patients with epilepsy: a review. *Epilepsy Res.* 2002;49(1):11–33.
2. Schwartz JM, Marsh L. The psychiatric perspectives of epilepsy. *Psychosomatics.* 2000;41(1):31–38.
3. Fisher RS, van Emde Boas W, Blume W, et al. Epileptic seizures and epilepsy: definitions proposed by the International League Against Epilepsy (ILAE) and the International Bureau for Epilepsy (IBE). *Epilepsia.* 2005;46(4):470–472.
4. Geschwind N. Behavioural changes in temporal lobe epilepsy. *Psychol Med.* 1979;9(2):217–219.
5. Engel J, Pedley TA, Aicardi J, eds. *Epilepsy: A Comprehensive Textbook.* 2nd ed. Lippincott Williams & Wilkins; 2007.
6. Engel J. *Seizures and Epilepsy.* FA Davis; 1989.
7. Williamson PD, Spencer SS. Clinical and EEG features of complex partial seizures of extratemporal origin. *Epilepsia.* 1986;27(suppl 2):46–63.
8. Sachdev P. Schizophrenia-like psychosis and epilepsy: the status of the association. *Am J Psychiatry.* 1998;155(3):325–336.
9. Williams D. The structure of emotions reflected in epileptic experiences. *Brain.* 1956;79(1):29–67.
10. Barry JJ. The recognition and management of mood disorders as a comorbidity of epilepsy. *Epilepsia.* 2003;44(suppl 4):30–40.
11. Delgado-Escueta AV, Mattson RH, King L, et al. Special report. The nature of aggression during epileptic seizures. *N Engl J Med.* 1981;305(12):711–716.
12. Scaramelli A, Braga P, Avellanal A, et al. Prodromal symptoms in epileptic patients: clinical characterization of the pre-ictal phase. *Seizure.* 2009;18(4):246–250.
13. Fenwick P. The basis of behavioral treatments in seizure control. *Epilepsia.* 1995;36(suppl 1):46–50.
14. Lancman M. Psychosis and peri-ictal confusional states. *Neurology.* 1999;53(5 suppl 2):33–38.
15. Kanner AM, Stagno S, Kotagal P, et al. Postictal psychiatric events during prolonged video-electroencephalographic monitoring studies. *Arch Neurol.* 1996;53(3):258–263.
16. Nadkarni S, Arnedo V, Devinsky O. Psychosis in epilepsy patients. *Epilepsia.* 2007;48(suppl 9):17–19.
17. Kanner AM, Balabanov A. Depression and epilepsy: how closely related are they? *Neurology.* 2002;58(8 suppl 5):27–39.
18. Standage KF, Fenton GW. Psychiatric symptom profiles of patients with epilepsy: a controlled investigation. *Psychol Med.* 1975;5(2):152–160.
19. Barraclough BM. The suicide rate of epilepsy. *Acta Psychiatr Scand.* 1987;76(4):339–345.
20. Mendez MF. Depression in epilepsy. *Arch Neurol.* 1986;43(8):766–770.
21. Currie S, Heathfield KWG, Henson RA, et al. Clinical course and prognosis of temporal lobe epilepsy: a survey of 666 patients. *Brain.* 1971;94(1):173–190.
22. Blumer D, Zielinski JJ. Pharmacologic treatment of psychiatric disorders associated with epilepsy. *J Epilepsy.* 1988;1(3):135–150.
23. Harris EC, Barraclough B. Suicide as an outcome for mental disorders. A meta-analysis. *Br J Psychiatry.* 1997;170(3):205–228.
24. Forsgren L, Nyström L. An incident case-referent study of epileptic seizures in adults. *Epilepsy Res.* 1990;6(1):66–81.
25. Kanner AM, Barry JJ. Is the psychopathology of epilepsy different from that of nonepileptic patients? *Epilepsy Behav.* 2001;2(3):170–186.
26. Blumer D, Montouris G, Hermann B. Psychiatric morbidity in seizure patients on a neurodiagnostic monitoring unit. *J Neuropsychiatry Clin Neurosci.* 1995;7(4):445–456.
27. Slater E, Beard AW. The schizophrenia-like psychoses of epilepsy: I. Psychiatric aspects. *Br J Psychiatry.* 1963;109(458):95–112.
28. Gastaut H, Roger J, Lesevre N. Differenciation psychologique des epileptiques en fonction des formes electrocliniques de leur maladie. *Rev Psychol Appl.* 1953;3:237–249.
29. Devinsky O, Najjar S. Evidence against the existence of a temporal lobe epilepsy personality syndrome. *Neurology.* 1999;53(5 suppl 2):13–25.
30. Patorno E, Bohn RL, Wahl PM, et al. Anticonvulsant medications and the risk of suicide, attempted suicide, or violent death. *JAMA.* 2010;303(14):1401–1409.
31. Schmitz B. Effects of antiepileptic drugs on mood and behavior. *Epilepsia.* 2006;47(suppl 2):28–33.
32. French JA, Krauss GL, Wechsler RT, et al. Perampanel for tonic-clonic seizures in idiopathic generalized epilepsy. A randomized trial. *Neurology.* 2015;85(11):950–957.
33. Kwan P, Brodie MJ, Laurenza A, et al. Analysis of pooled phase III trials of adjunctive perampanel for epilepsy: impact of mechanism of action and pharmacokinetics on clinical outcomes. *Epilepsy Res.* 2015;117:117–124.
34. Mula M, Sander JW. Suicide risk in people with epilepsy taking antiepileptic drugs. *Bipolar Disord.* 2013;15(5):622–627.
35. Major P, Greenberg E, Khan A, et al. Pyridoxine supplementation for the treatment of levetiracetam-induced behavior side effects in children: preliminary results. *Epilepsy Behav.* 2008;13(3):557–559.
36. Kanner AM, Kozak AM, Frey M. The use of sertraline in patients with epilepsy: is it safe? *Epilepsy Behav.* 2000;1(2):100–105.
37. Hovorka J, Herman E, Nemcová I. Treatment of interictal depression with citalopram in patients with epilepsy. *Epilepsy Behav.* 2000;1(6):444–447.
38. Post RM, Putnam F, Uhde TW, et al. Electroconvulsive therapy as an anticonvulsant. *Ann N Y Acad Sci.* 1986;462:376–388.
39. Sackeim HA. The anticonvulsant hypothesis of the mechanisms of action of ECT: current status. *J ECT.* 1999;15(1):5–26.
40. Fink M, Kellner CH, Sackeim HA. Intractable seizures, status epilepticus, and ECT. *J ECT.* 1999;15(4):282–283.
41. McConnell H, Duncan D. Treatment of psychiatric comorbidity in epilepsy. In: McConnell H, Snyder P, eds. *Psychiatric Comorbidity in Epilepsy: Basic Mechanisms, Diagnosis, and Treatment.* American Psychiatric Press; 1998:245–362.

42. Pisani F, Oteri G, Costa C, et al. Effects of psychotropic drugs on seizure threshold. *Drug Saf.* 2002;25(2):91–110.

43. Aybek S, Perez DL. Diagnosis and management of functional neurological disorder. *BMJ.* 2022;376:064.

44. Barry E, Krumholz A, Bergey GK, et al. Nonepileptic posttraumatic seizures. *Epilepsia.* 1998;39(4):427–431.

45. Krumholz A, Niedermeyer E. Psychogenic seizures: a clinical study with follow-up data. *Neurology.* 1983;33(4):498–502.

46. Kerr MP, Mensah S, Besag F, et al. International consensus clinical practice statements for the treatment of neuropsychiatric conditions associated with epilepsy. *Epilepsia.* 2011;52(11):2133–2138.

47. LaFrance WC, Baird GL, Barry JJ, et al. Multicenter pilot treatment trial for psychogenic nonepileptic seizures: a randomized clinical trial. *JAMA Psychiatry.* 2014;71(9):997–1005.

48. Alper K, Devinsky O, Perrine K, et al. Nonepileptic seizures and childhood sexual and physical abuse. *Neurology.* 1993;43(10):1950–1953.

49. Fiszman A, Alves-Leon SV, Nunes RG, et al. Traumatic events and posttraumatic stress disorder in patients with psychogenic nonepileptic seizures: a critical review. *Epilepsy Behav.* 2004;5(6):818–825.

50. Devinsky O, Fisher R. Ethical use of placebos and provocative testing in diagnosing nonepileptic seizures. *Neurology.* 1996;47(4):866–870.

51. Krumholz A, Ting T. Psychogenic nonepileptic seizures. In: Johnson RT, Griffin JW, McArthur JC, eds. *Current Therapy in Neurologic Disease.* 7th ed. Mosby Elsevier; 2006:49–53.

52. Krumholz A. Nonepileptic seizures: diagnosis and management. *Neurology.* 1999;53(5 suppl 2):76–83.

53. Bare MA, Burnstine TH, Fisher RS, et al. Electroencephalographic changes during simple partial seizures. *Epilepsia.* 1994;35(4):715–720.

54. Benbadis SR. Provocative techniques should be used for the diagnosis of psychogenic nonepileptic seizures. *Epilepsy Behav.* 2009;15(2):106–118.

55. Cragar DE, Berry DTR, Fakhoury TA, et al. A review of diagnostic techniques in the differential diagnosis of epileptic and nonepileptic seizures. *Neuropsychol Rev.* 2002;12(1):31–64.

56. Drane DL, Williamson DJ, Stroup ES, et al. Cognitive impairment is not equal in patients with epileptic and psychogenic nonepileptic seizures. *Epilepsia.* 2006;47(11):1879–1886.

57. Prigatano GP, Kirlin KA. Self-appraisal and objective assessment of cognitive and affective functioning in persons with epileptic and nonepileptic seizures. *Epilepsy Behav.* 2009;14(2):387–392.

58. Henrichs TF, Tucker DM, Farha J, et al. MMPI indices in the identification of patients evidencing pseudoseizures. *Epilepsia.* 1988;29(2):184–187.

59. Kutlubaev MA, Xu Y, Hackett ML, et al. Dual diagnosis of epilepsy and psychogenic nonepileptic seizures: systematic review and meta-analysis of frequency, correlates, and outcomes. *Epilepsy Behav.* 2018;89:70–78.

60. Dodick DW. Diagnosing headache: clinical clues and clinical rules. *Adv Stud Med.* 2003;3:S550–S555.

61. Stovner LJ, Hagen K, Linde M, et al. The global prevalence of headache: an update, with analysis of the influences of methodological factors on prevalence estimates. *J Headache Pain.* 2022;23:34.

62. Steiner TJ, Stovner LJ, Jensen R, et al. Migraine remains second among the world's causes of disability, and first among young women: findings from GBD2019. *J Headache Pain.* 2020;21:137.

63. International Headache Society.. The international classification of headache disorders: 3rd edition. *Cephalalgia.* 2018;38(1):1–211.

64. Cutrer FM, Bhasin P. Headache. In: Ballantyne J, ed. *The Massachusetts General Hospital Handbook of Pain Management.* 2nd ed. Lippincott Williams & Wilkins; 2002.

65. Lance JW, Goadsby PJ. *Mechanism and Management of Headache.* 7th ed. Elsevier; 2005.

66. Schain AJ, Agustin M, Strassman AM, et al. Cortical spreading depression closes paravascular space and impairs glymphatic flow: implications for migraine headache. *J Neurosci.* 2017;37(11):2904–2915.

67. Kruit MC, van Buchen MA, Hofman PAM, et al. Migraine as a risk factor for subclinical brain lesions. *JAMA.* 2004;291:427–434.

68. Palm-Meinders IH, Koppen H, Terwindt GM, et al. Structural brain changes in migraine. *JAMA.* 2012;308:1889–1897.

69. Kaufman DM, Geyer HL, Milstein MJ. *Clinical Neurology for Psychiatrists.* 8th ed. Elsevier; 2017.

70. Nestoriuc Y, Martin A, Rief W, et al. Biofeedback treatment for headache disorders: a comprehensive efficacy review. *Appl Psychophysiol Biofeedback.* 2008;33:125–140.

71. Steiner TJ. Evaluation and management of headache in primary care. *Expert Rev Neurother.* 2004;4(3):425–437.

72. Mathew NT. The prophylactic treatment of chronic daily headache. *Headache.* 2004;46(10):1552–1564.

73. Bendtsen L, Jensen R. Mirtazapine is effective in the prophylactic treatment of chronic tension-type headache. *Neurology.* 2004;62:1706–1711.

74. Freund B, Rao A. Efficacy of botulinum toxin in tension-type headaches: a systematic review of the literature. *Pain Pract.* 2019; Jun;19(5):541–551.

75. Bron C, Sutherland HG, Griffiths LR. Exploring the hereditary nature of migraine. *Neuropsychiatr Dis Treat.* 2021; Apr 22;17:1183–1194.

76. Campbell JK, Penzien DB, Wall EM, et al. *Evidence-Based Guidelines for Migraine Headache: Behavioral and Physical Treatments.* US Headache Consortium. Available at: <https://www.hpmaine.com/images/PDFs/aan-guidelines.pdf >; 2000.

77. Seng EK, Singer AB, Metts C, et al. Does mindfulness-based cognitive therapy for migraine reduce migraine-related disability in people with episodic and chronic migraine? A phase 2b pilot randomized clinical trial. *Headache.* 2019;59(9):1448–1467.

78. Evans RW, Tepper SJ, Shapiro RE, et al. The FDA alert on serotonin syndrome with use of triptans combined with selective serotonin reuptake inhibitors or selective serotonin-norepinephrine reuptake inhibitors: american headache society position paper. *Headache.* 2010;50(6):1089–1099.

79. Orlova Y, Rizzoli P, Loder E. Association of coprescription of triptan antimigraine drugs and selective serotonin reuptake inhibitor or selective norepinephrine reuptake inhibitor antidepressants with serotonin syndrome. *JAMA Neurol.* 2018;75(5): 566–572.

80. Schwenk ES, Walter A, Torjman MC, et al. Lidocaine infusions for refractory chronic migraine: a retrospective analysis. *Reg Anesth Pain Med.* 2022;47(7):408–413.

81. Fischera M, Marziniak M, Gralow I, et al. The incidence and prevalence of cluster headache: a meta-analysis of population-based studies. *Cephalalgia.* 2008;28(6):614–618.

82. Gooriah R, Buture A, Ahmed F. Evidence-based treatments for cluster headache. *Ther Clin Risk Manag.* 2015;11:1687–1696.

83. Saper JR, Lake III AE, Hamel RL, et al. Daily scheduled opioids for intractable head pain: long-term observations of a treatment program. *Neurology.* 2004;62:1687–1694.

84. Limmroth V, Katsarava Z, Fritsche G, et al. Features of medication overuse headache following different acute headache drugs. *Neurology.* 2002;59:1011–1014.

85. Medication overuse: diagnosis and treatment. In: Young W, Silberstein S, Nahas S, et al. eds. *Jefferson Headache Manual.* 1st ed. Demos; 2011. Available at: <https://www.r2library.com/Resource/Title/1933864702>

86. Evers S, Jensen R. Treatment of medication overuse headache—guideline of the EFNS headache panel. *Eur J Neurol.* 2011;18:1115–1121.

87. Pompili M, Di Cosimo D, Innamorati M, et al. Psychiatric comorbidity in patients with chronic daily headache and migraine: a selective overview including personality traits and suicide risk. *J Headache Pain.* 2009;10(4):283–290.

88. Louter MA, Wilbrink LA, Haan J, et al. Cluster headache and depression. *Neurology.* 2016;87(18):1899–1906.

89. Leo RJ, Singh J. Migraine headache and bipolar disorder comorbidity: a systematic review of the literature and clinical implications. *Scand J Pain.* 2016;11:136–145.

90. Fornaro M, De Berardis D, De Pasquale C, et al. Prevalence and clinical features associated to bipolar disorder-migraine comorbidity: a systematic review. *Compr Psychiatry.* 2015;56:1–16.

91. Ashina S, Serrano D, Lipton RB, et al. Depression and risk of transformation of episodic to chronic migraine. *J Headache Pain.* 2012;13(8):615–624.

92. Naomi B, Schultz L. Migraine headaches and suicide attempt. *Headache.* 2012;52(5):723–731.

93. Guglielmetti M, Serafini G, Amore M, et al. The relation between persistent post-traumatic headache and PTSD: similarities and possible differences. *Int J Environ Res Public Health.* 2020;17(11):4024.

94. Salem H, Vivas D, Cao F, et al. ADHD is associated with migraine: a systematic review and meta-analysis. *Eur Child Adolesc Psychiatry.* 2018;27(3):267–277.

95. Harmon KG, Drezner JA, Gammons M, et al. American Medical Society for Sports Medicine position statement: concussion in sport [published correction appears in. *Br J Sports Med.* 2013;47(1):15–26. Br J Sports Med. 2013;47(1):15–26.

96. Lau CI, Liu MN, Chen WH, et al. Clinical and biobehavioral perspectives: is medication overuse headache a behavior of dependence? *Prog Brain Res.* 2020;255:371–402.

97. Gordon-Smith K, Forty L, Chan C, et al. Rapid cycling as a feature of bipolar disorder and comorbid migraine. *J Affect Disord.* 2015;175:320–324.

98. Sachs GS, Lafer B, Stoll AL, et al. A double-blind trial of bupropion versus desipramine for bipolar depression. *J Clin Psychiatry.* 1994;55(9):391–393.

99. Riediger C, Schuster T, Barlinn K, et al. Adverse effects of antidepressants for chronic pain: a systematic review and meta-analysis. *Front Neurol.* 2017;8:307.

100. Telang S, Walton C, Olten B, et al. Meta-analysis: second generation antidepressants and headache. *J Affect Disord.* 2018;236:60–68.

101. Brewerton TD, Murphy DL, Mueller EA, et al. Induction of migraine-like headaches by the serotonin agonist m-chlorophenylpiperazine. *Clin Pharmacol Ther.* 1988;43(6): 605–609.

102. Leone M, Attanasio A, Croci D, et al. The serotonergic agent m-chlorophenylpiperazine induces migraine attacks: a controlled study. *Neurology.* 2000;55(1):136–139.

103. Rampello L, Alvano A, Chiechio S, et al. Evaluation of the prophylactic efficacy of amitriptyline and citalopram, alone or in combination, in patients with comorbidity of depression, migraine, and tension-type headache. *Neuropsychobiology.* 2004;50(4):322–328.

104. Evans RW, Burch RC, Frishberg BM, et al. Neuroimaging for migraine: the American Headache Society systematic review and evidence-based guideline. *Headache.* 2020;60(2):318–336.

105. Denninger JW, Norris ER, Samuels MA. Headache. In: Stern TA, Herman JB, eds. *Psychiatry Update and Board Preparation.* 2nd ed. McGraw-Hill; 2004.

106. Minyard AN, Parker JC. Intracranial saccular (berry) aneurysm: a brief overview. *South Med J.* 1997;90(7):672–677.

107. Stam J. Thrombosis of the cerebral veins and sinuses. *N Engl J Med.* 2005;352(17):1791–1798.

108. Tana C, Bentivegna E, Cho SJ, et al. Long COVID headache. *J Headache Pain.* 2022 Aug 1;23(1):93.

109. Feigin VL, Stark BA, Johnson CO, et al. Global, regional, and national burden of stroke and its risk factors, 1990-2019: a systematic analysis for the Global Burden of Disease Study 2019. *Lancet Neurol.* 2021;20(10):795–820.

110. Heron M. *Deaths: Leading Causes for 2018.* National Center for Health Statistics; 2021.

111. Murray CJL, Abbafati C, Abbas KM, et al. Five insights from the Global Burden of Disease Study 2019. *Lancet.* 2020;396: 1135–1159.

112. Jorge RE, Starkstein SE, Robinson RG. Apathy following stroke. *Can J Psychiatry.* 2010;55:350–354.

113. van Dalen JW, van Charante EPM, Nederkoorn PJ, et al. Poststroke apathy. *Stroke.* 2013;44:851–860.

114. Carod-Artal J, Egido JA, Gonzalez JL, et al. Quality of life among stroke survivors evaluated 1 year after stroke: experience of a stroke unit. *Stroke.* 2000;31:2995–3000.

115. Ayerbe L, Ayis S, Wolfe CD, et al. Natural history, predictors and outcomes of depression after stroke; systematic review and meta-analysis. *Br J Psychiatry.* 2013;202:14–21.

116. Kraeplin E. *Manic Depressive Insanity and Paranoia.* E and S Livingstone; 1921.

117. Bleuler EP. *Textbook of Psychiatry*. Macmillan; 1924.
118. Ironside R. Disorders of laughter due to brain lesions. *Brain*. 1956;79:589–609.
119. Schubert DS, Burns R, Paras W, et al. Increase in medical hospital length of stay by depression in stroke and amputation patients: a pilot study. *Psychother Psychosom*. 1992;57:61–66.
120. Langhorne P. Organisation of acute stroke care. *Br Med Bull*. 2000;56:436–443.
121. Rahkonen T, Makela H, Paanila S, et al. Delirium in elderly people without severe predisposing disorders: etiology and 1-year prognosis after discharge. *Int Psychogeriatr*. 2000;12:473–481.
122. McManus J, Pathansali R, Hassan H, et al. The course of delirium in acute stroke. *Age Ageing*. 2009;38:385–389.
123. Sheng AZ, Shen Q, Cordato D, et al. Delirium within three days of stroke in a cohort of elderly patients. *J Am Geriatr Soc*. 2006;54:1192–1198.
124. Reitz C, Luchsinger JA, Mayeux R, et al. Vascular disease and cognitive impairment. *Expert Rev Neurother*. 2008;8:1171–1174.
125. Desmond DW, Moroney JT, Paik MC, et al. Frequency and clinical determinants of dementia after ischemic stroke. *Neurology*. 2000;54:1124–1131.
126. Pendlebury ST, Rothwell PM. Prevalence, incidence, and factors associated with pre-stroke and post-stroke dementia: a systematic review and meta-analysis. *Lancet Neurol*. 2009;8:1006–1018.
127. Hackett ML, Yapa C, Parag V. Frequency of depression after stroke: a systematic review of observational studies. *Stroke*. 2005;36:1330–1340.
128. Hackett ML, Kohler S, O'Brien JT, et al. Neuropsychiatric outcomes of stroke. *Lancet Neurol*. 2014;13:525–534.
129. Hama S, Yamashita H, Shigenobu M, et al. Depression or apathy and functional recovery after stroke. *Int J Geriatr Psychiatry*. 2007;22:1046–1051.
130. Kohler S, Verhey F, Weyerer S, et al. Depression, non-fatal stroke and all-cause mortality in old age: a prospective cohort study of primary care patients. *J Affect Disord*. 2013;150:63–69.
131. Bartoli F, Lillia N, Lax A, et al. Depression after stroke and risk of mortality: a systematic review and meta-analysis. *Stroke Res Treat*. 2013;2013:862978.
132. Ouimet MA, Primeau F, Cole MG. Psychosocial risk factors in poststroke depression: a systematic review. *Can J Psychiatry*. 2001;46:819–828.
133. Eastwood MR, Rifat SL, Nobbs H, et al. Mood disorder following cerebrovascular accident. *Br J Psychiatry*. 1989;154:195–200.
134. Robinson RG, Kubos KL, Starr LB, et al. Mood disorders in stroke patients: importance of location of lesion. *Brain*. 1984;107:81–93.
135. Morris PL, Robinson RG, Raphael B. Lesion location and depression in hospitalized stroke patients: evidence supporting a specific relationship in the left hemisphere. *Neuropsychiatry Neuropsychol Behav Neurol*. 1992;3:75–82.
136. Fang J, Cheng Q. Etiological mechanisms of post-stroke depression: a review. *Neurol Res*. 2009;31:904–909.
137. Zhan Y, Yang YT, You HM, et al. Plasma-based proteomics reveals lipid metabolic and immunoregulatory dysregulation in post-stroke depression. *Eur Psychiatry*. 2014;29:307–315.
138. Tang CZ, Zhang YL, Wang WS, et al. Elevated serum levels of neopterin at admission predicts depression after acute ischemic stroke: a 6-month follow-up study. *Mol Neurobiol*. 2016;53:3194–3204.
139. Carson AJ, MacHale S, Allen K, et al. Depression after stroke and lesion location: a systematic review. *Lancet*. 2000;356:122–126.
140. Taylor-Pillae RE, Hepworth JT, Couli BM. Predictors of depressive symptoms among community dwelling stroke survivors. *J Cardiovasc Nurs*. 2013;28:460–467.
141. Parikh RM, Robinson RG, Lipsey JR, et al. The impact of post-stroke depression on recovery of activities of daily living over two-year follow-up. *Arch Neurol*. 1990;47:785–789.
142. American Psychiatric Association. *Diagnostic and Statistical Manual of Mental Disorders*. 5th ed. American Psychiatric Association; 2013.
143. Fruehwald S, Gatterbauer E, Rehak P, et al. Early fluoxetine treatment of post-stroke depression: a three month double-blind placebo-controlled study with an open-label long-term follow up. *J Neurol*. 2003;250:347–351.
144. Murray V, Von Arbin M, Varelius R, et al. Sertraline in poststroke depression—a controlled study. *Stroke*. 2002;33:292.
145. Andersen G, Vestergaard K, Lauritzen L. Effective treatment of poststroke depression with the selective serotonin reuptake inhibitor citalopram. *Stroke*. 1994;25:1099–1104.
146. Wiart L, Petit H, Joseph PA, et al. Fluoxetine in early poststroke depression: a double-blind placebo-controlled study. *Stroke*. 2000;31:1829–1832.
147. Lipsey JR, Robinson RG, Pearlson GD, et al. Nortriptyline treatment of poststroke depression: a double-blind study. *Lancet*. 1984;1:297–300.
148. Kimura M, Robinson RG, Kosier JT. Treatment of cognitive impairment after poststroke depression: a double-blind treatment trial. *Stroke*. 2000;31:1482–1486.
149. Robinson RG, Schultz SK, Castillo C, et al. Nortriptyline vs. fluoxetine in the treatment of depression and in short-term recovery after stroke: a placebo-controlled, double-blind study. *Am J Psychiatry*. 2000;157:351–359.
150. Kucukalic A, Bravo-Mehmedbasic A, Kulenovic AD, et al. Venlafaxine efficacy and tolerability in the treatment of post-stroke depression. *Psychiatr Danub*. 2007;19:56–60.
151. Hackett ML, Anderson CS, House A, et al. Interventions for treating depression after stroke. *Cochrane Database Syst Rev*. 2008;(4):CD003437.
152. Masand P, Murray GB, Pickett P. Psychostimulants in poststroke depression. *J Neuropsychiatry Clin Neurosci*. 1991;3:23–27.
153. Lingam VR, Lazarus LW, Groves L, et al. Methylphenidate in treating poststroke depression. *J Clin Psychiatry*. 1988;49:151–153.
154. Currier MB, Murray GB, Welch CC. Electroconvulsive therapy for poststroke depressed geriatric patients. *J Neuropsychiatry Clin Neurosci*. 1992;4:140–144.
155. Williams LS, Kroenke K, Bakas T, et al. Care management of poststroke depression: a randomized, controlled trial. *Stroke*. 2007;38:998–1003.

156. Oradei DM, Waite NS. Group psychotherapy with stroke patients during the immediate recovery phase. *Am J Orthopsychiatry*. 1974;44:386–395.

157. Watzlawick P, Coyne JC. Depression following stroke: brief, problem-focused family treatment. *Fam Process*. 1980;19:13–18.

158. Robinson RG, Jorge RE, Moser DJ, et al. Escitalopram and problem-solving therapy for prevention of poststroke depression. *JAMA*. 2008;299:2391–2400.

159. Lincoln NB, Flannaghan T. Cognitive behavioral psychotherapy for depression following stroke: a randomized controlled trial. *Stroke*. 2003;34:111–115.

160. Almeida OP, Waterreus A, Hankey GJ. Preventing depression after stroke: results from a randomized placebo-controlled trial. *J Clin Psychiatry*. 2006;67:1104–1109.

161. Rasmussen A, Lunde M, Poulsen DL, et al. A double-blind, placebo-controlled study of sertraline in the prevention of depression in stroke patients. *Psychosomatics*. 2003;44:216–221.

162. Niedermaier N, Bohrer E, Schulte K, et al. Prophylactic mirtazapine may help to prevent post-stroke depression in people with good cognitive function. *J Clin Psychiatry*. 2005;65:1619–1623.

163. Withall A, Brodaty H, Altendorf A, et al. A longitudinal study examining the independence of apathy and depression after stroke: the Sydney Stroke Study. *Int Psychogeriatr*. 2011:264–270.

164. Marin RS. Apathy: a neuropsychiatric syndrome. *J Neuropsychiatry Clin Neurosci*. 1991;3:243–254.

165. Caeiro L, Ferro J, Figueria M. Apathy in acute stroke patients. *Eur J Neurol*. 2012;19:291–297.

166. Castillo CS, Schultz SK, Robinson RG. Clinical correlates of early-onset and late-onset poststroke generalized anxiety. *Am J Psychiatry*. 1995;152:1174–1179.

167. Astrom M. Generalized anxiety disorder in stroke patients: a three-year longitudinal study. *Stroke*. 1996;27:270–275.

168. Starkstein SE, Robinson RG, Price TC. Comparison of cortical and subcortical lesions in the production of post-stroke depression matched for size and location of lesions. *Arch Gen Psychiatry*. 1988;45:247–252.

169. Chemerinski E, Levine SR. Neuropsychiatric disorders following vascular brain injury. *Mt Sinai J Med*. 2006;73:1006–1014.

170. Goyal R, Sameer M, Chandrasekaran R. Mania secondary to right-sided stroke responsive to olanzapine. *Gen Hosp Psychiatry*. 2006;28:262–263.

171. Wijeratne C, Malhi GS. Vascular mania: an old concept in danger of sclerosing? A clinical overview. *Acta Psychiatr Scand*. 2007;116(suppl 434):35–40.

172. Robinson RG, Boston JD, Starkstein SE, et al. Comparison of mania with depression following brain injury: causal factors. *Am J Psychiatry*. 1988;145:172–178.

173. Cummings JL, Mendez MF. Secondary mania with focal cerebrovascular lesion. *Am J Psychiatry*. 1984;141:1084–1087.

174. Starkstein SE, Mayberg HS, Berthier ML, et al. Secondary mania: neuroradiological and metabolic findings. *Ann Neurol*. 1990;27:652–659.

175. Robinson RG. Mood disorders secondary to stroke. *Semin Clin Neuropsychiatry*. 1997;2:244–251.

176. Rabins PV, Starkstein SE, Robinson RG. Risk factors for developing atypical (schizophreniform) psychosis following stroke. *J Neuropsychiatry Clin Neurosci*. 1991;3:6–9.

177. Levine DN, Finklestein S. Delayed psychosis after right temporoparietal stroke or trauma: relation to epilepsy. *Neurology*. 1982;32:267–272.

178. Starkstein SE, Fedoroff JP, Price TR, et al. Catastrophic reaction after cerebrovascular lesions: frequency, correlates, and validation of a scale. *J Neurol Neurosurg Psychiatry*. 1993;5:189–194.

179. Carota A, Rossetti AO, Karapanayiotides T, et al. Catastrophic reaction in acute stroke: a reflex behavior in aphasic patients. *Neurology*. 2001;57:1902–1905.

180. Morrison JH, Molliver ME, Grzanna R. Noradrenergic innervation of the cerebral cortex: widespread effects of local cortical lesions. *Science*. 1979;205:313–316.

181. Andersen G. Treatment of uncontrolled crying after stroke. *Drug Ther*. 1999;6:105–111.

182. Morris PLP, Robinson RG, Raphael B. Emotional lability after stroke. *Aust N Z J Psychiatry*. 1993;27:601–605.

183. Rosen HF, Cummings J. A real reason for patients with pseudobulbar affect to smile. *Ann Neurol*. 2007;61:92–96.

184. Lieberman A, Benson DF. Control of emotional expression in pseudobulbar palsy. A personal experience. *Arch Neurol*. 1977;34:717–719.

185. Starkstein SE, Federoff JP, Berthier ML, et al. Manic depressive and pure manic states after brain lesions. *Biol Psychiatry*. 1991;29:149–158.

186. Bakchine S, Lacomblez L, Benoit N, et al. Manic-like state after orbitofrontal and right temporoparietal injury: efficacy of clonidine. *Neurology*. 1989;39:778–781.

187. Filardi da Rocha F, Correa H, Teixeira AL. A successful outcome with valproic acid in a case of mania secondary to stroke of the right frontal lobe. *Prog Neuropsychopharmacol Biol Psychiatry*. 2008;32:587–588.

188. Robinson RG, Parikh RM, Lipsey JR, et al. Pathological laughing and crying following stroke: validation of measurement scale and double-blind treatment study. *Am J Psychiatry*. 1993;150:286–293.

189. Andersen G, Vestergaard K, Riis J. Citalopram for poststroke pathological crying. *Lancet*. 1993;342:837–839.

190. Burns A, Russell E, Stratton-Powell H, et al. Sertraline in stroke-associated lability of mood. *Int J Geriatr Psychiatry*. 1999;14:681–685.

191. Schiffer RB, Herndon RM, Rudick RA. Treatment of pathologic laughing and weeping with amitriptyline. *N Engl J Med*. 1985;312:1480–1482.

192. Pioro EP, Brooks BR, Cummings J, et al. Dextromethorphan plus ultra low-dose quinidine reduces pseudobulbar affect. *Ann Neurol*. 2010;68:693–702.

193. CDC1 Centers for Disease Control and Prevention, National Center for Injury Prevention and Control. *Report to Congress on Traumatic Brain Injury in the United States: Epidemiology and Rehabilitation*. Centers for Disease Control and Prevention; 2015.

194. Breiding MJ, Peterson A, Waltzman D, et al. Traumatic brain injury epidemiology and public health issues. In: Zasler ND,

Katz DL, Zafonte RD, eds. *Brain Injury Medicine: Principles and Practice*. 3rd ed. Springer Publishing Company; 2022:92–108.

195. Marik PE, Varon J, Trask T. Management of head trauma. *Chest*. 2002;122:699–711.

196. Kaufman DM, Milstein MJ. *Clinical Neurology for Psychiatrists*. 7th ed. Elsevier Saunders; 2013:527–543.

197. McCullagh S, Feinstein A. Cognitive changes. In: Silver JM, McAllister TW, Yudofsky SC, eds. *Textbook of Traumatic Brain Injury*. American Psychiatric Publishing; 2011.

198. Max JE, Robertson BA, Lansing AE. The phenomenology of personality change due to traumatic brain injury in children and adolescents. *J Neuropsychiatry Clin Neurosci*. 2001;13:161–170.

199. Koponen S, Taiminen T, Portin R, et al. Axis I and II psychiatric disorders after traumatic brain injury: a 30-year follow-up study. *Am J Psychiatry*. 2002;159:1315–1321.

200. Seel RT, Kreutzer JS, Rosenthal M, et al. Depression after traumatic brain injury: a National Institute on Disability and Rehabilitation Research Model Systems multicenter investigation. *Arch Phys Med Rehabil*. 2003;84:177–184.

201. Rapoport MJ, McCullagh S, Streiner D, et al. The clinical significance of major depression following mild traumatic brain injury. *Psychosomatics*. 2003;44:31–37.

202. Deb S, Lyons I, Koutzoukis C, et al. Rate of psychiatric illness one year after traumatic brain injury. *Am J Psychiatry*. 1999;156:374–378.

203. van Reekum R, Cohen T, Wong J. Can traumatic brain injury cause psychiatric disorders? *J Neuropsychiatry Clin Neurosci*. 2000;12:316–327.

204. Kuipers P, Lancaster A. Developing a suicide prevention strategy based on the perspectives of people with brain injuries. *J Head Trauma Rehabil*. 2000;15:1275–1284.

205. Robinson RG, Jorge RE. Mood disorders. In: Silver JM, McAllister TW, Yudofsky SC, eds. *Textbook of Traumatic Brain Injury*. American Psychiatric Publishing; 2011.

206. Dikman SS, Bombardier CH, Machamer JE, et al. Natural history of depression in traumatic brain injury. *Arch Phys Med Rehabil*. 2004;85:1457–1464.

207. Simpson G, Tate R. Clinical features of suicide attempts after traumatic brain injury. *J Nerv Ment Dis*. 2005;193:680–685.

208. Bryant RA, Moulds M, Guthrie R, et al. Treating acute stress disorder following mild traumatic brain injury. *Am J Psychiatry*. 2003;160:585–587.

209. Klein E, Caspi Y, Gil S. The relation between memory of the traumatic event and PTSD: evidence from studies of traumatic brain injury. *Can J Psychiatry*. 2003;48:28–33.

210. Stengler-Wenzke K, Muller U. Fluoxetine for OCD after brain injury. *Am J Psychiatry*. 2002;159:872.

211. Corcoran C, McAllister TW, Malaspina D. Psychotic disorders. In: Silver JM, McAllister TW, Yudofsky SC, eds. *Textbook of Traumatic Brain Injury*. American Psychiatric Publishing; 2011.

212. Fujii DE, Ahmed I. Risk factors in psychosis secondary to traumatic brain injury. *J Neuropsychiatry Clin Neurosci*. 2001;13:61–69.

213. Sloan R, Brown K, Pentland B. Fluoxetine as a treatment for emotional lability after brain injury. *Brain Inj*. 1992;6:315–319.

214. Perino C, Rago R, Cicolin A, et al. Mood and behavioural disorders following traumatic brain injury: clinical evaluation and pharmacological management. *Brain Inj*. 2001;15:139–148.

215. Meythaler J, Depalma L, Devivo M, et al. Sertraline to improve arousal and alertness in severe traumatic brain injury secondary to motor vehicle crashes. *Brain Inj*. 2001;15:321–331.

216. Kant R, Smith-Seemiller L, Zeiler D. Treatment of aggression and irritability after head injury. *Brain Inj*. 1988;12:661–666.

217. Silver JM, Arciniegas DB, Yudofsky SC. Psychopharmacology. In: Silver JM, McAllister TW, Yudofsky SC, eds. *Textbook of Traumatic Brain Injury*. American Psychiatric Publishing; 2011.

218. Deb S, Crownshaw T. The role of pharmacotherapy in the management of behavior disorders in traumatic brain injury patients. *Brain Inj*. 2004;18:1–31.

219. Bouvy P, van der Wetering B, Meerwaldt J, et al. Buspirone: neuropsychiatric effects. *J Head Trauma Rehabil*. 1991;6:90–92.

220. Pourcher E, Filteau M, Bouchard R, et al. Efficacy of the combination of buspirone and carbamazepine in early posttraumatic delirium (letter). *Am J Psychiatry*. 1994;151:150–151.

221. Ratey J, Leveroni C, Miller A, et al. Low-dose buspirone to treat agitation and maladaptive behaviour in brain-injured patients: two case reports (letter). *J Clin Psychopharmacol*. 1992;12:362–364.

222. Spritzer SD, Kinney CL, Condie J, et al. Amantadine for patients with severe traumatic brain injury: a critically appraised topic. *Neurologist*. 2015;19:61–64.

223. Elovic EP, Lansang R, Li Y, et al. The use of atypical antipsychotics in traumatic brain injury. *J Head Trauma Rehabil*. 2003;18:177–195.

224. Kim E, Bijlani M. A pilot study of quetiapine treatment of aggression due to traumatic brain injury. *J Neuropsychiatry Clin Neurosci*. 2006;18:547–549.

225. Carter CG, Sanders KM, et al. Traumatic brain injury. In: Stern TA, Rosenbaum JF, Fava M, eds. *Massachusetts General Hospital Comprehensive Clinical Psychiatry*. Mosby; 2008:1107–1121.

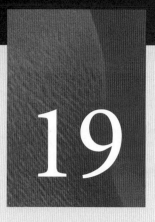

19

PATIENTS WITH ABNORMAL MOVEMENTS

OLIVER FREUDENREICH, MD ■ FELICIA A. SMITH, MD ■
ALICE W. FLAHERTY, MD, PHD

OVERVIEW

Psychiatrists encounter patients with abnormal movements in a variety of clinical settings. Recognizing and correctly labeling motor phenomena in each setting helps to create a differential diagnosis that serves as the basis for optimal treatment since abnormal movements can be the first indication of an unsuspected medical or neurologic disorder in a patient treated for psychiatric symptoms. A solid understanding of conditions that have prototypical abnormal movements (e.g., Huntington disease, Parkinson disease) or tremors will help psychiatrists to correctly categorize abnormal movements. All movement disorders, whether they are primary or drug induced, contribute to morbidity (with loss of independence) and mortality (e.g., secondary to falls or choking). Many of these disorders are stigmatizing, as abnormal movements are immediately obvious to others.

Movement disorders caused by basal ganglia damage or dysfunction create trouble starting or stopping movements. They differ from cerebellar disorders (that affect movement targeting) and stroke-related weakness. Abnormal movements from neuroleptic malignant syndrome (NMS) and catatonia are discussed in Chapter 21. Observing real patients and watching videos are excellent ways to learn to recognize abnormal movements. A word of caution: many of the free videos available on the internet show patients with functional movement disorders (FMDs) who have made videos of themselves and do not depict classic movement disorders; therefore one should select reputable sources, such as a video atlas.[1]

Gathering the History and Performing a Physical Examination

A movement disorder is a clinical diagnosis based on the patient's history and a physical examination; laboratory tests and brain imaging usually do not facilitate making the diagnosis. A family history can be informative if there is a history of a hereditary movement disorder. One should ask about the current and past use of prescribed medications as well as substances of abuse, as these are the most common causes of abnormal movements.

The examination begins with unobtrusive observation when meeting the patient in the waiting area or when approaching the patient's bedside. One should determine if the movements exist when unobserved and if the patient shuffles or writhes when walking. A patient who lies stiffly in bed might be parkinsonian or catatonic. The neurologic examination is focused on establishing deficits beyond their relationship to the motor strip and the basal ganglia; it also includes the assessment of cortical and cerebellar functioning, as well as the elicitation of other motor signs. Muscle tone should be evaluated (e.g., as being rigid, spastic, or hypotonic). If you suspect catatonia, you should perform an examination looking for other signs of catatonia. Some patients cannot relax while their limb is being examined for muscle tone, and as a result they seem to (voluntarily) resist each passive movement. This is called *gegenhalten* or paratonia.

Table 19.1 summarizes common abnormal movements. Overall, it is helpful to determine if your patient moves too much (hyperkinetic) or too little

TABLE 19.1
Motor Symptoms

Tremor (Rhythmic Involuntary Alternation of Agonist and Antagonist Muscles)

Action tremor—triggered by voluntary movement

Rest tremor—stops during voluntary movement

Postural tremor—seen with either action or rest tremor, not itself diagnostic

Movements That Can Look Like Tremor But Are Not

Cerebellar dysmetria (intention "tremor")—worsens as limb approaches target

Myoclonus—involuntary non-rhythmic jerk, moves only one joint

Asterixis (negative myoclonus, "flapping tremor")—arrhythmic lapses of sustained posture

Focal seizures—non-rhythmic trains of unilateral twitching, lasting seconds to minutes.

Fasciculations—visible contractions within a muscle that do not move a joint

The Hyperkinetic–Hypokinetic Spectrum—From Fast to Slow, in Descending Order

Chorea—brief, unpredictable, semi-purposeful movements

Choreoathetosis—when you cannot decide if it is chorea or athetosis

Athetosis—slow but continuous movements

Dystonia—abnormal postures held for at least several seconds

Lead-pipe rigidity—constant resistance throughout the range of passive motion

Bradykinesia—slow movements

Akinesia—sustained periods of no movement

Other Hyperkinetic Movements

Hemiballism—violent, unilateral, repetitive but non-rhythmic jerks of proximal limbs

Stereotypies—repetitive self-soothing movements (e.g., tapping foot, biting nails)

Tics—semi-voluntary fast movement, often multi-joint, usually urge driven

TABLE 19.2
Gait Syndromes

Parkinsonian: slow, shuffling, stooping with arms flexed, festinating (unable to stop); many falls

Choreic: posturing, writhing; fewer falls

Ataxic: wide based, lurching; fewer falls

Neuropathic: foot slaps, patient steps high to avoid tripping

Spastic: stiff, circumducted leg, toe walking

Functional (astasia-abasia): wild, seemingly poor balance but no falls

When examining a patient with a tremor, the main question is whether the tremor occurs mainly at rest (a resting tremor) or during action (an action tremor). Postural tremors can occur with either action or rest and are not in and of themselves diagnostic. Writing or drawing will reliably evoke an action tremor in the writing hand, whereas rest tremors can intensify with movement of the opposite hand. The phenomenological description of the tremor is followed by a search for other neurologic signs or symptoms to help refine the diagnostic possibilities. This is important since treatment depends on the etiology of tremors, although the treatment of some tremors can be non-specific and based on their severity and the patient's tolerance of them.

Table 19.2 summarizes manifestations of gait disorders. Observing a patient's gait and understanding the etiology of a gait disturbance are particularly important during a patient visit. Gait disturbances not only interfere with a patient's independence, but they can lead to dangerous falls (especially in the elderly). Hypokinetic movement disorders, including parkinsonism associated with the use of antipsychotics, lead to falls because patients react too slowly when they stumble. Those with ataxia or hyperkinetic movement disorders sustain fewer falls. A potentially reversible cause of a gait disturbance is normal-pressure hydrocephalus, which is manifest by a triad of (a parkinsonian) gait, incontinence, and dementia (the latter being a late-stage manifestation). Shunt placement can prevent symptom progression, and if this intervention is carried out early in the condition's course, some of the symptoms may even be reversed.

One should also ask about swallowing difficulties, which can result in aspiration pneumonia.

(hypokinetic), or if there are rhythmic tremors or non-rhythmic twitches. Myoclonus or asterixis can initially appear somewhat rhythmic, so one must observe carefully. Asterixis can suggest the presence of a serious metabolic disturbance, whereas myoclonus is non-specific and may be benign. Other phenomena that mimic tremors include focal seizures and cerebellar dysmetria. Some movements defy easy categorization but should be considered in patients with psychiatric conditions (e.g., catatonic symptoms, stereotypies, mannerisms).

IDIOPATHIC MOVEMENT DISORDERS

Parkinson Disease

Idiopathic Parkinson disease (PD) is a hypokinetic syndrome characterized by the triad of slow movement, rigidity, and tremor. The combination of tremor and rigidity leads to the cogwheeling on examination. Although a resting tremor is often the first sign of PD, up to one-fourth of patients have no tremor. Difficulties initiating movements, like starting to walk, are called freezing, where a patient's feet appear to be glued to the ground.

The mainstay of treatment for PD is the administration of the dopamine precursor levodopa.[2] Bradykinesia responds better to levodopa than does tremor. Unfortunately, while levodopa is highly effective early in the illness course (reversing dopamine loss-related akinesia), its long-term administration is complicated by levodopa-induced dyskinesias that arise due to striatal hyper-responsiveness to acute dopaminergic stimulation. In the later stages of the disease, patients experience periods of immobility that alternate with good symptom control (called "on-off phenomenon"). Some patients with parkinsonism have an *atypical* response to dopamine agonists (i.e., it is poor). Atypical parkinsonian syndromes (e.g., Parkinson-plus) occur in patients who experience not only parkinsonian symptoms but other symptoms as well. Such syndromes include Lewy body dementia (LBD) or multi-system atrophy (MSA), where, as the name implies, other brain systems are affected. Clinicians should consider that they will only know if a patient is poorly responsive to levodopa if it is tried.

PD is, for most patients, a multi-faceted disease; it is more than a pure movement disorder (by virtue of the biological nature of the illness, treatment side effects, or the psychological effects of having a progressive illness). Table 19.3 summarizes its core clinical symptoms.

Some patients who are eventually diagnosed with PD have a pre-morbid (i.e., prior to the onset of abnormal movements) personality style that is characterized by an affinity for high harm avoidance and low novelty.[3] Such patients are temperamentally conscientious, industrious, inflexible, and prone to dysthymia. On the other hand, a complication of PD progression is

TABLE 19.3
Clinical Symptoms in Parkinson Disease

Motor
Bradykinesia
Masked face
Stooped posture and festinating gait
Falls, especially backward
Atypical parkinsonism: spasticity, eye movement abnormalities

Neuropsychiatric
Pre-morbid personality (conscientious, inflexible, risk averse)
Depression: may precede motor symptoms
Dementia: if early, is a sign of atypical parkinsonism
Psychosis: if early, is a sign of atypical parkinsonism

a dopamine dysregulation syndrome, with impulsive behaviors that can take the form of gambling, hypersexuality, compulsive shopping, or binge eating,[4] all manifestations that were not characteristic of the patient. Punding (i.e., repetitive, prolonged, purposeless behavior) is another late complication that makes life difficult for PD patients and their families.[5] These problems are due, at least in part, to the use of medications and antipsychotics with partial dopamine agonist properties (e.g., aripiprazole) that carry some risk of inducing compulsions and impulsive urges to shop, eat, have sex, or gamble.

Fatigue, apathy, insomnia, and depression are very common in PD. Dementia and psychosis are late-stage problems of PD; when these complications begin early in the illness course, they usually indicate atypical parkinsonism. Autonomic dysfunctions, such as postural hypotension and drooling, are severe in MSA and are often problematic in PD. Muscle rigidity can cause pain, especially in the muscles of the shoulder and back.

At least one-third of patients with PD have depression and apathy (*abulia*). Apathy can be the first symptom of PD; it needs to be differentiated from depression (a treatable psychiatric disorder). Depression often goes undiagnosed due to its symptom overlap with PD, which includes psychomotor retardation, masked facies, poor sleep, and cognitive complaints. As in other medical disorders, depression, when present, is a major contributor to poor quality of life. Depression and motor fluctuations are poorly correlated. In a clinical trial that compared a placebo, paroxetine, and a noradrenergic tricyclic antidepressant, nortriptyline was effective but paroxetine was not.[6] The role of selective serotonin reuptake inhibitors (SSRIs) is therefore thought to be limited, and perhaps best reserved for those with a pseudobulbar affect, as SSRIs can worsen motor symptoms. A recent placebo-controlled trial, however, showed benefit from paroxetine and venlafaxine without exacerbating motor symptoms.[7] Other antidepressants to consider are bupropion or a stimulant; the latter is often used for the treatment of apathy. The dopamine agonist pramipexole has a direct antidepressant effect in patients with PD and is another therapeutic option.[8] In refractory depression, electroconvulsive therapy (ECT) and transcranial magnetic stimulation can be tried, although post-ECT delirium complicates its use. Mirtazapine is a good choice for those with anxiety and poor sleep.

In a large epidemiologic study, almost one-third of patients with PD who were receiving routine outpatient neurologic care met the criteria for dementia; higher rates of sub-syndromal cognitive impairment were found in this group.[9] Over time, most patients with PD develop dementia. In a cohort of newly diagnosed patients, 83% of patients who lived for 20 years with PD had dementia.[10] The dementia associated with PD is a subcortical dementia that is characterized by slowed mentation and processing (bradyphrenia), poor attention, and difficulties with executive function. The Mini-Mental State Examination (MMSE) is insensitive for the detection of these problems, and it should not be used as a screening tool in this population. However, co-morbidities with cortical dementias (e.g., Alzheimer dementia, LBD) lead to mixed cortical/subcortical pictures. On autopsy, LBD and PD with dementia look alike. They may represent the same disease, with dementia preceding motor problems in LBD and the reverse being true in PD dementia. Very poor tolerability of antipsychotics is a hallmark of both LBD[11] and late-stage PD dementia. The mainstay of treatment for PD with dementia is acetylcholinesterase inhibitors, which are also frequently used in LBD. Levodopa is ineffective and poorly tolerated; moreover, it can induce hallucinations in both conditions.

Psychosis is a complication of PD in about half of those with PD. Symptoms (that include vivid dreams, illusions, hallucinations, misidentification syndromes, and paranoid delusions) can result from the treatment of PD and from the disease itself, particularly if dementia develops. Early-onset hallucinations are a predictor of dementia, and they are primarily, but not exclusively, visual. They can be simple (seeing flashes), of the passage variety (i.e., seeing fleeting images in the periphery of vision), or take the form of presence hallucinations (i.e., feeling that someone is close by). More complex hallucinations include seeing small animals or children. Both hallucinations and delusions predict nursing home placement; therefore, attempts to treat these symptoms are important. The first step is to exclude other causes of psychosis, including polypharmacy. Next, modifying the PD regimen by reducing polypharmacy, lowering the levodopa dose, and dosing it more frequently can be helpful. Last, antipsychotics should be trialed, although the tolerability of most antipsychotics, including those with loose binding to the dopamine receptor (e.g., quetiapine), is poor, particularly in later disease stages. Moreover, efficacy has not been clearly established for quetiapine, an agent that is often used because of its perceived better tolerability. Low-dose clozapine (e.g., 6.25 mg or 12 mg/day) might be the best choice, as it can be used when other antipsychotics have not been tolerated.[12] Pimavanserin is a selective $5-HT_{2A}$ inverse agonist used for the treatment of PD-related psychosis.[13] While effective, its role in the management of psychosis in PD has yet to be established, particularly regarding its efficacy when compared with clozapine.[13]

Sleep disruption from restless legs syndrome (RLS) or obstructive sleep apnea is common in PD, can be debilitating, but is relatively treatable (with gabapentin and continuous positive airway pressure, respectively). Many individuals with PD have rapid eye movement behavior disorder (RBD), which can greatly disrupt their caregivers' sleep and contribute to caregiver stress. Of patients with RBD without PD, 50% will develop PD within a decade, and most of the rest will develop another neurodegenerative disorder.[14]

Huntington Disease

Huntington chorea or Huntington disease (HD) is a rare autosomal dominant progressive neuropsychiatric disorder. It typically begins in the fourth decade of life and leads to death in about a decade. Psychiatrists should keep in mind, however, that 10% of cases of HD (juvenile HD) begin during adolescence, and such patients may be misdiagnosed as having schizophrenia or another psychiatric disorder when neuropsychiatric symptoms precede motor symptoms. The age of onset is inversely correlated with the number of CAG repeat expansions in the pathogenic gene, a phenomenon known as genetic anticipation. Unfortunately, knowledge of the genetic mutation and its mechanism has not yet been translated into disease-modifying treatments for this single-gene disorder.

As the term chorea implies, HD is a hyperkinetic movement disorder with its hallmark choreiform movements. Psychiatrists might encounter patients with stimulant-induced chorea, which is a complication that arises in those with a long history of stimulant misuse; it is also known as "crack dancing," which can develop acutely during cocaine use or with chronic use.[15] The differential diagnosis of choreiform movements is provided in Table 19.4.

Other motor phenomena in HD include dysphagia, parkinsonism, and dystonia, particularly as the illness progresses. In addition, almost all patients with HD experience neuropsychiatric symptoms, ranging from dysphoria and irritability to anxiety and psychosis. Depression is also frequent, and the risk of suicide is high. The end-stage of HD is characterized by increased immobility and dementia. Patients with juvenile HD experience difficult-to-manage seizures and early psychiatric and cognitive symptoms in addition to bradykinesia, dystonia, rigidity, and oropharyngeal dysfunction. Purely behavioral problems, such as aggression, are other early signs. A diagnosis of HD should be suspected if the hallmark imaging findings of caudate and putamen degeneration are seen. Genetic testing confirms the diagnosis.

There are no disease-modifying treatments. Death typically occurs within 10 to 15 years of the initial diagnosis. Symptomatic treatments include the use of SSRIs for depression, low-dose antipsychotics for psychosis, and one of the vesicular monoamine transporter (VMAT)-2 inhibitors (i.e., tetrabenazine, deutetrabenazine, and valbenazine) for chorea. All treatments carry a risk of worsening the disease (e.g., worsening dysphagia) and must be adjusted to the disease stage.

A family history allows for early diagnosis, which can be facilitated by pre-symptomatic testing. However, in some families, the history might be unknown, or the parent might not have expressed symptoms yet. Genetic testing poses ethical challenges, particularly the testing of asymptomatic family members who might still be children.[16] The risk of suicide after the diagnosis is made needs to be considered.

TABLE 19.4
Differential Diagnosis of Choreiform Movements

Inherited Disorders
Huntington disease
Fahr syndrome (idiopathic basal ganglia calcification)
Neuroacanthocytosis
Wilson disease
Friedreich ataxia
Spinocerebellar ataxia

Acquired Disorders
Focal striatal lesion
Post-infectious: Sydenham chorea, PANDAS (pediatric autoimmune disorders associated with streptococcal infection)
Pregnancy: chorea gravidarum
Lupus erythematosus
Thyrotoxicosis
Acquired immunodeficiency syndrome
Paraneoplastic syndromes

Drug Induced
Tardive dyskinesia
Phenytoin
Cocaine ("crack dance")
Levodopa
Oral contraceptives

Tourette Syndrome

The hallmark of Tourette syndrome (TS) is the presence of tics that start before the age of 18 years and that consist of both multiple motor tics (e.g., eye blinking or shoulder shrugging) and vocal tics (e.g., throat clearing). Chronic tic disorders, with either motor or vocal tics but not both, are likely a *forme fruste* of TS. The male-to-female ratio for tic disorders is 3:1. Many children who develop TS in early childhood have complete resolution of their symptoms by early adulthood. Co-morbid psychiatric disorders, especially obsessive-compulsive disorder and attention-deficit disorder (ADD), are common. Other problems include depression and secondary social phobia that are related to the tics. As with other movements, tics worsen with stress, excitement, or fatigue. Tics are somewhat voluntary and can be suppressed when a patient experiences a premonitory urge, at least for a while. These features differentiate tics from myoclonus. An individual tic may move several joints, unlike myoclonus. Complex tics, like repeating phrases (echolalia) or shouting obscenities (coprolalia), are rare and often misperceived as volitional.

Treatment of tics is usually unnecessary unless they are persistent, impairing, or distressing. Social phobia that has developed in response to tics can be treated directly with therapy and SSRIs. Habit-reversal training is a psychological treatment for tics that can work.[17] ADD, which is highly co-morbid with tics, can probably be treated with stimulants without the risk of worsening tics, contrary to previous recommendations and fears.[18] Tic-suppressing medications include α_2-adrenergic receptor agonists (e.g., clonidine and guanfacine) and antipsychotics.[19] Clonidine or guanfacine should be tried first, as they are safer than, albeit not as effective as, antipsychotics. Antipsychotics can cause tardive dyskinesia (TD) and rebound tics on their withdrawal. While high-potency antipsychotics (e.g., haloperidol or pimozide) have been traditionally used to manage patients with TS, they are apt to induce extrapyramidal symptoms (EPS) (and in the case of pimozide, the QTc interval can be prolonged). Instead, clinicians should try using aripiprazole or risperidone. In severe presentations, patients may consider undergoing deep brain stimulation (DBS).

Wilson Disease

Wilson disease (WD) is a very rare disorder of copper elimination.[20] Its symptoms are the result of insidious copper accumulation in organs, most importantly the liver and the brain. Depending on which organ is affected most, patients may present to hepatologists (because of liver enzyme abnormalities or frank cirrhosis), to neurologists (because of a mix of movement problems, including dysarthria, dysmetria, chorea, and tremor), or to psychiatrists (because of mood and personality changes, or rarely psychosis or catatonia). Kayser-Fleischer rings in concert with a serum ceruloplasmin level of <100 mg/L are diagnostic for WD. However, 50% of patients with WD do not develop eye findings. A 24-hour copper excretion in the urine >100 μg per 24 hours, in the absence of cholestatic liver disease, is strong evidence for WD. Ultimately, the diagnosis of WD hinges not on a single test result but on accounting for all available clinical information.

Timely diagnosis is important since eliminating excess copper from the body by means of chelating and depleting agents, such as penicillamine, while also preventing the addition of copper to the body by means of copper-absorption inhibitors (e.g., zinc) is only effective when initiated early before tissue damage has occurred. Psychiatric treatments are not well studied but are like those of other disorders that affect the basal ganglia; antipsychotics tend to be poorly tolerated. Without treatment, WD is fatal.

Restless Legs Syndrome (Willis-Ekbom Disease)

Restless legs syndrome (RLS) is a common neurologic movement disorder that affects up to 10% of those in the general population. The core feature of RLS is the urge to move the legs in response to an increasingly unpleasant (often described as a "creeping") feeling that builds in the legs when patients are at rest. Moving the legs relieves this sensation. For most patients, RLS is worse at night, making it difficult for them to fall asleep or to sleep soundly. RLS should not be confused with mere positional discomfort, leg pain, or leg cramps. An important differential diagnostic consideration for psychiatrists is akathisia. Periodic limb movements in sleep (PLMS) is distinct from RLS, but almost all patients with RLS show such movements during polysomnography. RLS can be primary or secondary to other medical disorders, most importantly iron deficiency anemia and renal failure.[21] One should consider measuring the ferritin level to rule out iron deficiency in cases of suspected RLS. RLS is frequently co-morbid with depression, which can pose a dilemma since antidepressants can exacerbate RLS.

Treatment typically involves the use of dopamine agonists (e.g., pramipexole or ropinirole) or alpha$_2$ delta calcium-channel ligands (e.g., gabapentin or pregabalin).[22] Benzodiazepines and opiates can help in refractory cases of RLS, but clinicians need to use them judiciously to avoid falls in the elderly and to guard against misuse, respectively.

TREMORS

The frequencies of different types of tremors overlap too much to be helpful unless they are unusually slow (e.g., 4 Hz in PD) or high (e.g., 18 Hz in primary orthostatic tremor). To complicate matters, different types of tremors can co-exist in the same patient. A so-called "intention tremor" (dysmetria) associated with cerebellar disorders is often accompanied by other cerebellar signs (e.g., an ataxic gait or ocular nystagmus); however, as noted earlier, it is not a true tremor. Seizures with retained consciousness would be a very rare cause of bilateral tremor.

Because stress-induced adrenaline itself causes tremors, anxious people often have a tremor, and their awareness of it can worsen their anxiety. It is important to appropriately reassure patients if they perceive a mild tremor to be disabling or a new-onset tremor as a sign of things to come (e.g., a brain tumor or a disabling progressive neurological disease). The psychological responses to tremors need to be managed with support to help cope with the tremor; treatment includes appropriate management of both the tremor and the psychological response to it. A physiologic (i.e., normal) bilateral finger tremor can be made worse by stress, physical work, or anxiety, as well as from stimulants, such as nicotine and caffeine. Professionals with stage fright, for example, can use a beta-blocker prior to a public appearance to suppress their physiological tremors. Some people have a prominent ("enhanced") physiologic tremor independent from stress or another neurological disease.

A so-called "benign essential tremor" is an isolated action tremor in the absence of other neurological movements that almost always involve the upper limbs (as seen in 95% of cases), although the head and voice among other body parts can be affected. The tremor is bilateral and symmetric and is said to respond well to the use of alcohol and to run in families. However, it is usually over-diagnosed because additional neurological signs suggestive of other syndromes, like PD, are overlooked. Moreover, it is increasingly recognized as not "benign" in the sense that it can be progressive and include non-tremor symptoms.[23] Propranolol is the first-line treatment. Primidone can be helpful, but it must be titrated very slowly because of its propensity to induce severe sedation. Up to half of patients with an action tremor will show no clear benefit from pharmacotherapy.

DRUG-INDUCED MOVEMENT DISORDERS

Iatrogenic movement disorders and tremors are secondary to medication treatments, most often, but not always, due to the use of antipsychotics. For psychiatrists, the most important to consider are iatrogenic movement disorders that are related to antipsychotic-induced EPS and drug-induced tremors. These side effects are important because they can be life threatening (e.g., laryngeal dystonia), unpleasant (e.g., akathisia), functionally impairing (e.g., parkinsonism), and socially stigmatizing (e.g., tremor, TD). TD is also problematic, in that it is potentially irreversible, as opposed to the other drug-induced symptoms that usually subside once treatment with the offending agent has been stopped. Finally, current or recent drug use can lead to movement disorders and tremors, either during intoxication or withdrawal, depending on the substance. NMS, which is accompanied by motor abnormalities, is an iatrogenic form of malignant catatonia (it is discussed in Chapter 21).

Drug-Induced Tremors

Myriad medications, including but not limited to psychotropics, can cause tremors. A complete review of the patient's medication list, including over-the-counter drugs as well as alcohol and stimulants (e.g., caffeine and nicotine), is therefore critical for patients with a tremor. All major psychiatric medication groups (e.g., antidepressants, antipsychotics, and mood stabilizers [including lithium]) can cause a tremor at usual doses. Sedatives, including benzodiazepines and alcohol, can cause movements during withdrawal states, typically with a coarse tremor.

A resting tremor is almost always parkinsonian, including its drug-induced variant. On the other hand, lithium, many anti-epileptic drugs (e.g., valproate, lamotrigine), and stimulants cause action tremors. The lithium-induced tremor is an exaggerated physiologic tremor (postural tremor)[24]; it is symmetric and related to the dose and blood level of lithium. A more prominent and coarser tremor is the most common symptom of lithium intoxication that should alert clinicians to search for other signs of lithium toxicity (e.g., confusion, dysarthria, diarrhea) and to check the lithium level. If missed, prolonged lithium toxicity can cause an irreversible, poorly treatment-responsive cerebellar tremor.[25] Using the lowest effective lithium dose and removing aggravating factors (e.g., non-steroidal anti-inflammatory drugs, hyponatremia, diuretics) is often enough to manage lithium-induced tremor. The most commonly prescribed beta-blocker, propranolol, at doses between 60 and 320 mg/day, is effective in cases that require treatment. Primidone, gabapentin, or benzodiazepines (to reduce arousal) are other options.

Whenever possible, the tremors should be treated in the context of the psychiatric syndrome. For example, one can switch from most antipsychotics to clozapine in a patient with EPS, or one can avoid medications, such as valproate, that worsen tremors in depressed patients with a tremor.

Antipsychotic-Induced Extrapyramidal Symptoms

Patients who are treated with an antipsychotic can develop one of three types of iatrogenic movement disorders in the form of EPS; each follows a different time course. Early complications, after only a dose or so, include akathisia and acute dystonic reactions. Parkinsonism usually does not become apparent until after several weeks of treatment. By definition, a late-developing ("tardive") problem is TD. Tardive variants have also been described for akathisia and dystonia. The Pisa syndrome is a variant of dystonia that can also be medication induced, and as the name suggests leads to a sideways-leaning patient due to persistent truncal dystonia.[26] In populations with serious mental disorders, patients might display various admixtures of the three main complications from antipsychotic use. In a representative cohort of 99 chronically institutionalized patients with schizophrenia who received mostly first-generation antipsychotics (FGAs), only about 40% were free from motor symptoms when carefully examined, while 60% suffered from one of three side effects.[27] Despite the increased use of second-generation antipsychotics (SGAs) over the past decade, the same group found an almost unchanged number of movement disorder–free patients in their cohort when they were able to repeat their cross-sectional assessment 8 years later.[28] Antipsychotic-induced EPS remains a major clinical concern for any psychiatrist who prescribes antipsychotics, including newer agents, for longer periods. When assessing a patient who is taking an antipsychotic, one should examine for all three main manifestations of EPS, accounting for the possibility of overlap, as graphically depicted in Fig. 19.1[28].

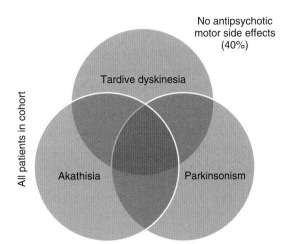

Fig. 19.1 ■ Overlap between antipsychotic-induced extrapyramidal symptoms (EPS) in a cohort of patients treated with antipsychotics. Based on Janno S, Holi M, Tuisku K, et al. Prevalence of neuroleptic-induced movement disorders in chronic schizophrenia inpatients. Am J Psychiatry. 2004;161(1):160–163.

Acute Dystonic Reactions

Patients can have an acute dystonic reaction after only a single antipsychotic dose, with most cases occurring within a week. Younger male patients are at the highest risk of developing this complication. Classically, it takes the form of an oculogyric crisis (with eyes rolling backward), opisthotonus (body arching), torticollis, or trismus (jaw locking). These acute-onset problems are frightening and painful. Many older patients with schizophrenia still remember and will tell you about the first time they received high-dose FGAs like haloperidol and had a dystonic reaction. High-potency antipsychotics are a poor choice for treatment initiation in antipsychotic-naive, first-episode psychosis patients; it is best to avoid inducing an acute dystonic reaction. While anxiety-provoking, dystonic symptoms are rarely life threatening, except when the dystonia affects the larynx.

One can treat acute dystonic reactions effectively with the use of a parenteral benztropine or diphenhydramine. When patients are sent home, they should receive several days of oral benztropine or diphenhydramine to prevent a return trip to the ED. In addition, one should keep in mind that cocaine and phencyclidine can cause dystonia.

Akathisia

Akathisia is an inability to sit still; afflicted patients fidget and may stand up and walk about during the interview. In mild akathisia, patients describe inner restlessness, but they can, with effort, suppress visible movements. Very severe akathisia can induce suicidal and homicidal behavior. As with acute dystonic reactions, akathisia can occur after a single antipsychotic dose. It is important to distinguish akathisia from anxiety-driven stereotypies and involuntary dyskinesias by asking patients what drives their movements. Dyskinetic patients feel that their movements are involuntary. Akathisic and anxious patients each describe their movements as voluntary, but patients with akathisia often feel irritable or bored, not frightened. If akathisia is misdiagnosed as psychotic anxiety, clinicians can worsen the patient's symptoms by increasing, rather than by decreasing, the antipsychotic.

Treatment of acute akathisia with a benzodiazepine (e.g., 10 mg diazepam) is reasonable, and, if possible, the antipsychotic dose should be lowered. As with RLS, akathisia may respond to the use of dopamine agonists and gabapentin. Although patients with akathisia sometimes tolerate a switch to a more sedating antipsychotic with a lower propensity for akathisia (e.g., quetiapine, clozapine), all antipsychotics, including SGAs and clozapine, can cause akathisia. In mild akathisia, low-dose mirtazapine (7.5 or 15 mg)[29] and high-dose propranolol (at a high-enough dose, starting with 10 mg tid) can suppress akathisia. Of note, anticholinergics—while they are often used in the mistaken belief that they treat all manifestations of EPS—are ineffective for akathisia.

Case 1

John, a 22-year-old college student, was brought to the emergency department (ED) by his friends, who had become increasingly concerned about him. He had been making illogical statements, not attending classes, and staying in his room all day. In the ED, he was found to be psychotic but neither depressed nor manic, and he was psychiatrically admitted. He had no medical problems and there was no substance use. Apparently, he had a similar episode 1 year ago, for which he was briefly admitted and treated with haloperidol.

On the unit, John was initially unwilling to start treatment because he had reacted badly to haloperidol. He remembered from his first hospitalization that he had "neck pulling" and "eyes rolling back into my head," which was frightening and painful. "Nobody warned me that this could happen." His treatment team told him he had an acute dystonic reaction and added benztropine to his haloperidol. He had stopped treatment shortly after being discharged because he "didn't feel right, kind of wired." With some hesitation, he agreed to try a different antipsychotic during this hospitalization. He was discharged on aripiprazole 10 mg/day, greatly improved after a 7-day hospitalization.

When John's outpatient psychiatrist saw him a week after discharge, John appeared visibly uncomfortable, and he was unable to sit still during the interview. He described general restlessness, and anxiety "all over," but he was not clearly psychotic. Walking helped transiently, but the restlessness was otherwise constant. His neurologic examination was normal, except for psychomotor agitation. He displayed no abnormal movement, had normal muscle tone and muscle strength, and there was no tremor. There were no signs of catatonia.

To manage acute akathisia, the psychiatrist prescribed 5 mg of diazepam twice daily and stopped aripiprazole. The patient's sensitivity to EPS suggested that he would need an antipsychotic with a very low risk of akathisia, that is, quetiapine, as opposed to trying to manage akathisia symptomatically with propranolol or low-dose mirtazapine. If quetiapine turned out to be insufficient to control his psychosis, he might need clozapine to manage his illness. Unfortunately, adherence might already be compromised by having had an acute dystonic reaction and acute akathisia.

Parkinsonism

Antipsychotic-induced parkinsonian symptoms should be managed if they are functionally impairing (e.g., increasing the fall risk or leading to difficulties swallowing) or distressing (e.g., tremors). Parkinsonian symptoms overlap with negative symptoms (the expressivity cluster) and can easily be mistaken for depression. The drug-induced parkinsonian tremor is a coarse, low-frequency, resting tremor that is indistinguishable from the idiopathic resting tremor of PD. Although psychiatrists often try to distinguish idiopathic parkinsonism from drug-induced parkinsonism by the predominance of a unilateral tremor, in the former, their main treatment response should be the same in either case: lower any dopamine blockers, if possible. Parkinsonism can cause a lip tremor—sometimes called a "rabbit tremor" because of its resemblance to a rabbit who is eating—and is more rhythmic than the orobuccal dyskinesia of TD. Unless a patient also has underlying PD, withdrawing the antipsychotic resolves drug-induced parkinsonism, but it may take months for the symptoms to resolve completely. Anticholinergics, such as benztropine (1 or 2 mg twice daily), can suppress parkinsonism in patients with EPS who are unable to tolerate levodopa. Because anticholinergics can cause delirium in the elderly, some clinicians try to use the milder drug, amantadine (100 mg twice daily)[30]; it is an *N*-methyl-D-aspartate receptor antagonist related to memantine. The risk of exacerbating psychosis is low in patients treated with antipsychotics.

Tardive Dyskinesia

TD is a late complication from treatment with dopamine-blocking agents, usually antipsychotics. One should remember that metoclopramide and prochlorperazine, used widely to manage nausea and migraine headaches, are dopamine antagonists that can cause TD. Risk factors for TD include cumulative antipsychotic exposure, advanced age, and previous experience of EPS. The risk of developing TD from exposure to FGAs is estimated to be 5% per year in young adults.[31] While somewhat lower for SGAs, the risk of TD remains a clinical concern given its usually irreversible nature.[32] Older adults have a much higher risk (25%) per year of developing this complication. Patients with a mood disorder are more likely than those with schizophrenia to develop TD.

The classical movements of TD are involuntary and choreiform; they begin insidiously. Sometimes, a dystonic element can be present. As noted earlier, TD can also co-exist with residual parkinsonian EPS. Movements of TD typically affect the face, but they can also affect the limbs and trunk. Symptoms of TD fluctuate with one's level of arousal. Although TD often does not worsen after the first few months, even mild TD

movements can cause social stigma. Voluntary movement can temporarily suppress mild TD; this should not be mistaken for the "distractibility" of a psychosomatic movement disorder. Severe TD is so disabling that its constant movements make patients unable to sit in a chair, feed themselves, or hold a book. TD can affect the diaphragm, thereby interrupting breathing.

The best treatment for TD is prevention. A clear indication for the use of antipsychotics should exist, and a low-risk antipsychotic should be chosen. Increasingly, SGAs are used in the management of treatment-resistant depression. The risk-benefit analysis of using this medication class for (non-psychotic) mood disorders must include consideration of TD.[33] Antipsychotics should also be used judiciously in elderly individuals with psychosis, particularly those with dementia where the risk-benefit may be unfavorable. The American Psychiatric Association has published guidelines regarding the use of antipsychotics to treat agitation or psychosis in a patient with dementia.[34] Key recommendations included a quantitative assessment of agitation and psychosis and a periodic assessment of the need for ongoing treatment. Patients who receive antipsychotics in acute care settings to manage delirium should not leave the hospital with an order for an antipsychotic unless ongoing treatment is indicated. Patients who are treated with a maintenance antipsychotic need to be appropriately monitored.[35] Clinicians must examine for TD at every visit, as part of the mental status examination. In addition, a formal examination for TD with the Abnormal Involuntary Movement Scale (AIMS) should be documented periodically. The AIMS should be administered at least annually in routine care and more often to high-risk antipsychotic-treated patients. Instructions for the use of the AIMS are nicely summarized in a classic paper by Munetz and Benjamin.[36] One should obtain a baseline assessment for abnormal motor abnormalities before starting an antipsychotic to document either the presence or absence of any pre-existing motor abnormalities.

The best treatment for TD, once it is recognized, is to stop the offending drug—and to do so slowly. Abrupt discontinuation of an antipsychotic can induce withdrawal dyskinesia that can be severe and even involve respiratory muscles. Any patient with mild TD can convert to having fulminant TD, with respiratory muscle involvement, because the clinician panicked and stopped the drug suddenly, causing a serious rebound.

If ongoing antipsychotic treatment is required, clozapine is the best choice, followed by quetiapine. The treatment of choice for TD is the use of the newer VMAT-2 inhibitors (i.e., valbenazine, deutetrabenazine) that have been shown in clinical trials to reduce the symptoms of TD.[37] However, this class of dopamine-depleting agents can be sedating, worsen mood, and cause parkinsonism. Patients should be monitored for thoughts of suicide if depression develops. VMAT-2 inhibitors do not cure TD; once stopped, the abnormal movements return. Vitamin E used to be given in the hope of preventing TD; however, its use has fallen out of favor as the promising response seen in initial trials failed to show benefit in subsequent larger trials.[38] For some patients with TD, particularly if there is a dystonic component or focal involvement (e.g., blepharospasm), botulinum toxin injections can help, but they need to be repeated every 3 months.[39] DBS is a treatment of last resort for TD.[40] The basic management principles for TD are summarized in Fig. 19.2[40].

FUNCTIONAL MOVEMENT DISORDERS

Up to 20% of patients in movement disorder clinics have functional movement disorders (FMDs). Such movements can mimic any of the known movement disorders but appear willful or motivated. The diagnosis of FMD is problematic. All movement disorders affect willed action and the motivation to move—the line between "real" and "psychogenic" disorders is not especially clear. While the *Diagnostic and Statistical Manual of Mental Disorders, Fourth Edition* (DSM-IV) definition of somatoform disorders included having a "non-organic" cause that reflected the intuitive dualism that even trained neuroscientists find hard to resist, the DSM-5 definition of somatic symptom disorder avoids this error.[41]

Observers typically suspect that patients with FMDs are malingering or acting to obtain unconscious secondary gain. However, patients with FMDs do not benefit from their symptoms; they are typically more disabled, more depressed, and more stigmatized than those whose symptoms have a clear physical cause. Patients who malinger typically have symptoms that are more traditional and convincing than the apparently willful symptoms of functional disorders. Classic clues of "psychogenicity," such as *la belle indifference* (lack of concern for the medical problem) are highly unreliable. Clinicians should also not depend on the perceived "bizarreness" of the movements. Sudden unexplained onsets and full remissions suggest an FMD. Not falling despite wild flailing movements (astasia-abasia) suggests a functional disorder. Improvement of the symptom with distraction is often misdiagnosed since most movement disorders are highly influenced by attention, anxiety, and movement of other body parts. A more reliable sign is the entrainment of a tremor to the voluntary tapping of another body part at a new frequency.

Mass psychogenic illness (also referred to as mass sociogenic illness) is an interesting phenomenon that can produce epidemics of FMDs. Such outbreaks are not only of historical interest (e.g., Saint Vitus dance in the Middle Ages during the Black Death or hysterical illnesses in the Salem witch trials) but continue to occur. For example, a recent outbreak affected about 20 teenagers in Le Roy, New York.[41] Mass psychogenic illnesses show us the importance of role expectations, social learning, and social networks, including social media.[42] In the specific context of a modern Western society, fears of toxins combined with distrust of industry and a cover-up by the state (all not necessarily unfounded) combine to produce psychogenic illness in a susceptible group, where an initial index case allows for spread to those in the social network. Recognizing mass psychogenic illness is as difficult at the level of a group as it is for individual patients, as one can "never be sure" that there is no toxin. Endless investigations can never clearly settle the case, just like more laboratory tests can never put to rest the idea that one might have a yet-to-be-discovered illness. Mass psychogenic illness requires recognition and prevention of spread. In many cases, opinion leaders need to be separated from the larger group. Media attention and rapid spread through social media unfortunately make containment next to impossible.

Neurologists typically perform exhaustive tests to rule out rare disorders that can cause abnormal movements and wait until all are negative to discuss

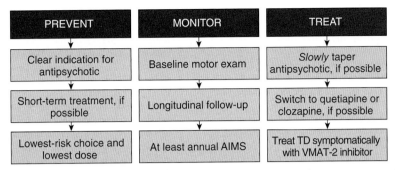

Fig. 19.2 ■ Prevention and treatment of tardive dyskinesia (TD). *AIMS*, Abnormal Involuntary Movement Scale.

psychiatric factors that may contribute to the symptoms. It is better for both neurologists and psychiatrists to be involved from the start if a functional disorder is likely. Neurology needs to be involved since it is difficult to ascertain the functional character of movements unless clinical experience is there to recognize functional unsteadiness (astasia-abasia). Psychiatry, on the other hand, can identify treatable psychiatric disorders and work with patients' psychological responses to their symptoms and build coping skills. However, quite frequently, patients resist referral to psychiatric practitioners, and one could argue that roughly 50% of those without psychiatric psychopathology or distress have a point (i.e., there does not seem to be a conversion from psychological conflict to bodily expression). Unfortunately, these patients get stuck if neurologists feel that they have little else to offer beyond offering a diagnosis.

When and how should you tell a patient that their movements are "functional?" One should not wait until "every possible test" has been done; instead, one should discuss anxiety and other psychiatric aspects of their symptoms at the beginning of their neurologic work-up. Most patients are firmly committed to finding a traditional medical explanation whose severity explains their subjective sense that there is something terribly wrong with their body. Rather than telling a patient "Don't worry, your tremor is just anxiety," consider re-framing your description physiologically, for example, "past stress has raised your adrenaline levels, and adrenaline causes tremors." Explain that their symptoms have "real" brain correlates (i.e., altered neurocircuitry)

in functional neuroimaging studies. The term "psychogenic" is best avoided as patients feel dismissed. Direct the patients to www.neurosymptoms.org, an excellent self-help website for patients who want to educate themselves about FMDs.[43]

Doctors become frustrated by patients with functional symptoms when they do not know how to help them and if they believe that the patient does not truly want to get better. Cognitive-behavioral therapy, however, is one psychological treatment modality that can help.[44] Specialized physical and occupational therapies have been developed.[45] Psychotropics can be used judiciously to address distress. A solid doctor-patient relationship that conveys sincere caring and a hopeful approach with symptom remission as a goal can prevent chronicity.

BIBLIOGRAPHY

1. Bhidayasiri R, Tarsy D. *Movement Disorders: A Video Atlas*. Humana Press; 2012.
2. Reich SG, Savitt JM. Parkinson's disease. *Med Clin North Am.* 2019;103:337–350.
3. Menza M. The personality associated with Parkinson's disease. *Curr Psychiatry Rep.* 2000;2:421–426.
4. O'Sullivan SS, Evans AH, Lees AJ. Dopamine dysregulation syndrome: an overview of its epidemiology, mechanisms and management. *CNS Drugs.* 2009;23:157–170.
5. Evans AH, Stegeman JR. Punding in patients on dopamine agonists for restless leg syndrome. *Mov Disord.* 2009;24:140–141.
6. Menza M, Dobkin RD, Marin H, et al. A controlled trial of antidepressants in patients with Parkinson disease and depression. *Neurology.* 2009;72:886–892.
7. Richard IH, McDermott MP, Kurlan R, et al. A randomized, double-blind, placebo-controlled trial of antidepressants in Parkinson disease. *Neurology.* 2012;78:1229–1236.

8. Ji N, Meng P, Xu B, et al. Efficacy and safety of pramipexole in Parkinson's disease with anxiety or depression: a meta-analysis of randomized clinical trials. *Am J Transl Res*. 2022;14:1757–1764.
9. Riedel O, Klotsche J, Spottke A, et al. Cognitive impairment in 873 patients with idiopathic Parkinson's disease. Results from the German Study on Epidemiology of Parkinson's Disease with Dementia (GEPAD). *J Neurol*. 2008;255:255–264.
10. Hely MA, Reid WG, Adena MA, et al. The Sydney multicenter study of Parkinson's disease: the inevitability of dementia at 20years. *Mov Disord*. 2008;23:837–844.
11. Walker Z, Possin KL, Boeve BF, et al. Lewy body dementias. *Lancet*. 2015;386:1683–1697.
12. Kyle K, Bronstein JM. Treatment of psychosis in Parkinson's disease and dementia with Lewy Bodies: a review. *Parkinsonism Relat Disord*. 2020;75:55–62.
13. Mansuri Z, Reddy A, Vadukapuram R, et al. Pimavanserin in the treatment of Parkinson's disease psychosis: meta-analysis and meta-regression of randomized clinical trials. *Innov Clin Neurosci*. 2022;19:46–51.
14. Howell MJ, Schenck CH. Rapid eye movement sleep behavior disorder and neurodegenerative disease. *JAMA Neurol*. 2015;72:707–712.
15. Brust JC. Substance abuse and movement disorders. *Mov Disord*. 2010;25:2010–2020.
16. Baig SS, Strong M, Rosser E, et al. 22 Years of predictive testing for Huntington's disease: the experience of the UK Huntington's Prediction Consortium. *Eur J Hum Genet*. 2016;24:1396–1402.
17. Dutta N, Cavanna AE. The effectiveness of habit reversal therapy in the treatment of Tourette syndrome and other chronic tic disorders: a systematic review. *Funct Neurol*. 2013;28:7–12.
18. Tourette's Syndrome Study Group.. Treatment of ADHD in children with tics: a randomized controlled trial. *Neurology*. 2002;58:527–536.
19. Pringsheim T, Okun MS, Muller-Vahl K, et al. Practice guideline recommendations summary: treatment of tics in people with Tourette syndrome and chronic tic disorders. *Neurology*. 2019;92:896–906.
20. Schilsky ML, Roberts EA, Bronstein JM, et al. A multidisciplinary approach to the diagnosis and management of Wilson disease: executive summary of the 2022 Practice Guidance on Wilson disease from the American Association for the Study of Liver Diseases. *Hepatology*. 2023;77:1428–1455.
21. Trenkwalder C, Allen R, Hogl B, et al. Restless legs syndrome associated with major diseases: a systematic review and new concept. *Neurology*. 2016;86:1336–1343.
22. Manconi M, Garcia-Borreguero D, Schormair B, et al. Restless legs syndrome. *Nat Rev Dis Primers*. 2021;7:80.
23. Louis ED, Okun MS. It is time to remove the 'benign' from the essential tremor label. *Parkinsonism Relat Disord*. 2011;17:516–520.
24. Baek JH, Kinrys G, Nierenberg AA. Lithium tremor revisited: pathophysiology and treatment. *Acta Psychiatr Scand*. 2014;129:17–23.

25. Niethammer M, Ford B. Permanent lithium-induced cerebellar toxicity: three cases and review of literature. *Mov Disord*. 2007;22:570–573.
26. Barone P, Santangelo G, Amboni M, et al. Pisa syndrome in Parkinson's disease and parkinsonism: clinical features, pathophysiology, and treatment. *Lancet Neurol*. 2016;15:1063–1074.
27. Janno S, Holi M, Tuisku K, et al. Prevalence of neuroleptic-induced movement disorders in chronic schizophrenia inpatients. *Am J Psychiatry*. 2004;161:160–163.
28. Parksepp M, Ljubajev U, Taht K, et al. Prevalence of neuroleptic-induced movement disorders: an 8-year follow-up study in chronic schizophrenia inpatients. *Nord J Psychiatry*. 2016;70:498–502.
29. Poyurovsky M, Weizman A. Treatment of antipsychotic-induced akathisia: role of serotonin 5-HT(2a) receptor antagonists. *Drugs*. 2020;80:871–882.
30. McEvoy JP. A double-blind crossover comparison of anti-parkinson drug therapy: amantadine versus anticholinergics in 90 normal volunteers, with an emphasis on differential effects on memory function. *J Clin Psychiatry*. 1987;48(suppl.):20–23.
31. Jeste DV, Caligiuri MP. Tardive dyskinesia. *Schizophr Bull*. 1993;19:303–315.
32. Carbon M, Hsieh CH, Kane JM, et al. Tardive dyskinesia prevalence in the period of second-generation antipsychotic use: a meta-analysis. *J Clin Psychiatry*. 2017;78:e264–e278.
33. Jha MK, Mathew SJ. Pharmacotherapies for treatment-resistant depression: how antipsychotics fit in the rapidly evolving therapeutic landscape. *Am J Psychiatry*. 2023;180:190–199.
34. Reus VI, Fochtmann LJ, Eyler AE, et al. The American Psychiatric Association Practice Guideline on the Use of Antipsychotics to Treat Agitation or Psychosis in Patients With Dementia. *Am J Psychiatry*. 2016;173:543–546.
35. Caroff SN, Citrome L, Meyer J, et al. A modified Delphi consensus study of the screening, diagnosis, and treatment of tardive dyskinesia. *J Clin Psychiatry*. 2020:81.
36. Munetz MR, Benjamin S. How to examine patients using the Abnormal Involuntary Movement Scale. *Hosp Community Psychiatry*. 1988;39:1172–1177.
37. Solmi M, Pigato G, Kane JM, et al. Treatment of tardive dyskinesia with VMAT-2 inhibitors: a systematic review and meta-analysis of randomized controlled trials. *Drug Des Devel Ther*. 2018;12:1215–1238.
38. Adler LA, Rotrosen J, Edson R, et al. Vitamin E treatment for tardive dyskinesia. Veterans Affairs Cooperative Study #394 Study Group. *Arch Gen Psychiatry*. 1999;56:836–841.
39. Anandan C, Jankovic J. Botulinum toxin in movement disorders: an update. *Toxins (Basel)*. 2021;13(1):42.
40. Szczakowska A, Gabryelska A, Gawlik-Kotelnicka O, et al. Deep brain stimulation in the treatment of tardive dyskinesia. *J Clin Med*. 2023;12(5):1868.
41. Mink JW. Conversion disorder and mass psychogenic illness in child neurology. *Ann N Y Acad Sci*. 2013;1304:40–44.

42. Muller-Vahl KR, Pisarenko A, Jakubovski E, et al. Stop that! It's not Tourette's but a new type of mass sociogenic illness. *Brain.* 2022;145:476–480.

43. *Functional Neurological Disorders.* Available from: https://neurosymptoms.org/en/.

44. Sharpe M, Walker J, Williams C, et al. Guided self-help for functional (psychogenic) symptoms: a randomized controlled efficacy trial. *Neurology.* 2011;77:564–572.

45. Maggio JB, Ospina JP, Callahan J, et al. Outpatient physical therapy for functional neurological disorder: a preliminary feasibility and naturalistic outcome study in a U.S. cohort. *J Neuropsychiatry Clin Neurosci.* 2020;32:85–89.

20

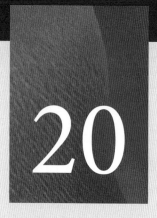

INFECTIOUS OR INFLAMMATORY NEUROPSYCHIATRIC IMPAIRMENT

G. KYLE HARROLD, MD ■ JENNY J. LINNOILA, MD, PHD

OVERVIEW

While there has always been a close association between neurologic and psychiatric disorders, in the past decade and a half, with the identification of a new class of autoimmune encephalitides that are associated with profound neuropsychiatric impairments,[1] and the realization that psychiatric disorders, such as schizophrenia, may be linked with deficient components of the immune system that are responsible for synaptic pruning,[2] the two disciplines have become increasingly interwoven. This overlap necessitates greater collaboration between neurologists and psychiatrists and a multi-disciplinary approach to shared patients. Similarly, there may be considerable overlap in the manifestations of infectious and inflammatory etiologies. The blending between "neurologic," "psychiatric," "infectious," and "inflammatory" disorders can make the diagnosis and treatment of these disorders daunting. This chapter aims to demystify these complex disorders and offer a practical approach to the diagnosis and treatment of infectious and inflammatory disorders that present with neuropsychiatric impairment.

POTENTIAL ETIOLOGIES OF ACUTE AND SUBACUTE NEUROPSYCHIATRIC IMPAIRMENT

Encephalitis Versus Encephalopathy

In the hospital setting, neuropsychiatric impairment is often secondary to similar, but distinct, entities—encephalitis and encephalopathy. In general, *encephalitis* (inflammation of the brain), can be thought of as

being due to direct involvement of the brain parenchyma, while *encephalopathy* is a more general term that refers to a non-specific confusional state that is not necessarily due to malfunction or inflammation of the brain. For instance, encephalopathy can stem from the dysfunction of other organs (e.g., the liver in hepatitis, the kidneys in uremia, and the entire body with sepsis). Although encephalitis can result in encephalopathy, the opposite is not necessarily true, that is, encephalopathy does not necessarily imply encephalitis. While encephalitis is common in hospital settings, in most cases, its cause remains unknow. Even in cases in which an infectious etiology is strongly suspected, the causative microbe often goes un-identified. However, this may change with the incorporation of next-generation gene sequencing[3] of body fluids, including cerebrospinal fluid (CSF), for any known pathogen. A bevy of previously cryptogenic cases of encephalitis has been identified as autoimmune, often mediated by pathogenic antibodies to neuronal cell surface antigens, such as N-methyl-D-aspartic acid receptors (NMDARs). Indeed, a retrospective analysis of nearly 500 cases of cryptogenic encephalitis demonstrated that roughly 1% of them were due to NMDAR encephalitis.[4] The pathophysiology underlying these autoimmune encephalitides remains unknown.

Causes of Encephalopathy

Encephalopathy has a broad differential diagnosis. High on the list are toxic (both endogenous and exogenous) and metabolic causes. Infectious etiologies include hepatitis, systemic infections, and especially in the elderly, common infections (e.g., pneumonia and urinary tract infections). Inflammatory causes (e.g., autoimmune hepatitis, primary biliary sclerosis, systemic lupus erythematosus, and immunoglobulin [Ig] A nephropathy) lead to encephalopathy primarily by contributing to end-organ dysfunction or failure. The medical literature also suggests that even celiac disease can lead to psychosis.[5] Encephalopathy is typically manifested as an altered mental status (e.g., delirium), with waxing and waning confusion, disorientation, hallucinations, and sometimes, seizures.

Evaluation for Encephalopathy

Laboratory tests of blood and urine for encephalopathy commonly reveal abnormalities, such as metabolic or electrolyte derangements (e.g., hyponatremia, hypercalcemia, hypercapnia, hyperammonemia, transaminitis, elevated creatinine and/or blood urea nitrogen levels, hyper/hypoglycemia), elevated white blood cell (WBC) counts, and/or positive toxicology screening results (e.g., a positive drug screen and/or an elevated anion gap). An electroencephalogram (EEG) can reveal generalized triphasic discharges, which are classically seen in cases of toxic/metabolic encephalopathy. Brain magnetic resonance imaging (MRI) is usually normal or reveals symmetric changes, indicative of a generalized process that adversely affects the brain. Since this chapter focuses on infectious and inflammatory causes of encephalitis rather than on the work-up for an altered mental status secondary to encephalopathy, the reader is referred to Chapter 9.

Encephalitic Neuropsychiatric Impairment
Clinical Features of Infectious Encephalitis

When encephalitis is suspected, distinguishing between infectious and inflammatory causes (Table 20.1) can

TABLE 20.1	
Clues to an Autoimmune Versus Infectious Etiology for Encephalitis	
Clues to an Autoimmune Etiology	**Clues to an Infectious Etiology**
Symptoms: predominantly psychiatric (especially early and at an unusual age for initial presentation)	*Symptoms*: broader, including fever,[a] headache, obtundation, meningismus
Onset: subacute (days to weeks)	*Onset*: often precipitous[a] (hours to days)
Medical history: personal or family history of organ- or non-organ-specific autoimmune disorder	*Medical history*: immunocompromised state
Serum: systemic markers of autoimmunity (e.g., elevated ANA or TPO antibodies) and/or identification of a neural autoantibody	*Serum*: markedly elevated[a] ESR and/or CRP, tests (cultures, ELISAs, PCR, Western blots, antibodies, blood smears) identifying specific microbes
Cancer status: history of or concurrent malignancy	*Cancer status*: generally N/A, unless immunocompromised (e.g., from chemotherapy)
CSF studies: elevated WBC (usually <100 cells/μL), protein (usually <100 mg/dL), IgG index, oligoclonal bands, synthesis rate, and/or identification of a neural autoantibody	*CSF studies*: elevated WBC (usually >100 cells/μL[a]), protein (often >100 mg/dL), elevated RBC and/or xanthochromia possible, decreased glucose, tests (cultures, ELISAs, PCR, western blots, antibodies, smears) identifying specific microbes
EEG: focal abnormalities	*EEG*: no particular pattern; could have triphasic waves
MRI brain: T2/FLAIR hyperintensities, rarely enhancement	*MRI brain*: T2/FLAIR hyperintensities (may be symmetric), more often has an enhancement, may have leptomeningeal or spinal cord involvement, may have a mass effect, may have blood
PET brain: areas of hyper/hypometabolism	*PET brain*: not typically done
Therapy: response to immunosuppression	*Therapy*: response to antimicrobials

[a]May not apply to immunocompromised patients.
ANA, Antinuclear antibody; *CRP*, C-reactive protein; *CSF*, cerebrospinal fluid; *EEG*, electroencephalogram; *ELISA*, enzyme-linked immunosorbent assay; *ESR*, erythrocyte sedimentation rate, *FLAIR*, fluid attenuation inversion recovery; *IgG*, immunoglobulin G; *MRI*, magnetic resonance imaging; *N/A*, not applicable; *PCR*, polymerase chain reaction; *PET*, positron emission tomography; *RBC*, red blood cell count; *TPO*, anti-thyroperoxidase antibody; *WBC*, white blood cell.

be challenging, as there is often overlap in the patient's initial clinical presentation. Regarding this chapter, inflammatory causes of encephalitis refer to autoimmune neurologic disorders, including those associated with cancer, which are termed "paraneoplastic disorders." In general, infectious etiologies of encephalitis are often associated with fever,[6] but this is not always true, especially in immunocompromised or elderly individuals, who may not be able to mount a robust immune response. If a headache is present, it is more likely to indicate an infection, as opposed to an inflammatory encephalitis. In addition, infectious encephalitis usually leads to a precipitous decline over a matter of hours to days, as opposed to the more gradual decline that is seen with inflammatory causes of encephalitis, which more often tend to manifest over weeks to months. Of course, exceptions exist (e.g., autoimmune encephalitis in children can present with an acute course).[7] The neuropsychiatric decline noted with syphilis can appear decades after the initial infection. Similarly, people living with the human immunodeficiency virus (HIV) can develop cognitive impairment (termed HIV-associated neurocognitive disorder) after living with a well-controlled HIV infection for several decades). Some infections (such as toxoplasmosis, which classically affects people with acquired immunodeficiency syndrome and can cause symptoms that progress over weeks) arise in immunocompromised individuals; these may develop subacutely.[8]

In addition to encephalitis, infections can also trigger meningitis, or inflammation of the meninges, the protective coverings of the brain. Signs of meningismus include fever, headache, nuchal rigidity (which may produce positive Kernig and Brudzinski signs), and vomiting with or without photophobia.[6] Meningitis is much less frequently associated with autoimmune causes.

Clinical Features of Autoimmune Encephalitis

Regardless of the specific manifestations, there are a few features that raise suspicion for autoimmune disorders.[9] There is usually a distinct change from a patient's baseline functional status over days to weeks. The patient's symptoms may have a fluctuating course. Family members often describe that the patient's behavioral or cognitive changes came "out of the blue" and are highly divergent from the patient's

baseline personality. When considering psychiatric presentations, the patient's age is important; for example, it is highly unusual for hallucinations to occur in a young child, or for schizophrenia to first manifest in a patient's later decades. Such circumstances would be less consistent with a primary psychiatric disorder and more consistent with autoimmune encephalitis. Additionally, a patient presenting primarily with isolated psychiatric symptoms is more likely to have an autoimmune disorder than an infectious encephalitis. However, it is exceedingly rare for patients with autoimmune encephalitis to remain with purely psychiatric symptoms over time, without accumulating other symptoms, such as confusion, movement disorders, or seizures. Patients with autoimmune encephalitis may have a personal or family history of a systemic autoimmune disease, such as Hashimoto thyroiditis, rheumatoid arthritis, and/or celiac disease. Moreover, as with systemic autoimmunity, patients may have overlapping autoimmune neurologic diseases, such as neuromyelitis optica and autoimmune encephalitis,[10] making diagnosis and treatment particularly challenging. Paraneoplastic disorders cause neurologic symptoms in patients with malignancy, commonly before the cancer is diagnosed.[11] A personal history of neoplasm in a patient with new neurologic symptoms should raise one's suspicion of a paraneoplastic disorder. It can be difficult to differentiate infectious from inflammatory encephalitides, especially early on in a patient's course, because many patients with autoimmune encephalitis present with a viral prodrome,[12] as in up to half of cases of NMDAR encephalitis.

Work-Up for Infectious and Inflammatory Causes

Bloodwork. The initial work-up for infectious and autoimmune causes of encephalitis should always include basic bloodwork, a urinalysis, and toxicology screens, to exclude readily diagnosed causes of encephalopathy. Serum markers that raise the suspicion of infectious or inflammatory encephalitis include an elevated erythrocyte sedimentation rate (ESR) and/or C-reactive protein (CRP). Markedly elevated values are more often associated with infectious, as opposed to inflammatory encephalitides, although CNS-isolated infections may not lead to elevations in systemic inflammatory markers. In autoimmune encephalitis, ESR and CRP values can be normal or elevated. Patients with infectious encephalitis may have an elevated serum WBC count. In the work-up for autoimmune encephalitis, elevated antinuclear antibodies or thyroid peroxidase (TPO) antibodies, although non-specific, can be considered as helpful markers for a patient's autoimmune tendency.[9] Specific infectious etiologies can be tested for in the serum, most often by growing cultures, testing for antibodies with enzyme-linked immunosorbent assays (ELISAs) or Western blots, or nucleic acids with polymerase chain reactions (PCRs).[6] A blood smear may be useful for detecting organisms and/or abnormal blood cells. Testing should be selected based on a patient's presentation and personal risk factors, accounting for their age, sex, medical history, location, behaviors, travel history, and immunocompromised status, if applicable. Consulting with an infectious disease specialist, either general or neurologic, can be useful to determine the specific tests to order.

CSF Analysis. Before performing a lumbar puncture (LP), it is imperative to obtain either a computed tomography (CT) or MRI imaging scan of the head, to rule out masses or hydrocephalus, which can be associated with infectious causes, and may create a risk for herniation from a LP. Central nervous system (CNS) infections can cause CSF to appear cloudy or yellow. Herpes infections are neurotropic[13,14] and both herpes simplex virus (HSV) and varicella-zoster virus (VZV) can cause necrosis and hemorrhage, potentially resulting in pink CSF, elevated CSF red blood cell counts, elevated CSF protein counts, and/or the presence of xanthochromia. Both infectious and inflammatory encephalitides can result in elevations of protein and WBC counts. However, the protein and WBC count elevations are typically much higher with infections, for instance, with protein >100 mg/dL and a WBC count >100/μL, as compared with <100 for each, on average, for autoimmune encephalitides.[9] The WBC differential is also important. Whereas infectious encephalitides can be associated with elevations in polymorphonuclear leukocytes (for bacterial more than viral causes), autoimmune encephalitides are overwhelmingly associated with elevated lymphocyte counts. However, viral meningitides can shift from a polymorphonuclear to a lymphocytic predominance.[6] CSF glucose is only rarely abnormal in autoimmune encephalitides. In contrast, especially with bacterial meningitis and tuberculous meningitis, CSF glucose may be decreased in CNS infections. In autoimmune encephalitides, an initial CSF pleocytosis often resolves and is replaced with alternative markers of inflammation, including an elevated immunoglobulin G (IgG) index and oligoclonal bands,[1] which are considered general markers of intrathecal antibody synthesis, but can also be elevated in infectious encephalitis. As with the serum (and other bodily fluids), microbes can also be tested for directly in the CSF. A Gram stain and smear may be useful for detecting organisms and/or abnormal immune cells. Consultation with an infectious disease specialist can help to determine which cultures and studies to order based on the patient's presentation, CSF markers, and personal risk factors (such as age, sex, medical history, location, behaviors, travel history, and immunocompromised status), if applicable. For example, the initial work-up for people from an area of the world where tuberculosis (TB) is endemic may be tailored differently than for someone who has become immunocompromised after a bone marrow transplant.

Neural Autoantibody Testing. The past decade and a half have seen the identification of a multitude of new neurally directed autoantibodies that have been linked with autoimmune encephalitis.[1,15] Many are now available for commercial testing and are available as part of panels that are grouped by symptomatology, including encephalitis, seizures, and dementia.[9] The current standard of care is to order these symptom-based panels, as opposed to more traditional paraneoplastic panels, which generally do not include newer antibodies. Rather, relevant paraneoplastic antibodies are now embedded within the newer panels. As there can be significant overlap between the clinical signs and symptoms associated with each neural autoantibody, it is prudent to order a comprehensive autoantibody evaluation, as opposed to testing for a single autoantibody or a small subset of them. Neural autoantibody testing is available for serum and CSF. It is important to analyze both, as they are complementary. For instance, some autoantibody tests, such as for voltage-gated calcium channel (VGCC) antibodies, have been validated only in serum. Additionally, testing for other antibodies, such as leucine-rich, glioma-inactivated 1 (LGI-1), is more sensitive from the serum, as compared to NMDAR antibody testing, which is more sensitive from the CSF. For example, an analysis of paired CSF and serum samples from 250 patients with NMDAR encephalitis showed that whereas all the CSF samples tested positive for NMDAR antibodies, between 6% and 13% (depending on the methodology used) of the corresponding paired serum samples tested negative for NMDAR antibodies.[16] Thus, testing both the serum and the CSF raises the overall sensitivity (and specificity) of the testing. It is important to note that neural autoantibody testing is not fool-proof; sometimes it can reveal the presence of antibodies that are poorly correlated with the patient's symptoms, while at other times the patient may test positive for a low level of an antibody, such as glutamic acid decarboxylase (GAD-65) autoantibodies, which may only indicate an autoimmune tendency, as opposed to a specific autoimmune encephalitis diagnosis. It is also important to test both serum and CSF because while earlier first-episode psychosis (FEP) literature reported that a small number of patients with isolated psychosis tested positive for neural autoantibodies, such as NMDAR from the blood,[17,18] and thus were felt to have autoimmune psychosis,[19] when a prospective analysis of patients with FEP was expanded to include routine analysis of the CSF, no patients tested positive for neural autoantibodies.[20] Thus, the results of neural autoantibody testing must be interpreted carefully, to determine whether they are clinically relevant. Table 20.2 lists neural autoantibodies that are commonly associated with autoimmune encephalitides.

Intracellular Versus Cell Surface–Targeted Neural Autoantibodies. Paraneoplastic disorders, such as myasthenia gravis linked with thymoma[21] (and acetylcholine receptor antibodies) and Lambert-Eaton myasthenic syndrome linked with small cell lung cancer (and VGCC antibodies),[22] have long been recognized. In the past few decades, many more paraneoplastic disorders have been identified, linked with conditions such as cerebellar degeneration and limbic encephalitis,[11] a disorder characterized by confusion, behavioral changes, and/or seizures. Many paraneoplastic disorders have been associated with antibodies targeting intracellular proteins. Studies have shown that many of these neural autoantibodies, while serving as markers of paraneoplasia, do not appear to be pathogenic themselves. Rather, they seem to reflect

cytotoxic effector T-cell-mediated CNS damage, which is generally poorly responsive to immunotherapy, resulting in limited neurologic recovery of patients, even with maximal treatment.[23]

However, the last nearly two decades have seen the identification of many new neural autoantibodies, especially ones associated with autoimmune encephalitis.[24–40] As opposed to many of the previously identified paraneoplastic antibodies, these antibodies' antigens are mostly on, or associated with, the neuronal cell surface. These autoantibodies are less often associated with malignancy. Moreover, many of them are themselves pathogenic.[24,30,32,38,41–43] The autoantibodies trigger processes, such as receptor downregulation, which are often reversible, in large part explaining the responsiveness of patients' symptoms to immunotherapy. In general, these neural antibodies predict better responses to immunotherapy. However, brain atrophy and other irreversible damage can also occur with these autoantibodies, necessitating rapid diagnosis and treatment for the best possible clinical outcomes.

Overlap Syndromes: Parainfectious Autoimmune Encephalitis

The identification of a neural autoantibody typically corresponds with a diagnosis of autoimmune encephalitis. However, reports of autoimmune (in particular NMDAR) encephalitis after HSV encephalitis (HSE) (and now COVID-19[44]) have complicated the diagnostic picture, as there appears to be overlap between infectious and autoimmune encephalitides.[45–48] Some patients who have been treated for HSE and either suffer a recurrence of neurologic symptoms or continue to deteriorate or fail to improve, rather than having a recurrence of HSE, as was originally thought, have been found to have subsequent autoimmune encephalitis. It is important to recognize this, as autoimmune encephalitides are often immunotherapy responsive, and thus the high morbidity typically associated with HSE may be modifiable. Many adult patients with post-HSE NMDAR encephalitis have predominantly neuropsychiatric symptoms, including behavior changes, agitation, aggression, suicidal ideation, confusion, and delusions, that were previously interpreted as sequelae of HSE.[49] It is possible that these symptoms may instead be attributable to autoimmune encephalitis. Moreover,

TABLE 20.2

Neural Autoantibodies Associated With Autoimmune Encephalitides

Antigen	Intracellular/Cell Surface	Clinical Features	Tumor Association
AGNA[90] (SOX1)	Intracellular	Lambert-Eaton myasthenic syndrome (LEMS), limbic encephalitis, neuropathy	Highly associated with small cell lung cancer, especially with LEMS
AMPAR[24]	Cell surface	Limbic encephalitis; may occur with pure psychiatric manifestations Relapses common	~70% (lung, breast, thymoma)
Amphiphysin[91]	Intracellular	Wide clinical spectrum: stiff person syndrome, cerebellar degeneration, limbic encephalitis, encephalomyelitis, myelopathy, peripheral neuropathy, opsoclonus myoclonus	~85% (breast, small cell lung cancer)
ANNA-1[92] (Anti-Hu)	Intracellular	Wide clinical spectrum: sensory neuronopathy, limbic encephalitis, cranial neuropathies, cerebellar degeneration, encephalomyelitis, partial epilepsy, status epilepticus, autonomic dysfunction including intestinal pseudo-obstruction, opsoclonus myoclonus	~80% (small cell lung cancer, neuroblastoma, prostate cancer)
ANNA-3[40]	Intracellular	Neuropathy, cognitive changes, cerebellar ataxia, dysautonomia	~90% (most commonly neuroendocrine tumors)
CASPR2[25,69]	Cell surface	Encephalopathy, Morvan syndrome, neuromyotonia. Relapses of encephalopathy are common	~0%–40% (thymoma)
CRMP-5[93] (anti-CV2)	Intracellular	Wide clinical spectrum: cerebellar degeneration, limbic encephalitis, optic neuritis, retinopathy, uveitis, chorea, encephalomyelitis, sensorimotor neuropathy	~75% (small cell lung cancer, thymoma)
DPPX[26]	Cell surface	Encephalopathy with CNS hyperexcitability: confusion, psychiatric manifestations, tremor, myoclonus, nystagmus, hyperekplexia, PERM-like symptoms, ataxia Diarrhea and profound weight loss are common	Rare B-cell neoplasms reported
GABA$_A$R[32,94]	Cell surface	Prominent seizures, status epilepticus	Infrequent, associated with thymoma
GABA$_B$R[27]	Cell surface	Limbic encephalitis, prominent seizures, status epilepticus	~50% (lung, neuroendocrine)
GFAP[39]	Intracellular	Wide clinical spectrum: encephalopathy, tremor, headache, myelopathic signs, meningeal signs, optic disc edema, psychiatric symptoms, ataxia, autonomic dysfunction, seizures, meningoencephalomyelitis	~1/3 (teratoma ≫ adenoma, CNS glioma, lung cancer)
GAD-65[95,96]	Intracellular	Wide clinical spectrum: encephalopathy, stiff person syndrome, cerebellar ataxia, seizure disorder With cancer more likely to see opsoclonus myoclonus syndrome and encephalomyelitis	~10% (lung cancer, neuroendocrine tumor, thymoma, breast cancer)[97]
GlyαR[28]	Cell surface	Wide clinical spectrum: stiff person syndrome, PERM, limbic encephalitis, cerebellar degeneration, and optic neuritis reported	Infrequent
IgLON5[33,98]	Cell surface	Sleep disorder, gait abnormalities, bulbar dysfunction, chorea, cognitive decline, papillitis[99]	None reported
Kelch11[34,100]	Intracellular	Rhomboencephalitis ≫ neuropsychiatric dysfunction, myeloneuropathy, and cervical amyotrophy. Associated with hearing loss and tinnitus	Germ cell testicular cancer common

TABLE 20.2
Neural Autoantibodies Associated With Autoimmune Encephalitides—cont'd

Antigen	Intracellular/Cell Surface	Clinical Features	Tumor Association
LGI-1[25,101]	Cell surface	Limbic encephalitis, faciobrachial dystonic seizures, REM sleep behavior disorder, myoclonus. ~60% with hyponatremia (adults)	≤10% (small cell lung cancer, thymoma)
LUZP4[36]	Intracellular	Rhomboencephalitis > limbic encephalitis, seizures/encephalitis, motor neuronopathy/polyradiculopathy. Often co-exists with Kelch11 antibodies	Germ cell testicular cancer common
Anti-Ma2 (Ta)[102]	Intracellular	Ma2 (only): limbic encephalitis, hypothalamic dysfunction, brainstem encephalitis	Germ cell testicular cancer common
mGluR5[29]	Cell surface	Ophelia syndrome: limbic encephalitis, myoclonus. Very few cases	Hodgkin lymphoma; may occur without tumor
MOG[37]	Cell surface	Mostly associated with demyelinating disease in adults, especially affecting optic nerves and spinal cord, and acute disseminated encephalomyelitis (ADEM) in children, but it is also associated with autoimmune encephalitis in children	Infrequent[103]
NIF[35,104]	Intracellular	Encephalopathy, cerebellar ataxia, myeloradiculopathy	~50% (most often small cell or other neuroendocrine)
NMDAR[12] (GluN1)	Cell surface	NMDAR encephalitis: progression through psychiatric manifestations, insomnia, reduced verbal output, seizures, amnesia, movement disorders, catatonia, hypoventilation, autonomic instability, coma. ~50% Viral prodrome ~30% with "delta brush pattern" on EEG Relapses 12% at 2 years	Age-dependent: ~10%–45%, most often ovarian teratomas, rarely carcinomas, rare in children
Neurexin-3α[30]	Cell surface	Confusion, seizures, altered consciousness Often follows viral prodrome (fever, headache, GI symptoms) Patients can deteriorate rapidly Few cases reported	None reported
Septin-7[38]	Intracellular	Encephalopathy with prominent neuropsychiatric symptoms, myelopathy, ataxia	Infrequent; breast cancer, lymphoma, carcinoid have been reported
VGCC (N-type, P/Q type)[105]	Cell surface	N: variable; includes encephalopathy, seizures. P/Q: cerebellar degeneration, seizures	Sometimes associated with small cell lung cancer

Percentage refers to the percentage of patients with particular antibodies that also have malignancy.

AGNA, Antiglial nuclear antibody; *AMPAR*, alpha-amino-3-hydroxy-5-methyl-4-isoxazolepropionic acid receptor; *ANNA*, antineuronal nuclear antibody; *CASPR2*, contactin-associated protein-like 2; *CNS*, central nervous system; *CRMP-5*, collapsin response mediator protein 5; *DPPX*, dipeptidyl-peptidase-like protein-6; *EEG*, electroencephalogram; *GABAR*, gamma-amino-butyric acid receptor; *GAD-65*, glutamic acid decarboxylase; *GI*, gastrointestinal; *GluN1*, ionotropic NMDA glutamate receptor 1; *GlyαR*, glycine alpha receptor; *IgLON5*, immunoglobulin-like cell adhesion molecule 5; *LEMS*, Lambert-Eaton myasthenic syndrome; *LGI-1*, leucine-rich, glioma-inactivated 1; *LUZP4*, leucine zipper 4; *mGluR*, metabotropic glutamate receptor; *NIF*, neuronal intermediate filament; *NMDAR*, N-methyl-D-aspartic acid receptor; *MOG*, myelin oligodendrocyte glycoprotein; *PERM*, progressive encephalomyelitis with rigidity and myoclonus; *REM*, rapid eye movement; *SOX1*, sex-determining region Y box 1 transcription factor; *VGCC*, voltage-gated calcium channel.

this phenomenon happens with other viral encephalitides, which can trigger the production of neural autoantibodies.[50,51] Thus, a clear distinction between infectious and inflammatory causes of encephalitis does not always exist.

Electroencephalography. Infectious and autoimmune encephalitides can both cause seizures. In contrast with the generalized discharges (such as triphasic waves) often associated with encephalopathy, encephalitides commonly cause localized, or focal, abnormalities on the EEG. It is important to recognize that seizure phenotypes are broader than generalized tonic-clonic, or "grand mal" seizures. This is particularly important when considering the neuropsychiatric manifestations of seizures; partial complex seizures can cause behavioral arrest, confusion, and a sense of "lost time"; temporal lobe seizures can lead to auditory hallucinations and behavioral changes (such as hyper-religiosity); seizures involving the amygdala can result in fear or anxiety; and occipital lobe seizures can present with visual hallucinations. Whereas it may be impossible to distinguish between infectious and autoimmune encephalitides based on the EEG alone, at least one distinctive EEG abnormality, termed "extreme delta brush" has been strongly associated with NMDAR encephalitis.[52] On the other hand, faciobrachial dystonic (FBD) seizures, brief dystonic contractions of the patient's face and/or arm (typically on the same side) that are often seen in LGI-1 encephalitis,[53] may not be picked up by standard EEG scalp electrodes, perhaps due to a deep seizure focus. If autoimmune encephalitis is suspected, it is important to make the reading neurologist aware, so that the patient's EEG can be interpreted in the appropriate context.

Brain Imaging. Brain imaging is an essential component of the work-up for encephalitis. Brain MRIs should be done with contrast, whenever possible. In general, MRI abnormalities, including T2/fluid attenuation inversion recovery (FLAIR) hyperintensities and contrast enhancement, are more often seen in infectious, as compared to autoimmune encephalitides. An exception can be seen with severe and/or frequent seizures, which can lead to T2/FLAIR hyperintensities, contrast enhancement, and

diffusion restriction on diffusion-weighted imaging.[54] Autoimmune encephalitides do not typically cause hydrocephalus, meningitis, ventriculitis, and the accumulation of material (proteinaceous debris) in the ventricles, each of which can be seen with infectious encephalitides. Autoimmune encephalitides, especially early in their course, may not produce any abnormalities on brain MRI. In these cases, abnormalities may instead be visible on positron emission tomography (PET) imaging, in the form of areas of hypo- or hypermetabolism.[55,56] While PET findings can be seen in both infectious and autoimmune encephalitides, there are particular PET patterns, such as a frontotemporal-to-occipital gradient, reported in severe cases of NMDAR encephalitis,[57] which raise the suspicion for autoimmune encephalitis. In addition, whereas the FBD seizures noted in LGI-1 encephalitis may not produce abnormalities on the EEG, in some cases, they are associated with changes in the basal ganglia on brain MRI and/or PET imaging.[58] Like focal EEG findings, discussed above, focal imaging abnormalities, seen either via MRI or PET scans, may sometimes correspond with a patient's neuropsychiatric impairments (e.g., hyperintensity or hypermetabolism in the amygdala corresponding with fearful preoccupations).

Malignancy Screening. As mentioned previously, some neural autoantibodies have been associated with neoplasms, particularly those that target intracellular proteins. This necessitates a search for malignancy, guided by a patient's particular neural autoantibodies and their personal risk factors for cancer (such as age, family or personal medical history, and smoking status).[9] Neoplasms are much less frequent in children than in adults.[59,60] Because neurologic symptoms frequently present before malignancy in paraneoplastic disorders (in up to 70% of cases),[11] neoplasms associated with autoimmunity are often detected early into their course and thus they can be small and have limited regional spread, to a single lymph node, for instance. Therefore, they may be difficult to identify on conventional imaging due to only subtle imaging abnormalities. Given this, pulmonary nodules or enlarged lymph nodes should be investigated further, when autoimmune encephalitides are diagnosed or suspected. There is sometimes controversy as

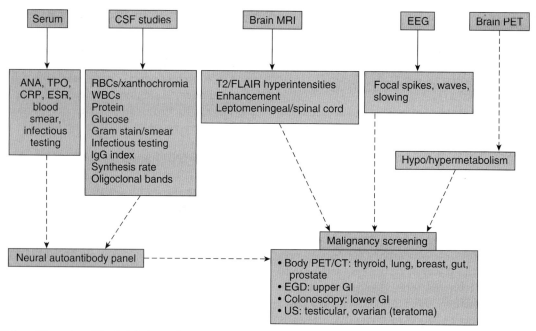

Fig. 20.1 ■ *Diagnostic workflow for infectious and/or autoimmune encephalitis.* Solid arrows indicate work-ups done for both infectious and autoimmune encephalitides. Dashed arrows indicate additional work-up done for autoimmune encephalitides. *ANA,* Antinuclear antibody; *CRP,* C-reactive protein; *CSF,* cerebrospinal fluid, *CT,* computerized tomography; *EEG,* electroencephalogram; *EGD,* esophagogastroduodenoscopy; *ESR,* erythrocyte sedimentation rate; *FLAIR,* fluid attenuation inversion recovery; *GI,* gastrointestinal; *IgG,* immunoglobulin G; *MRI,* magnetic resonance imaging; *PET,* positron emission tomography; *RBCs,* red blood cells; *TPO,* thyroid peroxidase antibody; *US,* ultrasound; *WBCs,* white blood cells. (Modified with permission from Linnoila J, et al. *Semin Neurol.* 2016;36:382–396.)

to whether PET scans of the body should be used routinely in autoimmune malignancy work-ups. A study examining the added benefit of PET in cases of suspected paraneoplastic disorders determined that PET detected malignancies in up to 20% of cases suspected of being paraneoplastic, but where CT imaging was negative.[61] This included cancers of the thyroid (papillary), tonsil (squamous cell), lung (small cell, non-small cell, and adenocarcinoma), and adenocarcinomas of the colon, prostate, and breast. However, the imaging modality is important to consider, depending on the targeted malignancy. For instance, for tumors of the testicles or ovaries, ultrasound and MRI are recommended, whereas for cancers of the gastrointestinal system, endoscopy and colonoscopy are preferred.[9] Certain neural autoantibodies are predictive of particular cancer types and can help to direct the malignancy search.[62] For patients with autoantibodies that are strongly associated with

malignancy, if no malignancy or a malignancy different from that which was expected is identified, it is prudent to do periodic cancer screening once or twice yearly for the next few years.

Fig. 20.1 outlines an overall diagnostic scheme for the work-up of infectious and autoimmune encephalitides. Diagnostic guidelines that incorporate the principles discussed above exist for the diagnosis of autoimmune encephalitis in adults[63] and children.[7]

ILLUSTRATIVE AUTOIMMUNE ENCEPHALITIC SYNDROMES MANIFESTING WITH NEUROPSYCHIATRIC IMPAIRMENT

In general, while the symptoms of infectious encephalitides are usually non-specific (such as fevers), they are often reflective of the underlying pathophysiology. An altered mental status and/or obtundation, headaches, and vomiting are frequently seen with increased intracranial pressure and hydrocephalus, as in CNS cryptococcal infections. However, headaches and vomiting can also be secondary to meningeal involvement, as seen with herpes, Lyme disease, or TB. Seizures can be due to general electrolyte imbalances, inflammation, or mass lesions, which can be seen in TB, toxoplasmosis, neurocysticercosis, or cryptococcal infections, among others.

What follows are examples of autoimmune encephalitides that can present with profound neuropsychiatric impairment.

NMDAR Encephalitis

NMDAR encephalitis (see Case 1) is the most common and likely the best known of the autoimmune encephalitides. It was the first of the newer neuronal cell surface-mediated autoimmune encephalitides to be described, in 2007.[31] This disorder is most common in young adults, predominantly in females. In adults, the syndrome often starts with a viral prodrome, which progresses to psychiatric/behavioral changes and insomnia, usually followed by decreased consciousness, seizures, unusual movements, and autonomic instability that may result in central hypoventilation.[12] As patients recover, symptoms typically resolve in the reverse order. The psychiatric changes typically include paranoid delusions, hallucinations, behavioral disinhibition, catatonia, and anxiety. Often, patient's families seek out psychiatric care initially, and indeed many patients have ended up in inpatient psychiatric units until they start to suffer from seizures, autonomic instability, and/or obtundation. The syndrome in children is similar, but the first symptoms are often behavioral changes, seizures, or movement disorders.[64] In children who develop NMDAR encephalitis after HSVE, they often develop choreoathetotic movements, which are generally not observed in adults with the disorder.[46,49,65,66] In NMDAR encephalitis, the CSF often shows a lymphocytic pleocytosis, with or without oligoclonal bands.[9] Only about one-third of patients have abnormal brain MRI findings, usually FLAIR hyperintensity in cortical or subcortical regions, or the cerebellum and/or brainstem. However, they may have the frontal to posterior gradient on PET imaging. Approximately 30% of patients have the "extreme

delta brush" EEG pattern. There is an age-related association with tumors, almost always ovarian teratomas, with a tumor found in 46% of all females, but in only 6% of those younger than 12 years.[12] In general, the best clinical outcomes are in cases where treatment was instituted early into the patient's course and where teratomas, if found, were resected.

Limbic Encephalitis

Limbic encephalitis is characterized by subacute short-term memory loss, confusion, sleep disturbances, and mood or behavioral changes, such as depression, irritability, and hallucinations occurring with or without seizures. Whereas initially thought to be associated with malignancy,[67] as historically many patients tested positive for paraneoplastic antibodies that have a strong correlation with cancer, it has recently become evident that many cell surface–targeted antibodies have also been linked with limbic encephalitis.[24,25,27] Limbic encephalitis is named based on the presenting symptoms, as well as on the underlying cerebral structures that are often disrupted, including the amygdala, hippocampus, and mesiotemporal lobes. Brain imaging often shows MRI T2 hyperintensity and/or contrast enhancement and/or PET hyper/hypometabolism in the mesiotemporal regions. If abnormal, the EEG often reveals focal temporal lobe seizures.

LGI-1 Encephalitis

LGI-1 antibodies are a more specific subset of voltage-gated potassium channel (a now obsolete term) antibodies, which are only rarely associated with malignancy (typically small cell lung cancer or thymomas).[25] Patients with LGI-1 antibodies are predominantly males, usually in their seventh decade of life. LGI-1 encephalitis usually presents with limbic encephalitis, seizures, and sleep disruptions. Rapid eye movement sleep behavior disorder has been described in patients with LGI-1 encephalitis.[68] Part of this dysfunction may be explained by antibodies that disrupt hypothalamic function,[69] which may also account for the hyponatremia that is seen in a little over half of adult patients. Some patients also have brief myoclonic-like FBD seizures, which are often not captured on the EEG. Less than half of the patients, have an abnormal CSF profile, although many of them have mesiotemporal FLAIR abnormalities consistent with limbic encephalitis on their brain MRI.[1] Patients often have profound short-term memory deficits, which can vary from case to case, depending upon the extent of mesiotemporal involvement, whether it is unilateral or bilateral, and whether atrophy has occurred. An analysis of 76 cases of patients with LGI-1 encephalitis showed that, while many cases are responsive to immunotherapy, including steroid treatment, treatment at sufficient doses (high-dose steroids, for instance) and for a sufficient amount of time (weeks to months) is necessary to prevent relapses.[70]

TREATMENT STRATEGIES FOR PATIENTS WITH INFECTIOUS OR INFLAMMATORY CAUSES OF ENCEPHALITIC NEUROPSYCHIATRIC IMPAIRMENT

Treatment strategies vary, depending upon whether an infectious or autoimmune encephalitis is being treated and whether the autoimmune encephalitis is paraneoplastic. For patients with multiple symptoms, including seizures, behavioral and/or mood changes, and movement disorders, an inter-disciplinary approach is often needed.[1] Successful treatment often stems from collaborations among neurologists, psychiatrists, infectious disease physicians, and/or oncologists, in addition to physical, speech, and occupational therapists, as well as social workers.

Treatment of Infectious Encephalitis or Meningitis

In general, treatment of infectious encephalitides must proceed rapidly once they are diagnosed or even suspected, as by the time the patient reaches medical attention, these conditions can proceed quickly, resulting in significant morbidity and mortality. If an infection is suspected, empiric treatment with antibiotics and/or antivirals is begun, until culture, PCR, and/or antibody results return.[6] Some of the morbidity associated with infectious encephalitis is secondary to a vigorous immune response, which can result in significant parenchymal edema. Thus, some infections, such as bacterial meningitis, tuberculous meningitis, and neurocysticercosis, are treated with steroids and antimicrobials. The timing can be critical, however, as

steroids have only shown benefit if given before antibiotics for bacterial meningitis, while in HSVE, animal studies have shown that giving steroids too early can interfere with the body's ability to fight the herpes infection.[71] In general, tuberculous, fungal, parasitic, and opportunistic infections require treatment for months with multiple agents. Treatment of cryptococcal and cytomegalovirus (CMV) infections requires different medications for the acute and maintenance phases. Some infections can co-exist, in particular in patients with HIV, who may have concurrent CMV, syphilis, TB, toxoplasmosis, and/or *Cryptococcus*. With the institution of antiretroviral treatment for HIV infection, as the immune system is restored, patients can paradoxically worsen, as the immune system starts fighting infections that have long been dormant in the host, resulting in immune reconstitution inflammatory syndrome (IRIS).[72] HIV requires life-long treatment to maintain viral suppression. For infections such as *Cryptococcus*, which can result in significant proteinaceous build-up and hydrocephalus, frequent LPs or CSF shunts may be required to manage increased intracranial pressure. Specific treatments are available for only certain viral encephalitides, including HSV, VZV, and CMV. For most viral infections, supportive care is provided, and co-morbidities are managed. Many viral meningitides or encephalitides remain undiagnosed and resolve on their own, with or without long-term sequela. Consultation with an infectious disease specialist is recommended.

Treatment of Autoimmune Encephalitis

Identification of Objective Measures to Follow Over Time

Treatment of autoimmune encephalitides often takes weeks to months. It is ideal to identify objective and validated markers of dysfunction that can be followed over time to assess response to treatment (Table 20.3).[9] For instance, standardized bedside neuropsychological tests, such as the Mini-Mental State Examination or the Montreal Cognitive Assessment should be performed to provide objective measurements of cognitive deficits. EEGs and seizure diaries can be used to track seizure frequency, location, and/or duration. Video can be useful for tracking adventitious movements. In general, antibody titers are not particularly

<table>
<tr><td colspan="2">TABLE 20.3
Objective Measures for Monitoring
Autoimmune Encephalitis Treatment Response</td></tr>
</table>

Symptom/ Finding	Objective Tests to Follow
Cognitive decline	MMSE, MoCA, and other neuropsychometric tests
Seizures	EEG (sleep deprived, EMU, or prolonged ambulatory), seizure diary
Brain inflammation	Brain MRI—T2/FLAIR, post-contrast sequences
	Brain PET—track areas of hypo/hypermetabolism
Movement disorder	Movement lab studies,[a] video
Autonomic dysfunction	Autonomic reflex testing, thermoregulatory sweat testing,[a] gastric emptying study, GI transit study

[a]Specialized studies are not available everywhere.
EEG, electroencephalogram; *EMU*, epilepsy monitoring unit; *FLAIR*, fluid attenuation inversion recovery; *GI*, gastrointestinal; *MMSE*, Mini-Mental Status Examination; *MoCA*, Montreal Cognitive Assessment; *MRI*, magnetic resonance imaging; *PET*, positron emission tomography.
Modified with permission from Linnoila J, et al. *Semin Neurol.* 2016;36:382–396.

useful in assessing clinical responses to treatment, although baseline titers drawn after clinical recovery may be useful for diagnosing a potential relapse.

General Treatment Goals

In general, treatment should aim to maximize the reversibility of symptoms and maintain the reversibility of symptoms while using a minimal therapeutic dose.[9] To maximize reversibility, it is imperative to make the diagnosis and to start treatment as early into the clinical course as possible. This may mean beginning treatment before antibody results have been received, or treating despite negative antibody results if there is a high suspicion of an autoimmune process. Having a neural autoantibody does not guarantee that the patient will respond to treatment, especially when it is an intracellular antibody. Successful treatment may be marked by stopping clinical progression, or deterioration, and not necessarily by reversal of symptoms. The overall initial goal of treatment is to determine whether there is a response to immunotherapy and then to maximize the reversibility of symptoms. To this end, a sufficient trial of immunosuppression

must be undertaken. However, if multiple immunotherapies have been tried with no signs of objective improvement, the disorder may not be immunotherapy responsive, and further trials may not be justified. Once a response to immunotherapy is demonstrated, the goal shifts to finding the minimal dose of immunotherapy that will best maintain the patient, if applicable. Whereas some autoimmune encephalitides can be monophasic, such as LGI-1 encephalitis,[73] others require longer-term treatment or maintenance immunotherapy to prevent relapse.

Treatment Strategies

The largest study of treatment outcomes for patients with a neuronal cell surface antibody thus far came from a meta-analysis of over 1500 patients with NMDAR encephalitis.[12,74] Most autoimmune encephalitides are treated similarly. Patients are generally treated with "first-line" therapy: steroids (typically intravenous [IV] × five daily doses), IV immunoglobulin (IVIg; five daily doses), and/or plasmapheresis (five sessions total, administered every other day), potentially followed by the second-line therapies, rituximab and cyclophosphamide. This is a reasonable strategy for the inpatient treatment of many of the cell surface–targeted neural autoantibodies, keeping in mind that recovery may take months. However, when there is little initial response to first-line agents, second-line therapies should be tried sooner rather than later, as opposed to trying multiple rounds of alternative first-line agents, particularly when the patient's symptoms are severe.[1] The second-line therapies are more likely to attack the pathophysiologic process underlying the patient's illness. For patients with intra-cellularly targeted antibodies, cyclophosphamide is generally preferable, as many of the other therapies are ineffective and there is an urgency to preserve brain function and structure, to attempt to prevent permanent brain atrophy. It is important to treat as early into the disease course as possible, as long-term studies have shown that even with treatment, patients are often left with lingering cognitive deficits and neuropsychiatric dysfunction.[70,75,76] This is especially true in LGI-1 encephalitis, where patients who are diagnosed and treated before the onset of cognitive decline fare better overall than those who are treated after its appearance.

Additionally, early treatment of patients with Ig-like cell adhesion molecule 5 (IgLON5) autoantibodies is associated with immunotherapy responsiveness,[77] whereas a prolonged course without treatment is associated with tauopathy and neurodegeneration.[33]

Paraneoplastic Disorders

For patients with a co-existing malignancy, it is important to treat both the tumor and the paraneoplastic disorder concomitantly, if possible.[1,9] Working closely with an oncologist is advised. Many people assume that cancer is more important to focus on initially. However, often malignancies associated with paraneoplastic disorders are small and localized. The longer the neurologic symptoms persist untreated and the more brain atrophy occurs, the less likely it is that the patient will return to a reasonable level of neurologic function. Without prompt treatment of the neurologic symptoms, the patient may be cured of their cancer. Still, they may require institutionalization regardless, as paraneoplastic disorders can be quite severe, leaving some patients markedly disabled and dependent on others. It is presumed that the malignancy is the source of the antigen and thus removing the cancer, if possible, along with immunotherapy, is the best strategy for treating the neurologic symptoms and preventing a relapse. Unfortunately, in practice, tumor removal may not result in dramatic clinical improvement. If possible, adding cyclophosphamide to the chemotherapy regimen may be helpful.

Psychiatric Considerations in the Treatment of Patients With Infectious or Inflammatory Neuropsychiatric Impairment

As mentioned above, treating patients with infectious or autoimmune encephalitides often involves a multidisciplinary team approach. While it is important to treat the etiology of their symptoms, if possible (e.g., treating a co-existing malignancy, using antimicrobials to treat infections, and using immunotherapy to treat autoimmune disorders) to bring about a long-term resolution or remission of their disorder, many of the manifesting symptoms require specialty management. Many patients with encephalitis are delirious, and general delirium precautions (including frequent re-orientation, surrounding the patient with familiar pictures or family members, and maintenance

of a normal day/night light cycle) are needed. Some autoimmune encephalitides have a direct effect on the hypothalamus, resulting in disruptive sleep patterns that often require treatment. Patients may have a combination of seizures and mood disruptions, in which case choosing an antiepileptic drug, such as valproic acid or lamotrigine, which are known to have dual actions, may be ideal. Sometimes patients may have co-existing agitation and movement disorders, for example, in NMDAR or LGI-1 encephalitis. In addition, some children with post-HSE NMDAR encephalitis and choreoathetotic movements have anti-dopamine receptor antibodies.[66] Particularly in NMDAR encephalitis, avoiding dopamine-blockers in favor of benzodiazepines may be preferred, as dopamine-blockers may result in rigidity, which, along with potential autonomic storming, may result in an incorrect diagnosis of neuroleptic malignant syndrome. Additionally, many patients with autoimmune disorders, including autoimmune encephalitis with catatonia and stiff person syndrome, can tolerate (and often need) high doses of benzodiazepines for successful symptomatic management, sometimes at doses that would ordinarily be over-sedating for most patients. Overall, while the patient's symptoms are being managed, it is also imperative to treat the underlying pathophysiology.

REMAINING QUESTIONS ON AUTOIMMUNE ENCEPHALITIDES

The field of autoimmune neurology is rapidly changing, and with the seemingly constant identification of new autoantibodies, it is difficult to know how to interpret test results and how best to apply that knowledge to helping patients. Here are some common questions encountered in the day-to-day course of diagnosing and treating autoimmune encephalitides.

What Should Be Done if There Are Low-Titer Autoantibodies?

A common concern is what to do about low-titer antibody results, which are only slightly above the negative cut-off value.[9] Some antibodies, including GAD-65,[78] can be found at low values in normal patients without neurologic disease. GAD-65 can also be elevated in patients with systemic autoimmune endocrinopathies, such as type I diabetes. In addition, antibody results must be carefully interpreted after IVIg, as treatment can result in false positives, which are typically present for many weeks after the last dose. In general, results must be examined within the clinical context, with the caveat that sometimes antibodies are only rarely associated with certain symptoms; if the test results are completely incongruent with the patient's presentation, they may be unrelated.

What Should Be Done About Late Diagnoses?

Sometimes the diagnosis has been only made after an extended period.[9] A corollary to this is whether there are cases of spontaneous remission. Spontaneous remissions are rare, as a large NMDAR encephalitis series has shown.[12] This same analysis also noted that in paraneoplastic NMDAR cases, prompt tumor removal is important, as it speeds recovery and prevents relapses. Autoimmune neurologic disorders typically require immunologic treatment. However, particularly in paraneoplastic cases that come to attention late, the neurologic symptoms may have plateaued, remaining stable without deterioration for many months. Without evidence of ongoing decline, these patients may be observed over time. While the best outcomes are seen with early diagnosis and treatment, even if a late diagnosis is made, if there is ongoing deterioration, a course of immunotherapy should be attempted, as responses to therapy are sometimes seen, and treating with immunotherapy addresses the etiology, as opposed to merely the symptoms of the disorder, which can be severe.

What Is Hashimoto Encephalitis, and Does It Truly Exist?

Antibodies against TPO have had an interesting trajectory in the history of autoimmune encephalitides.[1] This antibody, with or without anti-thyroglobulin antibodies, was initially thought to signify an autoimmune encephalitis known as Hashimoto encephalitis,[79] although the range of clinical presentations was highly variable, making it difficult to describe a specific Hashimoto encephalitis syndrome. Hashimoto encephalitis was eventually re-named steroid responsive encephalitis with associated autoimmune thyroiditis,[80] as patients with Hashimoto encephalitis were generally found to be responsive to steroids. However, this did not clarify the syndrome, as not all syndromes considered to be Hashimoto encephalitis have been responsive to steroids. A recent analysis of patients carrying the diagnosis of "Hashimoto encephalitis" found that about a quarter of the patients were not thought to have an autoimmune CNS disorder at all, but rather had alternative diagnoses, such as psychiatric disease, functional neurologic disorders, or a neurodegenerative disease.[81] With the identification of novel antibodies that recognize neuronal cell surface epitopes, as opposed to TPO antibodies that do not react with neurons, some patients with Hashimoto encephalitis have been re-classified with specific syndromes, such as NMDAR or limbic encephalitis.[82] The TPO antibodies may be better interpreted as markers of autoimmunity. Overall, the boundaries of Hashimoto encephalitis are unclear, and it should be considered only after excluding specific antibody-associated autoimmune encephalitides.[83]

Are Antibody Subtypes Important?

There have been many reports in the literature associating antibodies against neuronal surface antigens with several disorders, including neuropsychiatric lupus, bipolar disorder, and neurodegenerative conditions.[84–86] These antibodies must be distinguished from those that are syndrome-specific or pathogenic. For instance, in NMDAR encephalitis, the associated antibodies are IgGs that target the ionotropic NMDA glutamate receptor 1, or GluN1, a subunit of the NMDA receptor.[87] These are highly specific and pathogenic antibodies that, when well characterized in the serum and particularly in the CSF, are not found in other disorders. Other NMDAR subunit–targeted antibodies or IgA or IgM antibody subtypes are unrelated to NMDAR encephalitis; they have been reported in the sera of patients with a myriad of neurologic and psychiatric diseases[88] at the same frequency as in healthy subjects (~10%),[89] without clear pathogenic effects. Part of the problem is the over-simplified use of the term "NMDA receptor antibodies" for all subtypes of antibodies (IgA, IgM, IgG) and antibodies targeting different subunits. For all known (named) autoimmune encephalitides, pathogenic antibodies have been of the IgG class; these are the ones for which the commercial antibody panels test.

Case 1

Ms. B, a 24-year old without a prior psychiatric history, was admitted to a psychiatric ward for "anxiety." Before admission, she was paranoid, agitated, yelling, scared, and could not sleep. She called her mother with disorganized speech. She thought her mother responded through the TV. Ms. B was rigid and mute, with a mild fever, elevated blood pressure, and tachycardia; her parents took her to a nearby hospital. A head CT, brain MRI/A with and without contrast, an abdominal ultrasound, and two EEGs were normal. Toxicology and heavy metal screens were negative. An LP revealed 48 WBCs; 100% lymphocytes. ESR and CRP were mildly elevated. The infectious work-up was negative. Ms. B was given a 10-day course of acyclovir before HSV testing returned negative. She had a poor response to neuroleptics and benzodiazepines.

Ms. B's parents took her to a different psychiatric hospital. She was in and out of a confusional state, with labile emotions, bursts of seemingly volitional shaking episodes, disinhibited behavior, mutism, and preoccupations about dying. She had periods where she was more lucid, able to communicate, and less anxious. She had poor sleep, was noted to have jerky movements, and continued to run a low-grade fever. Ms. B was uncooperative with the neurologic examination and had an intermittently unstable gait. She was transferred to a large tertiary care hospital.

Ms. B was catatonic and spoke of "walking with God." Repeat infectious work-up, toxicology screen, EEG, MRI, and LP (WBC 2) were normal. Brain PET showed posterior symmetric occipital lobe hypometabolism. NMDA receptor encephalitis was suspected; IVIg was administered. Shortly thereafter, CSF and serum NMDA receptor antibody testing returned positive from samples collected before treatment with IVIg. A search for a teratoma was unrevealing. Her catatonic symptoms were treated with benzodiazepines. Three weeks later, she was minimally improved. She received rituximab every 6 months for 2 years and had a slow but complete recovery. Nearly a decade after her illness, she continues to do well and has had no signs of relapse.

CONCLUSION

Common causes of neuropsychiatric impairment encountered in the hospital setting include encephalopathy, usually a consequence of end-organ failure, and encephalitis, representing inflammation of the brain tissue itself. Encephalitis is often secondary to infectious and/or inflammatory causes. The past several decades have brought the realization that many inflammatory encephalitides are autoimmune, and associated with neural autoantibodies that serve as useful diagnostic markers, particularly in paraneoplastic cases. It has also been discovered that some infectious encephalitides can lead to subsequent autoimmune encephalitides, potentially clouding the diagnostic picture. Infectious and autoimmune encephalitides can have high morbidity. However, early diagnosis and treatment, usually from a multi-disciplinary perspective, can improve outcomes.

REFERENCES

1. Linnoila JJ, Rosenfeld MR, Dalmau J. Neuronal surface antibody-mediated autoimmune encephalitis. *Semin Neurol.* 2014; 34:458–466.
2. Sekar A, Bialas AR, de Rivera H, et al. Schizophrenia risk from complex variation of complement component 4. *Nature.* 2016;530(7589):177–183.
3. Wilson MR, Naccache SN, Samayoa E, et al. Actionable diagnosis of neuroleptospirosis by next-generation sequencing. *N Engl J Med.* 2014;370(25):2408–2417.
4. Pruss H, Dalmau J, Harms L, et al. Retrospective analysis of NMDA receptor antibodies in encephalitis of unknown origin. *Neurology.* 2010;75(19):1735–1739.
5. Jackson JR, Eaton WW, Cascella NG, et al. Neurologic and psychiatric manifestations of celiac disease and gluten sensitivity. *Psychiatr Q.* 2012;83(1):91–102.
6. Piquet AL, Lyons JL. Infectious meningitis and encephalitis. *Semin Neurol.* 2016;36(4):367–372.
7. Cellucci T, Van Mater H, Graus F, et al. Clinical approach to the diagnosis of autoimmune encephalitis in the pediatric patient. *Neurol Neuroimmunol Neuroinflamm.* 2020;7(2).
8. Luft BJ, Remington JS. Toxoplasmic encephalitis in AIDS. *Clin Infect Dis.* 1992;15(2):211–222.
9. Linnoila J, Pittock SJ. Autoantibody-associated central nervous system neurologic disorders. *Semin Neurol.* 2016;36(4):382–396.
10. Titulaer MJ, Hoftberger R, Iizuka T, et al. Overlapping demyelinating syndromes and anti-N-methyl-D-aspartate receptor encephalitis. *Ann Neurol.* 2014;75(3):411–428.
11. Darnell RB, Posner JB. Paraneoplastic syndromes involving the nervous system. *N Engl J Med.* 2003;349(16):1543–1554.
12. Titulaer MJ, McCracken L, Gabilondo I, et al. Treatment and prognostic factors for long-term outcome in patients with

anti-NMDA receptor encephalitis: an observational cohort study. *Lancet Neurol.* 2013;12:157–165.

13. Rabin ER, Jenson AB, Melnick JL. Herpes simplex virus in mice: electron microscopy of neural spread. *Science.* 1968;162(3849):126–127.

14. Braun E, Zimmerman T, Hur TB, et al. Neurotropism of herpes simplex virus type 1 in brain organ cultures. *J Gen Virol.* 2006;87(Pt 10):2827–2837.

15. Uy CE, Binks S, Irani SR. Autoimmune encephalitis: clinical spectrum and management. *Pract Neurol.* 2021;21(5):412–423.

16. Gresa-Arribas N, Titulaer MJ, Torrents A, et al. Antibody titres at diagnosis and during follow-up of anti-NMDA receptor encephalitis: a retrospective study. *Lancet Neurol.* 2014;13(2):167–177.

17. Scott JG, Gillis D, Ryan AE, et al. The prevalence and treatment outcomes of antineuronal antibody-positive patients admitted with first episode of psychosis. *Br J Psych Open.* 2018;4(2):69–74.

18. Lennox BR, Palmer-Cooper EC, Pollak T, et al. Prevalence and clinical characteristics of serum neuronal cell surface antibodies in first-episode psychosis: a case-control study. *Lancet Psychiatry.* 2017;4(1):42–48.

19. Pollak TA, Lennox BR, Muller S, et al. Autoimmune psychosis: an international consensus on an approach to the diagnosis and management of psychosis of suspected autoimmune origin. *Lancet Psychiatry.* 2020;7(1):93–108.

20. Guasp M, Gine-Serven E, Maudes E, et al. Clinical, neuroimmunologic, and CSF investigations in first episode psychosis. *Neurology.* 2021;97(1):e61–e75.

21. Hohlfeld R. Myasthenia gravis and thymoma: paraneoplastic failure of neuromuscular transmission. *Lab Invest.* 1990;62(3):241–243.

22. Roberts A, Perera S, Lang B, et al. Paraneoplastic myasthenic syndrome IgG inhibits 45Ca2+ flux in a human small cell carcinoma line. *Nature.* 1985;317(6039):737–739.

23. Bien CG, Vincent A, Barnett MH, et al. Immunopathology of autoantibody-associated encephalitides: clues for pathogenesis. *Brain.* 2012;135(Pt 5):1622–1638.

24. Lai M, Hughes EG, Peng X, et al. AMPA receptor antibodies in limbic encephalitis alter synaptic receptor location. *Ann Neurol.* 2009;65(4):424–434.

25. Irani SR, Alexander S, Waters P, et al. Antibodies to Kv1 potassium channel-complex proteins leucine-rich, glioma inactivated 1 protein and contactin-associated protein-2 in limbic encephalitis, Morvan's syndrome and acquired neuromyotonia. *Brain.* 2010;133(9):2734–2748.

26. Boronat A, Gelfand JM, Gresa-Arribas N, et al. Encephalitis and antibodies to dipeptidyl-peptidase-like protein-6, a subunit of Kv4.2 potassium channels. *Ann Neurol.* 2013;73(1):120–128.

27. Lancaster E, Lai M, Peng X, et al. Antibodies to the GABA(B) receptor in limbic encephalitis with seizures: case series and characterisation of the antigen. *Lancet Neurol.* 2010;9(1):67–76.

28. Hutchinson M, Waters P, McHugh J, et al. Progressive encephalomyelitis, rigidity, and myoclonus: a novel glycine receptor antibody. *Neurology.* 2008;71(16):1291–1292.

29. Lancaster E, Martinez-Hernandez E, Titulaer MJ, et al. Antibodies to metabotropic glutamate receptor 5 in the Ophelia syndrome. *Neurology.* 2011;77(18):1698–1701.

30. Gresa-Arribas N, Planaguma J, Petit-Pedrol M, et al. Human neurexin-3alpha antibodies associate with encephalitis and alter synapse development. *Neurology.* 2016;86(24):2235–2242.

31. Dalmau J, Tuzun E, Wu HY, et al. Paraneoplastic anti-N-methyl-D-aspartate receptor encephalitis associated with ovarian teratoma. *Ann Neurol.* 2007;61(1):25–36.

32. Petit-Pedrol M, Armangue T, Peng X, et al. Encephalitis with refractory seizures, status epilepticus, and antibodies to the GABAA receptor: a case series, characterisation of the antigen, and analysis of the effects of antibodies. *Lancet Neurol.* 2014;13(3):276–286.

33. Sabater L, Gaig C, Gelpi E, et al. A novel non-rapid-eye movement and rapid-eye-movement parasomnia with sleep breathing disorder associated with antibodies to IgLON5: a case series, characterisation of the antigen, and post-mortem study. *Lancet Neurol.* 2014;13(6):575–586.

34. Mandel-Brehm C, Dubey D, Kryzer TJ, et al. Kelch-like protein 11 antibodies in seminoma-associated paraneoplastic encephalitis. *N Engl J Med.* 2019;381(1):47–54.

35. Basal E, Zalewski N, Kryzer TJ, et al. Paraneoplastic neuronal intermediate filament autoimmunity. *Neurology.* 2018;91(18):e1677–e1689.

36. Dubey D, Kryzer T, Guo Y, et al. Leucine zipper 4 autoantibody: a novel germ cell tumor and paraneoplastic biomarker. *Ann Neurol.* 2021;89(5):1001–1010.

37. Armangue T, Olive-Cirera G, Martinez-Hernandez E, et al. Associations of paediatric demyelinating and encephalitic syndromes with myelin oligodendrocyte glycoprotein antibodies: a multicentre observational study. *Lancet Neurol.* 2020;19(3):234–246.

38. Hinson SR, Honorat JA, Grund EM, et al. Septin-5 and -7-IgGs: neurologic, serologic, and pathophysiologic characteristics. *Ann Neurol.* 2022;92(6):1090–1101.

39. Fang B, McKeon A, Hinson SR, et al. Autoimmune glial fibrillary acidic protein astrocytopathy: a novel meningoen-cephalomyelitis. *JAMA Neurol.* 2016

40. Zekeridou A, Yang B, Lennon VA, et al. Anti-neuronal nuclear antibody 3 autoimmunity targets Dachshund homolog 1. *Ann Neurol.* 2022;91(5):670–675.

41. Hughes EG, Peng X, Gleichman AJ, et al. Cellular and synaptic mechanisms of anti-NMDA receptor encephalitis. *J Neurosci.* 2010;30(17):5866–5875.

42. Moscato EH, Peng X, Jain A, et al. Acute mechanisms underlying antibody effects in anti-N-methyl-D-aspartate receptor encephalitis. *Ann Neurol.* 2014;76(1):108–119.

43. Landa J, Gaig C, Plaguma J, et al. Effects of IgLON5 antibodies on neuronal cytoskeleton: a link between autoimmunity and neurodegeneration. *Ann Neurol.* 2020;88(5):1023–1027.

44. Valencia Sanchez C, Theel E, Binnicker M, et al. Autoimmune encephalitis after SARS-CoV-2 infection: case frequency, findings, and outcomes. *Neurology.* 2021;97(23):e2262–e2268.

45. Prüss H, Finke C, Höltje M, et al. N-methyl-D-aspartate receptor antibodies in herpes simplex encephalitis. *Ann Neurol.* 2012;72:902–911.

46. Armangue T, Leypoldt F, Málaga I, et al. Herpes simplex virus encephalitis is a trigger of brain autoimmunity. *Ann Neurol.* 2014;75:317–323.

47. Armangue T, Spatola M, Vlagea A, et al. Frequency, symptoms, risk factors, and outcomes of autoimmune encephalitis after herpes simplex encephalitis: a prospective observational study and retrospective analysis. *Lancet Neurol.* 2018;17(9):760–772.

48. Schabitz WR, Rogalewski A, Hagemeister C, et al. VZV brainstem encephalitis triggers NMDA receptor immunoreaction. *Neurology.* 2014;83(24):2309–2311.

49. Armangue T, Moris G, Cantarin-Extremera V, et al. Autoimmune post-herpes simplex encephalitis of adults and teenagers. *Neurology.* 2015;85(20):1736–1743.

50. Linnoila J, Binnicker M, Klein C, et al. CSF herpes virus and autoantibody profiles in the evaluation of encephalitis. *Neurol Neuroimmunol Neuroinflamm.* 2016

51. Liu B, Liu J, Sun H, et al. Autoimmune encephalitis after Japanese encephalitis in children: a prospective study. *J Neurol Sci.* 2021;424:117394.

52. Schmitt SE, Pargeon K, Frechette ES, et al. Extreme delta brush: a unique EEG pattern in adults with anti-NMDA receptor encephalitis. *Neurology.* 2012;79(11):1094–1100.

53. Irani SR, Stagg CJ, Schott JM, et al. Faciobrachial dystonic seizures: the influence of immunotherapy on seizure control and prevention of cognitive impairment in a broadening phenotype. *Brain.* 2013;136(Pt 10):3151–3162.

54. Lansberg MG, O'Brien MW, Norbash AM, et al. MRI abnormalities associated with partial status epilepticus. *Neurology.* 1999;52(5):1021–1027.

55. Probasco JC, Solnes L, Nalluri A, et al. Abnormal brain metabolism on FDG-PET/CT is a common early finding in autoimmune encephalitis. *Neurol Neuroimmunol Neuroinflamm.* 2017;4(4):e352.

56. Baumgartner A, Rauer S, Mader I, et al. Cerebral FDG-PET and MRI findings in autoimmune limbic encephalitis: correlation with autoantibody types. *J Neurol.* 2013;260(11):2744–2753.

57. Leypoldt F, Buchert R, Kleiter I, et al. Fluorodeoxyglucose positron emission tomography in anti-N-methyl-D-aspartate receptor encephalitis: distinct pattern of disease. *J Neurol Neurosurg Psychiatry.* 2012;83(7):681–686.

58. Flanagan EP, Kotsenas AL, Britton JW, et al. Basal ganglia T1 hyperintensity in LGI1-autoantibody faciobrachial dystonic seizures. *Neurol Neuroimmunol Neuroinflamm.* 2015;2(6):e161.

59. Armangue T, Petit-Pedrol M, Dalmau J. Autoimmune encephalitis in children. *J Child Neurol.* 2012;27(11):1460–1469.

60. Hacohen Y, Wright S, Waters P, et al. Paediatric autoimmune encephalopathies: clinical features, laboratory investigations and outcomes in patients with or without antibodies to known central nervous system autoantigens. *J Neurol Neurosurg Psychiatry.* 2013;84(7):748–755.

61. McKeon A, Apiwattanakul M, Lachance DH, et al. Positron emission tomography-computed tomography in paraneoplastic neurologic disorders: systematic analysis and review. *Arch Neurol.* 2010;67(3):322–329.

62. Pittock SJ, Kryzer TJ, Lennon VA. Paraneoplastic antibodies coexist and predict cancer, not neurological syndrome. *Ann Neurol.* 2004;56(5):715–719.

63. Graus F, Titulaer MJ, Balu R, et al. A clinical approach to diagnosis of autoimmune encephalitis. *Lancet Neurol.* 2016; 15(4):391–404.

64. Armangue T, Titulaer MJ, Malaga I, et al. Pediatric anti N methyl-D-aspartate receptor encephalitis-clinical analysis and novel findings in a series of 20 patients. *J Pediatr.* 2013;162(4): 850–856. e852.

65. De Tiege X, Rozenberg F, Des Portes V, et al. Herpes simplex encephalitis relapses in children: differentiation of two neurologic entities. *Neurology.* 2003;61(2):241–243.

66. Mohammad SS, Sinclair K, Pillai S, et al. Herpes simplex encephalitis relapse with chorea is associated with autoantibodies to N-methyl-D-aspartate receptor or dopamine-2 receptor. *Mov Disord.* 2014;29(1):117–122.

67. Gultekin SH, Rosenfeld MR, Voltz R, et al. Paraneoplastic limbic encephalitis: neurological symptoms, immunological findings and tumour association in 50 patients. *Brain.* 2000;123(Pt 7): 1481–1494.

68. Iranzo A, Graus F, Clover L, et al. Rapid eye movement sleep behavior disorder and potassium channel antibody-associated limbic encephalitis. *Ann Neurol.* 2006;59(1):178–181.

69. Irani SR, Pettingill P, Kleopa KA, et al. Morvan syndrome: clinical and serological observations in 29 cases. *Ann Neurol.* 2012;72(2):241–255.

70. Arino H, Armangue T, Petit-Pedrol M, et al. Anti-LGI1-associated cognitive impairment: presentation and long-term outcome. *Neurology.* 2016;87(8):759–765.

71. Sergerie Y, Boivin G, Gosselin D, et al. Delayed but not early glucocorticoid treatment protects the host during experimental herpes simplex virus encephalitis in mice. *J Infect Dis.* 2007; 195(6):817–825.

72. Le LT, Spudich SS. HIV-associated neurologic disorders and central nervous system opportunistic infections in HIV. *Semin Neurol.* 2016;36(4):373–381.

73. Vincent A, Buckley C, Schott JM, et al. Potassium channel antibody-associated encephalopathy: a potentially immunotherapy-responsive form of limbic encephalitis. *Brain.* 2004;127(Pt 3): 701–712.

74. Nosadini M, Eyre M, Molteni E, et al. Use and safety of immunotherapeutic management of N-methyl-D-aspartate receptor antibody encephalitis: a meta-analysis. *JAMA Neurol.* 2021;78(11):1333–1344.

75. Yeshokumar AK, Gordon-Lipkin E, Arenivas A, et al. Neurobehavioral outcomes in autoimmune encephalitis. *J Neuroimmunol.* 2017;312:8–14.

76. van Sonderen A, Thijs RD, Coenders EC, et al. Anti-LGI1 encephalitis: clinical syndrome and long-term follow-up. *Neurology.* 2016;87(14):1449–1456.

77. Cabezudo-Garcia P, Mena-Vazquez N, Estivill Torrus G, et al. Response to immunotherapy in anti-IgLON5 disease: a systematic review. *Acta Neurol Scand.* 2020;141(4):263–270.

78. Walikonis JE, Lennon VA. Radioimmunoassay for glutamic acid decarboxylase (GAD65) autoantibodies as a diagnostic aid for stiff-man syndrome and a correlate of susceptibility to type 1 diabetes mellitus. *Mayo Clin Proc.* 1998;73(12):1161–1166.

79. Brain L, Jellinek EH, Ball K. Hashimoto's disease and encephalopathy. *Lancet.* 1966;2(7462):512–514.

80. Castillo P, Woodruff B, Caselli R, et al. Steroid-responsive encephalopathy associated with autoimmune thyroiditis. *Arch Neurol.* 2006;63(2):197–202.

81. Valencia-Sanchez C, Pittock SJ, Mead-Harvey C, et al. Brain dysfunction and thyroid antibodies: autoimmune diagnosis and misdiagnosis. *Brain Commun.* 2021;3(2):fcaa233.

82. Tuzun E, Erdag E, Durmus H, et al. Autoantibodies to neuronal surface antigens in thyroid antibody-positive and -negative limbic encephalitis. *Neurol India.* 2011;59(1):47–50.

83. Chong JY, Rowland LP, Utiger RD. Hashimoto encephalopathy: syndrome or myth? *Arch Neurol.* 2003;60(2):164–171.

84. Choe CU, Karamatskos E, Schattling B, et al. A clinical and neurobiological case of IgM NMDA receptor antibody associated encephalitis mimicking bipolar disorder. *Psychiatry Res.* 2013;208(2):194–196.

85. Pruss H, Holtje M, Maier N, et al. IgA NMDA receptor antibodies are markers of synaptic immunity in slow cognitive impairment. *Neurology.* 2012;78(22):1743–1753.

86. Steup-Beekman G, Steens S, van Buchem M, et al. Anti-NMDA receptor autoantibodies in patients with systemic lupus erythematosus and their first-degree relatives. *Lupus.* 2007;16(5): 329–334.

87. Gleichman AJ, Spruce LA, Dalmau J, et al. Anti-NMDA receptor encephalitis antibody binding is dependent on amino acid identity of a small region within the GluN1 amino terminal domain. *J Neurosci.* 2012;32(32):11082–11094.

88. Steiner J, Walter M, Glanz W, et al. Increased prevalence of diverse N-methyl-D-aspartate glutamate receptor antibodies in patients with an initial diagnosis of schizophrenia: specific relevance of IgG NR1a antibodies for distinction from N-methyl-D-aspartate glutamate receptor encephalitis. *JAMA Psychiatry.* 2013;70(3):271–278.

89. Hammer C, Stepniak B, Schneider A, et al. Neuropsychiatric disease relevance of circulating anti-NMDA receptor autoantibodies depends on blood-brain barrier integrity. *Mol Psychiatry.* 2014;19(10):1143–1149.

90. Graus F, Vincent A, Pozo-Rosich P, et al. Anti-glial nuclear antibody: marker of lung cancer-related paraneoplastic neurological syndromes. *J Neuroimmunol.* 2005;165(1-2):166–171.

91. Pittock SJ, Lucchinetti CF, Parisi JE, et al. Amphiphysin autoimmunity: paraneoplastic accompaniments. *Ann Neurol.* 2005;58(1):96–107.

92. Lucchinetti CF, Kimmel DW, Lennon VA. Paraneoplastic and oncologic profiles of patients seropositive for type 1 antineuronal nuclear autoantibodies. *Neurology.* 1998;50(3):652–657.

93. Yu Z, Kryzer TJ, Griesmann GE, Kim K, et al. CRMP-5 neuronal autoantibody: marker of lung cancer and thymoma-related autoimmunity. *Ann Neurol.* 2001;49(2):146–154.

94. Spatola M, Petit-Pedrol M, Simabukuro MM, et al. Investigations in GABA(A) receptor antibody-associated encephalitis. *Neurology.* 2017;88(11):1012–1020.

95. Pittock SJ, Yoshikawa H, Ahlskog JE, et al. Glutamic acid decarboxylase autoimmunity with brainstem, extrapyramidal, and spinal cord dysfunction. *Mayo Clin Proc.* 2006;81(9): 1207–1214.

96. Budhram A, Sechi E, Flanagan EP, et al. Clinical spectrum of high-titre GAD65 antibodies. *J Neurol Neurosurg Psychiatry.* 2021;92(6):645–654.

97. Arino H, Hoftberger R, Gresa-Arribas N, et al. Paraneoplastic neurological syndromes and glutamic acid decarboxylase antibodies. *JAMA Neurol.* 2015;72(8):874–881.

98. Gaig C, Graus F, Compta Y, et al. Clinical manifestations of the anti-IgLON5 disease. *Neurology.* 2017;88(18):1736–1743.

99. Varma-Doyle A, Chwalisz BK, Linnoila J. Anti-immunoglobulin-like cell adhesion molecule-5 (IgLON5) associated neurological disease presenting with bilateral intraocular optic neuritis as an initial presentation: expanding clinical phenotype of the disease. *J Neuroophthalmol.* 2024. https://doi.org/10.1097/WNO.0000000000002114.

100. Dubey D, Wilson MR, Clarkson B, et al. Expanded clinical phenotype, oncological associations, and immunopathologic insights of paraneoplastic kelch-like protein-11 encephalitis. *JAMA Neurol.* 2020;77(11):1420–1429.

101. Lai M, Huijbers MG, Lancaster E, et al. Investigation of LGI1 as the antigen in limbic encephalitis previously attributed to potassium channels: a case series. *Lancet Neurol.* 2010;9(8): 776–785.

102. Dalmau J, Graus F, Villarejo A, et al. Clinical analysis of anti-Ma2-associated encephalitis. *Brain.* 2004;127(Pt 8):1831–1844.

103. Trentinaglia M, Dinoto A, Carta S, et al. Investigating the association between neoplasms and MOG antibody-associated disease. *Front Neurol.* 2023;14 1193211.

104. McKeon A, Shelly S, Zivelonghi C, et al. Neuronal intermediate filament IgGs in CSF: autoimmune axonopathy biomarkers. *Ann Clin Transl Neurol.* 2021;8(2):425–439.

105. Zalewski NL, Lennon VA, Lachance DH, et al. P/Q- and N-type calcium-channel antibodies: oncological, neurological, and serological accompaniments. *Muscle Nerve.* 2016;54(2): 220–227.

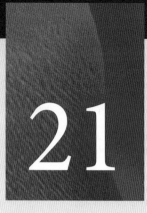

21

CATATONIA, NEUROLEPTIC MALIGNANT SYNDROME, AND SEROTONIN SYNDROME

NATHAN PRASCHAN, MD, MPH ■ SCOTT R. BEACH, MD ■ GREGORY L. FRICCHIONE, MD ■ JEFFERY C. HUFFMAN, MD ■ THEODORE A. STERN, MD

OVERVIEW

Each of the syndromes described in this chapter involves a complex interaction of motor, behavioral, and systemic manifestations that are derived from mechanisms that are not fully clear. What *is* clear is that neurotransmitters, such as dopamine (DA), gamma-aminobutyric acid (GABA), and glutamate, are of major importance in catatonia and neuroleptic malignant syndrome (NMS), whereas serotonin (5-hydroxytryptamine, 5-HT) is centrally involved in serotonin syndrome (SS). Many now believe that NMS represents a malignant catatonic state that results from the use of DA-blocking medications and that SS may also be within the spectrum of catatonic disorders. These syndromes have symptoms and treatments that certainly overlap. As our psychopharmacologic armamentarium grows and as drugs with potent effects on modulation of monoamines proliferate, the diagnosis and management of these complex disorders becomes even more important.

CATATONIA

Case 1: Catatonia

Mr. A, a 42-year-old male with a long history of epilepsy (status post a left temporal lobectomy with limited seizure control, despite the continued use of phenytoin and other anti-epileptics), developed catatonic withdrawal after his admission to the hospital following a seizure. After administration of intravenous (IV) lorazepam, he became alert, agitated, and aggressive; moreover, he was paranoid and reported nihilistic and religious delusions. Following several more doses of lorazepam, a higher dosage of phenytoin, and a low dose of an atypical antipsychotic (olanzapine), his psychosis gradually dissipated. At that point, he was able to state that he felt alone and dissociated, and he was unsure whether he even existed. He commented, "I feel separated from the human race, like I am on another planet."

Definition

Catatonia comprises a constellation of motor and behavioral signs and symptoms that occur in relation to neuro-medical or psychiatric insults. Structural brain disease, intrinsic brain disorders (e.g., epilepsy, toxic-metabolic derangements, infectious diseases), a variety of systemic disorders that affect the brain, and idiopathic psychiatric disorders (such as affective and schizophrenic psychoses) have all been associated with catatonia.[1] Catatonia was first defined by Karl Kahlbaum in 1847[2]; his work was among the first studies in the area of mental illness to use the symptom-based approach to diagnose disorders without a known etiopathogenesis. Kahlbaum believed that patients with catatonia passed through several phases of illness: a short stage of immobility (with waxy flexibility and posturing), a second stage of stupor or melancholy, a third stage of mania (with pressured speech, hyperactivity, and hyperthymic behavior), and finally, after repeated cycles of stupor and excitement, a stage of dementia.[2]

Kraepelin,[3] who was influenced by Kahlbaum, included catatonia in the group of deteriorating psychotic disorders named dementia praecox. Bleuler[4] adopted Kraepelin's view that catatonia was subsumed under severe idiopathic deteriorating psychoses, which he renamed *schizophrenias*. Kraepelin and Bleuler both recognized that catatonic symptoms could emerge as part of a mood disorder or a medical condition, but, as a result of a nosologic misconception, catatonia was overly associated with schizophrenia until the 1990s. Thanks in large part to the work of Fink and Taylor,[5] the *Diagnostic and Statistical Manual of Mental Disorders, Fourth Edition* (DSM-IV), finally included new criteria for mood disorders with catatonic features and for catatonic disorder secondary to a general medical condition, as well as the catatonic type of schizophrenia. In the DSM-5, the catatonic subtype of schizophrenia was removed, leaving diagnoses of catatonia associated with another mental disorder, catatonic disorder due to another medical condition, and unspecified catatonia. According to the DSM-5, a diagnosis of catatonia requires three or more of the following symptoms: stupor, catalepsy, waxy flexibility, mutism, negativism, posturing, mannerism, stereotypy, agitation, grimacing, echolalia, or echopraxia. In the case of catatonia due to another medical condition, the symptoms cannot occur exclusively during delirium.[6]

Epidemiology, Risk Factors, and Potential Etiologies

Primary catatonia refers to catatonia associated with psychiatric etiologies. Prospective studies on patients hospitalized with acute psychotic episodes place the incidence of catatonia in the range of 7% to 17%.[7] In patients who suffer from mood disorders, occurrence rates have ranged from 13% to 31% over the past century, and catatonia appears to be particularly common in those with bipolar disorder.[8] Some have contended that the incidence of catatonia has diminished in cases

of schizophrenia, but variations in diagnostic criteria and study design over time hamper interpretation. Personality disorders, post-traumatic stress disorder, and conversion disorder have also been cited as causes of catatonia. Catatonia is more common in patients with neurodevelopmental disorders and in those with autism-spectrum disorders, with up to 17% of patients with autism displaying symptoms in their lifetime.[9] Catatonia can also be idiopathic in many cases.

Non-psychiatric presentations may account for between 20% and 40% of all catatonia, with infections and autoimmune conditions accounting for 29% herein.[10] Table 21.1 includes an extensive, but not exhaustive, list of neuro-medical causes of catatonia. Notably, catatonic features are highly co-morbid with those of delirium.[11] Although the DSM-5 excludes the diagnosis of catatonia in the setting of delirium, there is no empirical basis for this exclusion.

Recent literature has highlighted that limbic encephalitis is frequently associated with catatonia and typically refers to an autoimmune response to neuronal antigens in the limbic and peri-limbic regions. Anti-*N*-methyl-D-aspartate (NMDA) receptor antibody encephalitis is most commonly associated with catatonia and other neuropsychiatric symptoms.[12] It is classically triggered by an ovarian teratoma but may also be associated with other tumors, a preceding viral illness, or even a previous bout of herpetic encephalitis.[12] The course typically begins with a viral infection–like prodrome over the course of a week, followed by subacute to acute-onset anxiety progressing rapidly to psychosis, agitation, and catatonia. From there, neurological complications arise, including dysautonomia, seizures, and coma.[12] Treatment involves identifying and removing the triggering tumor (if present) and otherwise treating with immunosuppressive agents. Symptomatic treatment of catatonia with lorazepam and electroconvulsive therapy (ECT) may be useful.[12] Other possible anti-neuronal antibodies presenting with limbic encephalitis include, but are not limited to, anti-Hu, anti-AMPA receptor, anti-leucine-rich glioma-inactivated 1 (LGI1), anti-contact-associated protein-like 2 (CASPR2), anti-glutamic acid decarboxylase 65 kD (GAD65), and anti-GABA B receptor. Viral encephalitis may also present with catatonia, as might occur with the herpes simplex virus and COVID-19 infection.[13] Other autoimmune conditions,

TABLE 21.1

Potential Etiologies of Catatonia

Psychiatric
Mood disorder (major depression or bipolar disorder)
Schizophrenia-spectrum disorder
Dissociative disorders
Obsessive-compulsive disorder
Personality disorders
Autism-spectrum disorders

Neurological
Infectious and autoimmune encephalitis
Cerebrovascular
Alcoholic degeneration
Wernicke encephalopathy
Cerebellar degeneration
Cerebral anoxia
Closed head trauma
Frontal lobe atrophy
Hydrocephalus
Lesions of the thalamus and globus pallidus
Posterior reversible encephalopathy syndrome
Parkinsonism
Seizure disorders
Surgical interventions
Tuberous sclerosis
CNS neoplasm

Toxic
Coal gas
Manganese
Organic fluorides
Tetraethyl lead poisoning

Infections
Acquired immunodeficiency syndrome
Bacterial meningoencephalitis
Bacterial sepsis
Syphilis
Malaria
Mononucleosis
Subacute sclerosing panencephalitis
Tuberculosis
Typhoid fever
Viral encephalitides (especially herpes)
Viral hepatitis

Metabolic and Other Medical Causes
Acute intermittent porphyria
Addison disease

Cushing disease
Diabetic ketoacidosis
Glomerulonephritis
Hepatic dysfunction
Hereditary coproporphyria
Homocystinuria
Hyperparathyroidism
Idiopathic hyperadrenergic state
Multiple sclerosis
Pellagra
Wilson disease
Peripuerperal
Systemic lupus erythematosus
Thrombocytopenic purpura
Uremia

Drug Related
Neuroleptics
Other dopamine-blocking agents (metoclopramide)
Dopamine withdrawal (e.g., levodopa)
Dopamine depleters (e.g., tetrabenazine)
Sedative-hypnotic withdrawal
Alcohol withdrawal
Antidepressants (tricyclic antidepressants, monoamine oxidase inhibitors, and others)
Anticonvulsants (e.g., carbamazepine, primidone)
Aspirin
Disulfiram
Baclofen
Antibiotics (macrolides, fluoroquinolones)
Steroids
Tacrolimus
Cyclosporine
Interferon
Ribavirin
Lithium carbonate
Morphine
Cannabinoids
Hallucinogens (e.g., mescaline, phencyclidine, lysergic acid diethylamide, and cathinones)
Synthetic cannabinoids
Cannabinoid withdrawal
Efavirenz
Levetiracetam

such as systemic lupus erythematosus, have also been associated with catatonia.[14]

Drug (including prescription medication)-related etiologies have also been identified as secondary causes of catatonia. Dopamine antagonist medications

(e.g., neuroleptics, metoclopramide) and dopamine-depleting medications (e.g., tetrabenazine) can lead to catatonia, as can the discontinuation of dopamine agonist medications, sedative-hypnotic medications, and clozapine.[15] Some medications, including hydroxyzine, have mild dopamine-blocking properties, of which most practitioners are unaware. Withdrawal from GABAergic agents, such as alcohol or benzodiazepines, also represents a common etiology for catatonia. In the case of long-acting benzodiazepines, other signs of withdrawal may be subtle at the outset, and the presentation may be delayed. Many other drugs have been associated with catatonia, including disulfiram, antibiotics, immunomodulatory agents, and drugs of abuse like phencyclidine, cocaine, and cannabis.[15]

There appears to be increased familial transmission with periodic catatonia that shows a pattern of anticipation from generation to generation as well as association with chromosome 15.[16] In addition, Prader-Willi syndrome, a genetic disorder due to the lack of gene expression from paternal chromosome 15q11-q13, is associated with catatonia, and data support GABA dysfunction in Prader-Willi syndrome, schizophrenia, and autism associated with catatonia.[16] Catatonia has also been associated with other genetic disorders, including fragile X[17] and DiGeorge syndrome (22q11.2 deletion syndrome).[18]

Furthermore, among families whose members are prone to catatonia, the phenotypic presentation (e.g., the presence of mutism and rigidity) and severity of catatonia have been reported to be highly similar, irrespective of the underlying psychiatric diagnosis, implying a genetic basis for catatonic presentations.[19]

Subtypes of Catatonia

Motoric subtypes of catatonia include stuporous catatonia (catatonic withdrawal; characterized by psychomotor hypoactivity) and excited catatonia (characterized by psychomotor hyperactivity), which may alternate during a catatonic episode.

Kraepelin, in 1908, identified a "periodic" catatonia with an onset in adolescence characterized by intermittent excited states, followed by catatonic stuporous stages and a remitting and relapsing course. More recently authors have argued that periodic catatonia supports the DSM-5 category of "unspecified catatonia," which can be used to diagnose idiopathic cases of catatonia not associated with primary psychiatric or secondary neuro-medical causes. These authors highlight that periodic catatonia is defined by a longitudinal course of cyclical relapsing and remitting psychomotor symptoms interrupted by periods of mild residual

symptoms and also report that periodic catatonia may respond better to treatment with antipsychotics than to conventional treatments for catatonia.[20] In 1934 Stauder[21] described lethal catatonia, distinguished by the rapid onset of manic delirium, high temperatures, and catatonic stupor; it was said to have a mortality rate of more than 50%. An overlapping syndrome, malignant catatonia, has been described more commonly, typically involving fever, autonomic instability, and elevated creatinine kinase. Malignant catatonia, regardless of etiology, is considered a psychiatric emergency and requires prompt treatment and early consideration of ECT.

Delirious mania is a syndrome with an acute onset of excitement, grandiosity, emotional lability, delusions, and insomnia characteristic of mania and the disorientation and altered consciousness characteristic of delirium, as well as fever, tachycardia, hypertension, and tachypnea. It overlaps significantly with descriptions of lethal catatonia, and many consider it a form of malignant, excited catatonia. Other hallmark features of delirious mania include denuding, water obsession, and inappropriate toileting.[22] A diagnostic evaluation, including careful assessment for catatonic symptoms, is essential. The onset of mania tends to be more rapid than in classic bipolar disorder, and the mania tends to wax and wane with the delirium. The use of lithium and neuroleptics, commonly used medications for the treatment of mania, may worsen the catatonic symptoms and lead to NMS. Higher-dose benzodiazepines are often needed at the outset, and ECT is considered the treatment of choice for patients with delirious mania.

Clinical Features and Diagnosis

Signs and symptoms of the catatonic syndrome are outlined in Table 21.2 (the Modified Bush-Francis Catatonia Rating Scale). The specific number and nature of signs and symptoms required to make a diagnosis of catatonia remain controversial. Some have contended that even one cardinal characteristic has as much clinical significance for diagnosis and treatment as the presence of seven or eight characteristics. The DSM-5-TR requires 3 of 12 symptoms, while the widely used Bush-Francis Catatonia Rating Scale requires 2 of 14 symptoms for diagnosis and lists 23 symptoms for severity rating.[23] When assessing the etiology of

TABLE 21.2
Modified Bush-Francis Catatonia Rating Scale[a]

Catatonia Can Be Diagnosed by the Presence of Two or More of the First 14 Signs Listed Below

■ Excitement	Extreme hyperactivity, and constant motor unrest, which is apparently non-purposeful; not to be attributed to akathisia or goal-directed agitation
■ Immobility/stupor	Extreme hypoactivity, immobility, and minimal response to stimuli
■ Mutism	Verbal unresponsiveness or minimal responsiveness
■ Staring	Fixed gaze, little or no visual scanning of the environment, and decreased blinking
■ Posturing/catalepsy	Spontaneous maintenance of posture(s), including mundane behavior (e.g., sitting/standing for long periods without reacting)
■ Grimacing	Maintenance of odd facial expressions
■ Echopraxia/echolalia	Mimicking of an examiner's movements/speech
■ Stereotypy	Repetitive, non-goal-directed motor activity (e.g., finger-play, or repeatedly touching, patting, or rubbing oneself); the act is not inherently abnormal but is repeated frequently
■ Mannerisms	Odd, purposeful movements (e.g., hopping or walking on tiptoe, saluting those passing by, or exaggerating caricatures of mundane movements); the act itself is inherently abnormal
■ Verbigeration	Repetition of phrases (like a scratched record)
■ Rigidity	Maintenance of a rigid position despite efforts to be moved; exclude if cogwheeling or tremors present
■ Negativism	Apparently motiveless resistance to instructions or attempts to move/examine the patient; contrary behavior; doing the exact opposite of the instruction
■ Waxy flexibility	During re-posturing of the patient, the patient offers initial resistance before allowing repositioning, like that of a bending candle; alternatively, slight, even resistance to positioning
■ Withdrawal	Refusal to eat, drink, or make eye contact
■ Impulsivity	Sudden inappropriate behaviors (e.g., running down a hallway, screaming, or taking off clothes) without provocation; afterward, gives no or only facile explanations
■ Automatic obedience	Exaggerated cooperation with the examiner's request or spontaneous continuation of the movement requested
■ *Mitgehen*	"Anglepoise lamp": arm raising in response to light pressure of a finger, despite instructions to the contrary
■ *Gegenhalten*	Resistance to a passive movement that is proportional to the strength of the stimulus; appears automatic rather than willful
■ Ambitendency	The appearance of being "stuck" in indecisive, hesitant movement
■ Grasp reflex	Per neurologic examination
■ Perseveration	Repeatedly returns to the same topic or persistence with movement
■ Combativeness	Usually aggressive in an undirected manner, with no, or only facile, explanation afterward
■ Autonomic abnormality	Abnormal temperature, blood pressure, pulse, or respiratory rate, and diaphoresis

[a]The full 23-item Bush-Francis Catatonia Rating Scale measures the severity of 23 signs on a 0 to 3 continuum for each sign. The first 14 signs combine to form the Bush-Francis Catatonia Screening Instrument (BFCSI). The BFCSI measures only the presence or absence of the first 14 signs, and it is used for case detection. Item definitions on the two scales are the same.
Modified from Bush G, Fink M, Petrides G, et al. Catatonia—I: rating scale and standardized examination. *Acta Psychiatr Scand.* 1996;93:129–136.

the catatonia, the psychiatrist should consider secondary causes of catatonia related to underlying neurologic, toxic, or metabolic abnormalities, as well as primary psychiatric causes (Table 21.1). An approach to examining patients for catatonia is outlined in Table 21.3. Because catatonia is often under-diagnosed,[24] it is important to maintain a high degree of suspicion and include a brief catatonia evaluation as part of all exams. A key is to differentiate catatonia from other syndromes with similar manifestations but with different etiologies, such as akinetic mutism (AM), locked-in syndrome, and malignant hyperthermia. AM, in particular, can be challenging to distinguish from catatonia. The noted Massachusetts General Hospital

TABLE 21.3
Standardized Examination for Catatonia

The method described here is used to complete the 23-item Bush-Francis Catatonia Rating Scale and the 14-item Bush-Francis Catatonia Screening Instrument (BFSCI). Item definitions on the two scales are the same. The BFCSI measures only the presence or absence of the first 14 signs.

Ratings are based solely on observed behaviors during the examination, except for completing the items for "withdrawal" and "autonomic abnormality," which may be based on directly observed behavior or chart documentation.

Generally, only items that are clearly present should be rated. If the examiner is uncertain as to the presence of an item, rate the item as "0."

Procedure
1. Observe the patient while trying to engage in a conversation.
2. The examiner should scratch his or her head in an exaggerated manner.
3. The arm should be examined for cogwheeling. Attempt to re-posture and instruct the patient to "keep your arm loose." Move the arm with alternating lighter and heavier force.
4. Ask the patient to extend his or her arm. Place one finger beneath his or her hand and try to raise it slowly after stating, "Do *not* let me raise your arm."
5. Extend the hand stating, "Do *not* shake my hand."
6. Reach into your pocket and state, "Stick out your tongue. I want to stick a pin in it."
7. Check for grasp reflex.
8. Check the chart for reports from the previous 24-hour period. Check for oral intake, vital signs, and any incidents.
9. Observe the patient indirectly, at least for a brief period each day, regarding the following:

   - Activity level
   - Abnormal movements
   - Abnormal speech
   - Echopraxia
   - Rigidity
   - Negativism
   - Waxy flexibility
   - *Gegenhalten*
   - *Mitgehen*
   - Ambitendency
   - Automatic obedience
   - Grasp reflex

neurologist, C. Miller Fisher, proposed that AM might represent a "pure motor catatonia," and that many features overlap, including immobility, mutism, and paratonia.[25] AM is characterized as the extreme end of the abulic spectrum, and patients typically develop AM in the setting of neurologic injury or infectious or inflammatory brain states. Unlike catatonia, AM does not typically involve fearful affect or hyperkinetic features.[26] Importantly, AM does not respond to benzodiazepines but may improve with the use of dopamine agonists, such as amantadine or zolpidem. Routine work-up for catatonia includes a metabolic panel; serum and urine toxicology screening; an infectious-disease workup, including human immunodeficiency virus and rapid plasma reagin testing; autoimmune screening (erythrocyte sedimentation rate, C-reactive protein, and antinuclear antibodies); and thyroid and micronutrient screening. Heavy metal testing may be considered for appropriate patients. Creatine phosphokinase (CPK) levels, though not indicative of etiology, should be monitored, as they may indicate a malignant subtype. Iron studies are also recommended, as a low serum iron level is a risk factor for catatonia and for conversion to malignant catatonia.

Magnetic resonance imaging (MRI) of the brain, with and without contrast, and an autoimmune encephalopathy panel in both the serum and the cerebrospinal fluid (CSF) (along with routine CSF testing) should be considered and pursued in appropriate cases (e.g., with the first presentation of catatonia or when the diagnosis is unclear).[24] In cases of limbic encephalitis, enhancement in the medial temporal lobes may be seen, although a negative MRI brain scan does not definitively rule out autoimmune encephalitis or another neuro-medical etiology. In suspected cases, abdominal imaging and/or whole-body positron emission tomography scans should be considered in the search for a tumor.

An electroencephalogram (EEG) may also be considered, as any abnormality on the EEG is 76% sensitive and 67% specific for ruling in a neuro-medical cause, with epileptiform activity and focal abnormalities having higher specificity.[27] Notably, features of encephalopathy (e.g., generalized slowing) may also be present in psychiatric illness as well.

Neuropathophysiology

Catatonia has been described as a disorder of the cortico-striato-thalamo-cortical loop tracts (including the motor circuit that produces rigidity; the anterior cingulate-medial orbitofrontal circuit that produces akinetic mutism and, perhaps through lateral hypothalamic connections, hyperthermia, and dysautonomia; and the lateral orbitofrontal circuit that produces imitative and repetitive behaviors) (Fig. 21.1).[7] Dopamine (DA) activity in the dorsal striatum, ventral striatum, and paralimbic cortex is thus reduced, perhaps secondary to reduced $GABA_A$ inhibition of $GABA_B$, substantia nigra, and ventral tegmental area interneurons. This would lead to a dampened DA outflow in the mesocortical and nigrostriatal tracts. $GABA_A$, through the use of agonists, such as lorazepam, would disinhibit DA cell

activity.[1] Another possible site of pathophysiologic action involves reduced $GABA_A$ inhibition of frontal cortico-striatal tracts, leading to NMDA changes in the dorsal striatum, and indirectly in the substantia nigra and ventral tegmental area.[1] Multiple etiologies, if they affect the basal ganglia, thalamus, or paralimbic or frontal cortices, have the potential to cause neurotransmitter alterations that disrupt basal ganglia-thalamo-cortical circuits, leading to the phenomenology of catatonia. These hypotheses are supported by structural imaging research that demonstrates that

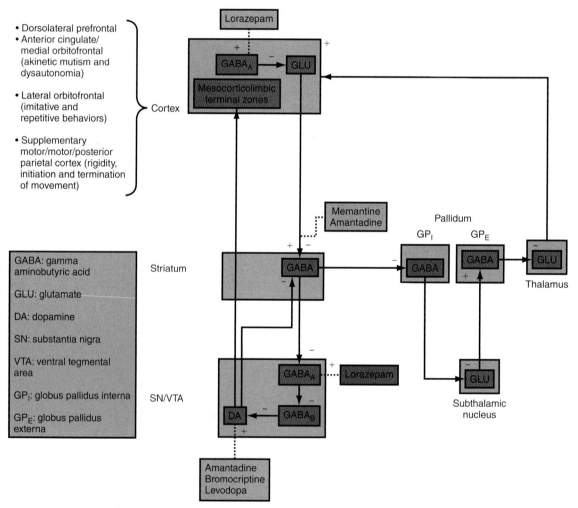

Fig. 21.1 ■ Basal ganglia-thalamo-cortical circuits and catatonia: a candidate loop. (From Fricchione GL, Huffman JC, Bush G, et al. Catatonia, neuroleptic malignant syndrome, and serotonin syndrome. In: Stern TA, Rosenbaum JF, Fava M, et al., eds. *Massachusetts General Hospital Comprehensive Clinical Psychiatry.* Mosby; 2008:761–771.)

catatonia-prone individuals with schizophrenia had reduced gray matter volume in the orbitofrontal cortex, anterior cingulate, thalamus, and amygdala compared to those with schizophrenia.[28]

In the mesostriatal and mesocorticolimbic systems, the long feedback loops from DA neurons are regulated by GABA pathways. Given its extensive projections on both limbic and motor structures, the nucleus accumbens (NAc) may be a hub for the linkage between motivation and movement.[29] By extrapolating from animal evidence (i.e., $GABA_A$ antagonists lead to catalepsy, and $GABA_A$ agonists protect against catalepsy), and from the hypothesis that neuroleptic-induced catatonia may result from reduced DA and $GABA_A$ activity in the mesostriatum, it has been proposed that primary psychogenic catatonia results from a similar destabilization.[30] $GABA_A$ agonists could be restorative by inhibiting the pars reticulata's inhibitory $GABA_B$ neurons, resulting in disinhibition of the neighboring pars compacta's DA cells with a resultant striatal DA agonism.[29]

The interactivity among the NAc, the ventral subiculum/hippocampus, and medial PFC areas, including the anterior cingulate cortex (ACC) and medial orbitofrontal cortex (MOFC), is important for our understanding of catatonia given their common modulation by DA and their importance in value-based decision making in the face of amygdalar-based threat. The NAc serves as a hub for the integration of cognitive information from the ACC/MOFC, affective information from the basolateral amygdala, and environmental context from the subiculum/hippocampus. It has this role primarily for the purpose of establishing a motivational valence (reward prediction error) in advance of translation into movement. The response selection itself is accomplished in the ACC-MOFC-supplementary motor area network, with the ACC serving as another transmodal hub for cortical and limbic information integration. This decision making is mediated with the help of modulatory aminergic flow in the medial forebrain bundle. Disruption in these systems associated with $GABA_A$ and DA reductions and an up-regulation of glutamatergic activity primarily in the ACC/MOFC basal ganglia-thalamo-cortical loop with nodes in the ventral striatum and medial dorsal nucleus of the thalamus will lead to pathological avoidance/approach decisions with catatonic overtones.

The ACC/MOFC projects motivational messaging to the ventral striatum and then to the ventral tegmentum, while the premotor and motor cortex send motor information to the dorsal striatum and then to the substantia nigra pars reticulata. The dorsolateral PFC sends frontal executive working memory and anticipated reward signal information into the central striatum and then to tegmental border zones between the ACC/MOFC (ventral) and motor cortical (dorsal) striatal and tegmental sites. There are non-reciprocal, feed-forward components that link up regions that are associated with different cortical-basal ganglia circuits. These feed-forward tracts serve an integrative function when all goes well, resulting in complex goal-directed movement. These connections terminate indirectly on a DA cell via a GABAergic interneuron, resulting in disinhibition and facilitation of DA cell burst firing. In this way, ventral striatal (motivational) regions influence more dorsal striatal (motor) regions via spiraling striatal-nigral-striatal projections. $GABA_A$ and DA deficiency syndromes and glutamatergic excess will present a phenotype of catatonia, and the use of $GABA_A$ agonists will disinhibit DA flow altering terminal zone motivational state in NAc and ACC/MOFC.

Neuroleptics reduce the conditioned avoidance response, which is thought to be secondary to decreased DA activity in the NAc and the striatum. Stress has been shown to increase medial pre-frontal cortical DA release, which in turn is thought to reduce DA activity in subcortical DA terminal fields in the mesolimbic and mesostriatal systems.[31] Friedhoff and co-workers[32] were able to show that rats undergoing twice-daily tail-shock stress for 8 days displayed conditioned avoidance response inhibition, along with a reduction in NAc DA use. The findings provided support for a restitutive hypothesis involving an endogenous DA-dependent system that mimicked the effects of neuroleptics in the context of repeated stress-induced medial PFC hyperdopaminergia. When such a system downregulates too much because of the neurologic or medical insult, primary psychiatric dysfunction, or neuroleptic medication, catatonic stupor may occur.

Early work took a top-down approach to understanding catatonia pathophysiology, with a particular focus on deficits in OFC functioning.[33] Indeed, during working memory tasks and with emotional-motor activation, the OFC appears to be hypoactive in subjects who previously had been catatonic when studied with functional magnetic resonance imaging during provocative testing.[7] However, research on regional blood flow has also shown basal ganglia asymmetry with left-sided hyper-perfusion, as well as hypoperfusion in the left medial temporal area, and decreased perfusion in the right parietal cortex.

It is probable that bottom-up dysfunction is just as important in the integration of basal ganglia-thalamo-cortical circuit mediation of motivation and movement in the catatonic syndrome.[29] And, by examining the nature of basal ganglia thalamo-limbic-cortical loops, we can hypothesize why such a wide array of neuro-medical and psychiatric etiologies can present with the catatonic syndrome and why the treatments (discussed later) may be therapeutic (Fig. 21.1).

An evolutionary model for catatonia has been proposed, suggesting that catatonia in humans may be akin to "playing dead" behavior in primitive mammals (e.g., Virginia opossum, duck-billed platypus).[34] In this way, catatonia may represent a maladaptive fear response in the setting of intense physiologic or psychological stress.

Fink and Taylor proposed that catatonia may represent a form of limbic epilepsy.[35] Subtle ictal events involving the pre-frontal cortex and the basal ganglia have been postulated as causing catatonia. They note that the same medications used to treat complex partial status epilepticus (IV benzodiazepines) are also the treatment of choice for catatonia.

Management and Treatment

Whatever its etiology, catatonia is accompanied by significant morbidity and mortality from systemic complications (Table 21.4). In addition, many of the physical illnesses responsible for catatonia can be debilitating. Thus, timely diagnosis and treatment are essential. If a neurologic or medical condition is found, then treatment for that specific illness is indicated. Agents thought to exacerbate catatonia, including antipsychotic medications and other dopamine-blocking drugs (e.g., metoclopramide), should be discontinued. If dopamine agonists were recently stopped, they should be re-started, and withdrawal from GABAergic agents should also be treated appropriately.

TABLE 21.4
Some Medical Complications Associated with Catatonia

Simple Non-Malignant Catatonia
Aspiration
Burns
Cachexia
Dehydration and its sequelae
Pneumonia
Pulmonary emboli
Thrombophlebitis
Urinary incontinence
Urinary retention and its sequelae

Malignant Catatonia
Acute renal failure
Adult respiratory distress syndrome
Cardiac arrest
Cheyne-Stokes respirations
Death
Disseminated intravascular coagulation
Dysphagia due to muscle spasm
Electrocardiographic abnormalities
Gait abnormalities
Gastrointestinal bleeding
Hepatocellular damage
Hypoglycemia (sudden and profound)
Intestinal pseudo-obstruction
Laryngospasm
Myocardial infarction
Myocardial stunning
Necrotizing enterocolitis
Respiratory arrest
Rhabdomyolysis and sequelae
Seizures
Sepsis

Data from Rogers et al. Evidence-based consensus guidelines for the management of catatonia: recommendations from the British Association for Psychopharmacology. *J Psychopharmacol.* 2023;37(4):327–369.

Lorazepam is the first-line treatment for catatonia, regardless of etiology, with response rates varying from 66% to 100%.[24] IV lorazepam is preferred over other benzodiazepines and routes of administration (because of its ease of administration, quick onset of action, and longer effective length of action).[36] With a drug distribution that is less rapid and less extensive, a relatively high plasma level can be maintained, thus prolonging the clinical benefit. Lorazepam also preferentially binds to the $GABA_A$ receptor, which may further account for its high efficacy. If IV access is unavailable, intramuscular

(IM) or sublingual routes are preferred over oral medication. It is important to keep in mind that because the main affective response in catatonia is one of intense fear, repeated administration of IM medications may be traumatizing for patients. Nonetheless, given IM in the deltoids, lorazepam is more reliably absorbed than other IM benzodiazepines.

A typical starting dose of lorazepam is 2 mg. Lower doses may occasionally be used in pediatric populations or frail, elderly patients but are not recommended in adults because of the likely equivocal response. In many cases, the response to lorazepam 2 mg will be immediate and dramatic, with patients who were previously mute and rigid sitting up in bed and conversing normally. In other cases, the response may take 30 to 120 minutes and may be more subtle. A lack of response to an initial dose of 2 mg of lorazepam does not rule out catatonia. If suspicion remains high, additional lorazepam should be given. Although individuals with catatonia have a higher threshold for sedation, falling asleep after a dose of lorazepam also does not rule out catatonia. Many patients will awaken later with significant improvement in symptoms.

Once a positive response to lorazepam has been established, or if suspicion for the diagnosis remains high despite a negative response, lorazepam should be instituted in a standing regimen, generally at a dose of 2 mg every 6 to 8 hours. Because medications are often held when patients are asleep, and because catatonia has a very high likelihood of recurrence as the lorazepam wears off, nursing staff should be instructed to give the medication if the patient is asleep and to hold only for respiratory depression. Regular doses of lorazepam generally maintain the therapeutic effect, and standing benzodiazepines are recommended for at least the first 24 to 48 hours. If improvement is significant over that time, consideration can be given to a slow taper of benzodiazepines. If lorazepam is unsuccessful within 5 days or if symptoms of malignant catatonia emerge, ECT should be considered.

ECT is considered the definitive and most effective treatment for catatonia in cases of partial or nonresponse to benzodiazepines or in cases of lethal or malignant catatonia. Response rates range from 59% to 100%.[24] Mann and associates[37] found that in one series of cases of lethal catatonia where ECT was used, 40 of 41 patients survived. These findings have been supported by other studies.[24] The message is clear: when a patient presents with malignant catatonia of any type, ECT should be used expeditiously, preferably bilateral, and at least twice weekly.[24]

In the past, neuroleptics were frequently used to treat catatonia, and more recently, case reports have emerged of atypical antipsychotics being used to treat catatonia. Clinical experience suggests a variable response to these drugs; however, neuroleptics are well described as precipitating catatonic reactions and NMS.[38] Among the 292 patients with malignant catatonia reviewed by Mann and associates,[39] for example, 78% of those treated with a neuroleptic alone died, compared with an overall mortality rate of 60%. Use of typical or atypical antipsychotics as a primary treatment strategy for catatonia is therefore not recommended, with the exception of clozapine for clozapine-withdrawal catatonia.[24] Aripiprazole and other partial D2 antagonist agents may be safer and have been shown to be effective in several case reports.[40] If antipsychotic agents are needed to manage psychosis and agitation, low-potency agents in combination with benzodiazepines should be administered at the lowest effective dose.

Alternatives and adjuncts to ECT and lorazepam in simple catatonias include zolpidem (5–10 mg orally), amantadine (100–200 mg twice a day orally), memantine (5–10 mg twice a day orally), valproate (125–500 mg three times daily orally or IV), and topiramate (100 mg twice a day orally).[40] Carbamazepine, calcium channel blockers, anticholinergics, minocycline, lithium, thyroid medication, corticosteroids, and adrenocorticotropic hormone have each had anecdotal success in catatonia.[24] While stimulants and carbidopa-levodopa have also been used, they reliably worsen psychosis and are therefore not recommended. Repetitive transcranial magnetic stimulation or transcranial direct current stimulation may also be useful if benzodiazepines are intolerable and ECT is not available.[41]

The treatment strategy for patients who have catatonia secondary to schizophrenia may be challenging because the catatonia found in those with schizophrenia can at times be less responsive to lorazepam.[42] In these patients, clozapine has been found to be useful, as well as to a lesser extent NMDA-receptor antagonists.[24]

Table 21.5 outlines recommendations for the treatment of simple and malignant (including NMS) catatonias, and Table 21.6 reviews management principles.

TABLE 21.5
Treatment of Simple and Malignant Catatonia

A. Test for catatonia. Lorazepam 2 mg IV (1 mg for adolescents or elderly patients) may result in temporary relief.

B. *Simple catatonia* (including neuroleptic-induced catatonia): lorazepam 1–4 mg IV/IM/SL/PO trial followed by 3–20 mg/day in divided doses.

   Monitor for respiratory depression.
   → If still catatonic, consider adding DA agonist.
   → If still catatonic, ECT.

C. Malignant catatonia (including NMS):

   1. Lorazepam IV trial expeditiously (effective in 75% of NMS cases). May add dantrolene ± DA agonist but less evidence for this.

   2. If still catatonic especially if the temperature is higher than 102°F, or if there is severe encephalopathy, ECT should be instituted before day 5 of the syndrome, if possible.

DA, Dopamine; *ECT,* electroconvulsive therapy; *IM,* intramuscular; *IV,* intravenous; *NMS,* neuroleptic malignant syndrome; *PO,* by mouth; *SL,* sublingual.
Modified from Fricchione G, Bush G, Fozdur M, et al. The recognition and treatment of the catatonic syndrome. *J Intensive Care Med.* 1997;12:135–147.

TABLE 21.6
Principles of Management of Catatonia

1. Early recognition is important. Once catatonia has been diagnosed, the patient must be closely observed and vital signs taken frequently.

2. Supportive care is essential. Such care involves hydration, nutrition, mobilization, anticoagulation (to prevent venous thromboembolism and thrombophlebitis), and precautions against aspiration.

3. Discontinue antipsychotics or other drugs, such as metoclopramide, which can cause or worsen catatonia.

4. Restart recently withdrawn dopamine agonists, especially in patients with parkinsonism.

5. Institute supportive measures (e.g., a cooling blanket if hyperthermia is present, or parenteral fluids and antihypertensives or pressors if autonomic instability emerges and if malignant catatonia is suspected).

6. Maintain a high index of suspicion for the development of medical complications and new medical problems.

Prognosis and Complications

For patients with catatonia, the long-term prognosis is good in almost half the cases.[7] Those with an acute onset and shorter duration of less than 1 month, a diagnosis of depression, or a family history of depression, have a better prognosis. Periodic catatonia can have a good short- and long-term prognosis. However, given its potential morbidity and mortality, concerted efforts at supportive care are essential to avoid the myriad complications that are associated with simple catatonia, and more so with malignant catatonia (see Table 21.4).

NEUROLEPTIC MALIGNANT SYNDROME (NMS)

Case 2: Neuroleptic Malignant Syndrome

Ms. B, a 56-year-old woman with a history of bipolar disorder, was admitted to the hospital after arguing with her husband. She became agitated and combative and required haloperidol (5 mg IM) on two occasions in the emergency room. Her psychiatric history was notable for depression, suicidal ideation, and auditory hallucinations as a teenager that required ECT and long-term treatment with perphenazine, lithium, and sertraline. Soon after her admission, she became withdrawn, hypokinetic, mute, and rigid. Her temperature reached 101.6°F and her CPK level was elevated (7260 U/L). An EEG revealed generalized slowing. A diagnosis of NMS was made, and her medications were discontinued. Her catatonic symptoms responded to lorazepam (2 mg IV, administered twice). Divalproex sodium and olanzapine were started 2 weeks after the resolution of her NMS.

Epidemiology and Risk Factors

NMS is temporally related to the use of a dopamine-blocking agent, or removal of a dopaminergic agent. It has been estimated that 0.16% of patients treated with neuroleptics develop NMS, although disparities across diagnostic criteria, survey instruments, prescribing habits, and catchment and population factors have historically complicated the epidemiology of NMS.[43] Cohort and drug registry studies have confirmed risk factors that include the use of high-potency neuroleptics (although low-potency and atypical agents also confer risk), prescription of multiple neuroleptics, and injected formulations. Patient-specific risk factors include a history of mood or psychotic disorder and a history of catatonia or NMS. Young adult males may be more likely to experience extrapyramidal symptoms, including NMS. Other factors include alcohol or sedative-hypnotic withdrawal, agitation, dehydration, exhaustion, and disorders of the basal ganglia (e.g., Parkinson, Wilson, and Huntington diseases, and tardive movement disorders). Low serum iron levels appear to be a state-specific finding in patients with NMS, and patients with a low serum iron level in the context of catatonia may be at increased risk for NMS if they are placed on a neuroleptic medication.[24] Studies have not supported any particular genetic predisposition, although case reports have implicated an association with cytochrome CYP 2D6.[44]

Clinical Features and Diagnosis

NMS is a syndrome of autonomic dysfunction with tachycardia, elevated blood pressure, and fever; as well as rigidity (including "lead-pipe" and cogwheeling variants), mutism, and stupor; associated with the use of neuroleptics.[44] Mental status changes occur in 97% of cases.[44] Notably, antipsychotics, often second-generation, have also been associated with cases of so-called "atypical NMS" that lack one or more features of NMS. Many such cases actually appear to represent non-malignant catatonia induced by neuroleptic use.[45] Indeed, many authors have noted the similarities between NMS and catatonia, and it is now commonly held that NMS is a form of malignant catatonia induced by neuroleptics.[24] Table 21.7 shows the symptoms of catatonia and NMS that overlap.

The diagnostic work-up is like that for catatonia, including consideration of an EEG and neuroimaging.[44] The EEG often demonstrates generalized slowing consistent with an encephalopathy. Neuroimaging and CSF are usually normal.

Diagnostic criteria for NMS remain under some debate, and various algorithms have been proposed. Prior algorithms de-emphasized certain features of NMS, including altered mental status and fever. The DSM-5-TR no longer lists specific criteria for NMS, instead favoring a descriptive approach. The latest criteria from the International Consensus study require recent dopamine antagonist exposure or dopamine agonist withdrawal; hyperthermia >100.4°F on at least two occasions; rigidity; mental status alteration; CK

TABLE 21.7		
Catatonia and Neuroleptic Malignant Syndrome (NMS): Shared Features		
	NMS	Catatonia
Clinical Signs		
Hyperthermia	Yes	Often
Motor rigidity	Yes	Yes
Mutism	Yes	Yes
Negativism	Often	Yes
Altered consciousness	Yes	Yes
■ Stupor or coma	Yes	Yes
Autonomic dysfunction	Yes	Often
■ Tachypnea	Yes	Often
■ Tachycardia	Yes	Often
■ Abnormal blood pressure	Yes	Yes
■ Diaphoresis	Yes	Yes
Laboratory Results		
Creatine phosphokinase elevated	Yes	Often
Serum iron reduced	Yes	Probable
Leukocytosis	Yes	Often

elevation at least four times the upper limit of normal; sympathetic nervous system lability including blood pressure elevation ≥25% above baseline, blood pressure fluctuation ≥20 mm Hg (diastolic) or ≥25 mm Hg (systolic) change within 24 hours; tachycardia ≥25% above baseline and tachypnea ≥50% above baseline; and a negative work-up for other causes.[46] An optimal cutoff score of 74 on the International Consensus Diagnostic Criteria for NMS was found to be 70% sensitive and 91% specific for NMS cases against expert opinion.[46]

Typically, NMS develops over several days, often beginning with rigidity and mental status changes followed by signs of hypermetabolism. The course is usually self-limited, lasting 2 days to 1 month (once neuroleptics are stopped and supportive measures are initiated).[44] Persistent cases are usually secondary to the use of depot neuroleptics, and ECT is highly effective in these cases. Although the mortality rate has been reduced through better recognition and management, there is an approximately 7.6% risk of death, with older age, continuation of neuroleptics, and severity of vital sign abnormalities conferring the greatest risk.[47]

Myoglobinuria and rhabdomyolysis may have long-term consequences for renal health.

Management

The first step in managing NMS is discontinuation of all dopamine antagonists, with additional consideration given to removing anticholinergic medications to avoid worsening hyperthermia. Supportive management, including administering IV fluids and monitoring vital signs and mental status, should be pursued given the high-risk of cardiorespiratory arrest, pneumonia, renal failure, and thromboembolism.[24] For moderate to severe NMS (moderate-to-severe rigidity, HR >100–120 beats per minute, temperature >38°–40°C), lorazepam and ECT should be strongly considered. Bromocriptine and amantadine may be beneficial in severe cases, although they may worsen underlying psychosis in vulnerable patients.[24] In clinical practice, they are less frequently used due to the high efficacy and lower rate of side effects of benzodiazepines.

Re-challenging a patient who has had NMS with an antipsychotic is controversial, as 30% of patients with a history of NMS may develop a recurrent episode.[24] Most investigators suggest that antipsychotics should not be given until at least 2 weeks after an episode of NMS has resolved and that re-challenge should be with a second-generation antipsychotic, with careful titration and monitoring.

SEROTONIN SYNDROME

Case 3: Serotonin Syndrome

Ms. C, a 69-year-old woman with a history of depression who was partially responsive to paroxetine 40 mg/day had her dose increased to 60 mg/day; 2 weeks later, buspirone 5 mg three times daily was added, along with trazodone 100 mg for sleep. She became confused, diaphoretic, febrile (to 101.2°F), hyperreflexic, and mildly rigid and was admitted to the hospital. Paroxetine, trazodone, and buspirone were discontinued. Over the next 2 days, her condition improved (with acetaminophen and supportive care).

Definition

Serotonin is a neurotransmitter involved in many neuropsychiatric disorders, and many pharmacologic agents have been designed to increase central serotonergic tone. Heightened clinical awareness is necessary to prevent, recognize, and intervene when a toxic syndrome secondary to serotonin excess emerges. Although serotonin syndrome (SS) has classically occurred due to an interaction between serotonergic agents and monoamine oxidase inhibitors (MAOIs), it is now far more common in cases of overdose on serotonergic agents or concomitant use of multiple serotonergic agents. Signs of SS include mental status changes (e.g., confusion, anxiety, irritability, euphoria, dysphoria); gastrointestinal symptoms (e.g., nausea, vomiting, diarrhea, incontinence); behavioral manifestations (e.g., restlessness, agitation); neurologic findings (e.g., ataxia or incoordination, tremors, myoclonus, hyperreflexia, ankle clonus, muscle rigidity); and autonomic nervous system abnormalities (e.g., hypertension, hypotension, tachycardia, diaphoresis, shivering, sialorrhea, mydriasis, tachypnea, hyperthermia).[48]

Epidemiology

The incidence of SS has been difficult to ascertain, although among US veterans who are psychiatric patients, an incidence of 0.07% and 0.09% has been reported.[49] Between 14% and 16% of selective serotonin reuptake inhibitor overdoses present with SS.[48] Given the overlap of symptoms with NMS, SS is often mistaken for it and thus may be under-reported. The existence of the syndrome in varying degrees also may confound its recognition, as can unawareness on the part of most physicians.[48] SS most often occurs in individuals being treated with psychotropics for a psychiatric disorder, although many medications have serotonergic effects of which many clinicians are unaware (e.g., meperidine).

Clinical Features and Diagnosis

As with NMS, taking a detailed history is crucial. The use of two or more serotonergic agents confers a greater risk of developing SS. Obtaining a history of neuroleptic use can be especially important because NMS shares many clinical features with SS, as do other toxic syndromes (Table 21.8).

TABLE 21.8

Comparison of Serotonin Syndrome with Neuroleptic Malignant Syndrome

Feature	Serotonin Syndrome	Neuroleptic Malignant Syndrome
Temperature	Hyperthermia variable	Hyperthermia
Mental status	■ Coma ■ Confusion ■ Delirium ■ Stupor ■ Euphoria ■ Irritability ■ Anxiety	■ Coma ■ Confusion ■ Delirium ■ Stupor
Neurologic	■ Muscle rigidity variable ■ Hyperreflexia ■ Tremor ■ Ankle clonus ■ Myoclonus ■ Incoordination	■ Muscle rigidity ■ Hyperreflexia (uncommon) ■ Tremor
Behavioral	■ Agitation ■ Restlessness	■ Agitation ■ Restlessness
Autonomic	■ Diaphoresis ■ Hypertension/hypotension ■ Incontinence ■ Mydriasis ■ Sialorrhea ■ Tachycardia ■ Tachypnea ■ Shivering	■ Diaphoresis ■ Hypertension/hypotension ■ Incontinence ■ Mydriasis ■ Sialorrhea ■ Tachycardia ■ Tachypnea
Gastrointestinal	Diarrhea Nausea Vomiting	
Laboratory	Elevated creatine phosphokinase (CPK) (uncommon) White blood cell count (WBC) elevated Liver function tests (LFTs) elevated	Elevated CPK (common) WBC elevated LFTs elevated

Modified from Keck PE, Arnold LM. The serotonin syndrome. *Psychiat Ann.* 2000;30:333–343; 339.

The syndrome ranges from mild to severe, with a mildly affected patient showing restlessness, tremors, tachycardia, shivering, diaphoresis, and the start of hyperreflexia. Moderately severe cases show tachycardia, hypertension, and fever, sometimes as high as 40°C (104°F). There is also mydriasis, strong bowel sounds, hyperreflexia, and clonus (greater in the lower extremities than the upper ones). Horizontal ocular clonus is also seen in moderately severe cases, as well as mental status changes of agitation, pressured speech, and autonomic hyperactivity. Head rotation with neck extension has also been reported. In severe cases, there are severe autonomic hyperactivity and severe hyperthermia with temperatures sometimes over 41.1°C (106°F). There is an agitated delirium accompanied by severe muscular rigidity, again greater in the lower extremities. This severe hypertonicity may obscure the appearance of clonus and hyperreflexia and thereby confound the diagnosis. Catatonic features are often present in SS and may be more prevalent in cases of moderate-to-severe SS. Rigidity, mutism, and waxy flexibility are often observed. The Hunter Serotonin Toxicity Criteria—that have replaced the older Sternbach criteria[50] in most clinical settings—emphasize that SS may be diagnosed with serotonergic exposure in combination with spontaneous clonus alone; with inducible clonus and agitation or diaphoresis; with inducible peripheral or ocular clonus, hypertonicity, and hyperthermia; or with tremors and hyperreflexia.[51]

Laboratory abnormalities are mostly non-specific or are secondary to the medical complications of the syndrome. A complete laboratory evaluation is nevertheless essential to rule out other causes for the signs and symptoms that are shared with SS. Leukocytosis, rhabdomyolysis, and liver function test abnormalities have all been reported in patients with SS, along with hyponatremia, hypomagnesemia, and hypocalcemia. Disseminated intravascular coagulation (DIC) has been reported in SS due to platelet dysfunction associated with serotonin activity. Acute renal failure secondary to myoglobinuria can occur and has been associated with fatalities. Urine toxicology may be useful to identify other substances that may contribute to serotonin excess.

Carcinoid syndrome and small-cell lung carcinoma, which may produce serotonin, have been associated with SS. Imaging of the abdomen and lung may sometimes be helpful in working up SS if no serotonergic agent has been identified. An EEG and neuroimaging are often useful in uncovering a seizure disorder or another neurologic condition. Drugs associated with SS are included in Table 21.9.

Pathophysiology

In both animal and human studies, the role of 5-HT has been implicated in the pathogenesis of SS. Nucleus raphe serotonin nuclei (located in the midbrain and arrayed in the midline down to the medulla) are involved in mediating thermoregulation, appetite, nausea, vomiting, wakefulness, migraines, sexual activity, and affective behavior. The animal model of SS seems to be associated with receptors in the lower brainstem and spinal cord. Ascending serotonergic projections are likely to play a role, particularly in hyperthermia, mental status, and autonomic changes. The 5-HT_{2A} and 5-HT_{1A} receptors appear to be overactive in SS. There also appears to be CNS norepinephrine overactivity. This is clinically significant because clinical outcomes may be associated with increased sympathetic tone.[48] The roles of catecholamines and 5-HT_2 and 5-HT_3 receptor interactions are unclear, as are the contributions of glutamate, GABA, and DA.

Management and Treatment

No prospective studies have looked at the treatment of SS. Recommendations for treatment are based solely on case reports and case series. SS is often self-limited, and removal of the offending agents frequently results in the resolution of symptoms within 24 hours. Therefore, the initial step in managing SS is to discontinue the suspected offending agent or agents. The next step is to provide supportive measures to prevent potential medical complications. These supportive measures include the use of antipyretics and cooling blankets to reduce hyperthermia, monitoring, and support of the respiratory and cardiovascular systems, IV hydration to prevent renal failure, use of clonazepam for myoclonic jerking, use of anticonvulsants if seizures arise, and use of hypertensive agents for significantly elevated blood pressures. The syndrome rarely leads to respiratory failure. When it does, it usually is because of aspiration and artificial ventilation may be required.

Benzodiazepine management of agitation, even when mild, is essential for patients with SS. This is because benzodiazepines, such as diazepam and lorazepam, can reduce autonomic tone and temperature and

TABLE 21.9
Central Nervous System Serotonergic Agents

Antidepressants
Monoamine oxidase inhibitors
Tricyclic antidepressants
Selective serotonin reuptake inhibitors
Serotonin-norepinephrine reuptake inhibitors
Other antidepressants
    Mirtazapine
    Nefazodone
    Trazodone
    Lithium
Atypical antipsychotics
    Quetiapine
    Olanzapine
    Clozapine
    Ziprasidone
    Caripiprazine (partial)
    Brexpiprazole (partial)
Other psychiatric medications
    Amphetamines
    Buspirone
    Lithium
Recreational drugs
    Cocaine
    Meta-chlorophenylpiperazine
    Methamphetamine
    Methylenedioxy-methamphetamine
    Some psychedelic compounds (e.g., lysergic acid diethylamide, psilocybin)
Opioids and opiate-like medications
    Meperidine
    Tramadol
Antibiotics
    Linezolid
Other medications
    Dextromethorphan
    Triptans
    Bromocriptine
    Pethidine
Supplements
    L-Tryptophan
    Fenfluramine
    Sibutramine
    Dihydroergotamine
    St. Johns wort

thus may have positive effects on survival.[52] Physical restraints should be avoided if at all possible because muscular stress can lead to lactic acidosis and elevated temperature.

Specific 5-HT receptor antagonism has occasionally been advocated for the treatment or prevention of the symptoms associated with SS, though these are rarely used in clinical practice. Cyproheptadine (4–24 mg/day) has been used.[48] Ketanserin, a $5\text{-}HT_2$ antagonist, and propranolol, which has $5\text{-}HT_{1A}$ receptor-blocking properties, have been used in a small number of cases. For the management of hypertension, nitroprusside and nifedipine are recommended, while esmolol is suggested for controlling tachycardia.[48] Dantrolene has also been used as a muscle relaxant. Because the temperature rise is muscular in origin, antipyretics are of no use in SS, and paralytics are required when fevers are high.

Care should be taken to avoid SS whenever possible. Non-selective MAOIs may interact with any medication acting on the monoamine system, and therefore a 2-week (5-week for fluoxetine) washout period is required whenever transitioning to, or from, MAOIs and other antidepressants.

Prognosis and Complications

SS is usually self-limited, with most cases resolving within 24 hours of discontinuing the offending agents.[52] Higher levels of monitoring may be needed for severe or prolonged cases. Rhabdomyolysis is the most common and serious complication; it occurs in roughly 25% of cases.[44] Generalized seizures occur in approximately 1%, with 39% of these patients dying. Myoglobinuric renal failure accounted for roughly 5% of medical complications, as did DIC. Nearly two-thirds of those with DIC died.

REFERENCES

1. Fricchione G, Bush G, Fozdar M. Recognition and treatment of the catatonic syndrome. *J Intensive Care Med.* 1997;12(3). https://doi.org/10.1177/088506669701200304.
2. Kahlbaum KL. *Catatonia.* Johns Hopkins University Press; 1973.
3. Kraepelin E. *Dementia Praecox and Paraphrenia.* Krieger Publishing; 1971.
4. Bleuler E. *Dementia Praecox and the Group of Schizophrenia.* International University Press; 1950.
5. Fink M, Taylor M. Catatonia: a separate category in DSM-IV? *Integr Psychiatry.* 1991;7(25).
6. American Psychiatric Association. *Diagnostic and Statistical Manual of Mental Disorders.* 5th ed. American Psychiatric Association Publishing; 2013.
7. Caroff SN, Mann SC, Francis A, Fricchione GL. *Catatonia: From Psychopathology to Neurobiology.* American Psychiatric Publishing, Inc; 2004:229. xiii.
8. Bräunig P, Krüger S, Shugar G. Prevalence and clinical significance of catatonic symptoms in mania. *Compr Psychiatry.* 1998;39(1):35–46. https://doi.org/10.1016/s0010-440x(98)90030-x.
9. Fink M, Taylor MA, Ghaziuddin N. Catatonia in autistic spectrum disorders: a medical treatment algorithm. *Int Rev Neurobiol.* 2006;72:233–244. https://doi.org/10.1016/S0074-7742(05)72014-6.
10. Oldham MA. The probability that catatonia in the hospital has a medical cause and the relative proportions of its causes: a systematic review. *Psychosomatics.* 2018;59:333–340.
11. Wilson JE, Carlson R, Duggan MC, et al. Delirium and catatonia in critically ill patients: the delirium and catatonia prospective cohort investigation. *Crit Care Med.* 2017;45(11):1837–1844. https://doi.org/10.1097/CCM.0000000000002642.
12. Dalmau J, Armangué T, Planagumà J, et al. An update on anti-NMDA receptor encephalitis for neurologists and psychiatrists: mechanisms and models. *Lancet Neurol.* 2019;18(11):1045–1057. https://doi.org/10.1016/S1474-4422(19)30244-3.
13. Vazquez-Guevara D, Badial-Ochoa S, Caceres-Rajo KM, et al. Catatonic syndrome as the presentation of encephalitis in association with COVID-19. *BMJ Case Rep.* 2021;14(6):e240550. https://doi.org/10.1136/bcr-2020-240550.
14. Grover S, Parakh P, Sharma A, et al. Catatonia in systemic lupus erythematosus: a case report and review of literature. *Lupus.* 2013;22(6):634–638. https://doi.org/10.1177/0961203313486951.
15. Duggal HS, Singh I. Drug-induced catatonia. *Drugs Today Barc Spain 1998.* 2005;41(9):599–607. https://doi.org/10.1358/dot.2005.41.9.899610.
16. Dhossche DM, Stoppelbein L, Rout UK. Etiopathogenesis of catatonia: generalizations and working hypotheses. *J ECT.* 2010;26(4):253–258. https://doi.org/10.1097/YCT.0b013e3181fbf96d.
17. Winarni TI, Schneider A, Ghaziuddin N, et al. Psychosis and catatonia in fragile X: case report and literature review. *Intractable Rare Dis Res.* 2015;4(3):139–146. https://doi.org/10.5582/irdr.2015.01028.
18. Faedda GL, Wachtel LE, Higgins AM, et al. Catatonia in an adolescent with velo-cardio-facial syndrome. *Am J Med Genet A.* 2015;167A(9):2150–2153. https://doi.org/10.1002/ajmg.a.37087.
19. Peralta V, Fañanás L, Martín-Reyes M, et al. Dissecting the catatonia phenotype in psychotic and mood disorders on the basis of familial-genetic factors. *Schizophr Res.* 2018;200:20–25. https://doi.org/10.1016/j.schres.2017.09.013.
20. Caroff SN, Hurford I, Bleier HR, et al. Recurrent idiopathic catatonia: implications beyond the Diagnostic and Statistical Manual of Mental Disorders 5th Edition. *Clin Psychopharmacol Neurosci Off Sci J Korean Coll Neuropsychopharmacol.* 2015;13(2):218–221. https://doi.org/10.9758/cpn.2015.13.2.218.
21. Stauder K. Die tödliche katatonie. *Arch Psychiatr Nervenkr.* 1934;102:614–634.
22. Karmacharya R, England ML, Ongür D. Delirious mania: clinical features and treatment response. *J Affect Disord.* 2008;109(3):312–316. https://doi.org/10.1016/j.jad.2007.12.001.
23. Bush G, Fink M, Petrides G, et al. Catatonia. I. Rating scale and standardized examination. *Acta Psychiatr Scand.* 1996;93(2). https://doi.org/10.1111/j.1600-0447.1996.tb09814.x.

24. Rogers JP, Oldham MA, Fricchione G, et al. Evidence-based consensus guidelines for the management of catatonia: recommendations from the British Association for Psychopharmacology. J Psychopharmacol Oxf Engl. 2023;37(4):327–369. https://doi.org/10.1177/02698811231158232.

25. Fisher CM. 'Catatonia' due to disulfiram toxicity. Arch Neurol. 1989;46(7):798–804. https://doi.org/10.1001/archneur.1989.00520430094024.

26. Fusunyan M, Praschan N, Fricchione G, et al. Akinetic mutism and coronavirus disease 2019: a narrative review. J Acad Consult-Liaison Psychiatry. 2021;62(6):625–633. https://doi.org/10.1016/j.jaclp.2021.08.009.

27. Hosseini P, Whincup R, Devan K, et al. The role of the electroencephalogram (EEG) in determining the aetiology of catatonia: a systematic review and meta-analysis of diagnostic test accuracy. eClinicalMedicine. 2023;56:101808. https://doi.org/10.1016/j.eclinm.2022.101808.

28. Walther S, Nadesalingam N, Nuoffer M. Structural alterations of the motor cortex and higher order cortical areas suggest early neurodevelopmental origin of catatonia in schizophrenia. Schizophr Res. 202210.1016/j.schres.2022.10.004 S0920-9964(22)00374-7.

29. Fricchione G, Beach S. Cingulate-basal ganglia-thalamo-cortical aspects of catatonia and implications for treatment, BA Vogt, Handbook of Clinical Neurology. Vol 166. Elsevier B.V.; 2019:223–252. http://doi.org/10.1016/B978-0-444-64196-0.00012-1.

30. Fricchione GL. Neuroleptic catatonia and its relationship to psychogenic catatonia. Biol Psychiatry. 1985;20(3):304–313. https://doi.org/10.1016/0006-3223(85)90060-5.

31. Bubser M, Schmidt WJ. Injection of apomorphine into the medial prefrontal cortex of the rat increases haloperidol-induced catalepsy. Biol Psychiatry. 1994;36(1):64–67. https://doi.org/10.1016/0006-3223(94)90065-5.

32. Friedhoff AJ, Carr KD, Uysal S, et al. Repeated inescapable stress produces a neuroleptic-like effect on the conditioned avoidance response. Neuropsychopharmacol Off Publ Am Coll Neuropsychopharmacol. 1995;13(2):129–138. https://doi.org/10.1016/0893-133X(95)00047-H.

33. Northoff G. What catatonia can tell us about "top-down modulation": a neuropsychiatric hypothesis. Behav Brain Sci. 2002;25(5):555–577. https://doi.org/10.1017/s0140525x02000109. discussion 578-604.

34. Moskowitz A. "Scared stiff": catatonia as an evolutionary-based fear response. Psychol Rev. 2004;111(4):984–1002. https://doi.org/10.1037/0033-295X.111.4.984.

35. Fink M, Taylor MA. The catatonia syndrome: forgotten but not gone. Arch Gen Psychiatry. 2009;66(11):1173–1177. https://doi.org/10.1001/archgenpsychiatry.2009.141.

36. Greenblatt DJ, Shader RI. Prazepam and lorazepam, two new benzodiazepines. N Engl J Med. 1978;299(24):1342–1344. https://doi.org/10.1056/NEJM197812142992405.

37. Mann SC, Caroff SN, Bleier HR, et al. Electroconvulsive therapy of the lethal catatonia syndrome. Convuls Ther. 1990;6(3):239–247.

38. Sienaert P, van Harten P, Rhebergen D. The psychopharmacology of catatonia, neuroleptic malignant syndrome, akathisia, tardive dyskinesia, and dystonia. Handb Clin Neurol. 2019;165:415–428. https://doi.org/10.1016/B978-0-444-64012-3.00025-3.

39. Mann SC, Caroff SN, Bleier HR, et al. Lethal catatonia. Am J Psychiatry. 1986;143(11):1374–1381. https://doi.org/10.1176/ajp.143.11.1374.

40. Beach SR, Gomez-Bernal F, Huffman JC, et al. Alternative treatment strategies for catatonia: a systematic review. Gen Hosp Psychiatry. 2017;48:1–19. https://doi.org/10.1016/j.genhosppsych.2017.06.011.

41. Hansbauer M, Wagner E, Strube W, et al. rTMS and tDCS for the treatment of catatonia: a systematic review. Schizophr Res. 2020;222:73–78. https://doi.org/10.1016/j.schres.2020.05.028.

42. Ungvari GS, Chiu HF, Chow LY, et al. Lorazepam for chronic catatonia: a randomized, double-blind, placebo-controlled cross-over study. Psychopharmacology (Berl). 1999;142(4):393–398. https://doi.org/10.1007/s002130050904.

43. Schneider M, Regente J, Greiner T, et al. Neuroleptic malignant syndrome: evaluation of drug safety data from the AMSP program during 1993-2015. Eur Arch Psychiatry Clin Neurosci. 2020;270(1):23–33. https://doi.org/10.1007/s00406-018-0959-2.

44. Mann SC, Keck PE, Lazarus A. Neuroleptic Malignant Syndrome and Related Conditions. 2nd ed. American Psychiatric Publishing, Inc; 2003.

45. Belvederi Murri M, Guaglianone A, Bugliani M, et al. Second-generation antipsychotics and neuroleptic malignant syndrome: systematic review and case report analysis. Drugs RD. 2015;15(1):45–62. https://doi.org/10.1007/s40268-014-0078-0.

46. Gurrera RJ, Mortillaro G, Velamoor V, et al. A validation study of the International Consensus Diagnostic Criteria for Neuroleptic Malignant Syndrome. J Clin Psychopharmacol. 2017;37(1):67–71. https://doi.org/10.1097/JCP.0000000000000640.

47. Guinart D, Misawa F, Rubio JM, et al. A systematic review and pooled, patient-level analysis of predictors of mortality in neuroleptic malignant syndrome. Acta Psychiatr Scand. 2021;144(4):329–341. https://doi.org/10.1111/acps.13359.

48. Boyer EW, Shannon M. The serotonin syndrome. N Engl J Med. 2005;352(11):1112–1120. https://doi.org/10.1056/NEJMra041867.

49. Nguyen CT, Xie L, Alley S, et al. Epidemiology and economic burden of serotonin syndrome with concomitant use of serotonergic agents: a retrospective study utilizing two large US claims databases. Prim Care Companion CNS Disord. 2017;19(6):17m02200. https://doi.org/10.4088/PCC.17m02200.

50. Sternbach H. The serotonin syndrome. Am J Psychiatry. 1991;148(6):705–713. https://doi.org/10.1176/ajp.148.6.705.

51. Dunkley EJC, Isbister GK, Sibbritt D, et al. The Hunter Serotonin Toxicity Criteria: simple and accurate diagnostic decision rules for serotonin toxicity. QJM Mon J Assoc Physicians. 2003;96(9):635–642. https://doi.org/10.1093/qjmed/hcg109.

52. Scotton WJ, Hill LJ, Williams AC, et al. Serotonin syndrome: pathophysiology, clinical features, management, and potential future directions. Int J Tryptophan Res IJTR. 2019;12 https://doi.org/10.1177/1178646919873925. 1178646919873925.

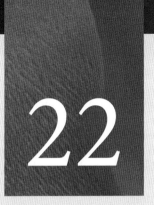

22

PATIENTS WITH DISORDERED SLEEP

AMIT CHOPRA, MBBS ■ JOHN W. WINKELMAN, MD, PHD ■ THEODORE A. STERN, MD

OVERVIEW

Sleep is an active biochemical process that is characterized by a variety of physiologic markers, stages, and patterns that, like vital signs, provide a basic indication of one's overall well-being. Sleep and psychiatry are intertwined due to the existence of myriad sleep disturbances associated with common psychiatric disorders. Increasing evidence suggests a bidirectional association between sleep disturbances and psychiatric disorders, as poor sleep worsens the clinical burden and outcomes of psychiatric disorders and is recognized as a risk factor for the development of common psychiatric disorders. In addition, sleep disturbances are increasingly recognized as modifiable risk factors for self-harm and suicide. Moreover, treatment of disturbed sleep can help to prevent psychiatric problems, as early recognition and management of sleep disorders, such as insomnia, can prevent the onset of major depressive disorder (MDD). Therefore, an understanding of clinical features and management of primary sleep disorders can facilitate better outcomes for psychiatric disorders. This chapter examines the biological and psychiatric aspects of normal and disordered sleep; it also discusses the clinical features, diagnosis, and treatment of common sleep disorders. Finally, key subjective and objective components of sleep disturbances and the effect of psychotropics on sleep are discussed.

NORMAL SLEEP

Normal sleep is comprised of *non-rapid eye movement* (NREM) and *rapid eye movement* (REM) sleep.

Aserinsky and Kleitman (1953) were the first to investigate rapid eye movements during sleep. They postulated that depth of sleep could be assessed through eye motility and tested this hypothesis through direct observation of infants' eye movements during sleep.[1] Moreover, they noted slow rolling eye movements during the early stages of sleep that disappeared as sleep progressed, and observed periods of rapid eye movements are associated with irregular breathing and increased heart rate.[1] Aserinsky and Kleitman coined the terms NREM (to indicate slow rolling rhythmic eye movements) and REM (to indicate fast erratic eye movements). In 1957 Kleitman and Dement discovered that REM and NREM sleep occurred cyclically throughout the night and named this overall NREM-REM pattern *sleep architecture*. NREM and REM sleep alternate in a rhythmic fashion known as the *NREM-REM cycle* approximately every 90 to 120 minutes. NREM sleep is further divided into stages including N1, N2, and N3. The proportion of each sleep stage during an average night's sleep is as follows: N1 (2%–5%); N2 (45%–55%); N3 (15%–25%); and REM sleep 20%–25%. Stage N3 is most prominent in the first half of the night, and it diminishes thereafter. In contrast to NREM sleep, REM sleep appears in longer blocks as the night progresses. The time from sleep onset to the first REM period is known as *REM latency*, which is usually 90 to 100 minutes. *Sleep efficiency* is the amount of sleep achieved per the total time in bed, multiplied by 100; it is typically ≥85% in individuals with normal sleep.

The average adult sleeps between 6 and 9 hours per night. However, the quantity and quality of sleep vary across the lifespan. Infants spend about two-thirds of the day sleeping, whereas this amount decreases to less than one-third of the day in adults. Sleep architecture becomes altered as people age; more time is spent in N1 sleep, nocturnal awakenings become more frequent, and N3 sleep and overall sleep efficiency decrease. [2]

SLEEP NEUROPHYSIOLOGY

The actual neurophysiological basis for the sleep-wake cycle remains unclear, but current research reveals that specific brain regions are critical for wakefulness and sleep. These neuronal systems (in the brainstem, hypothalamus, and basal forebrain) have neurons that project diffusely throughout the neocortex.[3] The major wake-promoting centers include the tuberomammillary nucleus (via histamine), the reticular activating system (via serotonin), the locus coeruleus (via norepinephrine), the basal forebrain (via acetylcholine), and the hypothalamus (via orexin). The major NREM sleep–promoting nucleus is the ventrolateral preoptic nucleus (VLPO) in the hypothalamus, which is thought to inhibit the main ascending monoaminergic arousal systems by releasing inhibitory neurotransmitters, mainly gamma amino-butyric acid (GABA) and galanin. The pedunculopontine and dorsolateral tegmental nuclei of the brainstem, which are both cholinergic, have projections predominantly to the thalamus; these structures play an important role in REM sleep circuitry.

The timing of sleep and wakefulness is largely determined by an internal biological cycle known as the *circadian rhythm*.[4] This biological clock serves as an endogenous rhythm of bodily functions that is influenced by environmental cues, or *zeitgebers*, of which the main one is daylight. The average circadian cycle is slightly longer than 24 hours for most people. The suprachiasmatic nuclei (SCN), located in the anterior hypothalamus, is the brain region that controls the human circadian rhythms. The SCN receives input from the eyes via the retinohypothalamic tract, and it sends information to the hypothalamus and the pineal gland. Melatonin, a hormone secreted by the pineal gland during darkness, is associated with the suppression of the SCN, thus facilitating sleep in diurnal mammals[5]; light suppresses melatonin production. Another mechanism (called homeostatic sleep drive) tracks how much sleep has occurred recently, such that as time spent awake increases, homeostatic pressure accumulates to increase the probability of falling asleep. The biological basis for this system is thought to reside in adenosine levels, which build during wakefulness and wane during sleep.[6] Caffeine is thought to enhance wakefulness by blocking adenosine signaling.

Sleep Investigations

Polysomnography

Polysomnography is the "gold standard" method for evaluating sleep physiology and many sleep disorders. It involves simultaneously recording multiple physiologic variables in a standardized fashion, known as the *polysomnogram* (PSG).[7] The parameters recorded by the PSG include, but are not limited to, the following:

- *Electroencephalogram (EEG)*: A recording of the electrical activity of cortical neurons via scalp electrodes that are placed in standardized positions, usually bilateral frontal, central, and occipital positions.
- *Electro-oculogram (EOG)*: A recording of eye movements bilaterally.
- *Electrocardiogram (ECG)*: A recording of heart rate and rhythm.
- *Electromyogram (EMG)*: A recording of the activity of the bilateral tibialis anterior muscles, and the submental (chin) muscles.
- *Respiration*: Recordings of nasal and oral airflow by means of pressure and thermal sensors, and recordings of thoracic and abdominal movements by means of respiratory inductance plethysmography.
- *Pulse oximetry*: A recording of blood oxygen hemoglobin saturation.
- *Snore monitor*: A tool to detect and record snoring by means of a vibration sensor placed on the neck.

Through analysis of the EEG, EMG, and EOG signals, the different sleep-wake stages are scored, typically by manual visual inspection by skilled technologists. From the epoch-by-epoch scoring, various metrics are presented in PSG reports, such as sleep-onset latency, NREM sleep, REM sleep, and awakenings that occur throughout the night.

The *waking state* is defined by the PSG tracings in the following manner: the EEG reveals low amplitude and mixed high frequencies with the eyes open, and an occipital predominant 8 to 13 Hz wave pattern known as *alpha waves* when the eyes are closed; the EMG reveals muscle tone and activity; and the EOG demonstrates variable eye movements, including blinking. Sleep is normally entered through NREM sleep. NREM sleep is divided into three stages identified by specific EEG criteria; REM is identified by a combination of findings on the EEG, EOG, and EMG.

- *Stage N1*: Alpha waves, present during wakefulness, account for less than 50% of an epoch (a 30-second interval on the PSG). The EEG frequencies are mixed but slower than those seen during wakefulness, usually with the emergence of theta waves (4–7 Hz).
- *Stage N2*: Theta activity continues in this stage, while two hallmark waveforms emerge: sleep spindles (rhythmic 12–14 Hz waves that last 0.5 seconds or more) and K-complexes (high-amplitude negative waves that are followed by a positive deflection, lasting 0.5 seconds or more).
- *Stage N3*: Delta waves (high-amplitude, slow-frequency 0.5–2.0 Hz waves) occur in at least 20% of an epoch. This stage is commonly called delta sleep or slow-wave sleep (SWS).
- REM sleep, also known as *paradoxical sleep* owing to its similarity to wakefulness, is defined by three principal features. First, the EEG demonstrates low-amplitude high-frequency waves that may resemble those of the waking state or NREM stage 1. Second, the chin EMG reveals an absence of, or a marked decrease in, muscle activity. Finally, conjugate rapid eye movements become evident, often in bursts (termed phasic REM) separated by quiescent periods (tonic REM), on the EOG.[8]

Home Sleep Apnea Testing

Home sleep apnea testing (HSAT) includes a limited-channel study with a minimum of four channels (including measurement of respiratory airflow, respiratory effort, heart rate, and oxygen saturation). Attendance of a sleep technologist is not required for HSATs; therefore it can be administered in the home setting. HSAT lacks EEG monitoring that is used to detect respiratory events associated with cortical arousals; it has a lower sensitivity than the PSG. Therefore, HSAT may lead to false-negative studies and an overall underestimation of sleep-disordered breathing.[9] The American Academy of Sleep Medicine (AASM) guidelines recommend obtaining a standard (in-lab) study when HSAT is negative for obstructive sleep apnea-hypopnea syndrome[10] and not using HSAT for general screening or for assessment of low-risk patients, for patients with significant medical co-morbidities, or those with sleep disorders, such as insomnia or parasomnia.

Multiple Sleep Latency Test

A multiple sleep latency test (MSLT) is obtained for the evaluation of hypersomnolence disorders, such as narcolepsy, in a sleep laboratory, after completing a PSG the night before. The MSLT procedure involves providing five nap opportunities, beginning 2 hours after awakening and every 2 hours afterward. Patients are awakened after napping for 20 minutes and then kept awake between nap opportunities. The average sleep latency is recorded, with values below 8 minutes regarded as consistent with pathological sleepiness. REM latency (i.e., the time from sleep onset to REM onset) is recorded; the presence of two or more sleep-onset REM (SOREM) periods, along with pathological sleepiness (with an average sleep onset latency <8 minutes) in the appropriate clinical setting, is considered diagnostic of narcolepsy. The results of an MSLT can be confounded by the use of certain medications. For example, most antidepressants suppress REM sleep, and patients who use stimulants can exhibit rebound sleepiness with their abrupt discontinuation. For these reasons, if it is clinically safe and appropriate to wean these drugs, they should be tapered at least 2 weeks before the MSLT. Patients are advised to maintain sleep diaries for 7 to 14 days before their MSLT to ensure that they have regular sleep patterns with sufficient sleep. Complete cessation of alcohol and substance use is recommended, and urine drug testing should be obtained to verify the drug use exposure on the day of the MSLT.[9]

Actigraphy

An actigraph is a small watch-like device that is worn on the non-dominant wrist and measures movement with a piezoelectric sensor. Periods of high activity are scored as wakefulness, whereas periods of relative absence of wrist movements are scored as sleep by an actigraph device. Actigraphy offers a distinct advantage, as the device can be worn 24 hours per day for 1 to 2 weeks; this can assist in the identification of irregular sleep-wake cycles in those with a unique home/work environment. Actigraphy is utilized to assist in the diagnosis of sleep disorders, including circadian rhythm sleep-wake disorders, insomnia, and hypersomnia.[9]

CLINICAL APPROACH TO THE PATIENT WITH DISORDERED SLEEP

Once a sleep complaint has reached clinical attention, it is important to conduct a careful evaluation to correctly assess, diagnose, and treat any potential underlying sleep disorder. The following discussion is based on a general approach to the proper diagnosis and management of sleep disorders.

The initial step in the diagnostic process is to obtain a detailed sleep history, either through direct inquiry of the patient and his or her bed partner or by means of sleep questionnaires. Table 22.1 provides a list of specific areas that should be addressed.[11] In addition to a detailed sleep history, patients are encouraged to keep a 2-week sleep diary that details the time and amount of sleep, the number and length of any naps, the number of awakenings, wake-up times, any medications taken, and subjective moods during the day. For those in whom hypersomnia is the major complaint, an Epworth Sleepiness Scale—a simple, self-administered, questionnaire that requires patients to rate their degree of sleepiness in a variety of routine situations— is often administered (Table 22.2).[12] In addition to the sleep history and screening examinations, a medical history that includes the past medical history, current medications, alcohol and drug history, family history, and psychiatric history should be completed.

After taking a comprehensive history, and if it is clinically indicated, patients should undergo a detailed physical examination. For those who have hypersomnia, this examination focuses on the distribution of obesity, the respiratory system, the cardiovascular system,

---

TABLE 22.1
Sleep History: Important Questions

- What time do you go to bed and wake up?
- How long does it take you to fall asleep?
- How often do you wake up overnight?
- Do you snore?
- Do you feel sleepy during the daytime?
- Do you experience any disturbing movement overnight including an urge to move your legs relieved by moving them? (restless legs syndrome)
- Trouble moving or rolling over in bed? (rigidity)
- Abnormal postures? (dystonia)
- Do you act out your dreams overnight?

From Ashbrook L, During EH. Chapter 5 - Sleep and movement disorders. In: Miglis M, ed. *Sleep and Neurologic Disease*. 1st ed. Elsevier; 2017:89–113.

TABLE 22.2
Epworth Sleepiness Scale

How likely are you to doze off or fall asleep in the following situations, in contrast to feeling just tired? This refers to your usual way of life in recent times. Even if you have not done some of these things recently, try to work out how they would have affected you. Use the following scale to choose the most appropriate number for each situation:

0 = no chance of dozing
1 = slight chance of dozing
2 = moderate chance of dozing
3 = high chance of dozing

Situation	Score
Sitting and reading	_____
Watching TV	_____
Sitting inactive in a public place (e.g., a theater or a meeting)	_____
As a passenger in a car for an hour without a break	_____
Lying down to rest in the afternoon when circumstances permit	_____
Sitting and talking to someone	_____
Sitting quietly after lunch without alcohol	_____
In a car, while stopped for a few minutes in traffic	_____
Total	_____

From Johns MW. A new method for measuring daytime sleepiness: the Epworth sleepiness scale. *Sleep*. 991;14(6):540–545.

and the oro-maxillofacial region, with careful attention to the tongue, tonsils, uvula, and pharynx. If indicated, laboratory examinations, including a complete blood cell count, arterial blood gas analysis, pulmonary function tests (PFTs), an ECG, thyroid function tests (TFTs), serum iron analysis, and electrolytes can be considered. Cephalometric x-rays of the skull and neck may be obtained to evaluate for skeletal discrepancies, if craniofacial malformations are suspected as a possible etiology for any breathing-related sleep disorder.[13]

Once a diagnosis has been confirmed, utilizing appropriate sleep investigations where needed, patients are offered appropriate treatment. Table 22.3 summarizes non-pharmacologic and pharmacologic treatments for the common primary sleep disorders.

SLEEP DISORDERS

Although several classification systems for sleep disorders exist, the *Diagnostic and Statistical Manual of Mental Disorders, 5th Edition* (DSM-5)[14] and the *International Classification of Sleep Disorders, 3rd Edition* (ICSD-3)[15] are the most widely used.

Insomnia Disorder

Clinical Features

The DSM-5 specifies that this sleep difficulty occurs on ≥3 nights for ≥3 months, despite an adequate opportunity for sleep, and the absence of another primary sleep disorder (such as sleep apnea) or substance use; in addition, it cannot be explained by a co-existing medical or psychiatric problem (such as mania or hyperthyroidism). The DSM-5 describes sleep-onset insomnia (or initial insomnia) as involving difficulty falling asleep, sleep maintenance insomnia (or middle insomnia) as involving frequent or prolonged awakenings throughout the night, and late insomnia as involving early-morning awakening with an inability to return to sleep. It defines difficulty falling asleep as a subjective sleep latency for ≥20 to 30 minutes, and difficulty maintaining sleep as waking after 20 to 30 minutes. Early morning awakening involves spontaneous waking >30 minutes before the desired wake time, and before the total sleep time reaches 6.5 hours.

Diagnosis

The diagnosis of insomnia is based exclusively on the clinical history, which involves difficulty falling asleep or staying asleep, associated with non-refreshing sleep or some other daytime sequelae. The etiology of insomnia is often multi-factorial, but the final common pathway is postulated to be a state of hyperarousal. There is evidence in neuroimaging studies of patients with insomnia of, increased arousal during sleep as well as during wakefulness.[16] A PSG is not typically recommended for the evaluation of patients with chronic insomnia, unless another sleep disorder, such as periodic limb movements of sleep (PLMS) or obstructive sleep apnea (OSA), is suspected.

Treatment

The treatment for insomnia disorder is often multimodal and it includes behavioral and pharmacological approaches to improve the subjective quality of sleep, relieve distress related to sleep, and improve daytime functioning.

Behavioral Treatments

Cognitive-behavioral treatment for insomnia (CBT-I) is a first-line treatment for the management of insomnia disorder that integrates several techniques (such as stimulus control, sleep restriction, cognitive restructuring, and relaxation). CBT-I is typically delivered in six to eight individual sessions; the efficacy of brief versions of CBT-I has been demonstrated.[17] More recently, a digital CBT-I has been approved by the US Food and Drug Administration (FDA) for the management of insomnia disorder based on the positive results of this intervention. The acute effects of CBT-I over a period of 6 to 10 weeks have been comparable or superior to those of hypnotic medications,[18] and these effects are maintained for up to 3 years of follow-up.[19] In addition, behavioral treatments are efficacious in patients who take hypnotics and help patients reduce the use of hypnotic agents.[20]

Medication Treatments

Hypnotics should be used with caution, and in the lowest effective dose; their use should be re-evaluated frequently and attempts to wean them should be made. Older patients, their families, and caregivers (e.g., nurses and aids in nursing homes) should be cautioned about their risks and fall precautions should be taken. Therefore alternatives to hypnotic agents, including CBT-I, should be used initially, whenever possible.[21]

TABLE 22.3
Treatment Options for Commonly Encountered Primary Sleep Disorders

Primary Sleep Disorder	Non-Pharmacologic Treatment	Pharmacologic Treatment
Dyssomnias		
Primary Insomnia	Sleep hygiene	*Benzodiazepines*
	Stimulus control	Triazolam 0.125–0.25 mg
	Sleep restriction	Temazepam 7.5–30 mg
	Biofeedback	
	Relaxation training	*Imidazopyridines*
	Paradoxical intention	Zolpidem 5–10 mg
	Cognitive therapy	Eszopiclone 1–3 mg
	Psychotherapy	
		Pyrazolopyrimidines
		Zaleplon 5–10 mg
		Dual Orexin Receptor Antagonists (DORAs)
		Suvorexant 5–20 mg
		Lemborexant 5–10 mg
		Daridorexant 25–50 mg
		Sedating Antidepressants
		Doxepin 3–6 mg
		Melatonin Agonists
		Ramelteon 8 mg
		Atypical Antipsychotics
		Quetiapine 12.5–100 mg
		Olanzapine 2.5–10 mg
Idiopathic Hypersomnia	Regular bedtime	*Amphetamines*
	Avoid daytime naps	Dextroamphetamine 5–60 mg/day
		Methylphenidate 5–60 mg/day
		Dexmethylphenidate 5–20 mg/day
		Amphetamine/dextroamphetamine 5–40 mg/day
		Lisdexamfetamine 20–70 mg/day
		Non-amphetamines
		Modafinil 100–400 mg/day
		Armodafinil 150–250 mg/day
Narcolepsy	Regular bedtime	*Non-amphetamines*
	Scheduled daytime naps	Modafinil 100–400 mg/day
		Armodafinil 150–250 mg/day
		GABA-B Agonists
		Sodium oxybate 3–9 g HS (in divided doses)
		Dopamine and Norepinephrine Reuptake Inhibitor
		Solriamfetol 75–150 mg/day
		H3 Antagonists
		Pitolisant 17.8–35.6 mg/day
		Amphetamines
		Dextroamphetamine 5–60 mg/day
		Methylphenidate 5–80 mg/day
		Dexmethylphenidate 5–20 mg/day
		Amphetamine/dextroamphetamine 5–40 mg/day
		Lisdexamfetamine 20–70 mg/day
		Antidepressants (for Cataplexy)
		Venlafaxine 75–150 mg
		Fluoxetine 20–60 mg

TABLE 22.3
Treatment Options for Commonly Encountered Primary Sleep Disorders—cont'd

Primary Sleep Disorder	Non-Pharmacologic Treatment	Pharmacologic Treatment
Breathing-Related Sleep Disorders	Weight loss Avoidance of sedating substances Positional therapy Oral appliance Nasal positive airway pressure Hypoglossal nerve stimulation UPPP Maxillomandibular advancement Tracheostomy CPAP/BiPAP	Acetazolamide (for central apnea) No drugs have been reliably shown to improve obstructive sleep apnea
PLMD and RLS	None	*Dopaminergic Agonists* Pramipexole 0.125–0.5 mg Ropinirole 0.25–4 mg Rotigotine patch (1–3 mg) *Alpha-2-delta Ligand Medications* Gabapentin 300–600 mg; gabapentin enacarbil 600 mg *Benzodiazepines* Clonazepam 0.5–2 mg *Opioids* Codeine 15–30 mg Oxycodone 5–10 mg
Parasomnias Sleepwalking Disorder	Reassurance Maintenance of a safe environment Psychotherapy Hypnosis	Clonazepam 0.5–2.0 mg
Sleep Terror Disorder	Reassurance Stress reduction	Clonazepam 0.5–2.0 mg
Nightmare Disorder	Reassurance Stress reduction Psychotherapy Desensitization Rehearsal therapy	Prazosin 2–5 mg
REM Sleep Behavior Disorder	Reassurance Maintenance of a safe bedroom environment	Clonazepam 0.5–2.0 mg Melatonin 3–12 mg

BiPAP, Bilevel positive airway pressure; *CPAP*, continuous positive airway pressure; *PLMD*, periodic limb movement disorder; *RLS*, restless leg disorder; *UPPP*, uvulopalatopharyngoplasty.

Benzodiazepine Receptor Agonists. Both benzodiazepines and non-benzodiazepine hypnotics (e.g., zolpidem, eszopiclone, and zaleplon) are often called benzodiazepine receptor agonists (BzRAs), as these medications work at the benzodiazepine receptor complex ($GABA_A$). The newer non-benzodiazepine agents may stimulate only a subset of benzodiazepine receptors ($GABA_A$ alpha$_1$ receptor), whereas the benzodiazepines may be less selective in their action.[22]

The short-term efficacy of BzRAs has been established in terms of significant improvements in sleep quality and sleep latency. In addition, wake after sleep onset (WASO), total sleep time (TST), and sleep efficiency (SE) also improve depending on the drug's duration of action. The newer BzRAs have been shown to be efficacious for up to 6 months after nightly[23] or intermittent use[24] in double-blind placebo-controlled studies, and they have a low potential for abuse and dependence; however, like the traditional benzodiazepines they are labeled as Class IV agents by the FDA. The tendency for abuse exists with the BzRAs, especially in those with a history of alcohol or other sedative abuse.[25]

Relative contraindications to BzRA use include severe pulmonary failure, untreated sleep apnea, hepatic failure, alcohol or sedative abuse/dependence, and use of other sedative drugs.[26]

Anterograde amnesia, sleepwalking, sleep-related eating disorders, and sleep-driving without conscious awareness have all been reported with the use of BzRAs. Evidence suggests that the BzRAs may increase the risk of falls (especially in the elderly) and the increased fall risk may extend to the day after hypnotic use.

Dual Orexin Receptor Antagonists. The neuropeptide, orexin, plays an important role in the stabilization and maintenance of wakefulness by reinforcing wake-promoting signaling in the brain via orexin receptors (OX1R and OX2R). Dual orexin receptor antagonists (DORAs), including suvorexant, lemborexant, and daridorexant, are Drug Enforcement Administration schedule IV medications that have been FDA-approved for the treatment of insomnia disorder.[27] Common side effects of DORAs include somnolence, abnormal dreams, fatigue, and dry mouth; these medications are contraindicated in individuals with narcolepsy, a condition characterized by a deficiency of orexin.[28]

Melatonin Agonists. Ramelteon is a specific agonist of melatonin receptors (MT1 and MT2) with properties like those of endogenous melatonin.[19] Ramelteon has been shown to reduce sleep-onset latency, but it does not improve sleep maintenance. Doses of 8 mg/day are effective, and they do not seem to produce rebound insomnia. Ramelteon is not a controlled substance, and it has minimal abuse potential.

H_1 Receptor Antagonists. Doxepin, a tricyclic antidepressant (TCA) with selective affinity for the H_1 receptor at low doses (3–6 mg), is FDA-approved

for insomnia at doses of 3 to 6 mg. In clinical trials, doxepin use has been associated with reduced WASO, increased SE, and TST for up to 5 weeks, with little effect on sleep latency.[29] Doxepin affects WASO and SE across the entire night; hence, it is recommended for use in sleep maintenance insomnia.

Off-Label Use of Medications. Trazodone is one of the most prescribed agents for insomnia in psychiatric settings, but the dose-related safety and efficacy of trazodone as a hypnotic has not been formally established.[30] Mirtazapine is an atypical antidepressant with sedative effects due to antihistaminergic activity; this explains its off-label use for insomnia, particularly at low doses (7.5 mg). TCAs are also prescribed frequently for insomnia, as they improve sleep continuity, reduce sleep latency, increase TST, and improve daytime function. Data on the optimal dosing for TCAs for insomnia is also limited. TCAs are toxic in overdose and have potent anticholinergic and antihistaminic effects; they may produce delirium, as well as cause problems with gait and cognition, especially in the elderly. Quetiapine and other atypical antipsychotics, such as olanzapine, should not be considered as first-line treatments for insomnia. When atypical antipsychotics are used to manage insomnia, doses far lower than doses for primary indications are typically prescribed, while closely monitoring for metabolic and extrapyramidal symptoms (EPS).

Over-the-Counter Sleep Aids. Over-the-counter (OTC) sleep aids, which usually contain a sedating antihistamine as the active component, are widely used by those in the general population.[31] However, sedating antihistamines may not reduce sleep latency, increase sleep duration, or improve daytime function.[32] These medications may also produce delirium and disturbances of gait and memory, especially in the elderly. Melatonin is available OTC in immediate- and sustained-release formulations in a variety of doses. Other supplements (including valerian, tryptophan, kava, chamomile, and passion flower) have had anecdotal claims for relief of insomnia. However, they are not well studied, except for valerian root, which did not show significant benefit for insomnia in a meta-analysis.

Breathing-Related Sleep Disorders

The most common breathing-related sleep disorder is obstructive sleep apnea (OSA)-hypopnea syndrome (OSAHS). Although OSAHS is a commonly encountered cause of hypersomnia, many patients with OSAHS lack objective or subjective sleepiness, which accounts in part for widespread under-diagnosis. OSAHS is characterized by repeated partial or complete obstructions of the airway during sleep, which are associated with oxygen desaturation and EEG arousal, as well as autonomic nervous system swings. The principal defect is repetitive occlusion of the upper airway at the level of the pharynx (that results from an abnormal decrease in oropharyngeal muscle tone), excessive tissue mass in the pharynx and tongue, malposition of the jaw or tongue, or a narrow airway.

The most significant risk factors for OSAHS include male sex, age >50 years, obesity, cigarette smoking, use or abuse of alcohol, poor physical health, and a neck circumference >17 inches.[33] Nocturnal signs and symptoms include snoring, gasping arousals, witnessed apneas, enuresis, gastroesophageal reflux, hypoxemia, hypercapnia, and cardiac dysrhythmias. Daytime signs and symptoms include headaches, hypersomnolence, neuropsychiatric abnormalities, and hypertension.

Diagnosis

The PSG is the gold standard diagnostic test to identify OSA as well as breathing-related sleep syndromes, such as central apnea, or obesity-related hypoventilation. Manual scoring of the PSG allows for quantification of the severity of OSA, based on the frequency of breathing events per hour of sleep. *Apnea* is defined as the cessation of airflow for >10 seconds. The most common form is obstructive apnea, based on ongoing respiratory effort. These obstructions can be so complete and the effort so powerful that the chest and abdomen can move in opposite directions, a phenomenon known as *paradoxical breathing*. Central apnea, by contrast, has no respiratory effort. Mixed apneas contain features of both central and obstructive patterns. Hypopneas are partial reductions in airflow of >30% amplitude, associated with ≥4% desaturation.

Treatment

Currently the apnea-hypopnea index (AHI) values in the mild range (5–15 events per hour) warrant therapy if symptoms attributable to poor sleep are present. For those with AHI values >15 per hour, treatment is recommended even if the patient is asymptomatic.

Conservative measures, such as weight loss, help but may not cure OSAHS. Evidence suggests that a 10-kg reduction in body weight can yield a reduction in the AHI index of roughly five events per hour.[34] Several studies suggest that OSAHS re-emerges or persists after surgical or non-surgical weight loss.[35] Nasal continuous positive airway pressure (CPAP) is the treatment of choice for adults with OSAHS. CPAP adherence is roughly 60% to 70% and interventions such as education and support, use of nasal decongestants, heated humidification for nasal issues, use of preferred CPAP face masks, and consolidation of fragmented sleep, have increased CPAP adherence in those with OSAHS.[34] Sedatives should be used with caution in individuals with OSAHS, as these medications change arousal thresholds, thereby delaying arousal and lengthening apneic spells; this may worsen oxygen desaturation and the other negative consequences of apnea. CPAP improves symptoms of hypersomnolence in those with OSAHS; stimulatory agents (e.g., modafinil) help those with excessive daytime sleepiness (EDS) (even when the symptom persists after CPAP treatment).

In patients with unsuccessful CPAP treatment, generally due to the inability to tolerate the device, the treatment alternatives for OSAHS include positional therapy, the use of adjustable oral appliances, and upper airway surgery. Adjustable oral appliances generally advance the mandible to prevent retroglossal collapse and are preferred to CPAP by some patients, particularly those with mild to moderate disease.[34] Surgical approaches to alleviate OSAHS include tonsillectomy and/or adenoidectomy (which is the first-line treatment for pediatric OSAHS), nasal surgery (turbinectomy or straightening of nasal septum), uvulopalatopharyngoplasty, and maxillomandibular advancement. Since 2014 hypoglossal nerve stimulation, using an implantable neurostimulator device, has been introduced as a novel strategy for the treatment of moderate-to-severe OSAHS based on significant reductions in the AHI and oxygen desaturation after device implantation in selected patients.[36]

Case 1

Mr. A, a 52-year-old man with chronic depression, managed with a stable dose of a selective serotonin reuptake inhibitor (SSRI), noted gradually worsening fatigue over the past year. On questioning about associated changes in his mood, he reported that he was concerned about his fatigue, and he could not be certain whether it was from his worsening mood, or if the mild worsening in his mood was from the fatigue. He had gained 10 pounds. Although he denied snoring and his wife has not noticed that he had any breathing problems, he had an elevated body mass index (BMI) and hypertension. Since he was at an elevated risk for OSA, a PSG was ordered. The test indicated moderate OSA, and Mr. A agreed to a CPAP trial, but he could not tolerate the mask. After consultation with a sleep physician to discuss alternatives, Mr. A was referred to a dental specialist who fitted an oral appliance. He returned to report that his mood and fatigue were both substantially improved.

Central Disorders of Hypersomnolence

Narcolepsy

Narcolepsy occurs in approximately 0.07% of the general population; it typically arises in the second decade of life. Symptoms usually begin with sleep and are associated with EDS. Cataplexy occurs in approximately 50% of cases with narcolepsy. The probability of developing narcolepsy is 40 times greater if an immediate family member suffers from it.[37] A strong association exists between narcolepsy with cataplexy and the human leukocyte antigen *HLA-DR2* and *DQ1* phenotypes. The most specific antigen associated with narcolepsy with cataplexy in all ethnicities is *HLA-DQB1*0602*.[38] Although 85% or more of patients with narcolepsy with cataplexy have this allele, fewer than half of patients with narcolepsy without cataplexy have it; however, it is non-specific, as it is also found in 25% of healthy controls. Although the exact abnormality of narcolepsy is unknown, leading theories for narcolepsy with cataplexy implicate a loss of neurons that synthesize the neurotransmitter *hypocretin* in the hypothalamus.[39] Also known as orexin, this neurotransmitter is produced in the posterior hypothalamus, has activating projections diffusely throughout the brain, and

inhibits activity in the sleep-inducing ventrolateral pre-optic area (VLPO). Hypocretin deficiency destabilizes sleep-wake partitioning, and in narcolepsy with cataplexy, there is a loss of hypothalamic hypocretin–secreting cells.[40]

Clinical Features

Narcolepsy is a primary hypersomnia associated with a pentad of symptoms:

- *Sleep attacks*: Irresistible and brief sleep episodes that occur several times a day, often at inappropriate times.
- *Cataplexy*: Sudden and brief loss of motor tone without impairment of consciousness, triggered by strong emotions (most often laughter, but also anger or surprise); the motor loss can be global or partial/unilateral.
- *Disturbed night sleep*: Disturbed and fragmented nocturnal sleep characterized by brief nightly awakenings with poor sleep quality.
- *Sleep paralysis*: Brief episodes of muscular paralysis associated with the transitions of sleep-onset or awakening.
- *Hypnagogic* or *hypnopompic hallucinations*: Vivid visual and auditory phenomena that are associated with the transitions to sleep-onset or awakening.

Diagnosis

The diagnosis of narcolepsy is made on the MLST, a series of five scheduled naps with EEG, EOG, and EMG recordings, 2 hours apart during the day, typically following an overnight PSG study. A short average sleep latency (<8 minutes) and two episodes of REM sleep or more during the naps are diagnostic for narcolepsy. However, the MSLT cannot be properly interpreted in the presence of stimulants or REM-suppressing agents, such as antidepressants, which should be discontinued at least 2 weeks before the study, if clinically feasible.

Treatment

General treatment strategies for the management of narcolepsy include patient and family education, counseling regarding good sleep hygiene, scheduled naps, discussion of safety issues (including driving recommendations), and vocational counseling. Medication treatments are aimed at improving wakefulness, reducing cataplexy attacks, and treating the symptoms of disturbed nocturnal sleep, sleep paralysis, and sleep-related hallucinations in narcolepsy.[41] Modafinil, a selective dopamine and norepinephrine reuptake inhibitor, is often used as a first-line therapy for EDS due to its favorable side-effect profile and low potential for abuse. It is typically administered twice daily (100–200 mg) on awakening and in the early afternoon. It is usually well tolerated, and its potential adverse effects include headache, nausea, dry mouth, anorexia, diarrhea, and, rarely, Stevens-Johnson syndrome. Armodafinil, a purified R-isomer of modafinil, requires once-daily dosing (150–250 mg). A traditional stimulant (such as methylphenidate or amphetamine) may be considered if modafinil or armodafinil is ineffective in the management of EDS.[42] Stimulants, including methylphenidate (10–60 mg daily), dextroamphetamine (10–60 mg daily), and amphetamine-dextroamphetamine (10–60 mg daily) can be effective for the treatment of EDS. More significant adverse effects of stimulants include anorexia, weight loss, hypertension, arrhythmias, and psychosis (particularly with the use of high doses). Drug-seeking behavior and addiction can develop, but they are unusual in those taking stimulants to treat narcolepsy. Solriamfetol, a dopamine and norepinephrine reuptake inhibitor, has been FDA-approved at doses of 75 to 150 mg/day for the treatment of EDS in narcolepsy. Common side effects associated with solriamfetol include headache, decreased appetite, nausea, anxiety, insomnia, dry mouth, constipation, palpitations, and dose-dependent increases in blood pressure and heart rate.[41]

Sodium oxybate, the sodium salt of gamma hydroxybutyrate, acts as a $GABA_B$ receptor agonist.[38] Sodium oxybate increases slow-wave sleep, improves sleep continuity, and helps to mitigate EDS and cataplexy. Due to its short half-life, it is administered in two divided doses; the first dose is taken before bedtime, and the second dose is administered 2.5 to 4 hours later.[42] Treatment usually starts at 3 g/night with doses gradually increasing to 4.5 to 9 g/night. Sodium oxybate's side effects include nausea, dizziness, confusion, and urinary incontinence. Occasionally, psychosis may arise, which can limit the use of the drug.[42] Sodium oxybate has respiratory depressant effects and therefore OSAHS can develop or worsen due to its use in a dose-dependent manner. Concomitant use of medications, such as benzodiazepines and opiates, increases the risk of respiratory depression and therefore these drugs should be avoided when using sodium oxybate.[43] Sodium oxybate should be used with caution in patients with heart failure, hypertension, or renal impairment due to its high salt content.[42] In July 2020, the FDA-approved the compound, JZP-258, which is a combination of sodium oxybate, potassium oxybate, calcium oxybate, and magnesium oxybate; it has 92% less sodium than the recommended dosage range of sodium oxybate for narcolepsy.[44] Sodium oxybate is distributed only through a central pharmacy to reduce its potential for abuse; therefore, the rates of diversion are extremely low (1 instance per 5,200 patients treated). The risk of abuse and dependence with the use of sodium oxybate has reportedly been rare (1 case for every 2600 and 6500 patients treated).[45]

Pitolisant is a first-in-class H_3R antagonist/inverse agonist with wake-promoting and anti-cataplectic effects.[41] Pitolisant blocks the inhibitory effect of histamine (or H_3R agonists) on endogenous histamine release and enhances histamine release throughout the central nervous system (CNS).[46] Pitolisant was approved by the FDA for the treatment of EDS in adults with narcolepsy; the recommended dose range is 17.8 to 35.6 mg/day. Its most common side effects include insomnia, headache, nausea, anxiety, irritability, dizziness, depression, tremor, fatigue, vomiting, vertigo, and dyspepsia.[41]

Medications that inhibit norepinephrine or serotonin reuptake have anti-cataplectic effects in the treatment of cataplexy due to their potent REM-suppressant effects. Venlafaxine (75–150 mg daily), a serotonin-norepinephrine reuptake inhibitor, is often used as a first-line treatment for cataplexy. SSRIs, including fluoxetine (20–60 mg) and sertraline (50–150 mg), and tricyclic antidepressants (TCAs), such as clomipramine (75–125 mg) and imipramine (75–125 mg), are also effective in the management of cataplexy. Common antidepressant side effects include nausea, dizziness, dry mouth, headache, insomnia, and sexual dysfunction.[42]

Idiopathic Hypersomnia

Idiopathic hypersomnia may resemble narcolepsy without cataplexy. Patients with this condition may routinely sleep >10 hours per night but remain excessively sleepy. Patients have periods of "sleep drunkenness" on arousal and may experience extreme difficulty waking up with external stimuli, such as an alarm. Patients may have long, non-restorative daytime naps. An MSLT confirms objective sleepiness, but afflicted patients do not have two or more SOREM periods that are typical of narcolepsy. Modafinil has been shown to improve subjective and objective measures of hypersomnolence in patients with idiopathic hypersomnia. Other treatments include the use of traditional stimulants. Treatment of hypersomnia in idiopathic hypersomnia follows the recommendations for narcolepsy, e.g., amphetamine class agents, modafinil, or the related drug armodafinil.

Kleine-Levin syndrome

Kleine-Levin syndrome (KLS) is a rare, often self-limiting condition that is characterized by relapsing-remitting episodes of hypersomnia. Symptoms of KLS include hypersomnia, hyperphagia, hypersexuality, and cognitive, and psychiatric symptoms (mood, anxiety, and psychotic symptoms). Episodes may last from 2 days to 5 weeks and occur at least once every 18 months. Patients with KLS have normal cognition and sleepiness between episodes. KLS often resolves spontaneously by age 30. The exact cause of KLS is unknown, however, it may have a genetic component to its etiology. No medication has been very efficacious for KLS episodes or to prevent its recurrence. Amphetamines or amantadine may be used for acute episodes, whereas lithium, gabapentin, carbamazepine, and valproic acid may be tried for relapse prevention.

Behaviorally Induced Insufficient Sleep Syndrome

Behaviorally induced insufficient sleep syndrome results from voluntary, but unintentional, chronic sleep deprivation. Patients do not appreciate the difference between the actual need for sleep and the amount they obtain. It is characterized by failure to meet the minimum sleep duration requirement necessary to maintain adequate wakefulness thus resulting in daytime hypersomnolence. Prescribing longer periods of sleep reverses its symptoms.

Circadian Rhythm Sleep-Wake Disorders

Circadian rhythm sleep-wake disorders (CRSWDs) emerge when societal expectations conflict with a person's endogenous sleep-wake cycle. Patients who have these disorders might complain of insomnia, hypersomnia, sleepiness, fatigue, or simply that their inherent timing of sleep does not align with social or work demands.

Clinical Features

The CRSWDs include jet lag syndrome, shift-work sleep disorder (SWSD), delayed sleep phase disorder (DSPD), advanced sleep phase disorder (ASPD), and non-24-hour sleep-wake disorder.

Jet lag occurs when a person rapidly crosses several time zones, often from western to eastern time zones. This results in an advancement in the sleep-wake cycle, leaving the person feeling tired earlier in the evening.[47] SWSD occurs when the circadian rhythm conflicts with a work schedule that does not coincide with a conventional day-night cycle. DSPD occurs in persons whose circadian rhythm is set for a later time than the conventional sleep-wake cycle. Considered "night owls," these persons are most alert in the evening and at night and become sleepy several hours after the conventional bedtime. If left undisturbed, these individuals can sleep 7 to 8 hours, with problems arising when they are required to adhere to conventional daytime schedules.

Advanced sleep phase disorder (ASPD) occurs in persons whose circadian rhythm is set for an earlier time than the conventional sleep-wake cycle.[48] Considered "larks," these persons (who are often elderly) are most alert in the early morning, and they become sleepy several hours earlier than the conventional bedtime. Although they sleep for 7 to 8 hours, they might awaken at 2 to 3 a.m. complaining of an inability to stay asleep all night.

The non-24-hour sleep-wake disorder is a phenomenon seen mostly in people who are totally blind and who are unable to perceive visual *zeitgebers*. These patients, who function on a natural circadian rhythm of 24.5 to 25.0 hours, go to sleep and wake up about 45 minutes later each day, and thus are referred to often as the "free running" phenotype.[47] As opposed to persons who follow a conventional sleep-wake schedule, their sleep-wake cycle will literally go "around the clock" in approximately 3 weeks, with increasing sleep complaints (insomnia) and daytime function complaints (fatigue) when their endogenous rhythm is anti-phase with conventional day-night scheduled activities or work.

Diagnosis

Current diagnostic guidelines from the AASM recommend obtaining sleep logs for at least 7 and preferably 14 days, along with actigraphy monitoring for assessment of patients with suspected CRSWDs. Questionnaires such as the Morning-Eveningness Questionnaire (MEQ) can be used to generate a chronotype, which is an individual's preference to be a night owl, early bird, or a neutral type. PSG is not routinely indicated for the diagnosis of CRSWDs but may be indicated to rule out another primary sleep disorder.[47]

Treatment

Optimization of sleep hygiene measures is key to the treatment of all CRSWDs. Oral melatonin can be used to advance or delay the phase of the circadian rhythm, depending on the timing of its administration relative to the position of the biological clock. Phase advance occurs when melatonin is given 2 to 7 hours before the dim light melatonin onset, which typically occurs approximately 2 hours before the onset of sleep. Administration of melatonin in the early morning hours (biological morning) causes a phase delay to occur. Relatively low doses of oral melatonin (0.5 mg) appear to be the most effective for phase-advancing effects. Light administration prevents melatonin release by inhibiting the activation of the pineal gland by the SCN. Depending on the prescribed time of administration and exposure to light therapy, the circadian rhythm can be phase shifted, with varying effects, using proper wavelength, duration, and light intensity.

The AASM Task Force recommendations suggested the use of evening light therapy for ASPD; strategically timed melatonin for DSPD; and light therapy for the treatment of irregular sleep-wake disorder in the elderly with dementia.[49] Tasimelteon, a melatonin receptor agonist (MT1 and MT2), is the only FDA-approved medication for the treatment of non-24-hour sleep-wake disorder that has been shown to improve nighttime sleep and daytime sleepiness.[50] For SWSD, hypnotic medications may be indicated to promote or improve daytime sleep among night-shift workers. Modafinil and armodafinil are both approved by the

FDA for EDS in SWSD. Armodafinil (150 mg), administered at the beginning of a night shift, has improved objective sleepiness and performance, as well as post-shift driving safety in those with SWSD.[51]

Parasomnias

Parasomnias are a group of primary sleep disorders in which abnormal behaviors or physiologic events arise during specific sleep stages or during transitions between wakefulness and sleep. These events occur across a spectrum from mild to bizarre, with clinical implications ranging from annoyance of bed partners to injurious behaviors. Parasomnias are subdivided into NREM arousal disorders, REM sleep disorders, and other parasomnias.

NREM Parasomnia Disorders

NREM parasomnias are noted in individuals with frequent arousals from slow-wave sleep (N3) and the transition from NREM sleep to wakefulness is thought to be compromised in NREM parasomnia disorders.

Clinical Features

In sleepwalking disorder or somnambulism, individuals experience episodic motor behaviors while emerging from delta sleep, most often during the first third of the night. Some arousal disorder behaviors are simple (e.g., walking, sitting up in bed, or picking at bed sheets), but more complex and serious behaviors can occur (e.g., running, eating, driving, or committing violent attacks).[52] Affected individuals are often unresponsive to efforts to wake them, confused and disoriented when awakened, and amnestic to the sleep-related event the next day. Sleepwalking is not uncommon in childhood; it is rare in adulthood, a fact that should prompt a search for a possible underlying medical, neurologic, or iatrogenic etiology.

As with sleepwalking disorder, sleep terrors occur during partial arousal from delta sleep, usually during the first third of the night. As in sleepwalking disorder, patients are difficult to awaken, they lack dream recall, and they are amnestic for the episodes. Caretakers are often bothered more by this disorder than are the patients. Symptoms include repeated awakenings followed by intense fear, screaming, flailing, and autonomic hyperarousal (e.g., tachycardia, tachypnea, and mydriasis). In adults, this disorder is associated with post-traumatic stress disorder (PTSD), generalized anxiety disorder (GAD), and borderline personality disorder. Confusional arousals, also known as sleep drunkenness, occur when persons are awakened from delta sleep, from a nap, or are induced to wake in the morning. They are characterized by disorientation, amnesia, and occasionally by violent or sexual behavior.

Diagnosis

An overnight video-PSG should be considered when the details of nocturnal events are not available if an atypical history is provided, and there is a concern for a primary sleep disorder or seizure activity.[53] In addition, dangerous behaviors in children or adults and de-novo NREM parasomnia episodes in adults warrant an overnight video-PSG. A typical nocturnal episode may not be captured during the overnight study; however, features suggestive of NREM instability, such as frequent arousals from N3 sleep, may be seen. In addition, the PSG can be used to rule out primary sleep disorders that increase sleep fragmentation and the use of an extended EEG and EMG channels can help to rule out seizure activity and REM parasomnia disorders.[53]

Treatment

Prevention of injury is the primary focus of treatment for NREM parasomnias, therefore, modifying the sleep environment is the initial and most important step in preventing sleep-related injuries. Factors that increase arousal during sleep and predispose to NREM parasomnias should be identified and optimally addressed. Sleep deprivation and irregular sleep-wake cycles should be avoided. Discontinuation of medications (e.g., hypnotics, antidepressants, atypical antipsychotics) that trigger parasomnias are advised to treat iatrogenic NREM parasomnias. Co-morbid sleep disorders, including OSAHS and restless legs syndrome (RLS), should be addressed for optimal outcomes.[53] Allowing enough time for disorientation to wear off is usually sufficient treatment for confusional arousals. In terms of medication management, clonazepam is a typical first-line pharmacological treatment for sleepwalking and sleep terrors. Clonazepam has been effective with long-term use without a dose escalation for the treatment of NREM

parasomnias. In addition to clonazepam, topiramate has helped with sleep-related eating.

REM Parasomnia Disorders

The hallmarks of this group of parasomnias are the occurrence in REM sleep, dreaming, and awareness of specific events. The most commonly encountered REM sleep disorders are nightmare disorder and REM sleep behavior disorder.

Nightmare Disorder

The essential feature of *nightmare disorder* is repeated episodes of terrifying dreams that awaken the patient. In contrast to patients with sleep terror disorder, patients with nightmare disorder often have vivid recall of the events, are atonic during the experience, lack autonomic arousal, and experience the events in the latter half of the night (when REM sleep is the longest and most dense). Prazosin, a centrally acting alpha$_1$-adrenergic receptor antagonist, is considered the first-line treatment for PTSD-associated nightmares. Prazosin (1–10 mg at bedtime) has been beneficial, and it is generally well tolerated; however, clinicians should monitor their patients for orthostatic hypotension. Placebo-controlled studies of prazosin have reported positive effects on nightmares, in both military and civilian samples.[54] Among cognitive-behavioral approaches, image rehearsal therapy (IRT) is a brief, effective, well-tolerated treatment for chronic nightmares. IRT is a modified CBT technique that utilizes recalling the nightmare, writing it down, changing the theme as well as its storyline and ending (or any part of the dream to a more positive one), and rehearsing the re-written dream scenario so that the patient can displace the unwanted content when the dream recurs. IRT provides a cognitive shift that empirically refutes the original premise of the nightmare and acts to inhibit the original nightmare. This technique is practiced for 10 to 20 minutes per day while awake.[55]

REM Sleep Behavior Disorder

REM sleep behavior disorder (RBD) presents as a dream enactment that ranges from simple to quite complex behaviors while asleep, including jumping out of bed, walking, or running.[56] RBD events are typically accompanied by vivid dream recall. Patients with RBD lack the muscle atonia that normally accompanies REM sleep; this results in the acting out of dream content.[57] The disorder often occurs in isolation, but longitudinal studies suggest that well over half of affected individuals will develop parkinsonian syndrome over subsequent decades of life. RBD is also seen with other underlying neurologic processes, such as vascular dementia and Alzheimer dementia (AD), as well as focal brainstem lesions of any cause. It is more common in the elderly, and it affects males nine times more frequently than females.

Treatment of RBD is important to reduce the risk of injury to patients and their bed partners. General recommendations include modification of the sleep environment to ensure safety; measures include lowering the bed mattress to the floor, padding any sharp bedside furniture surfaces, and removing firearms from the bedroom environment. Separate bedrooms may be necessary to prevent injuries to bed partners. Medications including antidepressants, beta-blockers, or tramadol, that may worsen the frequency and severity of RBD, should be either discontinued or reduced, when feasible. Alcohol abuse and withdrawal have been associated with RBD and the patients should be counseled about their use of alcohol.[55] Per the AASM Task Force recommendations, clonazepam (0.5–2 mg) is suggested for the treatment of RBD, but it should be used with caution in patients with dementia, gait disorders, or concomitant OSAHS. In addition, melatonin (3–12 mg) is suggested for treatment for RBD with the advantage of a better side effect profile.

Sleep-Related Movement Disorders

Restless Legs Syndrome. Restless legs syndrome (RLS) is characterized by intense aching or crawling sensations inside the legs and calves that occur while sitting or lying down; it causes an urge to move or rub the legs. Symptoms are typically worse at bedtime (or during the day at rest, such as in a car), and are relieved or improved by movement. For some, the symptoms interrupt sleep because the patient may repeatedly get out of bed to walk or stretch. RLS is associated with various medical problems, especially kidney failure, diabetes, iron-deficiency anemia, and peripheral nerve injury, as well as with the use of medications, particularly SSRIs and neuroleptics.

In many instances, symptoms are mild and sufficiently self-limited to require no treatment. In the cases where an etiologic factor is identified (e.g., iron deficiency), treatment should be directed at its correction. Oral or intravenous (IV) iron repletion may be beneficial for those in whom the serum ferritin is <75 g/L. Avoidance of alcohol and caffeine and the performance of moderate exercise can also be helpful. When RLS is caused by antidepressants or by the taper of opiates, switching to another antidepressant or revising a tapering schedule of opiates can be useful. Acupuncture may also be helpful.

RLS with mild symptoms are usually managed effectively by alpha$_2$ delta ligand medications (e.g., gabapentin, pregabalin), while moderate or severe symptoms may instead require dopaminergic therapy or consideration of an opioid medication.[58] Gabapentin enacarbil is FDA-approved for the treatment of RLS at a dose of 600 mg in the early evening. Dopamine agonists (including pramipexole, ropinirole, and rotigotine) have been the mainstays of therapy for RLS.[58] Pramipexole, starting at 0.125 mg orally may then be further titrated by 0.125 mg every 3 to 7 days toward a target dose in the range of 0.375 to 0.5 mg daily. Ropinirole, starting at 0.25 mg PO HS and titrating it at weekly intervals by 0.25 to 0.5 mg increments up to the maximum recommended dose of 4 mg/day, is an effective alternative. The rotigotine patch can provide daylong symptomatic control for RLS; given its prolonged duration of action and more continual release of dopamine into the bloodstream, it may minimize dopamine fluctuations at receptors and may be associated with a lower risk of augmentation syndrome.[59] Rotigotine may be started using a 1.0 mg patch strength and then titrated weekly to either a 2 or 3 mg maximal daily dose. Although effective, dopamine agonists have a high rate of discontinuation (up to 25%) not only due to inadequate response or bothersome side effects but also because of augmentation of symptoms (e.g., onset of symptoms earlier in the day with greater severity and possibly spread to the upper extremities). Impulse control disorders (e.g., compulsive shopping, gambling, eating, and hypersexuality) may occur, mainly in those with an underlying neurodegenerative disorder and/or with the use of higher doses. Patients should be cautioned about driving, as sudden sleep attacks have been reported by patients taking pramipexole or ropinirole.[58]

Opioids are used in the treatment of refractory or incapacitating RLS that fails to respond to other therapeutic modalities, but opiate dependence is a concern and the evidence for efficacy is based mostly on clinical experience rather than on controlled studies. Low-dose opioids (e.g., tramadol [50–200 mg], oxycodone [5–20 mg], and methadone [5–10 mg]) can be used in the treatment of refractory RLS or severe augmentation that fails to respond to other therapeutic modalities, but careful attention to the risks of misuse or abuse is required. In addition, these agents are associated with constipation, sedation, and, at higher doses, respiratory suppression.[58]

Periodic Limb Movement Disorder

Periodic limb movements of sleep (PLMS), sometimes called *nocturnal myoclonus*, is a common finding in up to 40% of people >65 years of age and in 11% of patients referred to sleep disorder clinics who complain of insomnia.[60] PLMS manifests as brief (0.5–5.0 seconds), stereotypic, and involuntary contractions of the lower limbs (often the dorsiflexion of the ankle), at intervals of 20 to 40 seconds. Contractions appear more commonly during NREM stages 1 and 2. Although patients are typically unaware of them, the EEG may demonstrate nocturnal arousals and actual awakenings. Sleep is often unrefreshing, with hypersomnia being the most common complaint. When no other cause of sleep-related symptoms is present, besides the PSG-based finding of an elevated level of PLMS, then the diagnosis of periodic limb movement disorder (PLMD) can be made.

The diagnosis is made by an overnight PSG and is confirmed when the *myoclonus index* (the number of leg jerks per hour of sleep) reaches ≥15. Although the pathogenesis of PLMD is unknown, it is associated with a variety of medical conditions (e.g., renal failure, diabetes, chronic anemia, peripheral nerve injuries, and even uncomplicated pregnancy). Medications (including antidepressants, neuroleptics, lithium, and diuretics) and narcotic withdrawal may induce or worsen PLMS. Treatment is symptomatic and includes the use of dopaminergic facilitating agents (e.g., pramipexole, ropinirole), and in severe or refractory cases, the use of benzodiazepines can be considered.

Case 2

Ms. B, a 45-year-old woman with GAD and mild obsessive-compulsive disorder, managed with an SSRI as well as a *pro re nata* (PRN) benzodiazepine, also has chronic insomnia and has noted that poor sleep can worsen her psychiatric symptoms; however, when her anxiety is elevated, her sleep is adversely impacted. Because of her prominent sleep symptoms, she had aggressive pharmacologic trials to control the insomnia, but Ms. B has been refractory to multiple hypnotic trials. Although CBT-I is the gold standard for chronic insomnia, there were no specialist providers near her home. And, although a PSG is not routinely indicated for insomnia, her chronic and refractory nature prompted you to discuss such testing with her, and she agreed. The PSG found that she had a combination of sleep-wake state misperception and an elevated PLMS. Although initially skeptical about the misperception finding, she was somewhat reassured by it. The growing number of validated online CBT-I options was reviewed with her, and she agreed to try them. Since relative iron deficiency (based on a ferritin level of 23) can be problematic, you recommended iron supplementation, as well as moving her SSRI to the morning instead of night-time dosing to help reduce her leg movements. These interventions improved the proportion of "good nights," and she avoided further hypnotic use.

Sleep and Psychiatric Disorders

Major Depressive Disorder. Sleep disturbances occur in up to 60% of outpatients and 90% of inpatients with major depressive disorder (MDD). Consequently, more is known about sleep disturbances in depressed patients than in any other psychiatric illness. Most patients with MDD complain of initial, middle, and terminal insomnia and early morning awakening; in addition, they experience restlessness and fatigue. Hypersomnia and neurovegetative reversal, however, tend to occur in atypical depression. A PSG is not recommended for the evaluation of sleep in MDD per se, except to the extent that a co-morbid sleep disorder of relevance may be diagnosed, such as OSA or PLMD. The objective PSG findings in MDD may show prolonged sleep latency, a decrease in delta sleep, a decreased delta sleep ratio, decreased REM latency, and increased duration and density of the first REM period. Evidence suggests that these abnormalities can persist after remission of MDD and that they precede the onset of another episode. In addition, some studies suggest that decreased REM latency or decreased delta sleep can predict relapse in depressed patients.[61]

Bipolar Disorder. Sleep disturbances are the most common prodrome of mania and can precede the onset of depressive episodes in patients with bipolar disorder (BPD). In addition, variability in sleep-wake cycles, insomnia, and hypersomnia have been reported between mood episodes in patients with BPD. During manic episodes, approximately 69% to 99% of patients report having sleep disturbances, including a decreased need for sleep and insomnia symptoms (including trouble falling asleep, sleep fragmentation, and waking up several hours before their preferred wake-up time). Findings on the PSG in patients with mania show a shorter REM latency, an increased REM density, and a decreased TST. Depressive episodes in BPD may be characterized by insomnia or hypersomnia with PSG findings suggesting reduced REM latency. As compared to healthy controls, patients with BPD have an increased likelihood of circadian rhythm abnormalities, such as lower levels and delayed onset of peaks of melatonin, and having an evening chronotype with a preference for functioning at night rather than during the day. Treatments for BPD, such as lithium and bright light therapy are known to alter circadian rhythms.[62]

Psychotic Spectrum Disorders. Sleep is usually markedly impaired with the onset of psychotic symptoms and with each subsequent relapse in patients with schizophrenia. Patients usually experience prolonged periods of total sleeplessness when experiencing severe psychotic agitation and pronounced insomnia during states of less severe psychotic agitation. Recurrence or exacerbation of psychotic symptoms is often preceded by increasing insomnia. Subjective sleep complaints, particularly early and middle insomnia, are common in clinically stable patients with schizophrenia who are taking medications. Patients with schizophrenia also complain of poor sleep quality, which is predictive of self-assessed poor quality of life and impaired coping skills. The PSG findings in patients with schizophrenia include poor sleep efficiency, abnormally short REM sleep latency, and slow-wave sleep deficits. Because many of the medications used for treating psychosis can cause similar disruptions in sleep architecture, medication side effects must be ruled out. Current evidence suggests, however, that many of these sleep abnormalities, particularly delta sleep deficits, are the function of a psychotic disorder rather than the result of medication use.[63]

Anxiety Disorders. GAD and insomnia are highly overlapping and co-morbid disorders. Difficulty initiating or maintaining sleep, or sleep that is restless and unsatisfying, is one of the features needed to establish the diagnosis of GAD. The differentiating feature between GAD and insomnia disorder may be the foci of worry at night as the foci of worry in insomnia disorder are insomnia itself, whereas the worry is focused on the multiple themes that are also preoccupations during the day (such as career, finances, relationships, finances). As compared to controls, patients with GAD have an increased sleep latency, an increased WASO time, lower sleep efficiency, and decreased TST based on PSG data. Importantly, reduced REM latency, as noted in patients with MDD, is not noted in non-depressed patients with GAD. Patients suffering from panic disorder can experience attacks during sleep, usually during the transition from NREM Stage 2 sleep and early delta sleep.[64]

Post-traumatic Stress Disorder. Sleep findings in those with PTSD often include heightened arousal, insomnia, nightmares (re-experiencing phenomenon), and increased sleep-related movements.[65] Insomnia complaints are very common symptoms of PTSD; however, nightmares are more specific to the disorder. It has been suggested that the severity of the sleep complaints mediates the association between PTSD and functional disability. PSG findings in PTSD patients include increased N1 sleep, decreased slow-wave sleep, increased REM density, and increased REM fragmentation. In addition, TST is often reduced owing to recurrent awakenings and impaired sleep maintenance. Evidence suggests that there is an increased sympathetic activation during REM sleep that may contribute to the development of PTSD. On the other hand, psychological treatments that focus on sleep impairments in PTSD can yield strong therapeutic effects across the full spectrum of PTSD symptoms.

Substance Use Disorders. Substances, whether prescribed or illicit, can have profound effects on sleep. These effects can arise during regular use, acute ingestion, or withdrawal and can masquerade as any primary sleep disorder. In general, if the substance is a CNS depressant, intoxication results in sedation and withdrawal results in insomnia. Similarly, if the substance is a CNS stimulant, intoxication results in insomnia, and withdrawal results in sedation. Diagnosis of these disorders can only be made if the sleep disturbance is severe enough to warrant independent clinical attention, it is caused by the direct physiologic effects of a substance, if it developed during or within a month of intoxication or withdrawal from the substance, and if it is not the result of a mental disorder or delirium. Once a substance-related sleep disorder is suspected, a thorough substance-abuse history must be obtained to identify the offending substance. Treatment consists of judicious discontinuation of the substance, management of any acute withdrawal, and treatment of any underlying co-morbid psychiatric disorders.

Alcohol is perhaps the most commonly used sleep aid, but its soporific value is limited by significant side effects, including dependence, addiction, and withdrawal. Its effects on sleep are well documented and depend on the pattern of use and the state of intoxication or withdrawal. During acute intoxication, alcohol alters sleep architecture by decreasing sleep latency, increasing delta sleep, and decreasing REM sleep for the first 3 to 4 hours of sleep. In the last 2 to 3 hours of sleep, wakefulness and REM are increased. OSA may be exacerbated by alcohol consumption. During acute withdrawal, however, its effects on sleep architecture are reversed; initial insomnia, decreased delta sleep, short REM latency, an increased percentage of REM sleep, decreased TST, and decreased SE all develop. Each of these features may be a contributing factor to alcohol relapse in dependent patients.[66] For individuals recovering from alcohol use disorder (AUD), insomnia, poor sleep continuity, and decreased delta sleep can persist for several years after detoxification.[67] The definitive treatment for alcohol-related sleep complaints is detoxification and abstinence, in addition to treatment of co-morbid psychiatric conditions. Benzodiazepines, hypnotics, and sedating antidepressants should, in general, be avoided due to cross-tolerance, risk of AUD relapse, and synergistic sedative effects that can lead to CNS depression, should the patient relapse.

The effects of non-alcoholic substances on sleep are not as well established as are the effects of alcohol. In general, intoxication with either amphetamine or cocaine prolongs sleep latency, decreases the amount of REM sleep, disrupts sleep continuity, and shortens TST. During the first week of withdrawal from these substances, patients often experience hypersomnia (a "crash") and excessive REM sleep, followed perhaps by several days of insomnia.[68]

Opioids are also known to increase sleep and reduce REM sleep, with rebound insomnia occurring on their discontinuation. Chronic opiate use has been associated with central sleep apnea syndrome (CSA) which appears to be associated with the effects of opioids on the respiratory rhythm generators in the medulla. Opioids affect respiration during sleep by decreasing central respiratory control sensitivity to hypercapnia and decreasing peripheral sensitivity to hypoxemia, leading to unstable ventilation and recurrent CSA. Patients having CSA co-morbid with opioid use suffer from sleep fragmentation, hypoxemia, and hypercapnia during sleep. The risk factors for the development of CSA co-morbid with opioid use, include morphine equivalent dose (MED) >200 mg, low or normal BMI, and concurrent use of benzodiazepines or hypnotics.[69] A dose-dependent relationship between the opioid dose and central apneas has been reported, such that with each 100 mg MED, the rate of central apneas has increased by 29.2%.[70]

Psychotropic Medications and Sleep

Sedative-hypnotics. Sedative-hypnotics, particularly BzRAs, shorten sleep latency, increase stage N2 sleep, and decrease REM sleep. Concerns regarding BzRA use include rebound insomnia and tolerance Rebound insomnia is observed, at times, during abrupt discontinuation, particularly from shorter-acting drugs, and refers to an increase in sleep symptoms beyond baseline levels. Early studies have suggested a lower potential for rebound insomnia with non-benzodiazepine drugs compared to benzodiazepines; however, it can occur with both.[71] Strategies including prior CBT-I and gradual dose reduction over weeks-months of BzRAs may reduce the risk of rebound insomnia.

Antidepressants. SSRIs are the most prescribed antidepressant medications. SSRIs can produce arousal and insomnia in some patients and sedation in others with MDD. The effects of SSRIs on sleep architecture include decreased REM latency, sleep, and REM sleep. The mechanism of action of SSRIs and other antidepressants' REM suppression is believed to be related to the reversal of monoaminergic-cholinergic imbalance characteristic of MDD. REM sleep onset is associated with a decline in monoaminergic activity and an increase in cholinergic activity; this explains REM disinhibition in MDD which is characterized by decreased REM latency, increased REM density, and increased REM sleep. Sedating antidepressants, such as trazodone and mirtazapine, have been associated with an increase in slow-wave sleep due to 5-HT$_{2A/C}$ receptor antagonism. Antidepressants can also cause or worsen primary sleep disorders, including RLS, sleepwalking, sleep-related eating, and RBD.[72]

Mood Stabilizers. The effects of lithium carbonate on sleep architecture in depressed individuals include increased SWS, decreased REM sleep, and increased REM latency. Plasma lithium levels have been negatively correlated with REM sleep percentage and positively correlated with REM sleep latency. In addition, evidence suggests that lithium affects cellular circadian rhythms and increases morningness behaviors in those with BPD, changes that may contribute to the therapeutic effects of lithium.[73]

Antipsychotic Medications. Like antidepressants, antipsychotics can lead to both activating and sedating effects. Based on PSG data, clozapine, olanzapine, quetiapine, and ziprasidone increase TST and/or SE in healthy individuals. Olanzapine and ziprasidone can augment SWS, while changes corresponding to REM sleep have been inconsistent. Furthermore, administration of clozapine, olanzapine, and paliperidone to patients with schizophrenia has been associated with a significant reduction of sleep latency and an increased TST and SE. In addition, olanzapine and paliperidone augmented SWS and REM sleep.[74] Antipsychotic medication use has been associated with causation or worsening primary sleep disorders including RLS and NREM parasomnias

(e.g., sleepwalking, sleep-related eating disorder), and worsening of OSAHS due to weight gain side effects.

REFERENCES

1. Aserinsky E, Kleitman N. Regularly occurring periods of eye motility and concomitant phenomena during sleep. *Science.* 1953;118(3062):273–274.
2. Williams RL, Gokcebay N, Hirshkowitz M, et al. Ontogeny of sleep. In: Cooper R, ed. *Sleep.* Chapman and Hall Medical; 1994:60–75.
3. Culebras A. Update on disorders of sleep and the sleep–wake cycle. *Psychiatric Clin North Am.* 1992;15(2):467–489.
4. Barion A, Zee PC. A clinical approach to circadian rhythm sleep disorders. *Sleep Med.* 2007;8(6):566–577.
5. King DP, Takahashi JS. Molecular genetics of circadian rhythms in mammals. *Annu Rev Neurosci.* 2000;23:713–743.
6. Landolt HP. Sleep homeostasis: a role for adenosine in humans? *Biochem Pharmacol.* 2008;75(1):2070–2079.
7. Carskadon MA, Roth T. Normal sleep and its variations. In: Kryger MH, Roth T, Dement WC, eds. *Principles and Practice of Sleep Medicine.* 2nd ed. WB Saunders; 1994:3–15.
8. Silber MH, Ancoli-Israel S, Bonnet MH, et al. The visual scoring of sleep in adults. *J Clin Sleep Med.* 2007;3(2):121–131.
9. Manis E, Shelgikar AV. Clinical applications of technical procedures in sleep medicine. In: Chopra *Management of Sleep Disorders in Psychiatry.* Oxford University Press; 2020.
10. Collop NA, Anderson WM, Boehlecke B, et al. Clinical guidelines for the use of unattended portable monitors in the diagnosis of obstructive sleep apnea in adult patients. Portable Monitoring Task Force of the American Academy of Sleep Medicine. *J Clin Sleep Med.* 2007;3(7):737–747.
11. Ashbrook L, During EH. Sleep and movement disorders. In: Miglis M, ed. *Sleep and Neurologic Disease.* 1st ed. Elsevier; 2017:89–113. (Table 5.1).
12. Johns MW. A new method for measuring daytime sleepiness: the Epworth Sleepiness Scale. *Sleep.* 1991;14(6):540–545.
13. Guilleminault C. Clinical features and evaluation of obstructive sleep apnea. In: Kryger MH, Roth T, Dement WC, eds. *Principles and Practice of Sleep Medicine.* 2nd ed. WB Saunders; 1994: 667–678.
14. American Psychiatric Association Diagnostic and Statistical Manual of Mental Disorders. 5th ed. American Psychiatric Association Publishing; 2004.
15. American Academy of Sleep Medicine International Classification of Sleep Disorders: Diagnostic and Coding Manual. 3rd ed. American Academy of Sleep Medicine; 2005.
16. Nofzinger EA, Buysse DJ, Germain A, et al. Functional neuroimaging evidence for hyperarousal in insomnia. *Am J Psychiatry.* 2004;161:2126–2128.
17. Buysse DJ, Germian A, Moul DE, et al. Efficacy of brief behavioral treatment for chronic insomnia in older adults. *Arch Intern Med.* 2011;171(10):887–895.
18. Mitchell MD, Gehrman P, Perlis M, et al. Comparative effectiveness of cognitive behavioral therapy for insomnia: a systematic review. *BMC Fam Pract.* 2012;13:40.

19. Buysse DJ. Insomnia. *JAMA*. 2013;309(7):706–716.

20. Morin CM, Bastien C, Guay B, et al. Randomized clinical trial of supervised tapering and cognitive behavior therapy to facilitate benzodiazepine discontinuation in older adults with chronic insomnia. *Am J Psychiatry*. 2004;161(2):332–342.

21. Boyle N, Naganathan V, Cumming RG. Medication and falls: risk and optimization. *Clin Geriatr Med*. 2010;26(4):583–605.

22. Bateson AN. The benzodiazepine site of the GABAA receptor: an old target with new potential? *Sleep Med*. 2004;5(suppl 1):S9–15.

23. Walsh JK, Krystal A, Amato D, et al. Nightly treatment of primary insomnia with eszopiclone for six months: effect on sleep, quality of life, and work limitations. *Sleep*. 2007;30(8):959–968.

24. Krystal AD, Erman M, Zammit G, et al. Long-term efficacy and safety of zolpidem extended-release 12.5 mg, administered 3 to 7 nights per week for 24 weeks, in patients with chronic primary insomnia: a 6-month, randomized, double-blind, placebo-controlled, parallel-group, multicenter study. *Sleep*. 2008;31(1):79–90.

25. Hajak G, Müller WE, Wittchen HU, et al. Abuse and dependence potential for the non-benzodiazepine hypnotics zolpidem and zopiclone: a review of case reports and epidemiological data. *Addiction*. 2003;98(10):1371–1378.

26. Sateia MJ, Buysse DJ, Krystal AD, et al. Clinical Practice Guideline for the Pharmacologic Treatment of Chronic Insomnia in Adults: an American Academy of Sleep Medicine Clinical Practice Guideline. *J Clin Sleep Med*. 2017;13(2):307–349.

27. Muehlan C, Vaillant C, Zenklusen I, et al. Clinical pharmacology, efficacy, and safety of orexin receptor antagonists for the treatment of insomnia disorders. *Expert Opin Drug Metab Toxicol*. 2020;16(11):1063–1078.

28. Doghramji K, et al. Pharmacological management of insomnia. In: Chopra A, ed. *Management of Sleep Disorders in Psychiatry*. Oxford University Press; 2020.

29. Krystal AD, Lankford A, Durrence HH, et al. Efficacy and safety of doxepin 3 and 6 mg in a 35-day sleep laboratory trial in adults with chronic primary insomnia. *Sleep*. 2011;34(10):1433–1442.

30. Walsh JK. Drugs used to treat insomnia in 2002: regulatory-based rather than evidence-based medicine. *Sleep*. 2004;27(8):1441–1442.

31. Basu R, Dodge H, Stoehr GP, et al. Sedative-hypnotic use of diphenhydramine in a rural, older adult, community-based cohort: effects on cognition. *Am J Geriatr Psychiatry*. 2003;11(2):205–213.

32. Richardson GS, Roehrs TA, Rosenthal L, et al. Tolerance to daytime sedative effects of H1 antihistamines. *J Clin Psychopharmacol*. 2002;22(5):511–515.

33. Partinen M, Telakivi T. Epidemiology of obstructive sleep apnea syndrome. *Sleep*. 1992;15:S1S4.

34. Jordan AS, McSharry DG, Malhotra A. Adult obstructive sleep apnoea. *Lancet*. 2014;383(9918):736–747.

35. Marien H, Rodenstein D. Morbid obesity and sleep apnea. Is weight loss the answer? *J Clin Sleep Med*. 2008;4(4):339–340.

36. Strollo Jr PJ, Soose RJ, Maurer JT, et al. Upper-airway stimulation for obstructive sleep apnea. *N Engl J Med*. 2014;370(2):139–149.

37. Mignot E, Wang C, Rattazzi C, et al. Genetic linkage of autosomal recessive canine narcolepsy with a mu immunoglobulin heavy-chain switch-like segment. *Proc Natl Acad Sci USA*. 1991;88:3475–3478.

38. Khan Z, Trotti LM. Central disorders of hypersomnolence: focus on narcolepsies and idiopathic hypersomnia. *Chest*. 2015;148(1):262–273.

39. Krahn LE, Black JL, Silber MH. Narcolepsy: new understanding of irresistible sleep. *Mayo Clin Proc*. 2001;76(2):185–194.

40. Thannickal T, Moore RY, Nienhuis R, et al. Reduced number of hypocretin neurons in human narcolepsy. *Neuron*. 2000;27:469–474.

41. Thorpy MJ. Recently approved and upcoming treatments for narcolepsy. *CNS Drugs*. 2020;34(1):9–27.

42. Golden EC, Lipford MC. Narcolepsy: Diagnosis and management. *Cleve Clin J Med*. 2018;85(12):959–969.

43. Alhifzi S, Zaki N, Almeneesier AS, et al. Hypersomnolence disorders. In: Chopra A, ed. *Management of Sleep Disorders in Psychiatry*. Oxford University Press; 2020.

44. Bogan RK, Thorpy MJ, Dauvilliers Y, et al. Efficacy and safety of calcium, magnesium, potassium, and sodium oxybates (lower-sodium oxybate [LXB]; JZP-258) in a placebo-controlled, double-blind, randomized withdrawal study in adults with narcolepsy with cataplexy. *Sleep*. 2021;44(3).

45. Wang YG, Swick TJ, Carter LP, et al. Safety overview of postmarketing and clinical experience of sodium oxybate (Xyrem): abuse, misuse, dependence, and diversion. *J Clin Sleep Med*. 2009;5(4):365–371.

46. Schwartz JC. The histamine H3 receptor: from discovery to clinical trials with pitolisant. *Br J Pharmacol*. 2011;163(4):713–721.

47. Morganthaler TI, Lee-Chiong T, Alessi C, et al. Practice parameters for the clinical evaluation and treatment of circadian rhythm sleep disorders. American Academy of Sleep Medicine Report. *Sleep*. 2007;30(11):1445–1459.

48. Richardson GS. Circadian rhythms and aging. *Biol Aging*. 1990;13:275–305.

49. Auger RR, Burgess HJ, Emens JS, et al. Clinical Practice Guideline for the Treatment of Intrinsic Circadian Rhythm Sleep-Wake Disorders: Advanced Sleep-Wake Phase Disorder (ASWPD), Delayed Sleep-Wake Phase Disorder (DSWPD), Non-24-Hour Sleep-Wake Rhythm Disorder (N24SWD), and Irregular Sleep-Wake Rhythm Disorder (ISWRD). An Update for 2015: an American Academy of Sleep Medicine Clinical Practice Guideline. *J Clin Sleep Med*. 2015;11(10):1199–1236.

50. Lockley SW, Dressman MA, Licamele L, et al. Tasimelteon for non-24-hour sleep-wake disorder in totally blind people (SET and RESET): two multicentre, randomised, double-masked, placebo-controlled phase 3 trials. *Lancet*. 2015;386(10005):1754–1764.

51. Howard R, Roth T, Drake CL. The effects of armodafinil on objective sleepiness and performance in a shift work disorder sample unselected for objective sleepiness. *J Clin Psychopharmacol*. 2014;34(3):369–373.

52. Ebrahim IO. The nonrapid eye movement parasomnias: recent advances and forensic aspects. *Curr Opin Pulm Med*. 2013;19(6):609–615.

53. Jung J, Louis EKS. Parasomnias. In: Chopra A, ed. *Management of Sleep Disorders in Psychiatry*. Oxford University Press; 2020.

54. Raskind MA, Peskind ER, Hoff DJ, et al. A parallel group placebo-controlled study of prazosin for trauma nightmares and sleep disturbance in combat veterans with post-traumatic stress disorder. *Biol Psychiatry*. 2007;61(8):928–934.

55. Aurora RN, Zak RS, Maganti RK, et al. Best practice guide for the treatment of REM sleep behavior disorder (RBD). *J Clin Sleep Med*. 2010;6(1):85–95.

56. Schenck CH, Mahowald MW. REM sleep behavior disorder: clinical, developmental, and neuroscience perspectives 16 years after its formal identification in SLEEP. *Sleep*. 2002;25(2):120–138.

57. Gagnon JF, Postuma RD, Mazza S, et al. Rapid eye movement sleep behavior disorder and neurodegenerative disorders. *Lancet Neurol*. 2006;5(5):424–432.

58. Gossard TR, Trotti LM, Videnovic A, et al. Restless legs syndrome: contemporary diagnosis and treatment. *Neurotherapeutics*. 2021;18(1):140–155.

59. Garcia-Borreguero D, Allen R, Hudson J, et al. Effects of rotigotine on daytime symptoms in patients with primary restless legs syndrome: a randomized, placebo-controlled study. *Curr Med Res Opin*. 2016;32(1):77–85.

60. Allen RP. Restless legs syndrome/Willis Ekbom disease: evaluation and treatment. *Int Rev Psychiatry*. 2014;26(2):248–262.

61. Giles DE, Jarrett RB, Roffwarg HP. Reduced REM latency: a predictor of recurrence in depression. *Neuropsychopharmacology*. 1988;1:33–39.

62. Plante DT, Winkelman JW. Sleep disturbance in bipolar disorder: therapeutic implications. *Am J Psychiatry*. 2008;165(7):830–843.

63. Keshavan MS, Matcheri S, Reynolds III CF, et al. Delta sleep deficits in schizophrenia: evidence from automated analyses of sleep data. *Arch Gen Psychiatry*. 1998;55:443–448.

64. Uhde TH. The anxiety disorders. In: Kryger MH, Roth T, Dement WC, eds. *Principles and Practice of Sleep Medicine*. 2nd ed. WB Saunders; 1994:871–898.

65. Mellman TA, Kulick-Bell R, Ashlock LE, et al. Sleep events among veterans with combat-related posttraumatic stress disorder. *Am J Psychiatry*. 1995;152:110–115.

66. Brower KJ. Alcohol's effects on sleep in alcoholics. *Alcohol Res Health*. 2001;25(2):110–125.

67. Landolt HP, Gillin JC. Sleep abnormalities during abstinence in alcohol-dependent patients: aetiology and management. *CNS Drugs*. 2001;15(5):413–425.

68. Watson R, Bakos L, Compton P, et al. Cocaine use and withdrawal: the effect on sleep and mood. *J Drug Alcohol Abuse*. 1992;18:21–28.

69. Sinha S, Kolla BP, Mansukhani MP. Substance use disorders. In: Chopra A, ed. *Management of Sleep Disorders in Psychiatry*. Oxford University Press; 2020.

70. Walker JM, Farney RJ, Rhondeau SM, et al. Chronic opioid use is a risk factor for the development of central sleep apnea and ataxic breathing. *J Clin Sleep Med*. 2007;3(5):455–461.

71. Licata SC, Rowlett JK. Abuse and dependence liability of benzodiazepine-type drugs: GABA(A) receptor modulation and beyond. *Pharmacol Biochem Behav*. 2008;90(1):74–89.

72. Sharpley AL, Cowen PJ. Effect of pharmacologic treatments on the sleep of depressed patients. *Biol Psychiatry*. 1995;37(2):85–98.

73. Rohr KE, McCarthy MJ. The impact of lithium on circadian rhythms and implications for bipolar disorder pharmacotherapy. *Neurosci Lett*. 2022;786:136772.

74. Monti JM, Torterolo P, Pandi Perumal SR. The effects of second-generation antipsychotic drugs on sleep variables in healthy subjects and patients with schizophrenia. *Sleep Med Rev*. 2017;33:51–57.

23

SEXUAL DISORDERS AND SEXUAL DYSFUNCTION

LINDA C. SHAFER, MD

OVERVIEW

A comprehensive psychiatric evaluation of any patient in the general hospital setting should include close attention to complaints, impairments, and deviations of sexual function. Although on occasion, sexual problems are the primary reason for consultation, more often they may provide important clues about an underlying medical or psychological condition. Consider the "difficult" patient on obstetrics who repeatedly refuses gynecologic exams, the formerly mild-mannered elderly gentleman who now shouts obscenities and gropes at nurses, or the sexually provocative patient who evokes strong reactions from the medical team. Could the patient on obstetrics have a history of sexual trauma, the elderly male a frontal lobe tumor, or the provocative patient a personality disorder? These are a few of many examples that serve to highlight the role that understanding sexuality plays in caring for patients both compassionately and effectively.

The consulting psychiatrist should also be reminded of the importance that being able to maintain a healthy sexual life holds for many patients, regardless of the reason for hospitalization. Sexuality may take on even greater significance for patients suffering from illnesses that directly impair sexual function, because of the difficulties both real and perceived. Psychiatric consultants should be alert to high rates of sexual problems in patients with chronic diseases (especially cardiovascular disease, cancer, diabetes, neurologic problems, end-stage renal disease [ESRD], and pain). Many chronic diseases result in depression, which in

turn contributes to decreased sexual desire. Moreover, psychological reactions to existing illnesses run the gamut, from fear that sex can kill (post-myocardial infarction [MI]) to distress over low sexual self-image (post-disfiguring surgery), to avoidance of sex, to fear of pain during sex, to fear that sexual advances will be rejected, all leading to decreased sexual intimacy.[1]

When offering suggestions for patient management, such as prescribing a new psychotropic medication, care should be taken to minimize or treat sexual side effects as much as possible. This may also help to improve patient rapport and adherence to treatment regimens. In cases where sexual dysfunction appears to have a psychological component, or where longer-term behavioral, psychotherapeutic, or pharmacologic therapy may be warranted, referral for outpatient psychiatric care can be arranged. The consulting psychiatrist may be the first to diagnose a sexual problem and can facilitate the transition from inpatient to outpatient care.

EPIDEMIOLOGY AND RISK FACTORS

Sexual disorders are extremely common. It has been estimated that 43% of females and 31% of males in the United States suffer from sexual dysfunction.[2] In addition, lack of sexual satisfaction is associated with significant emotional (including depression and marital conflict) and physical (e.g., cardiovascular disease and diabetes mellitus) problems.[3]

Sexual disorders affect individuals across the epidemiologic spectrum. Risk factors include female sex, older age, and co-existing psychiatric or medical (e.g., cardiovascular) disease.[4] It has been estimated that 10% to 54% of patients do not resume sexual activity after MI; 45% to 100% of patients with uremia or who are undergoing hemodialysis experience low sexual desire; and 26% to 50% of patients with untreated depression experience erectile dysfunction (ED).[5] Worldwide, the recent coronavirus disease 2019 (COVID-19) pandemic has likely led to long-lasting effects on sexual health, which continue to be studied.[6]

Among those with obesity and a sedentary lifestyle, weight loss and increased physical activity are associated with improved sexual function.[7] The association between race and sexual dysfunction is more variable.[2] There is a strong association between ED and vascular diseases. In fact, ED may be the presenting symptom of cardiovascular disease.[8] ED may be more frequent among individuals with specific genetic mutations (e.g., polymorphisms in genes for nitric oxide synthase) in molecular pathways responsible for resisting endothelial dysfunction.[9] Sexual trauma for both sexes is associated with long-term negative changes in sexual function.[10] A strong association exists between paraphilic disorders and childhood attention-deficit/hyperactivity disorder (ADHD), substance use, major depression or dysthymia, and phobic disorder.[11] The prototypical patient with a paraphilic disorder is young, white, and male. Anxiety, depression, and suicidal thoughts or actions, as well as homosexual or bisexual orientation, are commonly associated with gender dysphoria.[12]

PATHOPHYSIOLOGY

The ability to maintain adequate sexual function depends on complex interactions among the brain, peripheral nerves, hormones, and the vascular system. Disease states in these systems are associated with sexual dysfunction. However, no single comprehensive view has been established.

Brain regions involved in sexual arousal include the anterior cingulate gyrus, prefrontal cortex, thalamus, temporo-occipital lobes, hypothalamus, and amygdala.[13] Neurotransmitters dopamine, and norepinephrine appear to stimulate sexual function, whereas serotonin may inhibit orgasm. Testosterone, estrogen, progesterone, oxytocin, and melanocortin

hormones have a positive effect on sex, but prolactin is an inhibitor.[14]

Data suggest a central role for nitric oxide (NO) at the vascular level. In females, NO is thought to control vaginal smooth muscle tone; higher levels of NO are associated with increased vaginal lubrication. In males, NO allows for increased intra-penile blood flow, which facilitates erection. NO acts via the generation of cyclic guanosine monophosphate (cGMP), which has vasodilatory properties. Phosphodiesterase type 5 (PDE-5) inhibitors (the prototype of which is sildenafil) act to inhibit the degradation of cGMP, which prolongs the effects of NO.[15] Cholinergic fibers, prostaglandin E, vasoactive intestinal peptide (VIP), and possibly neuropeptide Y and substance P may also improve vasocongestion.[16]

Sexual dysfunction may be best understood by having knowledge of the stages of the normal sexual response; these vary with age and physical status. Medications, diseases, injuries, and psychological conditions can affect the sexual response in any of its component phases and can lead to different dysfunctional syndromes (Table 23.1).

Three major models of the human sexual response have been proposed. Masters and Johnson developed the first model of the human sexual response, consisting of a linear progression through four distinct

TABLE 23.1
Classification of Sexual Dysfunctions

Impaired Sexual Response Phase	Female	Male
Desire	Female sexual interest/arousal disorder	Male hypoactive sexual desire disorder
	Other specified sexual dysfunction: sexual aversion	Other specified sexual dysfunction: sexual aversion
Excitement (arousal, vascular)	Female sexual interest/arousal disorder	Erectile disorder
Orgasm (muscular)	Female orgasmic disorder	Delayed ejaculation/premature ejaculation
Sexual pain	Genito-pelvic pain/penetration disorder	Other specified or unspecified sexual dysfunction

phases: (1) excitement (arousal), (2) plateau (maximal arousal before orgasm), (3) orgasm (rhythmic muscular contractions), and (4) resolution (return to baseline).[17] Following resolution, a refractory period exists in males.

Kaplan modified the Masters and Johnson model by introducing a desired stage; this model emphasizes the importance of neuropsychological input in the human sexual response.[18] The Kaplan model consists of three stages: (1) desire, (2) excitement/arousal (including an increase in peripheral blood flow), and (3) orgasm (muscular contraction).

Basson, who recognized the complexity of the female sexual response, more recently proposed a biopsychosocial model of female sexuality that consists of four overlapping components: (1) biology, (2) psychology, (3) sociocultural factors, and (4) interpersonal relationships.[19] Notably, this conceptualization suggests that females may be receptive to, and satisfied with, sex even in the absence of intrinsic sexual desire if other conditions are met (such as emotional closeness). The fact that physical measurements of female arousal (such as increased vaginal secretions) are poorly correlated with sexual satisfaction lends support to Basson's view.

Aging is associated with changes in the normal human sexual response. Males are slower to achieve erections and require more direct stimulation of the penis to achieve erections. Females have decreased levels of estrogen, which leads to decreased vaginal lubrication and narrowing of the vagina. Testosterone levels in both sexes decline with age, which may result in decreased libido.[20]

CLINICAL FEATURES AND DIAGNOSIS

The *Diagnostic and Statistical Manual of Mental Disorders, Fifth Edition, Text Revision* (DSM-5-TR) classifies sexual disorders into three major categories.[21] *Sexual dysfunction* is characterized by a clinically significant disturbance in the ability to respond sexually or to experience sexual pleasure. *Paraphilic disorders* are characterized by recurrent, intense sexual urges that involve unusual objects or activities and cause personal distress or harm to self or others. *Gender dysphoria* involves conflict between one's assigned and experienced genders, resulting in personal distress or functional impairment.

The diagnosis of a sexual problem relies on a thorough medical and sexual history. Physical examination and laboratory investigations may be crucial to the identification of organic causes of sexual dysfunction. Primary psychiatric illness may present with sexual complaints (Table 23.2). However, most sexual disorders have both an organic and a psychological component. Physical disorders, surgical conditions (Table 23.3), medications, and use or abuse of drugs (Table 23.4) can affect sexual function directly or cause secondary psychological reactions that lead to a sexual problem. Psychological factors may predispose, precipitate, or maintain a sexual disorder (Table 23.5).

TABLE 23.2
Psychiatric Differential Diagnosis of Sexual Dysfunction

Psychiatric Disorder	Sexual Complaint
Depression (major depression or dysthymic disorder)	Low libido, erectile dysfunction
Bipolar disorder (manic phase)	Increased libido
Generalized anxiety disorder, panic disorder, posttraumatic stress disorder	Low libido, erectile dysfunction, lack of vaginal lubrication, anorgasmia
Obsessive-compulsive disorder	Low libido, erectile dysfunction, lack of vaginal lubrication, anorgasmia, "anti-fantasies" focusing on the negative aspects of a partner
Schizophrenia	Low desire, bizarre sexual desires
Paraphilic disorder	Deviant sexual arousal
Gender dysphoria	Dissatisfaction with one's own birth-assigned gender and sexual phenotype, causing distress and/or harm
Personality disorder (passive-aggressive, obsessive-compulsive, histrionic)	Low libido, erectile dysfunction, premature ejaculation, anorgasmia
Marital dysfunction/interpersonal problems	Varied
Fears of intimacy/commitment	Varied, intrapsychic issues

TABLE 23.3
Medical and Surgical Conditions Causing Sexual Dysfunctions

Organic Disorders	Sexual Impairment
Endocrine	
Hypothyroidism, adrenal dysfunction, hypogonadism, diabetes mellitus	Low libido, (early) erectile dysfunction, decreased vaginal lubrication
Vascular	
Hypertension, atherosclerosis, stroke, venous insufficiency, sickle cell disorder	Erectile disorder with intact ejaculation and libido
Neurologic	
Spinal cord damage, diabetic neuropathy, herniated lumbar disc, alcoholic neuropathy, multiple sclerosis, temporal lobe epilepsy	Sexual disorder (early sign), low libido (or high libido), erectile dysfunction, impaired orgasm
Local Genital Disease	
Male: Priapism, Peyronie disease, urethritis, prostatitis, hydrocele	Low libido, erectile dysfunction
Female: Imperforate hymen, vaginitis, pelvic inflammatory disease, endometriosis	Genito-pelvic pain, low libido, decreased arousal
Systemic Debilitating Disease	
Renal, pulmonary, or hepatic diseases, advanced malignancies, infections	Low libido, erectile dysfunction, decreased arousal
Surgical Postoperative States	
Male: Prostatectomy (radical perineal), abdominal-perineal bowel resection	Erectile dysfunction, no loss of libido, ejaculatory impairment
Female: Episiotomy, vaginal repair of prolapse, oophorectomy	Genito-pelvic pain, decreased lubrication
Male and female: Amputation (leg), colostomy, and ileostomy	Mechanical difficulties in sex, low self-image, fear of odor

TABLE 23.4
Drugs and Medicines That Cause Sexual Dysfunction

Drug	Sexual Side Effects
Cardiovascular	
Methyldopa	Low libido, erectile dysfunction, anorgasmia
Thiazide diuretics	Low libido, erectile dysfunction, decreased lubrication
Clonidine	Erectile dysfunction, anorgasmia
Propranolol, metoprolol	Low libido, erectile dysfunction
Digoxin	Gynecomastia, low libido, erectile dysfunction
Clofibrate	Low libido, erectile dysfunction
Psychotropics	
Sedatives	
Alcohol	Higher doses cause sexual problems
Barbiturates	Erectile dysfunction
Anxiolytics	
Alprazolam, diazepam	Low libido, delayed ejaculation
Antipsychotics	
Thioridazine	Delayed or retrograde ejaculation
Haloperidol	Low libido, erectile dysfunction, anorgasmia
Risperidone	Erectile dysfunction
Antidepressants	
MAOIs (phenelzine)	Erectile dysfunction, delayed ejaculation, anorgasmia
TCAs (imipramine)	Low libido, erectile dysfunction, delayed ejaculation
SSRIs (fluoxetine, sertraline)	Low libido, erectile dysfunction, delayed ejaculation
Atypical (trazodone)	Priapism, delayed or retrograde ejaculation
Lithium	Low libido, erectile dysfunction
Hormones	
Estrogen	Low libido in males
Progesterone	Low libido, erectile dysfunction
Gastrointestinal	
Cimetidine	Low libido, erectile dysfunction
Methantheline bromide	Erectile dysfunction
Opiates	Orgasmic dysfunction
Anticonvulsants	Low libido, erectile dysfunction, priapism

MAOIs, Monoamine oxidase inhibitors; *SSRIs,* selective serotonin reuptake inhibitors; *TCAs,* tricyclic antidepressants.

APPROACH TO SEXUAL HISTORY-TAKING

The sexual history provides an invaluable opportunity to uncover sexual problems (Case 1). Because patients are often embarrassed to discuss their sexuality with physicians or view sex as outside the realm of medicine, and because physicians are often reluctant to broach the topic of sex for fear of offending

TABLE 23.5
Psychological Causes of Sexual Dysfunction

Predisposing Factors
Lack of information/experience
Unrealistic expectations
Negative family attitudes to sex
Sexual trauma: rape, incest
Precipitating Factors
Childbirth
Infidelity
Dysfunction in the partner
Maintaining Factors
Interpersonal issues
Family stress
Work stress
Financial problems
Depression
Performance anxiety
Gender dysphoria

their patients, the need to make sexual history-taking a routine part of the practice is paramount. Physicians should always attempt to be sensitive, unbiased, and non-judgmental in their interviewing techniques, moving from general topics to more specific ones. Questions about sexual function may follow naturally from aspects of the medical history (such as introduction of a new medication, or investigation of a chief complaint that involves a gynecologic or urologic problem).

Case 1

Ms. K, a 28-year-old administrative assistant without a psychiatric history, was admitted with lower abdominal and pelvic pain of unclear etiology. However, she refused a pelvic exam and pelvic ultrasound, which were deemed essential for her work-up. She threatened to leave against medical advice, and psychiatry was consulted to help elucidate her thought process and capacity to make this decision.

On interview, Ms. K was alert, oriented, lucid, and irritable. She stated, "The doctors have no right to do this to me. It's my body. They should find another way." Her angry words then gave way to tears and sadness. On taking a social and sexual history, Ms. K revealed that she had dated briefly several males,

but her fears of sexual intimacy coupled with her partners' infidelities and physical and verbal abuse usually ended her relationships. Over the course of the interview, Ms. K revealed that she had been sexually molested by her stepfather beginning at the age of 12. She expressed resentment toward her mother, who "knew what was going on but stood by and did nothing."

After this history was revealed, the goal of the consultant was to gain the patient's trust and give the patient some control over her situation. The consultant took time to explain the importance of the pelvic exam and ultrasound in excluding potentially serious conditions. Eventually, the patient agreed to undergo the exams with the condition that only female providers be present and that a small speculum/ultrasound probe be used. With Ms. K's permission, the consultant brought Ms. K's suggestions to the team, who agreed with this plan. Ms. K underwent the exams uneventfully. Her work-up was unrevealing, and she was deemed medically safe to be discharged home. The consultant checked back frequently during Ms. K's hospital stay and helped arrange for outpatient psychiatric care.

Screening questions include: Are you sexually active? If so, with males, females, or both? Is there anything you would like to change about your sex life? Have there been any changes in your sex life? Are you satisfied with your present sex life? To maximize its effectiveness, the sexual history may be tailored to the patient's needs and goals. Physicians should recognize that paraphilics are often secretive about their activities, in part because of legal and societal implications. Patients should be reassured about the confidentiality of their interaction (except in cases where their behavior requires mandatory legal reporting, e.g., as with child abuse).[22]

In taking a sexual history, the consulting psychiatrist should recognize that chronic illness often contributes to sexual dysfunction, whether by direct physical damage or associated psychological effects. Patients with cancer, ESRD, coronary artery disease, multiple sclerosis, and diabetes are all at increased risk of sexual problems. To explore the role physiologic illness may play in sexual dysfunction, consultants should ask questions about diseases, procedures, and medications that might affect hormone balance, disrupt normal anatomic genitalia, cause central nervous system dysfunction, damage vascular or peripheral nerve supply to sexual organs, or contribute to pain during sexual activity.[1]

With online pornography and "cybersex" activities now available on-demand, anytime, and the growing availability of artificial intelligence (AI)-driven erotic chatbots and robots, psychiatrists should be aware of increasing patient concerns about "sexual addiction" (although not a formal diagnosis in DSM-5-TR) and screen for excessive and/or compulsive sexual activities.[23,24] "Hypersexuality" may be a primary problem. However, if behaviors are new or rapidly escalating, an underlying medical or neurological problem should be excluded first, particularly in the inpatient setting.

Physical Examination and Laboratory Investigation

Although history-taking is often the most important tool in the diagnosis of sexual disorders, the physical examination may reveal a clear medical or surgical basis for sexual dysfunction. Special attention should be paid to the endocrine, neurologic, vascular, urologic, and gynecologic systems. Similarly, laboratory studies may be indicated, depending on the degree to which an organic cause is suspected. There is no "routine sexual panel."

Screening tests can be guided by the history and physical examination. Tests for systemic illness include complete blood count, urinalysis, creatinine, lipid profile, thyroid function tests, and fasting blood sugar. Endocrine studies (including testosterone, prolactin, luteinizing hormone [LH], and follicular stimulating hormone), can be performed to assess low libido and ED. An estrogen level and microscopic examination of a vaginal smear can be used to assess vaginal dryness. A cervical culture and pap smear can be performed to investigate a diagnosis of dyspareunia (pain during intercourse). The nocturnal penile tumescence (NPT) test is valuable in the assessment of ED. If NPT occurs regularly (as measured by a RigiScan monitor), problems with erection are unlikely to be organic. Penile plethysmography is used to assess paraphilias by measuring an individual's sexual arousal in response to visual and auditory stimuli. Genetic or chromosomal testing may be pertinent in the evaluation of gender dysphoria with ambiguous genitalia. For example,

heritable disorders of abnormal sexual development (e.g., congenital adrenal hyperplasia, 5-alpha reductase-2 deficiency) are in some cases associated with gender dysphoria later in life.

DIAGNOSTIC CRITERIA OF SPECIFIC SEXUAL DISORDERS

Male Disorders of Sexual Function

Erectile Disorder

ED (previously referred to colloquially as "impotence") is defined as the inability of a male to obtain or maintain an erection sufficient to complete sexual activity in more than 75% of sexual encounters.[21] It affects up to 30 million American males and increases in prevalence with age.[25] Primary (life-long) ED occurs in 1% of males under the age of 35 years. Secondary (acquired) ED occurs in 40% of males over the age of 60 years; this figure increases to 73% of males over the age of 80 years. A number of risk factors for the disorder have been identified (see Table 23.6), and more than 86% of ED cases have an organic basis.[26] ED may be generalized (i.e., occurring in all circumstances) or situational (i.e., limited to certain types of stimulation, situations, and partners). It may be a symptom of a generalized vascular disease and should prompt further investigation.[25] Bicycle riding also may be linked to penile numbness (associated with perineal nerve

TABLE 23.6
Risk Factors Associated With Erectile Dysfunction

Hypertension
Diabetes mellitus
Smoking
Coronary artery disease
Peripheral vascular disorders
Blood lipid abnormalities
Peyronie disease
Priapism
Pelvic trauma or surgery
Renal failure and dialysis
Hypogonadism
Alcoholism
Depression
Lack of sexual knowledge
Poor sexual technique
Interpersonal problems

damage) and to ED (due to decreased oxygen pressure in the pudendal arteries), although research is ongoing. Depression is a common co-morbidity.

Delayed Ejaculation

This disorder (previously referred to as "retarded ejaculation") is defined as a persistent infrequency of, delay in, or absence of ejaculation following normal sexual excitement in at least 75% of sexual encounters. Delayed ejaculation is rare; fewer than 1% of males meet DSM-5-TR criteria.[21] Risk factors include sexual inexperience and young age (under 35 years). Delayed ejaculation is usually restricted to failure to reach orgasm during intercourse with an intravaginal ejaculation latency time >10 minutes.[27] Orgasm can usually occur with masturbation and/or from a partner's manual or oral stimulation. The condition must be differentiated from retrograde ejaculation, in which the bladder neck does not close off properly during orgasm, causing semen to spurt backward into the bladder. Delayed ejaculation may also be an unsuspected cause of a couple's infertility problems. The male may not have admitted his lack of ejaculation to his partner.

Premature (Early) Ejaculation

This disorder is defined as recurrent ejaculation with minimal sexual stimulation before, on, or shortly after penetration (within 1 minute) and before the person wishes it. Early ejaculation is common and was reported in nearly one-third of males aged 18 to 70 in an international cohort. However, less than 3% of males meet DSM-5-TR criteria, which specify that symptoms must cause clinically significant distress and occur for 6 months or more in at least 75% of sexual encounters.[21] Prolonged periods without sexual activity increase the risk of premature ejaculation. If the problem is chronic and untreated, secondary erectile dysfunction may occur.[28]

Male Hypoactive Sexual Desire Disorder

This disorder is characterized by persistent or recurrent absence of sexual thoughts or fantasies and desire for sexual activity. Symptoms must be present for 6 months or more.[21] In males, sexual desire declines with increasing age. In fact, more than two in five males aged 66 to 74 report decreased sexual desire, compared with 6% of males aged 18 to 44. Yet, low sexual desire is usually not associated with clinically significant distress; less than 2% of males aged 16 to 44 meet DSM-5-TR criteria for male hypoactive sexual desire disorder.[21,29]

Female Disorders of Sexual Function

Female Sexual Interest/Arousal Disorder

This disorder (FSIAD) is defined by reduced or absent sexual interest, thoughts, arousal, excitement, genital sensation, and/or activity (with reluctant participation in and initiation of sex). Three or more of these components must be present for at least 6 months and cause significant personal distress to meet the criteria.[21] Decreased sexual interest is reported in 20% to 40% of females.[30] However, the exact prevalence of FSIAD as per DSM-5-TR criteria remains unknown.

Female Orgasmic Disorder

This disorder (FOD) is defined as a recurrent delay in, or absence of, orgasm following a normal sexual excitement phase, in at least 75% of sexual encounters.[21] Some females who can have orgasms with direct clitoral stimulation find it impossible to reach orgasm during intercourse; however, this is a normal variant. While as many as 30% of females in the United States experience difficulties with orgasm, few report significant associated distress, which is necessary to meet DSM-5-TR criteria for FOD. The ability to reach orgasm increases with sexual experience. Claims that stimulation of the Grafenberg spot, or G-spot, in a region in the anterior wall of the vagina, will cause orgasm and female ejaculation have never been substantiated, despite ongoing research. Premature ejaculation in the male may contribute to female orgasmic dysfunction.[31]

Genito-Pelvic Pain/Penetration Disorder

This disorder is defined as recurrent and persistent vulvovaginal pain or fear of pain during penetration or intercourse. The prevalence is unknown, but approximately 15% of North American females report recurrent pain with sexual intercourse.[21] Contraction of the vaginal outlet as an examining finger or speculum is introduced during routine gynecologic examination may be a clue to the diagnosis. Sexual trauma and co-existing medical/pelvic conditions are important associations and potential precipitants. Lack of vaginal lubrication and other physiologic contributors to sexual pain should be first excluded.[32]

Sexual Dysfunction Disorders Affecting Both Genders

Substance/Medication-Induced Sexual Dysfunction

This disorder is characterized by clinically significant sexual impairment that is immediately temporally related to the ingestion of a specific substance or medication. The disorder should not be diagnosed during a state of delirium.

Other Specified and Unspecified Sexual Dysfunction

These diagnoses refer to sexual dysfunction not meeting DSM-5-TR criteria for other named disorders. The "other specified" modifier should be used if the clinician chooses to state the reason that criteria for another disorder are not met; otherwise, the "unspecified" modifier should be used. Of note, "sexual aversion" (marked disinclination toward partnered genital sexual contact) is not a discrete entity in DSM-5-TR but can be acknowledged as an "other specified" disorder if appropriate.[21]

Paraphilic Disorders

Paraphilias refer to any persistent, intense sexually arousing fantasies, urges, or behaviors other than genital stimulation or fondling with a mature, consenting, human partner. They may involve non-human objects or the suffering or humiliation of one's partner, children, or other non-consenting persons. Paraphilias may involve a conditioned response in which non-sexual objects become sexually arousing when paired with a pleasurable activity (masturbation). Some individuals always require paraphilic fantasies, while others rely on them during times of stress. Paraphilias run the gamut from exhibitionism (exposure of genitals to an unsuspecting stranger) to masochism (pleasure from abuse), to pedophilia (sex with a prepubescent child).[21]

Under DSM-5-TR, paraphilias are considered disorders when they have been present for at least 6 months; the individual has acted on the underlying urges; and the associated behaviors cause marked personal distress or harm to self or others. Most paraphilic disorders are thought to have a psychological basis.

Individuals with these conditions often have difficulty forming more socialized sexual relationships. An interest in non-consenting partners may have legal and societal implications. Co-occurring ADHD, substance use, major depression or dysthymia, and phobic disorder are common.[33]

Gender Dysphoria

This group of disorders is characterized by discordance between one's assigned and one's experienced gender (inclusive of non-binary gender), causing marked personal distress or impaired function for at least 6 months.[21] It is subclassified into childhood and adult/adolescent forms, depending on the age of onset. The childhood form is typified by gender-atypical play and behavior. In contrast, adolescents and adults usually express a strong desire to rid themselves of assigned secondary sexual characteristics. By late adolescence or adulthood, 75% of birth-assigned boys with a history of gender dysphoria as a child will have a homosexual or bisexual orientation. Children with gender dysphoria may have co-existing separation anxiety, generalized anxiety, and depression. Adolescents and adults have a propensity for suicidal thoughts and actions as well as anxiety, depression, and paraphilic behaviors. Associated personality disorders are also common in male patients. One in 30,000 males and 1 in 100,000 females have gender-affirming (sex-reassignment) surgery.[21,34]

DIFFERENTIAL DIAGNOSIS OF SEXUAL DISORDERS

The differential diagnosis of sexual disorders includes medical and surgical conditions (Table 23.3), adverse effects of medications (Table 23.4), and other psychiatric disorders (Table 23.2). Before a primary sexual disorder is diagnosed, it is important to identify potentially treatable conditions (both organic and psychiatric) that manifest as problems with sexual function. For example, treatment for depression may improve erectile function. Although paraphilic disorders often have a psychological basis, an organic cause should be considered if the behavior begins in middle age or later; there is a regression from previously normal sexuality; there is excessive aggression; there are reports of auras or seizure-like symptoms before or during the sexual behavior; there is an abnormal body habitus; or there is an abnormal neurologic examination. See Table 23.7 for the psychiatric differential diagnosis of paraphilic disorders. Patients who present with gender dysphoria generally have normal physical findings and normal laboratory studies. The differential diagnosis includes non-conformity to stereotypical sex role behaviors, transvestic fetishism (cross-dressing), and schizophrenia (e.g., with the delusion that one belongs to a different sex). It should be stressed that gender incongruence without associated distress or impaired function is not considered pathological and has increased in prevalence with greater social awareness and acceptance.[35]

TREATMENT

Organically Based Treatment

The essence of treatment for sexual disorders involves the treatment of pre-existing illnesses (e.g., diabetes); discontinuation or substitution of offending medications; reduction of alcohol, smoking, and other psychoactive substances (illicit or non-illicit) as applicable; increase in exercise; improvement in the diet; and addition of medications for psychiatric conditions (e.g., depression). Although many medications for the treatment of hypertension inhibit sexual function, the angiotensin II receptor blockers (e.g., losartan), are not associated with sexual side effects and

may actually help prevent or correct sexual problems (such as sexual dissatisfaction, low frequency of sex, or ED).[36] Any hormone deficiency should be corrected (e.g., the addition of testosterone for hypogonadism, thyroid hormone for hypothyroidism, estrogen/testosterone for postmenopausal females, or bromocriptine for elevated prolactin after neuroimaging of the pituitary). Many medical illnesses are associated with physiologic and psychological impairments that when treated improve sexual function; selected examples are shown in Table 23.8.[5]

TABLE 23.7
Psychiatric Differential Diagnosis of Paraphilic Disorders

Intellectual disability
Dementia
Substance intoxication
Manic episode (bipolar disorder)
Schizophrenia
Obsessive-compulsive disorder
Gender dysphoria
Personality disorder
Sexual dysfunction
Non-paraphilic compulsive sexual behaviors
Compulsive use of erotic videos, magazines, or cybersex
Uncontrolled masturbation
Unrestrained use of prostitutes
Numerous brief and superficial sexual affairs
Hypersexuality/sexual addiction

TABLE 23.8
Specific Treatments for Sexual Dysfunction Attributable to Medical Illness

Disease	Associated Impairment Causing Sexual Dysfunction	Treatment
Coronary artery disease	Fear of recurrent MI Fear of nitrate-PDE-5 interaction Concurrent depression	Reassure, encourage exercise Switch from nitrate to trimetazidine (not FDA approved) Treat depression
Renal failure	Low testosterone (males) Hyperprolactinemia Low zinc levels Anemia Uremic menorrhagia Concurrent depression Estrogen deficiency	Consider testosterone Try bromocriptine, 25(OH)D Consider zinc replacement Erythropoietin Consider cyclic or daily progesterone Treat depression Local estrogen therapy
Urinary incontinence	Urinary leakage during sex	Consider surgery
Diabetes	Hyperglycemia	Improve glycemic control
Elevated prolactin	Hyperprolactinemia	Treat underlying cause
Adrenal disease	Diminished adrenal hormones	Consider DHEA

25(OH)D, 25-Hydroxy-vitamin D; *DHEA*, dehydroepiandrosterone; *MI*, myocardial infarction; *PDE*, phosphodiesterase type 5.

Psychotropic Medication–Induced Sexual Dysfunction

Antidepressants. Sexual dysfunction is a commonly reported side effect of selective serotonin reuptake inhibitors (SSRIs). According to some estimates, as many as 80% of SSRI users experience sexual side effects.[37] Strategies to treat SSRI-induced sexual dysfunction are presented in Table 23.9. Monoamine oxidase inhibitors and tricyclic antidepressants (TCAs) also cause sexual problems. Because of their inhibitory sexual properties, SSRIs have been used with success to treat premature ejaculation and reduce compulsive sexual acts associated with Alzheimer disease, paraphilic behavior, and sexual obsessions in patients with obsessive-compulsive disorder spectrum.

Antipsychotics. First-generation (typical) antipsychotics (e.g., haloperidol, thioridazine) as well as second-generation (atypical) agents (e.g., risperidone, clozapine) are all associated with adverse sexual effects and usually inhibit sexual function.[38] Hyperprolactinemia may play a causal role. Most second-generation antipsychotics (e.g., olanzapine, quetiapine, aripiprazole, ziprasidone) are associated with fewer sexual side effects. Antipsychotics have also been used to dampen sexually inappropriate behaviors and paraphilic behaviors.

Premature Ejaculation

There is no US Food and Drug Administration (FDA)-approved treatment for premature ejaculation. However, the SSRIs (e.g., fluoxetine, sertraline, paroxetine) used continuously or intermittently (2–12 hours before sex), can cause delayed ejaculation, in turn treating premature ejaculation. Low doses may be effective. Clomipramine (a TCA) may be more effective in delaying ejaculation than SSRIs. Dapoxetine, an SSRI with a rapid onset and short half-life, was developed as an on-demand treatment for premature ejaculation and has been approved in many countries but not in the United States. On-demand tramadol also demonstrates promise but may be limited by potential dependency given the agent's weak opioid properties. Topical anesthetic creams (such as lidocaine derivatives including EMLA cream) appear to be successful in slowing ejaculation without inducing the systemic side effects of antidepressants; however, they can cause local skin irritation and penile numbing that sometimes lead to erectile problems. When premature ejaculation is secondary to ED, PDE-5 inhibitors should be used to treat ED first.[39]

Erectile Dysfunction

The mainstay of treatment for ED is the use of oral PDE-5 inhibitors (e.g., sildenafil, vardenafil, tadalafil, and most recently avanafil), which can help males with a wide range of conditions; they are easy to use and have few adverse effects (Table 23.10). An important

---

TABLE 23.9

Treatment Strategies for SSRI-Induced Sexual Dysfunction

Strategy	Comments
Decrease the dose	May diminish antidepressant effect Consider in patients on high doses
Switch SSRIs	Paroxetine linked to highest rates of sexual dysfunction Fluvoxamine may have fewer sexual side effects No clear evidence to support this strategy
Switch to a non-SSRI agent	Data support bupropion, mirtazapine, vortioxetine, vilazodone, nefazodone (brand name Serzone withdrawn in the United States) Consider transdermal selegiline Not FDA approved: tianeptine, reboxetine, moclobemide, agomelatine, gepirone Venlafaxine and desvenlafaxine are *not* superior to SSRIs
Add "antidote" drug	Best evidence to support PDE-5 inhibitors (sildenafil, tadalafil, vardenafil, avanafil), next bupropion, then buspirone (high dose) PDE-5 inhibitors not only improve erectile dysfunction but also arousal and orgasm even in some females on SSRIs Small studies support maca root (herbal agent) Consider amantadine, dextroamphetamine, methylphenidate, ginkgo biloba, granisetron, cyproheptadine, yohimbine, and atomoxetine (data mixed)
Take a drug holiday	Limited studies show no clear benefit to this approach May precipitate withdrawal and encourage noncompliance
Await spontaneous remission	Rarely occurs

FDA, US Food and Drug Administration; *SSRI*, selective serotonin reuptake inhibitor.

TABLE 23.10

First-Line Treatment for Erectile Dysfunction: Comparison of PDE-5 Inhibitors

Medication	Dose	Onset	Duration	Food Interaction	Advantages	Side Effects	Contraindications
Sildenafil (Viagra)	25–100 mg Max—one dose per day	30–60 min	4 h (up to 12 h)	Delayed absorption with high-fat foods	50%–85% efficacy Longest track record	Headache, low BP, flushing, dyspepsia, vasodilation, diarrhea, visual changes (blue tinge to vision), hearing loss (rare) NAION—not proven	Active CAD, hypotension No nitrates for 24 h after dose Caution with α-blockers
Vardenafil (Levitra)	2.5–20 mg Max—one dose per day	15–30 min	4 h (up to 12 h)	Delayed absorption with high-fat foods	75% efficacy No visual side effects Available as ODT preparation (Staxyn)	Headache, low BP, flushing, dyspepsia, vasodilation, diarrhea, visual changes, hearing loss (rare) NAION—not proven	Active CAD, hypotension May prolong QTc May increase LFTs Avoid nitrates for 24 h after the dose Avoid α-blockers (terazosin and doxazosin). Use cautiously with tamsulosin or alfuzosin
Tadalafil (Cialis)	5–20 mg	15–45 min	24–36 h	None	75% efficacy No visual side effects Can be taken with food More PDE-5 selective	Headache, low BP, flushing, dyspepsia, vasodilation, diarrhea, back pain, myalgias, hearing loss (rare) NAION—not proven	Active CAD, hypotension Avoid nitrates for 48 h after the dose Avoid α-blockers (terazosin and doxazosin). Use cautiously with tamsulosin or alfuzosin
Avanafil (Stendra)	50–200 mg Max—one dose per day	15 min	Up to 6 h	Delayed absorption with high-fat foods	Shortest onset of action Shortest duration Fewer drug interactions More PDE-5 selective	Headache, low BP, flushing, nasal congestion, dizziness, hearing loss (rare) NAION—not proven	Active CAD, hypotension No nitrates for 12 h after dose (weaker and briefer effect compared with other PDE-5s) Start at a lower dose (50 mg) if on (stable) α-blocker

CAD, Coronary artery disease; NAION, non-arteritic anterior ischemic optic neuropathy; QTc, corrected QT interval; LFTs, liver function tests; ODT, orally disintegrating tablet.

absolute contraindication is the recent concurrent use of nitrates, which can lead to profound hypotension.[40] Other potential risks include hypotension with concurrent use of an α-blocker (e.g., for benign prostate hypertrophy or hypertension) and possibly hearing loss and development of non-arteritic anterior ischemic optic neuropathy (NAION). The PDE-5 inhibitors are effective in the treatment of antidepressant-induced ED and delayed ejaculation. Of note, these agents are metabolized by P450 3A4 and 2C9 isoenzyme systems. Patients who take potent inhibitors (including grapefruit juice, cimetidine, ketoconazole, erythromycin, and ritonavir) of these P450 isoenzyme systems, should have a lower starting dose of a PDE-5 inhibitor. Statins may also help improve the efficacy of PDE-5 inhibitors.

Other oral agents are used to treat ED. Yohimbine, an α_2-adrenergic inhibitor, has been available for many years, and it may be useful in the treatment of psychogenic ED; however, its efficacy is uncertain. Phentolamine is an α-blocker (not FDA approved) that may produce erections by dilation of blood vessels. Apomorphine is a centrally acting D_1/D_2 dopamine receptor agonist administered sublingually. Although efficacious in stimulating erections, the drug is limited by its side effects, especially nausea and vomiting, and

is only FDA-approved for Parkinson disease. Centrally acting melanocortin receptor agonist bremelanotide appears to be effective, but it is currently only FDA approved for subcutaneous use in females, and side effects may limit its utility. The amino acid L-arginine (an NO precursor) appears promising in males.[41] Other agents under study include naltrexone, an opioid antagonist, clavulanic acid, a serotonin/dopamine modulator, and trazodone, a 5-HT_{2C} serotonin receptor. Herbal agents and supplements have overall demonstrated limited benefit, with *Panax ginseng*, *Butea superba*, and *Lepidium meyenii* (maca root) showing more promise. Some "natural agents" in fact contain traces of PDE-5 inhibitors.[42]

Non-approved topical agents include alprostadil cream, minoxidil solution, and nitroglycerine ointment. In hypogonadal males, transdermal testosterone or clomiphene citrate may be considered. Testosterone therapy has also been show to improve ED in elderly males with initially low testosterone levels.[43] Second-line treatment for ED includes the use of intra-penile injection therapy, intraurethral suppository therapy, and vacuum-assisted devices (Table 23.11). The third-line treatment for ED is the surgical implantation of an inflatable or malleable rod or penile prosthesis. Endarterectomy or drug-eluting stents may correct

TABLE 23.11
Second-Line Treatments for Erectile Dysfunction

Treatment	Effects	Advantages	Disadvantages
Intraurethral suppository: MUSE (alprostadil)	Prostaglandin E_1 gel delivered by applicator into the meatus of the penis. Induces vasodilation to cause erection	60% Efficacy. Less penile fibrosis and priapism than with penile injections. Can be used twice daily	Not recommended with pregnant partners. Mild penile/urethral pain
Penile self-injection: alprostadil (Caverject and Edex)	Prostaglandin E_1 injected into the base of the penis. Induces vasodilation to cause erection	50%–87% efficacy. Few systemic side effects	Can cause penile pain, priapism, fibrosis. Not recommended for daily use
Intracavernosal injection: vasoactive intestinal polypeptide (VIP) + phentolamine: aviptadil (Senatek)	VIP causes veno-occlusion while phentolamine increases arterial flow	Associated with less pain than alprostadil and therefore preferred by patients	Less effective than alprostadil
Vacuum constriction device (pump)	Creates a vacuum to draw blood into the penile cavernosa. Elastic band holds blood in the penis	67% efficacy. No systemic side effects. Safe if erection not maintained more than 1h	May not be acceptable to partner. Erection hinged at base; does not allow for external ejaculation

ED in certain patients with underlying vascular disease. Extracorporeal low-intensity shock wave lithotripsy, low-intensity pulsed ultrasound, and injectable gene and platelet-rich plasma therapies are in investigational stages.[25,41]

Female Sexual Dysfunction

Flibanserin became the first FDA-approved medication for treating female dysfunction in 2015, indicated for premenopausal females with "hypoactive sexual desire disorder" (HSDD), as defined by the fourth edition of DSM (DSM-IV). The term HSDD was removed from the DSM-5/DSM-5-TR but it most closely resembles FSIAD. The drug remains controversial, given its only modest benefit with a potential for serious side effects, such as marked hypotension when combined with alcohol. In 2019 a second agent, subcutaneous bremelanotide (as previously discussed), also received FDA approval for premenopausal HSDD. Potential adverse effects include nausea, flushing, injection site reactions, and localized gum and skin hyperpigmentation that may persist even after stopping the medication. Besides these agents, the only other FDA-approved medication relevant to the treatment of female sexual dysfunction is ospemifene, an oral selective estrogen receptor modulator indicated for postmenopausal dyspareunia (genital pain associated with sex). Dyspareunia is also not a discrete diagnosis in DSM-5-TR but is encompassed under genito-pelvic pain/penetration disorder. An alternative non-medication but approved intervention is EROS-CTD, a clitoral suction device, which is used to increase vasocongestion and engorge the clitoris for better sexual arousal and orgasm.[44]

Numerous drug trials are in progress using medications approved or being studied for male sexual dysfunction (such as PDE-5 inhibitors), hormone-based therapies, and novel agents. In general, PDE-5 inhibitors are not effective in improving female sexual function, but they may benefit some females who exhibit greatly diminished genital vasocongestion.[44] PDE-5 inhibitors also appear to be effective for females with SSRI-induced sexual dysfunction.[45] Bupropion (a dopamine and noradrenergic agonist) may increase arousability and sexual response in females. Other investigational agents include yohimbine, apomorphine, L-arginine, and various herbals.[46]

Transdermal testosterone with or without estrogen appears to be effective in treating postmenopausal HSDD, but no agents are currently FDA approved for this indication.[44] Tibolone, a steroid hormone with estrogenic, androgenic, and progestogenic metabolites, has been shown to increase vaginal lubrication, arousability, and sexual desire. However, it is also associated with an increased risk of stroke in females with osteoporosis over the age of 60 and has been rejected by the FDA.[47] In general, once fervent interest in hormonal therapies has been tempered by associated risks of cardiovascular disease and breast cancer highlighted by landmark Women's Health Initiative studies.

Additional novel therapies for female sexual dysfunction include intranasal oxytocin for improving sexual satisfaction. Onabotulinum toxin A injections may help ameliorate vaginismus (involuntary vaginal muscular tightening on attempted penetration). Vaginal diazepam may also decrease sexual pain. In addition, sacral neuromodulation, currently indicated for overactive bladder, has been shown in small pilot studies to increase sexual desire, lubrication, orgasm, and satisfaction. Micro-ablative vaginal carbon-dioxide laser is another trending therapy that appears safe and possibly effective for treating postmenopausal vaginal symptoms.[48]

Paraphilic Disorders

Pharmacologic therapy for paraphilias is aimed at the suppression of compulsive sexual behavior. The antiandrogen drugs, cyproterone (CPA) and medroxyprogesterone acetate (MPA), which act by competitive inhibition of androgen receptors, may be used off-label to reduce aberrant sexual tendencies by decreasing androgen levels. Treatment with a synthetic GnRH analog (FDA-approved for prostate cancer but not paraphilic disorders), including leuprorelin, triptorelin, and goserelin, decreases testosterone to chemically castrating levels (after an initial transient increase), and may completely abolish deviant sexual tendencies. The SSRIs and clomipramine may lower aberrant sexual urges by decreasing the compulsivity/impulsivity of the act and by decreasing aggressive behaviors. Psychostimulants, such as methylphenidate sustained release, may be helpful when co-morbid ADHD is present. Antipsychotics have also been used to treat paraphilic disorders.[49]

Gender Dysphoria

The definitive treatment for gender dysphoria is gender-affirming surgery (formerly known as sex-reassignment surgery), in combination with hormonal therapies to suppress secondary characteristics. Such hormonal agents include LH-releasing hormone agonists, gonadotropin-releasing hormone agents (GnRH), spironolactone, CPA, estrogens, and testosterone, with associated risks of cardiovascular and thromboembolic disease and osteoporosis. Of note, hormonal therapy alone is in general associated with significantly improved psychological symptoms and quality of life. In contrast, gender-confirming surgery may lead to significant regret and not significantly affect objective measures of psychological functioning. Treatment for gender dysphoria, especially in young children, has recently become entangled in much sociopolitical controversy. Nonetheless, with the high risk of self-harm and suicidality among untreated individuals, a personalized approach to maximizing expected benefit over harm is likely prudent.[50]

Psychologically Based Treatments

Sexual Dysfunction

General principles of treatment include improving communication (verbally and physically) between partners, encouraging experimentation, decreasing the pressure of performance by changing the goal of sexual activity away from erection or orgasm to feeling good about oneself, and relieving the pressure of the moment (by suggesting that there is always another day to try). The PLISSIT model provides a useful framework for approaching the treatment of sexual problems and can be tailored to the desired level of intervention. The stages are as follows: (1) P, permission; (2) LI, limited information; (3) SS, specific suggestions; and (4) IT, intensive therapy. Permission-giving involves reassuring the patient about sexual activity, alleviating guilt about activities the patient feels are "bad" or "dirty," and reinforcing the normal range of sexual activities. Limited information includes providing basic knowledge about anatomy and physiology and correcting myths and misconceptions. Specific suggestions include techniques of behavioral sex therapy (Table 23.12). Intensive therapy may be useful for patients with chronic sexual problems, complex psychological

issues, or both. Whereas the first three stages (P, LI, SS) may be implemented by any healthcare provider, the last stage (IT) usually requires an expert with special training in sex therapy.[18]

Paraphilic Disorders

Paraphilic disorders are often refractory to treatment, and recidivism is high, but several non-pharmacologic modalities have been used with varying success. Insight-oriented or supportive psychotherapy is relatively ineffective. Cognitive-behavioral therapy can be used to help patients identify aberrant sexual tendencies, alter their behavior, and avoid sexual triggers to prevent relapse.[49] Aversive therapy, via conditioning with ammonia, is used to reduce paraphilic behavior. Orgasmic re-conditioning is used to teach the paraphilic how to become aroused by more acceptable mental images. Social skills training (individual or group) is used to help the paraphilic form better interpersonal relationships. Surveillance systems (using family members to help monitor patient behavior) may be helpful. Lifelong maintenance is required.

Gender Dysphoria

Individual psychotherapy is useful both in helping patients understand their gender dysphoria and in addressing other psychiatric issues. A thorough psychological evaluation is generally required before gender-affirming surgery can be performed.[50] Marital and family therapy can help with adjustment to a new gender, including the possibility of intense and under-anticipated stigmatization and discrimination.

CONCLUSION

Sexual problems are common in the general population, and in medically ill, hospitalized patients, the prevalence is even greater. Even when a sexual problem is not the primary reason for consultation, the consulting psychiatrist should feel comfortable and well equipped to take a sexual history as a routine part of the evaluation. Although time and privacy are important limitations in the inpatient setting, the sexual history may reveal an unrecognized sexual concern; uncover an underlying medical or psychiatric illness; or at the very least help better understand the

TABLE 23.12
Specific Behavioral Techniques of Sex Therapy

Sexual Disorder	Suggestions
Male hypoactive sexual desire disorder	Sensate focus exercises (non-demand pleasuring techniques) to enhance enjoyment without pressure
	Erotic material, masturbation training
Female sexual interest/arousal disorder	Sensate focus exercises
	Lubrication: saliva, KY jelly for vaginal dryness
Other specified sexual dysfunction: sexual aversion	Sensate focus exercises
	For phobic/panic symptoms, use anti-anxiety/antidepressant meds
Erectile disorder	Sensate focus exercises (non-demand pleasuring techniques)
	Use a female superior position (heterosexual couple) for non-demanding intercourse
	The female manually stimulates the penis, and if an erection is obtained, she inserts the penis into the vagina and begins the movement
	Learn ways to satisfy your partner without penile/vaginal intercourse
Female orgasmic disorder	Self-stimulation
	Use of fantasy materials
	Kegel vaginal exercises (contraction of pubococcygeus muscles)
	Use of controlled intercourse in a female superior position
	"Bridge technique"—male stimulates the female's clitoris manually after insertion of the penis into the vagina
Delayed ejaculation (during intercourse)	Female stimulates male manually until orgasm becomes inevitable
	Insert penis into the vagina and begin thrusting
Premature ejaculation	Increased frequency of sex
	"Squeeze technique"— the female manually stimulates the penis until ejaculation is approaching, then the female squeezes the penis with her thumb on the frenulum. The pressure is applied until the male no longer feels the urge to ejaculate (15–60s). Use the female superior position with gradual thrusting and the "squeeze" technique as excitement intensifies "Stop-start technique"— the female stimulates the male to the point of ejaculation and then stops the stimulation. She resumes the stimulation for several stop-start procedures until ejaculation is allowed to occur
Genito-pelvic pain/penetration disorder	Treat any underlying gynecologic problem first
	Treat insufficient lubrication using, e.g., KY jelly
	Female is encouraged to accept larger and larger objects into her vagina (e.g., her fingers, her partner's fingers, Hegar graduated vaginal dilators, syringe containers of different sizes)
	Recommend the use of the female superior position allowing the female to gradually insert the erect penis into the vagina
	Practice Kegel vaginal exercises to develop a sense of control

patient in a functional context, and in turn, improve the patient-doctor relationship.

With our population growing older, the potential for sexual problems is on the rise. Patients both in and out of the hospital are living with complex medical problems and taking multiple medications. At the same time, with the shifting focus of medicine from improving not only the length of life but also the *quality* of life, a physician's responsibility to recognize and treat sexual problems is ever greater. Consulting psychiatrists can be helpful in discerning the biological, psychological, and social factors that contribute to a sexual problem. Recognizing the sexual side effects of psychotropics and other medications is a key part of the evaluation. Fortunately, many effective treatment strategies now exist (e.g., the use of PDE-5 inhibitors for SSRI-induced sexual dysfunction). With an increasing understanding of the biological basis for sexual dysfunction, the opportunity to treat sexual problems should only continue to expand.

Some sexual problems may be the result of an acute illness or require only short-term treatment or medication adjustment. By seeing patients in the hospital setting and obtaining an appreciation of the psychological and physical limitations that patients face, consultant psychiatrists may offer creative solutions to facilitate a sexual life. The inpatient setting also provides a unique opportunity to assemble a multi-disciplinary specialty team (e.g., urology, gynecology, endocrinology) as necessary to provide comprehensive care. Ultimately, the consultant psychiatrist may play a pivotal role in connecting the patient to an outpatient provider for longer-term management.

REFERENCES

1. McInnes RA. Chronic illness and sexuality. *Med J Aust.* 2003;179:263–266.
2. Laumann EO, Paik A, Rosen RC. Sexual dysfunction in the United States: prevalence and predictors. *JAMA.* 1999;281:537–544.
3. Bahnsen MK, Graugaard C, Andersson M, et al. Physical and mental health problems and their associations with interpersonal sexual inactivity and sexual dysfunctions in Denmark: baseline assessment in a national cohort study. *J Sex Med.* 2022;19:1562–1579.
4. McCabe MP, Sharlip ID, Lewis R, et al. Risk factors for sexual dysfunction among women and men: a consensus statement from the Fourth International Consultation on Sexual Medicine 2015. *J Sex Med.* 2016;13:153–167.
5. Basson R, Schultz WW. Sexual sequelae of general medical disorders. *Lancet.* 2007;369:409–424.
6. Pennanen-Iire C, Prereira-Lourenço M, Padoa A, et al. Sexual health implications of COVID-19 pandemic. *Sex Med Rev.* 2021;9:3–14.
7. Rowland DL, McNabney SM, Mann AR. Sexual function, obesity, and weight loss in men and women. *Sex Med Rev.* 2017;5:323–338.
8. Diaconu CC, Manea M, Marcu DR, et al. The erectile dysfunction as a marker of cardiovascular disease: a review. *Acta Cardiol.* 2020;75:286–292.
9. Patel DP, Pastuszak AW, Hotaling JM. Genetics and erectile dysfunction: leveraging early foundations for new discoveries. *Int J Impot Res.* 2022;34:252–259.
10. O'Driscoll C, Flanagan E. Sexual problems and post-traumatic stress disorder following sexual trauma: a meta-analytic review. *Psychol Psychother.* 2016;89:351–367.
11. Soldati L, Bianchi-Demicheli F, Schockaert P, et al. Association of ADHD and hypersexuality and paraphilias. *Psychiatry Res.* 2021;295:113638.
12. Dhejne C, Van Vlerken R, Heylens G, et al. Mental health and gender dysphoria: a review of the literature. *Int Rev Psychiatry.* 2016;28:44–57.
13. Rees PM, Fowler CJ, Maas CP. Sexual function in men and women with neurological disorders. *Lancet.* 2007;369:512–525.
14. Bhasin S, Enzlin P, Coviello A, et al. Sexual dysfunction in men and women with endocrine disorders. *Lancet.* 2007;369:597–611.
15. Lue TF. Erectile dysfunction. *N Engl J Med.* 2000;342:1802–1813.
16. Clayton AH. Sexual function and dysfunction in women. *Psychiatr Clin North Am.* 2003;26:673–682.
17. Masters WH, Johnson VE.*Human Sexual Inadequacy.* Bantam Books; 1970.
18. Kaplan HS.*The Evaluation of Sexual Disorders.* Brunner/Mazel; 1983.
19. Basson R. A model of women's sexual arousal. *J Sex Marital Ther.* 2002;28:1–10.
20. Sinković M, Towler L. Sexual aging: a systematic review of qualitative research on the sexuality and sexual health of older adults. *Qual Health Res.* 2019;29:1239–1254.
21. American Psychiatric Association… *Diagnostic and Statistical Manual of Mental Disorders, Text Revision.* 5th ed. American Psychiatric Publishing; 2022.
22. Brookmeyer KA, Coor A, Kachur RE, et al. Sexual history taking in clinical settings: a narrative review. *Sex Transm Dis.* 2021;48:393–402.
23. Jacobs T, Geysemans B, Van Hal G, et al. Associations between online pornography consumption and sexual dysfunction in young men: multivariate analysis based on an international web-based survey. *JMIR Public Health Surveill.* 2021;7:e32542.
24. Dubé S, Anctil D. Foundations of erobotics. *Int J Soc Robot.* 2021;13:1205–1233.
25. Irwin GM. Erectile dysfunction. *Prim Care.* 2019;46:249–255.
26. Pozzi E, Fallara G, Capogrosso P, et al. Primary organic versus primary psychogenic erectile dysfunction: findings from a real-life cross-sectional study. *Andrology.* 2022;10:1302–1309.
27. Abdel-Hamid IA, Ali OI. Delayed ejaculation: pathophysiology, diagnosis, and treatment. *World J Mens Health.* 2018;36:22–40.
28. Pereira-Lourenço M, Brito DVE, Pereira BJ. Premature ejaculation: from physiology to treatment. *J Family Reprod Health.* 2019;13:120–131.
29. McCarthy B, McDonald D. Assessment, treatment, and relapse prevention: male hypoactive sexual desire disorder. *J Sex Marital Ther.* 2009;35:58–67.
30. Laumann EO, Nicolosi A, Glasser DB, et al. Sexual problems among women and men aged 40-80 y: prevalence and correlates identified in the Global Study of Sexual Attitudes and Behaviors. *Int J Impot Res.* 2005;17:39–57.
31. Marchand E. Psychological and behavioral treatment of female orgasmic disorder. *Sex Med Rev.* 2021;9:194–211.
32. Dias-Amaral A, Marques-Pinto A. Female genito-pelvic pain/penetration disorder: review of the related factors and overall approach. *Rev Bras Ginecol Obstet.* 2018;40:787–793.
33. Soldati L, Bianchi-Demicheli F, Schockaert P, et al. Association of ADHD and hypersexuality and paraphilias. *Psychiatry Res.* 2021;295:113638.

34. Zucker KJ, Lawrence AA, Kreukels BP. Gender dysphoria in adults. *Annu Rev Clin Psychol.* 2016;12:217–247.

35. Claahsen-van der Grinten H, Verhaak C, Steensma T, et al. Gender incongruence and gender dysphoria in childhood and adolescence-current insights in diagnostics, management, and follow-up. *Eur J Pediatr.* 2021;180:1349–1357.

36. Ismail SB, Noor NM, Hussain NHN, et al. Angiotensin receptor blockers for erectile dysfunction in hypertensive men: a brief meta-analysis of randomized control trials. *Am J Mens Health.* 2019;13 1557988319892735.

37. Atmaca M. Selective serotonin reuptake inhibitor-induced sexual dysfunction: current management perspectives. *Neuropsychiatr Dis Treat.* 2020;16:1043–1050.

38. Stępnicki P, Kondej M, Kaczor AA. Current concepts and treatments of schizophrenia. *Molecules.* 2018;23:2087.

39. Gul M, Bocu K, Serefoglu EC. Current and emerging treatment options for premature ejaculation. *Nat Rev Urol.* 2022;19:659–680.

40. Krzastek SC, Bopp J, Smith RP, et al. Recent advances in the understanding and management of erectile dysfunction. *F1000Res.* 2019;8 F1000 Faculty Rev-102.

41. Kim S, Cho MC, Cho SY, et al. Novel emerging therapies for erectile dysfunction. *World J Mens Health.* 2021;39:48–64.

42. Fleshner N, Harvey M, Adomat H, et al. Evidence for contamination of herbal erectile dysfunction products with phosphodiesterase type 5 inhibitors. *J Urol.* 2005;174:636–641.

43. Snyder PJ, Bhasin S, Cunningham GFR, et al. Effects of testosterone in older men. *N Engl J Med.* 2016;374:611–624.

44. Lee JH, Lee JE, Harsh V, et al. Pharmacotherapy for sexual dysfunction in women. *Curr Psychiatry Rep.* 2022;24:99–109.

45. Nurnberg HG, Hensley PL, Heiman JR, et al. Sildenafil treatment of women with antidepressant-associated sexual dysfunction: a randomized controlled trial. *JAMA.* 2008;300:395–404.

46. Dording CM, Sangermano L. Female sexual dysfunction: Natural and complementary treatments. *Focus (Am Psychiatr Publ).* 2018;16:19–23.

47. Cummings SR, Ettinger B, Delmas PD, et al. The effects of tibolone in older postmenopausal women. *N Engl J Med.* 2008;359 697-670.

48. Weinberger JM, Houman J, Caron AT, et al. Female sexual dysfunction: a systematic review of outcomes across various treatment modalities. *Sex Med Rev.* 2019;7:223–250.

49. Assumpção AA, Garcia FD, Garcia HD, et al. Pharmacologic treatment of paraphilias. *Psychiatr Clin North Am.* 2014;37:173–181.

50. Bizic MR, Jeftovic M, Pusica S, et al. Gender dysphoria: bioethical aspects of medical treatment. *Biomed Res Int.* 2018;2018:9652305.

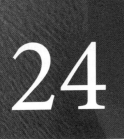

24

THE PSYCHIATRIC MANAGEMENT OF PATIENTS WITH CARDIAC DISEASE

JULIANA ZAMBRANO, MD, MPH ■ SCOTT R. BEACH, MD ■ CHRISTOPHER M. CELANO, MD ■ JEFFERY C. HUFFMAN, MD ■ JAMES L. JANUZZI, JR., MD, FACC, FESC ■ THEODORE A. STERN, MD

OVERVIEW

Caring for patients with cardiac conditions can present a host of dilemmas for the general hospital psychiatrist. Moreover, care is often complicated when those with psychiatric conditions also exhibit cardiac symptoms, when psychotropic agents induce electrocardiographic abnormalities, and when psychiatric symptoms result from cardiac conditions. Because the overlap between psychiatry and cardiology is so great, knowledge of ways to manage specific problems can be of tremendous benefit. For instance, knowing how to deal with chest pain in the setting of a psychiatric syndrome, an electrocardiographic complication from a psychotropic medication, or delirium due to cerebral hypoperfusion, can facilitate comprehensive and compassionate care.

This chapter focuses on the core psychiatric syndromes and issues that arise in those with cardiac conditions: anxiety, depression, delirium, severe mental illness, and management of psychiatric medications and their cardiac side effects. For each of the disorders, we will consider epidemiology, clinical manifestations, differential diagnosis, psychopharmacologic approaches, and practical management strategies for patients with cardiac disease in the general hospital. Additional information relevant to the interface between psychiatric and cardiac care will also be provided in other chapters.

ANXIETY IN PATIENTS WITH CARDIAC CONDITIONS

The assessment of anxiety in patients with cardiac issues is often complex. First, it may be difficult to ascertain whether the patient is experiencing distress as a result of a myocardial event, an acute confusional state, a primary anxiety disorder, or a complex interaction among these factors. Furthermore, anxiety may result from an adjustment reaction to a serious cardiac event, the physiologic sequelae of myocardial dysfunction, or the anxiogenic effects of cardiac medications. Among inpatients, the threshold for the treatment of anxiety tends to be lower than it is in the outpatient setting.

Epidemiology

Anxiety in Patients With Cardiac Problems

Anxiety is common in patients with cardiovascular (CV) disease, such as coronary artery disease (CAD) or heart failure (HF). Following an acute coronary syndrome (ACS), 20% to 30% of patients experience elevated levels of anxiety, and 10% to 14% have anxiety levels higher than in the average psychiatric inpatient.[1] Half of these patients continue to experience anxiety 1 year after their cardiac event, suggesting that many have an underlying anxiety disorder. Similarly, clinically significant anxiety occurs in up to one-fourth of patients awaiting coronary artery bypass grafting (CABG), although in most cases this anxiety resolves within 3 months of the procedure.[2] Anxiety is also highly prevalent in patients with more chronic cardiac conditions, such as HF, where 28% experience clinically significant anxiety and 13% meet the criteria for an anxiety disorder.[3]

Patients who receive invasive cardiac devices (e.g., implantable cardioverter defibrillators [ICDs] and left ventricular assist devices), may also experience anxiety, panic, and fear, oftentimes associated with these devices. A systematic review suggested that clinically significant anxiety arises in 27% to 63% of patients before ICD implantation and in 8% to 59% of patients after ICD placement.[4]

Anxiety Disorders in Patients With Cardiac Conditions

In addition to high levels of free-floating anxiety, patients with cardiac problems also develop formal anxiety disorders, with rates of approximately 15.5% in a recent meta-analysis.[5] Generalized anxiety disorder (GAD) is commonly encountered in patients with CV disease. Among patients hospitalized for an ACS, arrhythmia, or HF, GAD was as common as major depressive disorder (MDD).[1] GAD has also been found in 8% of patients with CAD,[5] a substantially higher prevalence than in the general population.

Patients with CV disease frequently develop panic disorder (PD). In a systematic review and meta-analysis of 29 studies, the prevalence of PD was 6.8%. Other studies have suggested that patients with CAD have PD at approximately four times the rate of those in the general population.[6] While some patients with PD and chest pain may not have underlying structural cardiac disease, clinicians must remain open to the possibility of co-morbid cardiac illness in this patient population.

Finally, patients with cardiac problems who experience life-threatening events (e.g., intensive care, cardiac arrest) as traumatic during their hospitalization may exhibit symptoms of post-traumatic stress disorder (PTSD). Recent studies have found that 8% to 16% of patients who sustain a myocardial infarction (MI) develop symptoms of PTSD; such symptoms also arise at a similar rate among patients who undergo CABG.[7] Some studies have suggested that PTSD may be even more prevalent among cardiac patients in intensive

care units (ICUs). Finally, patients who have received an ICD also appear to be at higher risk for PTSD. In this population, 10% to 25% have elevated PTSD symptoms[8] and approximately 8% meet criteria for PTSD. PTSD may result specifically from the firing of their automatic implantable cardioverter defibrillator (AICD), which has been compared to being kicked in the chest by a mule.

Association Between Anxiety and Cardiac Illness

Anxiety and anxiety disorders may also be associated with an increased risk of developing CV disease and having poor cardiac outcomes, although the evidence for these relationships is not as strong as that for depression. Epidemiologic studies suggest that cardiac illness may lead to increased anxiety and that anxiety may also exacerbate cardiac illness. Both acute and chronic emotional stress have been linked to the development of ventricular arrhythmias and the exacerbation of silent myocardial ischemia.[9]

Among those without pre-existing heart disease, anxiety has been associated with the development of CAD. In a meta-analysis involving 249,846 healthy individuals, anxious persons were at significantly elevated risk for the development of CAD and for cardiac-related mortality over the next 11 years, independent of health behaviors and sociodemographic and medical covariates.[10] This suggests that among healthy individuals, significantly elevated levels of anxiety may be associated with physiologic changes that predispose to a higher risk for the development and progression of CAD.

Among patients with established heart disease, the association between anxiety and CV outcomes is less clear. Among individuals with CAD, anxiety is associated with higher rates of adverse cardiac events and mortality in unadjusted analyses.[11] However, after adjusting for potential confounding variables, the relationships were less clear. While one recent meta-analysis found that anxiety was associated with increased risks of both short- and long-term cardiac events following MI,[12] a second study found that the relationships between anxiety and CV outcomes were present in individuals with stable CAD but not in those whose anxiety was assessed within 2 months of the cardiac event.[11] Among patients with HF, prospective, observational studies have failed to find a significant relationship between anxiety (as a symptom) and mortality when controlling for relevant medical and psychological covariates.[13] Taken together, these findings suggest that while anxiety may be a useful marker for poor outcomes in patients with heart disease, its relationship with health outcomes may be accounted for by other psychiatric, medical, and sociodemographic factors.

While the relationship between anxiety and cardiac outcomes is not entirely clear, there is evidence that specific anxiety disorders are associated with adverse cardiac outcomes. When anxiety reaches the threshold of a disorder, it is more persistent, pervasive, and limiting, and carries a more significant risk in terms of cardiac outcomes. GAD has also been associated with higher rates of smoking, diabetes, and hypercholesterolemia, which may increase the risk of developing CV diseases. Following MI, GAD has been associated with higher mortality and cardiac re-admission rates.[14] Similarly, in patients with stable CAD, GAD diagnosis predicts major cardiac events in the subsequent 2 years.[10] PD also has been associated with the development and progression of CV disease. In a systematic review and meta-regression involving >1 million patients, PD was associated with incident CAD, MI, and major adverse cardiac events.[15,16]

While less research has been completed on the relationship between PTSD and cardiac health, preliminary evidence suggests that PTSD may be harmful to cardiac health. PTSD has been associated with an increased incidence of CAD and HF, independent of relevant medical factors.[17,18] In patients who have experienced an ACS, PTSD has been linked to a greater risk of major adverse cardiac events and all-cause mortality.[19]

In sum, cardiac patients have high rates of situational anxiety and formal anxiety disorders (e.g., PD, GAD, and PTSD). While the links between anxiety (as a symptom) and CV outcomes remain unclear, anxiety disorders have been associated with an increased risk of developing cardiac disease, as well as worse cardiac outcomes and higher rates of mortality in patients with established cardiac disease. This highlights the importance of identifying and treating these disorders in a timely fashion in those at risk for, or with, existing CV disease.

The Differential Diagnosis of Anxiety in Patients With Cardiac Problems

Anxiety experienced in the general hospital is often due to a primary psychiatric problem caused by stressful medical events. However, anxiety in patients with cardiac problems can also be caused by myriad medications and general medical conditions that are commonly associated with cardiac care (Table 24.1).

Not uncommonly, cardiac events cause anxiety. Myocardial ischemia, arrhythmias, and HF can each cause anxiety owing to the sympathetic discharge associated with these conditions *and* because of what they may represent to the patient (e.g., the fear of dying, the worsening of medical illness, the loss of role identity). Other general medical conditions may cause or exacerbate anxiety; important among these is pulmonary embolism in the sedentary cardiac patient. Anxiety may also be a medication side effect (e.g., of sympathomimetics). Anxiety can also result from substance intoxication or withdrawal that may cause or exacerbate acute cardiac issues (e.g., cocaine intoxication, and alcohol withdrawal). Finally, impaired sleep in the hospital (as the result of an unfamiliar setting, frequent medical interventions, and significant noise) can lead to or exacerbate anxiety.

TABLE 24.1

Selected Medical Causes of Anxiety Among Cardiac Patients in the General Hospital

Cardiac Events
Myocardial ischemia
Atrial and ventricular arrhythmias
Congestive heart failure

Other Medical Conditions
Pulmonary embolism
Asthma/chronic obstructive pulmonary disease exacerbation
Hyperthyroidism
Hypoglycemia
Delirium

Medications
Sympathomimetics
Thyroid hormone
Bronchodilators
Stimulants
Corticosteroids

Illicit Substances
Cocaine or amphetamine intoxication
Alcohol or benzodiazepine withdrawal

The general hospital psychiatrist should consider general medical causes of anxiety when evaluating patients with cardiac problems; this is especially true when anxiety has developed during an uneventful hospitalization, when the patient has no history of anxiety, or when anxiety persists despite appropriate treatment.

Approach to the Anxious Patient With Cardiac Problems

The psychiatric consultant is frequently called to cardiology services to assess and treat anxiety. A careful, stepwise approach to these consultations can ensure that an accurate diagnosis and appropriate treatment can be made and delivered.

Consider a Broad Differential Diagnosis for the Patient's Distress. A primary role of the general hospital psychiatrist is to accurately characterize a patient's distress as anxiety, denial, depression, delirium, or another psychiatric phenomenon. Patients who appear anxious and tremulous may, in fact, be disoriented, paranoid, and frightened—that is, delirious. Therefore the consultant should be careful in the interview to assess affect, behavior, and cognition. If the patient's primary psychiatric symptom appears to be anxiety, the consultant should then consider the potential contribution of medications or medical symptoms to this anxiety. As noted earlier, there is a long list of conditions that can cause or exacerbate anxiety, and the consultant should carefully consider these and recommend appropriate diagnostic studies, if appropriate. It may be especially useful to identify correlations between anxiety levels and the initiation or discontinuation of potentially offending medications or substances. Finally, generating an accurate timeline of the onset and progression of anxiety symptoms is essential to determining whether the anxiety arose in the setting of a cardiac event or whether the patient has a long-standing anxiety disorder—this distinction may influence prognosis and guide treatment recommendations.

Evaluate Sources of Anxiety and Assess How the Patient Has Dealt With Difficult Situations Before. A careful psychiatric interview of the anxious patient will help determine what factors are causing his or her anxiety. Is the patient awaiting CABG surgery anxious because a relative died during cardiac surgery

years ago? Is the patient with an AICD fearful that his defibrillator will discharge again? By determining the sources of anxiety, the consultant will be able to address these worries through education, reassurance, medication, or brief psychotherapy.

A related task is to determine the patient's coping style and coping strengths. How does he or she manage anxiety outside of the hospital? How has he or she managed difficult situations in the past? The consultant can use this information to identify the patient's strengths and determine the best approach to the patient's concerns and fears.

Another question for patients involves stimulation and control. Some individuals with cardiac problems crave control and wish to know every detail of their care; they feel anxious when they lack comprehensive information about their illness and when they are not part of all treatment decisions. In contrast, other patients find such information and the pressure to make decisions over-stimulating and feel less anxious when told only the general details of their condition.

Recommend Appropriate Behavioral and Therapeutic Interventions. Having learned about the patient's sources of anxiety, coping strengths, and preferences regarding control, the consultant is in an excellent position to design a treatment plan that reduces the patient's anxiety. For example, if a patient reports that the hospitalization is overwhelming, members of the treatment team can be encouraged to limit detailed information and reassure the patient that they see this condition frequently (if true) and that they plan to provide excellent care to the patient. On the other hand, for the patient whose anxiety increases with the perceived lack of control, the treatment team can be encouraged to provide the patient with detailed information and written materials. The patient should also be included in treatment decisions; inclusion in even small decisions (e.g., the best time for dressing changes) can allay anxiety and allow the patient to feel in control.

In other cases, patients who are worried simply need to express their anxieties to someone. If the consultant, treating physician, and nursing staff can set aside short periods to reflectively listen to the patient's fears, this time investment often results in significantly less anxiety, greater adherence to treatment, and less chaos for the patient and staff alike. If the patient seems to have an insatiable desire to discuss his or her fears, staff can consistently set aside time to listen to the patient while setting limits on his or her time; for example, a nurse may tell the patient that she will sit with him or her for 5 minutes at the beginning, middle, and end of the shift to talk about his or her worries. If the patient attempts to engage the nurse in further conversation about this topic, the nurse can calmly tell the patient that they can discuss it at their next visit.

Thoughtfully Use Psychiatric Medications to Treat Specific Target Symptoms. Agents used to treat anxiety in the general hospital include benzodiazepines, antidepressants, and antipsychotics. *Please refer to the section on Critical Issues in at the end of the chapter for a more in-depth discussion.*

Benzodiazepines are commonly used to treat anxiety in those hospitalized with cardiac problems. These medications rapidly relieve anxiety and have several beneficial CV effects. Although some clinicians shy away from the use of benzodiazepines due to their perceived risks, they can typically be used safely over the short term with good effects. If the anxiety appears to be situation specific (e.g., whenever a procedure is performed), a rapidly acting and short-to-moderate-lasting benzodiazepine can be used on an as-needed basis (e.g., lorazepam 0.5–1.0 mg as needed for acute anxiety). However, for most patients, longer-lasting benzodiazepines that are given on a standing basis provide the smoothest and most consistent path to anxiety reduction. Most anxious patients with cardiac problems can be started on clonazepam 0.5 mg at night or twice per day; doses can be titrated upward if this dose is well tolerated and anxiety persists. In general, these agents can be discontinued on hospital discharge if they are only used on a short-term basis.

Benzodiazepines may not be the agents of choice for those with acute or chronic organic brain syndromes (e.g., delirium, dementia, traumatic brain injury), tenuous respiratory function (including obstructive sleep apnea), or a history of substance use disorders. For these patients low-dose antipsychotics or gabapentin are often useful, alleviating agitation and confusion in delirious patients while also reducing anxiety. Dosing of quetiapine (at 12.5–25 mg at night) or gabapentin (at 100 mg three times daily) is often initiated. Although

no antipsychotics have received US Food and Drug Administration (FDA) approval for use in anxiety disorders, their use as an adjunctive treatment for anxiety in non-medical populations is now standard clinical practice. These agents may also offer additional benefits for the management of co-morbid delirium, and they do not induce the paradoxical disinhibition that is sometimes associated with the use of benzodiazepines. However, antipsychotics can cause orthostasis and anticholinergic effects (most often associated with low-potency agents), and many are associated with prolongation of the corrected QT (QTc) interval. Most atypical antipsychotic agents also increase the risk of weight gain and metabolic derangements, which may further predispose patients to adverse cardiac outcomes.

Both gabapentin and pregabalin have been used for the acute treatment of anxiety. They have essentially no risk of physiologic dependence and do not cause orthostasis or anticholinergic effects. However, their efficacy in the treatment of acute anxiety in patients hospitalized for cardiac problems has not been formally studied.

Antidepressants may be useful in the treatment of primary anxiety disorders and when depression is co-morbid with anxiety, although no randomized clinical trials (RCTs) have examined this. Notably, these agents often take several weeks to work and are best used to treat primary anxiety disorders (e.g., PD, GAD, or PTSD). For acutely anxious patients with cardiac problems, it is often wise to co-administer a benzodiazepine when antidepressants are prescribed, to acutely reduce anxiety during a vulnerable CV state.

Return Frequently to See the Patient. Anxious patients are, in general, relieved to see a familiar face, especially one who has attempted to understand and address their anxiety. Such frequent follow-up, which is itself therapeutic, allows for careful monitoring of behavioral and pharmacological interventions.

Case 1

Mr. A, a 53-year-old executive without a psychiatric history, was admitted for CABG after his cardiac catheterization revealed three-vessel cardiac disease. Initially, he had an uneventful perioperative course.

However, on the day after his operation, psychiatry was consulted to assess his capacity to leave the hospital against medical advice.

On interview, Mr. A was alert, oriented, lucid, and initially quite angry. He reported, "I have no assurance that I'm getting the right care; the doctors and nurses come in and out of my room and bark orders to one another, but they don't include me at all. They haven't even listened to the fact that I always take my sleeping pill at 9 p.m. every night instead of 11 p.m. like they give it to me. I'm fed up." By the end of his tirade, Mr. A's anger had changed to fear and anxiety.

The consultant told Mr. A that he would bring his concerns to the team. The consultant met with members of the treatment team and encouraged them to provide as much information as possible about his care and to allow him to contribute to some aspects of his treatment when possible (e.g., getting his sleeping pill at 9 p.m.). The consultant, nurse, and Mr. A then met together so that Mr. A could express his concerns and the nurse and consultant could outline the ways their procedures would change so that he could have more information and more control. Mr. A agreed to this plan and agreed to use clonazepam (0.5 mg twice per day) to reduce his anxiety.

The consultant checked back frequently with Mr. A to assess his response to this treatment plan. Small changes in the plan were instituted at his request, and his anxiety steadily decreased. He was discharged to cardiac rehabilitation after 3 days without a prescription for clonazepam and he thanked the nursing staff for their "compassionate care."

DEPRESSION IN PATIENTS WITH CARDIAC PROBLEMS

Over the past few decades, substantive research has firmly established a bidirectional link between depression and cardiac disease; patients with depression are more likely to develop cardiac disease, and patients with cardiac disease are more likely to suffer from depression.[18] Multiple studies have also demonstrated that patients with depression and cardiac disease have worse outcomes than those without depression. These findings underscore the importance of the general

hospital psychiatrist's role in identifying depression in patients with cardiac problems and considering appropriate treatments.

Depression in Patients With Established Cardiac Illness

Depression is common among patients with CAD, with prevalence rates of MDD hovering around 20%.[20] This rate of MDD is greater than the prevalence of depression in the general population (which is approximately 10%–15%), and it is even higher for those with more serious cardiac disease. Roughly 15% to 30% of post-ACS patients; 20% to 35% of patients with HF; and 24% to 33% of patients with an AICD meet criteria for MDD.[21,22] Rates of suicidal ideation are also increased among patients with cardiac disease.[23] Furthermore, studies indicate that most patients who are found to have MDD during a cardiac hospitalization have a history of MDD that predates their cardiac event, and depressive symptoms often persist following discharge,[24] with more than half of patients with post-ACS depression remaining depressed after 1 year.

Despite the high prevalence of MDD and the risks it carries for cardiac patients, fewer than 15% of post-MI depressed patients are recognized as such.[25] Several factors likely account for these low rates of recognition. The pattern of depression (with hostility, listlessness, and withdrawal being more common than sad mood) is often somewhat atypical. Furthermore, depression is often seen as a normal consequence of having a serious medical event, such as an ACS. Finally, most patients with ACS have brief inpatient stays, and it may be difficult to assess a patient's mood or to obtain psychiatric consultation during this brief time frame.

In short, depression is common among patients with cardiac conditions, and it has been best studied in those with recent ACS. In inpatient cardiology services, depression is highly prevalent, frequently persistent, and under-recognized by clinicians.

Depression as a Risk Factor for Cardiac Disease

Evidence from many community studies over the past 20 years indicates that depression is an independent risk factor for CV disease. Several studies have found that patients with depressive symptoms are 1.5 to 3.5 times more likely to have an ACS than those without such symptoms, while those with MDD have an even greater risk.[26] This increased vulnerability holds true for females as well as for those >65. In a meta-analysis, van der Kooy and colleagues examined 28 relevant studies comprising more than 80,000 subjects and demonstrated that depression was associated with an increased risk of CV disease (risk ratio 1.46).[27] This analysis found that the strongest association was made when patients were diagnosed by a clinical interview and that studies using depression scales demonstrated a dose-response relationship between depressed mood and the development of CV disease.

In addition to predicting the development of CAD in healthy people, depression has also been associated with significantly higher rates of cardiac death and overall mortality among those with established CAD. Numerous studies have found that depressive symptoms after ACS are associated with higher rates of morbidity and mortality in the subsequent 5 years. These effects on mortality appear to be largely independent of the severity of cardiac disease, demographic variables, medications, or other confounding factors. Bush and colleagues found that even minimal depressive symptoms were associated with an elevated risk of cardiac mortality, although more severe depressive symptoms more strongly predicted cardiac mortality.[28] A meta-analysis of 22 studies of post-MI subjects found that post-MI depression was associated with a 2- to 2.5-fold increased risk of negative CV outcomes.[29] Patients experiencing a first episode of depression in the aftermath of an ACS may be at the highest risk for negative cardiac outcomes. Considering this overwhelming evidence, the American Heart Association identified depression as a risk factor for adverse events following an ACS.[30]

Depressive symptoms also appear to predict cardiac morbidity and mortality in other cardiac populations. In depressed patients hospitalized for cardiac illness, each additional point on the Patient Health Questionnaire-9 (PHQ-9) depression rating scale was independently associated with a 9% greater risk of cardiac re-admission over the next 6 months.[31] Pre-CABG depressive symptoms have also been associated with an increase in cardiac morbidity at 6- or 12-month follow-up.[32] Among patients undergoing cardiac transplantation, persistent depression was associated with higher rates of incident CAD and mortality.[33] Depression is a risk factor for incident HF, and several studies have shown that depression predicts higher mortality, independent of demographic factors or clinical status.[34] Patients with depression at the time of AICD placement have higher rates of all-cause mortality over the subsequent 4 years, and depressed patients with atrial fibrillation (AF) have higher rates of recurrence following cardioversion.[35]

Numerous mechanisms have been offered to explain the link between depression and CV disease. Behavioral hypotheses include poor health habits (e.g., smoking, lack of exercise) and non-adherence to medical care. Depressed patients appear to have less adherence to medication regimens, and depressed cardiac patients attend cardiac rehabilitation programs less often than their non-depressed peers. Furthermore, patients who are depressed after ACS are less likely to follow recommendations about diet, exercise, and smoking cessation.[20]

Proposed physiologic mediators of the links between depression and worsened outcomes in cardiac disease include inflammation, endothelial dysfunction, platelet activation and aggregation, and autonomic nervous system dysfunction. Specifically, depression has been linked to elevated blood levels of markers of inflammation (e.g., C-reactive protein [CRP], interleukin-6) and endothelial dysfunction (e.g., endothelin-1), increased platelet aggregation, reduced heart-rate variability (a marker of increased sympathetic and reduced parasympathetic activity), elevated levels of catecholamines, and exaggerated catecholamine responses to stress. These physiologic changes may increase stress on the heart and have been linked to poor CV outcomes. Perhaps the most obvious example of the link between depression, increased sympathetic drive, and cardiac illness is the phenomenon of stress (Takotsubo) cardiomyopathy, in which negative psychological factors, such as depression, grief, or acute loss can directly lead to a reversible cardiomyopathy that mimics an acute MI and can be fatal.[36]

The link between depression in cardiac patients and increased cardiac morbidity is likely mediated by multiple factors. One crucial, yet unanswered, question is whether treatment of depression among cardiac patients improves cardiac prognosis. While most RCTs have failed to find a significant association between antidepressant use and CV outcomes,[20] they were not powered to do so and had relatively short follow-up periods.

More recent registry-based studies have suggested that depression treatment leads to improved health outcomes, and a recent meta-analysis of eight RCTs of 1148 post-ACS patients with depression found a 44% lower risk of non-fatal MI in patients treated with antidepressants.[37] Finally, data from the EsDEPACS study, a randomized, placebo-controlled trial of escitalopram for the management of post-ACS depression, found that individuals randomized to receive escitalopram had a significantly lower risk of major adverse cardiac events over a 12-year follow-up period.[38]

Differential Diagnosis of Depression in Patients With Cardiac Problems

As with anxiety, there are several medical conditions and medications that can cause or exacerbate depressive symptoms in those with cardiac problems. Table 24.2 lists several medical influences on mood. Common conditions associated with depressed mood in those with cardiac problems include hypothyroidism (both idiopathic and secondary to amiodarone, which is frequently prescribed to cardiac patients), Cushing syndrome (Cushing disease or symptoms secondary to steroid administration), neoplasm (especially pancreatic cancer), vitamin B_{12} and folate deficiencies,

TABLE 24.2
Selected Medical Causes or Mimics of Depression Among Cardiac Patients in the General Hospital

Medical Conditions
Hypothyroidism (idiopathic or amiodarone induced)
Cushing syndrome
Vitamin B_{12} or folate deficiency
Neoplasm (especially pancreatic, lung, or central nervous system tumors)
Major neurocognitive disorder
Hypoactive delirium (mimic)
Movement disorders (e.g., Parkinson disease or Huntington disease)

Medications
Methyldopa
Reserpine
Corticosteroids
Interferon

Illicit Substances
Chronic alcohol or benzodiazepine abuse
Cocaine or amphetamine withdrawal

hypoactive delirium, and depressive symptoms associated with major neurocognitive disorders. Substances can also influence mood; chronic alcohol use and withdrawal from cocaine or amphetamines commonly lead to depression. β-Blockers have long been associated with depression; however, that connection has recently been re-examined.

Because depression can have significant effects on cardiac and psychosocial outcomes in cardiac patients and because the causes of depression are often reversible or treatable, the general hospital psychiatrist should consider these in all depressed cardiac patients.

Approach to the Management of the Depressed Cardiac Patient

The approach to the depressed cardiac patient is in many ways like the approach to the anxious cardiac patient. The consultant must first confirm that depression is the primary psychiatric symptom and evaluate for co-morbid psychiatric conditions. Furthermore, the psychiatrist must consider the presence of medical conditions or medications that can cause or exacerbate mood symptoms. Once these steps have been completed, an approach to treatment involves the identification of the patient's coping strengths and support network; it may also involve weighing the risks and benefits of antidepressant treatment.

Routine Screening

One of the biggest obstacles to diagnosing depression in patients with cardiac disease is the failure to adequately screen. Since 2008, the American Heart Association has recommended routine screening for depression using the PHQ-2 and PHQ-9 in patients with cardiac disease in all settings.[39] Given the resource burden and lack of evidence that screening alone improves outcomes, we recommend screening only in the setting of adequate treatment options. It is important to remember that patients with cardiac problems are also at increased risk for thoughts of suicide, and screening for thoughts of suicide is a crucial component of depression screening.

Consider Appropriate Psychiatric and Medical Differential Diagnoses

A positive screen for depression should be followed by consideration of alternative explanations. As with consultations on cardiac floors for apparent anxiety, we also find that consultations for apparent depression often reveal that a patient's distress is caused by another psychiatric syndrome, such as hypoactive delirium or somatic symptoms secondary to cardiac illness. Demoralization is exceedingly common in cardiac patients and can mimic depression, with prominent neurovegetative symptoms, hopelessness, and helplessness. However, demoralized patients are rarely anhedonic. Distinguishing demoralization from depression in patients with cardiac problems is of utmost importance because demoralization responds to supportive therapy and education, but not to antidepressant medications.

The consultant should also note the course of depressive symptoms to see if the onset or worsening of such symptoms correlates with the administration of a new medication or new physical symptoms or if there are other indications that a physical disorder might be implicated in the evolution of the depressive symptoms. The general hospital psychiatrist should also order laboratory tests and other studies as indicated.

Attempt to Identify the Patient's Coping Style and the Triggers for Depressive Symptoms

Determining the external factors that exacerbate depressive symptoms may help the consultant reduce the patient's stressors. The consultant can use this information to implement solutions that are psychotherapeutic in nature (e.g., discussing mortality and life goals) or more concrete (e.g., having family members call the patient to let him know he is missed and important to them). Identification of the patient's coping strengths—especially, how the patient has previously managed difficult situations—will inform the treatment team's approach to the patient.

Make Use of Existing Social Supports or Help Develop a Network

Social support has been associated with superior medical outcomes in depressed patients after MI; therefore, if such social support does not exist, the consultant can work with the treatment team to consider options to improve the patient's support system. Such options could include participation in cardiac rehabilitation, having visiting nurses, or joining a support group.

Carefully Consider the Use of Medication

Please refer to the section on Critical Issues in Psychopharmacology and Cardiac Health at the end of the chapter for a more in-depth discussion. Antidepressants are effective in the treatment of depression for patients with CAD. Selective serotonin reuptake inhibitors (SSRIs), particularly sertraline, appear to be both safe and effective for patients with CAD, with few CV side effects. SSRIs appear to be less effective for the treatment of depression in the setting of HF. Two large RCTs found SSRIs to be equivalent to placebo for reducing depressive symptoms, although both studies enrolled patients with moderate to severe HF, and most patients did not have a history of MDD, raising questions as to whether their symptoms could have been attributed to HF alone.[40,41] Citalopram may carry a slightly higher risk of QTc prolongation and therefore should be used more thoughtfully in this population. Bupropion also has few drug-drug interactions and may be the agent of choice in patients with co-morbid MDD and a desire to stop smoking. Mirtazapine is also an appropriate alternative in some cases, as it has few effects on cardiac conduction or vital signs, but may cause weight gain, which may be important to monitor in this population.

The risks and benefits of antidepressant medications should be more carefully considered in patients with recent MI and probably by extension all patients with severe cardiac disease. For most patients who have just had an MI or a CABG, we typically do not prescribe antidepressants for the onset of depressive symptoms within days after having an MI, both because such patients have not yet met the criteria for MDD and because extensive data establishing the safety of these agents in the post-MI or post-cardiac surgery period do not exist. These patients should be encouraged to follow-up with a psychiatrist for further monitoring; alternatively, direct coordination with their primary care physician or cardiologist may allow for repeat screening in 2 weeks, with a plan for intervention, if indicated. For patients who have evidence of pre-existing but untreated MDD, however, initiation of an SSRI in the immediate post-ACS period may be indicated. Severe depression that impairs one's ability to adequately participate in rehabilitation or self-care, or the return of depressive symptoms in a patient with a history of severe depression, may also be indications for more aggressive medication treatment. If available, involvement in collaborative care or blended care programs also appears to be an excellent treatment strategy for patients.

Psychostimulants have also been shown to be rapidly acting and efficacious antidepressants in medically hospitalized patients. Although they may slightly elevate blood pressure or heart rate, stimulants may be indicated in cardiac patients whose depression requires rapid treatment (e.g., depression that is severe, is negatively affecting rehabilitation owing to anergia or minimal oral intake, or that is affecting the patient's capacity to make medical decisions). Stimulants are relatively contraindicated in patients with a history of ventricular tachycardia (VT), current angina, recent MI, HF, uncontrolled hypertension, or persistent tachycardia.

Other Treatment Modalities for the Depressed Cardiac Patient

Several studies have also examined the efficacy of psychotherapy to treat depression in cardiac patients. Though both cognitive-behavioral therapy and interpersonal therapy have been shown to reduce depressive symptoms in patients with cardiac disease, the effects are typically short lived.[42]

Increasing evidence suggests that collaborative care, stepped care, and blended care models are highly effective in treating depression in cardiac populations. These programs use a non-physician care manager to identify and monitor psychiatric conditions while transmitting care recommendations from a study team psychiatrist to primary medical providers. Both pharmacologic and psychotherapeutic approaches are often utilized. Collaborative care programs have been successful for depressed patients undergoing CABG, for patients with recent ACS or HF, and even when started in the hospital during admission for an acute cardiac illness. In addition to improving depression, these programs have been shown to be cost-effective and possibly even cost-saving, and they have resulted in reduced rates of cardiac readmissions and death in some studies.[42]

Case 2

Ms. B, a 52-year-old female with a history of MDD, was admitted to the hospital with chest pain. Her electrocardiogram (ECG) showed ST-segment depression in the anterolateral leads, her cardiac enzymes were elevated, and she was diagnosed as having an MI. Although she had not been depressed in the year before admission, she developed depressive symptoms in the days after her MI; psychiatric consultation was obtained.

On interview, Ms. B was dysphoric but alert, oriented, and able to actively engage in conversation with the interviewer. She reported depressed mood, anhedonia, and low energy, along with disturbed concentration and appetite; she denied significant anxiety. She denied feeling suicidal or being unable to care for herself. Ms. B reported one episode of relatively mild MDD 3 years earlier that responded well to sertraline (100 mg/day for 1 year); she had also had several episodes of "feeling low" for 3 to 5 days that spontaneously resolved. She appeared to be invested in getting better, had a strong social support network, and planned to follow up with her cardiologist shortly after her hospitalization.

Given Ms. B's relatively mild current depressive symptoms, her history of having only one mild episode of MDD, and her ability and willingness to follow up with her cardiologist, the consultant decided to defer antidepressant treatment while Ms. B was in the hospital. The consultant contacted Ms. B's cardiologist and they agreed that sertraline should be started (given Ms. B's history of good response to this medication) if she continued to be depressed at the follow-up appointment in 2 weeks.

Ms. B had an uneventful medical course and was discharged 3 days after her MI. She followed up in 2 weeks with her cardiologist; she remained depressed and was started on sertraline. She tolerated the sertraline (ultimately titrated to 100 mg per day) well, and her depressive symptoms subsided over the next 8 weeks.

DELIRIUM IN CARDIAC PATIENTS

Despite advances in the treatment of cardiac illness and the use of non-invasive procedures, general hospital patients with cardiac disease continue to suffer delirium at high rates (ranging from 3% to 72% depending on the specific illness and type of procedure).[43] The general hospital psychiatrist should be aware of the special issues in the diagnosis and management of delirium in cardiac patients.

Epidemiology

Reports of risk factors for the development of delirium in cardiac patients have varied, but it is universally agreed that the etiology of delirium in cardiac patients is multi-factorial, with different factors varying in importance from patient to patient. Pre-morbid risk factors for delirium include a history of MI or stroke, diabetes, aortic insufficiency, decreased cardiac output, dehydration, electrolyte imbalance, and the use of anticholinergic drugs. Hospital risk factors include sleep deprivation, use of narcotic and anticholinergic or sedative-hypnotic medications, and medication toxicity (e.g., from digoxin). Patients undergoing cardiac procedures, including surgery, may also be at elevated risk. Intraoperatively, the use of on-pump CABG surgery is associated with an increased rate of intracerebral micro-emboli and dysfunction of several neurotransmitter systems (serotonergic, noradrenergic, dopaminergic, and anticholinergic), which may contribute to delirium. Delirium in cardiac patients has been associated with longer ICU stays, ICU re-admission, longer hospital stays, a greater prevalence of falls, a greater chance of discharge to a nursing facility, and an increased mortality rate at 30 days and 1 year. Older individuals who develop delirium in the setting of cardiac surgery have poorer short-term function in terms of independent activities of daily living (ADLs).

Differential Diagnosis of Delirium in the Cardiac Patient

In the delirious cardiac patient, several specific causes should be carefully considered (Table 24.3). Central nervous system (CNS) hypoperfusion is a common mechanism of delirium in the cardiac population; this can result from poor cardiac output caused by HF or myocardial ischemia, from co-morbid carotid disease, from CNS bleeding (in the setting of anticoagulation), or relative hypotension.

Other common causes of delirium in cardiac patients include hypoxia during HF, hypertensive encephalopathy, electrolyte abnormalities (e.g., hyponatremia in the context of diuretic therapy), medication effects, and substance withdrawal. The general

---

TABLE 24.3

Selected Causes of Delirium Among Cardiac Patients in the General Hospital

Central Nervous System Hypoperfusion
Myocardial infarction/ischemia
Cerebrovascular accident (ischemic or hemorrhagic)
Hypovolemia (due to dehydration or bleeding)
Relative hypotension

Other Medical Conditions
Electrolyte abnormalities (especially sodium with diuretic administration)
Thyroid abnormalities
Hypertensive encephalopathy
Hypoxia (during pulmonary edema)
Infections (e.g., pneumonia, urinary tract infections)
Alcohol withdrawal
Cardiopulmonary bypass

Medication-Related Causes
Digoxin toxicity
Narcotic analgesics
Benzodiazepines
Anticholinergic medications

---

hospital psychiatrist should rule out each of these potential etiologies of delirium in the cardiac patient.

The Practical Management of the Delirious Cardiac Patient

As with other conditions involving cardiac patients, the management of delirium involves careful diagnosis and consideration of co-morbid conditions. Once the diagnosis and etiology have been established, the general hospital psychiatrist can implement optimal behavioral and non-pharmacologic strategies and intelligently use psychotropic agents that reduce medical risk while effectively decreasing symptoms.

Make an Informed Diagnosis of Delirium, and Carefully Consider Potential Etiologies. Delirium is characterized by acute onset, disorientation, poor attention, fluctuation of levels of consciousness, and alterations in the sleep-wake cycle. Psychotic symptoms, anxiety, worry, and reports of depressed mood may be present. A careful review of the chart and cognitive evaluation (that considers orientation, attention, and executive function) can allow the consultant to use these factors to distinguish delirium from other psychiatric illnesses. Once a diagnosis has been made, the psychiatrist should work to consider all possible causes of delirium. The cause of delirium is frequently multi-factorial; therefore, the identification of one potential contributing factor of delirium should not preclude the search for further potential abnormalities leading to an acute confusional state. The consultant should pay special attention to the initiation and termination of medications and their relationship to the onset of delirium; a careful review of nursing medication sheets often reveals a wealth of information that can provide important answers regarding delirium of unknown etiology.

Aggressively Treat All Potential Etiologies of Delirium. Treating the core etiology of delirium is the only way to definitively reverse delirium; all other behavioral and pharmacologic remedies are symptomatic treatments that reduce risk and increase comfort until the primary etiologies of the delirium resolve. Therefore treatment of a urinary tract infection, vitamin B_{12} deficiency, mild metabolic abnormalities, and other seemingly minor contributing factors to delirium is crucial.

Use Non-Pharmacologic Strategies to Minimize Confusion and Ensure Safety. Situating a patient near the nursing station or in other areas where the patient can be monitored frequently can reduce the risk of falls, wandering, or other dangerous actions. Placing the patient in a room with a window and a clock—to help orient him or her to day-night cycles—can also be useful. The use of mittens, sitters, or locked restraints may be required when a delirious patient's inability to safely navigate places him or her at risk; in almost all cases, medication should be given in combination with physical restraint to reduce discomfort and risk of harm while in restraints. The presence of reassuring family members or friends at the bedside can mitigate paranoia and agitation, whereas visitors who over-stimulate the patient may worsen symptoms. The consultant may recommend that the team either encourage or dissuade interaction with certain visitors depending on the response of the patient's symptoms to the visitors. The use of the ABCDEF bundle and early mobilization following surgery has been shown to reduce the rates of delirium in ICU settings.

Use Antipsychotic Medications to Reduce Agitation and Psychotic Symptoms and Regulate the Sleep-Wake Cycle. The use of medications is an important component of a multi-pronged approach to the psychiatric management of delirium.

Large studies have suggested that antipsychotics do not necessarily treat delirium or reduce the amount of time that patients are delirious, but they remain a vital resource for managing the sequelae of delirium. They can reduce agitation and may help normalize the sleep-wake cycle. In addition, they can reduce the risk of patient harm and alleviate patient distress until the etiology is identified and effectively treated. They may also be used to mitigate psychotic symptoms in delirium and therefore reduce the risk of post-delirium PTSD or post-ICU syndrome (PICS). In general, they are quite safe. *Please refer to the section on Critical Issues in Psychopharmacology and Cardiac Health at the end of the chapter for a more in-depth discussion.*

Pharmacologic management should be strongly considered in those with hyperactive delirium or in those with significant psychotic symptoms, such as paranoia or hallucinations. Intravenous (IV) haloperidol remains the "gold standard" for managing delirium. The protocol used at the MGH (Table 24.4) for the use of IV haloperidol considers risk factors for *torsades de pointes* (TdP) and uses a progressive dosing schedule. An initial dose (from 0.5 to 10 mg based on the age and size of the patient and the extent of agitation) is selected and administered to the patient. If the patient is not calm within 20 to 30 minutes, the dose is doubled and continues to be doubled every 20 to 30 minutes until the patient is calm. This effective dose is then used when and if the patient becomes agitated again. Although most patients require standard doses of haloperidol (2–10 mg), some patients have safely received thousands of milligrams for agitation. *Please refer to the section on Critical Issues in Psychopharmacology and Cardiac Health at the end of the chapter for an in-depth discussion of the risk of QTc prolongation and TdP with IV haloperidol.*

Atypical antipsychotics, such as quetiapine and olanzapine, are also commonly used in the management of delirium. Importantly, whereas olanzapine achieves D_2-blockade even at low doses (2.5–5 mg), quetiapine does not and effectively serves as an anti-histaminergic and anticholinergic agent at commonly-used doses of

TABLE 24.4

Massachusetts General Hospital Protocol for IV Haloperidol in Agitated Delirious Patients

Check Pre-Haloperidol QTc Interval and Determine the Presence of Other Risk Factors for TdP

Check Potassium and Magnesium and Correct Abnormalities

Aim for potassium >4 mEq/L, magnesium >2 mEq/L.

Give a Dose of Haloperidol (0.5–10 mg) Based on the Level of Agitation and the Patient's Age and Size

The goal is to have the patient calm and awake.

Haloperidol precipitates with phenytoin and heparin; flush the line before giving haloperidol if these agents have been used in the same intravenous tubing.

Wait 20–30 minutes. If the patient remains agitated, double the dose.

Continue to double the dose every 30 minutes until the patient is calm.

Follow QTc Interval to Ensure That QTc Is Not Prolonging

If QTc increases by 25% or becomes >500 ms, consider alternative treatments.

Once an Effective Dose Has Been Determined, Use That Dose for Future Episodes of Agitation

Depending on the likely course of delirium, may schedule haloperidol or give it on an as-needed basis.

For example, may divide the previous effective dose over the next 24 hours, giving it every 6 hours.

Or may simply give an effective dose as needed for agitation.

Consider a small dose at night to regulate the sleep-wake cycle in all delirious patients.

ECG Monitoring

If the total dose is <5 mg and there are one or no risk factors, no monitoring is needed.

If the total dose is >5 mg OR there are two or more risk factors, check baseline and follow-up ECG.[a]

If the total dose is >25 mg, check a daily ECG.

If the total dose is >100 mg or the QTc >500 ms, use continuous telemetry.

[a]Because the total dose required is often not predictable, baseline and follow-up ECG are reasonable in standard practice for any dose when feasible. *ECG*, Electrocardiogram; *IV*, intravenous; *TdP, torsades de pointes.*

25 to 100 mg. Most antipsychotics carry a risk for QTc prolongation and TdP, with the possible exceptions being aripiprazole and lurasidone. Aside from these two medications, there is no evidence to suggest that atypical antipsychotics have any lower risk of QTc prolongation compared to IV haloperidol, and some (e.g., ziprasidone) likely are associated with a higher risk of QTc prolongation than IV haloperidol. Additionally, antipsychotics may be associated with other side effects, such as orthostasis or tachycardia.

When QTc prolongation or other concerns preclude the use of antipsychotic medications, other second-line medications may be used for the management of delirium in cardiac patients. Valproic acid is often helpful in reducing agitation and frontal disinhibition and is relatively safe in cardiac patients. Usual doses are between 500 and 2000 mg daily, with target levels between 60 and 100. Increasingly, α_2-agonists, such as clonidine and dexmedetomidine, are being used to manage delirium. These agents should be used cautiously in cardiac patients, given their risk of hypotension and bradycardia, respectively. Bradycardia is a major risk factor for TdP in patients with QTc prolongation. Clonidine is typically dosed three times daily, with total daily doses between 0.3 and 0.9 mg. Dexmedetomidine, a potent and highly selective α_2-agonist, is being used increasingly for delirium management and prophylaxis. Trazodone (25–50 mg q6h as needed) is another agent sometimes used to mitigate agitation, though it also carries a risk of orthostasis and QTc prolongation. Finally, benzodiazepines (e.g., IV lorazepam 0.5 mg q6h) are sometimes given in combination with an antipsychotic to reduce the dose of the antipsychotic needed; although these agents may worsen confusion, they are effective when sedation is needed urgently.

Once the agitated delirious patient has been safely and adequately sedated, there is often a question of whether to schedule antipsychotic medication or to use it on an as-needed basis for agitation. Such a decision may depend on the likely duration of the delirium if this can be determined. For example, if the delirium is secondary to CNS hypoperfusion in a patient with low cardiac output, such delirium may well be prolonged, and scheduling of an antipsychotic would be reasonable. In contrast, delirium in an elderly cardiac patient resulting from narcotic administration may be short lived once the narcotic has been eliminated, and standing antipsychotics may not be needed. In most cases of delirium, it is often reasonable to schedule a low dose of IV haloperidol or an oral atypical antipsychotic at bedtime to help regulate the sleep-wake cycle, which is often seriously perturbed in delirious patients. We have found that by ensuring adequate sleep at appropriate hours, delirious cardiac patients have the best possible chance to recover.

Case 3

Mr. C, a 64-year-old man with three-vessel CAD and no significant psychiatric history, was admitted for CABG. Though he was alert, oriented, pleasant, and cooperative before his surgery, he became angry and threatening 2 days later, reporting that the nurses were the "minions of the devil" and that he needed to leave the hospital immediately; notes revealed that he had not slept for 24 hours. Psychiatry was urgently consulted for "psychosis and capacity to leave against medical advice."

The psychiatrist found Mr. C sitting on his bed, wearing only his pajama top. He angrily reported that the nurses were stealing money from him and had injected "poisons" into him. He was disoriented to time and place, and he was unable to attend to conversation for more than a few seconds. He had pulled off his telemetry leads and was not allowing the nurses to check his vital signs. The psychiatrist was able to get Mr. C to agree to stay for the moment, and after confirming a normal postoperative QTc interval and normal electrolyte levels, he persuaded Mr. C to accept an injection of 3 mg IV haloperidol. After 10 minutes, Mr. C calmed, and he fell asleep after 45 minutes.

When Mr. C's leads were reattached and vital signs checked, he was noted to have new-onset AF with a ventricular rate of 119 beats per minute. His heart rate was slowed with the use of β-blockers, and he returned to normal sinus rhythm within 12 hours. He received two further doses of IV haloperidol, and 25 mg of quetiapine each night. His delirium slowly resolved over the next 6 days, coinciding with the resolution of his AF and with the treatment of a urinary tract infection, and the quetiapine was discontinued on his discharge to a cardiac rehabilitation facility.

SEVERE MENTAL ILLNESS AND CARDIAC DISEASE

Individuals with serious mental illness (e.g., bipolar disorder and schizophrenia) have shorter life expectancies than those in the general population. Although the attribution of unnatural deaths (such as suicide) is high, medical conditions account for approximately

70% of deaths. CV disease is the worst offender, contributing 17.4% to 22.0% of the reduction in overall life expectancy. Known risk factors for CV disease (such as smoking, low exercise, and an unhealthy diet) are common in this patient population, often higher than healthy adults. In addition, antipsychotic drugs (often the first-line treatment), although associated with reduced overall mortality, are linked with an increased risk of weight gain, dyslipidemia, and the development of diabetes mellitus, all known risk factors for CV disease. These patients have higher risks of CAD, ACS, and stroke than those in the general population, but they are less likely to access appropriate medical and surgical care.[44]

Although behavioral interventions have been largely ineffective in these populations, classic pharmacologic interventions (such as the use of statins, aspirin, antihypertensives, and diabetes medications) reduce cardiac risk factors and should be used early in secondary prevention.[44]

CRITICAL ISSUES IN PSYCHOPHARMACOLOGY AND CARDIAC HEALTH

Antidepressants

Antidepressants are effective in the treatment of depression and anxiety for patients with cardiac disease. However, older antidepressants (i.e., tricyclic antidepressants and monoamine oxidase inhibitors) have effects that make their use in cardiac patients problematic.

SSRIs are now considered as first-line medications for treating depression in patients with cardiac disease. None cause problematic orthostasis, and, except for paroxetine, they are generally not associated with significant anticholinergic effects. The safety of SSRIs, particularly sertraline, has been well established in post-MI populations. RCTs of sertraline, citalopram, and escitalopram have found that all are safe and effective at reducing depressive symptoms in patients with CAD.[45,46] In contrast, two trials found that sertraline and escitalopram were not effective at reducing depressive symptoms in patients with HF, although patients in those studies had substantial HF symptoms and frequently were experiencing their first episode of depression, raising concerns that their symptoms may have been due primarily to HF.[40–42] Our clinical experience with the use of SSRIs in cardiac patients has also found SSRIs to be safe, and we have safely prescribed SSRIs in post-MI patients earlier than 1 month post-MI when indicated by the severity of depression or the follow-up circumstances. We would also consider using SSRIs in individuals with HF, particularly when there is evidence to suggest that the symptoms being experienced are not solely related to HF itself (e.g., there is a history of depression that precedes the diagnosis of HF).

Although SSRIs had long been considered safe from the standpoint of cardiac conduction, the FDA in 2011 issued a warning regarding the potential for citalopram to prolong the QTc interval and increase the risk for lethal ventricular arrhythmias such as TdP. This warning was based on a thorough QT study ordered by the FDA, which showed a dose-dependent increase in the QTc with citalopram, with an absolute increase of 18.5 ms at doses of 60 mg daily. Although a dose-dependent increase was also shown for escitalopram, the magnitude was smaller (10.7 ms at 30 mg), and no warning was issued. In 2012 the warning was downgraded to note that citalopram is not recommended at doses >40 mg in the general population, is not recommended at doses >20 mg in patients over the age of 65 or with pre-existing liver disease, is not recommended for patients with congenital long-QT syndrome, and should be discontinued in patients with a QTc >500 ms. Several subsequent studies, as well as a meta-analysis, have suggested that citalopram does indeed separate out from other SSRIs in its propensity to prolong the QTc.[47] From a clinical standpoint, the magnitude of the increase is small and likely to be insignificant for most patients; however, many no longer use citalopram as a first-line agent in those with a history of, or significant risk factors for, heart disease, preferring sertraline instead, given its established safety.

Non-SSRI antidepressants are less well-studied than SSRIs in cardiac patients. Venlafaxine can elevate blood pressure, which may preclude its use as a first-line agent in patients with cardiac disease. Duloxetine has not been associated with QTc prolongation or other cardiac side effects and may be a reasonable second-line agent. Bupropion, at therapeutic doses, does not have adverse effects on blood pressure, heart rate, or other CV parameters, and has been shown to reduce rates of smoking.[42] Mirtazapine has

few effects on cardiac conduction or vital signs, even in overdose. The Myocardial Infarction Depression Intervention Trial (MIND-IT), a 24-week randomized, placebo-controlled study, found mirtazapine to be safe in 209 post-MI patients with depression, and mirtazapine often has more immediate effects on sleep than do other antidepressants.[48] However, mirtazapine is highly associated with weight gain as a result of its interaction with histamine receptors, limiting its use in patients with cardiac disease.

Benzodiazepines

Among patients with myocardial ischemia or infarction, benzodiazepines reduce catecholamine levels and decrease coronary vascular resistance.[49] Although β-blockers have similar effects, anxious patients tend to have elevations in vital signs, catecholamines, and coronary pressures as the result of their anxiety, despite the use of β-blockers; benzodiazepines can effectively treat these abnormalities. Furthermore, benzodiazepines are generally well tolerated; low rates of hypotension, virtually no anticholinergic effects, and very low rates of respiratory compromise develop when standard doses of benzodiazepines are used. Benzodiazepines also appear to be safe even in seriously ill patients, with low rates of adverse events. Although clinicians may be concerned about the development of benzodiazepine dependence, when these agents are used in the acute care setting, at adequate doses and for appropriate indications, the risk of dependence is minimal. Benzodiazepines may even have beneficial effects on CV outcomes in specific populations, such as those with cocaine-induced chest pain.

One important caveat for the use of benzodiazepines is that they can exacerbate confusion and paradoxically worsen agitation in patients with delirium or dementia; therefore, other agents (e.g., antipsychotics) may be more appropriate for the treatment of anxiety, fear, and distress in the delirious or demented cardiac patient.

Antipsychotics

In general, antipsychotic agents are used for the management of primary psychotic illnesses and bipolar disorder, as adjuvants for depression, in the management of delirium, and increasingly as anxiolytics. They can reduce agitation and psychotic symptoms and may help normalize the sleep-wake cycle. In general, they are quite safe.

Haloperidol has been the agent most widely used in the management of delirium. This agent can be given orally or intramuscularly, but the IV form is both more rapidly acting and much less associated with the development of extrapyramidal symptoms.[50] Haloperidol generally has no significant effects on heart rate, blood pressure, or respiratory status, and it has essentially no anticholinergic effects.

Haloperidol has been associated with QTc prolongation and development of TdP, though this relationship has likely been exaggerated. In 2007 the FDA issued a warning regarding the potential for IV haloperidol to cause TdP and recommended continuous telemetry with any use of the drug. Subsequent evidence, however, suggests that low to moderate doses of haloperidol are rarely associated with QTc prolongation. Many studies show that IV haloperidol does not separate from placebo in terms of QTc prolongation, and reported cases of QTc prolongation and TdP are often confounded by the agent being used commonly in the sickest patients and those at greatest risk for such outcomes. No thorough QT study has been conducted with IV haloperidol, and little head-to-head evidence suggests that IV haloperidol is more likely than either other forms of haloperidol or atypical antipsychotics to prolong the QTc interval. The only study associating IV haloperidol with higher rates of QTc prolongation than atypical agents did not control for indication.[51] A systematic review of 11 prospective studies involving over 1500 patients identified only one study finding marginal QTc prolongation in 9 of 177 patients,[52] with the other 10 prospective studies demonstrating no evidence of QTc prolongation with IV haloperidol in doses up to 20 mg.[53] TdP appears more common at high doses (>35 mg/day) of haloperidol, and patients who developed TdP were more likely to have QT_C >550 ms (85.7% vs. 15.4%, odds ratio = 33 [95% confidence interval: 6, 135]) prior to TdP.[54] While it is important for psychiatrists to be aware of the potential risks with IV haloperidol, behavioral risks inherent in delirium often outweigh these concerns in a careful risk-risk analysis.

MGH psychiatrists have developed a stratified algorithm based on the patient's risk factors and the dose of IV haloperidol.[53] No ECG monitoring is necessary

for total doses <5 mg daily and in patients with 1 or no risk factors. For patients with 2 or more risk factors or when using doses >5 mg daily, a baseline and follow-up ECG are recommended. Daily ECGs are reasonable for total cumulative doses >25 mg, with the use of telemetry reserved for total doses >100 mg or when the QTc exceeds 500 ms.[55] Given the lack of evidence suggesting that other antipsychotics are safer than IV haloperidol, if physicians are sufficiently concerned about QTc prolongation or TdP to warrant cessation of IV haloperidol, non-antipsychotic agents, such as valproate, should be used.

More recently, atypical antipsychotics (especially risperidone, quetiapine, and olanzapine) have been used in the management of delirium. Although these agents are generally considered safe in cardiac populations, risperidone, and quetiapine can cause orthostatic hypotension, and quetiapine and olanzapine have strong anticholinergic effects. Many atypical antipsychotics also cause weight gain and predispose patients to metabolic syndrome, although the risk is likely lower with short-term use. There have also been concerns about the potential for atypical antipsychotics to cause QTc prolongation in patients with cardiac disease, and no evidence suggests that they are safer than IV haloperidol in this regard. In healthy volunteers, ziprasidone causes the greatest mean QTc prolongation of the atypical antipsychotics, and although it has only been associated with TdP in a handful of cases, its use in cardiac patients is not recommended. In a meta-analysis comparing the side effects of antipsychotic agents, ziprasidone and iloperidone caused the most QTc prolongation, while aripiprazole and lurasidone performed the best.[55] While aripiprazole is occasionally used for hypoactive delirium with perceptual disturbances, it is associated with higher rates of akathisia, and its very long half-life and partial dopamine agonism prevent the binding of other antipsychotics to the D_2 receptor for up to 2 weeks. Lurasidone is not widely used for delirium.

Because hypokalemia and hypomagnesemia have been associated with the development of TdP, patients receiving antipsychotics for delirium or other causes should have these electrolytes monitored and repleted, as needed. When feasible, for patients with risk factors, an ECG should be checked prior to the initial antipsychotic dose and checked again 30 to 60 minutes following the dose. If the QTc is >500 ms or increases by more than 25%, a careful risk-benefit analysis is recommended before proceeding with further dosing. Nonetheless, because TdP is a very low base-rate phenomenon and difficult to predict even in the setting of a prolonged QTc interval, and because agitation in delirium may predispose patients to even greater risks (such as removing central lines and other devices), there may be an indication for ongoing use of antipsychotic agents even with significantly lengthened QTc intervals.

Finally, in elderly patients with dementia, atypical antipsychotics have been associated with mortality related to cardiac events (some of which may represent episodes of ventricular arrhythmia such as TdP); this has led to an FDA black box warning for these medications and highlights the caution needed when prescribing these medications in certain populations.[47]

Clozapine is never used to manage delirium, but for patients taking the medication for other indications, psychiatrists should be aware of the potential for unique cardiac side effects. Although its incidence is low (<1%), clozapine carries a risk of myocarditis and cardiomyopathy, especially in the first 1 to 2 months.[56] The diagnosis is often difficult to make due to vague symptom presentation. Clinical findings include fever, tachycardia, tachypnea, hypotension, or abnormal heart sounds. It is usually associated with elevated systemic inflammatory markers (such as CRP, white blood cells, and/or an increased erythrocyte sedimentation rate) and evidence of cardiac involvement (elevated creatine phosphokinase, troponins, or B-type natriuretic peptide). If suspected, clozapine should be discontinued promptly until further evaluation is done, including consulting a cardiologist. It is important to always obtain an ECG, a chest x-ray, and an echocardiogram if indicated.[56]

REFERENCES

1. Hanssen TA, Nordrehaug JE, Eide GE, et al. Anxiety and depression after acute myocardial infarction: an 18-month follow-up study with repeated measures and comparison with a reference population. *Eur J Cardiovasc Prev Rehabil.* 2009;16(6):651–659.
2. Koivula M, Tarkka M-T, Tarkka M, et al. Fear and anxiety in patients at different time-points in the coronary artery bypass process. *Int J Nursing Studies.* 2002;39(8):811–822.
3. Easton K, Coventry P, Lovell K, et al. Prevalence and measurement of anxiety in samples of patients with heart failure: meta-analysis. *J Cardiovasc Nurs.* 2016;31(4):367–379.
4. Magyar-Russell G, Thombs BD, Cai JX, et al. The prevalence of anxiety and depression in adults with implantable cardioverter defibrillators: a systematic review. *J Psychosomatic Res.* 2011;71(4):223–231.
5. Tully PJ, Cosh SM, Baumeister H. The anxious heart in whose mind? A systematic review and meta-regression of factors associated with anxiety disorder diagnosis, treatment and morbidity risk in coronary heart disease. *J Psychosom Res.* 2014;77(6):439–448.
6. Todaro JF, Shen B-J, Raffa SD, et al. Prevalence of anxiety disorders in men and women with established coronary heart disease. *J Cardiopulm Rehabil Prev.* 2007;27(2):86–91.
7. Huffman JC, Pollack MH. Predicting panic disorder among patients with chest pain: an analysis of the literature. *Psychosomatics.* 2003;44(3):222–236.
8. Stoll C, Schelling G, Goetz AE, et al. Health-related quality of life and post-traumatic stress disorder in patients after cardiac surgery and intensive care treatment. *J Thorac Cardiovasc Surg.* 2000;120(3):505–512.
9. von Kanel R, Baumert J, Kolb C, et al. Chronic posttraumatic stress and its predictors in patients living with an implantable cardioverter defibrillator. *J Affect Disord.* 2011;131(1–3):344–352.
10. Roest AM, Martens EJ, de Jonge P, et al. Anxiety and risk of incident coronary heart disease: a meta-analysis. *J Am Coll Cardiol.* 2010;56(1):38–46.
11. Celano CM, Millstein RA, Bedoya CA, et al. Association between anxiety and mortality in patients with coronary artery disease: a meta-analysis. *Am Heart J.* 2015;170(6):1105–1115.
12. Wen Y, Yang Y, Shen J, Luo S. Anxiety and prognosis of patients with myocardial infarction: a meta-analysis. *Clin Cardiology.* 2021;44(6):761–770.
13. Celano CM, Villegas AC, Albanese AM, Gaggin HK, Huffman JC. Depression and anxiety in heart failure: a review. *Harv Rev Psychiatry.* 2018;26(4):175–184. https://doi.org/10.1097/HRP.0000000000000162.
14. Friedmann E, Thomas SA, Liu F, et al. Relationship of depression, anxiety, and social isolation to chronic heart failure outpatient mortality. *Am Heart J.* 2006;152(5):940.
15. Pelle AJ, Pedersen SS, Schiffer AA, et al. Psychological distress and mortality in systolic heart failure. *Circ Heart Fail.* 2010;3(2):261–267.
16. Tully PJ, Turnbull DA, Beltrame J, et al. Panic disorder and incident coronary heart disease: a systematic review and meta-regression in 113,1612 persons and 581,11 cardiac events. *Psychol Med.* 2015;45(14):2909–2920.
17. O'Donnell CJ, Longacre LS, Cohen BE, et al. Posttraumatic stress disorder and cardiovascular disease: state of the science, knowledge gaps, and research opportunities. *JAMA Cardiology.* 2021;6(10):1207–1216.
18. Roy SS, Foraker RE, Girton RA, Mansfield AJ. Posttraumatic stress disorder and incident heart failure among a community-based sample of US veterans. *Am J Public Health.* 2015;105(4):757–763. https://doi.org/10.2105/AJPH.2014.302342.

19. Edmondson D, Rieckmann N, Shaffer JA, et al. Posttraumatic stress due to an acute coronary syndrome increases risk of 42-month major adverse cardiac events and all-cause mortality. *J Psychiatr Res.* 2011;45(12):1621–1626.

20. Celano CM, Huffman JC. Depression and cardiac disease: a review. *Cardiol Rev.* 2011;19(3):130–142.

21. Moradi M, Doostkami M, Behnamfar N, et al. Global prevalence of depression among heart failure patients: a systematic review and meta-analysis. *Curr Prob Cardiol.* 2022;47(6).

22. Strik JJ, Honig A, Maes M. Depression and myocardial infarction: relationship between heart and mind. *Prog Neuropsychopharmacology Biol Psychiatry.* 2001;25(4):879–892.

23. Larsen KK, Agerbo E, Christensen B, et al. Myocardial infarction and risk of suicide: a population-based case-control study. *Circulation.* 2010;122(23):2388–2393.

24. Martens E, Smith O, Winter J, et al. Cardiac history, prior depression and personality predict course of depressive symptoms after myocardial infarction. *Psychol Med.* 2008;38(02):257–264.

25. Huffman JC, Smith FA, Blais MA, et al. Recognition and treatment of depression and anxiety in patients with acute myocardial infarction. *Am J Cardiol.* 2006;98(3):319–324.

26. Wulsin LR, Singal BM. Do depressive symptoms increase the risk for the onset of coronary disease? a systematic quantitative review. *Psychosom Med.* 2003;65(2):201–210.

27. Van der Kooy K, van Hout H, Marwijk H, et al. Depression and the risk for cardiovascular diseases: systematic review and meta-analysis. *Int J Geriatric Psychiatry.* 2007;22(7):613–626.

28. Bush DE, Ziegelstein RC, Tayback M, et al. Even minimal symptoms of depression increase mortality risk after acute myocardial infarction. *Am J Cardiology.* 2001;88(4):337–341.

29. Van Melle JP, De Jonge P, Spijkerman TA, et al. Prognostic association of depression following myocardial infarction with mortality and cardiovascular events: a meta-analysis. *Psychosom Med.* 2004;66(6):814–822.

30. Lichtman JH, Froelicher ES, Blumenthal JA, et al. Depression as a risk factor for poor prognosis among patients with acute coronary syndrome: systematic review and recommendations: a scientific statement from the American Heart Association. *Circulation.* 2014;129(12):1350–1369.

31. Beach SR, Januzzi JL, Mastromauro CA, et al. Patient Health Questionnaire-9 score and adverse cardiac outcomes in patients hospitalized for acute cardiac disease. *J Psychosom Res.* 2013;75(5):409–413.

32. Connerney I, Shapiro PA, McLaughlin JS, et al. Relation between depression after coronary artery bypass surgery and 12-month outcome: a prospective study. *Lancet.* 2001;358(9295):1766–1771.

33. Zipfel S, Schneider A, Wild B, et al. Effect of depressive symptoms on survival after heart transplantation. *Psychosom Med.* 2002;64(5):740–747.

34. Friedmann E, Thomas SA, Liu F, et al. Relationship of depression, anxiety, and social isolation to chronic heart failure outpatient mortality. *Am Heart J.* 2006;152(5):940.e1–940.e8.

35. Lange HW, Herrmann-Lingen C. Depressive symptoms predict recurrence of atrial fibrillation after cardioversion. *J Psychosomatic Res.* 2007;63(5):509–513.

36. Beach SR, Wichman CL, Canterbury RJ. Takotsubo cardiomyopathy after electroconvulsive therapy. *Psychosomatics.* 2010;51(5):432–436.

37. Fernandes N, Prada L, Rosa MM, et al. The impact of SSRIs on mortality and cardiovascular events in patients with coronary artery disease and depression: systematic review and meta-analysis. *Clin Res Cardiology.* 2021;110(2):183–193.

38. Kim JM, Stewart R, Lee YS, et al. Effect of escitalopram vs placebo treatment for depression on long-term cardiac outcomes in patients with acute coronary syndrome: a randomized clinical trial. *JAMA.* 2018;320(4):350–358. [published correction appears in JAMA 2018 Nov 27;320(20):2154].

39. Lichtman JH, Bigger JT, Blumenthal JA, et al. Depression and coronary heart disease recommendations for screening, referral, and treatment: a science advisory from the American Heart Association Prevention Committee of the Council on Cardiovascular Nursing, Council on Clinical Cardiology, Council on Epidemiology and Prevention, and Interdisciplinary Council on Quality of Care and Outcomes Research: endorsed by the American Psychiatric Association. *Circulation.* 2008;118(17):1768–1775.

40. Angermann CE, Gelbrich G, Störk S, et al. Effect of escitalopram on all-cause mortality and hospitalization in patients with heart failure and depression: the MOOD-HF Randomized Clinical Trial. *JAMA.* 2016;315(24):2683–2693.

41. O'Connor CM, Jiang W, Kuchibhatla M, et al. Safety and efficacy of sertraline for depression in patients with heart failure: results of the SADHART-CHF (Sertraline Against Depression and Heart Disease in Chronic Heart Failure) trial. *J Am Coll Cardiol.* 2010;56:692–699.

42. Zambrano J, Celano CM, Januzzi JL, et al. Psychiatric and psychological interventions for depression in patients with heart disease: a scoping review. *J Am Heart Assoc.* 2020;9(22):e018686.

43. Noriega FJ, Vidan MT, Sanchez E, et al. Incidence and impact of delirium on clinical and functional outcomes in older patients hospitalized for acute cardiac diseases. *Am Heart J.* 2015;170(5):938–944.

44. Nielsen RE, Banner J, Jensen SE. Cardiovascular disease in patients with severe mental illness. *Nat Rev Cardiol.* 2021;18(2):136–145.

45. Shapiro PA, Lesperance F, Frasure-Smith N, et al. An open-label preliminary trial of sertraline for treatment of major depression after acute myocardial infarction (the SADHART Trial). Sertraline Anti-Depressant Heart Attack Trial. *Am Heart J.* 1999;137(6):1100–1106.

46. Lespérance F, Frasure-Smith N, Koszycki D, et al. Effects of citalopram and interpersonal psychotherapy on depression in patients with coronary artery disease: the Canadian Cardiac Randomized Evaluation of Antidepressant and Psychotherapy Efficacy (CREATE) trial. *JAMA.* 2007;297(4):367–379.

47. Beach SR, Celano CM, Noseworthy PA, et al. QTc prolongation, torsades de pointes, and psychotropic medications. *Psychosomatics.* 2013;54(1):1–13.

48. Honig A, Kuyper AM, Schene AH, et al. Treatment of post-myocardial infarction depressive disorder: a randomized, placebo-controlled trial with mirtazapine. *Psychosom Med.* 2007;69(7):606–613.

49. Melsom M, Andreassen P, Melsom H, et al. Diazepam in acute myocardial infarction. Clinical effects and effects on catecholamines, free fatty acids, and cortisol. *Br Heart J*. 1976;38(8):804–810.

50. Menza MA, Murray GB, Holmes VF, et al. Controlled study of extrapyramidal reactions in the management of delirious, medically ill patients: intravenous haloperidol versus intravenous haloperidol plus benzodiazepines. *Heart Lung*. 1988;17(3):238–241.

51. Ozeki Y, Fujii K, Kurimoto N, et al. QTc prolongation and antipsychotic medications in a sample of 1017 patients with schizophrenia. *Prog Neuropsychopharmacol Biol Psychiatry*. 2010;34(2):401–405.

52. van den Boogaard M, Schoonhoven L, van Achterberg T, van der Hoeven JG, Pickkers P. Haloperidol prophylaxis in critically ill patients with a high risk for delirium. *Crit Care*. 2013;17(1):R9.

53. Beach SR, Gross AF, Hartney KE, et al. Intravenous haloperidol: A systematic review of side effects and recommendations for clinical use. *Gen Hosp Psychiatry*. 2020;67:42–50.

54. Sharma ND, Rosman HS, Padhi ID, et al. Torsades de pointes associated with intravenous haloperidol in critically ill patients. *Am J Cardiol*. 1998;81(2):238–240.

55. Leucht S, Cipriani A, Spineli L, et al. Comparative efficacy and tolerability of 15 antipsychotic drugs in schizophrenia: a multiple-treatments meta-analysis. *Lancet*. 2013;382(9896):951–962.

56. Bellissima BL, Tingle MD, Cicović A, et al. A systematic review of clozapine-induced myocarditis. *Int J Cardiol*. 2018;15(259):122–129.

25 PATIENTS WITH KIDNEY DISEASE

SAMUEL I. KOHRMAN, MD ▪ ANA IVKOVIC, MD ▪ THEODORE A. STERN, MD

OVERVIEW

General hospital psychiatrists are frequently consulted on patients with kidney disease, a patient population that accounts for approximately 15% (i.e., 37 million) of those in the United States. Many of those consultations are requested for patients undergoing dialysis who develop depression and anxiety. Furthermore, a host of neuropsychiatric conditions are triggered by psychological reactions to having kidney failure, the need for kidney transplantation, and the biological effects of renal impairment or its treatment. In addition, psychiatric management of patients with kidney disease requires consideration of renal clearance of medications, the potential for renal toxicity, the neuropsychiatric side effects of medications (e.g., immunosuppressants), and the timing of medications in relation to hemodialysis (HD).

PATIENTS WITH NORMAL KIDNEY FUNCTION

Clearance of Toxins and Homeostasis

The kidneys serve to clear waste material from the bloodstream and to maintain homeostasis of water, salt, and acid/base states. More than one-fifth of a person's cardiac output is delivered to the kidneys every minute, generating roughly 180 L of filtrate every day. Only a small portion of this filtrate is excreted. This tight control is achieved by orchestrated structures called *nephrons*, the basic functional units of the kidney. Each nephron is composed of a highly differentiated vascular tuft, the glomerulus, which is entangled with a tubule that is lined by specialized epithelial cells arranged in a unique order. The glomeruli oversee the filtration of the blood through closely knit podocytes, which line the glomerular basement membrane and ensure that cellular elements as well as large macromolecules are not filtered. Renal tubules selectively re-absorb solutes and water, secrete toxins and acids, and concentrate the filtrate, resulting in a urine output that varies in volume and concentration according to one's daily intake of water and solutes. Levels of sodium, potassium, bicarbonate, calcium, phosphate, and magnesium are tightly maintained by these structures.

Volume Control

The ability of the kidneys to continuously filter a large blood volume each minute leads to its central role in controlling blood pressure.[1] The juxtaglomerular apparatus detects states of hyper- or hypofiltration and either decreases or increases the filtration rate via the activity of the renin-angiotensin system. The collecting duct can further fine-tune the body's volume status via the epithelial sodium channels, which are regulated by aldosterone secretion[2] that are triggered by a variety of stimuli (e.g., angiotensin II).

Endocrine Function

In addition to toxin clearance, electrolyte homeostasis, and volume status regulation, the kidneys also have an endocrine function. Interstitial fibroblasts within the kidney secrete erythropoietin in response to a decrease in oxygen tension in the blood,[3] which stimulates bone marrow erythropoiesis. Aldosterone secretion by the adrenal glands maintains euvolemia as an end result of renin secretion by the kidneys. Additionally, the kidneys activate vitamin D (via the 1-alpha-hydroxylase enzyme), which is important for calcium and phosphorus absorption from the gut, serotonin activation in the brain, and mediation of the cross-talk between the kidneys and the parathyroid glands.[4]

All things considered—between toxin clearance, electrolyte homeostasis, blood pressure control, hypoxemia responsiveness, and vitamin D activation—it becomes clear that healthy kidney function supports optimal brain function. Conversely, the presence of kidney disease should alert medical teams and consultants to the possibility of neuropsychiatric dysfunction.

KIDNEY DISEASE

Acute Kidney Injury

Acute kidney injury (AKI), previously known as acute renal failure, is defined by an acute increase in the serum creatinine level; this abnormality is accompanied by a decreased urinary output.[5] Pre-renal, renal, and post-renal categorizations of the etiologies continue to be used. Pre-renal azotemia results from a decrease in the effective circulatory volume that is associated with hypovolemia, shock, as well as cardiorenal or hepatorenal syndrome. Intrinsic renal causes of AKI include ischemic or toxic acute tubular necrosis (ATN), vasculitis, glomerulonephritides, and tubulo-interstitial disorders.[6] Important causes of kidney injury with relevance to the general hospital psychiatrist include drug-induced nephrotoxicity from non-steroidal anti-inflammatory drugs (NSAIDs) and certain drugs of abuse (e.g., heroin crystal nephropathy), as well as ATN secondary to rhabdomyolysis from a variety of causes (e.g., cocaine use, neuroleptic malignant syndrome, and other malignant catatonias). Post-renal etiologies of AKI include obstructive uropathy from nephrolithiasis, bladder outlet obstruction, pelvic tumors, or less commonly, retroperitoneal fibrosis. AKI is widely associated with increased morbidity, length of hospital stays, and mortality rates.[7] In addition, AKI is a risk factor for the development of chronic kidney disease (CKD).[5]

Chronic Kidney Disease and End-Stage Renal Disease

CKD occurs on a spectrum up to end-stage renal disease (ESRD) and it is defined by markers of kidney damage (e.g., albuminuria, abnormal urine sediment, abnormal imaging results) for more than 3 months or a glomerular filtration rate (GFR) <60 mL/min per 1.73 m^2 for ≥ 3 months, with or without kidney damage. ESRD or kidney failure is defined as a GFR <15 mL/min/1.73 m^2 or the need for dialysis.[8] Kidney disease is a major public health problem. According to the US Renal Data System's (USRDS) 2022 report,[9] the overall prevalence of CKD in the general population is 14%, and the prevalence of ESRD is 2271 per million persons. Obesity, hypertension, and diabetes are the most common risk factors for developing CKD. Genetics also plays a role. For example, steroid-resistant nephrotic syndrome, one of the most intractable kidney diseases, results from podocin mutations in about 25% of childhood cases and in 15% of adult cases.[10] Additionally, autosomal dominant polycystic kidney disease (PKD) affects 1 in 1000 individuals and results from mutations in *PKD1* and *PKD2* that affect renal tubular cell differentiation.[11]

Lithium and Kidney Disease: Nephrogenic Diabetes Insipidus and CKD

Widely and successfully used for the treatment of bipolar disorder (BPD), this alkali metal is known for its potential nephrotoxicity. Chronic lithium exposure is associated with an increased incidence of nephrogenic diabetes insipidus (NDI) and CKD; although both complications are uncommon, they are not rare. NDI results from lithium's inhibition of the translocation of aquaporin 2 to the apical membrane of the principal cell of the collecting duct, leading to decreased tubular permeability to water and the excretion of large volumes of dilute urine.[12] The accompanying hypernatremia stimulates thirst and polydipsia. The prevalence of lithium-induced NDI is 50% to 73% in long-term lithium users, and the extent of the urine concentration deficit correlates with the duration of treatment. Lithium-induced CKD is manifested by a slowly progressing (over decades) kidney dysfunction with pathologic features of chronic tubulo-interstitial nephropathy including interstitial fibrosis, tubular atrophy, and the development of microcysts. The duration of lithium treatment is a principal factor in the development of kidney disease, in as much the prevalence of CKD and ESRD increase in those treated chronically with lithium, with a mean duration of lithium treatment 16.5 to 31 years and 23 years, respectively.[13] Finally, lithium's narrow therapeutic window mandates frequent monitoring of lithium levels and educating patients about the risk of lithium intoxication. A 2015 Extracorporeal Treatments in Poisoning Workgroup (EXTRIP) systematic review of lithium poisoning recommended that HD is warranted when kidney function is impaired and the lithium level is >4.0 mEq/L, or when the level of consciousness is decreased, or when seizures or life-threatening dysrhythmias (irrespective of the lithium level) occur.[14] Of note, although lithium is contraindicated for patients with AKI, it may be used with caution in those with CKD. In fact, some patients who have required kidney transplantation because of lithium-induced nephrotoxicity decide, in consultation with their nephrologist and psychiatrist, to resume lithium post-transplantation since it is often the only medication that is effective for their BPD symptoms.

Paradoxically, recent data suggest that lithium may have nephro-protective properties in several animal models of AKI.[15] This has yet to be substantiated in clinical settings.

Complications of Kidney Disease

In addition to the increased morbidity and mortality associated with both CKD and ESRD, a wide array of symptoms and pathologies are linked to kidney disease. The most common cause of death in this patient population is related to cardiovascular (CV) disease. Chronic inflammation, frequent shifts in hemodynamics, and disrupted calcium/phosphate metabolism are thought to contribute to the increase in CV events; CV disease is the leading cause of death in patients with ESRD.[16]

Furthermore, kidney disease leads to a bevy of other complications. Anemia stems mainly from decreased erythropoietin synthesis by diseased kidneys in addition to perturbed iron transport. Lower hemoglobin levels predict lower quality-of-life scores in patients with kidney disease as compared with healthy controls.[17] Metabolic acidosis occurs frequently with

progressive kidney disease, and it leads to loss of bone mass, potential acceleration of kidney disease, and altered metabolism leading to impaired nutritional status.[18] Perturbed calcium-phosphate metabolism and parathyroid hormone (PTH), vitamin D, and fibroblast growth factor-23 (FGF-23) pathways are thought to contribute to vascular calcification and more frequent CV events in patients with CKD.[19]

Cognitive decline has also been associated with a decreasing GFR[20] and is attributed to white matter lesions that have variable phenotypic presentations.[21] Furthermore, depression is highly prevalent in ESRD, and depressive affect has been related to death, CV disease, and dialysis non-adherence.[22]

Therapeutic Options for Advanced Kidney Disease

Once kidney disease progresses to ESRD there will likely be evidence of progressive anemia, acidosis, and a decreased functional and nutritional status that prompts the initiation of dialysis. In 2022 according to the last USRDS data report,[9] there were more than 800,000 cases of ESRD in the United States. Among these 59.8% were receiving HD, 8.1% utilized peritoneal dialysis (PD), and 30.6% had a functioning kidney transplant. Among new cases of ESRD, 83.9% initiated therapy with HD, 12.7% with PD, and 3.1% received a pre-emptive kidney transplant.

Dialysis

More than 85% of patients who receive dialysis to manage ESRD are receiving HD. HD replaces kidney function by allowing the diffusion of small molecules across a semi-permeable membrane and by simultaneously removing body water through ultra-filtration.[23] Access to the circulation is obtained by an arteriovenous (AV) fistula or synthetic graft that is typically placed in the non-dominant upper extremity or less often via an intra-jugular dialysis catheter. HD is most often conducted in dialysis units, three times per week for 3 to 4.5 hours per session. More frequent HD with longer sessions is supported by data suggesting better outcomes compared to standard HD.[23] Home HD has also been gaining popularity, due to its convenience, flexibility, and its potential for better survival rates[24,25] compared with in-center HD. However, it remains the least prevalent mode of dialysis. PD is a popular home dialysis modality that relies on the surface area and permeability of the peritoneal membrane to provide clearance and volume removal. Continuous ambulatory PD requires significant motivation on behalf of the patient, who must manually exchange their dialysate at set intervals, while automated PD assures that dialysis occurs at a pre-set frequency and is typically performed over the course of the night while the patient is sleeping, offering a convenient option, especially for younger patients.[26] Unfortunately, PD is often limited to relatively short-term use, since it relies on the preservation of low but residual kidney function as well as on the preservation of the integrity of the peritoneal membrane, which can be affected each time PD is complicated by peritonitis.[27] The latter is a major source of morbidity and mortality in patients treated with PD, and interestingly, depression has been shown to be a risk factor for its development.[28,29]

Overall the time commitment of HD can be quite disruptive to a patient's life, and it is frequently demoralizing. Depression frequently arises with HD treatments, prompting psychiatric involvement. The symbolism of being dependent on a machine for survival can also generate significant anxiety. Occasionally, patients refuse HD, prompting psychiatric consultation for capacity assessments, which can be challenging since refusing HD is tantamount to a death sentence. This is illustrated by the following case.

Case 1

Mr. C, a 62-year-old man with ESRD, was brought to the hospital by his family in the context of his refusal of HD for the past week; he was admitted for emergency dialysis in the context of uremic encephalopathy. On clearing his mental state, he informed the medical team that he wanted to stop HD, which prompted psychiatric consultation for determination of the "capacity to refuse HD."

The psychiatric interview revealed that prior to initiating HD several months earlier, he had been an active and independent man. He had hoped for a pre-emptive transplant, but he had no living donors, and his renal function deteriorated quickly, necessitating HD, which he had wanted to avoid. Although he was listed for a deceased donor, he knew that he could be waiting for several years before being transplanted. He described having a difficult time adjusting to being dependent on a machine, which was in marked contrast to the independence he valued. He felt demoralized by being surrounded by sick people on HD. In this context, he developed multiple neurovegetative symptoms of depression, including anhedonia. In recent weeks, this had been intensifying, but he was too ashamed to seek psychiatric treatment and felt it would be easier to let nature "take its course." The consulting psychiatrist diagnosed him as having depression and initiated a trial of methylphenidate (for more rapid onset and his profound anergia) as well as sertraline. Mr. C felt better quickly, became more hopeful, and agreed to continue HD on hospital discharge. With continued treatment of his depression, he remained adherent to HD and years later underwent successful transplantation.

Kidney Transplantation

Compared with dialysis, kidney transplantation is the best therapeutic modality for ESRD in terms of cost-effectiveness, quality of life, and survival.[30-32] It is also associated with improved cognitive function[33] compared with HD.

Currently in the United States, there are about 75,000 patients with ESRD registered and awaiting a kidney transplant.[34] Annually, about 24,000 kidney transplants are performed across the nation; over 75% of these originate from deceased donors, and less than 25% come from living donors. As wait times on dialysis increase pre-transplantation, they are associated with worse patient and graft survival post-transplant,[35] and as a result pre-emptive kidney transplantation is encouraged in patients with advanced stages of CKD when a living donor is available. The advantages of kidney transplantation come at the cost of life-long immunosuppressive medications required to prevent graft rejection. The most commonly used regimen is a triple immunosuppression with a calcineurin inhibitor (CNI), e.g., tacrolimus, an anti-proliferative agent (e.g., mycophenolic acid derivatives), and steroids.[34] CNIs have a wide array of side effects, prompting the emergence of new CNI-sparing regimens with promising outcomes.[36] Steroid-free regimens are used in about 30% of patients after kidney transplantation; this offers metabolic advantages[37] and neuropsychiatric benefits (e.g., a decreased risk of affective psychosis by avoiding high-dose steroids post-transplant). Unfortunately, improved short-term outcomes with kidney transplantation are not yet aligned with a similar improvement in long-term outcomes. Most patients, particularly younger ones, must cope with progressive CKD and they undergo kidney transplantation more than once during their lives. Non-adherence to immunosuppressive medications is prevalent in adolescent transplant recipients and is thought to be the cause of worse long-term outcomes in this age group.[38,39] Depression has been correlated with intentional non-adherence to immunosuppressive medications[40] and is a relative contraindication for kidney transplantation if untreated.

PSYCHIATRIC DISORDERS IN CKD AND ESRD

General hospital psychiatrists should be familiar with the array of psychiatric syndromes that arise in patients with ESRD. Accumulating evidence points to the role of biological stress mediators, especially hormones that affect the central nervous system (CNS) and hypothalamus-pituitary-adrenal axis, in precipitating and exacerbating mental disturbances in individuals with medical illnesses.[41] Patients with kidney disease are no exception. Indeed, the abnormal peptide and steroid metabolism that occurs in ESRD creates a milieu of chronic stress. This, in conjunction with psychosocial factors, can precipitate and exacerbate psychiatric conditions that involve depression, anxiety, serious mental illness (SMI) (e.g., schizophrenia and BPD), and cognitive impairment. Multiple treatments have been studied and continue to be assessed for their efficacy in treating psychiatric co-morbidities in the context of ESRD.

Depression and Anxiety

Depressive disorders and anxiety disorders are the best-studied and most commonly encountered psychiatric illnesses in patients with ESRD. Depression rates generally range from 20% to 30% [22,41] in patients with ESRD depending on the population assessed and the questionnaire used; anxiety rates range from 12% to 52% in ESRD (with approximately 30%–45% of those on HD suffering from generalized anxiety disorder).[22,42] Evidence suggests that patient self-rated scales

overestimate the prevalence of depression as compared to those from clinician-administered scales.[22]

Of the numerous screening instruments available to assess depression, the Beck Depression Inventory has been validated in patients on HD; a cut-off score of 14 to 16 has been suggested to have the highest sensitivity and specificity for a clinical diagnosis of depression.[22] Multiple reliable instruments exist for the measurement of anxiety symptoms, but there is no consensus yet on the best screening tool for use in patients with ESRD.

Depression is a well-known condition linked with increased morbidity and mortality, and it has been linked to poor outcomes in adults with CKD (e.g., patients with CKD with depression were more likely to progress to adverse events, such as initiation of dialysis, hospitalization, and death than were non-depressed patients with CKD)[22,43]; anxiety and anxiety co-morbid with depression less consistently trend toward poorer outcomes in this population. Treatment options available to depressed individuals with ESRD mirror those for the general population and include psychotherapeutic and pharmacotherapeutic modalities. Few trials have been conducted to assess medications for depression in ESRD, and the data for therapy are even more limited. Selective serotonin reuptake inhibitors (SSRIs) are recommended as first-line agents due to their efficacy in patients with ESRD as well as their favorable side effect profiles compared with other antidepressants. Serotonin norepinephrine reuptake inhibitors (SNRIs) are regarded similarly. Tricyclic antidepressants (TCAs) and monoamine oxidase inhibitors (MAOIs) should be used with caution, if at all, due to their potential adverse effects (e.g., arrhythmias, drug-drug interactions, orthostatic hypotension) that are exacerbated in patients undergoing dialysis. Few clinical trials have assessed treatment options for anxiety disorders in patients with ESRD. Clinical practice has shifted away from the use of benzodiazepines and barbiturates and toward newer agents (such as SSRIs, SNRIs, and buspirone). The same cautions for dose adjustments in renal impairment exist as for depression.

CKD and Serious Mental Illness (SMI)

Individuals with SMI, including those with schizophrenia and BPD, experience significant inequalities in access to health care and in health outcomes.

Individuals with SMI are at higher risk for developing CKD, due to a number of factors (such as engaging in adverse health behaviors of cigarette smoking, having an unhealthy diet and a sedentary lifestyle, using substances, as well as receiving treatments for SMI that increase one's risk of developing diabetes/metabolic syndrome [e.g., antipsychotics and mood stabilizers, such as lithium]).[44] There is a lack of evidence supporting the rates of SMI in individuals with CKD; however, having SMI and co-morbid CKD is associated with poor health outcomes, higher mortality rates, and higher hospitalization rates.

Neurologic Complications in Kidney Failure

Neurologic complications contribute to the morbidity and mortality in patients with kidney failure and are related directly to renal impairment itself and to its treatments (e.g., renal replacement therapy [RRT], kidney transplantation, and associated immunosuppression).

Mild Cognitive Impairment and Dementia

Cognitive impairment in CKD and ESRD is both common and under-recognized, with an estimated prevalence of 10% to 40% depending on the stage of CKD and the study method employed. Disorders of cognition found in CKD and ESRD range in acuity and severity; the prevalence of cognitive impairment increases as individuals progress toward dialysis, with one study showing that 50% of patients on HD demonstrated mild-moderate cognitive impairment while 37% demonstrated severe impairment.[45] As in most cases of cognitive impairment, causes are often multi-factorial. Patients with CKD and ESRD suffer disproportionate levels of clinical and subclinical CV and cerebrovascular diseases. Patients with CKD are prone to developing atherosclerosis and are at increased risk for ischemic stroke. Anemia and ultra-filtration-related arterial hypotension that occurs with HD can result in cerebral hypoperfusion and ischemia. Patients with kidney failure suffer bleeding disorders from a combination of anticoagulation and uremia that leads to platelet dysfunction. As such, they are at increased risk for intra-cranial bleeding (e.g., subdural, subarachnoid, and intracerebral hematomas). Hemorrhagic stroke may also result from hypertension. Patients with PKD are also vulnerable to CNS

bleeds due to their increased risk for cerebrovascular malformations. Suboptimal clearance of medication and neurotoxic uremic toxins, hormonal balance, and hemodynamic shifts with HD also contribute to cognitive changes. Frontal executive function deficits are commonly present. Presentations include mild cognitive impairment (MCI), delirium, and dementia, and some manifestations (e.g., dialysis dementia) specific to ESRD are associated with aluminum toxicity, delirium syndromes of uremic encephalopathy, and dialysis disequilibrium.

Many screening tools are available for the assessment of cognitive status, and one can be selected based on the amount of time it takes to administer and the degree of diagnostic accuracy required. The Mini-Mental State Exam and the Montreal Cognitive Assessment are two brief and popular instruments. Shorter exams tend to sacrifice specificity for sensitivity, and more extensive neuropsychological testing may be necessary when assessing complicated cases, decision-making capacity, or transplant candidacy.

Recognizing cognitive impairment in patients with chronic illness, including ESRD, helps to rule out and treat reversible causes of declining cognition. Even in instances when the cause is irreversible, identifying impaired cognition can allow families and treatment teams to plan around deficits in self-care and decision-making, including planning for end-of-life care. Moreover, dementia is associated with poor outcomes, including withdrawal from dialysis as well as increased morbidity and a higher mortality rate.[45]

For patients with diagnosed Alzheimer disease (AD) and CKD/ESRD, treatment options with disease-modifying potential in AD fall into two drug classes, the cholinesterase inhibitors (e.g., donepezil, rivastigmine) and the N-methyl-D-aspartate receptor antagonists (e.g., memantine). While the benefit of these medications is modest (i.e., delaying cognitive decline by perhaps 4–6 months), there is a paucity of data on their safety or efficacy in ESRD. Since memantine is excreted renally, the dose should be reduced in the context of renal impairment.

Management of behavioral symptoms in patients with ESRD and dementia or delirium involves a stepped approach: environmental modifications, psychosocial interventions, and use of pharmacologic agents. Based on studies that have shown an increased risk of stroke and death in patients with dementia treated with antipsychotics, these medications should be used with caution.

Specific to patients receiving HD, dialysis is known to reverse uremic encephalopathy, but it is unclear whether more extensive dialysis would further improve cognition. In general, treatment decisions in MCI, dementia, and delirium for patients with ESRD should be individualized, as there is a lack of relevant literature and clinical guidelines.

Delirium in ESRD

Encephalopathy in ESRD is the most common debilitating CNS complication; it is often multi-factorial and results from a combination of uremic toxins (i.e., uremic encephalopathy), other metabolic abnormalities (e.g., acidosis, hyponatremia, hypocalcemia), and the underlying disorders that led to kidney failure (e.g., hypertension).

Uremic encephalopathy presents with a variety of mental status changes including mild confusional states, personality changes, and deep coma.[46] Motor findings (e.g., asterixis, focal motor signs, and the "uremic twitch-convulsive" syndrome) are often present. Its presentation is most dramatic in the context of superimposed AKI. Milder insidious manifestations of chronic uremic encephalopathy found in CKD are manifested by subtle cognitive deficits and personality changes. This diagnosis is often missed as these manifestations can resemble other conditions (e.g., hypertensive encephalopathy, medication side effects, or depression). Patients with uremic encephalopathy typically improve with dialysis; however, the degree of encephalopathy correlates poorly with the degree of azotemia. Electroencephalogram findings in this condition are non-specific and typically include generalized slowing.[47] The diagnosis of uremic encephalopathy is made clinically and supported by improvement with dialysis or successful kidney transplantation.

For patients undergoing dialysis, Wernicke encephalopathy (from accelerated loss of thiamine with dialysis) often goes unrecognized since clinicians may overlook the diagnosis when the classical clinical triad is absent; Wernicke encephalopathy often presents solely with confusion. Other forms of encephalopathy associated with dialysis include dialysis encephalopathy (or, "dialysis dementia," a now rare

but progressive syndrome of dysarthria, mental status changes, myoclonus, and seizures arising from the use of aluminum-based phosphate binders or aluminum-containing dialysate); hypertensive encephalopathy (characterized by confusion, headaches, nausea, and visual disturbances and rarely associated with the use of recombinant human erythropoietin for treatment of renal anemia); disequilibrium syndrome (a short-lived state attributed to dialysis-related fluid and electrolyte shifts and characterized by altered mentation, headache, nausea, cramps, and seizures within 24 hours post-dialysis); other metabolic encephalopathies (e.g., from acidosis, hypercalcemia, hypermagnesemia, hypo- and hypernatremia); and drug toxicity (e.g., from the accumulation of renally excreted drugs, altered protein-binding in kidney failure).[48,49] Furthermore, encephalopathy in ESRD is an independent predictor of mortality; encephalopathy in elderly patients initiating HD in the hospital is independently associated with early mortality.[50]

For the kidney transplant patient, immunosuppressant-related encephalopathy is another frequently overlooked cause of confusion that can be seen at both toxic and therapeutic drug levels. Other signs of toxicity (e.g., tremors, insomnia, headache, visual changes) help steer the clinician toward the correct diagnosis. Rejection encephalopathy (a confusional state occurring in the context of transplant rejection, presumably from excess cytokine production) is also a risk. Most importantly, posterior reversible leukoencephalopathy syndrome (PRES) may develop and present a clinical emergency.

Movement Disorders in CKD and ESRD

Movement disorders are frequently seen with kidney failure. Most commonly, involuntary movements, including asterixis and myoclonus, seen in other forms of metabolic encephalopathy occur. The uremic "twitch-convulsive" syndrome consists of pronounced asterixis and myoclonic jerks accompanied by fasciculations and seizures. Dexmedetomidine has been reported to provide relief and should be considered for agitated delirious patients with kidney failure and this motor disturbance.[51] Choreiform movements in patients receiving HD have been associated with thiamine deficiency, possibly due to basal ganglia dysfunction.[52] Restless legs syndrome (RLS) occurs in 15% to 30% of patients undergoing dialysis (as compared to

5%–10% of those in the general population).[53] RLS is characterized by prickling, crawling, and aching sensations in the legs and an overwhelming urge to move the legs during rest, which can be relieved temporarily by movement. If left untreated, RLS leads to significant psychological distress with insomnia and depression, which often warrants psychiatric involvement. Treatment with dopamine agonists, benzodiazepines, gabapentin (typically 200–300 mg three times per week after dialysis), clonidine, or opioids is often useful. Correction of iron deficiency, anemia, and vitamin D deficiency is also important. Newer guidelines recommend treating with vitamin E (400 mg) and with vitamin C (important to iron metabolism and monoamine synthesis; orally or parenterally 200–250 mg for optimal renal clearance).[53] Kidney transplantation has been reported to result in significant improvement. The paresthesia of RLS can mimic uremic neuropathy. Patients with RLS may also be confused and have akathisia, as the following case illustrates.

Case 2

A psychiatric consultation was requested for Ms. K, a 57-year-old woman with BPD and ESRD on long-term HD who developed paranoid delusions directed toward staff at her HD center; this led to HD refusal. Although family members indicated that the delusions were present for at least several months, the delusions had never previously resulted in HD refusal. Her medication list was notable for quetiapine, sertraline, and ropinirole for "RLS"; ropinirole had been increased weeks previously to a dose of 4 mg/day. On interview, Ms. K described her RLS as a constant feeling as if she needed to jump from her skin, and the sensation was not clearly relieved by rest. Akathisia from the use of an SSRI and quetiapine was considered, prompting the replacement of ropinirole with clonazepam. She reported subjective improvement on this regimen. Her paranoia eventually diminished, and she was able to resume HD at her previous HD center.

Hyponatremia is a common electrolyte derangement that develops in patients with renal impairment. If corrected too aggressively with dialysis, central pontine myelinolysis (characterized by acute progressive quadriplegia, dysarthria, and altered consciousness) may arise. Extra-pontine regions of the brain can also be involved and result in a varied clinical spectrum (e.g., parkinsonism with basal ganglia involvement or ataxia with cerebellar involvement).

Peripheral Nervous System Complications

Peripheral nervous system complications in kidney failure include uremic polyneuropathy, mononeuropathies, and autonomic disturbances. Uremic polyneuropathy is a distal symmetric sensorimotor axonal neuropathy that typically occurs in patients with advanced kidney failure, usually with GFRs <12 mL/min, with a prevalence varying from 50% to 100%.[54] The etiology is thought to be related to various nutritional deficiencies (e.g., thiamine, biotin, zinc) as well as to an accumulation of neurotoxic uremic toxins and associated oxidative stress–related free radical activity.[54] Sensory disturbances and decreased or absent tendon reflexes are common. Milder forms typically resolve with RRT, whereas severe forms may not be reversible. Physical therapy and medications that target neuropathic pain can be useful as adjunctive agents. Kidney transplantation is perhaps the most effective treatment.

Several mononeuropathies can be seen with uremic intoxication and as complications of RRT. Most commonly, nerves of the forearm are affected. Carpal tunnel syndrome occurs in nearly 90% of patients receiving chronic dialysis, often on the side used for vascular access for dialysis (although the contralateral arm may also be affected).

Autonomic neuropathy is also common in kidney failure. It is typically manifested by marked orthostatic hypotension and dialysis-related hypotension secondary to impaired baroreflex responses. There is some literature supporting the use of SSRIs in the management of dialysis-related hypotension. The best treatment, however, is successful kidney transplantation.

Finally, calciphylaxis arising from kidney failure is a rare cause of painful myopathy that can significantly interfere with a patient's sleep and quality of life.

Neurologic Findings in Pediatric Populations

Children with ESRD are also at increased risk for neurologic complications. A retrospective review of 68 children with ESRD revealed that neurological complications occurred in roughly one-third of affected children, with seizures being the most common event.[55] Uncontrolled hypertension was the leading cause of neurological events, indicating that more effective control of hypertension is needed in this population.

PSYCHIATRIC TREATMENT CONSIDERATIONS FOR PATIENTS WITH CKD AND ESRD

Pharmacotherapy and psychotherapy are the mainstays of treatment for patients with CKD, depression, and anxiety. Cognitive-behavioral therapy has substantial empirical support for its efficacy in treating these conditions. Exercise training programs have led to reductions in depressive symptoms in several studies.[22] Other treatment considerations including psychosocial factors that impact mental health in chronic illness can benefit patients. Studies have shown that social support is linked to improved adherence and greater survival rates in patients receiving HD.[22] The quality of marital relationships also differentially impacts the course of medical illnesses, with marital conflict being related to worse outcomes and marital satisfaction to better outcomes. Finally, societally and institutionally mediated factors should be kept in mind: minority race, lower socioeconomic status, and residence in poorer neighborhoods have been associated with worse outcomes in those with chronic illness as well as in those with ESRD. Kidney transplantation and the modality of RRT have also been shown to impact depression, anxiety, and cognition in patients with ESRD, with kidney transplantation proving more effective at modifying these measures than either PD or HD, while patients receiving PD scored higher than those on HD on the cognitive functioning scale.

PSYCHOPHARMACOLOGIC CONSIDERATIONS

Kidney disease can alter the pharmacokinetics of most medications.[56–58] Renal-induced changes in fluid balance and volume of distribution may change the bioavailability of hydrophilic medications. Uremic compounds may displace protein-bound drugs, thereby increasing the amount of free drug that

circulates in the plasma. Kidney disease may also modify hepatic drug metabolism by altering gene expression and the function of cytochrome P450 enzymes. Phase II metabolic reactions (such as glucuronidation, methylation, sulfation, and acetylation) aimed at making medications more water soluble are impaired in kidney disease. Changes in the absorption of medications from the gastrointestinal (GI) tract are also seen in kidney disease due to changes in gut motility (seen in gastroparesis due to diabetes) and edema in the GI tract due to volume overload.

The ratio of free drug levels versus total drug levels (free drug plus protein-bound drug) is altered in kidney disease. Furthermore, drug monitoring methods may only indicate the total drug level that is often reduced due to decreased protein-binding. Highly protein-bound medications, such as valproic acid, may therefore yield results that appear to be sub-therapeutic and doses may be erroneously increased, possibly due to toxic levels. Therefore, free drug levels should be obtained whenever possible in patients with kidney disease.

Creatinine clearance (CrCl), as measured by the estimated glomerular filtration rate (eGFR), can be used to guide adjustments in medication dosage. Psychotropic medications that are primarily metabolized or eliminated by the kidney include: lithium, gabapentin, pregabalin, topiramate, risperidone, paliperidone, paroxetine, desvenlafaxine, venlafaxine, and memantine. Duloxetine is also renally eliminated. Doses of these medications should be reduced depending on the level of renal insufficiency. Mild renal insufficiency is defined as a CrCl >50 mL/min, moderate RI 10 to 50 mL/min, and severe RI <10 mL/min.

Whether a medication is effectively removed with HD or PD is determined by its level of protein-binding, lipophilicity, and volume of distribution. High amounts of lipophilicity and protein-binding, as well as a large volume of distribution make substantial removal by dialysis unlikely. If dialysis clearance is <30% of the total drug clearance, it is likely that significant drug accumulation can occur, and decreasing the dose of medication or avoiding it altogether may be warranted. Dialysis will cause significant fluid shifts both during and after each treatment, and it may take many hours to reach equilibrium. Medications associated with orthostasis should be used cautiously (or avoided when possible) in patients undergoing dialysis. Dialyzable medications include carbamazepine, gabapentin, lamotrigine, lithium, pregabalin, topiramate, and valproate.

Most other psychotropic medications do not require drastic dose changes in patients with kidney disease or even kidney failure (Table 25.1). However, consideration of possible accumulation or overlapping synergetic effects with other medications or organ failure should be considered.

Indications and considerations for medication use in patients with kidney disease by medication class are provided below.

Antidepressants

A recent review of patients with stage 3–5 CKD undergoing treatment for depression found that drug clearance was markedly reduced for the MAOI selegiline, the TCAs amitriptyline and tianeptine, the SNRIs venlafaxine, desvenlafaxine and milnacipran,

---

TABLE 25.1

Medications Known to Require Dosage Adjustment in Renal Insufficiency (RI) Based on Estimated Glomerular Filtration Rate

	Mild RI (>50 mL/min)	Moderate RI (10–50 mL/min)	Severe RI (<10 mL/min)
Antidepressants			
Mirtazapine	None	Reduce by 30%	Reduce by 50%
Paroxetine	None	Reduce by 25%–50%	Max dose 40 mg daily
Venlafaxine	Reduce by 25%	Reduce by 50%	Reduce by 50%
Desvenlafaxine	None	Do not exceed 50 mg daily	Do not exceed 50 mg every other day
Antipsychotics			
Paliperidone	Start ≤3 mg daily Max dose ≤6 mg daily	Start ≤1.5 mg daily Max dose ≤3 mg daily	Start ≤1.5 mg daily Max dose ≤3 mg daily
Risperidone	Start 0.25–0.5 mg once or twice a day Beyond 1.5 mg, increase the dose at weekly or longer intervals	Start 0.25–0.5 mg once or twice a day Beyond 1.5 mg, increases in dose should take place at weekly or longer intervals	Start 0.25–0.5 mg once or twice a day Beyond 1.5 mg, increases in dose should take place at weekly or longer intervals
Benzodiazepines			
Chlordiazepoxide	None	None	Reduce by ≥50%
Anticonvulsants			
Carbamazepine	None	None	Reduce by 25%
Gabapentin	Creatinine clearance (CrCl) >60 mL/min: max dose 1200 mg daily CrCl 30–60 mL/min: max dose 600 mg daily	CrCl 15–30 mL/min: max dose 300 mg daily	CrCl <15 mL/min: max dose 150 mg daily
Pregabalin	Reduce by 50%	Reduce by 75%	Reduce by 87.5%
Topiramate	None	Reduce by 50%	Reduce by 75%
Lithium			
	None	Reduce by 25%–50%	Consider further decrease and dosing on alternate days
Cholinesterase Inhibitors			
Galantamine	None	Max dose: 16 mg daily	Use not recommended
Memantine	None	None	Max dose 5 mg twice a day

Data from Owen JA. Psychopharmacology. In: Levenson JL, ed. *Textbook of Psychosomatic Medicine Psychiatric Care of the Medically Ill*. American Psychiatric Publishing; 2010:957–1019.

norepinephrine dopamine reuptake inhibitor bupropion, as well as the selective noradrenaline reuptake inhibitor reboxetine.[59]

TCAs have been used in patients with ESRD for decades, often with good effects. However, certain TCAs should generally be avoided due to their anticholinergic properties, and propensity to induce orthostatic hypotension or QT-prolongation.[59–62] Amitriptyline may have a decreased drug clearance in patients with CKD. Nortriptyline and desipramine are less likely to cause these effects and can be considered for use in patients with ESRD. No dose adjustments were recommended for nortriptyline or for doxepin regardless of the severity of renal insufficiency.

SSRIs have been safe in patients with ESRD, however, certain side effects as well as individual medications warrant special attention. SSRIs may be associated with serotonin-related platelet dysfunction and an increased risk of bleeding.[60] Moreover, the bleeding risk may be elevated in those with kidney disease due to uremia-induced platelet dysfunction. While not considered an absolute contraindication, bleeding risk should be monitored in patients with renal insufficiency receiving SSRIs. Paroxetine clearance is significantly reduced in renal insufficiency (up to 50%) and doses should be reduced by 25% to 50% in moderate renal insufficiency. Potential anticholinergic effects (e.g., urinary retention, orthostasis, and QT-prolongation) are also possible with paroxetine and its use should be limited in patients with severe kidney disease. Citalopram doses >40 mg/day have been associated with significant QT interval prolongation. Given the uncertainty and unpredictability of possible drug accumulation, electrolyte changes, and co-morbid CV conditions, an alternative SSRI is advisable in patients with renal insufficiency.

SNRIs (venlafaxine, desvenlafaxine, and duloxetine) are renally eliminated. Venlafaxine is not significantly removed by dialysis and may cause increases in hypertension. In mild-to-moderate renal insufficiency, a 25% decrease in dosage is suggested for patients with an eGFR <30 mL/min a 50% reduction is recommended. When discontinuing venlafaxine in patients with renal insufficiency, a slow taper over 2 to 4 weeks is recommended to avoid uncomfortable withdrawal and discontinuation effects. Desvenlafaxine is also not substantially removed by dialysis and dose reduction by 50% is recommended for mild, moderate, and severe renal insufficiency. Duloxetine should be reduced by up to 75% of the total maximum dose in normal kidney function, no higher than 40 mg/day for patients with an eGFR of <30 mg/mL. Other sources suggest not prescribing duloxetine to patients with an eGFR <30 mg/mL.

Bupropion's water-soluble metabolites, hydroxybupropion and threohydroxybupropion, are increased in patients with ESRD. Toxic levels of bupropion may be associated with an increased risk of seizures, agitation, anxiety, and psychosis. In patients with renal insufficiency, the initial dose should be reduced and titrated with caution.

Mirtazapine's clearance is reduced in patients with renal insufficiency by 30% in those with moderate renal insufficiency and by 50% in those with severe renal insufficiency. It is also highly protein-bound and therefore not readily removed by dialysis. Initial and subsequent doses should therefore be reduced in patients with moderate-to-severe renal insufficiency.

There are very few data regarding the pharmacokinetics of trazodone in patients with kidney disease. No dose adjustments were suggested in patients with an eGFR >15 mL/min, whereas for patients with an eGFR <15 mL/min, doses should not exceed 150 mg.

There are very few data on the use of MAOIs in patients with renal insufficiency. The suggested dosing for selegiline in patients with an eGFR of <30 mg/mL was half of the dose used with normal renal functioning (5 mg). Similarly, a 50% decrease in the total daily dose is suggested for tranylcypromine. Little or no data exist to inform prescribers about recommending isocarboxazid or phenelzine.

While not directly an antidepressant, the common anxiolytic and antidepressant augmenter buspirone is impacted in cases of renal insufficiency. Levels of this serotonergic 5-HT_{1A} partial agonist were increased up to four times in patients with an eGFR <60 mg/mL, and a dose reduction was recommended.

Benzodiazepines

The use of benzodiazepines is common in patients with renal insufficiency due to higher rates of anxiety, RLS, and sleep disorders. Medications with active metabolites which are renally excreted (including chlordiazepoxide, diazepam, flurazepam, and clorazepate), should be avoided. Drug accumulation is likely with most if not all benzodiazepines as these medications are not effectively removed by dialysis. In severe renal insufficiency, the chlordiazepoxide dose should be reduced by 50%. Lorazepam and oxazepam are the preferred agents of this class as they do not have active metabolites. Yet, levels of lorazepam and oxazepam may increase four-fold and smaller doses with increased interval of administration are recommended.

Non-benzodiazepine sedatives-hypnotics, such as zaleplon, zolpidem, and zopiclone, are generally under-studied in patients with kidney disease. While dose requirements may not be necessary, more data are needed.

Mood Stabilizers

No dose adjustments are suggested for carbamazepine in mild-to-moderate renal insufficiency. A 25% dose reduction is recommended in patients with severe renal insufficiency.

No dose adjustment is necessary for valproic acid in patients with renal insufficiency though it is prudent to monitor the free level, as opposed to the total level as mentioned previously, given its high affinity for protein binding.

Gabapentin is extensively excreted by the kidney and dose reductions are recommended: for a CrCl of 30 to 60 mL/min a maximum dosage of 300 mg twice a day is recommended, for a CrCl of 15 to 30 mL/min a dose of 300 mg/day is recommended, and for a CrCl of <15 mL/min the maximum suggested dosage is 300 mg every other day.

Lamotrigine levels have not been extensively studied in patients with renal insufficiency.

Oxcarbazepine dosing should be reduced by 50% in patients with an eGFR of <30 mL/min and the starting dose should not exceed 150 mg twice a day.

Suggestions for dosing of topiramate are as follows: reduce the total daily dose by 50% in patients with moderate renal insufficiency and reduce it by 75% in patients with severe renal insufficiency.

Lithium is almost entirely excreted by the kidneys. Its use is contraindicated in AKI but not in CKD. Lithium is completely dialyzed and can be given as a single oral dose of 200 to 600 mg following HD, guided by levels checked immediately before dialysis. Polyuria is common during treatment with lithium.

Severe polyuria, as seen in NDI, may occur in up to 40% of patients taking lithium and if present, discontinuation or starting the potassium-sparing amiloride (typically 5 mg twice a day) is recommended. NSAIDs may be used cautiously to reduce urinary free water loss though this should be done in consultation with a nephrologist. During long-term treatment with lithium, creatinine should be monitored approximately every 6 months. If the serum Cr is >1.5 mg/dL or increases by >25% from its baseline, further investigation is warranted, including an estimation of CrCl and eGFR or consultation with a nephrologist.

Antipsychotics

No dose adjustments are generally required for conventional or first-generation antipsychotics (including haloperidol, perphenazine, and chlorpromazine), however, there are very few data on the use of conventional antipsychotics in patients with ESRD. Haloperidol undergoes extensive hepatic metabolism and only 1% is excreted unchanged in the urine. It is extensively bound to plasma proteins and has a large volume of distribution, making it difficult to remove by dialysis. When prescribing conventional antipsychotics, it is pertinent to account for relevant medication effects, including the potential for QTc-prolongation, the development or worsening of movement disorders, and other side effects that patients with ESRD are more prone to experience.

Like conventional antipsychotics, most atypical or second-generation antipsychotics do not require dose adjustments in this patient population. The notable exceptions to this include paliperidone and risperidone. Paliperidone is a metabolite of risperidone and is extensively eliminated by the kidney. Its clearance is significantly decreased in all degrees of renal impairment. If these agents are utilized in patients with advanced kidney disease, they should be started at a low dose, titrated slowly and cautiously, and the target dose should be lower than in patients without significant kidney disease. For patients with mild renal impairment, paliperidone can be started at 3 mg daily with a maximum of 6 mg daily, whereas in moderate-to-severe impairment, it should be started at 1.5 mg daily with a maximum dose of 3 mg daily. Risperidone can be started at 0.25 to 0.5 mg twice a day with slow titration and cautious monitoring. As with conventional antipsychotics, patients with ESRD are at an increased risk for the development or exacerbation of class-related side effects and caution and close monitoring are warranted. For atypical antipsychotics, this usually includes: weight gain, hyperlipidemia, insulin resistance and hyperglycemia, CV morbidity, anticholinergic side effects, and movement disorders.

Access the reference list online at https://expertconsult.inkling.com/.

REFERENCES

1. Guyton AC. Kidneys and fluids in pressure regulation. Small volume but large pressure changes. *Hypertension.* 1992;19 (1 suppl):12–18.
2. Barbry P, Hofman P. Molecular biology of Na⁺ absorption. *Am J Physiol.* 1997;273(3 Pt 1):G571–G585.
3. Zeisberg M, Kalluri R. Physiology of the renal interstitium. *Clin J Am Soc Nephrol.* 2015;10(10):1831–1840.
4. Melamed ML, Thadhani RI. Vitamin D therapy in chronic kidney disease and end stage renal disease. *Clin J Am Soc Nephrol.* 2012;7(2):358–365.
5. Chawla LS, Eggers PW, Star RA, et al. Acute kidney injury and chronic kidney disease as interconnected syndromes. *N Engl J Med.* 2014;371:58–66.
6. Thadhani R, Pascual M, Bonventre JV. Acute kidney injury. *N Engl J Med.* 1996;334:1448–1460.
7. Chertow GM, Burdick E, Honour M, et al. Acute kidney injury: mortality, length of stay, and costs in hospitalized patients. *J Am Soc Nephrol.* 2005;16:3365–3370.
8. Levin A, Stevens PE. Summary of KDIGO 2012 CKD Guideline: behind the scenes, need for guidance, and a framework for moving forward. *Kidney Int.* 2014;85(1):49–61.
9. United States Renal Data System.. *2022 USRDS Annual Data Report: Epidemiology of Kidney Disease in the United States.* National Institutes of Health, National Institute of Diabetes and Digestive and Kidney Diseases; 2022.
10. Hildebrandt F. Genetic kidney diseases. *Lancet.* 2010;375(9722):1287–1295.
11. Torres VE, Harris PC, Pirson Y. Autosomal dominant polycystic kidney disease. *Lancet.* 2007;369(9569):1287–1301.
12. Bedford JJ, Weggery S, Ellis G, et al. Lithium-induced nephrogenic diabetes insipidus: renal effects of amiloride. *Clin J Am Soc Nephrol.* 2008;3(5):1324–1331.
13. Schoot TS, Molmans THJ, Grootens KP, et al. Systematic review and practical guideline for the prevention and management of the renal side effects of lithium therapy. *Eur Neuropsychopharmacology.* 2020;31:16–32. https://doi.org/10.1016/j.euroneuro.2019.11.006.
14. Decker BS, Goldfarb DS, Dargan PI, et al. Extracorporeal treatment for lithium poisoning: systematic review and recommendations from the EXTRIP workgroup. *Clin J Am Soc Nephrol.* 2015;10(5):875–887.
15. Alsady M, Baumgarten R, Deen PM, et al. Lithium in the kidney: friend and foe? *J Am Soc Nephrol.* 2016;27(6):1587–1595.
16. London GM. Cardiovascular disease in chronic renal failure: pathophysiologic aspects. *Semin Dial.* 2003;16(2):85–94.
17. Perlman RL, Finkelstein FO, Liu L, et al. Quality of life in chronic kidney disease (CKD): a cross-sectional analysis in the Renal Research Institute-CKD study. *Am J Kidney Dis.* 2005;45(4):658–666.
18. De Brito-Ashurst I, Varagunam M, Raftery MJ, et al. Bicarbonate supplementation slows progression of CKD and improves nutritional status. *J Am Soc Nephrol.* 2009;20(9):2075–2084.
19. Heine GH, Nangaku M, Fliser D. Calcium and phosphate impact cardiovascular risk. *Eur Heart J.* 2013;34(15):1112–1121.
20. Halipern SM, Melamed ML, Cohen HW, et al. Moderate chronic kidney disease and cognitive function in adults 20 to 59 years of age: third National Health and Nutrition Examination Survey (NHANES III). *J Am Soc Nephrol.* 2007;18(7):2205–2213.
21. Wei C-S, Yan C-Y, Yu X-R, et al. Association between white matter hyperintensities and chronic kidney disease: a systematic review and meta-analysis. *Front Med.* 2022;9:770184. https://doi.org/10.3389/fmed.2022.770184.
22. Ma TK-W, Li PK-T. Depression in dialysis patients. *Nephrology.* 2016;21:639–646. https://doi.org/10.1111/nep.12742.
23. Himmelfarb J, Ikizier TA. Hemodialysis. *N Engl J Med.* 2010;363(19):1833–1845.
24. Walker RC, Hanson CS, Palmer SC, et al. Patient and caregiver perspectives on home hemodialysis: a systematic review. *Am J Kidney Dis.* 2015;65(3):451–463.
25. Weinhandl ED, Liu J, Gilbertson DT, et al. Survival in daily home hemodialysis and matched thrice-weekly in-center hemodialysis patients. *J Am Soc Nephrol.* 2012;23(5):895–904.
26. Rabindranath KS, Adams J, Ali TZ, et al. Continuous ambulatory peritoneal dialysis versus automated peritoneal dialysis for end-stage renal disease. *Cochrane Database Syst Rev.* 2007(2):CD006515.
27. Kendrick J, Teitelbaum I. Strategies for improving long-term survival in peritoneal dialysis patients. *Clin J Am Soc Nephrol.* 2010;5(6):1123–1131.
28. Troidle L, Watnick S, Wuerth DB, et al. Depression and its association with peritonitis in long-term peritoneal dialysis patients. *Am J Kidney Dis.* 2003;42(2):350–354.
29. Perez Fontan M, Rodriguez-Carmona A, Garcia-Naveiro R, et al. Peritonitis-related mortality in patients undergoing chronic peritoneal dialysis. *Perit Dial Int.* 2005;25(3):274–284.
30. Laupacis A, Keown P, Pus N, et al. A study of the quality of life and cost-utility of renal transplantation. *Kidney Int.* 1996;50(1):235–242.
31. Neipp M, Karavul B, Jackobs S, et al. Quality of life in adult transplant recipients more than 15 years after kidney transplantation. *Transplantation.* 2006;81(12):1640–1644.
32. Wolfe RA, Ashby VB, Milford EL, et al. Comparison of mortality in all patients on dialysis, patients on dialysis awaiting transplantation, and recipients of a first cadaveric transplant. *N Engl J Med.* 1999;341(23):1725–1730.
33. Dixon BS, VanBuren JM, Rodrigue JR, et al. Cognitive changes associated with switching to frequent nocturnal hemodialysis or renal transplantation. *BMC Nephrol.* 2016;17:12.
34. Lentine KL, Smith JM, Hart A, et al. OPTN/SRTR 2020 Annual Data Report: kidney. *Am J Transplantation.* 2022;22:21–136. https://doi.org/10.1111/ajt.16982.

35. Meier-Kriesche HU, Port FK, Ojo AO, et al. Effect of waiting time on renal transplant outcome. *Kidney Int.* 2000;58(3):1311–1317.

36. Vincenti F, Rostaing L, Grinyo J, et al. Belatacept and long-term outcomes in kidney transplantation. *N Engl J Med.* 2016;374(4):333–343.

37. Vincenti F, Schena FP, Paraskevas S, et al. A randomized, multicenter study of steroid avoidance, early steroid withdrawal or standard steroid therapy in kidney transplant patients. *Am J Transplant.* 2008;8(2):307–316.

38. Dobbels F, Van Damme-Lombaert R, Vanhaecke J, et al. Growing pains: non-adherence with the immunosuppressive regimen in adolescent transplant recipients. *Pediatr Transplant.* 2005;9(3):381–390.

39. Berquist RK, Berquist WE, Esquivel CO, et al. Non-adherence to post-transplant care: prevalence, risk factors and outcomes in adolescent liver transplant recipients. *Pediatr Transplant.* 2008;12(2):194–200.

40. Griva K, Davenport A, Harrison M, et al. Non-adherence to immunosuppressive medications in kidney transplantation: intent vs. forgetfulness and clinical markers of medication intake. *Ann Behav Med.* 2012;44(1):85–93.

41. Cukor D, Cohen SD, Peterson RA, et al. Psychosocial aspects of chronic disease: ESRD as a paradigmatic illness. *J Am Soc Nephrol.* 2007;18(12):3042–3055.

42. Cukor D, Ver Halen N, Fruchter Y. Anxiety and quality of life in ESRD. *Semin Dial.* 2013;36(3):265–268.

43. Loosman WL, Rottier MA, Honig MA, et al. Association of depressive and anxiety symptoms with adverse events in Dutch chronic kidney disease patients: a prospective cohort study. *BMC Nephrol.* 2015;16:155.

44. Cogley C, Carswell C, Bramham K, et al. Chronic kidney disease and severe mental illness: addressing disparities in access to health care and health outcomes. *CJASN.* 2022;17:1413–1417. https://doi.org/10.2215/CJN.15691221.

45. Drew DA, Weiner DE, Sarnak MJ. Cognitive impairment in CKD: pathophysiology, management, and prevention. *Am J Kidney Diseases.* 2019;74:782–790. https://doi.org/10.1053/j.ajkd.2019.05.017.

46. Seifter JL, Samuels MA. Uremic encephalopathy and other brain disorders associated with renal failure. *Semin Neurol.* 2011;31(2):139–143.

47. Brouns R, De Deyn PP. Neurological complications in renal failure: a review. *Clin Neurol Neurosurg.* 2004;107(1):1–16.

48. Baumgaertel MW, Kraemer M, Berlit P. Neurologic complications of acute and chronic renal disease. *Handb Clin Neurol.* 2014;119:383–393.

49. Anghel D, Tanasescu R, Campeanu A, et al. Neurotoxicity of immunosuppressive therapies in organ transplantation. *Maedica (Buchar).* 2013;8(2):170–175.

50. Arai Y, Shioji S, Tanaka H, et al. Delirium is independently associated with early mortality in elderly patients starting hemodialysis. *Clin Exp Nephrol.* 2020;24:1077–1083. https://doi.org/10.1007/s10157-020-01941-5.

51. Nomoto K, Scurlock C, Bronster D. Dexmedetomidine controls twitch-convulsive syndrome in the course of uremic encephalopathy. *J Clin Anesth.* 2011;23(8):646–648.

52. Hung SC, Hung SH, Tarng DC, et al. Chorea induced by thiamine deficiency in hemodialysis patients. *Am J Kidney Dis.* 2011;37(2):427–430.

53. Safarpour Y, Vaziri ND, Jabbari B. Restless legs syndrome in chronic kidney disease: a systematic review. *Tremor Other Hyperkinetic Mov.* 2023;3:10. https://doi.org/10.5334/tohm.752.

54. Camargo CRSD, Schoueri JHM, Alves BDCA, et al. Uremic neuropathy: an overview of the current literature. *Rev Assoc Med Bras.* 2019;65L:469–474. https://doi.org/10.1590/1806-9282.65.3.469.

55. Albaramki JH, Al-Ammouri IA, Akl KF. Neurological and cardiac complications in a cohort of children with end-stage renal disease. *Saudi J Kidney Dis Transpl.* 2016;27(3):507–511.

56. Nolin TD. A synopsis of clinical pharmacokinetic alterations in advanced CKD. *Semin Dial.* 2015;28(4):325–329.

57. Pichette V, Leblond FA. Drug metabolism in chronic renal failure. *Curr Drug Metab.* 2003;4(2):91–103.

58. Eyler RF, Unruh ML, Quinn DK, et al. Psychotherapeutic agents in end-stage renal disease. *Semin Dial.* 2015;28(4):417–426.

59. Nagler EV, Webster AC, Vanholder R, et al. Antidepressants for depression in stage 3–5 chronic kidney disease: a systematic review of the pharmacokinetics, efficacy, and safety with recommendations by European Renal Best Practice (ERBP). *Nephrol Dial Transplant.* 2012;27(10):3736–3745.

60. Jeong BO, Kim SW, Kim SY, et al. Use of serotonergic anti-depressants and bleeding risk in patients undergoing surgery. *Psychosomatics.* 2014;55(3):213–220.

61. Funk KA, Bostwick JR. A comparison of the risk of QT prolongation among SSRIs. *Ann Pharmacother.* 2013;47(10):1330–1341.

62. Gillman PK. Tricyclic antidepressant pharmacology and therapeutic drug interactions updated. *Br J Pharmacol.* 2007;151(6):737–748.

26

PATIENTS WITH GASTROINTESTINAL DISEASE

ELIZABETH N. MADVA, MD ■ SAMUEL I. KOHRMAN, MD

INTRODUCTION

Psychiatric and gastrointestinal (GI) diseases have a robust bi-directional relationship that reflects a complex interplay between the central and enteric nervous systems. The assorted symptoms, sensations, and syndromes resulting from this reciprocal relationship are associated with alterations in immune system functioning and modulation of neurotransmitters that are common to both systems. Psychological states of anxiety or fear may be experienced as "butterflies" in one's stomach, and high rates of psychiatric co-morbidity are present in both "functional" and "organic" GI diseases.[1] In addition, psychotropic medications can cause GI side effects, and their efficacy depends on the integrity of the GI system's ability to absorb, metabolize, and distribute medications to the rest of the body. In the following sections, these complex relationships are explored with an emphasis on the relationships and treatment considerations that affect both disciplines.

DISORDERS OF THE ESOPHAGUS, STOMACH, AND UPPER INTESTINES

Dysphagia

Dysphagia can arise secondary to the use of antipsychotic medications (first and second generations) as a result of drug-induced parkinsonism, dystonia, and tardive dyskinesia (TD).[2] Case reports and case series have implicated various agents, including: haloperidol, loxapine, trifluoperazine, olanzapine, risperidone, quetiapine, clozapine, and aripiprazole. When

the symptom develops, treatment should address the underlying etiology. Dysphagia due to drug-induced dystonia should be treated with intravenous (IV) or intramuscular (IM) benztropine or diphenhydramine. Dysphagia due to drug-induced parkinsonism is typically not responsive to anticholinergic medications and is best managed by reducing or discontinuing the suspected agent.[2] Notably, regardless of the primary etiology, care should be taken when prescribing sedating medications to those with dysphagia, as over-sedation in this population may result in aspiration and other adverse events.

Globus Hystericus

The feeling that something is lodged in one's throat is an oft-reported symptom that requires medical attention. When pertinent diseases, including gastroesophageal reflux disease (GERD), airway masses, or esophageal masses have been ruled out, "psychogenic" causes are often considered. Functional dysphagia, classically known as *globus hystericus*, has a wide differential diagnosis as well as a high rate of co-morbidity with other medical and psychiatric conditions.[3] Management includes treating co-morbid conditions, and when applicable, the use of psychotherapy and/or medication for co-morbid anxiety.[3] If globus is thought to be due to a functional disorder, then reassurance, psychoeducation, and psychotherapy are recommended, although occasionally, there is also a role for the use of psychotropic medications to reduce visceral hypersensitivity.[4]

Gastroesophageal Reflux Disease

GERD is associated with increased rates of many psychiatric disorders including depression, anxiety, and sleep disorders.[1] A variety of mechanisms may account for the correlations between psychiatric illness and GERD, including increased production of pro-inflammatory cytokines from the esophageal mucosa and increases in autonomic (sympathetic) nervous system activation during coughing and arousal from sleep.[5] Most psychotropic medications can be used in patients with GERD without worsening symptoms; an exception is the use of anticholinergic medications that affect the lower esophageal sphincter and should be avoided, if possible.[2] Benzodiazepines and serotonin-norepinephrine reuptake inhibitors (SNRIs) have been associated with improvements in sleep, greater well-being, and even reduction in core GERD symptoms.[2]

Nausea and Vomiting

Nausea is a common side effect of serotonergic antidepressants due to agonism of 5-HT_3 receptors in the gut.[6] Medications that antagonize 5-HT_3 receptors (especially mirtazapine, olanzapine, and ondansetron) are less likely to cause GI distress and may be useful in patients with nausea and co-morbid depression or anxiety.[6] Blockade of dopamine (D_2) receptors, particularly in the chemoreceptor trigger zone, is also helpful in alleviating nausea and vomiting. Metoclopramide and prochlorperazine (a phenothiazine antipsychotic) are D_2-receptor antagonists marketed as anti-emetics.[6] While they are often effective over the short-term, their use may be limited by extrapyramidal symptoms (EPS), such as akathisia, and long-term effects, such as TD (see below, under Gastroparesis).

For patients with depression or anxiety co-morbid with chemotherapy-induced nausea and vomiting (CINV), hyperemesis gravidarum (HG), or other conditions, the anti-emetic properties of mirtazapine, certain antipsychotics (e.g., olanzapine, perphenazine, chlorpromazine, prochlorperazine, and other antipsychotics), and benzodiazepines can be considered if contraindications are not present. In a randomized, double-blind, placebo-controlled trial of patients scheduled to receive emetogenic chemotherapy, the addition of olanzapine 5 mg daily was associated with significant reductions in nausea and vomiting as well as with increases in quality of life over those in the control group.[7] The psychotropic medications shown to be efficacious in CINV include lorazepam (rather than other benzodiazepines), butyrophenone antipsychotics (including haloperidol and droperidol), phenothiazine antipsychotics (e.g., prochlorperazine and promethazine), olanzapine, gabapentin, and mirtazapine.[2,7] Anticipatory nausea and vomiting may cause a considerable amount of distress in cancer patients who are receiving chemotherapy. Psychological models for chemotherapy-related anticipatory nausea and vomiting include classical conditioning (e.g., associating chemotherapy with environmental cues or other physical sensations), demographic factors (including younger age, female gender, and the propensity to experience certain physical symptoms, such as dizziness), and beliefs and negative expectations related to treatment and symptom formation.[8] Adjunctive lorazepam has been shown to be helpful in anticipatory nausea and vomiting in this population.[8] Several therapies (including systematic desensitization, hypnosis, biofeedback, imagery, and relaxation) have also been shown to be helpful.[8]

Hyperemesis gravidarum (HG) is associated with high degrees of psychological stress and with elevated rates of depression and anxiety disorders, even after pregnancy. A study of 52 women with HG found that the prevalence of mood disorders was 15.4% and the prevalence of anxiety disorders was 36.5%. A sizable percentage of patients (36.5%) with HG have at least one personality disorder diagnosis (particularly an avoidant or obsessive-compulsive personality disorder). Additionally, most mood and anxiety disorders pre-date pregnancy in women with HG.[9] Treatment of HG typically involves vitamin supplementation (especially thiamine to avoid Wernicke encephalopathy), pyridoxine (vitamin B_6) with or without doxylamine, and for more severe cases, use of metoclopramide or steroids.[10] Mirtazapine and chlorpromazine have also been used successfully.[2,10]

Cyclic vomiting syndrome (CVS) is a condition consisting of recurrent episodes of incapacitating nausea and vomiting that are interspersed with symptom-free intervals lasting anywhere from a few days to several months.[11] While it is most common in children, it also occurs in adults and may be associated with specific triggers or environmental cues (e.g., migraines, seizures, stress, menstrual cycles).[11] There have been many proposed etiologies; more recent plausible causes include sympathetic and parasympathetic dysfunction, stress/anxiety/depression, and a central mechanism of nausea/vomiting involving corticotropin-releasing factors.[11] Treatment of CVS is multi-factorial, complex, and involves both pharmacologic and non-pharmacologic strategies. Interventions include identification and avoidance of any known triggers, use of prophylactic drug therapy to prevent recurrent episodes, use of abortive treatment and/or supportive care to ameliorate acute episodes, and provision of psychological support to the patient and their family.[11] Various medications (including prokinetics, anti-emetics, erythromycin, sumatriptan, tricyclic antidepressants (TCAs), benzodiazepines, and anticonvulsants) have been used with varying degrees of success.[2] Episodes of acute vomiting may require high-dose IV anti emetics and benzodiazepines. Long-term management with TCAs was found to be effective in most patients (i.e., decreasing the duration and frequency of episodes, emergency visits, and hospitalization in adults with CVS); although TCA's side effects were common, they were generally mild and well-tolerated.[11] Neuropsychiatric consultation and intervention may be particularly valuable to these patients; the major risk factors for non-response to treatment are co-existing and poorly controlled migraine headaches, a psychiatric disorder, and chronic use of narcotics or marijuana.[11] Additionally, a personal or family history of migraine and the presence of co-morbid psychiatric disorders is thought to be associated with an increased risk of CVS.

Cannabis hyperemesis syndrome (CHS) is like CVS but can be distinguished by a history of chronic cannabis use and by pathognomonic behavior of frequently bathing in hot water.[12] Paradoxically, although cannabis usually functions as an anti-emetic, it is thought that with chronic use, toxic levels accumulate and activate peripheral CB_1 receptors in the gut. This peripheral CB_1 binding over-rides the common anti-emetic properties of CB_1 receptors in the central nervous system (CNS) and CB_2 receptors in glial cells, resulting in decreased GI motility and emesis.[12] The mitigating mechanism of bathing in hot water is unknown but may include CB_1 activation by tetrahydrocannabinol in the hypothalamus as well as by a "cutaneous steal syndrome," which is thought to occur when blood flow

is re directed from the gut to the skin.[12] The most effective treatment of CHS is the cessation of cannabis use; indeed, the diagnosis of CHS is supported by symptom remission after cannabis use has been discontinued and its reappearance when cannabis use is resumed.[12] Otherwise, management, in addition to replenishing fluids and nutrients, often involves the judicious and cautious use of benzodiazepines. Anti-emetics have not been shown to be effective.[12]

Nausea and GI distress are the most common reasons for discontinuation of selective serotonin reuptake inhibitors (SSRIs) by patients.[2,13] SSRI-induced nausea is generally benign and transient, and it can be managed with over-the-counter anti-emetics. Nausea is also a common early side effect of psychostimulants, mood stabilizers, and acetylcholinesterase inhibitors.[2,6] Lithium is associated with nausea and vomiting although longer-acting formulations (e.g., Eskalith CR) or lithium citrate may reduce this effect (though lower GI tract symptoms may emerge).[6] For patients taking sodium valproate, switching to divalproex sodium may help to reduce nausea and vomiting.[13] For patients taking carbamazepine, dividing the total daily dose by twice daily administration may also alleviate nausea.[13] If nausea occurs in the setting of other side effects associated with drug toxicity, such as neurologic or other GI symptoms, consideration of drug toxicity and prompt evaluation should ensue.

Gastroparesis

Gastroparesis is characterized by delayed gastric emptying without an identifiable bowel obstruction. Patients with gastroparesis may experience abdominal pain, nausea, vomiting, bloating, and early satiety.[1] Common causes of gastroparesis include complications from diabetes mellitus, post-surgical complications, neurologic injury, and medication side effects. Anticholinergic medications (including those used for prophylaxis and/or treatment of EPS or dystonic reactions [such as benztropine and diphenhydramine]), as well as antipsychotic medications (such as clozapine and low-potency first-generation agents, e.g., chlorpromazine) worsen gastroparesis and should be avoided. Pharmacologic treatment for gastroparesis involves the use of prokinetic agents such as erythromycin, bethanechol, and metoclopramide. Metoclopramide is a dopamine-$_2$ receptor antagonist that is used in a variety of GI disorders. Its long-term use has been historically associated with an increased risk of TD, with rates ranging from 1% to 10% in different studies; however, a 2010 review showed the risk of TD to be <1%.[14] As with other D_2-receptor antagonists, metoclopramide may also be associated with other adverse reactions, including akathisia, dystonic reactions, and rarely neuroleptic malignant syndrome.[2] A 2015 meta-analysis found that continuous IV administration of metoclopramide was associated with a reduced rate of EPS when compared with bolus administration, and this may be an option for patients prone to these conditions.[15]

Gastric Bypass

Increasingly, patients are receiving gastric bypass surgery, with annual rates estimated at 580,000 worldwide, representing a 70% increase over the past two decades, with further increases expected to continue.[16] Anti-obesity surgeries are typically classified into: procedures that promote intestinal malabsorption (e.g., jejunoileal and jejunocolic bypass), gastric restrictive surgeries (e.g., vertical-banded gastroplasty, gastric band, gastric stapling, or sleeve gastrectomy), surgeries that combine restriction and malabsorption (e.g., Roux-en-Y gastric bypass), and surgeries that combine maldigestion, malabsorption, and gastric restriction (e.g., biliopancreatic diversion with partial gastrectomy, distal gastric bypass, or duodenal switch).[16] Regardless of the procedure, patients have less surface area to absorb nutrients and medications and have altered bowel transit times, often requiring adjustments in diet and medications.[17] Roughly 20% to 50% of patients who undergo bariatric surgery have a history of a mood disorder,[16] which is the most common co-morbid psychiatric condition, followed by binge-eating disorder, in this population. Changes in GI physiology occur after weight-loss surgical procedures and they influence the type and amount of medications that can be effectively administered to patients post-procedure. This may have significant implications for psychiatric treatment regimens.

In one analysis of medication absorption after Roux-en-Y gastric bypass surgery,[18] both lithium and bupropion demonstrated increased absorption in patients versus controls, whereas many medications (e.g., amitriptyline, clonazepam, clozapine, fluoxetine, olanzapine, paroxetine, quetiapine, risperidone, sertraline, and ziprasidone) showed reduced absorption. The medications with unchanged absorption pre- and post-surgery were buspirone, citalopram, diazepam, haloperidol, lorazepam, methylphenidate, oxcarbazepine, trazodone, venlafaxine, and zolpidem.[2,18] In a retrospective study of 439 patients who received the Roux-en-Y procedure, 23% of patients had increased antidepressant use after surgery; of these, 40% retained the same class of antidepressants and 18% started on a new class of antidepressants. Only 16% of patients had a decreased need for antidepressant treatment after surgery.[19] Notably, by 1 month after Roux-en-Y gastric bypass, it appears that the bioavailability of SSRIs is reduced.[20]

Patients who have had gastric bypass surgery or a gastrectomy can absorb medications dissolved in acidic solutions, whereas those with significant alterations in their intestines are less likely to absorb alkaline-soluble medications.[16] Drug poisoning from highly lipophilic medications may also occur, as anti-obesity surgeries may result in loss of body fat percentage and distribution.[16] Reductions in the size and area of the small intestine that are necessary for the absorption of nutrients, vitamins, and medications complicate the effective use of psychotropics in these patients. Medications dissolved in aqueous solution may help circumvent this, as they are absorbed faster than medications in solid form.[2] Thus, dissolving medications in water before ingestion may result in improved absorption and more predictable drug levels. Transit times through the intestine may be decreased, limiting the time of contact between medications and the small intestine essential for proper absorption. When large portions of the stomach and proximal small intestine are removed, long-lasting medications become less effective as they pass unchanged into the large intestine without losing their protective coating.[2] Therefore, immediate-release formulations are preferred over extended-release formulations in patients following gastric bypass surgery. Additional strategies that may produce more reliable drug levels and hence treatment efficacy include using: medications that are available as orally disintegrating tablets, liquid preparations of medications, transdermal patches, and IM long-acting formulations. Checking blood levels of medications may have more utility in post-bypass than in non-bypass patients due to the unpredictable absorption of many agents.

DISORDERS OF THE LOWER GASTROINTESTINAL TRACT

Constipation

Constipation is a common side effect of anticholinergic medications, such as benztropine, TCAs, many second-generation (atypical) antipsychotics, low-potency first-generation (typical) antipsychotics (e.g., chlorpromazine), and some SSRIs (e.g., paroxetine).[2,6] Paroxetine, which has high anticholinergic activity, much like many atypical antipsychotics (such as quetiapine, olanzapine, and especially clozapine), may be associated with constipation in up to one-fourth of patients.[21] Medications with anticholinergic properties may cause constipation by a variety of mechanisms, including alteration of duodenal motility, small and large bowel contractions, delay of colonic transit times, and the gastrocolic reflex.[21] Patients with medical and psychiatric conditions associated with a sedentary lifestyle or patients taking sedating medications (leading to a sedentary lifestyle) may be at higher risk for medication-induced constipation.[21] US Food and Drug Administration (FDA) registration trials report rates of constipation between approximately 3% and 16% for SSRIs, SNRIs, bupropion, and mirtazapine.[6]

Constipation is a common side effect for patients taking clozapine with reported rates of 25% to 60%.[21] Studies examining colonic transit time in patients on clozapine (alone and/or with other antipsychotics) versus other antipsychotics have shown that clozapine induces significantly more gut hypomotility than other antipsychotics.[21] Because reduced motility, constipation, and pseudo-obstruction may lead to disastrous complications, such as bowel ischemia or perforation, clozapine-treated patients should be monitored closely and treated with laxatives, as needed.[21] Importantly, bulk-forming laxatives are relatively contraindicated for patients treated with clozapine; instead, use of osmotic laxatives is preferred.[21]

Diarrhea

Diarrhea is reported to occur in approximately 6% to 20% of patients on SSRIs in FDA registration trials.[6] Rates of >1% to 2% (comparable with placebo) are found with bupropion XL, mirtazapine, and venlafaxine XL, and rates with duloxetine and desvenlafaxine are approximately 10%. Approximately 30% of patients develop diarrhea with vilazodone,[22] which is the highest rate among those taking antidepressants. While common, SSRI-induced diarrhea is typically short-lived. Population-based studies of patients taking lithium and carbamazepine have demonstrated high rates of diarrhea (33% and 25%, respectively) although the relationship to the dose or duration of treatment is unclear. If diarrhea persists with the use of lithium, carbamazepine, or divalproex, drug toxicity should be considered, and drug levels should be obtained.[6] Use of slow-release formulations of these medications may reduce the rates of diarrhea as a side effect.[2]

Irritable Bowel Syndrome

Irritable bowel syndrome (IBS) is a common functional GI disorder (FGID), also known as a disorder of gut-brain interaction,[8] which affects approximately 11% of the population worldwide.[23] Diagnostic criteria for FGID, including IBS, are provided by the Rome Foundation, a panel of international experts that continues to serially refine the diagnostic criteria based on ongoing research since their inception in the late 1980s.[8] IBS has been classified based on the presence of abdominal pain with prevailing irregular bowel movements with three main subtypes: predominant diarrhea (IBS-D), predominant constipation (IBS-C), mixed (IBS-M), or an unclassified type. More recently, the definition of FGIDs (including IBS) is based on pathophysiologic mechanisms including motility disturbance, visceral hypersensitivity, altered pain perception, altered mucosal and immune function, altered gut microbiota, and altered CNS functioning (i.e., altered brain-gut axis).[8] Additionally, environmental factors and triggers are prominent in the disease and include early life stressors (e.g., abuse and significant psychosocial stress), food intolerance, antibiotic use, and enteric infection (gastroenteritis).[23] The Rome criteria emphasize a biopsychosocial approach to understanding the complex interplay of host and environmental factors in the pathogenesis and treatment of IBS.[8] IBS tends to have a relapsing-remitting course with symptoms that vary over time.[23] Psychiatric co-morbidity is high: anxiety disorders are the most common psychiatric co-morbidity (nearly 50%), and depressive disorders are the second most common (approximately 25%).[1] Other common co-morbidities in patients with IBS include chronic pain syndromes (including fibromyalgia and chronic pelvic pain), sleep disturbances, GERD, functional dyspepsia, and headache.[1]

Treatment for IBS includes both pharmacologic and non-pharmacologic interventions. Non-pharmacologic interventions, referred to as brain-gut behavior therapies, which focus on remediation of GI symptoms over psychological co-morbidity, have a growing evidence base and include interventions such as cognitive-behavioral therapy (CBT), hypnotherapy, psychodynamic psychotherapy, and mindfulness-based interventions.[23] Pharmacotherapy for IBS includes the use of medications directed at specific GI symptoms (e.g., laxatives, anti-diarrheals), gut motility (e.g., prokinetics), and in some cases, the gut-brain axis (e.g., antidepressants, antipsychotics, and anti-epileptics).[23] A meta-analysis examining the efficacy of psychotropic medications for IBS found a collective number-needed-to-treat of 4.5 for antidepressants.[24] Consideration of the predominant pattern of bowel movements is key when selecting an antidepressant; for example, TCAs are often preferred in patients with IBS-D due to possible constipating effects, and SSRIs may be more useful in IBS-C due to possible prokinetic effects. Similarly, for patients with anorexia, weight loss, insomnia, or severe pain symptoms, TCAs may be preferable.[4]

Inflammatory Bowel Disease

Inflammatory bowel disease (IBD) is a chronic disease characterized by relapsing intestinal inflammation.[25] It is thought to be due to genetic factors, atypical immune responses to intestinal microbes, and loss of tolerance to typical gut microbiota.[26] The role of inflammation and abnormal levels of pro-inflammatory cytokines in various psychiatric disorders, particularly depression, is well-established and provides a putative link between many medical and psychiatric ailments, including autoimmune diseases.[27] Environmental factors are also instrumental and include psychological stress, dietary factors (e.g., vitamin D deficiency), and air pollution.[26] The two main types of IBD are Crohn's disease (CD) and ulcerative colitis (UC). Both UC and CD are associated with extraintestinal manifestations (e.g., oral ulcers, oligoarticular or polyarticular non-deforming peripheral arthritis, episcleritis or uveitis, erythema nodosum) in up to 50% of patients.

Although the prevalence of IBD is often described as being approximately 1% of the general population, current research indicates that both the incidence and prevalence of IBD are increasing globally, even among pediatric populations.[1]

UC and CD are chronic debilitating conditions that are commonly associated with psychiatric symptoms, which in turn adversely affect disease course and severity. The rate of anxiety symptoms among IBD patients ranges from 19% to 35% and the rate of depressive symptoms is approximately 27%.[1] Both anxiety and depression increase the risk and severity of disease recurrence and their prevalence also appears to increase after the diagnosis of IBD is made; whether co-morbid psychiatric symptoms in IBD are secondary to the disease burden or are reflective of systemic inflammatory processes is still under investigation.[1]

Due to the growing appreciation for the brain-gut axis and the associations between psychiatric symptoms and IBD, a variety of psychotherapeutic interventions (including CBT, psychodynamic psychotherapy, relaxation training, and psychoeducation) have been trialed. Limited studies have demonstrated that psychotherapeutic interventions and psychoeducation do not appear to impact the course of the disease, although they do mitigate psychological factors (such as coping, health-related quality of life, and anxiety related to the illness), suggesting further research is needed.[28]

Relatedly, additional evidence suggests that antidepressants (used for depression or anxiety) may have a positive effect on the course of illness in patients with IBD. Patients with IBD and a co-morbid anxiety or depressive disorder who were treated with an antidepressant (e.g., an SSRI, SNRI bupropion, mirtazapine) for at least 6 months showed a significant improvement in their quality-of-life scores, CD activity index, and ratings of depression and anxiety.[29] Approximately 7.5% of patients discontinued their medications due to side effects, most commonly due to new-onset sexual dysfunction. Those who were untreated or undertreated with antidepressants reported worse quality-of-life, psychiatric symptoms, and IBD symptoms.[30]

Early research also suggests that immunosuppressive medications used to treat core IBD symptoms may be effective in treating depression in patients with IBD. A small study of 14 patients with IBD found that depressive symptoms improved after two infusions of infliximab.[30] A retrospective study investigating the efficacy of immunosuppressive medication on depressive symptoms found significant decreases in the severity of depression as well as in overall depression scores in patients with IBD treated with immunosuppressive medications.[30] However, it should be noted that the aforementioned findings should be viewed with caution, as the relationship between inflammation and psychiatric symptoms is complex and many potential confounders to the evaluation of immunosuppressive treatment response exist. One such factor is the significant overlap of non-specific symptoms, such as fatigue and malaise, across many disorders, which is often not accounted for in depression rating scales. Additional investigation is needed to clarify whether patients with IBD and co-morbid psychiatric conditions do indeed experience relief from psychiatric symptoms when immunologic treatment is aimed at their IBD symptoms.

PSYCHIATRIC ISSUES RELATED TO CANCERS OF THE UPPER AND LOWER INTESTINES

GI Cancer

Psychiatric disorders are associated with poorer cancer detection and treatment, as well as an increased mortality rate. Approximately 50% of patients with advanced cancer meet the criteria for a psychiatric disorder, most commonly an adjustment disorder, major depression, or an anxiety disorder.[2] Additionally, patients with psychiatric illness (particularly schizophrenia) often do not utilize preventative care and screening procedures, such as colonoscopy, which is associated with a worse prognosis and outcomes.[31] Elderly patients diagnosed with colon cancer who have pre-existing mental illness are more likely to be diagnosed with cancer at autopsy, to be diagnosed at an unknown or later stage of cancer, or to receive no treatment at any stage of colon cancer.[32] Patients with pre-existing mental illness have a higher overall mortality rate and a higher cancer-related mortality rate than do controls. This has been found with all major psychiatric diagnoses, but it is especially pronounced in those with dementia or with a psychotic disorder, and it persists after adjusting for sociodemographic

factors, the stage of the diagnosis, and co-morbid conditions. Co-morbid depression is also an independent risk factor for lower survival rates and increased rates of disease recurrence among patients with oropharyngeal cancer.[33]

Whether (or the degree to which) GI cancers and depression share common biological pathways that adversely affect outcomes remains unknown. Poorer outcomes in depressed patients with cancer may be associated with abnormal chronic activation of the hypothalamic-pituitary axis, with prolonged inflammatory responses and weakened immunity, or with noradrenergic-driven tumor angiogenesis.[33] Other mechanisms may be that depression is linked with poorer healthy behaviors, such as decreased physical activity or increased use of tobacco and alcohol.[33]

Consistent with the putative role of altered immunologic function, increased levels of circulating interleukin (IL)-2R among patients with advanced colorectal cancer with liver metastases predict higher rates of depression.[34] A prospective controlled study identified a positive association between scores on the Hospital Anxiety and Depression Scale and levels of IL-1β, IL-6, IL-8, and TNF-α, and a negative correlation with IL-10 when comparing patients with colorectal cancer admitted for tumor resection to healthy controls.[35]

Approximately 10% of all cancer patients develop brain metastases; the vast majority of these occur in melanoma, and cancer of the lungs or breasts.[36] The incidence of brain metastases in cancers of GI origin is much lower (<1% in pancreatic and gastric cancer and <4% in esophageal and colorectal cancer).[36] Like other cancers, brain metastases associated with GI cancers are typically associated with a poorer prognosis, although there are reports of prolonged survival after neurosurgical resection. Limited information is available regarding the neuropsychiatric manifestations and sequelae of GI-associated brain metastases.

LIVER DISORDERS

Hepatitis C Virus

Approximately 3% of the world's population is infected with the hepatitis C virus (HCV).[37] The most common means of transmission is via IV drug use, and, while less common, HCV can also be transmitted via sexual contact and to infants by HCV-infected mothers.[37]

Other forms of transmission include blood transfusions, needle-stick injuries, and the application of tattoos[37]; fortunately, awareness, and prevention as well as treatment protocols have made these forms of transmission less common in the modern era.

HCV infection is associated with reduced quality of life and functioning.[37] Approximately half of patients with HCV infection have a history of a psychiatric illness and approximately 90% have a history of a substance use disorder (SUD).[38] HCV is associated with multiple medical co-morbidities including fibromyalgia, arthritis, peripheral neuropathy, and other pain-related disorders.[37] Each of these may have bi-directional relationships with neuropsychiatric symptoms, further complicating the successful management of these patients. Despite the high rates of co-morbid psychiatric and SUDs in patients infected with HCV, patients with such co-morbid conditions are less likely to receive treatment for HCV infection.[37] Traditional therapies for HCV infection, most notably interferon (IFN)-based treatments, are associated with higher rates of neuropsychiatric disorders, including increased rates of depression and/or exacerbation of other underlying psychiatric conditions, such as bipolar disorder.[37] Such concerns previously resulted in premorbid psychiatric conditions representing relative contraindications to treatment. Prophylactic antidepressant use, effective screening for psychiatric co-morbidity and symptoms, and multi-disciplinary team approaches have all been demonstrated to improve the treatment of many patients with psychiatric disorders (particularly depression and anxiety) receiving treatment for HCV infection.[37] In recent years, HCV treatment strategies have changed to include the use of direct-acting antivirals (e.g., protease inhibitors), and thus far, these treatments have been associated with significantly fewer side effects, including neuropsychiatric side effects.[37,38] While the initial findings are promising, clinicians should remain cautious about not over-interpreting these early discoveries meaning that there are no associated neuropsychiatric risks. Protease inhibitors may inhibit cyclooxygenase P450 enzymes (especially CYP P450 3A4) and thus interfere with the metabolism of many psychotropic medications. Furthermore, medications that stimulate P450 enzymes, such as carbamazepine, may reduce the levels of these medications, interfering with effective treatment.[39] Although these medications are better tolerated and the rates of neuropsychiatric effects are lower, caution should be exercised as pre-existing psychiatric and substance use issues may still affect therapy, including treatment adherence.[39] Thus, psychiatrists and other clinicians are still faced with the task of understanding complex drug-drug interactions, monitoring treatment effects and outcomes, and optimizing psychiatric care before, during, and after treatment for HCV infection.

IFN-induced hypomania or mania have been reported at varying time points after initiating treatment (weeks or months), after major dose reductions, or after abrupt discontinuation.[25] In such cases, symptoms typically resolve with discontinuation of IFN and initiation of psychotropic medications: for hypomania, mania and psychosis, atypical antipsychotics are considered the best treatment options.[25] Mood lability or irritability are more common than frank hypomania or mania and may not require discontinuation or marked changes in treatment; IFN-induced psychosis is a rarely reported treatment side effect. A retrospective analysis suggested that HCV infection among patients with bipolar disorder should still be treated, given similar rates of psychiatric complications and treatment adherence to those with unipolar depression.[40]

IFN-treated patients with HCV infection often report impairment of memory and concentration, as well as other cognitive concerns.[2,25] These symptoms occur independently from depression or other psychiatric disorders and are thought to increase with the dose and duration of IFN treatment. Patients receiving IFN for HCV infection demonstrate notable decreases in performance of multiple neurocognitive tasks, which typically reverses after completion of treatment.[41] Frank delirium is a rarely reported side effect of IFN.[25]

Hepatic Encephalopathy

Hepatic encephalopathy (HE) is characterized by the onset of neuropsychiatric symptoms and neuromuscular signs in patients with cirrhosis and/or porto-systemic shunting. Afflicted individuals may present with mild neurocognitive deficits only elicited with specific tests or show increasingly severe manifestations, such as frank delirium or coma.[25] Psychometric tests examining executive and other neurocognitive functions may be necessary for mild or subtle presentations, although there do not appear to be any gold standard bedside tests for this purpose, and the validity of some tests is questionable. Serum ammonia levels are elevated in many but not all patients with HE, and caution is required when interpreting laboratory test results, as some patients may have elevated and compensated baseline ammonia levels.[25] An electroencephalogram may be of help in establishing the diagnosis, although findings of generalized slowing and triphasic waves, which are not always present, are non-specific indicators of delirium secondary to various toxic-metabolic pathologic states.[42] Neuromuscular manifestations can include myoclonus, asterixis, and focal neurologic deficits (such as hemiplegia in the absence of stroke).[25]

Common precipitating events for HE include infections, GI bleeding, overuse of diuretics, electrolyte imbalance, and constipation.[43] HE may also result from aberrant protein breakdown leading to increased levels of serum ammonia.[43] Typically, protein is broken down into ammonia by gut bacteria, and ammonia is broken down into glutamine and urea by the liver; however, in the setting of severe liver disease, ammonia is not metabolized and thus a surplus of ammonia develops. In the brain, ammonia is metabolized by glutamine synthase to form glutamine.[43] Astrocytes play a prominent role in responding to increased levels of ammonia and glutamate. In acute liver disease, sudden increases in ammonia may lead to intracranial edema that leads to increased intracranial pressure. In chronic disease, astrocytes may adapt to elevated ammonia levels, resulting in a downregulation of glutamate.[43] Other mechanisms for HE include increased blood-brain barrier permeability to gamma amino butyric acid (GABA) and other small non-lipid polar compounds; decreased activity of GABA-transaminase (resulting in increased GABA levels); accumulation of endogenous compounds that bind to benzodiazepine binding sites on GABA receptors.[43]

Treatment of HE includes correction of precipitating factors (such as infections, electrolyte abnormalities, constipation, GI bleeding, and use of psychoactive medications). In addition, it is helpful to maintain regular bowel movements with non-absorbable disaccharide compounds (e.g., lactulose) that trap ammonia in the gut lumen. Finally, modification of nutrition and diet to include increased branched-chain amino acids, acetyl-L-carnitine, and probiotics can be helpful.[25]

DISORDERS OF THE PANCREAS

Pancreatic Cancer

Neuropsychiatric symptoms have long been associated with tumors of the pancreas. In 1931, Yaskin[44] reported that "nervous symptoms" appeared early in the course of pancreatic cancer and that disease manifestation was strongly linked to pre-morbid personality, as well as socioeconomic and psychogenic features. Clinical and academic findings have corroborated Yaskin's early report, and numerous studies have demonstrated an increased prevalence of psychiatric disturbances in those with pancreatic cancer.[44] Moreover, studies over the years have found that depressive symptoms and psychological distress may precede the diagnosis of pancreatic cancer by up to 6 months.[44] This points to a possible biological culprit linking these diseases, as depression related to psychological and coping reactions to illness would occur after a diagnosis is made. Interleukins, including IL-6, IL-18, TNF-α, as well other inflammatory cytokines, are elevated in pancreatic cancer,[44] and elevated IL-6 levels have been associated with various neuropsychiatric disturbances including major depressive disorder (MDD).[27] Moreover, IL-6 appears to be particularly elevated in patients with pancreatic cancer and co-morbid MDD.[44]

The reported prevalence of MDD in patients with pancreatic cancer varies widely, from 14% to 76%.[44] This variability appears to be related to the instruments used and the timing of the evaluation in the illness course, among other factors. Additionally, the type and stage of pancreatic cancer are often not included in analyses of psychiatric symptoms, which may impact the interpretation of self-reported or observed symptom severity and/or prognosis.[44]

Pancreatitis

Valproic acid (VPA) is rarely associated with drug-induced acute pancreatitis but does carry a "black box warning" for this reason. The estimated prevalence is 1:40,000, and it may develop at any time; it most commonly occurs, however, within the first year of treatment or after a dosage increase.[45] There is no dose-response relationship.[25] Benign transient hyperamylasemia occurs in up to 20% of adults on VPA and does not confer a greater risk of developing pancreatitis.[25,45]

Routine screening of serum amylase or lipase is not recommended in the absence of symptoms suggestive of possible pancreatitis (abdominal pain, nausea, vomiting, diarrhea, and anorexia).[6] Discontinuation of the offending agent often results in the resolution of symptoms within 10 days[2]; however, the mortality rate of VPA-induced pancreatitis is reported to be as high as 21%.[45] If drug-induced pancreatitis occurs, re-challenging with the same medication is absolutely contraindicated.[2,6,45]

MEDICATION CONSIDERATIONS IN GASTROINTESTINAL ILLNESS

Oral administration of medications may not be possible in patients with severe nausea or vomiting, esophageal disorders, or GI malabsorption syndromes. Challenges may also arise in patients who are delirious or unconscious, combative or uncooperative, or in the peri-operative period. In such cases, alternative routes of administration are often required. Many psychotropic medications, however, are only available in oral form, complicating management. Patient factors, such as adequate tissue perfusion and venous access must also be considered. Additionally, side effect profiles of the same medication may differ between different routes of administration. Another key point is that the bioavailability and potency of medications may differ significantly between different administration routes, and many medications require different dosing strategies among different formulations. Therefore, clinicians should refer to trusted sources to prescribe the correct dosing strategy. A summary of psychotropic medications available in IV, IM, sublingual, buccal, rectal, and transdermal formulations is summarized in Table 26.1. These data pertain to formulations available in the United States (US).

Liquid preparations or orally disintegrating formulations of psychotropic medication may be a viable option for patients who can tolerate oral dosing but have difficulty swallowing tablets or capsules. Liquid formulations must still pass through the GI tract and undergo first-pass metabolism; thus they still may not be suitable for patients with malabsorption, hepatic, or other GI diseases affecting drug metabolism. Orally disintegrating tablets may be an option for some patients who are non-adherent, or who "cheek" their

medication; once the tablet is placed on buccal or lingual mucosa, it will dissolve, thus making it difficult to spit out or hide.

While conferring certain advantages, liquid formulations and orally disintegrating tablets also have some disadvantages. Doses for liquid formulations may be difficult to calculate and convert from capsule or tablet form, which may increase the risk of dosing errors.[46] Additionally, orally disintegrating tablets are often more expensive than tablets or capsules, limiting their use.[46] A summary of psychotropic medications available in liquid form or oral disintegrating form is provided in Table 26.2. Clinicians should refer to packaging information or speak to a pharmacist, as many potential issues related to compatibility or incompatibility with other agents (such as caffeine, certain foods, or other medications) may negatively impact treatment. Furthermore, many formulations contain other compounds that may cause side effects or be contraindicated in certain patient populations (e.g., alcohol, propylene glycol).[46]

SSRI-Related Upper GI Bleeding

SSRIs are associated with an almost 55% increase in the risk for upper GI bleeding (UGIB). [47] Bleeding is much more likely in patients who are also taking non-steroidal anti-inflammatory drugs (NSAIDs) or anti-platelet medications, whereas the risk of bleeding is almost eliminated by the use of acid-suppressing medication.[47] SSRI-induced GI bleeding is thought to be due to the depletion of serotonin in platelets, which do not synthesize their own serotonin and therefore require reuptake from plasma. This results in decreased platelet aggregation and clotting.[25,47] Particular caution should be exercised with SSRI use in patients with pre-existing clotting or other bleeding disorders, as well as patients at risk for GI bleeding, particularly those taking NSAIDs.

MEDICATION CONSIDERATIONS IN LIVER DISEASE

Since most psychotropics are metabolized by the liver, impaired hepatic function will negatively impact various aspects of pharmacokinetics, including drug absorption (due to vascular congestion) as well as first-pass metabolism and biotransformation (due to

TABLE 26.1

Non-oral Preparations of Psychotropic Medication

Medications	Intravenous	Intramuscular	Sublingual	Rectal	Transdermal
Anxiolytics	Diazepam Lorazepam Midazolam	Chlordiazepoxide Diazepam Lorazepam Midazolam		Diazepam	
Hypnotics			Zolpidem		
			Selegiline	Amitriptyline Doxepin	Selegiline
Typical Antipsychotics	Chlorpromazine Haloperidol	Chlorpromazine Fluphenazine Haloperidol Prochlorperazine Thiothixene Depot medications: Fluphenazine Haloperidol		Prochlorperazine	
Atypical Antipsychotics	Olanzapine	Olanzapine Ziprasidone Depot medications: Aripiprazole Olanzapine Paliperidone Risperidone	Asenapine		
Mood Stabilizers	Valproate			Carbamazepine Valproate	
Psychostimulants				Dextroamphetamine	Methylphenidate
Cognitive Enhancers					Rivastigmine

Medications that are available in the United States are listed.
Data from Owen JA, Crone CC, Marcangelo M, Lackamp J, et al. Gastrointestinal disorders. In: Ferrando SJ, Levenson JL, Owen JA, eds. *Clinical Manual of Psychopharmacology in the Medically Ill*. American Psychiatric Publishing; 2010:103–148.

damaged hepatocytes and altered cytochrome P450 enzyme function).[2] Oral bioavailability of medications may be increased due to prolonged biotransformation, metabolism, and clearance, and may also be increased in porto-systemic shunting where the medication is passed untransformed to the systemic circulation and brain. Changes in total body water and volume of distribution in moderate to severe liver disease result in altered distribution of water-soluble drugs, and drug levels may shift drastically with fluid redistribution.[2] Therefore, medications with narrow therapeutic windows, even those not metabolized by the liver, such as lithium, should be used with caution.

Because moderate to severe hepatic disease results in decreased plasma proteins and interferes with protein binding, total drug-level monitoring for medications that are highly protein bound, such as VPA, may be misleading, and the unbound or free portion should be measured.

Regardless of the presence of hepatic dysfunction, many psychotropic medications can be continued unless liver enzymes exceed three times the upper limit of normal.[6] Initial doses of hepatically metabolized medications should be lowered and dose increases should occur over longer intervals. Medications that undergo complex multi-step biotransformation and

TABLE 26.2
Liquid and Orally Disintegrating Formulations of Psychotropic Medications

Medication	Liquid Formulations and Dose (mg/mL)	Orally Disintegrating Formulations and Dose (mg)
Antidepressants		
SSRIs	Citalopram 10 mg/5 mL (240 mL)	
	Escitalopram 1 mg/mL (240 mL)	
	Fluoxetine 20 mg/5 mL (5 mL, 120 mL)	
	Paroxetine 10 mg/5 mL (250 mL)	
	Sertraline 20 mg/mL (60 mL)	
TCAs	Doxepin 10 mg/mL (120 mL)	
	Nortriptyline 10 mg/mL (240 mL)	
NaSSA		Mirtazapine 15, 30, 45 mg
Antipsychotics		
	Aripiprazole 1 mg/mL	Aripiprazole 10, 15 mg
	Risperidone 1 mg/mL	Clozapine 12.5, 25, 100 mg
	Fluphenazine 2.5 mg/5 mL, elixir 5 mg/mL	Olanzapine 5, 10, 15, 20 mg
	Thioridazine 100 mg/mL	Risperidone 0.5, 1, 2, 3, 4 mg
Anxiolytics (Benzodiazepines)		
	Alprazolam 1 mg/mL (30 mL)	Alprazolam 0.25, 0.5, 1, 2 mg
	Diazepam 5 mg/mL (500 mL)	Clonazepam 0.125, 0.25, 0.5, 1, 2 mg
	Lorazepam 2 mg/mL (1 mL, 10 mL)	
Cholinesterase Inhibitors		
	Galantamine 4 mg/mL (100 mL)	Donepezil 5, 10 mg
	Rivastigmine 2 mg/mL (in 120 mL bottle)	
NMDA Receptor Antagonists		
	Memantine 2 mg/mL (in 360 mL bottle)	
Mood Stabilizers		
	Carbamazepine 100 mg/5 mL	Lamotrigine 25, 50, 100 mg
	Valproic acid 250 mg/5 mL (473 mL)	
Stimulants		
	Dextroamphetamine 5 mg/5 mL	
	Methylphenidate 5 mg/5 mL (500 mL)	

NaSSA, Noradrenergic and selective serotonin antagonist; *NMDA*, N-methyl-D-aspartate; *SSRI*, selective serotonin reuptake inhibitor; *TCA*, tricyclic antidepressant.
Data from Muramatsu RS, Litzinger MH, Fisher E, et al. Alternative formulations, delivery methods, and administration options for psychotropic medications in elderly patients with behavioral and psychological symptoms of dementia. *Am J Geriatr Pharmacother.* 2010;8(2):98–114.[46]

those that are metabolized into active metabolites (such as amitriptyline, imipramine, venlafaxine, and bupropion) may pose greater challenges in this population than would medications with simpler pharmacokinetics.[2] Medications with long half-lives (e.g., fluoxetine, aripiprazole) or extended- or slow-release formulations (e.g., venlafaxine XR) should be avoided if possible as their pharmacokinetics are less predictable.[2]

Dosing changes and recommendations can be made while considering hepatic severity as measured by the Child-Pugh score (CPS) which considers total bilirubin, serum albumin, ascites, international normalized ratio, and the presence or absence of hepatic encephalopathy.[2,6] Patients with mild (CPS-A) liver failure can usually tolerate 75% to 100% of the standard medication dose, those with moderate (CPS-B) disease may require a 50% to 75% reduction in dose, and for those with severe disease (CPS-C), (particularly those with HE), conservative dosing schedules and close monitoring are required.[2]

Certain psychotropics may be associated with drug-induced liver injury. Drug-induced liver injury is often idiosyncratic and cannot be predicted accurately by specific risk factors or drug dosage.[2,48] With the exception of carbamazepine and divalproex, there are no specific or formal manufacturer's guidelines for monitoring liver enzymes.[6] Medication-induced hepatotoxicity is associated with alanine aminotransferase (ALT) levels in excess of aspartate aminotransferase (AST). Caution is required when interpreting laboratory results in patients who have pre-existing liver disease and in obese patients with steatohepatitis and non-alcoholic fatty liver disease.[6] Mild to modest increases in transaminases may occur with carbamazepine, divalproex, certain TCAs, SNRIs, and atypical antipsychotics.[6] One review found that 0.5% to 3% of patients treated with antidepressants experienced asymptomatic and mild elevations of transaminases. Cases are generally not associated with dosage, and most reactions occur anywhere from several days to 6 months after initiating the medication. Elderly patients and patients taking multiple medications carry the highest risk. The highest risks of hepatotoxicity are associated with nefazodone, phenelzine, imipramine, amitriptyline, duloxetine, bupropion, trazodone, and agomelatine. Antidepressants with the lowest potential for hepatotoxicity are citalopram, escitalopram, paroxetine, and fluvoxamine.[48] Severe hepatotoxicity has been reported with duloxetine, nefazodone, carbamazepine, and divalproex; divalproex and nefazodone both carry FDA black box warnings.[6] The overall incidence of hepatoxicity of antiepileptic drugs has been estimated at 1/26,000 to 1/36,000. Of the antiepileptics, VPA is associated with the greatest potential for liver toxicity, with an onset of liver injury ranging from 3 days to 2 years after treatment initiation. Chlorpromazine and other phenothiazines may cause reversible cholestatic hepatotoxicity in up to 2% of cases; patients with primary biliary cirrhosis should not receive these medications.[2]

There are no specific guidelines for hepatic monitoring, and it is likely that none is needed for most patients who are receiving hepatically metabolized medications. If a patient has pre-existing liver disease or develops symptoms after starting a medication, it is reasonable to investigate further. If no clinical symptoms accompany elevated serum transaminases up to two times the normal limit, watchful waiting with laboratory monitoring versus drug discontinuation is reasonable. If transaminase levels exceed two to three times the normal limit, it is advisable to discontinue the medication.[2,6] Certain medications known to be associated with severe hepatotoxicity (e.g., duloxetine, nefazodone, carbamazepine, and divalproex) should be discontinued even in milder cases, as they are known to be associated with severe hepatotoxicity. Finally, if patients present with specific signs of liver disease, such as right upper quadrant pain, dark urine, lightly colored stool, itching, jaundice, nausea, or anorexia, medications should be stopped immediately, and expert consultation sought.

In contrast to ALT > AST patterns seen in drug- (and viral-) induced hepatotoxicity, in patients with alcohol-induced hepatotoxicity, AST:ALT ratios of 2:1 or 3:1 may be seen.[6] Carbohydrate-deficient transferrin and gamma-glutamyl transpeptidase (GTT) are both non-specific but sensitive markers of hepatic dysfunction and can be used to aid in the detection of recent (2-week) heavy drinking patterns. Elevated GTT distinguishes between liver-based as opposed to bone-based elevations in alkaline phosphatase; however, it may also be elevated in congestive heart failure and may not be useful in this patient population.[6]

Some patients metabolize medications differently due to varying isoforms of cytochrome P450 genes. This may further complicate effective management in the presence of hepatic disease. At times, genetic testing may help indicate whether psychotropics are being metabolized differently in patients who can be considered rapid metabolizers, ultra-rapid (0%–30% of the population) metabolizers, or poor (slow) metabolizers (0%–14% of the population) due to the presence or absence of CYP P450 isoforms.[49] Additionally, medications that increase or inhibit the metabolism of medications (such as carbamazepine [a potent CYP P450 inducer] or paroxetine [a potent CYP P450 inhibitor]) need to be accounted for, as their presence may require further dosing adjustments in patients with or without liver disease. Knowledge of medications that are minimally metabolized or undergo no metabolism by hepatic CYP P450 enzymes can aid in appropriate medication selection. These medications include pregabalin, lorazepam, oxazepam, temazepam, desvenlafaxine, milnacipran, paliperidone, gabapentin, levetiracetam, lamotrigine, lithium, and memantine.[49]

REFERENCES

1. Person H, Keefer L. Psychological comorbidity in gastrointestinal diseases: update on the brain-gut-microbiome axis. *Prog Neuropsychopharmacol Biol Psychiatry*. 2021;107:1–28.

2. Crone CC, Marcangelo M, Lackamp J, et al. Gastrointestinal disorders. In: Ferrando SJ, Levenson JL, Owen JA, eds. *Clinical Manual of Psychopharmacology in the Medically Ill*. American Psychiatric Association Publishing; 2010:103–148.

3. Ouyang A, Locke GR. Overview of neurogastroenterology-gastrointestinal motility and functional GI disorders: classification, prevalence, and epidemiology. *Gastroenterol Clin N Am*. 2007;36:485–498.

4. Sorbin WH, Heinrich TW, Drossman DA. Central neuromodulators for treating functional GI disorders: a primer. *Am J Gastroenterol*. 2017;112:693–702.

5. You ZH, Perng CL, Hu LY, et al. Risk of psychiatric disorders following gastroesophageal reflux disease: a nationwide population-based cohort study. *Eur J Intern Med*. 2015;26(7):534–539.

6. Goldberg JF, Ernst CL. Gastrointestinal system. In: Goldberg JF, Ernst CL, eds. *Managing the Side Effects of Psychotropic Medications*. American Psychiatric Association Publishing; 2012:187–199.

7. Navari RM, Aapro M. Antiemetic prophylaxis for chemotherapy-induced nausea and vomiting. *N Engl J Med*. 2016;374(14):1356–1367.

8. Drossman DA. Functional gastrointestinal disorders: history, pathophysiology, clinical features and Rome IV. *Gastroenterology*. 2016.

9. Uguz F, Gezginc K, Kayhan F, et al. Is hyperemesis gravidarum associated with mood, anxiety and personality disorders: a case-control study. *Gen Hosp Psychiatry*. 2012;34(4):398–402.

10. Kim DR, Connolly KR, Cristancho P, et al. Psychiatric consultation of patients with hyperemesis gravidarum. *Arch Womens Ment Health*. 2009;12:61.

11. Hejazi RA, McCallum RW. Cyclic vomiting syndrome: treatment options. *Exp Brain Res*. 2014;232(8):2549–2552.

12. Ruffle JK, Bajgoric S, Samra K, et al. Cannabinoid hyperemesis syndrome: an important differential diagnosis of persistent unexplained vomiting. *Eur J Gastroenterol Hepatol*. 2015;27(12):1403–1408.

13. Drossman DA, Dumitrascu DL. Rome III. New standard for functional gastrointestinal disorders. *J Gastrointestin Liver Dis*. 2006;15(3):237–241.

14. Rao AS, Camilleri M. Review article: metoclopramide and tardive dyskinesia. *Aliment Pharmacol Ther*. 2010;31(1):11–19.

15. Cavero-Redondo I, Álvarez-Bueno C, Pozuelo-Carrascosa DP, et al. Risk of extrapyramidal side effects comparing continuous vs. bolus intravenous metoclopramide administration: a systematic review and meta-analysis of randomised controlled trials. *J Clin Nurs*. 2015;24(23–24):3638–3646.

16. Geraldo Mde S, Fonseca FL, Gouveia MR, et al. The use of drugs in patients who have undergone bariatric surgery. *Int J Gen Med*. 2014;7:219–224.

17. Miller AD, Smith KM. Medication and nutrient administration considerations after bariatric surgery. *Am J Health Syst Pharm*. 2006;63(19):1852–1857.

18. Seaman JS, Bowers SP, Dixon P, et al. Dissolution of common psychiatric medications in a Roux-en-Y gastric bypass model. *Psychosomatics*. 2005;46(3):250–253.

19. Cunningham JL, Merrell CC, Sarr M, et al. Investigation of antidepressant medication usage after bariatric surgery. *Obes Surg*. 2012;22(4):530–535.

20. Hamad GG, Helsel JC, Perel JM, et al. The effect of gastric bypass on the pharmacokinetics of serotonin reuptake inhibitors. *Am J Psychiatry*. 2012;169(3):256–263.

21. Xu Y, Amdanee N, Zhang X. Antipsychotic-induced constipation: a review of the pathogenesis, clinical diagnosis, and treatment. *CNS Drugs*. 2021;35:1265–1274.

22. McCormack PL. Vilazodone: a review in major depressive disorder in adults. *Drugs*. 2015;75(16):1915–1923.

23. Enck P, Aziz Q, Barbara G, et al. Irritable bowel syndrome. *Nat Rev Dis Primers*. 2016;2(1):24.

24. Ford AC, Lacy BE, Harris LA, et al. Effect of antidepressants and psychological therapies in irritable bowel syndrome: an updated systematic review and meta-analysis. *Am J Gastroenterol*. 2019;114:21–39.

25. Crone CC, Dobbelstein CR. Gastrointestinal disorders. In: Levenson JL, ed. *Textbook of Psychosomatic Medicine-Psychiatric Care of the Medically Ill*. 2nd ed. American Psychiatric Association Publishing; 2011:463–490.

26. Seyedian SS, Nokhostin F, Malamir MD. A review of the diagnosis, prevention, and treatment methods of inflammatory bowel disease. *J Med Life*. 2019;12(2):113–122.

27. Najjar S, Pearlman DM, Alper K, et al. Neuroinflammation and psychiatric illness. *J Neuroinflammation*. 2013;10:43.

28. Gracie DJ, Hamlin PJ, Ford AC. The influence of the brain-gut axis in inflammatory bowel disease and possible implications for treatment. *Lancet Gastroenterol Hepatol*. 2019;4(8):632–642.

29. Yanartas O, Kani HT, Bicakci E, et al. The effects of psychiatric treatment on depression, anxiety, quality of life, and sexual dysfunction in patients with inflammatory bowel disease. *Neuropsychiatr Dis Treat*. 2016;12:673–683.

30. Horst S, Chao A, Rosen M, et al. Treatment with immunosuppressive therapy may improve depressive symptoms in patients with inflammatory bowel disease. *Dig Dis Sci*. 2015;60(2):465–470.

31. Lord O, Malone D, Mitchell AJ. Receipt of preventive medical care and medical screening for patients with mental illness: a comparative analysis. *Gen Hosp Psychiatry*. 2010;32(5):519–543.

32. Baillargeon J, Kuo YF, Lin YL, et al. Effect of mental disorders on diagnosis, treatment, and survival of older adults with colon cancer. *J Am Geriatr Soc*. 2011;59(7):1268–1273.

33. Shinn EH, Valentine A, Jethanandani A, et al. Depression and oropharynx cancer outcome. *Psychosom Med*. 2016;78(1):38–48.

34. Allen-Mersh TG, Glover C, Fordy C, et al. Relation between depression and circulating immune products in patients with advanced colorectal cancer. *J R Soc Med*. 1998;91(8):408–413.

35. Oliveira Miranda D, Soares de Lima TA, Ribeiro Azevedo L, et al. Proinflammatory cytokines correlate with depression and anxiety in colorectal cancer patients. *Biomed Res Int*. 2014; 2014:739650.

36. Lemke J, Scheele J, Kapapa T, et al. Brain metastases in gastrointestinal cancers: is there a role for surgery? *Int J Mol Sci*. 2014;15(9):16816–16830.

37. Hauser P, Kern S. Psychiatric and substance use disorders co-morbidities and hepatitis C: diagnostic and treatment implications. *World J Hepatol*. 2015;7(15):1921–1935.

38. Sockalingam S, Sheehan K, Feld JJ, et al. Psychiatric care during hepatitis C treatment: the changing role of psychiatrists in the era of direct-acting antivirals. *Am J Psychiatry*. 2015;172(6): 512–516.

39. Kiser JJ, Burton JR, Everson GT. Drug–drug interactions during antiviral therapy for chronic hepatitis C. *Nat Rev Gastroenterol Hepatol*. 2013;10(10):596–606.

40. Kelly EM, Corace K, Emery J, et al. Bipolar patients can safely and successfully receive interferon-based hepatitis C antiviral treatment. *Eur J Gastroenterol Hepatol*. 2012;24(7):811–816.

41. Kraus MR, Schäfer A, Wissmann S, et al. Neurocognitive changes in patients with hepatitis C receiving interferon alfa-2b and ribavirin. *Clin Pharmacol Ther*. 2005;77(1):90–100.

42. Kaplan PW. The EEG in metabolic encephalopathy and coma. *J Clin Neurophysiol*. 2004;21:307–318.

43. Jawaro T, Yang A, Dixit D, et al. Management of hepatic encephalopathy: a primer. *Ann Pharmacother*. 2016;50(7): 569–577.

44. Mayr M, Schmid RM. Pancreatic cancer and depression: myth and truth. *BMC Cancer*. 2010;10:569.

45. Zaccara G, Franciotta D, Perucca E. Idiosyncratic adverse reactions to antiepileptic drugs. *Epilepsia*. 2007;48(7):1223–1244.

46. Muramatsu RS, Litzinger MH, Fisher E, et al. Alternative formulations, delivery methods, and administration options for psychotropic medications in elderly patients with behavioral and psychological symptoms of dementia. *Am J Geriatr Pharmacother*. 2010;8(2):98–114.

47. Jiang HY, Chen HZ, Hu XJ, et al. Use of selective serotonin reuptake inhibitors and risk of upper gastrointestinal bleeding: a systematic review and meta-analysis. *Clin Gastroenterol Hepatol*. 2015;13(1):42–50.

48. Telles-Correia D, Barbosa A, Cortez-Pinto H, et al. Psychotropic drugs and liver disease: a critical review of pharmacokinetics and liver toxicity. *World J Gastrointest Pharmacol Ther*. 2017;8(1):26–38.

49. Andrade C. Drugs that escape hepatic metabolism. *J Clin Psychiatry*. 2012;73(7):e889–e890.

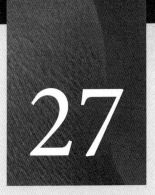

27

ORGAN FAILURE AND TRANSPLANTATION

LAURA M. PRAGER, MD

OVERVIEW

Solid organ transplantation is an accepted, successful, and commonly employed treatment option for patients with end-organ failure. Transplantation recipients of a heart, liver, kidney, lung(s), pancreas, or small intestine now live longer with an overall improved quality of life. Transplantation now also offers hope to patients with severed upper limbs and to those who have suffered facial disfigurement. Progress in the development of immunosuppressive medications and methods of organ procurement and distribution has also enabled transplantation. Former contraindications to transplant, such as a history of cancer or human immunodeficiency virus infection, are no longer absolute barriers.

In the United States, the United Network for Organ Sharing (UNOS), a non-profit organization endowed by Congress but reporting to the Department of Health and Human Services (HHS), regulates the allocation and distribution of donor organs. Since 1986, UNOS has overseen its two branches: the Organ Procurement and Transplant Network (OPTN) and the Scientific Registry of Transplant Recipients. The OPTN divides the country into 11 distinct geographical regions or donation service areas (DSAs); each region has its own waiting list. Allocation of organs generally follows a local, regional, and national progression, where local refers to the boundaries of the DSA. The length of time spent on the waiting list often differed greatly among regions. In addition, each DSA had Organ Procurement Organizations that, in conjunction with UNOS, determined the best patient match

for a given organ. In 2000, the Department of HHS issued a "final rule" that encouraged DSAs to distribute available organs outside of their own geographic boundaries based on the gravity of a given patient's clinical presentation. This "final rule" underwent some amendments, but it remains in effect today with the goal of offering organs more broadly given the persistent mismatch between those who need an organ transplant and the number of available organs.[1] More recently, physicians and public health researchers have called for eradicating the geographic boundaries of the DSAs and creating a "borderless distribution" network that incorporates both medical needs and geographic practicality.[2]

The determination of priority remains organ specific. For kidneys, the length of time on the waiting list is the primary determining factor, although patients listed simultaneously for transplant of a kidney and another solid organ have greater priority. In addition, full human leukocyte antigen (HLA) compatibility (zero antigen mismatch) as measured by panel-reactive antibodies (PRAs) confers priority. Pediatric recipients (those 18 years and under) of kidneys and livers take priority over adults. In 2011 the OPTN/UNOS Kidney Transplantation Committee reviewed this allocation procedure and drafted new guidelines that accounted for a candidate's ability to survive on the waiting list and created a measure of kidney quality that would optimize the match between donors and recipients.[3] In January 2023 OPTN rolled out a new policy affecting HLA compatibility measures. It approved a reworking of way the Calculated PRA is determined, which used technological advances and a much larger data set of potential donors, to increase the sensitivity of HLA matching.[4]

For many years, the Lung Allocation Score (LAS) conferred priority for lung transplantation and determined waiting-list placement for potential lung transplant recipients. The LAS is a calculated score for patients >12 years of age that involves several factors, including the severity of illness and the likelihood of a successful transplant outcome (e.g., age, blood type, and geographical location). This was an important change as more patients with acute respiratory failure were placed on a mechanical circulatory support device, an extracorporeal membrane oxygenator (ECMO), as a bridge to transplant and could not tolerate prolonged waiting times.[5] The score subsequently underwent frequent modifications based on shifts in the characteristics of the candidate cohort, with the consistent goal of reducing time spent on the waiting list. In 2021, OPTN again modified the way that the LAS was calculated. The planned implementation of this new policy was in early 2023; it allows for a single matching score rather than one with several components and will include geographical reasonableness that allows for donor organs from outside of the DSA.[6] The OPTN limits the allocation of lungs to patients <12 years of age to those donors within the same age range. This policy came under scrutiny a decade ago due to a highly publicized case in which the parents of a 10-year-old girl appealed to a federal judge to allow the patient access to lungs from the adult donor pool.[7] Based on that case, there have been some exceptions made to the OPTN; adult deceased donor lungs have been trimmed to fit a child, but those cases remain uncommon.

The Model for End-stage Liver Disease (MELD) is also a calculated score that predicts how urgently a patient >12 years of age will need a transplant within the next 3 months. The only exception to the MELD system is a special category known as "Status 1." Status 1 A patients have suffered acute hepatic failure and might die within hours or days without a transplant (Tables 27.1 and 27.2 list the LAS and MELD criteria, respectively).

Since 1999 heart transplant recipients have received organs based on medical urgency. Guidelines from 2006 dictate local and regional allocation and allow critically ill patients within a 500-nautical mile radius of the donor's hospital to take priority over patients

TABLE 27.1
Criteria for Lung Allocation Score (LAS) (Age 12 and Older)

- Diagnosis
- Age
- Body mass index
- Presence of diabetes
- New York Heart Association Functional Classification
- Distance walked in 6 minutes
- Forced vital capacity
- Pulmonary artery pressure
- Pulmonary capillary wedge pressure
- Creatinine and changes in creatinine
- Total bilirubin and change in bilirubin
- Amount of oxygen needed at rest
- Requirement for ventilatory support
- Current, highest, and lowest pCO_2 (partial pressure of carbon dioxide)

Adapted from UNOS. www.unos.org. https://unos.org/wp-content/uploads/unos/Lung_Patient.pdf

TABLE 27.2
Model for End-Stage Liver Disease (MELD) (Age 12 and Older)

Serum bilirubin
International normalized ratio
Serum creatinine
Scores range from 6 to 40
Represents urgency for need for transplant within 3 months of calculation

Adapted from UNOS. https://optn.transplant.hrsa.gov/resources/allocation-calculators/meld-calculator/

who are less ill but are within the local zone. In 2018 UNOS updated the scoring system for heart transplantation with a shift from a three-part ranking to a six-part ranking to decrease time on the waiting list.[8] Previously patients in cardiogenic shock were ranked as Status 1A[9]; now such patients are triaged into one of three groups—Status 1, 2, and 3—depending on how much other support (e.g., ECMO) the patient requires. Evaluation of the success of this change has suggested mixed results, as time on the waiting list has decreased but patients have not done as well post-transplant. More research is needed to assess whether the new allocation system will prove equitable or require additional adjustments.[10]

Several factors limit the success of organ transplantation, most significantly allograft rejection and the complications of antirejection therapy. In addition, immunocompromised hosts are vulnerable to bacteria, viruses, and fungi that are not considered pathogenic in the normal population. Finally, the side effects of immunosuppressive medications that are used to manage rejection can be debilitating, disfiguring, or life threatening, and increase the risk for neoplasms, problems with bone metabolism, a cushingoid body habitus, nephrotoxicity, posterior-reversible encephalopathic syndrome (PRES), and the development of diabetes mellitus. Initially, the COVID-19 pandemic adversely affected the number of solid-organ transplants due to the strain on hospitals to care for patients infected with SARS-CoV-2. However, after a sharp drop in transplants during the first COVID surge, by the fall of 2020 that volume increased and, in many cases, exceeded prior levels.[11]

The most pressing challenge, however, remains the shortage of available deceased donor and living donor organs. The scarcity of cadaveric organs creates a mismatch between the number of patients who need an organ transplant and the number who can undergo transplantation. Although the number of organ transplants done nationwide has increased significantly over recent decades, currently there are 104,528 active waiting-list candidates for solid organ transplantation and 42,887 transplants performed between January and December of 2022 compared with 118,725 on the list with 14,105 transplanted in 2013.[12] Transplant centers have attempted to expand the donor pool by harvesting organs from donors after circulatory (cardiac) death and expanded criteria donors in addition, to harvesting organs from persons who have been declared dead by neurological criteria, or donation after brain death.[13] In response to this problem, the Institute of Medicine, renamed in 2015 as the National Academy of Medicine, created a committee to study ways in which the supply of transplantable organs could be increased. The committee's report, released in May 2006, recommended the following: vigorous public education about organ donation; provision of more opportunities for registration as an organ donor; easier access to state donor registries; and renewed attention to improvement of organ procurement systems.[14] Other efforts included

the establishment of the Transplant Growth and Management Collaborative in 2007,[13] and in 2008 legislation that gave the Department of HHS a mandate to issue a National Medal honoring organ donors.[15] Some European countries follow the doctrine of "presumed consent" for post-mortem donation, but the United States has not embraced this idea. Internet platforms, such as MatchingDonors.com, have enabled patients to find living organ donors online, but many transplant centers have concerns about whether donors using these platforms truly provided informed consent and whether they received any form of compensation.[16] Most recently, in 2021 the National Institutes of Health convened an ad hoc committee from within the National Academies of Sciences, Engineering, and Medicine to study the issues of equity in deceased donor organ procurement systems, distribution networks, and decisions regarding allocation.[17] That report, published in 2022, contained 14 recommendations for improving equitable access to deceased donor organs, including, but not limited to, creating national performance goals, facilitating the ease with which transplant centers can accept donor organs, bolstering the continuous distribution framework, and improving the function of the system.

Organ donation by living donors is an increasingly important potential source of transplantable kidneys, livers, and lungs. This is especially true in Japan, where there are no defined criteria for the determination of brain death and therefore few cadaveric organs are available for harvest.[18,19] In the United States, living donors may be related to the recipient; unrelated but emotionally connected; or anonymous, altruistic strangers. According to data from OPTN (from 2023) 36,420 transplanted organs came from deceased donors and 6467 organ transplants (kidney, liver, and lung) came from live donors.[12] Parent-to-child liver transplantation (of the left lateral lobe) is an option, as is adult-to-adult transplantation of the right hepatic lobe.[20] Pediatric living donor recipients do better postoperatively. Living-lung donation is also an option for carefully selected candidates, but it requires a lower lobe from two different donors for each potential recipient. The source of the donated lung (i.e., from a deceased donor or a living donor) does not affect the recipient's outcome.

Living organ donation raises several ethical issues related to beneficence, non-maleficence, and autonomy. These include: What is the benefit to the donor? What level of risk is acceptable for a healthy, altruistic donor? What is true informed consent regarding both short- and long-term risks for the donor? Is the donor's offer (be it from an emotionally connected or unrelated person) truly voluntary?[21]

Several retrospective studies of the long-term medical and psychological sequelae of living organ donors have been conducted. Benefits generally include the satisfaction gained from improving another person's quality of life. Short-term risks for live kidney donors include the morbidity associated with surgery and anesthesia (e.g., bleeding, infection) and salary loss during the weeks of recovery. For kidney donors, long-term health risks include the development of microalbuminuria and the small but potential risk of renal failure in the remaining kidney; the mortality rate for kidney donors is 0.03%.[22]

With adult-to-adult liver donation, there is significant morbidity and a higher potential for mortality. In a recent retrospective study, the mortality rate (per 1000 person/year) was 0.91 up to 8 years following donation,[23] while mortality estimates approached 0.1% for those who donated a left lateral lobe and 0.5% for those who donated a right lateral lobe.[24] Morbidity following liver donation includes incisional pain, gastrointestinal (GI) distress, and lower exercise tolerance for several years following transplantation. Notwithstanding, donors generally express satisfaction with their decision and feel good about improving another person's life.

To date, no deaths have resulted from living lobar lung donation (LLLD), and it remains an option for those who cannot survive the projected waiting time for deceased donor lungs such as pediatric patients with cystic fibrosis (CF).[25] However, there is significant morbidity associated with LLLD, which limits the feasibility of this option, particularly because each recipient requires two donors.[26] One study found that donors lose 15% to 20% of their total lung volume and often experience a decrease in exercise capacity.[27] Another study demonstrated that both the forced vital capacity and forced expiratory volume at 1 minute decreased post-operatively but returned to 90% of baseline 1 year post-lobectomy.[28]

PSYCHIATRIC EVALUATION OF THE TRANSPLANT PATIENT

Psychiatrists and other mental health professionals are involved in many different aspects of the transplantation process. In some centers, a designated psychiatrist works with a specific team (e.g., the kidney transplant team). Other transplant centers rely on general hospital psychiatric consultation services, psychologists, or social workers to provide case-by-case consultation. The involvement of mental health professionals ranges from the preoperative evaluation of candidates and living donors, to the short- and long-term post-operative management of solid organ recipients.

The psychiatrist or other mental health professional plays an important role in the evaluation of the patient who is approaching a transplant. Initially, the psychiatrist conducts a thorough psychiatric evaluation of the potential recipient to determine "suitability" for transplant. The psychiatrist must be familiar with medical and surgical problems facing the patient (both before and after transplantation) to educate both the patient and the family members about the risks and benefits of transplantation.

The psychiatrist may also act as a liaison between the patient (and family members) and the transplant team. The patient will need support, direction, and clarification of the transplant team's expectations and concerns. The transplant team may require help interpreting a patient's behavior. The psychiatrist can direct the team's attention to ethical dilemmas that may arise, particularly in the area of directed living donation by a related or unrelated donor.

After transplantation, the psychiatrist will be instrumental in guiding the family through the patient's often difficult and unpredictable post-operative course, as well as in managing the potential neuropsychiatric sequelae secondary to graft rejection, infection, and immunosuppression.

Pre-Transplant Psychiatric Evaluation

There are no universally accepted guidelines for the psychiatric evaluation of candidates for organ transplantation and little reliable or predictive data regarding "suitability for transplantation." Some centers routinely offer a face-to-face clinical interview with a mental health provider, whereas other centers administer formal psychological testing or offer a structured or semi-structured interview. There are several tools, such as the Psychosocial Assessment of Candidates for Transplantation, the Transplant Evaluation Rating Scale, and the Stanford Integrated Psychosocial Assessment for Transplantation that were developed to help evaluators predict which transplant candidates are at highest risk for poor outcomes based on their psychosocial limitations. All three of these rating scales have strengths but are also limited by a paucity of validity and reliability. Currently, national consensus guidelines recommend that transplant centers that use rating scales do so as a component of a more comprehensive evaluation, rather than using a single score to predict how patients will do following transplantation.[29]

Transplant centers differ in their determination of who is an "acceptable" candidate and what degree of risk they are willing to assume. Common psychosocial and behavioral exclusion criteria include active substance use, active psychotic symptoms, thoughts of suicide (with intent or a plan), dementia, or a felony conviction. Relative contraindications include poor social support with an inability to arrange for pre-transplant or post-transplant care, personality disorders that interfere with a working relationship with a transplant team, non-adherence to a medication regimen, and neurocognitive limitations.[30]

The pre-transplantation psychiatric evaluation should be primarily diagnostic, but it can also be both educational and therapeutic. General objectives of the psychiatric evaluation include screening potential recipients for the presence of significant diagnoses that might complicate management or interfere with the patient's ability to comply with the treatment team's recommendations after transplantation. A diagnosis of, for example, major depressive disorder (MDD), schizophrenia, or bipolar disorder should not be a contraindication to transplant if the patient has been stable for an extended period on appropriate medications and has adequate outpatient care and support. However, pre-transplant depression in potential liver transplant recipients has been associated with long hospital stays, discharge to a facility rather than to home, and a shorter period of post-transplant survival.[31]

Case 1

Mr. A, a 40-year-old man with diabetes mellitus and end-stage renal disease (ESRD), was referred for psychiatric evaluation of depression because he wanted to discontinue hemodialysis (HD). There was no personal or family history of depression. He reported a depressed mood in association with chronic pain from diabetic neuropathy and from the severe headaches that often follow HD sessions. Mr. A agreed to a trial of an antidepressant and an analgesic after HD. His pain remitted, his mood lifted, and he subsequently chose to undergo renal transplantation.

Transplantation is possible even in pre-morbid cognitively impaired individuals with end-organ failure. Such patients may have family members who will assume legal responsibility for medical decision-making and oversee adherence to post-transplant protocols. Personality disorders are sometimes more difficult to diagnose in a cross-sectional interview, but, when present, can complicate the patient's interactions with members of the treatment team. Patients with borderline personality disorder or antisocial personality disorder are particularly problematic given their affective dysregulation, unstable personal relationships, and potential for impaired impulse control. Transplant psychiatrists must carefully assess the individual patient's history of interpersonal relationships, a substance use disorder (SUD), potential for self-injurious behavior, adherence to treatment recommendations, and interactions with caregivers, before deciding whether such a patient can work successfully with the team.[32]

Psychiatrists are often asked to predict a patient's motivation for transplantation and risk for non-adherence to medication regimens. Life following a transplant requires diligent attention to, and compliance with, medical protocols. Post-transplant patients often take as many as 20 medications daily and must attend regularly scheduled clinic appointments, self-monitor blood pressure and blood sugar, maintain good nutrition, and endure frequently uncomfortable procedures and tests.

Evaluators may also wish to assess the patient's resilience and ability to persevere despite setbacks, as well as the availability of social supports that will allow for continued care in the community and easy transportation to and from the hospital. There is controversy as to whether the transplant team should explore social media sites to verify the patient's report of his/her lifestyle choices. Most mental health professionals who work with this population do not engage in what some have referred to as "patient-targeted" googling,[33] but others feel strongly that they must use whatever means they have to decide about a candidate's ability to comply with the demands of transplantation (personal communication, TransplantPsychiatry@googlegroups.com, 2013).

Frequently, the question arises as to whether there is a conflict of interest if, as is often the case, the psychiatrist who conducts the initial screening for transplant candidacy is the same psychiatrist who works with the multi-disciplinary transplant team to decide which candidates can be listed. Again, there are no national guidelines, and individual transplant teams must address and resolve this ethical issue. The psychiatrist may choose to handle this situation by informing the patient and the family at the beginning of the evaluation that the information presented will be shared with other members of the team and will be considered in the team's decision regarding candidacy.

The issue of SUDs in the pre-transplant population is particularly challenging because of the risk of relapse with possible non-adherence post-transplant. Most transplant programs require 6 months to 1 year of sustained sobriety before initiation of the transplant evaluation, although this policy has not been shown to affect outcomes.[34] Some programs require patients to participate in a SUD counseling program in addition, to Alcoholics Anonymous or Narcotics Anonymous as a prerequisite for listing if they appear to be at high risk for relapse. However, a recent review of alcohol use disorder in transplant patients suggests that patients with acute alcoholic hepatitis and only a short period of sobriety can undergo liver transplantation and maintain sobriety post-operatively when managed longitudinally by a multi-disciplinary team that includes medical and surgical input as well as a psychologist and a psychiatrist familiar with SUDs and transplantation.[35] Likewise, whereas opioid use disorder was often an absolute contraindication to solid organ transplantation, even when the patient

had achieved sobriety using opioid agonist therapy (OAT), some transplant teams now accept these candidates and offer careful management of the OAT pre-, peri-, and post-transplant.[36] Use of cannabinoids in pre-transplant candidates is relatively common given its increasingly easy availability. According to a recent review, eight states have laws that prohibit the denial of transplantation candidacy based on the use of cannabinoids.[37] There is some evidence to suggest that cannabinoids increase the toxicity of immunosuppressive medications, specifically tacrolimus, due to CYP34A inhibition.[35] Cigarette smoking or any form of tobacco use is an absolute contraindication to lung transplantation. Patients must demonstrate sustained abstinence from cigarettes and undergo random measurements of urinary cotinine and/or serum carboxyhemoglobin as part of the evaluation process. Some centers also consider cigarette smoking as a contraindication for potential liver transplantation, as it increases the likelihood of post-operative vascular problems and the overall mortality rate.[38] In the end, there are no nationally defined guidelines for patients with SUDs, and individual transplant centers determine what degree of risk they are willing to tolerate.

PSYCHIATRIC CONSIDERATIONS IN PATIENTS WITH END-ORGAN FAILURE

Many psychiatric disorders (such as depression, anxiety, adjustment disorders, post-traumatic stress disorder [PTSD], and SUDs) are common in the pre-transplant candidate population, regardless of the type of end-stage organ failure. Other disorders are unique to patients who suffer from a specific type of end-organ failure. Usually, there is a significant wait between the time of listing for a transplant and undergoing a transplant. Many patients with heart failure must wait in a hospital's intensive care unit (ICU) attached to a cardiac monitor or an intra-aortic balloon pump (IABP); others live outside the hospital with a left ventricular assist device. Years can go by while the patient with lung disease waits at home, sometimes far from a transplant center, becoming gradually sicker and more sedentary, all the while tethered to an oxygen tank. The wait is stressful. A call from a member of the transplant team saying that an organ is available can come at any time or not at all. Sometimes a patient arrives at the hospital only to learn that the quality of the harvested organ is not good enough—the so-called "false start" or "dry run." Loss of physical strength and productivity (with accompanying role changes within the family or community) can lead to an adjustment disorder or depression.

A study of 103 patients published in 2022 found that >58% of patients with chronic kidney disease (CKD) (but who were not dialysis dependent) suffered from depression, as measured by the Patient Health Questionnaire-9, and ~50% met the criteria for generalized anxiety disorder (GAD), as measured by the GAD-7.[39] Another earlier study showed that as many as 25% of dialysis-dependent patients with ESRD manifest symptoms of MDD.[40] Disorders in endocrine function (e.g., hyperparathyroidism) and chronic anemia can also contribute to depression. The dialysis-dysequilibrium syndrome with resultant cerebral edema, as well as uremia, can precipitate a change in mental status or even a frank encephalopathy. Patients with renal failure are also prone to delirium from the accumulation of toxins (e.g., aluminum) or from prescribed medications that are normally cleared by the kidney.

Patients with heart failure are also at risk for depression and delirium. These patients can spend long periods in the ICU awaiting transplantation, with little contact with the outside world.[41] Delirium can be caused by decreased cerebral blood flow, multiple small ischemic events, or by IABP treatment.[42] The development of the ventricular assist device (VAD) as a bridge to heart transplantation offers a chance for improved quality of life and functional status in this population.

Hepatic failure (e.g., from cirrhosis) is also associated with a high degree of depression and with subclinical or frank encephalopathy.[43] Treatment of the mood disorder can result in a more positive outlook and better self-care. Acute hepatic failure can occur following a suicide attempt by toxic ingestion (e.g., of acetaminophen), which could require an immediate transplant. If these patients are sedated and on ventilators, conducting an interview is challenging. Therefore, the psychiatric consultant must rely on collateral sources of information about the patient's pre-morbid function.

Patients with end-stage lung disease are likely to suffer from an anxiety disorder, especially panic disorder, as well as an adjustment disorder, depression, and delirium. Most patients who were not anxious before they developed organ failure become anxious in the setting of increasing shortness of breath. They often describe anticipatory anxiety (in the setting of planned exertion), panic attacks, and agoraphobia, despite adequate oxygen supplementation. A decreasing radius of activity leads to an adjustment disorder and, sometimes, to depression, as patients struggle to cope with their relentless and progressive inability to perform even simple activities of daily living. Extremely compromised patients with pulmonary failure may become delirious from hypoxia or hypercapnia or from medications (such as intravenous [IV] benzodiazepines and narcotics) used to treat their anxiety and pain. Patients placed on ECMO as a bridge to transplantation pose a new challenge. These patients are awake and alert, but aware of their tenuous condition and their total dependence on the machine and the staff. In this setting, they often (understandably) become demanding and angry, and they test the energy and patience of the ICU team.

Case 2

Ms. E, a 21-year-old married woman with pulmonary fibrosis, was referred by her pulmonologist for lung transplantation. She had no other medical problems and had no formal psychiatric history. A college graduate, she had worked full time for several years. During the year before her evaluation, she had to work fewer hours because of worsening pulmonary function. Although she described herself as "even-keeled," she had become increasingly anxious as her pulmonary function worsened. Even when her pulmonologist started her on continuous oxygen treatment, she remained anxious. At the time of her evaluation, she felt overwhelmed and was having panic attacks, particularly when she anticipated leaving her apartment to go to work. She also had trouble socializing with her husband and her friends. Her discomfort was so profound that she considered leaving her job. Panic disorder secondary to pulmonary decline was diagnosed, and a selective serotonin reuptake inhibitor (SSRI) and a benzodiazepine (in a low dose) were prescribed. She did extremely well on this regimen, began a pulmonary rehabilitation program, kept her job, and resumed her social life with her friends.

Psychiatric Care of the Pre-Transplant Patient

Psychiatric care of the pre-transplant patient is based on the bio-psycho-social approach. Psychotropic medications are often a mainstay of treatment. Psychotherapeutic intervention can be helpful as well. Enhancement of a network of social support from family members, neighbors, and friends is crucial. Substance use counseling may be required for at-risk patients. Transplant centers may offer support groups run by mental health professionals or clinical nurse specialists who welcome both pre-transplant and post-transplant patients. Psychopharmacologic management of the pre-transplant patient follows the adage, "start low and go slow." The choice of medication and dosage depends on the patient's diagnosis, as well as the type and degree of organ failure.

SSRIs are usually the first-line treatment for depressive disorders, given their generally benign side-effect profile and anxiolytic effects. For patients who also struggle to refrain from cigarette smoking, bupropion may be a good choice. Antidepressants are metabolized in the liver, and it is wise to use lower doses for patients with hepatic disease. In addition, there is some evidence to suggest that SSRIs can put patients at increased risk for upper GI bleeding and therefore should be used with caution in patients with portal vein hypertension and cirrhosis.[44] Previously, clinicians were advised to use caution when prescribing SSRIs if the patient with a bacterial infection also required linezolid (an antibiotic that is also a weak monoamine oxidase inhibitor) because of the risk of serotonin syndrome.[45] However, a recent study of >1000 patients found that simultaneous use of SSRIs and linezolid did not increase the risk of serotonin syndrome, and the authors of the study advised providers to remain vigilant but not to withhold the antidepressant therapy.[46] Overall, SSRIs are well tolerated in patients with ESRD, although studies have been too small to draw definitive conclusions. Because the half-life of paroxetine is prolonged in patients with ESRD, it should be started at a very low dose, and the dose should be increased extremely slowly. Patients with ESRD may be at increased risk for bleeding due to ongoing platelet dysfunction; therefore, clinicians must account for this when prescribing an SSRI. Clearance of the selective serotonin-norepinephrine inhibitor venlafaxine is reduced in renal failure, and the metabolites of bupropion hydrochloride (which are excreted by the kidney) may accumulate and cause seizures in these vulnerable patients.[47]

Benzodiazepines are a mainstay of anxiety management; nonetheless, some transplant teams are unwilling to use them because of their addictive potential. Shorter-lasting agents (such as lorazepam) are preferable because longer-lasting agents (such as chlordiazepoxide) have active metabolites that can accumulate (particularly in patients with hepatic failure) and cause toxicity. Low-dose atypical antipsychotics (such as risperidone or olanzapine) can also be helpful in the treatment of anxiety in those patients who cannot tolerate benzodiazepines because of the risk of respiratory depression or abuse. However, there is a small risk of worsening CKD with second-generation antipsychotics (SGAs), with olanzapine and clozapine conferring the highest risk. In addition, SGAs can worsen pre-existing conditions, such as diabetes mellitus, so these agents should be used with caution in patients who are approaching kidney transplantation.[48]

Patients who require mood stabilizers (such as lithium, valproic acid, or carbamazepine) and neuroleptics can continue to take them before transplantation. Because mood-stabilizing medications have a high level of plasma protein binding, much lower doses are required in patients with ESRD. Lithium is eliminated by dialysis; therefore, serum levels should be obtained just before dialysis, and a dose should be given just after dialysis. For patients with hepatic failure, one should adjust the dose of valproic acid or carbamazepine, both of which are metabolized in the liver.

Psychotherapy can also be an extremely important therapeutic intervention for patients approaching a transplant. Even the relatively brief psychiatric pre-transplant evaluation can serve as a good opportunity for patients to share their hopes and dreams for the future, as well as their fears of ongoing illness and death, either before or after the transplant. Some psychiatrists will refer pre-transplant patients to other mental health providers for therapy because they feel that they cannot maintain the patients' confidentiality and continue to report to other members of the transplant team (personal communication, TransplantPsychiatry@googlegroups.com, 2006).

Common issues raised in psychotherapy include grief over the loss of productivity, guilt of being dependent, adaptation to a changing role within the family and community, potential risk of sexual dysfunction, concern about cognitive slowing secondary to immunosuppressive medications, and internal conflict between the reluctance to wish anyone ill and the desire for a deceased donor's organ.

Care of the Post-transplant Patient

The post-operative period is unpredictable. Some patients recover rapidly and can leave the hospital within several weeks. Others can be less fortunate and spend many weeks or even months in the ICU, endure lengthy stays in the transplant unit, and face discharge to a rehabilitation facility. Common sequelae in the immediate post-operative period include delirium, anxiety, and depression. Over the long term, patients can manifest continued anxiety and depression, develop problems with body image, fail to adhere to post-transplant medication regimens, and even revert to active substance abuse.

Short-Term Care

The hallmark of the early post-operative period for almost all transplant patients is delirium. The etiology can be multi-factorial but it usually represents a combination of medication effects or withdrawal states, metabolic changes, or infectious processes. Heart transplantation patients are at risk for intraoperative cerebral ischemia that may predispose them to delirium in the very early post-operative period. Lung transplantation patients may become hypoxic. Each of the immunosuppressive medications can cause psychotic symptoms (such as paranoid delusions and auditory and visual hallucinations, with or without accompanying delirium). Cyclosporine and tacrolimus can also cause PRES. High-dose steroids can precipitate hypomanic or manic behaviors with or without psychotic symptoms.

The management of delirium demands a search for the etiology and treatment of the underlying disorder. Cautious use of neuroleptics (such as haloperidol) can offer relief from disabling and frightening symptoms. Haloperidol is usually the first choice because it can be given intravenously, and it is primarily metabolized by the process of glucuronidation rather than by the CYP-450 isoenzymes. If the patient can tolerate oral medications, olanzapine is also a good choice. Gabapentin can be helpful in the management of steroid-induced psychosis (if the patient can take oral medication), with a dosage adjustment that accounts for renal insufficiency. When patients are unable to tolerate haloperidol, an infusion of dexmedetomidine, an alpha agonist, can be a good choice for the management of refractory delirium. Resting the patient overnight with an IV infusion and then turning it off and waking him up during the day can help reset a normal sleep-wake cycle and assist in the management of delirium.

Early symptoms of depression (e.g., mood changes, sleep disturbance, irritability, poor concentration) may be secondary to medications (such as beta-blockers or steroids) or may represent a recurrence of a pre-morbid mood disorder. Sometimes, new symptoms of depression herald the development of infectious processes (such as cytomegalovirus or *Mycobacterium avium* complex). Treatment with an SSRI can be helpful for its antidepressant and anxiolytic effects.

Anxiety symptoms in the early post-operative period can result from rapid adjustments in benzodiazepines or narcotics, early immunosuppressive toxicity, or sepsis. In lung transplant patients, anxiety can accompany acute rejection, pneumonia, or a pleural effusion. Treatment strategies include a gradual tapering of high-dose IV or oral benzodiazepines and/or narcotics, followed by maintenance with a low-dose, short-lasting benzodiazepine (such as lorazepam). Patients who have pre-morbid generalized anxiety or a panic disorder that recurs may be managed with a combination of an SSRI and a benzodiazepine.

Long-Term Care

Patients undergoing solid organ transplantation are effectively exchanging one set of problems (i.e., those related to end-organ failure) for another (e.g., rejection of the allograft, side effects of immunosuppressive medications, and possible progression of underlying systemic disease). Although transplant teams certainly inform potential recipients of the risks and benefits of the procedure, many of those recipients (and their families) have unrealistic expectations of their rate of recovery and their overall quality of life following transplantation.

Disappointment and dashed hopes can precipitate mood changes. Frequent medical setbacks, understood by the treatment team as part of the normal course of events, are discouraging for patients and family members. Family members can aggravate the situation by expecting too much, too soon, from the transplant recipient. Alternatively, family members or friends who have served as caretakers for many years may be unable to relinquish control, even when the recipient is stronger and better able to care for himself or herself.

Transplant recipients have spent many years in and around hospitals. After a transplant, they gradually move back into their community. Initially, clinic visits can be bi-weekly. As time passes, patients come into the hospital less frequently. Many transplant patients become anxious as they transition from the close monitoring provided by the medical and surgical teams to a more independent status. Phone contact with a member of the team can be helpful in such circumstances. These patients also benefit from regular attendance at a transplantation support group, where (under the guidance of a knowledgeable team leader) they can share their experiences with other transplant recipients.

All transplant patients require immunosuppressive agents including those used for induction, which act by depleting T cells, and those used for maintenance, which involves a combination of three drugs, including a corticosteroid, a calcineurin inhibitor or an mTOR (mammalian target of rapamycin), a protein kinase encoded by the mTOR gene that regulates cellular metabolic functions, and an antimetabolite.[49] Commonly used immunosuppressive agents used for maintenance and their neuropsychiatric side effects are listed in Table 27.3.

Corticosteroids remain a mainstay of treatment, and side effects include physical changes, specifically a Cushingoid distribution of body fat, hirsutism, easy bruising, insomnia, and mood changes that may require a psychopharmacologic intervention.[50] Young female patients often struggle with these bodily changes and may be more likely than other transplant recipients to refuse to take the steroids as prescribed. This level of nonadherence is extremely worrisome because it can result in potentially life-threatening acute or chronic rejection. Prompt psychiatric evaluation of the non-adherent transplant recipient for the presence of an underlying mood or adjustment disorder is essential to prevent rejection of the allograft. Ideally, the use of supportive

psychotherapy helps such patients understand the potentially self-destructive nature of their actions and devise strategies that can ensure better adherence.

SUDs can also re-emerge in the post-transplant period, even though the patient may have had years of sobriety before transplantation. Members of transplant teams often have difficulty managing the liver transplant recipient who has begun drinking again or the lung transplant recipient who picks up a cigarette, not only because of their concern regarding the risk to the allograft but also because of their tremendous disappointment in the patient's behavior.

PEDIATRIC TRANSPLANTATION

As of February 2022, nearly 2000 patients under the age of 18 (1918) were waiting for a solid organ transplant.[51] Pediatric transplant patients differ from adult transplant patients in several ways. A parent or appointed legal guardian makes the medico-legal decisions for the child; the children (infants, toddlers, and school-age children) are not responsible for the decision to proceed with the transplant or for pre-transplant and post-transplant care. Most young patients require a transplant because of a congenital disorder (such as biliary atresia, cardiac malformations, or pulmonary atresia) and are not held responsible for their disease in the same way that adults who are chronic drinkers and who develop cirrhosis may be. A child's ability to understand the serious nature of his or her illness and the risks and benefits of a transplant depends on the child's age and developmental stage. Many transplant patients have never had the chance to enjoy age-appropriate activities. The severity of their illness might have imposed limitations on school attendance and social interactions and bred a profound dependence on parents and other caregivers.

The primary goal of the psychiatrist who cares for a pediatric transplant patient is to help the child maintain a normal developmental trajectory in the face of a life-threatening illness. The psychiatrist must also attempt to balance the needs of the child with the needs of parents, siblings, and involved members of the extended family. No one wants to deny a child the chance for a longer life. However, some children, like some adults, may not be appropriate candidates for transplantation. Sometimes a child is disqualified for transplantation because of the inability of adult

---

TABLE 27.3

Psychiatric Side Effects of Immunosuppressive Medications

Immunosuppressant Agent	Description	Potential Psychiatric Side Effects	Laboratory Findings
Cyclosporine ■ *Neoral* ■ *Sandimmune*	Polypeptide fungal product	Delirium, auditory hallucinations, visual hallucinations, other psychotic symptoms, periventricular leukoencephalopathy	Side effects more prominent at high doses and serum values and tend to resolve as serum levels decrease, SSRIs may increase levels, carbamazepine may decrease levels, herbal agents such as St. Johns wort may decrease levels
Tacrolimus ■ *Prograf*	Also called *FK506* or *5FK*; macrolide antibiotic	Delirium, auditory and visual hallucinations, other psychotic symptoms, seizures, akinetic mutism	Side effects more prominent at high serum values and tend to resolve as serum levels decrease, MRI may reveal white matter changes in toxic patients
Mycophenolate ■ *Mofetil CellCept*	Suppresses T- and B-cell proliferation as an adjunct immunosuppressant or for patients who cannot tolerate cyclosporine or tacrolimus	Anxiety, depression, sedation	
Muromonab-CD3 ■ *OKT3*	Given immediately post-operatively to prevent rejection, a monoclonal antibody that suppresses CD3 T-cell function	Aseptic meningitis, hallucinations during administrations	
Corticosteroids	The mainstay of most transplant regimens usually starts high and tapered over weeks to months, though many patients remain on low doses indefinitely	Increased appetite, anxiety, depression, hypomania, mania, paranoia	Often dose related and resolved with lower dose

MRI, Magnetic resonance imaging; *SSRIs*, selective serotonin reuptake inhibitors.

caregivers to provide adequate monitoring or to follow the instructions of the treatment team. The psychiatrist who works with young patients with end-organ failure must also be able to understand and withstand the anger and disappointment of members of the treatment team when faced with such a situation.

Pre-Transplant Evaluation

Unlike with adults, however, the order and style of the pre-transplant psychiatric interview depend on the child's age and developmental stage. With a prepubertal child, it is appropriate to meet first with the parents or guardians to obtain a coherent, chronological history and to assess the parents' understanding of the risks and benefits, as well as their history of compliance in obtaining care for their child. For an adolescent, it is helpful to interview the child alone, before speaking with the parents, to support his or her independence and wish for autonomy. Again, the psychiatric evaluation should address the following issues: presence of mood disorders, anxiety disorders, attentional issues, and/or learning disabilities in the patient or a caregiver; history of past or current substance abuse; relationship with caregivers; the patient's and the family's motivation for transplant; ability of the caregivers to help the patient adhere to treatment recommendations (medication regimen and appointments); adequacy of social supports; and assessment of stressors within the family, such as marital discord or financial problems.

Although parents or guardians must be the ones to give "consent" for the surgery and post-operative care, a verbal child must be able to "assent" to the surgery and be willing to participate in treatment. Both parents and children must be fully engaged in preparation for transplant, as well as be able and willing to work together toward a common goal.

Case 3

An 11-year-old boy with advanced CF and no past psychiatric history was brought by his mother for a living donor pre-transplantation psychiatric evaluation. His mother was worried that her son would die before his LAS would be high enough to allow him to qualify for a transplant. She volunteered to be a living lobar lung donor, and she aggressively pursued other potential donors until she found one. On initial interviews, the patient was cheerful and appeared to have a good understanding of why his mother and a friend each wished to donate a lung lobe. In his meeting with the transplant team psychiatrist, however, the patient was not able to talk at all about the potential for transplantation and did not appear to have any understanding of why the two adults would need surgery. Ultimately, the team decided that it was the patient's mother and not the patient who was the motivating force for the transplant. The child did not feel ready to have an elective transplant with his mother and a friend as a donor. The team put the process on hold and encouraged the family to wait for a deceased donor transplant.

The dilemma of the adolescent transplant candidate with an SUD is particularly important. Adolescents are less likely than adults to have longstanding struggles with SUDs, but they are often recreational users of alcohol or street drugs, particularly in social situations. The normal adolescent's need for autonomy and independence often leads to substance use, despite a cognitive understanding of the grave risks. Some teens with liver disease drink alcohol, and some teens with lung disease smoke cigarettes or vape nicotine or cannabis. This behavior usually stops as the illness progresses and the patient becomes more medically compromised. It is difficult to know, however, whether this change reflects a true understanding of the risks, or whether it is simply a short-term response to the fear of jeopardizing their transplant candidacy.

In addition, adolescents often struggle to comply with medication regimens and treatment recommendations before transplantation. They are seeking to forge their own identity and to separate themselves from their parents. At the same time, they desperately want to be part of their peer group and to look just like

everyone else. Often this translates into, for example, a teenager with CF who refuses to take enzymes at lunch in the cafeteria or go to the nurse for an insulin injection in the middle of the day. Because non-adherence is a major cause of graft rejection, a history of this kind of behavior pattern in a pre-transplant adolescent candidate is worrisome—even though it is consistent with the patient's age and developmental stage.

In some instances, the evaluator may use the 17-item Pediatric Transplant Rating Instrument (P-TRI) to assess an adolescent's understanding of the transplant process, history of adherence to medication regimens, the recommendations of his/her treatment team, presence or absence of psychiatric problems and/or substance use, and degree of family engagement.[52] The P-TRI has not been used to determine eligibility for transplantation because the data linking patients' scores to transplant outcomes were lacking and limited by poor inter-rater reliability among providers.[53] A recent study using the P-TRI in a cohort of Turkish adolescents requiring kidney transplants determined that the P-TRI can distinguish adolescents who may be at risk for post-psychosocial outcomes following transplant.[54] Another group of researchers created a revised P-TRI that would help them look at risk factors and the relationship of those risk factors to the patient's transplant status 1 year following evaluation. This study was small, but it concluded that the results from this revised P-TRI, which placed patients in one of three groups—high, medium, and low risk—demonstrated an association with transplant listing at 1 year. Patients who were judged to be at high risk were less likely to have been transplanted 1 year following the evaluation.[55] These studies suggest that this rating instrument may at some point help transplant teams create therapeutic interventions for those pediatric patients deemed at high risk to expedite the time to transplant and facilitate better post-transplant outcomes.

Post-Transplant Care

The post-operative care of the pediatric transplant patient is like that of an adult. Delirium is a common complication. Immunosuppressive medications can cause neuropsychiatric symptoms such as hallucinations, and high-dose steroids can precipitate manic symptoms and psychosis. Cautious use of IV haloperidol remains the mainstay of treatment.

Evidence suggests that the extent to which pediatric patients with life-threatening illnesses feel traumatized both by the procedure and by its sequelae correlates with the parents' sense of stress.[56] In fact, although parents (and primary caregivers) have a relatively high rate of PTSD in the first few years following their child's transplant,[57] the transplant recipients themselves experience symptoms of PTSD at rates comparable to those of children with other life-threatening conditions. Interestingly, the likelihood of experiencing such symptoms (e.g., re-experiencing, having flashbacks, or manifesting avoidance) does not seem to be related to the type of organ being transplanted, and it is more common in those adolescents with relatively mild complications, or in those whose organ failure occurred abruptly.[58] In one more recent study, the authors found that children and parents differed in their assessment of psychological health following the transplant. Children generally under-reported their psychological distress, and parents reported that their children were more distressed than a normal cohort.[59]

In general, however, pediatric transplant patients do well. They feel better, return to school, and resume many of their activities. They do not demonstrate significant new psychopathology, although pre-morbid psychiatric illness may recur. Pediatric liver transplantation patients demonstrate significant neuropsychological deficits and developmental delays in intellectual and academic functioning, both before and after transplantation, thought to be related to the effect of elevated levels of bilirubin pre-transplant and the total number of days in the hospital in the first year following transplant.[60] Some studies have shown persistent cognitive deficits in pediatric heart transplant recipients,[57] but others found that 89% of children who underwent heart transplantation following VAD bridging demonstrated normal cognitive function.[61] A more recent study of 25 school-age children who underwent neuropsychological testing within several years of post-cardiac transplant, found that half demonstrated a learning disability. The mean full-scale intelligence quotient in the entire sample was low-average. Factors determined to place patients at greater risk were congenital heart disease and pre-transplant neurological problems. One limitation of the study was its small patient sample. Further research is needed in this area to help parents and guardians understand the potential for neuropsychiatric consequences of childhood heart transplantation and the educational and community resources that their children may need following the transplant.[62]

CONCLUSION

The patients with end-organ failure who are approaching transplantation have few real options. These patients are profoundly physically disabled and emotionally drained. They are often depressed and anxious, and at times quite desperate. Recognition and treatment of psychiatric disorders, both before and after transplant, can improve their quality of life.

The role of the transplant psychiatrist is challenging but also immensely rewarding. It requires a sophisticated appreciation of the medical and surgical issues facing patients with end-organ failure, an understanding of the mechanism of action and side-effect profiles of their medications, and the ways in which those medications interact with psychotropic medications. As a member of a multi-disciplinary team, the psychiatrist must act as a liaison to the patient, the family, and other medical providers, and serve as a resource for other team members. The transplant psychiatrist plays a central role in the selection of transplant candidates and potential living donors, necessitating an understanding of the ethical issues inherent in a system where resources are limited.

REFERENCES

1. Duda L. National organ allocation policy: the final rule. *Virtual Mentor.* 2005;7(9):604–607.10.1001/virtualmentor.2005.7.9.h law1-0509

2. Snyder JJ, Salkowski N, Wey A, et al. Organ distribution without geographic boundaries: a possible framework for organ allocation. *Am J Transplant.* 2018;18(11):2635–2640. https://doi. org/10.1111/ajt.15115. Epub 2018 Sep 29. PMID: 30203912.

3. Smith JM, Biggins SW, Hasselby DG, et al. Kidney, pancreas and liver allocation and distribution in the United States. *Am J Transplant.* 2012;12:3191–3212.

4. https://unos.org/news/update-cpra-calculation/.

5. Mattar A, Chatterjee S, Loor G. Bridging to lung transplantation. *Crit Care Clin.* 2019;35(1):11–25. https://doi.org/10.1016/j. ccc.2018.08.006. PMID: 30447774.

6. https://optn.transplant.hrsa.gov/professionals/by-organ/heart-lung/lung-continuous-distribution-policy/.

7. Ladin K, Hanto DW. Rationing lung transplants—procedural fairness in allocation and appeals. *N Engl J Med.* 2013;369:599–601.

8. https://optn.transplant.hrsa.gov/media/2414/adult_heart_infographic.pdf.

9. JD Estep, E Soltesz, R Cogswell. The new heart transplant allocation system: early observations and mechanical circulatory support considerations. *J Thorac Cardiovasc Surg.* 2020;S0022-5223(20)32638-6. https://doi.org/10.1016/j.jtcvs.2020.08.113. Epub ahead of print. PMID: 34756380.

10. Cogswell R, John R, Estep JD, et al. An early investigation of outcomes with the new 2018 donor heart allocation system in the United States. *J Heart Lung Transplant.* 2020;39(1):1–4. https://doi.org/10.1016/j.healun.2019.11.002. Epub 2019 Nov 20. PMID: 31810767.

11. Bartelt L, van Duin D. An overview of COVID-19 in solid organ transplantation. *Clin Microbiol Infect.* 2022;28(6):779–784. https://doi.org/10.1016/j.cmi.2022.02.005. Epub 2022 Feb 18. PMID: 35189336; PMCID: PMC8855607.

12. https://optn.transplant.hrsa.gov/data/.

13. Wynn JJ, Alexander DE. Increasing organ donation and transplantation: the U.S. experience over the past decade. *Transpl Int.* 2011;24:324–332.

14. http://www.iom.edu/Reports/2006/Organ-Donation-Opportunities-for-Action.aspx.

15. <http://organdonor.gov/legislation/timeline.html>.

16. Lewis A, Koukoura A, Tsianos GI, et al. Organ donation in the US and Europe: the supply vs demand imbalance. *Transplant Rev (Orlando).* 2021;35(2):100585. https://doi.org/10.1016/j.trre.2020.100585. Epub 2020 Oct 11. PMID: 33071161.

17. National Academies of Sciences, Engineering, and Medicine; Health and Medicine Division; Board on Health Care Services; Board on Health Sciences Policy; Committee on A Fairer and More Equitable, Cost-Effective, and Transparent System of Donor Organ Procurement, Allocation, and Distribution. In: M Hackmann, RA English, KW Kizer, eds. *Realizing the Promise of Equity in the Organ Transplantation System.* National Academies Press (US); 2022. PMID:35226429.

18. Nudeshima J. Obstacles to brain death and organ transplantation in Japan. *Lancet.* 1991;338:1063–1066.

19. Date H. Current status and problems of lung transplantation in Japan. *J Thorac Dis.* 2016 Aug;8(suppl 8):S631–636. https://doi.org/10.21037/jtd.2016.06.38. PMID: 27651939; PMCID: PMC5009071.

20. Goldaracena N, Barbas AS. Living donor liver transplantation. *Curr Opin Organ Transplant.* 2019;24(2):131–137. https://doi.org/10.1097/MOT.0000000000000610. PMID: 30694993.

21. Venkat KK, Eshelman AK. The evolving approach to ethical issues in living donor kidney transplantation: a review based on illustrative case vignettes. *Transplant Rev (Orlando).* 2014;28(3):134–139. https://doi.org/10.1016/j.trre.2014.04.001. Epub 2014 Apr 13. PMID: 24849414.

22. Lentine KL, Lam NN, Segev DL. Risks of living kidney donation: current state of knowledge on outcomes important to donors. *Clin J Am Soc Nephrol.* 2019;14(4):597–608. https://doi.org/10.2215/CJN.11220918. Epub 2019 Mar 11. PMID: 30858158; PMCID: PMC6450354.

23. Choi JY, Kim JH, Kim JM, et al. Outcomes of living liver donors are worse than those of matched healthy controls. *J Hepatol.* 2022;76(3):628–638. https://doi.org/10.1016/j.jhep.2021.10.031. Epub 2021 Nov 14. PMID: 34785324.

24. Wakade VA, Mathur SK. Donor safety in live-related liver transplantation. *Indian J Surg.* 2011;74(1):118–126.

25. LaPointe Rudow D, DeLair S, Feeley T, et al. Long-term impact of living liver donation: a self-report of the donation experience. *Liver Transpl.* 2019;25(5):724–733. https://doi.org/10.1002/lt.25402. Epub 2019 Mar 26. PMID: 30589993.

26. Yusen RD, Hong BA, Messersmith EE, RELIVE Study Group., et al. Morbidity and mortality of live lung donation: results from the RELIVE study. *Am J Transplant.* 2014;14(8):1846–1852. https://doi.org/10.1111/ajt.12771. PMID: 25039865; PMCID: PMC4152404.

27. Prager LM, Wain JC, Roberts DH, et al. Medical and psychological outcome of living lobar lung transplant donors. *ISHLT.* 2006;25(10):1206–1212.

28. Chen F, Fujinaga T, Shoji T, et al. Outcomes and pulmonary function in living lobar lung transplant donors. *Transpl Int.* 2012;35:153–157.

29. Bailey P, Vergis N, Allison M, et al. Psychosocial evaluation of candidates for solid organ transplantation. *Transplantation.* 2021;105(12):e292–e302. https://doi.org/10.1097/TP.0000000000003732.

30. Dobbels F, Verleden G, Dupont L, et al. To transplant or not? The importance of psychosocial and behavioral factors before lung transplantation. *Chron Respir Dis.* 2006;3(1):39–47.

31. Rogal SS, Mankaney G, Udawatta V, et al. Pre-transplant depression is associated with length of hospitalization, discharge disposition, and survival after liver transplantation. *PLoS One.* 2016;11(11):e0165517. https://doi.org/10.1371/journal.pone.0165517. PMID: 27820828; PMCID: PMC5098732.

32. Wessels-Bakker MJ, van de Graaf EA, Kwakkel-van Erp JM, et al. The relation between psychological distress and medication adherence in lung transplant candidates and recipients: a cross-sectional study. *J Clin Nurs.* 2022;31(5-6):716–725. https://doi.org/10.1111/jocn.15931. Epub 2021 Jul 2. Erratum in: *J Clin Nurs.* 2022 Oct;31(19-20):2981. PMID: 34216066; PMCID: PMC9292052.

33. Clinton BK, Silverman BS, Brendel DH. Patient-targeted googling: the ethics of searching on line for patient information. *Harv Rev Psychiatry.* 2009;18(2):103–112.

34. Parker R. Armstrong MJ, Corbett C, et al. Alcohol and Substance Abuse in Solid-Organ Transplant Recipients. <www.transplantjournal.com>;2013.

35. Winder G, Clifton E, Mellinger J. Substance use disorders in organ transplantation: perennial challenges and interprofessional opportunities. *Curr Opinion in Organ Transplantation.* 2022;27(6):495–500. https://doi.org/10.1097/MOT.0000000000001026.

36. Joyal K, Peckham AM, Wakeman SE, et al. Management of opioid agonist treatment for opioid use disorder in the setting of solid organ transplant. *Transplantation.* 2022;106(5):900–903. https://doi.org/10.1097/TP.0000000000003926. May 2022.

37. Melaragno J, Bowman L, Park J, et al. The clinical conundrum of cannabis: current practices and recommendations for transplant clinicians: an opinion of the Immunology/Transplantation

PRN of the American College of Clinical Pharmacy. *Transplantation*. 2021;105(2):291–299. https://doi.org/10.1097/TP.0000000000003309.

38. Carrion AF, Aye L, Martin P. Patient selection for liver transplantation. *Expert Rev Gastroenterol & Hepatol*. 2013;7(6):571–579. https://doi.org/10.1586/17474124.2013.824701. To link to this article.

39. Alshelleh S, Alhouri A, Taifour A, et al. Prevalence of depression and anxiety with their effect on quality of life in chronic kidney disease patients. *Sci Rep*. 2022;12(1):17627. https://doi.org/10.1038/s41598-022-21873-2. PMID: 36271287; PMCID: PMC9587015.

40. Zalai D, Szeifert L, Novak M. Psychological distress and depression in patients with chronic kidney disease. *Semin Dial*. 2012;25(4):428–438.

41. Correale M, Altamura M, Carnevale R, et al. Delirium in heart failure. *Heart Fail Rev*. 2020;25(5):713–723. https://doi.org/10.1007/s10741-019-09842-w. PMID: 31377979.

42. Sanders KM, Stern TA, O'Gara PT, et al. Delirium during IABP therapy: incidence and management. *Psychosomatics*. 1992;33:35–44.

43. Mullish BH, Kabir MS, Thursz MR, et al. Review article: depression and the use of antidepressants in patients with chronic liver disease or liver transplantation. *Aliment Pharmacol Ther*. 2014;40(8):880–892. https://doi.org/10.1111/apt.12925. Epub 2014 Sep 1. PMID: 25175904.

44. Andrade C, Sandarsh S, Chethan KB, et al. Serotonin reuptake inhibitor antidepressants and abnormal bleeding: a review for clinicians and a reconsideration of mechanisms. *J Clin Psychiatry*. 2010;71(12):1565–1575. https://doi.org/10.4088/JCP.09r05786blu. PMID: 21190637.

45. Taylor JJ, Wilson JW, Estes LL. Linezolid and serotonergic drug interactions: a retrospective survey. *Clin Infect Dis*. 2006;43(2):180–187.

46. Bai AD, McKenna S, Wise H, et al. Association of linezolid with risk of serotonin syndrome in patients receiving antidepressants. *JAMA Network Open*. 2022;5(12):e2247426. https://doi.org/10.1001/jamanetworkopen.2022.47426.

47. Cohen LM, Tessier EG, Germaine MJ, et al. Update on psychotropic medication use in renal disease. *Psychosomatics*. 2004;45:34–48.

48. Højlund M, Lund LC, Herping JLE, et al. Second-generation antipsychotics and the risk of chronic kidney disease: a population-based case-control study. *BMJ Open*. 2020;10(8):e038247. https://doi.org/10.1136/bmjopen-2020-038247. PMID: 32784262; PMCID: PMC7418669.

49. Holt CD. Overview of immunosuppressive therapy in solid organ transplantation. *Anesthesiol Clin*. 2017;35(3):365–380. https://doi.org/10.1016/j.anclin.2017.04.001. PMID: 28784214.

50. Zhang W, Egashira N, Masuda S. Recent topics on the mechanisms of immunosuppressive therapy-related neurotoxicities. *Int J Mol Sci*. 2019;20(13):3210. https://doi.org/10.3390/ijms20133210. PMID: 31261959; PMCID: PMC6651704.

51. https://www.organdonor.gov/learn/organ-donation-statistics.

52. Fung E, Shaw RJ. Pediatric Transplant Rating Instrument—a scale for the pretransplant psychiatric evaluation of pediatric organ transplant recipients. *Pediatr Transplant*. 2008;12:57–68.

53. Fisher M, Storfer-Isser A, Shaw RJ, et al. Inter-rater reliability of the pediatric transplant rating instrument (P-TRI): challenges to reliably identifying adherence risk factors during pediatric pre-transplant evaluations. *Pediatr Transplant*. 2011;15:142–147.

54. Taner HA, Sarı BA, Baskın E, et al. Can we identify "at-risk" children and adolescents for poor transplant outcomes in the psychosocial evaluation before solid organ transplantation? The reliability and validity study of Pediatric Transplant Rating Instrument (P-TRI) in Turkish pediatric renal transplant patients. *Pediatr Transplant*. 2022:e14444. https://doi.org/10.1111/petr.14444. Epub ahead of print. PMID: 36447352.

55. West KB, Plevinsky JM, Amaral S, et al. Predicting psychosocial risk in pediatric kidney transplantation: an exploratory cluster analysis of a revised Pediatric Transplant Rating Instrument. *Pediatr Transplant*. 2022:e14454. https://doi.org/10.1111/petr.14454. Epub ahead of print. PMID: 36518059.

56. Stuber ML, Kazak AE, Meeske K, et al. Predictors of posttraumatic stress symptoms in childhood cancer survivors. *Pediatrics*. 1997;100:958–964.

57. Stuber ML. Psychiatric issues in pediatric organ transplantation. *Child Adolesc Psychiatr Clin N Am*. 2010;19(2):285–300.

58. Mintzer LL, Stuber ML, Seacord D, et al. Traumatic stress symptoms in adolescent organ transplant recipients. *Pediatrics*. 2003;115:1640–1644.

59. Wu YP, Aylward BS, Steele RG, et al. Psychosocial functioning of pediatric renal and liver transplant recipients. *Pediatr Transplant*. 2008;12:582.

60. Krull K, Fuchs C, Yurk H, et al. Neurocognitive outcome in pediatric liver transplant recipients. *Pediatr Transplant*. 2003;7:111–118.

61. Stein ML, Bruno JL, Konopack KL, et al. Cognitive outcomes in pediatric heart transplant recipients bridged to transplantation with ventricular assist devices. *J Heath Lung Transplant*. 2013;32(2):212–220.

62. Gold A, Bondi BC, Ashkanase J, et al. Early school-age cognitive performance post-pediatric heart transplantation. *Pediatr Transplant*. 2020;24(8):e13832. https://doi.org/10.1111/petr.13832. Epub 2020 Oct 26. PMID: 33105067.

28

HIV INFECTION AND AIDS

ASHIKA BAINS, MD ■ FELICIA A. SMITH, MD

OVERVIEW

As recently as the 1990s, being infected with the human immunodeficiency virus (HIV) meant that you had a terminal illness. The advent of antiretroviral therapy (ART) has made HIV a manageable chronic illness for many, while adequate treatment necessitates that patients have frequent examinations and laboratory tests and are at risk for a bevy of medication side effects. Psychiatric care of patients with HIV infection is complex and requires recognition of at-risk populations, identification of barriers to attaining and maintaining treatment, knowledge of potential psychiatric symptoms that are due to the infection, knowledge of the neuropsychiatric side effect profiles of ART, and analysis of the multi-faceted interplay between psychiatric illness and infection. HIV infection is more prevalent among those with mental illness,[1] and psychiatric illnesses are more prevalent in those who are HIV positive.[2] Stigma, shame, socioeconomic and culture/lifestyle barriers continued to interfere with HIV detection and care. In addition, with improved overall survival, a new cohort of aging patients with HIV infection is emerging and a range of cognitive difficulties and chronic diseases, not necessarily related to HIV itself, is being identified.

HIV is a blood-borne, sexually transmitted retrovirus that contains RNA as its genetic material and the enzyme reverse transcriptase, which facilitates the (reverse) transcription of RNA to double-stranded DNA in infected human cells. This virion-derived DNA moves to the host cell nucleus, where it randomly integrates into host chromosomes, catalyzed by the virion-encoded enzyme, integrase. Once within the host chromosome, the pro-viral DNA can remain inactive (latent) or express a range of genetic activity, including functional virus production. Within the first 6 weeks of infection, a burst of viral replication accounts for wide dissemination of the virus throughout the body, particularly in lymphoid tissue and within the central nervous system (CNS).[3] Functional viruses can go on to infect other cells, preferentially the CD4 subpopulation of T-lymphocytes, thereby causing severe (primarily cell-mediated) immune dysfunction for which the virus and the resulting syndrome were named. This infection cycle repeats billions of times, the host mounts an immune response, and a set point (or dynamic equilibrium) is eventually reached. The set point varies from person to person, and it has been found to be of prognostic significance.[4] Acquired immunodeficiency syndrome (AIDS) is defined as a CD4 cell count below 200, having less than 14% of total lymphocytes, or having an AIDS-defining condition. Immunodeficiency, a predilection for certain opportunistic infections, and AIDS-defining conditions correlate with a decline in CD4 lymphocyte count (Table 28.1).

The general tenets of this chapter should provide a framework for the safe and comprehensive psychiatric evaluation and care of adults at risk for, or infected with, HIV, or having AIDS. Four general questions help set the context for such an evaluation: At what stage of HIV infection is the patient in terms of symptomatic disease and their CD4 lymphocyte count? Is there evidence of HIV-associated psychiatric sequelae or CNS infection?

TABLE 28.1

AIDS-Defining Conditions That Emerge With Advancing Immunosuppression

CD4 Cell Count (Cells/mm³)	Condition
200–500	Thrush
	Kaposi sarcoma
	Tuberculosis reactivation
	Herpes zoster
	Herpes simplex
	Bacterial sinusitis/pneumonia
100–200	*Pneumocystis jirovecii* pneumonia
50–100	Systemic fungal infections
	Primary tuberculosis
	Cerebral toxoplasmosis
	Progressive multi-focal leukoencephalopathy
	Peripheral neuropathy
	Cervical carcinoma
0–50	Cytomegalovirus disease
	Disseminated *Mycobacterium avium-intracellulare* complex
	Non-Hodgkin lymphoma
	Central nervous system lymphoma
	HIV-associated dementia

Modified from American Psychiatric Association. *Practice Guideline for the Treatment of Patients with HIV/AIDS*. American Psychiatric Press; 2000.

Does the patient have a pre-morbid psychiatric history? How did the patient become infected with HIV? The important implications of the first three questions might seem more obvious and should be clear by the completion of the chapter. The fourth question is often a highly personal story, one that reveals the patient as a person. The answer to this question foreshadows how the patient will relate to illness and to receiving medical care. This knowledge informs not only the psychiatrist's evaluation but also the patient's individualized treatment and management.

EPIDEMIOLOGY

Despite the existence of effective therapies, HIV/AIDS remains a terminal illness in much of the world; it cuts across all ages and socioeconomic groups, each with specific characteristics and considerations.[5] According to the United Nations AIDS data, the global prevalence of people living with HIV was 37.7 million in 2020, which is an increase from 33.3 million in 2010 and 36.7 million in 2015.[6,7] Females made up about half of the infected adults worldwide, and roughly 1.7 million children younger than 15 years are infected.[6] The incidence of new HIV infections was estimated to be 1.5 million, and the incidence of AIDS-related deaths was estimated at 680,000.[6] Fortunately, the total number of AIDS deaths has decreased since the 1990s and continues to do so in the past few decades (1.1 million in 2015)[7] which means the number of persons living with HIV has increased, although the prevalence (measured over a growing global population) has stabilized. Eastern and Southern Africa remain the most heavily infected regions, accounting for 55% of all people living with HIV, 46% of all AIDS deaths, and 45% of all new cases in 2020.[6] In the United States an estimated 1.2 million people were infected with the virus at the end of 2021, of whom more than 150,000 (13%) were unaware of their status.[8] The annual number of new diagnoses of HIV infection decreased by 7% between 2017 and 2021, with 36,136 people receiving a new diagnosis in 2021.

On a global scale, the populations most vulnerable to HIV infection are those who inject drugs (35 times higher risk), transgender females (34 times greater risk), female sex workers (26 times greater risk), and males who have sex with males (MSM) (25 times greater risk). These populations and their sexual partners accounted for 65% of HIV infections worldwide in 2020.[6] In 2021 male-to-male sexual contact accounted for most (67%) of the new HIV diagnoses in the United States, followed by heterosexual contact (22%) and injecting drug use (7%).[8] A disproportionate number of the newly infected cases in the United States are from ethnic and racial minorities (primarily Black and Hispanic population). Observing trends in the United States from 2014 to 2018, new HIV diagnoses among MSM have decreased by 7% while transmission via injection drug use increased by 10%; most age groups in males have seen either a stable incidence or a decrease, except for the group 25 to 34 years of age, which demonstrated an increase of 7%.[8] Recreational drug use (particularly methamphetamine) and unsafe sexual practices among younger males may account for some of the increasing trends. Reportedly, unprotected anal sex at least once in the past 12 months increased from 48% in 2005 to 57% in 2011.[9] Prevention strategies to reduce the risk of HIV transmission include pre-exposure prophylaxis (PrEP) and post-exposure prophylaxis (PEP). PrEP is antiretroviral therapy which, if taken as prescribed, reduces the risk of HIV infection from sex by about 99% and reduces the risk of getting HIV from injection drug use by at least 74%.[8] PEP is the use of anti-retroviral drugs after a single high-risk event to stop HIV seroconversion; it must be taken within 72 hours of exposure. Despite the availability of PrEP, including an injectable form, it is under-utilized with only 24.7% of people who might benefit from receiving a PrEP prescription in 2020.[6,8]

MEDICATIONS FOR HIV INFECTION

Early treatment is now the "gold standard" for patients with HIV infection. ART initiation at the time of diagnosis, regardless of one's CD4 count, is recommended to reduce clinically relevant morbidity and mortality. Due to the latent viral infection, patients must remain on ART indefinitely. In a large multi-site, multi-continent study known as the "START study," early treatment was shown to significantly reduce the risk of serious AIDS-related events, serious non-AIDS-related events, or death from any cause, compared with a deferred-treatment initiation arm, in which subjects were not treated until the CD4 count dropped below 350.[10] The US Department of Health and Human Services (DHHS) guidelines recommended immediate ART initiation for all persons with HIV.[11] Goals of ART are to achieve sustained virologic suppression of HIV, recover immune function, and thereby reduce HIV-associated morbidity and mortality and reduce community transmission. US Food and Drug Administration (FDA)-approved classes of antiretroviral medications include: nucleoside reverse transcriptase inhibitors (NRTIs); non-nucleoside reverse transcriptase inhibitors (NNRTIs); protease inhibitors (PIs); integrase strand transfer inhibitors (INSTIs); entry inhibitors; capsid inhibitors, and fusion inhibitors.[12] There are also pharmacokinetic enhancer medications used to increase the effectiveness of HIV treatment regimens. Drugs target various stages of the HIV replication cycle. Antiretroviral medications are used in combinations, typically three agents from more than one class. Single-drug therapy is ineffective because of the rapid development of resistance to that agent and in turn, to an entire class of medications. Similarly, incomplete adherence to a multi-drug combination regimen allows the HIV to continue replicating, again allowing for a mutation to occur and class-wide resistance to develop. Adherence to medications and engagement of patients in therapy is critical for treatment success.

The US DHHS provides recommendations for the treatment-naive patient, of which first-line treatment consists of two NRTIs plus either an INSTI, NNRTI, or PI boosted with either cobicistat or ritonavir.[11] There are currently several one-pill once-daily options[12]; several studies and a meta-analysis have shown better adherence in populations receiving once-daily regimens (Table 28.2).[13] Extended-release injectable suspension medications have also become available.

TABLE 28.2
Antiretroviral Recommended First-Line Regimen Options

Antiretroviral-naive (no PrEP)

DTG/ABC/3TC[a,b]

BIC/TAF/FTC[b]

DTG with (TAF or TDF) plus (FTC or 3TC)

DTG/3TC[b,c]

History of PrEP use and treatment is begun prior to INSTI genotypic resistance testing results:

DRV/c[d] or DRV/r with (TAF or TDF) plus (FTC or 3TC)

[a]Only for patients who are HLA-B*5701 negative.
[b]One pill once-daily regimen.
[c]Do not use if HIV RNA >500,000 copies/mL, HBV co-infection, or before the results of HIV genotypic resistance testing for reverse transcriptase or HBV testing are available.
[d]Cobicistat should be avoided in pregnancy.
3TC, lamivudine; *ABC,* abacavir; *BIC,* bictegravir; *DTG,* dolutegravir; *DRV/c,* cobicistat-boosted darunavir; *DRV/r,* ritonavir-boosted darunavir; *FTC,* emtricitabine; *HBV,* hepatitis B virus; *HIV,* human immunodeficiency virus; *HLA,* human leukocyte antigen; *PrEP,* pre-exposure prophylaxis; *TAF,* tenofovir alafenamide fumarate; *TDF,* tenofovir disoproxil fumarate.
Adapted from Panel on Antiretroviral Guidelines for Adults and Adolescents. *Guidelines for the Use of Antiretroviral Agents in Adults and Adolescents With HIV.* Department of Health and Human Services. Available at: https://clinicalinfo.hiv.gov/en/guidelines/adult-and-adolescent-arv/whats-new-guidelines.

Nucleoside (and Nucleotide) Reverse Transcriptase Inhibitors

Nucleoside and nucleotide reverse transcriptase inhibitors (NRTIs) are nucleoside analogs that inhibit the action of the enzyme reverse transcriptase which slows or prevents viral replication. This class forms the backbone of most of the current combination regimens. While older NRTIs were associated with challenging pharmacokinetics that required multiple daily doses and had numerous drug interactions and complications (such as pancreatitis, bone marrow toxicity, or disfiguring lipodystrophy), newer drugs are better tolerated and easier to take.

Non-nucleoside Reverse Transcriptase Inhibitors

As with the NRTIs, the NNRTIs also interfere with reverse transcriptase. The NNRTIs are potent agents that are active against viral strains of HIV that are resistant to NRTIs and sometimes to PIs. However, if NNRTIs are used alone or with a single NRTI, resistance develops quickly, and the resistance usually generalizes to the entire class. Drug interactions can occur because of their metabolism by the cytochrome P450 (CYP) hepatic isoenzyme system. Efavirenz is an NNRTI noteworthy for its greater potential for neuropsychiatric side effects (e.g., somnolence, agitation, insomnia, abnormal or vivid dreams, impaired concentration and attention, psychosis, and suicidality). Such side effects are thought to be related to plasma levels that are pharmacogenetically predisposed.[14] Importantly, the risk of developing thoughts of suicide or attempting suicide, or taking one's own life, may be twice as high for those taking an efavirenz-containing regimen compared with an efavirenz-free regimen.[15] The NNRTIs as a class can also cause a rash in the early phase of treatment; it is thought to be more common and severe (including Stevens-Johnson syndrome) with nevirapine, which is less commonly used in the United States but it is still a common component of treatment in developing countries.[16] Potential psychiatric side effects of ART are listed in Table 28.3.

Protease Inhibitors

Protease inhibitors (PIs) are another potent class of medications, and unlike NNRTIs they have a higher barrier to resistance. The initiation of 3-drug therapy

(NRTI backbone and either NNRTI or PI agents) heralded the "highly active" ART or HAART era. For the first time, HIV RNA was suppressed below the limit of detection, immune recovery occurred, and patients' survival increased dramatically.[16]

PIs interfere with viral replication, maturation, and new infection of cells by inhibiting the enzymatic cleavage of necessary viral protein precursors. The PIs have undergone significant drug development and have matured from requiring handfuls of pills several times each day and associated with prominent side effects to being well-tolerated once-daily regimens. PIs are metabolized by CYP enzymes, leading to significant drug interactions among antiretroviral agents. PIs can cause gastrointestinal (GI) side effects and liver transaminase elevations. In addition, PIs can worsen or cause diabetes, insulin resistance, lipodystrophy, and hyperlipidemia.[16]

Integrase Inhibitors

Integrase is the viral enzyme that catalyzes the integration of virally derived DNA into the host cell DNA in the nucleus, forming a provirus that can be activated to produce viral proteins. The initiation of INSTIs in 2007 brought a new class of medications, which was found to be incredibly effective and well tolerated.

TABLE 28.3

Neuropsychiatric Side Effects of Antiretroviral Therapy

Efavirenz	Somnolence, insomnia, abnormal dreams, dizziness, impaired concentration, depression, psychosis, suicidal ideation, ataxia, and encephalopathy. Some symptoms may be transient (subside or diminish after 2–4 weeks). Bedtime dosing and taking without food may reduce symptoms.
Rilpivirine	Depression, suicidality, sleep disturbances.
Doravirine	Sleep disorders and disturbances, dizziness, altered sensorium; depression and suicidality, and self-harm.
Integrase strand transfer inhibitors (INSTIs)	Insomnia, depression, and suicidality have been reported with INSTI use, primarily in patients with pre-existing psychiatric conditions.

Adapted from National Institutes of Health. *FDA-Approved HIV Medicines.* Available at: https://hivinfo.nih.gov/understanding-hiv/fact-sheets/fda-approved-hiv-medicines

A trial with treatment-naive HIV-infected patients demonstrated a more rapid decline in viral load (as compared with efavirenz), which helped to make INSTIs, initially used for multi-drug-resistant HIV infection, a key component of first-line regimens for treatment-naive individuals.[17]

Entry Inhibitors

Moving away from the replication cycle, the next class of agents acts to prevent viral entry into the host cell. For the HIV virion to enter the CD4 cell, it must bind to the cell at two binding sites. Viral protein gp120 forms a complex with the CD4 receptor that exposes CD4 cell co-receptors, either CCR5, CXCR4, or both. The virus can use either co-receptor to bind to gp120 to enter the host cell; some strains of the virus are predisposed to CCR5 and others to CXCR4.

Maraviroc selectively targets CCR5 and blocks the binding of HIV to CCR5 co-receptors in CCR5-tropic (R5 virus) HIV infection. Hence, if the virus can use CXCR4 as a co-receptor instead, maraviroc is ineffective. Therefore, before the use of maraviroc, viral tropism testing must be performed to determine if it is solely a CCR5-tropic virus. Though well tolerated, this tropism makes maraviroc a limited option.

Fostemsavir binds the gp120 protein on the outer surface of the virus, preventing the virus from entering CD4 cells.[12] Thus, fostemsavir can target CCR5, CXCR4, and dual tropic strains of HIV. In initial trials, fostemsavir has been well tolerated.[18]

Fusion Inhibitors

Enfuvirtide interferes with viral fusion to the host cell membrane by inhibiting the necessary conformational change in a particular viral envelope protein (gp41) that would allow viral entry into a host cell. Administered subcutaneously, enfuvirtide requires twice-daily injections. It is commonly associated with injection-site reactions, an increased incidence of bacterial pneumonia, and rare hypersensitivity reactions. The drug is now rarely used for treatment-experienced patients who develop viral replication despite continuous antiretroviral therapy.[19]

Capsid Inhibitors

Lenacapavir interferes with the protein shell that protects the virus' genetic material and enzymes needed for replication (capsid).[12] In a recent trial of patients with multi-drug-resistant HIV, the use of lenacapavir showed greater reductions from baseline in viral load as compared to placebo and did not demonstrate any serious adverse effects.[20]

Pharmacokinetic Enhancers

Use of ritonavir, a PI, was limited due to high pill burden and reduced tolerability; it was transitioned to an enhancing agent for other PIs due to its pharmacokinetic properties of inhibition of CYP isoenzymes 3 A4, 2D6, C19, 2C8, and 2C9.[21] Cobicistat is a structural analog of ritonavir without any antiretroviral activity, which is now being utilized as a pharmacokinetic booster for integrase inhibitors and PIs due to its activity as a selective inhibitor of CYP P450 isoenzymes, the main metabolizing pathway of several antiretrovirals, and it has been better tolerated thus far.[22] Due to the pharmacokinetics of each, there is potential for drug-drug interactions with psychotropics, particularly substrates of the 3A pathway (see Table 28.4 for relevant drug interactions).

HIV INFECTION AND THE CENTRAL NERVOUS SYSTEM

Within days of the initial infection, HIV enters the brain through migrating monocytes and lymphocytes that cross the blood-brain barrier (BBB), which can become active perivascular macrophages and facilitate infection of microglial cells.[23] Astrocytes may also be infected. Both cells can lead to excessive secretion of inflammatory substances, causing demyelination and cell death. That is, HIV infection causes neuronal destruction without infecting neurons. The CNS appears to be an independent reservoir of HIV replication; CSF viral load does not consistently correlate with plasma levels.[24] HIV in the CNS might also have different characteristics, such as mutations with increased viral resistance or neurotoxicity, than those of the peripherally observed virus. Current antiretrovirals have variable BBB penetrance, they may be less potent inhibitors of viral replication within the CNS, and some are themselves neurotoxic. The optimal antiretroviral drug regimen to combat HIV in the brain remains to be determined, but peripheral suppression of viral replication needs to be coupled

TABLE 28.4
Relevant Potential Drug-Drug Interactions between ART, Antidepressants, and Antipsychotics

	Antiretroviral	Potential Effect	Recommendation
Antidepressant			
Bupropion	Efavirenz	↓Bupropion levels	Monitor
Bupropion	Ritonavir	↓Bupropion levels[a]	Monitor, bupropion may need a dose increase
Fluoxetine	Ritonavir/PIs	↑Fluoxetine levels, potential for serotonin syndrome[b]	Consider fluoxetine dose reduction; monitor
Fluoxetine	Nevirapine	↓Fluoxetine level	Monitor, fluoxetine may need a dose increase
Paroxetine	Fosamprenavir/ritonavir	↓Paroxetine levels	Monitor, paroxetine may need a dose increase
TCAs	PIs	↑TCA level	Monitor for toxicity
Trazodone	PIs	↑Trazodone level	Use the lowest dose possible of trazodone for clinical effect
Venlafaxine	PIs	↑Venlafaxine levels	Monitor
Antipsychotics			
Antipsychotics (Ziprasidone)	Saquinavir, lopinavir/ritonavir	QTc prolongation[c]	Avoid combination if possible, otherwise monitor
Atypical Antipsychotics (Clozapine, Olanzapine)	Antiretrovirals (NRTI, PI)	Hyperglycemia, hypercholesterolemia, weight gain[c]	Evaluate risk, encourage lifestyle modifications, consider alternative agents
Aripiprazole	PI	↑Aripiprazole levels[b]	Monitor, aripiprazole may need dose reduction
Clozapine	Zidovudine	Myelosuppression[c]	Use caution
Olanzapine	Ritonavir	↓Olanzapine levels	Monitor
Risperidone	Indinavir/ritonavir	↑risperidone levels[b]	Consider risperidone dose reduction; monitor

[a]Effect may be dose dependent.
[b]Based on case reports.
[c]Overlapping toxicities.
NRTI, Nucleoside reverse transcriptase inhibitor; *PI*, protease inhibitors; *TCAs*, tricyclic antidepressants.
Adapted from Hill L, Lee KC. Pharmacotherapy considerations in patients with HIV and psychiatric disorders: focus on antidepressants and antipsychotics. *Ann Pharmacother*. 2013;47(1):75–89.

with neuroprotection. New therapies might target regulatory human genes that are involved in viral replication,[24] the identification and exploitation of brain HIV-inhibitory factors,[25] and the enhancement of intrinsic brain defenses that favor neuroprotective, as opposed to neurotoxic, responses to the virus.[25]

HIV has a predilection for subcortical structures, such as the hippocampus and basal ganglia, with lower concentrations in the cerebellum and mid-frontal cortices.[23] This distribution, further differentiation of viral burden within particular basal ganglia regions, and concomitant structural changes in the brain (including ventricular enlargement, hippocampal atrophy, decreased basal ganglia volume, and white matter lesions), might explain the more characteristic cognitive and behavioral impairments associated with CNS HIV infection, as well as the sensitivity of patients with HIV to the extrapyramidal symptoms (EPS) of certain psychiatric medications.[24,26]

When evaluating neurocognitive impairment in HIV-positive patients, HIV infection of the CNS should be a diagnosis of exclusion, made only after a thorough investigation of other etiologies for neuro-cognitive impairment, especially if symptoms are new or of acute onset. Opportunistic infection, neoplasm, other systemic illnesses, medication side effects, drug-drug interactions, use of recreational drugs, withdrawal syndromes, and metabolic and nutritional derangements should be considered. Primary psychiatric disease should be at the bottom of the list, especially if there is not a significant pre-infection history.

Although neuropsychologic testing might not be specific,[27] it helps to localize and quantify cognitive impairments. Recommended neuropsychological tests include an HIV-specific test battery that is based on measures found by the AIDS Clinical Trials Group and the Multi-center AIDS Cohort Study to be sensitive to HIV-related cognitive deficits. These measures include Trail Making A and B, Wechsler Adult Intelligence Scale—Revised digit span and digit symbol, grooved pegboard, finger tapping, Stroop color, and word test, F-A-S test of verbal fluency, Odd Man Out test, and computer-based measures of complex reaction time.[28-31] Other measures are added as clinically indicated. Test battery times of less than 60 minutes are less likely to produce patient fatigue, which confounds test interpretation and creates significant patient frustration or humiliation. Despite these recommendations, there is no ideal test, and it is important to keep in mind that mild deficits on testing can have significant functional consequences.

HIV-ASSOCIATED NEUROCOGNITIVE DISORDERS

HIV-associated neurocognitive disorders (HAND) encompass three conditions, including HIV-associated dementia (HAD), HIV-associated mild neurocognitive disorder (MND), and asymptomatic neurocognitive impairment (ANI).[32] Current hypotheses for the pathogenesis of HAND include early CNS invasion and latent CNS reservoir, chronic neuroinflammation, side effects from ART, and enhanced effects of co-morbid conditions (e.g., hepatitis C co-infection, and substance use disorders [SUDs]).[26,33,34] HAND presents with executive dysfunction, memory impairment, attention deficits, and poor impulse control, and can be associated with motor dysfunction including brady-kinesia, loss of coordination, and gait imbalance. These conditions are all diagnosed using neuropsychological

testing and functional status assessments and are thought to affect 15% to 55% of HIV-positive individuals.[32] HAND is a diagnosis of exclusion.

HIV-Associated Dementia

HIV-associated dementia (HAD), a subcortical dementia, is severe enough to cause functional impairment and marked impairment (>2 standard deviations [SDs] below demographically corrected norms) in at least two cognitive domains. HAD is an AIDS-defining condition with a prevalence in the United States of 21% to 25% before the advent of HAART; since then, it has decreased to less than 5%.[32] HAD is associated with pathologic changes in the brain that include generalized atrophy/leukoencephalopathy with reduced white matter volume, microglial nodules typical of viral encephalitis, atrophy of the basal ganglia (reduced gray matter volume), and multi-nucleated giant cells that appear to be directly infected by HIV by antigen staining.[26,35] Clinically, HAD is characterized by slowed information processing, deficits in attention and memory, and impairments in abstraction and fine motor skills.[27,36] Behavioral changes are wide ranging, including apathy, hypomania, and disinhibition and they can complicate management. Although the prevalence has decreased dramatically, HAD is now seen in patients with less severe immunosuppression and less evidence of structural brain changes, such as HIV encephalitis, as compared with 20 years ago. This condition carries a poor prognosis if left untreated.

HIV-Associated Mild Neurocognitive Disorder

MND involves mild-to-moderate cognitive impairment (1 SD), in at least two cognitive domains, that at least mildly interfere with daily activities.[37] For patients in cognitively taxing jobs, however, even "mild" problems may be significant enough to interfere with and preclude continued employment. MND may lead to poorer ART adherence and impairments in quality of life that could lead to an increased risk of death.

Asymptomatic Neurocognitive Impairment

Asymptomatic neurocognitive impairment (ANI), which may affect up to one-third of patients with HIV infection and two-thirds of all cases of HAND, also involves mild-to-moderate cognitive impairment

(1 SD) in at least two cognitive domains but without obvious impairment in daily function.[38] It is extremely difficult to determine that there are no obvious functional impairments without extensive third-person observation. ANI may be a risk factor for progression to more severe forms of HAND.[39]

HAND in the Era of ART

Before ART, most patients with HIV infection developed cognitive problems. The persistence of neurocognitive impairment despite ART and control of viral load had led to a broader spectrum of classification of HAND (HAD, MND, ANI). Hypotheses for the pathogenesis of HAND include early CNS invasion and latent CNS reservoir, chronic neuroinflammation, side effects from ART, and enhanced effects of co-morbid conditions.[26,33,34]

Ongoing HIV replication in the brain can persist even in the setting of systemic viral suppression. As many as 5% to 10% of patients on ART experience a discordant elevation of HIV RNA in the CSF despite relatively intact immune function; this can correlate with the incidence of neuropsychiatric symptoms. This phenomenon is known as CSF viral escape. Patients present acutely to sub-acutely, with symptoms of encephalitis, myelitis, or meningitis, and they may manifest psychiatric symptoms, including depressive features. The CSF usually demonstrates a lymphocyte-predominant pleocytosis and mild-to-moderately elevated protein levels, while magnetic resonance imaging (MRI) scans often show bilateral, confluent white matter hyperintensities.[32,40] CSF viral escape is thought to be influenced by either independent development of viral resistance in the CSF and/or inadequate CNS penetration of ART.

Chronic neuroinflammation from persistent CNS infection may contribute to the development of HAND. Numerous in vitro and in vivo studies have demonstrated a link between HIV-induced inflammation and neurodegeneration with macrophage proinflammatory cytokine/chemokine production, excitotoxic neuronal injury, and oxidative stress.[33,34,41]

Antiretroviral drugs, particularly NRTIs, can be neurotoxic and they have been associated with neuropathy. In addition, some clinical studies have suggested indirect neurodegenerative effects of ART in the CNS with insulin resistance, lipodystrophy, atherosclerosis, and coronary artery disease. Therefore direct and indirect side effects of ART should also be considered with possible links to impaired neurocognitive performance.

The presence of co-morbid conditions may also be linked to the development of neurocognitive impairment in persons living with HIV infection. Hepatitis C virus (HCV) has been shown to be neurotropic.[42] Substance use can contribute to the development of HAND through enhanced HIV replication, neuroinflammation, and an increase in disinhibition leading to medication non-adherence. Methamphetamine use has increased the expression of CXCR4 and CCR5, and alterations in BBB integrity by cocaine and methamphetamine have been proposed as a mechanism for enhancing neurodegeneration, based on in vitro studies.[34]

Markers that remain strongly correlated with the development of HAND include a CD4+ T cell count low nadir and a history of clinically defined AIDS (toxoplasmosis). Other risk factors for the development of HAND include older age, diabetes, hyperlipidemia, use of tobacco and other substances, and HCV co-infection. Cognitive reserve is also important—those with a higher education level appear to be less likely to develop HAND.

There remains no definitive treatment for HAND. Formerly, there was hope that early treatment with ART would prevent the onset of HAND, but the recent START trial failed to show a major effect of early ART treatment.[10] There is consensus that peripheral viral suppression is necessary to lower the risk of progression to HAND, although it remains unclear if regimens that penetrate the CNS confer some benefit. In fact, a large cohort study of over 50,000 patients found that those receiving a regimen with high CPE were 74% more likely to develop HAD compared to a regimen with low CPE.[43]

DIFFERENTIAL DIAGNOSIS OF PSYCHIATRIC DISTRESS

Psychiatric symptoms are common in HIV-infected individuals often reaching a severity level that meets the criteria for *Diagnostic and Statistical Manual for Mental Disorders*, 5th edition (DSM-5) disorders. Psychiatric symptoms may also be sub-syndromal; underlying causes should be identified and treated whenever possible, although it is often necessary to treat the psychiatric symptoms.

Mental Disorder Due to Another Medical Condition

When evaluating a person infected with HIV, the differential diagnosis should always begin with a mental disorder due to another medical condition. HIV-associated CNS infections should be considered along with opportunistic infections and neoplasms (Table 28.5). Other considerations include medication side effects; drug-drug interactions, such as with herbal and over-the-counter (OTC) preparations; nutritional effects; and effects of chronic substance use, as well as intoxication or withdrawal. Nutritional effects include nutritional deficits, such as of thiamine, folate, zinc, cobalamin (vitamin B_{12}), and pyridoxine (vitamin B_6); poor intake resulting from medication or disease-induced nausea, painful oral lesions; poor absorption; abnormal losses, such as from gastritis, diarrhea, vomiting, or nephropathy; or increased demand resulting from hypermetabolic state due to infection, stress, or neoplasm.[44] Metabolic derangements (e.g., electrolyte abnormalities), renal or hepatic dysfunction, and endocrinopathies (e.g., glucose intolerance, hyperadrenalism, hypocalcemia, or thyroid dysfunction) can also cause psychiatric symptoms.

Delirium

Delirium is a common neuropsychiatric complication in patients hospitalized with AIDS, and it may be a predictor of significantly decreased survival.[45] In patients with asymptomatic HIV infection or with lymphocyte counts greater than 500/μL, it is rare for an HIV-related condition to cause delirium; substance intoxication or withdrawal is a more likely cause. This includes drug side effects (such as those of steroids) used as alternative HIV therapies.

Among those with symptomatic HIV infection or a CD4 lymphocyte count less than 500/μL, HIV-related conditions and iatrogenic causes (Table 28.5) should be high on the list of differential diagnoses for delirium and should be at the top of the list for patients who are at an advanced stage of AIDS or when the CD4 lymphocyte count falls below 100/μL. There should be a continued high index of suspicion for substance intoxication and withdrawal. Seizure disorder should

---

TABLE 28.5
Differential Diagnosis of Neuropsychiatric Symptoms in Patients With HIV Infection and AIDS

Psychiatric disorders

Psychoactive substance intoxication or withdrawal

Primary HIV-associated syndromes
- Seroconversion illness
- HIV CNS infection
- HIV-associated neurocognitive disorders

CNS opportunistic infections
- Fungi: *Cryptococcus neoformans, Coccidioides immitis, Candida albicans, Histoplasma capsulatum, Aspergillus fumigatus*, and mucormycosis
- Protozoa/parasites: *Toxoplasma gondii* and amoebas
- Viruses: CJD virus (progressive multi-focal leukoencephalopathy), CMV, adenovirus type 2, herpes simplex virus, and varicella zoster virus
- Bacteria: *Mycobacterium avium–intracellulare, M. tuberculosis, Listeria monocytogenes*, gram-negative organisms, *Treponema pallidum*, and *Nocardia asteroides*

Other neurotropic infective agents
- Hepatitis C virus

Neoplasms
- Primary CNS non-Hodgkin lymphoma
- Metastatic Kaposi sarcoma (rare)
- Burkitt lymphoma

Medication side effects
- Endocrinopathies and nutrient deficiencies
- Addison disease (CMV, *Cryptococcus*, HIV-1, and ketoconazole)
- Hypothyroidism
- Vitamins A, B_6, B_{12}, and E deficiencies
- Hypogonadism

Anemia

Metabolic abnormalities: hypoxia; hepatic, renal, pulmonary, adrenal, and pancreatic insufficiency; hypomagnesemia; hypocalcemia; water intoxication, dehydration; hypernatremia; hyponatremia; alkalosis; and acidosis

Hypotension

Complex partial seizures

Head trauma

Non-HIV-related conditions

CJD, Creutzfeldt-Jakob disease; *CNS*, central nervous system; *CMV*, cytomegalovirus; *HIV*, human immunodeficiency virus. Adapted from Querques J, Worth JL. HIV infection and AIDS. In: Stern TA, Herman JB, eds. *Psychiatry Update and Board Preparation*. McGraw-Hill; 2000:208.

also be considered, as HIV-infected patients are at an increased risk for new-onset seizures, especially partial complex seizures.[46] A sudden change in mental status is not characteristic of HAD. Patients with advanced HAD experience symptomatic worsening with mild states of delirium during the late afternoon when they are increasingly fatigued, or during the night (i.e., sundowning).

The primary goal in the management of delirium is the identification and treatment of causative factors. The need for laboratory tests (including brain imaging, electroencephalogram, cerebrospinal fluid [CSF] examination, and blood tests) must be guided by history and clinical examination. If delirium is a treatment-emergent adverse effect, the suspected medication should be discontinued, or an alternative agent substituted for it.

Depression

The most common psychiatric complication of HIV infection or AIDS is depression; a diagnosis of depression should never be considered as being appropriate. When a person suffers from clinical depression (i.e., experiences sufficient symptoms to meet the DSM-5 criteria), the patient deserves to be treated. The same criteria for a diagnosis of depression in a person without HIV infection should be used in a person with HIV infection. As is the case with other medical illnesses, it may be difficult to interpret the somatic neurovegetative symptoms (e.g., fatigue, loss of appetite, altered sleep patterns, or difficulty with concentration). Evidence suggests that the prevalence of clinical depression is two- to four-fold higher in persons living with HIV infection.[47]

Low testosterone in HIV-positive males has been linked to symptoms of depression, including low mood, irritability, and decreased libido. Testosterone replacement has been helpful in some males with HIV infection and depressive symptoms, even in the absence of hypogonadism.[48] Checking total testosterone levels in the morning should be considered in this population.

Fatigue

Clinically impairing fatigue affects at least one-third of patients with HIV/AIDS.[49] Although the etiology may be multi-factorial, a search for remediable causes

is an important first step. Pain and sleep deprivation contribute to fatigue in many patients. Importantly, fatigue is not pathognomonic for depression. In fact, fatigue is associated with advanced HIV disease. It can also be disproportionate to apparent disease status.

Bereavement

Patients with HIV infection or AIDS often suffer multiple losses (including the loss of friends, health, physical ability, career, income, housing, child custody, independence, or a sense of freedom or autonomy). Mood and related symptoms require careful evaluation in the setting of loss or bereavement. If the patient meets the criteria for major depression and is not responding to supportive interventions, pharmacologic treatment is warranted.

Trauma

Patients living with HIV infection are vulnerable to traumatic events. Patients diagnosed before the advent and distribution of ART experienced the threat of death with the diagnosis, and many witnessed loved ones dying from AIDS and suffered from survivor's guilt. Even with ART, the possibility of treatment resistance, the chance of exposing others or being exposed to different strains of HIV, and the likelihood of debilitating sequala from infection or medication side effects continue to impact patients. Furthermore, exploration of the event that led to infection can reveal a story of trauma that includes sexual violence or child abuse. Patients living with HIV infection should be screened for symptoms of post-traumatic stress disorder (PTSD) that may precede or emerge post-HIV diagnosis. Untreated PTSD adversely impacts a patient's quality of life and may contribute to harmful health behaviors (such as reduced adherence to ART).

Suicide

Thoughts of suicide should always be assessed; they are more prevalent in patients with asymptomatic HIV infection than in those with AIDS and they may be seen in the setting of being given the diagnosis.[50] The incidence of suicide in patients with HIV infection or AIDS has decreased since the advent of ART; it is now similar to that seen with other medical illnesses. The incidence of suicide in this population and those with other medical illnesses, however, is still higher than in the general population. Risk factors include symptomatic depression, persistent pain, drug use (specifically injection drug use) or alcohol use, domestic violence, altered cognition (i.e., delirium or HAD), social isolation, multiple losses, hopelessness, being transgender, and personality disorders.[51,52] There is no consensus on the relationship between the stage of the disease and the highest risk for suicidal behavior. Serious thoughts of self-harm usually indicate the need for inpatient care. Electroconvulsive therapy may be a life-saving procedure for severely depressed and suicidal individuals, especially when they are medically compromised and unable to tolerate medications or a delay in their effectiveness.

Anxiety

Anxiety is prevalent in those with HIV infection; anxiety symptoms range from acute response to receiving the diagnosis and having an anxiety disorder. Patients with a history of an anxiety disorder are at increased risk, as are those with few social supports and poor coping skills. In susceptible patients, onset or recrudescence of anxiety symptoms may be predictably related to disease milestones or to signs of disease progression, such as the initial diagnosis, a declining CD4 count, an increased viral load, onset of opportunistic infections, chronic pain or paresthesias, wasting, or physical changes that make the disease more public. The somatic symptoms often associated with anxiety (e.g., tremor, muscle tension or spasm, shortness of breath, dizziness, headache, sweating, flushing, palpitations, nausea, vomiting, or diarrhea) need to be carefully investigated for possible medical causes, medication side effects, drug interactions, use of activating recreational drugs, or withdrawal from opiates or sedative-hypnotics.

Mania

Mania in the setting of a personal history of recurrent mood episodes is a core feature of bipolar disorder and is considered a primary (idiopathic) mania. Without such a history or a strong family history of bipolar disorder, any first episode of mania in the setting of HIV infection should be considered secondary (organic) mania as a result of the physiologic effects of HIV-related CNS infection, opportunistic infections, neoplasm, medications, or substance use.[53] Zidovudine

at high doses has also been associated with the development of mania by case report.[54] HIV-associated structural brain lesions might not be more common in patients who develop mania.[55] HIV-related mania is clinically distinct from primary mania, in that HIV-related mania typically manifests with more irritability and psychosis rather than euphoria, and patients are more cognitively impaired.[56]

Psychosis

A pre-existing psychotic disorder may be a risk factor for HIV infection, and it is positively associated with psychosis in HIV-positive patients. The literature suggests that a history of substance abuse, depressive episodes, or certain personality disorders might also correlate with the onset of psychotic symptoms in HIV-associated disease and that ART may be protective against the development of psychosis.[57-59] Secondary causes include more immediate psychoactive substance use (particularly methamphetamine use), CNS HIV infection (usually a late-stage manifestation), opportunistic infections, neoplasms, nutritional deficits, metabolic derangements, or delirium. HIV-infected patients with psychosis tend to exhibit greater cognitive impairment.[59] Efavirenz use has been associated with neuropsychiatric side effects, such as delusions and hallucinations.[60]

Sleep

Sleep problems are highly prevalent (30%–40%) in HIV infection for a variety of reasons.[61] Sleep disturbances may be related to the stage of HIV disease, persistent pain (e.g., from peripheral sensory neuropathy), or psychosocial issues.[61] Lack of structure (e.g., from unemployment), daytime napping, and other contributions to disordered sleep hygiene can lead to a reversal of the sleep-wake cycle. Other related medical conditions can include sleep apnea, congestive heart failure, paroxysmal nocturnal dyspnea, gastroesophageal reflux, polyuria, or delirium. Related movement disorders associated with sleep include restless legs syndrome and periodic limb movement disorder.

Medications (such as antivirals, interferon, psychostimulants, antidepressants, and bronchodilators) and substances (such as alcohol, caffeine, nicotine, cannabis, and opiates) can interfere with restorative sleep. Psychiatric disorders (such as depression, anxiety, adjustment disorders, acute stress, and coping with life events) can also disrupt normal sleep. Insufficient or inefficient sleep negatively affects energy, mood, memory, cognition and cognitive speed, work performance, quality, enjoyment, and safety. Insomnia and fatigue also appear to be associated with increased morbidity and disability. One-fourth of patients try OTC sleep aids (e.g., diphenhydramine, valerian root, or melatonin) or use alcohol and less than 15% take prescribed sedative-hypnotics.

Substance Use

Drug and alcohol abuse increases the risk of infection through injection use, unsafe sexual practices, drug-induced hypersexuality, disinhibition, impulsiveness, altered cognition, impaired judgment, or sex work to obtain drugs or money for drugs. Injection drug use may also increase the chance of becoming infected through heterosexual and mother-to-child transmission. HIV infection in those who use substances is associated with younger age, homelessness, ethnic minority status, and a history of sexual victimization. Prior psychiatric illness is also common. A multi-site study of HIV-positive people reported a 48% prevalence rate of SUD with 20% of the sample reporting polysubstance use. Specific rates were 31% for marijuana, 19% for alcohol, 13% for methamphetamine, 11% for cocaine, and 4% for opiates, with younger age and male gender being strong predictors for SUDs.[62]

Chronic drug use can speed the patient's decline in several ways: suppressed immune function, enhanced HIV replication, increased risk for infections (e.g., STIs, HCV, pneumonia, abscesses, endocarditis, and tuberculosis [TB]), drug interactions with antiretroviral agents, poor ability to adhere to complicated medical regimens, and difficulty with medical follow-up. This population is also at risk for impaired cognitive function from neurotoxic substances, neuroinflammation, poor nutrition, metabolic encephalopathies, ischemia, stroke, seizures, and head trauma.

Among MSM with HIV infection, crystal meth use represents a major co-morbidity. The use of crystal meth fuels unsafe sex practices in a culture known as "party and play," leading to increased rates of transmission. Chronic crystal meth use can also lead to manic symptoms as well as psychosis, and these symptoms often develop with shorter lengths of use in

HIV-positive individuals as compared to those in the general population. Long-term methamphetamine use can also lead to dyskinesias. Due to pharmacokinetic interactions with the CYP system, co-administration of substances and antiretrovirals can have harmful consequences, PIs (such as ritonavir) may inhibit the metabolism of amphetamines and ketamine increasing their risk for toxicity.[63]

Pain

The evaluation and treatment of pain are essential to the care of patients with HIV infection or AIDS. In a systematic literature review of pain in HIV patients, the point prevalence of pain ranged from 54% (based on 1-week recall) to 83% (based on 3-month recall).[64] Pain is a common reason for psychiatric consultation and, rather than death, is often what patients fear most. Pain control is one of the cornerstones in the care of patients with end-stage AIDS. Pain syndromes, including neuropathy, myopathies, and headaches, are common among patients with HIV infection, particularly those who have received older antiretroviral drugs. The psychiatrist might need to intervene when hospital staff who care for a patient with a history of SUD fail to distinguish between the management of the patient's addiction and adequate pain treatment.

Peripheral sensory neuropathy, the most common source of pain in patients with HIV-associated disease, affects up to 35% of patients with AIDS.[65] Most commonly, the neuropathy manifests as a distal, symmetric polyneuropathy that can be caused by HIV infection or by the "d" antiretroviral drugs (ddI, ddC, and stavudine [d4T]). Peripheral neuropathy due to antiretrovirals is typically seen in older individuals who have been treated with these medications. The diagnosis is confirmed by the neurologic examination and laboratory tests, including an electromyogram and nerve conduction studies. Treatment includes a change in the antiretroviral regimen to avoid nerve-toxic agents and the avoidance of other aggravating factors, such as alcohol.

Case 1

Mr. C, a 55-year-old male, who was diagnosed with HIV infection 10 years earlier and treated in the clinic for the last 4 years with ART, presented with new-onset paranoia regarding his downstairs neighbor. He started to believe that his neighbor was breaking into his apartment during the day and had placed recording equipment throughout the apartment. Mr. C reported that he was sleeping much less than normal and that he was not leaving the house. His history was notable for depression, treated for many years with fluoxetine, and a history of alcohol use disorder, in remission for the past 7 years. Consultation with the patient's primary care physician revealed that his CD4 count has remained high and his viral load undetectable over the last 3 years on his current regimen. Cognitive testing reveals mild deficits in attention and focus, with some mild executive dysfunction.

The differential diagnosis included major depression with psychotic features, a schizophrenia-spectrum disorder e.g., delusional disorder, alcohol-induced psychosis in the setting of possible relapse, another substance-induced psychosis, an unrecognized bipolar disorder presenting as a mania with psychosis, HIV-associated dementia with psychosis, opportunistic infection in the CNS, antiretroviral medication-induced psychosis, and CSF viral escape leading to mental disorder due to HIV infection.

Medication review revealed that the patient does not take any ART associated with prominent neuropsychiatric effects and the regimen had not changed, making an ART side effect unlikely. Laboratory tests revealed high CD4 counts which when combined with no focal neurologic deficits make an opportunistic infection less likely. The patient's bedside cognitive testing was not severely impaired enough to suggest an HIV-dementia; his deficits were mild. Aside from insomnia, the patient denies other prominent symptoms of mania or depression. Prior to further neurologic work-up, a urine toxicology was obtained, and it revealed the presence of amphetamines, which were not prescribed. On confrontation, the patient acknowledged having a pattern over the last several years, of bingeing on crystal meth in association with unsafe sexual practices. The diagnosis of amphetamine-induced psychosis was confirmed. Via counseling, engagement in a support group, and ongoing psychiatric treatment, Mr. C was able to achieve sobriety, and his psychotic symptoms gradually reduced in sever-

ity over the next several months, though he continued to have some lingering paranoia.

APPROACH TO PSYCHIATRIC CARE

Screening and Prevention

Roughly 13% of those infected with HIV in the United States are unaware of their seropositivity. In 2006 the Centers for Disease Control and Prevention (CDC) Division of HIV/AIDS Prevention took steps to address this by issuing new recommendations advocating for universal HIV screening in all healthcare settings: medical inpatient and outpatient, mental health, and substance abuse settings. The recommendations require no special patient consent for screening, which is performed once the patient is so notified unless the patient specifically declines consent; this is universal opt-out screening.[66] However, two states (New York and Nebraska) still have statutes that require written informed consent. In 2013 the United States Preventative Services Task Force recommended universal screening for HIV, which resulted in insurance companies having to cover the cost of screening.[67]

Psychiatrists should strongly consider screening their patients for HIV, consistent with the CDC recommendations, especially given that they care for at-risk populations. Screening is critical not just for secondary infections, but also to ensure that patients receive early treatment, as recommended. Screening should also take place routinely at substance-use treatment sites. Studies have shown that patients at such sites often have not been tested recently for HIV infection, and a small but significant minority has never been tested.[68]

Of the 45,000 HIV transmissions in 2009, 91.5% were attributable to patients with HIV who were undiagnosed (18% of the population) or not retained in medical care (45% of the population).[69] These figures illustrate that screening is necessary but insufficient for prevention. After screening, the next step in prevention is the assessment of the patient for risk factors and problematic behaviors. Prevention models with individuals and groups having chronic mental illness and SUDs must be specific and tailored to the population being addressed. Programs with counselors whose cultural backgrounds are like those of the patient population they are working with have proved most effective. Programs geared toward the injection drug use community have enlisted community members as prevention leaders.

Pre-exposure prophylaxis (PrEP) was approved by the FDA in 2012 as a strategy to prevent new infections in patients engaging in high-risk behaviors. Several randomized controlled trials as well as real-world observational studies have demonstrated a substantial decline in new infections when PrEP was used regularly.[70] Unfortunately, the use of PrEP is correlated with decreased use of condoms and increased rates of transmission of other STIs. Psychiatrists should be aware of the option of PrEP for patients engaged in high-risk behaviors.

Collaboration

Although several demonstration projects have shown the efficacy of wrap-around services for HIV-infected patients,[71] it is the exception rather than the rule to have medical, mental health, and addiction services, including opiate replacement therapy, in one coordinated site.[72] More commonly, patients with multiple diagnoses have complicated treatment regimens and have multiple providers at different sites of care, a situation that can parallel the chaos for the rest of their lives. In the absence of single-site treatment, intensive management of care can keep all treaters informed, provide outreach to improve attendance at appointments, assist with concrete services (e.g., housing, transportation, child care), and help devise and implement an individualized medication adherence plan. Consultation psychiatrists have a unique opportunity to facilitate communication and coordinate care among members of the patient's care team.

Adherence

Adherence is the cornerstone of successful therapy for HIV infection. Missed doses lead to treatment resistance and sometimes resistance to whole classes of medication. This, in turn, is correlated with greater morbidity and higher mortality rates, as well as the development of more treatment-resistant viral strains. Active substance use, homelessness, a lack of social support, domestic violence, personality disorders, and psychiatric illness, especially major depression, have long been recognized as risk factors for poor adherence.[73,74]

However, the presence of one or more of these factors is not justification for exclusion from ART. Rather, these factors are challenges to be addressed in preparation for initiating ART, which may be postponed for several months while active treatment is initiated for addictions or psychiatric problems, along with readiness for concurrent medications and education about adherence. The patient hospitalized with HIV infection presents a unique opportunity for the initiation or reinforcement of this preparation for ART.

Effective adherence programs are tailored to the patient in terms of language, education, culture, lifestyle, and personality. Individualized adherence programs capitalize on, or enhance, the patient's social supports (e.g., family, intimate partners, friends, and groups), cognitive abilities, and personality style. They require accessibility, flexibility, and positively framed incentives (i.e., rewards, not punishments).[75] Adherence is further promoted when the patient has a high level of satisfaction with the physician, understands the importance of taking every dose, believes that missed doses lead to resistance, knows and recognizes each specific medication, and is informed about possible side effects.[75]

Simplifying the regimen (e.g., reducing the number of doses and food restrictions) and minimizing the pill burden helps fit the regimen into the patient's lifestyle. Clearly written instructions are helpful if the patient is literate. Tying pill-taking to daily routines, along with pill boxes, alarms, pagers, directly-observed therapy, or new smartphone application reminder systems, can also increase adherence. Patients who are comfortable taking medications in front of other people also have an easier time incorporating ART into their lives.

Adherence is not static; it needs to be asked about, and promoted by, each provider at every visit. Pill fatigue, complacency, transient or prolonged relapse of substance abuse or depression, onset of morphologic or metabolic side effects, onset or exacerbation of other medical conditions, hospitalization, or psychosocial stressors (e.g., financial, housing, insurance issues or changes, family or relationship issues, and travel) can interrupt or decrease the patient's previous level of adherence.

In addition to medication adherence, adherence to appointments is also an important component of treatment. Adherence to scheduled medical appointments is associated with optimal viral suppression and might warrant appropriate outreach efforts. A recent study showed an increase in all-cause mortality for patients who failed to achieve retention in clinical care, while missed visits independently increased mortality rates in those considered to be retained in care.[76]

TREATMENT

Non-Pharmacologic Treatments

Case Management

Case management is often necessary to help with basic needs (such as food, shelter, transportation, childcare, medical coverage, and other entitlements), which may be needed in this population and are powerful barriers to adequate treatment. In particular, patients with cognitive impairment (executive dysfunction and memory problems) are at risk of falling through the cracks unless appropriate help and supervision are provided.

Groups

Groups of various types, often provided in the community or by AIDS activist organizations, offer a supportive, social network and positive affiliations for members of an often disenfranchised and stigmatized population. Self-help, 12-step, and peer-counseling groups are examples of such community-based programs. Therapy groups and other more formalized groups might focus on aspects of living with HIV infection (e.g., disclosure, adherence, parenting), participant characteristics (e.g., females, particular ethnic minorities, MSM, those with SUDs), or mission (e.g., risk reduction or prevention).[77]

Individual Psychotherapy

Individual psychotherapy can help patients cope with HIV infection or AIDS-related issues and distress with approaches, such as coping strategies, problem-solving, disclosure of HIV status, discrimination, relationships, sexuality, and bereavement. For patients whose infection was diagnosed more than a decade ago, issues of facing a foreshortened life span may be replaced by issues of living with a chronic illness. There may be themes of remorse and longing for missed opportunities referent to this erroneous life view. The focus and goals of therapy may be specific to the stage of HIV-associated disease; late in the course of AIDS, therapy may focus on end-of-life issues (such as concerns about ongoing childcare and guardianship, coping with loss, progressive disability, and unremitting pain).

For specific diagnoses, including depression or anxiety disorders, proven therapies, such as interpersonal psychotherapy or cognitive-behavioral therapy, have been shown to be effective in this population.[77] Self-hypnosis, guided imagery, meditation, muscle relaxation, massage, yoga, aerobic exercise, or acupuncture may be therapeutic for selected patients.

Adherence to medications for HIV infection and psychotropic medications should be reinforced or explored. It should be stressed that the therapist is a member of the patient's treatment team, and appropriate releases should be obtained to allow all team members to communicate and coordinate care.

Pharmacologic Treatment

Drug-Drug Interactions

Patients with HIV infection or AIDS may be taking ART, psychotropic drugs, OTC and herbal preparations, alcohol or drugs of abuse, and drugs to treat those addictions. Such drug combinations are prone to interactions, overlapping side effects, and toxicities. Drug side effects, such as diarrhea (common to many antiretroviral agents), can decrease the absorption of other drugs. Potential drug interactions do not necessarily preclude the concomitant use of such medications but require a careful risk-to-benefit assessment, possible dose adjustment, periodic drug level monitoring, and monitoring for, or treatment of, side effects.

Effects on the CYP enzyme system in the liver account for many of the drug-drug interactions. Of the key CYP isoenzymes involved in the metabolism of psychotropics and antiretrovirals (1A2, 2C9/19, 2D6, and 3A4), 3A4 and 2D6 account for most of the metabolism of psychiatric medications. Allelic differences cause 10% of White population and 1% of Asians to slowly metabolize 2D6 substrates,[78] while 20% of African-Americans and Asians and 5% of White people slowly metabolize 2C19 substrates.[79,80] Medications can rely on more than one metabolic pathway, which acts as a safeguard against drug interactions. In vitro studies of drug metabolism do not adequately portray the human experience that is complicated by individual genetic and nutritional differences and multi-drug and substance regimens.[78] As a rule of thumb, the PIs, followed by the NNRTIs, have the broadest effects on the CYP system. The PI ritonavir also induces glucuronyl transferase, a non-CYP metabolic enzyme.

For a variety of reasons, patients with HIV infection are very sensitive to small doses of psychiatric medications, like what is seen in geriatric patients. Helping patients tolerate medications is ultimately more important than raising the dose quickly. General principles for medications in this population are: "start low and go slow," avoid complex regimens, reduce pill burden where possible, and anticipate drug-drug interactions. Patients still need to receive an appropriate dose of any psychotropic. Due to the pill burden and complicated schedules that patients with HIV infection often endure, once-a-day medication therapy is generally preferable. Anticholinergic medications should be avoided or minimized because of their deleterious effects on cognition and the possibility of delirium or even seizures. Decreased saliva can also predispose to the development of thrush.

Depression

Selective serotonin reuptake inhibitors (SSRIs) remain the drugs of choice for depressive disorders in HIV patients because of established efficacy in this patient population and a favorable risk-to-benefit profile. SSRIs are largely metabolized by 2D6 and 3A4. Ritonavir, and to a lesser extent indinavir, inhibit the metabolism of 2D6 substrates; all of the PIs inhibit 3A4 metabolism to varying degrees.[81] Inhibition of the metabolism of the SSRIs and venlafaxine by ritonavir and PIs may increase the levels of the antidepressants, which might allow a therapeutic response at a low or moderate dose. Although high doses of the antidepressants could lead to serotonin syndrome or other toxicities, a wide range of concentrations are generally well tolerated.

All SSRIs are associated with sexual side effects, akathisia-like activation, and GI symptoms. Fluoxetine, with the longest half-life in this drug class, is a good option for patients who might miss doses. The use of fluoxetine weekly is also an option. Sertraline, citalopram, and escitalopram have the least potential for clinically significant drug interactions. While citalopram was once considered the initial SSRI of choice for

patients with HIV/AIDS, concerns about the potential for greater QT prolongation coupled with evidence suggesting HIV patients are themselves at higher risk for QT prolongation has somewhat limited its use as a first-line agent.[82]

Serotonin-Norepinephrine Reuptake Inhibitors. Venlafaxine, its metabolite desvenlafaxine, and duloxetine are serotonin and norepinephrine reuptake inhibitors (SNRIs). The extended-release form of venlafaxine is a reasonable first-line medication because of its once-a-day dosing and paucity of drug interactions. Because of inhibition by PIs noted above, lower doses may be sufficient. Duloxetine can induce liver enzymes, so close monitoring is required when patients are co-infected with HIV and HCV or have impaired liver function. SNRIs can be initially stimulating, and some patients have difficulty tolerating them. SNRIs can raise blood pressure unacceptably in hypertensive patients, and blood pressure monitoring is required. Milnacipran is an SNRI marketed in the United States for fibromyalgia.

Bupropion. Bupropion's stimulating effect, if tolerable, can benefit patients with fatigue or apathy, although, unlike psychostimulants, bupropion may not improve HIV-related cognitive slowing.[83] Bupropion lowers the seizure threshold in a dose-dependent manner, which is a concern in patients with a history of seizures, poorly controlled seizure disorders, head trauma, or other threshold-lowering pathology (e.g., space-occupying lesions, infections, or alcohol or psychoactive substance use). Patients with an eating disorder or metabolic derangements from drug side effects (such as vomiting or diarrhea) may be at increased risk for seizures. The slow-release forms may be safer regarding seizure risk, and lower doses (100–300 mg) are often used in patients with HIV infection. The actual risk of seizures in those with HIV infection treated with bupropion seems much less than previously thought.[84] Ritonavir has been shown to lower bupropion levels.[85] A prospective study that included the administration of bupropion to patients on PIs reported no serious adverse events and, specifically, no seizures.[86]

Trazodone. Primarily used for its major side effect, trazodone demonstrates a sedating effect within 20 to

30 minutes of ingestion, usually at a low dose (25 or 50 mg). In low doses, it is minimally anticholinergic. Males of all ages should be informed of its rare but serious side effect, priapism (with a prevalence of about 1/7000). In healthy volunteers, ritonavir increased trazodone plasma levels; therefore the recommendation is to use the lowest dose of trazodone required for clinical effect.[85]

Mirtazapine. At low doses, mirtazapine is useful for patients who have difficulty eating and sleeping, even in the absence of clear depression. At higher doses, it is also an effective antidepressant, albeit with histaminergic side effects (e.g., daytime drowsiness and significant weight gain). Patients who receive mirtazapine should be weighed at regular intervals. Mirtazapine appears to have no significant drug interactions with ART.

Tricyclic Antidepressants. Tricyclic antidepressants (TCAs) are often used in small doses for neuropathic pain, insomnia, or headaches. TCAs have a narrow therapeutic window; metabolic inhibition at 2D6, from PIs (or most SSRIs), can lead to serious toxicity, including death. Safe concurrent use of these medicines requires therapeutic drug monitoring and monitoring electrocardiograms (ECGs), particularly if the patient is on other QTc-prolonging medications.[82,84] The side effects of constipation may be helpful in some HIV-infected patients with diarrhea. TCAs can be lethal with ingestion of a 2-week supply. The least anticholinergic agents, nortriptyline and desipramine, are recommended given that anticholinergic can worsen cognition.

Monoamine Oxidase Inhibitors. Due to the myriad of drugs that patients with HIV infection might need over time, monoamine oxidase inhibitors are relatively contraindicated in these patients. They should specifically not be co-administered with zidovudine.

Psychostimulants. Psychostimulants, such as methylphenidate and dextroamphetamine, may be used to target co-morbid attention-deficit hyperactivity disorder, augment antidepressant therapy, or treat the symptoms of fatigue and cognitive decline associated with HIV infection. Methylphenidate can inhibit 2C9 and 2C19 metabolism, leading to increased levels of certain TCAs (i.e., desipramine, clomipramine, and imipramine), barbiturates, and warfarin. Dextroamphetamine, however, is a 2D6 substrate that neither inhibits nor induces the CYP isoenzymes, although it can compete at active sites.[84]

In low doses, psychostimulants can improve appetite, energy, and mood. They work quickly, often within hours, and have few side effects or interactions. Especially useful in patients who are unresponsive to or intolerant of other antidepressants, stimulants also help patients attend and stay more focused and organized. In late HAD, however, they can become toxic. Stimulants should also be avoided in the presence of psychotic symptoms or those with a history of seizures. Abuse is rare in patients who have no history of SUD. A history of a SUD is not a contraindication to the use of stimulants but it does require that the prescriber be more cautious. Modafinil and armodafinil are related wakefulness-promoting nonstimulant psychotropics that are sometimes used instead of a psychostimulant for HIV-related fatigue and depression.

Anxiety

Anxiolytic Antidepressants. For prolonged use in anxiety disorders, SSRIs as well as SNRIs are beneficial, and they decrease the required benzodiazepine dose when these medications are co-administered.

Benzodiazepines. For more time-limited episodes of intolerable anxiety, short- to medium-acting benzodiazepines without active metabolites and with the fewest drug-drug interactions should be used. Benzodiazepines are primarily 3A4 substrates, except for oxazepam, temazepam, and lorazepam (so-called "OTL", "outside the liver"), which are metabolized by glucuronyl transferase. Triazolobenzodiazepines (e.g., alprazolam, midazolam, and triazolam) are metabolized by CYP 3A4, an isoform inhibited by PIs, which can enhance the effects of the anxiolytics, possibly leading to dangerous respiratory depression. For this reason, OTL benzodiazepines are the drugs of choice when patients are on (3A4-inhibiting) PIs and for those with hepatic impairment. However, the use of these glucuronyl transferase substrates with ritonavir can require higher benzodiazepine doses. The NNRTIs, efavirenz, and nevirapine, along with the PI ritonavir, have the potential to induce the 3A isoenzymes. This 3A induction may be delayed and cause a drop in previously elevated benzodiazepine levels, resulting in decreased efficacy or withdrawal. This unpredictability further precludes the regular use of such short-acting agents (e.g., alprazolam) because of the risk that withdrawal will precipitate seizures. Benzodiazepines should be avoided in patients with HAND due to an increased risk of adverse effects (confusion, sedation, cognitive impairment, disinhibition).[87]

Buspirone. An option for patients on PIs, buspirone unfortunately takes several weeks to become effective. Concomitant use of benzodiazepines may be necessary to help the patient through the initiation and titration period. In advanced systemic illness, but not less symptomatic disease, buspirone has worsened cognition and triggered mania.[83]

Antipsychotics. Although generally not recommended for anxiety because of potentially serious long-term metabolic effects, low doses of atypical antipsychotics may be effective if fear or pain are prominent. See the section, "Psychosis" below for more information on the use of antipsychotics in patients with HIV.

Bipolar Disorder

Beyond optimizing the antiretroviral regimen, treatment of HIV-related secondary mania should be tailored to the patient's HIV status and general medical condition. In advanced HIV/AIDS, patients might find lithium or carbamazepine less tolerable. Although lithium does not interact with the CYP system, it should be avoided in HIV-positive patients with advanced illness because of its potential for toxicity with fluid and electrolyte shifts.[87] Carbamazepine induces CYP 3A4, lowering levels of the PIs and other antiretrovirals, a situation that could foster resistance, possibly to a whole class of medications.[84] It might be possible in certain instances to avert this resistance by using higher doses of the antiretroviral. However, carbamazepine is also relatively contraindicated in immune-suppressed patients because of its potential to cause leukopenia.

Valproate increases the risk of liver toxicity (especially in patients with chronic HCV or other liver disease) and bone marrow suppression (especially in combination with zidovudine, whose levels may be increased via glucuronyl transferase inhibition).[88] Nonetheless, valproic acid may be more effective for patients with secondary mania and brain abnormalities detected on MRI.[89] When valproate is prescribed, monitoring for liver function, platelet count, hyperammonemia, and weight gain is recommended.

Lamotrigine bypasses the CYP system, but it is a glucuronyl transferase substrate and needs to be titrated slowly to reduce the risk of Stevens-Johnson syndrome. Nonetheless, lamotrigine is often the mood stabilizer of choice in patients with HIV and bipolar disorder, especially those with a history of recurrent depression and less severe mania.

Although benzodiazepines have anti-manic properties, they carry the risk of disinhibition, anterograde amnesia, and confusion; they are generally not considered as primary pharmacologic treatment of mania. For medically complex patients with HIV disease, antipsychotics are often preferred over standard mood stabilizers.

Psychosis

Antipsychotics are the treatment of choice for psychotic symptoms from almost any cause. Patients with HIV infection, however, are extremely sensitive to the side effects of antipsychotics and are at risk for EPS and neuroleptic malignant syndrome with high-potency agents and confusion or seizures with low-potency agents.[85,87] In addition, overlapping toxicities, such as QT prolongation, from ziprasidone and saquinavir[82,85]; risk of weight gain and hypercholesterolemia from clozapine/olanzapine and NRTI, PI[85]; and, risk of myelosuppression from clozapine and ziprasidone[85] should be considered when selecting an agent.

Second-generation antipsychotics (SGAs) are often selected because of better tolerability, particularly regarding EPS. Use of very low starting doses and cautious titration are recommended. Risperidone and olanzapine have each been used effectively for HIV-related psychosis without causing undue sedation or cognitive impairment.[90] The deleterious effect of many SGAs on glucose metabolism, however, can limit their usefulness, especially in patients already at risk for diabetes, such as those taking PIs.[85] Aripiprazole has fewer metabolic side effects but still causes weight gain, while ziprasidone and lurasidone also have good metabolic profiles. Metformin is increasingly used for metabolic syndrome induced by antipsychotics, and it may be an option for HIV-positive patients who develop such side effects. Lurasidone toxicity has been reported in combination with atazanavir in at least one report.[91]

Plasma levels of clozapine, which has a complex metabolic pathway involving 1A2, 2C9/19, 3A4, and 2D6, can increase with concomitant use of PIs. Despite its relative contraindications given the potential for drug interactions and added bone marrow toxicity, clozapine may still be used, particularly because it is possible to monitor clozapine serum levels.

Substance Use Disorders

The treatment and management of patients hospitalized for HIV infection and SUDs has five main features, depending on the patient's level of addiction or recovery: prophylaxis against or treatment of withdrawal; encouragement to enter a recovery program that includes referral to a comprehensive addictions program; maintenance of recovery during the stress of hospitalization; adequate pain control including the use of narcotic medications, if appropriate; and careful monitoring for drug-drug interactions, especially for those on methadone maintenance.

Prescribed medications that are being abused probably need to be discontinued. There are limitations to the model of harm reduction used in many addiction-treatment programs, and prescribing oral forms of abused injection drugs does not promote recovery from a SUD. Maintenance medications, such as methadone, should be continued during the hospitalization, if possible. For patients on methadone maintenance with symptomatic HIV infection or with CD4+ lymphocyte counts below 500/μL, the initiation of some antimicrobial agents or ART can have pharmacologic consequences. For example, methadone increases zidovudine serum levels, which can lead to increased toxicity. Treatment with rifampin, amprenavir, darunavir, efavirenz, fosamprenavir, nelfinavir, nevirapine, and ritonavir can increase methadone metabolism and potentially precipitate acute opiate withdrawal. In this instance, the daily methadone dose needs to be increased. The discharge plan should include notification of the patient's methadone clinic about this dosage change. Methadone can prolong the QT interval,

placing patients with HIV at increased risk for lethal ventricular arrhythmias, such as *torsades de pointes*, especially when methadone is administered along with other QT-prolonging agents.

Patients prescribed Suboxone as an opiate replacement therapy also face challenges surrounding pain treatment. In some cases, Suboxone may block the effects of full μ-opioid agonists, leading to inadequate pain control with typical regimens. Suboxone has been used safely in many patients with HIV infection.

Another important substance-medication interaction to be aware of is that ritonavir inhibits the metabolism of ecstasy, ketamine, cocaine, and other stimulants, as well as γ-hydroxybutyrate. Fatal interactions between ecstasy and ritonavir have been reported.

Pain

The treatment of HIV-related neuropathy is like the approach used with chronic pain syndromes. Low doses of TCAs can be effective, either alone or in combination with other analgesic therapies. No systematic studies have been conducted to compare the efficacy of different TCAs, and no evidence exists for the superiority of amitriptyline for HIV-related neuropathy. Desipramine and nortriptyline are better tolerated and appear to be as effective.

Anticonvulsants, used in low doses, can be effective for neuropathic pain, either alone or in combination with other analgesic therapies. Both carbamazepine and valproic acid have been effective, but hematopoietic and hepatic side effects and drug interactions must be monitored. Gabapentin may be effective for neuropathic pain; its use avoids hematopoietic and hepatic side effects. Low-dose clonazepam can be particularly effective for hyperpathia. Lamotrigine has support for its use for HIV-related sensory neuropathy from a controlled trial.[92]

Some antiarrhythmics also have local anesthetic properties and can be useful for the management of some pain syndromes. Post-herpetic neuralgia can be highly disabling in HIV-infected patients, particularly those who have had multi-dermatomal herpes zoster. Intravenous lidocaine can offer relief, often with once- or twice-weekly infusions, and a significant dose reduction in narcotic analgesics.

Opiates are beneficial for short-term use or periods of pain exacerbation, but they can induce tolerance and abuse or dependence. A history of an SUD does not preclude the use of opiates that are required for adequate analgesia, but opiates require careful monitoring to prevent unauthorized escalation of the dosage. In discharge planning for patients with advanced HIV disease, psychiatrists should remember that cognitive impairment can make adherence to as-needed dosing schedules difficult, and patients can accidentally overuse analgesics. The use of a pill alarm or box can be helpful. If long-term therapy with opiates is needed, psychiatrists should consider the use of long-acting oral or transdermal formulations. The latter is particularly helpful in the care of terminally ill individuals, many of whom have odynophagia or dysphagia.

Opiates also interface with hepatic metabolism, affecting and being affected by interactions with antiretroviral medications. Meperidine may be cleared more quickly, leaving a higher concentration of its neurotoxic metabolite that causes delirium and possibly seizures. Clearance of fentanyl, a 3A4 substrate, is decreased by ritonavir, which can cause nausea, dizziness, and possibly respiratory depression. Codeine and its derivatives are prodrugs that need to be converted to analgesics. PIs can block this conversion and make pain control more difficult.

CONCLUSION

Neuropsychiatric symptoms are common in those with HIV infection and AIDS and they have multiple etiologies. HIV CNS infection and primary psychiatric disorders should always be considered. Other CNS infections or lesions, medications, drugs of abuse, drug-drug interactions, and metabolic derangements also need to be explored. When the source has been identified, underlying causes should be treated, but the psychiatric symptoms can require more immediate, symptomatic treatment.

Patients with HIV infection are often sensitive to small amounts of medication, and they should generally be given in geriatric doses with careful monitoring and slow dosage titration; ultimately, however, an effective dose must be prescribed. The PIs, and to a lesser extent the NNRTIs, are responsible for most of the drug-drug interactions with psychotropics. These interactions occur largely because of interference with the hepatic CYP enzyme system. Optimal psychiatric care (e.g., effective remission of depression) can help patients achieve sufficient adherence to antiretroviral treatment and even improve the prognosis. Some general principles and frequently updated resources (Table 28.6) can aid in the safe pharmacologic treatment of these patients.

TABLE 28.6		
Clinically Useful HIV/AIDS Resources on the Internet		
Program	**URL**	**Comments**
AIDS Clinical Trials Information Service (ACTIS)	www.actis.org	Provides quick and easy access to information on federally and privately funded clinical trials for adults and children
The Body Pro	www.thebodypro.com	Provides news updates and the latest treatment guidelines
Centers for Disease Control and Prevention	www.cdc.gov/hiv/	Comprehensive database with epidemiology, guidelines, latest research, and advocacy
HIV/AIDS Treatment Information Service	www.hivatis.org	Allows you to view and download HIV treatment guidelines, general HIV treatment information, and more
New York State Department of Health AIDS Institute	www.health.ny.gov/ diseases/aids/	Coordinates state programs, services, and activities relating to HIV/AIDS
UCSF HIV InSite	https://targethiv.org/	Includes a drug-interaction database by drug class, drug profiles, fact sheets, and links to treatment guidelines
United Nations Programme on HIV/AIDS	www.unaids.org	International epidemiology, news, and recommendations
US FDA HIV/AIDS Program	www.fda.gov/oashi/aids/ HIV.html	Includes information about approved antiretroviral drugs and treatment guidelines

AIDS, Acquired immunodeficiency syndrome; *HIV*, human immunodeficiency virus.

REFERENCES

1. Cournos F, McKinnon K, Rosner J. HIV among individuals with severe mental illness. *Psychiatr Ann.* 2001;31(1):50–56.
2. Pence BW, Miller WC, Whetten K, et al. Prevalence of DSM-IV-defined mood, anxiety, and substance use disorders in an HIV clinic in the Southeastern United States. *J AIDS.* 2006;42(3):298–306.
3. American Psychiatric Association. *Practice Guideline for the Treatment of Patients with HIV/AIDS.* American Psychiatric Publishing; 2000.
4. Geskus RB, Prins M, Hubert J-B, et al. The HIV RNA setpoint theory revisited. *Retrovirology.* 2007;4:65.
5. Mayer KH, Beyrer C. HIV epidemiology update and transmission factors: risks and risk contexts—16th International AIDS Conference epidemiology plenary. *Clin Infect Dis.* 2007;44(7):981–987.
6. Joint United Nations Programme on HIV/AIDS. *UNAIDS Data*; 2021. Available at: https://www.unaids.org/sites/default/files/media_asset/JC3032_AIDS_Data_book_2021_En.pdf. (Accessed 12 June 2023).
7. Joint United Nations Programme on HIV/AIDS. *Global AIDS*; Update 2016. Available at: http://www.unaids.org/sites/default/files/media_asset/global-AIDS-update-2016_en.pdf. (Accessed 12 June 2023).
8. Centers for Disease Control and Prevention. *HIV in the United States: HIV Basics.* Available at: https://www.cdc.gov/hiv/basics/statistics.html. (Accessed 12 June 2023).
9. Centers for Disease Control and Prevention HIV testing and risk behaviors among gay, bisexual, and other men who have sex with men—United States. *MMWR.* 2013;62(47):958.
10. Insight Start Study Group Initiation of antiretroviral therapy in early asymptomatic HIV infection. *N Engl J Med.* 2015;373:795–807.
11. U.S. Department of Health and Human Services, Panel on Antiretroviral Guidelines for Adults and Adolescents. *Guidelines for the Use of Antiretroviral Agents in Adults and Adolescents with HIV*; 2016. Available at: https://clinicalinfo.hiv.gov/en/guidelines/adult-and-adolescent-arv/whats-new-guidelines. (Accessed 12 June 2023).
12. National Institutes of Health. *FDA-Approved HIV Medicines.* 2023. Available at: https://hivinfo.nih.gov/understanding-hiv/fact-sheets/fda-approved-hiv-medicines. (Accessed 12 June 2023).
13. Nachega JB, Parienti J-J, Uthman OA, et al. Lower pill burden and once-daily dosing antiretroviral treatment regimens for HIV infection: a meta-analysis of randomized controlled trials. *Clin Infect Dis.* 2014;58(9):1297–1307.
14. Rodriguez-Novoa S, Barreiro P, Rendón A, et al. Influence of 516G> T polymorphisms at the gene encoding the CYP450-2B6 isoenzyme on efavirenz plasma concentrations in HIV-infected subjects. *Clin Infect Dis.* 2005;40(9):1358–1361.
15. Mollan KR, Smurzynski M, Eron JJ, et al. Association between efavirenz as initial therapy for HIV-1 infection and increased risk for suicidal ideation or attempted or completed suicide: an analysis of trial data. *Ann Intern Med.* 2014;161(1):1–10.
16. Pau AK, George JM. Antiretroviral therapy: current drugs. *Infect Dis Clin North Am.* 2014;28(3):371–402.
17. Markowitz M, Nguyen BY, Gotuzzo E, et al. Rapid and durable antiretroviral effect of the HIV-1 Integrase inhibitor raltegravir as part of combination therapy in treatment-naive patients with HIV-1 infection: results of a 48-week controlled study. *J Acquir Immune Defic Syndr.* 2007;46(2):125–133.
18. Gravatt LAH, Leibrand CR, Patel S, et al. New drugs in the pipeline for the treatment of HIV: a review. *Curr Infect Dis Rep.* 2017;19:1–9.
19. Bean P. New drug targets for HIV. *Clin Infect Dis.* 2005;41(suppl 1):96–100.
20. Segal-Maurer S, DeJesus E, Stellbrink HJ, et al. Capsid inhibition with lenacapavir in multidrug-resistant HIV-1 infection. *N Engl J Med.* 2022;386(19):1793–1803.
21. Tseng A, Hughes CA, Wu J, et al. Cobicistat versus ritonavir: similar pharmacokinetic enhancers but some important differences. *Ann Pharmacother.* 2017;51(11):1008–1022.
22. Shah BM, Schafer JJ, Priano J, et al. Cobicistat: a new boost for the treatment of human immunodeficiency virus infection. *Pharmacotherapy.* 2013;33(10):1107–1116.
23. Sanmarti M, Ibáñez L, Huertas S, et al. HIV-associated neurocognitive disorders. *J Mol Psychiatry.* 2014;2:1–10.
24. Schrager LK, D'souza MP. Cellular and anatomical reservoirs of HIV-1 in patients receiving potent antiretroviral combination therapy. *JAMA.* 1998;280(1):67–71.
25. Kramer-Hämmerle S, Rothenaigner I, Wolff H, et al. Cells of the central nervous system as targets and reservoirs of the human immunodeficiency virus. *Virus Res.* 2005;111(2):194–213.
26. Clifford DB, Ances BM. HIV-associated neurocognitive disorder. *Lancet Infect Dis.* 2013;13(11):976–986.
27. Wilkie FL, Goodkin K, Van Zuilen M, et al. Cognitive effects of HIV-1 infection. *CNS Spectr.* 2000;5(5):33–51.
28. Stern Y, Marder K, Bell K, et al. Multidisciplinary baseline assessment of homosexual men with and without human immunodeficiency virus infection: III. Neurologic and neuropsychological findings. *Arch Gen Psychiatry.* 1991;48(2):131–138.
29. Portegies P, Enting RH, de Gans J, et al. Presentation and course of AIDS dementia complex: 10 years of follow-up in Amsterdam, the Netherlands. *AIDS.* 1993;7(5):669–676.
30. Miller EN, Satz P, Visscher BC. Computerized and conventional neuropsychological assessment of HIV-1-infected homosexual men. *Neurology.* 1991;41(10):1608.
31. Worth JL, Savage CR, Baer L, et al. Computer-based neuropsychological screening for AIDS dementia complex. *AIDS.* 1993;7(5):677–682.
32. Bhatia NS, Chow FC. Neurologic complications in treated HIV-1 infection. *Curr Neurol Neurosci Rep.* 2016;16(7):1–10.
33. Eggers C, Arendt G, Hahn K, et al. HIV-1 associated neurocognitive disorder: epidemiology, pathogenesis, diagnosis, and treatment. *J Neurol.* 2017;264(8):1715–1727.
34. Gannon P, Khan MZ, Kolson DL. Current understanding of HIV-associated neurocognitive disorders pathogenesis. *Curr Opinion Neurol.* 2011;24(3):275.
35. Goodkin K, Baldewicz T, Wilkie FL, et al. HIV-1 infection of the brain: a region-specific approach to its neuropathophysiology and therapeutic prospects. *Psychiatr Ann.* 2001;31(3):182–192.

36. Goodkin K, Baldewicz TT, Wilkie FL, et al. Cognitive-motor impairment and disorder in HIV-1 infection. *Psychiatr Ann.* 2001;31(1):37–44.

37. Antinori A, Arendt G, Becker J, et al. Updated research nosology for HIV-associated neurocognitive disorders. *Neurology.* 2007;69(18):1789–1799.

38. Heaton R, Clifford D, Franklin D, et al. HIV-associated neurocognitive disorders persist in the era of potent antiretroviral therapy: CHARTER Study. *Neurology.* 2010;75(23):2087–2096.

39. Grant I, Franklin DR, Deutsch R, et al. Asymptomatic HIV-associated neurocognitive impairment increases risk for symptomatic decline. *Neurology.* 2014;82(23):2055–2062.

40. Saylor D, Dickens AM, Sacktor N, et al. HIV-associated neurocognitive disorder—pathogenesis and prospects for treatment. *Nat Rev Neurol.* 2016;12(4):234–248.

41. Lindl KA, Marks DR, Kolson DL, et al. HIV-associated neurocognitive disorder: pathogenesis and therapeutic opportunities. *J Neuroimmune Pharmacol.* 2010;5:294–309.

42. Laskus T, Radkowski M, Adair DM, et al. Emerging evidence of hepatitis C neuroinvasion. *AIDS.* 2005;19(suppl 3):140–144.

43. Caniglia EC, Cain LE, Justice A, et al. Antiretroviral penetration into the CNS and incidence of AIDS-defining neurologic conditions. *Neurology.* 2014;83(2):134–141.

44. Baldewicz TT, Brouwers P, Goodkin K, et al. Nutritional contributions to the CNS pathophysiology of HIV-1 infection and implications for treatment. *CNS Spectr.* 2000;5(4):61–72.

45. Uldall KK, Ryan R, Berghuis JP, et al. Association between delirium and death in AIDS patients. *AIDS Patient Care STDS.* 2000;14(2):95–100.

46. Kellinghaus C, Engbring C, Kovac S, et al. Frequency of seizures and epilepsy in neurological HIV-infected patients. *Seizure.* 2008;17(1):27–33.

47. Nanni MG, Caruso R, Mitchell AJ, et al. Depression in HIV infected patients: a review. *Curr Psychiatry Rep.* 2015;17(1):1–11.

48. Johnson JM, Nachtigall LB, Stern TA. The effect of testosterone levels on mood in men: a review. *Psychosomatics.* 2013;54(6):509–514.

49. Sullivan PS, Dworkin MS. Adult and adolescent spectrum of HIV disease investigators: prevalence and correlates of fatigue among persons with HIV infection. *J Pain Symptom Manage.* 2003;25(4):329–333.

50. O'Dowd MA, Biderman DJ, McKegney FP. Incidence of suicidality in AIDS and HIV-positive patients attending a psychiatry outpatient program. *Psychosomatics.* 1993;34(1):33–40.

51. Gielen AC, McDonnell KA, O'Campo PJ, et al. Suicide risk and mental health indicators: do they differ by abuse and HIV status? *Womens Health Issues.* 2005;15(2):89–95.

52. Grassi L, Mondardini D, Pavanati M, et al. Suicide probability and psychological morbidity secondary to HIV infection: a control study of HIV-seropositive, hepatitis C virus (HCV)-seropositive and HIV/HCV-seronegative injecting drug users. *J Affect Disord.* 2001;64(2):195–202.

53. Lyketsos CG, Schwartz J, Fishman M, et al. AIDS mania. *J Neuropsychiatry Clin Neurosci.* 1996;9(2):277–279.

54. Wright JM, Sachdev PS, Perkins RJ, et al. Zidovudine-related mania. *Med J Aust.* 1989;150(6):339–341.

55. Mijch AM, Judd FK, Lyketsos CG, et al. Secondary mania in patients with HIV infection: are antiretrovirals protective? *J Neuropsychiatry Clin Neurosci.* 1999;11(4):475–480.

56. Lyketsos CG, Treisman GJ. Mood disorders in HIV infection. *Psychiatr Ann.* 2001;31(1):45–49.

57. Susser E, Colson P, Jandorf L, et al. HIV infection among young adults with psychotic disorders. *Am J Psychiatry.* 1997;154(6):864–866.

58. De Ronchi D, Faranca I, Forti P, et al. Development of acute psychotic disorders and HIV-1 infection. *Int J Psychiatry Med.* 2000;30(2):173–183.

59. Sewell DD, Jeste DV, Atkinson JH, et al. HIV-associated psychosis: a study of 20 cases. San Diego HIV Neurobehavioral Research Center Group. *Am J Psychiatry.* 1994;151(2):237–242.

60. Zareifopoulos N, Lagadinou M, Karela A, et al. Efavirenz as a psychotropic drug. *Eur Rev Med Pharmacol Sci.* 2020;24(20):10729–10735.

61. Vosvick M, Gore-Felton C, Ashton E, et al. Sleep disturbances among HIV-positive adults: the role of pain, stress, and social support. *J Psychosomatic Res.* 2004;57(5):459–463.

62. Hartzler B, Dombrowski JC, Crane HM, et al. Prevalence and predictors of substance use disorders among HIV care enrollees in the United States. *AIDS Behav.* 2017;21(4):1138–1148.

63. Antoniou T, Tsen AL. Interactions between recreational drugs and antiretroviral agents. *Ann Pharmacother.* 2002;36:1598–1613.

64. Parker R, Stein DJ, Jelsma J. Pain in people living with HIV/AIDS: a systematic review. *J Int AIDS Soc.* 2014;17:18719.

65. Verma A, Bradley WG. HIV-1-associated neuropathies. *CNS Spectr.* 2000;5(5):66–72.

66. Branson BM, Handsfield HH, Lampe MA, et al. Revised recommendations for HIV testing of adults, adolescents, and pregnant women in health-care settings. *J Nat Med Assoc.* 2008;100(1):131–147.

67. U.S. Preventive Services Task Force. *Human Immunodeficiency Virus (HIV) Detection: Screening*; 2013. Available at: http://www.uspreventiveservicestaskforce.org/page/document/updatesummaryfinal/human-immunodeficiency-virus-hiv-infection-screening. (Accessed 30 June 2016).

68. Hernández D, Feaster DJ, Gooden L, et al. Self-reported HIV and HCV screening rates and serostatus among substance abuse treatment patients. *AIDS Behav.* 2016;20(1):204–214.

69. Skarbinski J, Rosenberg E, Paz-Bailey G, et al. Human immunodeficiency virus transmission at each step of the care continuum in the United States. *JAMA Int Med.* 2015;175(4):588–596.

70. Volk JE, Marcus JL, Phengrasamy T, et al. No new HIV infections with increasing use of HIV preexposure prophylaxis in a clinical practice setting. *Clin Infect Dis.* 2015;61(10):1601–1603.

71. Gomez MF, Klein DA, Sand S, et al. Delivering mental health care to HIV-positive individuals: a comparison of two models. *Psychosomatics.* 1999;40(4):321–324.

72. Kuehn BM. Integrated care needed for patients with HIV, drug abuse, and mental illness. *JAMA.* 2008;300(5):494–495.

73. Singh N, Squier C, Sivek C, et al. Determinants of compliance with antiretroviral therapy in patients with human immunodeficiency

virus: prospective assessment with implications for enhancing compliance. *AIDS Care.* 1996;8(3):261–270.

74. Chesney MA. Factors affecting adherence to antiretroviral therapy. *Clin Infect Dis.* 2000;30(suppl 2):171–176.

75. Godin G, Cote J, Naccache H, et al. Prediction of adherence to antiretroviral therapy: a one-year longitudinal study. *AIDS Care.* 2005;17(4):493–504.

76. Mugavero MJ, Westfall AO, Cole SR, et al. Beyond core indicators of retention in HIV care: missed clinic visits are independently associated with all-cause mortality. *Clin Infect Dis.* 2014;59(10):1471–1479.

77. Kelly JA, Murphy DA, Bahr GR, et al. Outcome of cognitive-behavioral and support group brief therapies for depressed, HIV-infected persons. *Am J Psychiatry.* 1993;150(11):1679–1686.

78. Pollock BG. Newer antidepressants and the cytochrome P450 system. *Am J Psychiatry.* 1996;153(3):311–320.

79. Greenblatt DJ, von Moltke LL, Harmatz JS, et al. Drug interactions with newer antidepressants: role of human cytochromes. *J Clin Psychiatry.* 1998;59(suppl 15):19–27.

80. Richelson E. Pharmacokinetic drug interactions of new antidepressants: a review of the effects on the metabolism of other drugs. *Mayo Clin Proc.* 1997;72(9):835–847.

81. Deeks SG, Smith M, Holodniy M, et al. HIV-1 protease inhibitors: a review for clinicians. *JAMA.* 1997;277(2):145–153.

82. Beach SR, Celano CM, Noseworthy PA, et al. QTc prolongation, torsades de pointes, and psychotropic medications. *Psychosomatics.* 2013;54(1):1–13.

83. Martin L, Tummala R, Fernandez F. Psychiatric management of HIV infection and AIDS. *Psychiatr Ann.* 2002;32(2):133–140.

84. Gillenwater DR, McDaniel JS. Rational psychopharmacology for patients with HIV infection and AIDS. *Psychiatr Ann.* 2001;31(1):28–34.

85. Hill L, Lee KC. Pharmacotherapy considerations in patients with HIV and psychiatric disorders: focus on antidepressants and antipsychotics. *Ann Pharmacol.* 2013;47(1):75–89.

86. Currier MB, Molina G, Kato M. A prospective trial of sustained-release bupropion for depression in HIV-seropositive and AIDS patients. *Psychosomatics.* 2003;44(2):120–125.

87. Ferrara M, Valero IP, Moore DJ, et al. Treatment of psychiatric disorders in HIV. In: Joska JA, Stein DJ, Grant I, eds. *HIV and Psychiatry.* 1st ed. John Wiley & Sons, Ltd; 2014:157–210.

88. Akula SK, Rege AB, Dreisbach AW, et al. Valproic acid increases cerebrospinal fluid zidovudine levels in a patient with AIDS. *Am J Med Sci.* 1997;313(4):244–246.

89. Halman MH, Worth JL, Sanders KM, et al. Anticonvulsant use in the treatment of manic syndromes in patients with HIV-1 infection. *J Neuropsychiatry Clin Neurosci.* 1993;5(4):430–434.

90. Repetto MJ, Evans DL, Cruess DG, et al. Neuropsycho-pharmacologic treatment of depression and other neuro-psychiatric disorders in HIV-infected individuals. *CNS Spectr.* 2003;8(01):59–63.

91. Naccarato M, Hall E, Wai A, et al. A case of a probable drug interaction between lurasidone and atazanavir-based antiretroviral therapy. *Antivir Ther.* 2016;21(8):735–738.

92. Simpson DM, McArthur J, Olney R, et al. Lamotrigine for HIV-associated painful sensory neuropathies: a placebo-controlled trial. *Neurology.* 2003;60(9):1508–1514.

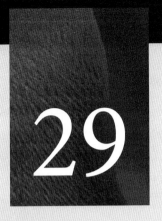

29

COVID-19 INFECTION

SCOTT R. BEACH, MD ▪ AMY L. NEWHOUSE, MD ▪ JULIA M. PROBERT, MD ▪ ANASTASIA B. EVANOFF, MD ▪ MARIE D. BOMM, MD, PHD ▪ FELICIA A. SMITH, MD

OVERVIEW

The coronavirus disease 2019 (COVID-19) pandemic dramatically changed the healthcare landscape starting in late 2019, with over one million deaths worldwide now estimated to have occurred as a result of the virus. While early reports emphasized devastating effects on the respiratory system, it quickly became clear that COVID-19 could affect the brain as well. Indeed, neuropsychiatric manifestations are common in the setting of COVID-19 infection and have been described in the acute, subacute, and chronic phases. This chapter explores both short-term and long-term neuropsychiatric sequelae of COVID-19 and summarizes the current understanding of these phenomena. However, it is important to keep in mind that the literature on neuropsychiatric manifestations of COVID-19 continues to evolve rapidly. Most large studies have been based on early infection waves and early variants, and their findings may not be generalizable to infections with new variants. Unfortunately, as of this writing, there remain little data on the neuropsychiatric sequelae of Omicron subvariants, which have been dominant since late 2021.

ACUTE NEUROPSYCHIATRIC SEQUELAE OF COVID-19 INFECTION

Early reports of the COVID-19 infection highlighted the unusual symptoms of anosmia (loss of smell) and ageusia (loss of taste) that suggested the possibility of neurologic involvement. Studies showed that 88% of people infected with early variants developed one of these two symptoms. With the evolution of newer variants, the rates of these symptoms have decreased significantly, with fewer than 10% to 20% of individuals infected with the Omicron variant reporting a loss of taste or smell. Studies that have examined the cause of anosmia in COVID-19 infection have yielded conflicting results, although more recent studies suggest that the virus attacks support cells leading to changes in olfactory sensory neurons.[1] The prominence of these symptoms in early variants suggests that the virus makes its way close to the brain, if not actually penetrating olfactory neurons or the blood-brain barrier. Other neurologic features described in association with COVID-19 infection include tinnitus, cerebrovascular accidents (CVAs), posterior reversible encephalopathy syndrome, and dysautonomia.[2] Acute hemorrhagic necrotizing encephalitis and acute disseminated encephalomyelitis have also been reported. However, no causal relationship has been established for many of these neurological syndromes. Guillain-Barre syndrome and transverse myelitis were initially thought to be caused by COVID-19 infection but were later determined to be coincidental findings. The same may be true for other of the above-mentioned syndromes.

Large studies of neurologic work-ups in the setting of acute COVID-19 infection have suggested that electroencephalograms (EEGs) are typically abnormal, but in a non-specific manner, most often showing diffuse background slowing.[3] Other common abnormalities identified include burst attenuation, generalized periodic discharges, and generalized rhythmic delta activity. Few reports of seizure activity have been forthcoming. Some research suggests that COVID-19 infection may increase the risk of epilepsy in those with an underlying neurological issue that predates their illness. Studies of cerebrospinal fluid (CSF) in patients with COVID-19 infection are generally normal. When the CSF is abnormal, it most commonly demonstrates oligoclonal bands and/or elevated protein levels, suggesting inflammation and possible encephalitis. Severe acute respiratory syndrome coronavirus 2 (SARS-CoV-2) virus has been isolated from the CSF in a minority of patients—approximately 6% of those tested in one series of patients having neuropsychiatric sequelae. Neuroimaging in those with an acute COVID-19 infection is typically normal, although several abnormal patterns have been described. Abnormal magnetic resonance imaging (MRI) findings include evidence of microvascular disease in various brain regions (e.g., cortical and subcortical structures). A pattern involving signal abnormalities in the mesial temporal lobe has been identified as being like the findings sometimes seen in anti-N-methyl-D-aspartate (NMDA)-receptor antibody encephalitis. A small series of patients undergoing magnetic resonance spectroscopy demonstrated a pattern consistent with delayed post-hypoxic leukoencephalopathy. Finally, most autopsy studies have not detected virus in brain tissue.[4] The most consistent findings at autopsy are acute hypoxic injuries, hemorrhages, and mild-to-moderate non-specific inflammation.[5]

Delirium

The COVID-19 pandemic led to high rates of hospitalizations around the globe. Altered mental status was a typical presentation of COVID-19 infection in emergency departments (EDs) and inpatient settings, with delirium representing the most common syndrome of altered mental status in hospital settings. This section addresses some of the unique features of delirium associated with COVID-19 infection, including its prevalence, etiology, distinct clinical phenomenology, and the relationship between neuropsychiatric symptoms of delirium in acute COVID-19 infection and post-acute sequelae of COVID-19 (PASC) or "long COVID."

Epidemiology and Risk Factors

Early in the pandemic, delirium was thought to be common in COVID-19-infected individuals, with a higher prevalence than in the general hospital population. Rates of delirium have been highest in those who arc critically ill with COVID-19 infection. Khan and colleagues[6] found that the prevalence of delirium was 83% within a cohort of 268 critically ill inpatients with COVID-19 infection, whereas typical prevalence rates of delirium in intensive care units (ICUs) are 25% to 30%. Delirium has been identified by the World Health Organization (WHO) as a core symptom of COVID-19, and one study found that altered mental status was the sixth most common presenting sign of COVID-19 infection, with 37% of patients lacking other core signs of infection.[7] Multiple variables appear to be related to the increased incidence of delirium in COVID-19 infection. Some of these (such as advanced age, illness severity, and a pre-existing neurocognitive disorder) are related to one's pre-morbid baseline. Others (such as mechanical ventilation and administration of certain medications, like benzodiazepines and opioids) are related to hospital care. While many of these risk factors are related to the development of delirium in the general population, there is some evidence to support unique risk factors in those who are infected with COVID-19. For example, one study found that social isolation may be a unique risk factor for delirium in the setting of COVID-19.[8] This finding highlights the inter-related and complex explanations for a relatively higher incidence of delirium in patients with COVID-19 infection.

As the COVID-19 virus has evolved through different variants, delirium has remained a common complication. Anecdotal reports have suggested that COVID-19 delirium is less prevalent with more recent waves of infection, such as those due to the Omicron variant. This may be attributable to several factors, including the vaccine's ability to reduce the prevalence of severe disease, widespread accessibility to testing allowing earlier disease detection, and treatment with oral antiviral agents and monoclonal antibody therapies.

Pathophysiology

The reason for the high prevalence of delirium in COVID-19 remains uncertain, but theories have included dysfunction due to systemic inflammation, direct viral entry into neural tissue, gross cerebral and systemic metabolic dysfunction, vascular events, and iatrogenic factors.[8] Direct viral invasion by SARS-CoV-2 has now been largely disproven. Infection with

COVID-19, especially with severe symptoms, is typically associated with signs of systemic inflammation (including fever, distributive shock, leukocytosis or leukopenia, and an elevation in inflammatory markers, including C-reactive protein [CRP]). This systemic inflammation leads to the breakdown of the blood-brain barrier, which allows cytokines, such as interleukin-6 to cross the blood-brain barrier.

Cerebral metabolic dysfunction is also prevalent with COVID-19 infection, either related to hypoxia and hypoperfusion or to multi-organ failure that affects the liver or kidneys and the accumulation of metabolically toxic substances. An elevated risk of stroke in COVID-19 infection has been widely observed, which likely contributes to an increased risk of delirium. Iatrogenic factors have also been considered relevant in those with COVID-19 infection. Non-pharmacologic prevention strategies for delirium often rely on the presence of staff and family members at the bedside; due to the restrictive visitor and infection control policies associated with the pandemic, these may not be possible. The use of personal protective equipment may further minimize the ability to communicate, thereby worsening patient isolation.[9] Other iatrogenic factors include the widespread administration of corticosteroids and other neuroactive medications (including antibiotics, such as cefepime [a posited γ-aminobutyric acid-A (GABA-A) antagonist]) in those with symptomatic COVID-19 infections. During the initial waves of the pandemic, midazolam and fentanyl were more commonly used due to concerns about the supply lines of newer sedative agents, which may have contributed to the observed higher rates of delirium.

Clinical Presentation

In addition to the multiple etiologies for delirium associated with COVID-19 infection, delirium may be heralded by unique clinical phenomena. Given the high incidence of delirium in COVID-19 infection much research has sought to identify specific clinical phenotypic findings in those with delirium. The core features of delirium—an acute onset of disturbed consciousness with a waxing and waning course along with specific disturbances in attention—remain essential to make the diagnosis. However, delirium is a heterogeneous syndrome with significant variability in its features (e.g., hypoactive, hyperactive, mixed subtypes),

the presence of perceptual disturbances, and linguistic dysfunction.

One area of heterogeneity relates to the motoric subtype of delirium. Khan and co-workers[6] found that 80% of critically ill patients with delirium and COVID-19 infection had a predominately hypoactive subtype of delirium. In contrast, a second study, by Velasquez-Tirado and associates,[10] found that 80% of COVID-19-infected patients had a hyperactive or mixed motoric subtype. This disparity across multiple studies may result from methodologic and institutional variance, e.g., how often patients are brought to the attention of psychiatry. Given this clinical heterogeneity and variability in the involvement of psychiatry, the universal use of a validated tool for the detection of delirium (such as the Confusion Assessment Method or Delirium Diagnostic Tool-Provisional) by clinical staff would be useful going forward.

The predominance of neuropsychiatric symptoms in those with COVID-19 infection has been widely appreciated. An early case series by Helms and colleagues[3] highlighted specific neurologic findings (including diffuse corticospinal tract signs [such as enhanced tendon reflexes, ankle clonus, and bilateral extensor plantar reflexes]) in two-thirds of critically ill patients with COVID-19 infection.[3] This study also identified a dysexecutive syndrome characterized by inattention and difficulty following commands. A study by Beckwith and co-workers[11] of 109 patients with delirium during the first wave of the pandemic examined the neuropsychiatric features of delirium in patients with and without COVID-19 infection. The authors found that several physical examination findings (including myoclonus [28% vs. 4%; $P = .002$], hypertonia [36% vs. 10%; $P = .003$], withdrawal [36% vs. 15%; $P = .011$], akinesia [19% vs. 6%; $P = .034$], abulia [19% vs. 3%; $P = .004$], and alogia [25% vs. 8%; $P = .012$]), were significantly more common in the COVID-19-infected group. These unique features are summarized in Table 29.1. No significant differences were noted in the occurrence of tremors, restlessness, paranoia, delusions, agitation, or perceptual disturbances. The presence of neuropsychiatric symptoms in the setting of delirium and COVID-19 infection appears to be distinct and potentially mediated by the etiologic neurobiological mechanisms outlined above.

Approach to the Delirious Patient With COVID-19

Regarding the management of COVID-19 delirium, unique features, and co-morbidities should be considered when planning a treatment approach. Several groups have published algorithms for the medical management of delirium.[12,13] Table 29.2 lists some of the agents that have been used to manage COVID-19 delirium as well as their potential risks and benefits. Given the high number of medications used by most inpatients with COVID-19 infection, medication consolidation is often

recommended. Agents with the potential to worsen delirium should be minimized, and environmental interventions, including early mobilization, should be prioritized, whenever possible. Medications should be considered for patients who are hyperactive, as such behavior can lead to an elevated risk of harming oneself or others, or for those experiencing distressing perceptual disturbances, such as hallucinations, which may increase their risk for post-delirium post-traumatic stress disorder (PTSD) or post-ICU syndrome. Finally, delirious patients may benefit from the use of melatonin to help restore the sleep-wake cycle. In COVID-19, melatonin may have the additional benefit of helping to suppress an overactive immune response. Melatonin should be used with caution in those who are immunocompromised or in those who appear to be unable to mount an appropriate immune response, given its immune-suppressing properties.

Whereas antipsychotic agents would often be considered first-line medications for the management of agitated delirium, some groups have recommended the use of alpha-2 agonists, such as clonidine, for

---

TABLE 29.1

Atypical Neuropsychiatric Features of Delirium in COVID-19 Infection

Myoclonus
Hypertonia
Withdrawal
Akinesia
Abulia
Alogia

TABLE 29.2

Agents for the Symptomatic Management of Delirium in COVID-19

Agent	Available Routes	Potential Benefits in COVID-19	Potential Drawbacks in COVID-19
Melatonin	PO: tablet, SL, gtt	May help to suppress an overactive immune response	Could inhibit appropriate immune response in immunocompromised patients
Alpha-2 Agonists			
Dexmedetomidine	IV	Evidence of benefit in COVID-19 hyperactive delirium in ICU setting	
Clonidine	PO, transdermal patch		
Antipsychotics			Risk of QTc prolongation in COVID-19 polypharmacy
Haloperidol	PO, IV, IM	IV formulation less likely to exert a hemodynamic effect and has a lower risk of EPS	Higher potency may increase the risk of EPS with COVID-19-related neuropsychiatric symptoms
Olanzapine	PO, ODT, IV, IM	Lower relative risk of EPS	
Chlorpromazine	PO, IV, IM	Lower relative risk of EPS	
Quetiapine	PO	Lower relative risk of EPS	
Other Agents			
Valproic Acid	PO, IV	Especially effective in the post-stroke population	Risk of thrombocytopenia compounded during sepsis; risk of drug-induced liver injury in COVID-19 polypharmacy (e.g., remdesivir)
Trazodone	PO	Especially effective and safe in elderly populations	Can cause QTc prolongation

EPS, Extrapyramidal symptoms; *gtt*, drop; *IM*, intramuscular; *IV*, intravenous; *ODT*, oral disintegrating tablet; *PO*, by mouth; *SL*, sublingual.

COVID-19 delirium. This is based partly on evidence suggesting a benefit from dexmedetomidine in COVID-19 delirium in the ICU setting, including decreased rates of delirium seen in patients who have been sedated with dexmedetomidine.[14] For agitated patients who are refractory to alpha-2 agonists, or for those experiencing perceptual disturbances, antipsychotics have been used safely in the setting of COVID-19 delirium. Considerations should include the potential for increased sensitivity to extrapyramidal symptoms (EPS) given some of the neuropsychiatric features described above, as well as the potential for QTc prolongation given the use of concomitant medications, such as azithromycin. Olanzapine, haloperidol, and chlorpromazine have been used safely and effectively in the setting of COVID-19 infection. Each of these agents has the advantage of being available in a parenteral form, for patients who cannot take orally administered medications easily. Valproic acid and trazodone have also been used effectively to manage agitation and may avoid some of these side effects. Moreover, trazodone has also been shown to safely manage anxiety and agitation due to delirium in the elderly, a population who are especially vulnerable to both delirium and severe infection with COVID-19.

Sequelae of Delirium in COVID-19

Finally, the relationship between delirium in the setting of an acute COVID-19 infection and the subsequent development of PASC remains unclear. Many PASC symptoms are neuropsychiatric; they include fatigue, difficulty concentrating, depression, and anxiety. It has been well-established that delirium is associated with relatively impaired post-discharge cognition, particularly in those with pre-existing neurocognitive or psychiatric morbidity. One study determined the estimated incidence of a neurological or psychiatric diagnosis in the 6 months following a COVID-19 diagnosis was 34%.[15] Given the high prevalence of delirium in those with a COVID-19 infection and the likelihood of severe infection associated with increasing age, some post-COVID-infection symptoms may be attributable to the long-lasting effects of delirium. This is especially true for those with a more vulnerable neurologic substrate, and pre-existing cognitive or psychiatric diseases.[16]

Case 1

Mr. C, a 75-year-old male with Alzheimer disease who was living in a nursing home, presented to the ED with 24 hours of an altered mental status marked by increasing aggression toward staff and his appearing to engage with people who were not present. In the ED, vital signs, initial bloodwork, and urine samples were all within normal limits. His presentation with an altered mental status prompted testing for COVID-19 infection; he tested positive. Given the clinical suspicion of delirium in the setting of a new COVID-19 infection, he was admitted to the medical service.

Psychiatry was consulted to assist with the management of his agitation. The mental status examination revealed irritability, inattention, disorientation, poor tolerance of cognitive testing, and reports of recent visual hallucinations. The psychiatrist recommended melatonin at bedtime (to help with the regulation of his sleep-wake cycle) and olanzapine (2.5 mg) at night (given his ongoing and bothersome perceptual disturbances). Mr. C also received intramuscular (IM) haloperidol (5 mg at night) because he attempted to get out of bed. After the administration of haloperidol, he slept well, but the following day he was minimally interactive with staff. He did not speak spontaneously, which represented a change from his baseline, and the motor exam by the psychiatric consultant revealed increased tone in his upper extremities, with cogwheeling. Concern was raised for catatonia, but a lorazepam challenge resulted in sedation with minimal change in his symptoms on awakening. Over the next 2 days, Mr. C remained withdrawn and minimally interactive. Given his concern for hypoactive delirium with features of akinetic mutism, his medications were minimized. On the fourth hospital day, Mr. C began to show gradual improvement, and after 3 more days, he returned to his baseline.

Psychosis

New-onset psychosis has been described in the setting of COVID-19 infection. Although less common than delirium, non-delirious psychoses can occur.[17] Patients who experience psychosis are out of touch with reality (e.g., with delusions and/or hallucinations, and often manifest disorganized thinking). Psychotic symptoms may impair an individual's judgment and interfere with their ability to work, maintain relationships, and meet their basic needs, increasing their risk to themselves or others. Psychosis may be due to a primary psychiatric disorder, substance use, or a general medical condition, including COVID-19. COVID-19 can trigger new-onset psychosis in those without a psychiatric history, and it has been linked with a higher rate of psychosis than with influenza or other respiratory tract infections.[15,18,19]

Of note, much of the literature surrounding psychosis with COVID-19 infection is based on case reports and case series, which are notoriously difficult to interpret given that they carry a significant risk of sampling bias. Case reports are also limited in their ability to infer causality. Using available evidence, this section explores the epidemiology and risk factors of COVID-19 psychosis, the clinical presentation and course of symptoms, the pathophysiology, the differential diagnosis, and the management and treatment options.

Epidemiology and Risk Factors

A large retrospective study found that the incidence of psychosis in the 6 months following COVID-19 infection was 1.4%.[15] This rate is twofold higher for patients hospitalized with COVID-19 infection (2.9%) and is significantly higher than the rate for patients diagnosed with other respiratory tract infections (hazard ratio 1.27, $P < .0001$).[15,17] This increased rate of psychosis persisted throughout the 2-year study period, whereas an elevated risk of mood and anxiety disorders was more transient.[17] This suggests that the mechanism behind the development of psychosis may persist long after the resolution of the acute infection. It should be kept in mind that these studies relied on claims data, which runs an inherent risk of ascertainment bias—that is, physicians treating patients who were diagnosed with COVID-19 and especially patients who were hospitalized for COVID-19 infection may be more likely to look for and report outcomes in the aftermath of a COVID-19 infection.

Many patients with new-onset psychosis have no psychiatric history. A review of 57 cases of COVID-19 psychosis found that two-thirds of patients had no prior psychiatric diagnoses, with only 2.5% (two patients) of those with a prior psychiatric illness reporting a history of a psychotic disorder.[19] Only two patients had a known family history of psychiatric illness, although many of the studies (61.4%, 35 patients) did not comment on a family history.[19] The mean age of patients with new-onset COVID-19 psychosis is 40 to 44 years old, with females having a slightly younger age of onset than males (40.3 years vs. 43.4 years, respectively).[18,19] This average age is older than one would expect for new-onset psychosis, and there does not seem to be a bi-modal peak, suggesting that middle age is in fact the time of greatest risk.

Risk factors for the development of psychosis in COVID-19 include certain medications, and some treatments for the medical sequelae of COVID-19 infection that may provoke psychosis. COVID-19 treatment can involve the use of high-dose steroids to modulate the inflammatory response, which can trigger manic and psychotic symptoms. In addition, antibiotics (including azithromycin, doxycycline, amoxicillin, and levofloxacin, as well as the antimalarial hydroxychloroquine, none of which are effective treatments for COVID-19 but were commonly prescribed during the first wave of the pandemic) have been shown to increase the odds of developing psychosis.[20]

Interestingly, some evidence suggests that patients with serious mental illness who adhere to antipsychotics were less likely to contract COVID-19, and they had better outcomes following infection than did those in the general population, with data suggesting that antipsychotics themselves have immunomodulatory properties that have been protective during the COVID-19 pandemic.[21] However, these data are limited.

Clinical Features

Patients with COVID-19-associated psychosis have varied presentations with the onset of psychiatric symptoms, the range of medical symptoms, and the time course of symptoms. Overall, it is difficult to characterize a typical course for COVID-19 psychosis, although some generalizations have been offered. The most common presenting symptoms of new-onset psychosis associated with COVID-19 infection have been delusions (92%–93%), followed by hallucinations (69%–73%).[18,19] Auditory hallucinations were more common than visual hallucinations. Many patients also exhibited disorganized behaviors and disorganized speech, as well as signs of catatonia.[18]

COVID-19-associated psychosis may also present with mania. A review of 23 patients with new-onset mania and concurrent COVID-19 infection had a significant burden of psychotic symptoms, with 83%[19] presenting with delusions (most frequently grandiose and religious), and 40%[9] with hallucinations (auditory, or auditory plus visual).[22] Only 4 of the 23 patients had a previous psychiatric disorder; none had a history of psychosis. However, 70% of them had risk factors for the development of bipolar disorder, including their own psychiatric history, a family history of bipolar disorder, or a pharmacologic trigger (including cannabis), suggesting that these triggers may have played a role in the development of psychiatric symptoms with COVID-19.

For some patients, psychosis can be the sole symptom of a COVID-19 infection, although, for most, it is associated with medical symptoms.[23] Medical symptoms range from mild to moderate (e.g., fever, cough, malaise, headaches, loss of taste and smell, myalgia, shortness of breath, diarrhea), to severe hypoxic respiratory failure, with most patients experiencing an uncomplicated medical course. Psychotic symptoms can appear at the onset of medical symptoms, or weeks after medical symptoms have resolved.[23]

Pathophysiology

It remains unclear whether psychosis is caused by COVID-19 infection or whether it is merely associated with infection. COVID-19 infection could impact the development of psychotic disorders both through an inflammatory response, molecular mimicry, or from secondary effects of medication treatment and psychosocial stress that accompany a pandemic. A well-documented history has linked pandemics to the development of psychosis, including during the Russian, Spanish, and Asian influenza outbreaks.[23]

Multiple hypotheses exist for the mechanism of COVID-19-induced psychosis, including neuroinflammation, hypercoagulability defects, and autoimmune pathways. Neuroinflammation and cytokine storm during COVID-19 infection may also play a role in the development of psychotic disorders,

triggering a chain of events that cause an imbalance in excitatory and inhibitory circuits.[22,23] Some evidence suggests that hypercoagulability and defects in coagulation pathways are possible biomarkers of psychosis, suggesting another possible link to COVID-19. Finally, the SARS-CoV-2 virus may cause cross-reactivity with self-antigens, and an autoimmune pathway may be responsible for the development of psychosis. Indeed, at least one case has been reported involving a novel autoantibody isolated in the setting of a COVID-induced psychosis, and a second case responded completely to steroid therapy, suggesting a possible underlying encephalitis.[24,25] Furthermore, cases of anti-NMDA-receptor antibody encephalitis in the weeks following COVID-19 infection have also been reported and are thought to result from molecular mimicry.

Differential Diagnosis

When evaluating a patient with COVID-19 psychosis, providers must consider a wide differential diagnosis, especially because many patients have not had a psychiatric history or risk factors for a psychotic disorder. The differential diagnosis for COVID-induced psychosis is provided in Table 29.3.

Given the frequency of delirium in COVID-19 infection, a top priority is to distinguish delirium from new-onset psychosis. In many case reports, newly diagnosed psychosis was more common in the elderly, in patients hospitalized with COVID-19 symptoms, and in those with encephalopathy, raising the concern that delirium may be under-reported, and that misdiagnosis of psychosis may occur in many clinical situations.[17] One review found that a sizable number of patients with new-onset psychosis (15.8%, 9 out of 57 patients) were found to have an "altered mental status," raising the concern that these patients were experiencing delirium and not psychosis.[19] Many of the case reports published on COVID-19-associated psychosis did not list delirium in the differential diagnosis, even when symptoms commonly associated with delirium, such as visual hallucinations, were present.[18] Therefore delirium must be thoroughly investigated and ruled out in patients with COVID-19 psychosis.

Along with delirium, other medical and neurologic causes of psychosis in patients with COVID-19

TABLE 29.3

Differential Diagnosis for Symptoms of Psychosis in Patients With COVID-19

Primary psychotic disorder	– Schizophrenia – Schizoaffective disorder – Delusional disorder – Brief psychotic disorder	Consider patients with a history of psychosis or with a family history of a psychotic disorder
Primary mood disorder	– Bipolar I disorder – Depression with psychotic features	Consider patients with a history of depression or mania or with a family history of a mood disorder
Other psychiatric disorders	– Complex PTSD – Personality disorders – Peri-partum psychosis	Consider patients with a history of trauma. Consider patients with current or recent pregnancies.
Substance/medication-induced psychotic disorder	– Recreational substance–induced psychosis – Medication/drug-induced psychosis	Consider patients who use recreational substances or patients who received steroids, antidepressants, or antimicrobial drug treatment
Delirium	– Delirium	Consider all patients with COVID-19 psychosis. Consider if the patient is having attentional deficits and visual hallucinations
Psychotic symptoms in neurocognitive disorders	– Alzheimer disease – Lewy body dementia – Parkinson disease	Consider patients with a history of memory loss, visual hallucinations, and motor symptoms. These patients are also highly susceptible to delirium
Psychotic disorder secondary to general medical condition	– COVID-19 psychosis – Autoimmune encephalitis – Cerebrovascular accident – Brain mass – HSV encephalitis	Consider patients with focal neurologic deficits. Consider those with an older age of onset and no personal or family history of psychiatric illness

HSV, Herpes simplex virus; *PTSD,* post-traumatic stress disorder.

should be considered. Providers must assess whether the medical and psychosocial stress of COVID-19 may have triggered a first episode of a primary psychotic or mood disorder or exacerbated an underlying trauma or personality disorder. Finally, substance-induced psychosis, both from recreational substances as well as from prescribed drugs, must be considered.

Given the significant risk of unrecognized delirium, a thorough medical and neurologic work-up should be performed in patients with COVID-19 psychosis. Medical studies should be ordered early, including neuroimaging and a lumbar puncture if neurologic deficits raise suspicion for autoimmune encephalitis or another neuro-medical condition.[22] If psychotic symptoms are thought to be secondary to delirium or another medical/neurologic cause, the underlying condition should be treated before a diagnosis of a primary psychotic illness is made. A thorough review of medications must be performed carefully in patients

with COVID-19 psychosis (including steroids, antidepressants, and antibiotics), all of which can worsen psychotic symptoms.

Management and Treatment

Once other conditions have been ruled out, the "gold-standard" treatment for COVID-19 psychosis is the administration of antipsychotics. Reviews of patients treated for COVID-19 psychosis show that almost all patients (96%) received antipsychotics, and more than half (60%) received benzodiazepines.[18] A wide array of antipsychotics (including haloperidol, quetiapine, olanzapine, ziprasidone, aripiprazole, clozapine, and risperidone) were used. A recent review of case reports of patients with COVID-19 psychosis found that more than half (53%) of patients improved on very low or low doses of antipsychotics, and two-thirds (67%) had significant improvement of symptoms within 5 days of treatment or hospitalization.[26] Some patients also received mood stabilizers, antidepressants, and electroconvulsive therapy (ECT). Almost three-fourths (72%) of patients improved or had their psychotic symptoms resolved completely with antipsychotic administration, while the remainder had residual depression, anxiety, or psychosis with limited information on their follow-up.[19] However, the timeline for resolution of psychotic symptoms is variable (between 2 and 90 days).

Much remains unknown about the prognosis and long-term psychiatric effects of COVID-19 psychosis. Given that an elevated risk of psychotic symptoms persists for more than 2 years after COVID-19 infection[17] psychiatric monitoring should be considered for patients with risk factors for developing psychosis even after symptom resolution.

Psychosocial Considerations

In addition to the sequelae of infection, the COVID-19 pandemic caused increased psychosocial stress for those vulnerable to, or already diagnosed with a psychotic illness. The pandemic caused fear and anxiety and minimized social interactions, including those with medical providers. Decreased social connectedness may have a more substantial effect on those with psychotic disorders than on those in the general population, and social distancing made it more difficult to obtain laboratory testing and attend in-person visits, causing interruptions in pharmacologic therapy. These factors may contribute to an increased risk of worsening psychotic symptoms in vulnerable populations.

It is also important to note that pre-morbid schizophrenia has been associated with a higher mortality rate from COVID-19 infection, with older age and smoking significantly influencing the mortality rate in these patients (Relative risk [RR] 2.22; 95% confidence interval: 1.54–3.20).[27] This is thought to be due to lower vaccination rates, higher rates of medical co-morbidities, limited access to health care, less adherence to treatment, and immune dysregulation found in this population.[27]

Summary

COVID-19 psychosis has been described in many patients after infection, and it can present with delusions, hallucinations, and disorganized thinking. However, the mechanisms remain unknown. Medications used to treat COVID-19 and the

psychosocial stressors that accompanied the pandemic likely contributed to cases of psychosis. Strikingly, COVID-19 psychosis was diagnosed in many patients older than 40 years and without a psychiatric history, many of whom also had no risk factors for psychosis. This suggests that the differential diagnosis of COVID-19 psychosis must be expanded from the virus triggering a first episode of a primary psychiatric disorder, such as bipolar disorder or schizophrenia, to include delirium and other secondary effects of medical or neurologic illness. While many patients with COVID-19 treated with antipsychotics had remission of their symptoms, the risk of psychosis following COVID-19 infection remains elevated 2 years after the diagnosis of the viral infection. More evidence is needed on the impact of COVID-19 on psychosis, including the prognosis and long-term consequences of the illness.

Case 2

Ms. B, a previously healthy 41-year-old female with no psychiatric history, and a medical history notable for hypertension and obesity, presented to the ED with a 3-day history of delusions that her wife had been poisoning her morning coffee. She also described having auditory hallucinations (of God speaking to her about her purpose on Earth to "save all the children."). Her wife reported that she had been having disorganized behaviors at home, which included rearranging all of the furniture in a bizarre manner and shredding many of their important financial documents. She has never seen her like this before. Ms. B had no family history of psychiatric illness, although she has used recreational cannabis several times per week. On physical examination, Ms. B was found to have a mild cough, and her wife reported that she had a fever and malaise 10 days prior, though it was mild and resolved without treatment. A COVID-19 PCR test was performed; Ms. B was positive for COVID-19. Basic bloodwork was normal, urine toxicology was negative for substances other than cannabis, and her brain MRI was unremarkable. An EEG did not demonstrate slowing. The patient was diagnosed with a brief psychotic disorder and treated with olanzapine. After 3 days, she improved dramatically. She was discharged to her home with psychiatric follow-up.

Catatonia

Since the beginning of the COVID-19 pandemic, case reports have emerged describing patients who have developed catatonia during the acute phase of the infection.[28,29] Many of these patients have also suffered from underlying psychosis.

Epidemiology and Risk Factors

The occurrence of catatonia in the setting of COVID-19 is being explored using larger databases. One study, utilizing the National Inpatient Sample, identified 610 cases of catatonia that occurred in close temporal proximity to COVID-19 infection in 2020.[30] This represents 3.7% of all catatonia cases identified that year, and 0.04% of discharges involving a COVID-19 diagnosis. Not surprisingly, the median length of stay was longer for those with catatonia in the setting of COVID-19 than it was for catatonia that occurred without COVID-19 (11 days vs. 10 days), and hospital charges were higher. When adjusting for other variables for COVID-19, but not for catatonia or the interaction between catatonia and COVID-19, there was an increased mortality rate. Among those with COVID-19-associated catatonia, diagnoses of acute brain dysfunction were common; roughly 20% of them also had a diagnosis of metabolic encephalopathy, 13.1% had an unspecified encephalopathy, 12.3% had delirium, and 11.5% had a toxic encephalopathy. This overlap between catatonia and delirium reflects the frequent co-morbidity of these syndromes despite their remaining mutually exclusive in the *Diagnostic and Statistical Manual of Mental Disorders, Fifth Edition, Revised* (DSM-5-TR).

Clinical Presentation

Typically, patients who present with catatonia in the setting of a COVID-19 infection, are described as having features consistent with stuporous catatonia (including immobility, mutism, rigidity, waxy flexibility, and withdrawal). Some cases manifest stereotypies, mannerisms, echo-phenomena, and automatic obedience. Many of the cases are responsive to lorazepam, which is often considered diagnostic of catatonia. More recently, several reviews have summarized and characterized the case report literature. A 2022 scoping review identified 42 patients cited in 27 articles with catatonia in the setting of COVID-19.[31] Among patients for whom demographic information was available, ages ranged from 12 to over 70 years, with 17 (40.4%) over the age of 50, and 9 (21.4%) over the age of 60. Males and females were represented equally. A substantial proportion had pre-morbid psychiatric illness, including many with a schizophrenia-spectrum illness. Ten (23.8%) had no known pre-morbid psychiatric illness. Lorazepam resolved catatonia in 18 of 22 patients in whom it was tried, and ECT was successful in the four remaining patients. Taken together, these findings suggest that catatonia occurs in the setting of COVID-19, although it is not yet possible to definitively say that COVID-19, itself, causes catatonia, given the numerous confounders inherent in case report literature.

Pathophysiology

The literature on COVID-19 and catatonia does not allow us to draw conclusions about causation. Many reasons can help to explain why catatonia might develop in the setting of COVID-19 infection. Catatonia sometimes occurs in response to severe psychological stress. In this context, one could imagine that the stress of the pandemic as well as the stress of isolation during an acute COVID-19 infection predisposes to the development of catatonia. Many patients with catatonia cited in the literature had a pre-morbid psychiatric illness, suggesting that catatonia may have occurred in the context of an exacerbation of an underlying illness, including depression, schizophrenia, or substance use. Access to medications may also be limited in the setting of COVID-19 infection. Patients experiencing an abrupt cessation of dopamine agonists or benzodiazepines are at increased risk for catatonia. Conversely, COVID-19 infection has been linked to increased blood levels of certain psychiatric medications, including clozapine, which could increase the risk of catatonia for those who take this medication.[32] Medications used to treat COVID-19 infection and its sequelae (including azithromycin, favipiravir, and steroids) have also been linked to adverse neuropsychiatric effects and may predispose some individuals to catatonia. Finally, COVID-19 infection may cause catatonia. Possible mechanisms would be like those described for delirium and psychosis. With regard to catatonia, an intriguing hypothesis is the idea of molecular mimicry. Some evidence has temporally linked cases of COVID-19 infection to NMDAR antibody encephalitis.[25] It has been observed that structural similarities exist between certain proteins on the

NMDA receptor and the SARS-CoV-2 molecule, which might lead to immune-mediated cross-reactivity to the NMDAR. Indeed, catatonia is a common symptom of NMDA-receptor antibody encephalitis, and some cases described may represent this phenomenon.

Akinetic Mutism

Akinetic mutism is a syndrome in which patients are awake but mute and have a profound motivational deficit. It has been thought to exist at the end of the abulic spectrum as a deficit of movement and motivation. C. Miller Fisher suggested that akinetic mutism may represent a pure "motor catatonia."[33] Indeed, akinetic mutism shares many of the motoric components of catatonia, including immobility, mutism, and withdrawal. On the other hand, akinetic mutism typically lacks behavioral features (such as echo-phenomena, stereotypies, and mannerisms), as well as the intense fear that is commonly seen in those with catatonia. Classically, akinetic mutism has been associated with brain injuries, but it has also been described in toxic/metabolic insults. It can manifest as a subtype of delayed post-hypoxic leukoencephalopathy and it may be the most common presentation of this illness. A vulnerability to akinetic mutism is thought to occur in states of dopamine depletion.

A study of patients with COVID-19 infection suggested that as many as 13% of patients may display features consistent with akinetic mutism, most commonly following extubation.[34] Most cases appear to be time limited, lasting 1 to 2 weeks on average, with a good recovery. Notably, medications that are sometimes used to treat akinetic mutism, such as amantadine, often do not appear to meaningfully alter the course of patients with COVID-19-induced akinetic mutism. Patients who appear to be most vulnerable to developing akinetic mutism in the setting of COVID-19 include those with severe respiratory illness requiring ventilation, those with meningoencephalitis, and those with pre-existing neuropsychiatric vulnerability.[35] Finally, as described above, patients with delirium in the setting of COVID-19 often exhibit atypical features that overlap significantly with akinetic mutism, including immobility, alogia, abulia, rigidity, and withdrawal.[11] This suggests an over-representation of signs of akinetic mutism in the setting of COVID-19 delirium, which may have important management implications.

Hypotheses regarding the association between COVID-19 infection and akinetic mutism include hypoxic-ischemic injury, coagulopathy, and metabolic disturbances. Several authors have suggested that COVID-19 infection may predispose patients to develop akinetic mutism because of the downstream effects of the inflammatory response. States of high systemic inflammation may disrupt dopamine synthesis and function, leading to impairment of dopaminergic meso-cortico-limbic pathways required for motivation and movement.

Work-up for Acute Neuropsychiatric Symptoms

For patients who present with neuropsychiatric symptoms in the setting of an acute COVID-19 infection, psychiatrists should be thoughtful about the appropriate work-up. Given that delirium is the sixth most common presentation of COVID-19 infection and is recognized by the WHO as a core symptom, testing for COVID-19 should be pursued in any patient who presents with a newly altered mental status. Thirty-seven percent of patients who present with delirium in the setting of a COVID-19 infection have no other symptoms of infection. For patients who present with delirium, basic bloodwork, including a CRP, should be obtained. EEG and CSF studies have low yields in the setting of delirium. In older patients, neuroimaging is recommended to rule out a CVA, a subdural hemorrhage, and an underlying neurodegenerative disease that may be unmasked by COVID-19 infection. Other testing should be guided by the occurrence of associated symptoms.

For patients who present with new-onset psychosis or mania, a full work-up for first-episode psychosis should be undertaken. Given the hypotheses about molecular mimicry with COVID-19 infection, special consideration should be given to ordering an autoimmune panel, including NMDA-receptor antibodies. For those who present with features of catatonia or akinetic mutism, it is reasonable to pursue standard tests for catatonia, including iron studies. A lorazepam challenge using intravenous (IV) lorazepam (typically 2 mg) should be undertaken unless there is significant concern for respiratory suppression. If improvement occurs in the setting of IV lorazepam, consideration should be given to the use of standing lorazepam. ECT should also be considered early in the course of catatonia. COVID-19 infection may pose specific complications with ECT, and involvement of anesthesiology is essential. If the lorazepam challenge is unsuccessful and the presentation appears consistent with akinetic mutism, it is reasonable to add amantadine, although caution is warranted as amantadine can lower the seizure threshold.

SUBACUTE TO LONG-TERM SEQUELAE OF COVID-19 INFECTION

Many people have symptoms that persist beyond the acute COVID-19 infection. If symptoms persist beyond 4 weeks, they can be considered a post-COVID-19 condition. These can be further categorized into short term (1 month), intermediate term (2–5 months), and long term (6 months or more).[36] Many terms have been used to describe this condition, including long COVID, long-haul COVID, post-acute COVID-19, post-acute sequelae of SARS-CoV-2 (PASC), and chronic COVID-19.

Epidemiology and Risk Factors

PASC can occur after a mild or severe initial infection, and it has been reported at rates up to 69%, although rates of 5% to 10% may be more accurate.[36] Risk appears to increase with each subsequent COVID-19 infection, and some evidence suggests that rates are lower among vaccinated individuals.[37] Antivirals, such as nirmatrelvir/ritonavir, have also led to decreased rates in some studies. It is not yet known whether Omicron variants are associated with a lower risk of PASC as compared to earlier variants, although some evidence suggests that this might be the case.[37] Female gender, older age, pre-existing asthma and diabetes, autoimmune conditions, more severe COVID-19 symptoms, smoking, a higher body-mass index, and several initial symptoms have all been identified as risk factors for the development of a post-COVID-19 condition.[38]

Clinical Features

PASC is a heterogeneous condition that can include a myriad of symptoms across several organ systems. The most commonly reported neuropsychiatric symptoms are fatigue, post-exertional malaise, and brain fog. Common peripheral symptoms include lingering shortness of breath, cough, palpitations, gastrointestinal symptoms and autonomic dysfunction. Depression and anxiety are often included as PASC symptoms, and patients with these symptoms commonly represent to long-COVID clinics, though they tend to be more subacute in onset, peaking within the first 1 to 2 months after infection.

Depression and Anxiety

During the first year of the pandemic, rates of major depressive disorder and anxiety disorders were observed to increase globally by 27.6% and 25.6%, respectively.[39] This correlated with a rise in infections and a decrease in functional mobility. While there may have been an element of acute reaction to the early phase of the pandemic, a higher frequency of depression and anxiety continued to be reported in the mid- to long-term follow-up even after several years.[40] In at least one meta-analysis rates of depression and anxiety increased the farther out people were from their initial infection; in other words, rates were higher in the long-term group compared to the mid-term, which raises the question of whether some of these symptoms may develop post-infection, rather than persist.[40] However, some evidence suggests that rates of anxiety and depression return to baseline 60 days after infection.[17] The severity of the initial infection has not correlated with post-COVID-19 depression and anxiety.[41]

PTSD, while technically falling under the umbrella of anxiety disorders, warrants special mention given its high prevalence rates in prior coronavirus outbreaks (such as SARS and Middle East respiratory syndrome) and similar findings in post-COVID-19 conditions. Studies have demonstrated rates of 14% to 48% in those assessed after hospitalization,[41] and the trajectory of symptoms has been mixed.[41] One study found that those with PTSD were more likely to experience persistent physical symptoms (such as shortness of breath, myalgias, and anorexia).[42] These co-morbidities are relevant to quality of life (QoL) and should be considered when planning for a successful return to work.[43]

Sleep Disturbances and Fatigue

Sleep disturbances and fatigue are also common with post-COVID-19 infection with rates up to 53% and 48%, respectively.[41] Residual fatigue has not been associated with the initial severity of the disease.[44] Functional imaging studies have demonstrated hypometabolism in the frontal lobe and cerebellum in those with post-COVID-19 fatigue, which may be driven by systemic inflammation.[45] Negative psychological and social factors have also been associated with fatigue.[46] Most studies have assessed insomnia broadly; however, breaking this down to early, middle, or late insomnia can help guide treatment. Finally, fatigue has been reported as the most common post-COVID-19 symptom and a major contributor to disability and reduced QoL.[47] In addition to fatigue, which is more generalized, many patients experience postexertional malaise, with physical or cognitive tiredness increasing following effort. Parallels have been made between post-COVID-19 postexertional malaise fatigue and myalgic encephalomyelitis or chronic fatigue syndrome as patients often experience significant fatigue in response to activities (physical or mental) that they previously were able to do without issue.

Neurocognitive Impairment

Cognitive symptoms, often referred to as "brain fog" are particularly common in post-COVID-19 conditions, even in patients who did not experience delirium during the acute phase. One meta-analysis found that 26% of those infected had post-COVID-19 cognitive symptoms at 6 months or later after acute infection; they also found that the rates and severity of cognitive impairment increased with age (greater than 60% in those older than 65 years).[47] Data are limited regarding risk factors for post-COVID-19 cognitive symptoms, although pre-morbid hypertension, sleep apnea, depression, anxiety, mild traumatic brain injury, and abnormal CSF findings have all been associated.[48]

While many individuals have a chief complaint of memory problems, neuropsychological testing typically shows deficits in attention, processing speed, and executive function.[49] This pattern is frequently seen with disruption of the frontal subcortical systems, which include the frontal cortex, striatum, globus pallidus, and thalamus. Notably, the frontal subcortical systems are relevant not only in cognitive functioning but also in mood, language, and motor functioning. Depending on the neurocircuitry involved, there can be disruptions in different clinical domains. For example, a dysexecutive syndrome with associated poor problem solving, apathy, and perseveration can occur with damage to the dorsolateral system. Emotional lability, disinhibition, and olfactory changes can occur with damage to the orbitofrontal system. As described above, akinetic mutism can occur from damage to the medial frontal system. Notably, many of those experiencing neuropsychiatric post-COVID-19 conditions may demonstrate a constellation of these symptoms.

Pathophysiology

Multiple hypotheses have been offered regarding the etiologies of post-COVID-19 conditions. Broadly speaking, these can be divided into direct effects of the viral infection and indirect psychological sequelae. Direct effects include lingering symptoms from the acute infection (such as hypoxic insult and thrombotic events) and persistent heightened neuroinflammatory response from the cytokine storm. Indirect effects include the impact of the huge uncertainty of what the future will bring, grief over personal losses, social isolation, fear of infection, and socioeconomic sequelae. Many consider the COVID-19 pandemic a traumatic event with associated consequences. In many cases of post-COVID-19 conditions, both direct and indirect factors are at play.

Although the host's response to the virus is highly individualized, direct viral invasion into the CNS has not been proven or seen on autopsy. Some studies have found CSF SARS-CoV-2 RNA and protein in the brain specimens; however, these did not correlate with the presence of neurological symptoms.[50,51] However, there is increasing belief that patients who suffer from PASC have a persistent viral reservoir, possibly in the gut, which drives ongoing inflammation. It is possible that the persistent viral presence leads to an aberrant complement activation cascade and thromboinflammation. Furthermore, inflammatory cytokines (such as interleukin 1, 6, and 10 and tumor necrosis factor) may cross the blood-brain barrier and cause further damage to microglia and astrocytes.[52] Another unifying theory posits that viral persistence leads to serotonin depletion, resulting in reduced vagal signaling and hippocampal dysfunction. Many believe that patients who suffered from severe complications of COVID during the acute infection may have a distinct, though phenotypically similar, variety of long COVID that is more related to end-organ damage.[44]

Differential Diagnosis

PASC is diagnosed based on the history and the examination. There is no single test that can diagnose it, nor is there a single treatment. Post-COVID-19 symptoms should always be considered in the broader context of the patient as in some cases the infection may not be acting in isolation. For example, those with prior headache syndromes or psychiatric disorders may experience exacerbation of these symptoms. Alternatively, it is been theorized that COVID-19 may accelerate the development of neurodegenerative disorders.

Similarly, there is no standardized diagnostic work-up. Bloodwork can be useful to evaluate for co-morbid vitamin deficiencies or metabolic disturbances. Trending serum inflammatory markers are not usually recommended. Several neuroimaging studies have demonstrated structural changes in the brain pre- and post-COVID-19 infection. One notable study showed a reduction in gray matter thickness in the orbitofrontal cortex and the parahippocampal gyrus in addition to a greater reduction in overall brain size.[53] In another study of 100 long-COVID-19 patients (including 87 confirmed and 13 presumed cases), the most common neuroimaging findings were subcortical and/or white matter hyperintensities.[54] Functional imaging has shown hypometabolism in the frontoparietal regions, and EEG studies have shown slowing.[55,56] The clinical utility of these findings has yet to be determined.

Management and Treatment

The broad array of post-COVID-19 symptoms likely reflects the Venn diagram of pre-morbid conditions, COVID-19 pathophysiologic mechanisms, and psychological responses. Many patients seem to improve gradually over time, even without treatment. There is no US Food and Drug Administration–approved post-COVID-19 treatment, nor any approved treatments to decrease rates of long COVID, though metiormin has shown early promise in this regard. The only medication thus far shown to improve cognitive symptoms compared to placebo for patients already experiencing brain fog is famotidine. A symptom-based approach can be useful as it allows for prioritizing the treatment of patients' primary symptoms. For example, if a patient primarily suffers from apathy, fatigue, and impaired attention, a trial of bupropion may be useful as it targets the

TABLE 29.4

Interventional Trials for Symptoms of PASC

Study	Study Design	Sample Size (n)	PASC Target Symptom	Intervention/ Treatment	Comparator	Outcomes
Daynes[57]	Cohort study	30	Fatigue, cognitive dysfunction	Physical rehabilitation and educational sessions	None	Improvement in physical/mental fatigue in intervention group
Taquet[58]	Cohort study	668	Cognitive dysfunction (prevention)	Phenytoin	None	Improvement in physical/mental fatigue in intervention group
Priyamvada[59]	Cohort study	30	Anxiety	Psychoeducation, relaxation exercises	None	Significant improvement in anxiety
Karosanidze[60]	Randomized, quadruple blind	100	Anxiety, depression, fatigue	Adaptogens	Placebo	Improvement of cognitive function, anxiety, and depression; however, these findings were also noted in the control group
Farahani[61]	Randomized, double blind	85	Fatigue, depression, anxiety, cognitive dysfunction, insomnia (prevention)	Fluvoxamine	Placebo	Improvement in fatigue
Oliver-Mas[62]	Randomized, double blind	47	Fatigue (physical and mental), depressive symptoms	Transcranial direct current stimulation	Sham	Improvement in physical fatigue and depressive symptoms
Rathi[63]	Randomized, double blind	200	Fatigue	Enzymes, systemic and probiotic	Placebo	Improvement in physical/mental fatigue in intervention group

meso-cortical dopaminergic system. If insomnia and headaches are the prominent symptoms, a trial of a tricyclic antidepressant may help target both complaints. The implication of serotonin depletion in the potential mechanism for PASC suggests that selective serotonin reuptake inhibitors may be a reasonable starting point for many patients. Importantly, evidence suggests that actual skeletal muscle damage can occur during exertion in patients with postexertional malaise, and exercise programs are therefore contraindicated in these patients, with a recommendation instead for pacing. Collaborating with ancillary services for physical and occupation therapy or cognitive rehabilitation can also be particularly helpful. Although many therapies have been tried, evidence is limited regarding post-COVID-19 treatments. Table 29.4 summarizes the findings of several treatment studies.

Neuromodulation techniques, such as transcranial direct current stimulation (tDCS), are also being investigated as treatment options. There is one published randomized, controlled double-blind study in which the effects of anodal tDCS (2 mA, 20 min/day) on the left dorsolateral prefrontal cortex were studied in patients with post-COVID-19 fatigue.[62] Patients ($n = 47$) were evaluated at baseline, immediately after treatment, and 1 month after receiving eight sessions of tDCS or a sham treatment. The primary endpoint was fatigue as measured by the Modified Fatigue Impact Scale. Treatment with tDCS was associated with a statistically significant improvement in physical fatigue at the end of treatment and the 1-month mark; however, there was no significant improvement in cognitive fatigue. Improvements were also noted in secondary endpoints of depressive symptoms but not QoL. Another case series demonstrated benefits in depressive symptoms and executive functioning in those with post-COVID-19 depression or cognitive decline treated with tDCS.[64] Overall, tDCS may represent a promising and well-tolerated treatment for patients with PASC, but further high-quality randomized controlled studies are needed.

CONCLUSIONS

In summary, both direct and indirect effects likely contribute to the vast array of symptoms in post-COVID-19 conditions. Common neuropsychiatric symptoms include fatigue, sleep disturbances, depression, anxiety, and cognitive impairment. Residual damage from the initial cytokine storm, ongoing neuroinflammation, and autoimmunity are leading pathophysiologic theories. Evidence-based treatments are limited, and while we are all still learning, clinical experience suggests that many patients do improve gradually over time. Validating patients' experiences, providing education, and recommending safe treatments are recommended.

REFERENCES

1. Zazhytska M, Kodra A, Hoagland DA, et al. Non-cell-autonomous disruption of nuclear architecture as a potential cause of COVID-19-induced anosmia. *Cell.* 2022;185(6):1052–1064. e1012.
2. Ellul MA, Benjamin L, Singh B, et al. Neurological associations of COVID-19. *Lancet Neurol.* 2020;19(9):767–783.
3. Helms J, Kremer S, Merdji H, et al. Neurologic features in severe SARS-CoV-2 infection. *N Engl J Med.* 2020;382(23):2268–2270.
4. Solomon IH, Normandin E, Bhattacharyya S, et al. Neuropathological features of Covid-19. *N Engl J Med.* 2020; 383(10):989–992.
5. Mukerji SS, Solomon IH. What can we learn from brain autopsies in COVID-19? *Neurosci Lett.* 2021;742:135528.
6. Khan SH, Lindroth H, Perkins AJ, et al. Delirium Incidence, duration, and severity in critically ill patients with coronavirus disease 2019. *Crit Care Explor.* 2020;2(12):e0290.
7. Kennedy M, Helfand BKI, Gou RY, et al. Delirium in older patients with COVID-19 presenting to the emergency department. *JAMA Netw Open.* 2020;3(11):e2029540.
8. Kotfis K, Williams Roberson S, Wilson JE, et al. COVID-19: ICU delirium management during SARS-CoV-2 pandemic. *Crit Care.* 2020;24(1):176.
9. White L, Jackson T. Delirium and COVID-19: a narrative review of emerging evidence. *Anaesthesia.* 2022;77(suppl 1):49–58.
10. Velasquez-Tirado JD, Trzepacz PT, Franco JG. Etiologies of delirium in consecutive COVID-19 inpatients and the relationship between severity of delirium and COVID-19 in a prospective study with follow-up. *J Neuropsychiatry Clin Neurosci.* 2021;33(3):210–218.
11. Beckwith N, Probert J, Rosenbaum BL, et al. Demographic features, physical examination findings, and medication use in hospitalized, delirious patients with and without COVID-19 Infection: a retrospective study. *J Acad Consult Liaison Psychiatry.* 2022
12. Baller EB, Hogan CS, Fusunyan MA, et al. Neurocovid: pharmacological recommendations for delirium associated with COVID-19. *Psychosomatics.* 2020;61(6):585–596.
13. Sher Y, Rabkin B, Maldonado JR, et al. COVID-19-associated hyperactive intensive care unit delirium with proposed pathophysiology and treatment: a case report. *Psychosomatics.* 2020; 61(5):544–550.

14. Ostuzzi G, Gastaldon C, Papola D, et al. Pharmacological treatment of hyperactive delirium in people with COVID-19: rethinking conventional approaches. *Ther Adv Psychopharmacol.* 2020;10:2045125320942703.

15. Taquet M, Geddes JR, Husain M, et al. 6-month neurological and psychiatric outcomes in 236 379 survivors of COVID-19: a retrospective cohort study using electronic health records. *Lancet Psychiatry.* 2021;8(5):416–427.

16. Krishnan K, Miller AK, Reiter K, et al. Neurocognitive profiles in patients with persisting cognitive symptoms associated with COVID-19. *Arch Clin Neuropsychol.* 2022;37(4):729–737.

17. Taquet M, Sillett R, Zhu L, et al. Neurological and psychiatric risk trajectories after SARS-CoV-2 infection: an analysis of 2-year retrospective cohort studies including 1 284 437 patients. *Lancet Psychiatry.* 2022;9(10):815–827.

18. Smith CM, Gilbert EB, Riordan PA, et al. COVID-19-associated psychosis: a systematic review of case reports. *Gen Hosp Psychiatry.* 2021;73:84–100.

19. Chaudhary AMD, Musavi NB, Saboor S, et al. Psychosis during the COVID-19 pandemic: a systematic review of case reports and case series. *J Psychiatr Res.* 2022;153:37–55.

20. Moccia L, Kotzalidis GD, Bartolucci G, et al. COVID-19 and new-onset psychosis: a comprehensive review. *J Pers Med.* 2023;13(1):104.

21. Tang SW, Leonard BE, Helmeste DM. Long COVID, neuropsychiatric disorders, psychotropics, present and future. *Acta Neuropsychiatr.* 2022;34(3):109–126.

22. Russo M, Calisi D, De Rosa MA, et al. COVID-19 and first manic episodes: a systematic review. *Psychiatry Res.* 2022;314:114677.

23. Mourani SC, Khoury R, Ghossoub E. Mechanisms of new-onset psychosis during the COVID-19 pandemic: what ignited the fire? *Ann Clin Psychiatry.* 2022;34(2):123–135.

24. McAlpine LS, Lifland B, Check JR, et al. Remission of subacute psychosis in a COVID-19 patient with an antineuronal autoantibody after treatment with intravenous immunoglobulin. *Biol Psychiatry.* 2021;90(4):e23–e26.

25. Vasilevska V, Guest PC, Bernstein HG, et al. Molecular mimicry of NMDA receptors may contribute to neuropsychiatric symptoms in severe COVID-19 cases. *J Neuroinflammation.* 2021;18(1):245.

26. O'Leary KB, Keenmon C. New-onset psychosis in the context of COVID-19 infection: an illustrative case and literature review. *J Acad Consult Liaison Psychiatry.* 2023;64(4):383–391.

27. Pardamean E, Roan W, Iskandar KTA, et al. Mortality from coronavirus disease 2019 (Covid-19) in patients with schizophrenia: a systematic review, meta-analysis and meta-regression. *Gen Hosp Psychiatry.* 2022;75:61–67.

28. Caan MP, Lim CT, Howard M. A case of catatonia in a man with COVID-19. *Psychosomatics.* 2020;61(5):556–560.

29. Fricchione GL, Paul AB, Chemali Z, et al. Case 34-2022: a 57-year-old woman with Covid-19 and delusions. *N Engl J Med.* 2022;387(19):1795–1803.

30. Luccarelli J, Kalinich M, McCoy Jr. TH, et al. Co-occurring catatonia and COVID-19 diagnoses among hospitalized individuals in 2020: a national inpatient sample analysis. *J Acad Consult Liaison Psychiatry.* 2023;64(3):209–217.

31. Dawood AS, Dawood A, Dawood S. Catatonia after COVID-19 infection: scoping review. *BJPsych Bull.* 2022:1–12.

32. Dotson S, Hartvigsen N, Wesner T, et al. Clozapine toxicity in the setting of COVID-19. *Psychosomatics.* 2020;61(5):577–578.

33. Fisher CM. Catatonia' due to disulfiram toxicity. *Arch Neurol.* 1989;46(7):798–804.

34. Nersesjan V, Amiri M, Lebech AM, et al. Central and peripheral nervous system complications of COVID-19: a prospective tertiary center cohort with 3-month follow-up. *J Neurol.* 2021; 268(9):3086–3104.

35. Fusunyan M, Praschan N, Fricchione G, et al. Akinetic mutism and coronavirus disease 2019: a narrative review. *J Acad Consult Liaison Psychiatry.* 2021;62(6):625–633.

36. Groff D, Sun A, Ssentongo AE, et al. Short-term and long-term rates of postacute sequelae of SARS-CoV-2 infection: a systematic review. *JAMA Netw Open.* 2021;4(10):e2128568.

37. Perlis RH, Santillana M, Ognyanova K, et al. Prevalence and correlates of long COVID symptoms among US adults. *JAMA Netw Open.* 2022;5(10):e2238804.

38. Chen C, Haupert SR, Zimmermann L, et al. Global prevalence of post-coronavirus disease 2019 (COVID-19) condition or long COVID: a meta-analysis and systematic review. *J Infect Dis.* 2022;226(9):1593–1607.

39. Collaborators C-MD. Global prevalence and burden of depressive and anxiety disorders in 204 countries and territories in 2020 due to the COVID-19 pandemic. *Lancet.* 2021;398(10312):1700–1712.

40. Premraj L, Kannapadi NV, Briggs J, et al. Mid and long-term neurological and neuropsychiatric manifestations of post-COVID-19 syndrome: a meta-analysis. *J Neurol Sci.* 2022;434 120162.

41. Efstathiou V, Stefanou MI, Demetriou M, et al. Long COVID and neuropsychiatric manifestations (review). *Exp Ther Med.* 2022;23(5):363.

42. Naidu SB, Shah AJ, Saigal A, et al. The high mental health burden of "long COVID" and its association with on-going physical and respiratory symptoms in all adults discharged from hospital. *Eur Respir J.* 2021;57(6):2004364.

43. Praschan N, Josephy-Hernandez S, Kim DD, et al. Implications of COVID-19 sequelae for health-care personnel. *Lancet Respir Med.* 2021;9(3):230–231.

44. Crook H, Raza S, Nowell J, et al. Long covid-mechanisms, risk factors, and management. *BMJ.* 2021;374:n1648.

45. Guedj E, Campion JY, Dudouet P, et al. 18F-FDG brain PET hypometabolism in patients with long COVID. *Eur J Nucl Med Mol Imaging.* 2021;48(9):2823–2833.

46. Morgul E, Bener A, Atak M, et al. COVID-19 pandemic and psychological fatigue in Turkey. *Int J Soc Psychiatry.* 2021;67(2):128–135.

47. Hartung TJ, Neumann C, Bahmer T, et al. Fatigue and cognitive impairment after COVID-19: a prospective multicentre study. *EClinicalMedicine.* 2022;53:101651.

48. Apple AC, Oddi A, Peluso MJ, et al. Risk factors and abnormal cerebrospinal fluid associate with cognitive symptoms after mild COVID-19. *Ann Clin Transl Neurol.* 2022;9(2):221–226.

49. Jaywant A, Vanderlind WM, Alexopoulos GS, et al. Frequency and profile of objective cognitive deficits in hospitalized patients

recovering from COVID-19. *Neuropsychopharmacology.* 2021; 46(13):2235–2240.

50. Proal AD, VanElzakker MB. Long COVID or post-acute sequelae of COVID-19 (PASC): an overview of biological factors that may contribute to persistent symptoms. *Front Microbiol.* 2021;12:698169.

51. Cosentino G, Todisco M, Hota N, et al. Neuropathological findings from COVID-19 patients with neurological symptoms argue against a direct brain invasion of SARS-CoV-2: a critical systematic review. *Eur J Neurol.* 2021;28(11):3856–3865.

52. Newhouse A, Kritzer MD, Eryilmaz H, et al. Neurocircuitry hypothesis and clinical experience in treating neuropsychiatric symptoms of postacute sequelae of severe acute respiratory syndrome coronavirus 2. *J Acad Consult Liaison Psychiatry.* 2022;63(6):619–627.

53. Douaud G, Lee S, Alfaro-Almagro F, et al. SARS-CoV-2 is associated with changes in brain structure in UK Biobank. *Nature.* 2022;604(7907):697–707.

54. Gutierrez-Martinez L, Karten J, Kritzer MD, et al. Post-acute sequelae of SARS-CoV-2 infection: a descriptive clinical study. *J Neuropsychiatry Clin Neurosci.* 2022;34(4):393–405.

55. Hosp JA, Dressing A, Blazhenets G, et al. Cognitive impairment and altered cerebral glucose metabolism in the subacute stage of COVID-19. *Brain.* 2021;144(4):1263–1276.

56. Toniolo S, Di Lorenzo F, Scarioni M, et al. Is the frontal lobe the primary target of SARS-CoV-2? *J Alzheimers Dis.* 2021;81(1):75–81.

57. Daynes E, Gerlis C, Chaplin E, et al. Early experiences of rehabilitation for individuals post-COVID to improve fatigue, breathlessness exercise capacity and cognition - a cohort study. *Chron Respir Dis.* 2021;18:14799731211015691.

58. Taquet M, Harrison PJ. Exposure to phenytoin associates with a lower risk of post-COVID cognitive deficits: a cohort study. *Brain Commun.* 2022;4(4):fcac206.

59. Priyamvada R, Ranjan R, Chaudhury S. Efficacy of psychological intervention in patients with post-COVID-19 anxiety. *Ind Psychiatry J.* 2021;30(suppl 1):S41–S44.

60. Karosanidze I, Kiladze U, Kirtadze N, et al. Efficacy of adaptogens in patients with long COVID-19: a randomized, quadruple-blind, placebo-controlled trial. *Pharmaceuticals (Basel).* 2022;15(3):345.

61. Farahani RH, Ajam A, Naeini AR. Effect of fluvoxamine on preventing neuropsychiatric symptoms of post COVID syndrome in mild to moderate patients, a randomized placebo-controlled double-blind clinical trial. *BMC Infect Dis.* 2023;23(1):197.

62. Oliver-Mas S, Delgado-Alonso C, Delgado-Alvarez A, et al. Transcranial direct current stimulation for post-COVID fatigue: a randomized, double-blind, controlled pilot study. *Brain Commun.* 2023;5(2):fcad117.

63. Rathi A, Jadhav SB, Shah N. A randomized controlled trial of the efficacy of systemic enzymes and probiotics in the resolution of post-COVID fatigue. *Medicines (Basel).* 2021;8(9):47.

64. Noda Y, Sato A, Fujii K, et al. A pilot study of the effect of transcranial magnetic stimulation treatment on cognitive dysfunction associated with post COVID-19 condition. *Psychiatry Clin Neurosci.* 2023; 77(4):241–242.

PATIENTS WITH CANCER

EMILY M. SORG, MD ■ GRETA JANKAUSKAITE, MA, MS ■ JAMIE M. JACOBS, PHD ■ JOSEPH A. GREER, PHD ■ CARLOS G. FERNANDEZ-ROBLES, MD, MBA ■ KELLY EDWARDS IRWIN, MD, MPH AND DONNA B. GREENBERG, MD

PSYCHO-ONCOLOGY

Psycho-oncology, sometimes also called *psychosocial oncology*, is a subspecialty concerned with the psychological, social, and behavioral aspects of cancer. It is a relatively new field, having only been formally established in the mid-1970s; it aims to provide comprehensive and humanistic support for people with cancer. Psycho-oncology is inter-disciplinary and often involves close collaboration among psychiatrists, psychologists, social workers, nurses, and oncologists. *psychosocial oncology*

To understand psycho-oncology's origins, it is crucial to appreciate that at the start of the 20th century "cancer" was almost an unspeakable diagnosis, rarely shared with patients due to its terminality (fatalism) and our limited understanding of how it developed (fear of transmission). Fortunately, as more effective treatments emerged in the decades that followed, so did optimism and hope that coincided with a growing societal focus on patients' rights and autonomy. The stigma surrounding cancer eventually diminished; this enabled patients to disclose their cancer diagnoses, although a second layer of stigma related to mental illness contributed to the psychological dimensions of cancer being minimized or ignored. Fortunately, the impact that these dimensions had on treatment engagement, quality of life, and disease outcomes was recognized, and psycho-oncology emerged.

Since then, psycho-oncology has grown rapidly, bolstered by robust research and clinical innovations around the globe. Now, 50 years after the field's beginnings, most cancer centers in the United States routinely provide psychosocial support to patients with

cancer, and many institutions also feature research and training programs.

Recent Advances in Cancer Treatment

Over the past decade, significant changes have been seen in the way that many cancers are approached and treated. For example, genetic testing can provide meaningful information about the risk of inherited cancers, which can guide preventive efforts. Targeted and biologic therapies for cancer have revolutionized treatment and brought hope to patients with diseases that were previously considered untreatable. Current cancer treatments often involve using these drugs, alone or in combination with older agents (like cytotoxic chemotherapy). Along with optimism, these advances have also increased uncertainty about side effects, life expectancy, and long-term plans. In addition, while many patients may live beyond active cancer treatment, the physical and emotional sequelae that follow continue to be a source of distress and an area in need of ongoing attention and management.

Role of Psychiatry in the Care of Patients With Cancer

The seriousness of a cancer diagnosis challenges the capacity of patients to survive, to set a course for living, and to fulfill hopes and dreams. Despite recent treatment advances and heterogeneous prognoses, "cancer" continues to evoke myriad emotions at the time of diagnosis and wields considerable psychological power. Moreover, a diagnosis of cancer does not occur in a vacuum: it is superimposed on one's life, with whatever supports, stressors, systems, conditions, strengths, and vulnerabilities exist at that time. Surgery and other cancer treatments, while potentially life saving, further compound and tax the patient's ability to cope with cancer as a chronic stressor. Psychiatrists can play a crucial role in helping patients cope more effectively with their cancer by addressing psychological and physical symptoms, developmental losses, changing relationships, existential distress, and the impact of cancer on their families and caregivers (refer to Table 30.1 for concerns raised surrounding specific types of cancer).

Coping and Hope

Psychiatrists can convey respect by exploring patients' wishes and by evaluating their coping strategies, which in turn, allows patients to nurture courage and resilience. Trust between patients and their psychiatrists is borne out of mutual respect. Patients gain a sense of control as they appraise and re-appraise the choices they make. Moreover, presenting the facts about an illness does not damage the trust that has been established between a patient and a physician; it facilitates understanding and empowerment. Fortunately, hope is not driven by one's prognosis; the capacity to hope is associated with one's personal identity, and the ability to direct one's life and to participate in meaningful relationships. As patients learn that having cancer does not strip them of their sense of self and their values, a sense of purpose adds value to their lives. The psychiatrist's capacity and commitment to listen to patients non-judgmentally allows patients to express their doubts and fears, to accept who they are, and to learn why they see things as they do. The presence of caring clinicians can assure patients that they are not alone amidst their crises and that they can explore what matters most to them.

Medical Choices and Care

Using a patient-centered and collaborative approach, psychiatrists can support patients by clarifying their understanding of the disease and its impact, as well as feasible and available medical choices. Although diagnostic, treatment, and prognostic decisions are complex, psychiatrists are in an excellent position to understand personalized medical plans and facilitate treatment adherence. As a psychiatrist learns more

about how their patient thinks and approaches the world, they can help their patients clarify goals, set priorities, and address obstacles to treatment to facilitate a better quality of life. Meanwhile, working alongside the rest of the care team, psychiatrists can create broad differential diagnoses as psychological symptoms arise and as the medical condition and treatments progress. Psychiatrists also educate and support caregivers and family members. Effective communication between psychiatrists and patients often facilitates acceptance, improves adherence, reduces distress, and helps patients face facets of the disease that cannot be controlled or changed.[1]

Psychiatric Diagnosis and Medication Management

Psychiatrists can offer an expert approach to the diagnosis and management of psychiatric conditions so that treatable symptoms do not stand in the way of a person's cancer care, interfere with goals of preferences for treatment, nor cause undue suffering. Psychotropic medications may be harnessed for their ability to address cancer-related side effects (such as nausea, insomnia, or hot flashes). Since polypharmacy is the norm in patients with cancer, psychiatrists must pay careful attention to drug-drug interactions when considering the use of psychotropics. Patients may be at increased risk of certain adverse side effects due to their cancer and/or its treatment. Finally, psychiatrists can identify and guide the treatment of specific cancer-related or cancer treatment–related neuropsychiatric symptoms (Table 30.2).

Disparities in Cancer Care and Outcomes

Cancer health disparities exist based on racial or ethnic backgrounds, disabilities, gender identity, sexual orientation, and socioeconomic factors (such as income and education).[2] Certain patient populations are at increased risk for psychiatric symptoms and they face additional barriers to cancer care, which results in disparities in clinical outcomes. Patients with serious mental illness (SMI), such as schizophrenia or bipolar disorder, experience delays in cancer diagnosis and care, as do patients with pre-existing cognitive impairments. Patients with SMI are less likely to receive cancer treatments and palliative care, and more likely to experience postoperative complications and to die

TABLE 30.1
Concerns of Patients With Specific Cancer Types

Cancer Type	Likely Concerns
Prostate Cancer	Significance of serum prostate-specific antigen test results: anxiety
	Once diagnosed, the initial choices are watchful waiting, surgery, or radiation treatment
	Side effects of surgery or radiation: incontinence or erectile dysfunction
	Sexual function and dysfunction
	Androgen blockade and its effects on fatigue and loss of sexual interest
Breast Cancer	Body image related to mastectomy or to reconstruction
	Adjuvant chemotherapy and its side effects: alopecia, weight gain, fatigue, and impaired concentration
	Menopausal symptoms: insomnia, sexual dysfunction, and hot flashes related to hormonal therapies
	Question of genetic risk and prophylactic mastectomy, oophorectomy
	Sexual health and fertility concerns
Colon Cancer	Adjustment to surgery or an ostomy
	Body image and sexual function
	Bowel dysfunction
Lung Cancer	Physical limitations of reduced lung capacity
	Post-thoracotomy neuralgia
	Cough
Ovarian Cancer	Anxiety about the tumor marker CA125
	Sexual health and fertility concerns
	Pain and recurrent bowel obstruction
Pancreatic Cancer	Maintenance of adequate nutrition
	Poor appetite
	Bowel function (and the need for pancreatic enzymes and laxatives)
	Pain
	Diabetes
	Depressed mood
Head and Neck Cancer	Facial deformity
	Dry mouth
	Poor nutrition
	Communication issues
	Post-treatment hypothyroidism
	Co-morbid substance use disorder(s)
Lymphoma	Corticosteroid-induced mood changes
	The need for recurrent chemotherapy and its effects
Hodgkin Disease	Post-treatment hypothyroidism
	Fatigue
Osteosarcoma	Amputation/prosthesis vs. bone graft
	Impaired mobility
	Post-thoracotomy neuralgia

from their cancer.[3] These underserved groups are also less likely to access and receive appropriate psycho-pharmacological and/or psychotherapeutic support due to perceived stigma, institutionalized racism, and mistrust of the healthcare system.[3] Working within an inter-disciplinary team, psychiatrists can intervene

TABLE 30.2
Possible Neuropsychiatric Side Effects of Cancer Drugs[a]

Hormonal Treatments

Class	Medication	Side Effects	Interactions With Psychiatric Medications	Cardiac Risk
Anti-estrogens	Tamoxifen	Hot flashes, insomnia, mood changes, confusion possible at high doses	Pro-drug, therefore cytochrome (CYP) 2D6 inhibitors and to a lesser extent 3A4 inhibitors may decrease its efficacy. Avoid use with bupropion, fluoxetine, duloxetine, paroxetine as able.	Mild QTc prolongation, not considered clinically significant
Aromatase Inhibitors	Anastrazole, letrozole, exemestane	Hot flashes, insomnia, fatigue, mood changes (including depression, anxiety, irritability, mood swings), cognitive changes (including difficulty concentrating, forgetfulness, and confusion), sexual dysfunction	CYP 3A4 and 1A2 inhibitors can decrease their metabolism	Insufficient and conflicting evidence
Androgen Blockers	Leuprolide, goserelin	Hot flashes, insomnia, fatigue, mood changes (including depression, anxiety, irritability, mood swings), cognitive changes (including difficulty concentrating, forgetfulness, and confusion), sexual dysfunction	Susceptible to CYP 3A4 inhibitors and inducers	Mild QTc prolongation, not considered clinically significant
	Flutamide, bicalutamide, nilutamide	Hot flashes, insomnia, fatigue, mood changes (including depression, anxiety, irritability, mood swings), cognitive changes (including difficulty concentrating, forgetfulness, and confusion), sexual dysfunction		
Glucocorticoids	Dexamethasone, prednisone, prednisolone, methylprednisolone	Insomnia, increased appetite, mood changes (including depression, anxiety, irritability, mood swings, mania), psychosis (particularly at doses equivalent to ≥60 mg of prednisone)		

Biological Agents

Class	Medication	Side Effects	Interactions with Psychiatric Medications	Cardiac Risk
Biologicals	Interleukin-2	Depression, anxiety, delirium, cognitive impairment, insomnia, psychosis	Can inhibit CYP 3A4	Cardiac dysrhythmias in 9% of patients, predominantly atrial fibrillation or supraventricular tachycardia

(Continued)

TABLE 30.2
Possible Neuropsychiatric Side Effects of Cancer Drugs[a]—Cont'd

Chemotherapies

Class	Medication	Side Effects	Interactions With Psychiatric Medications	Cardiac Risk
Vinca Alkaloids	Vincristine, vinblastine, vinorelbine	Neurotoxicity is dose related and usually reversible Peripheral neuropathy, cognitive impairment (including changes in memory, attention, concentration), mood changes, headaches, Rarely, seizures, hallucinations, and SIADH. Postural hypotension may be an aspect of autonomic neuropathy Less toxicity is noted with vinblastine and vinorelbine	Vinorelbine is primarily metabolized by the hepatic CYP P450 enzyme system, specifically by CYP 3A4 and CYP 3A5. It is also metabolized by other enzymes, including CYP 1A2, CYP 2C9, and CYP 2D6. Vinblastine and vincristine are not metabolized by the cytochrome P450 enzyme system. It undergoes hepatic metabolism through a non-P450-mediated process and is primarily excreted unchanged in the bile.	No QTc prolongation, however, can cause other arrhythmias, bradycardia, and hypotension
Alkylating Agents	Procarbazine	Mood changes (anxiety, irritability), delirium/confusion, cognitive impairment, fatigue, and rarely psychosis	Weak MAO inhibitor, anticholinergic drugs, CNS depressant, disulfiram	Limited information, however, some studies have suggested that procarbazine may have a mild QTc-prolonging effect
	Thiotepa	Mood changes, insomnia, headaches, ataxia, delirium, visual disturbances, and tinnitus	Not metabolized by P450 enzymes	Unknown
	Ifosfamide	Transient delirium, lethargy, seizures, parkinsonism, and cerebellar signs that improve within days of treatment Risk factors include liver and kidney impairment Leukoencephalopathy; thiamine or methylene blue may be antidotes	Metabolized by CYP 3A4 and CYP 2B6	Moderate QTc prolongation
	Fludarabine	Delirium, insomnia, dizziness, headache, somnolence, visual disturbances, mood changes, and rare progressive leukoencephalopathy	No significant interactions Fludarabine is not metabolized by the cytochrome P450 system. It is primarily metabolized in the plasma to an inactive metabolite, 2-fluoro-ara-A, by adenosine deaminase	Some studies have reported cases of QTc prolongation and ventricular arrhythmias in patients treated with fludarabine, but the incidence appears to be rare
	Cytarabine	Confusion, seizures, headaches, visual disturbances, loss of coordination, mood changes, anxiety, and agitation	It is not known to significantly inhibit or induce the activity of any cytochrome P450 enzymes	Moderate QTc prolongation
	5-Fluorouracil (5-FU)	Rarely, depression, delirium/confusion, and agitation. Most severe presentation is an acute cerebellar syndrome, presenting as ataxia, lack of coordination, and nystagmus. Seizures can occur with incidence between 0.1% and 1%	No significant interactions. 5-FU is primarily metabolized in the liver by the hepatic enzyme dihydropyrimidine dehydrogenase	No evidence for QTc prolongation

Chemotherapies

Class	Medication	Side Effects	Interactions With Psychiatric Medications	Cardiac Risk
	Methotrexate	Headache, dizziness, confusion, cognitive impairment, insomnia, and depression. Cumulative doses of intrathecal administration increase the risk of developing leukoencephalopathy presenting with confusion, cognitive impairment, motor deficits, seizures, and vision changes	Methotrexate can reduce the renal clearance of lithium. Also possible are additive hepatotoxicity with valproic acid and carbamazepine	No evidence for QTc prolongation
	Pemetrexed	Mood changes, insomnia, sedation, confusion, forgetfulness, difficulties concentrating. Rarely, hallucinations, delirium, and seizures can occur	Caution should be exercised when pemetrexed is used concurrently with lithium, as both drugs have the potential to cause renal toxicity and dehydration, which could lead to elevated lithium levels and lithium toxicity	No evidence for QTc prolongation
	Gemcitabine	Fatigue, flu-like syndrome, and a rare autonomic neuropathy	Not metabolized by P450 enzymes	Unknown
Topoisomerase Inhibitor	Etoposide	Postural hypotension and rare disorientation	Not metabolized by P450 enzymes	Unknown
Nitrosoureas	Carmustine	Delirium (high doses), rare leukoencephalopathy	Not metabolized by P450 enzymes	Unknown
Platinum-Containing Agents	Cisplatin	Rare reversible posterior leukoencephalopathy, parietal, occipital, frontal with cortical blindness Peripheral neuropathy, poor proprioception, and rarely autonomic symptoms Vitamin E and amifostine may limit peripheral toxicity Hearing may be decreased due to dose-related sensorineural hearing loss	Not metabolized by P450 enzymes. Increased risk of nephrotoxicity with lithium	Low risk for QTc prolongation
	Carboplatin	Neurotoxicity, but only at high doses.	Not metabolized by P450 enzymes. Increased risk of nephrotoxicity with lithium	Low risk for QTc prolongation
	Oxaliplatin	Acute dysesthesias of hands, feet, perioral region, jaw tightness, and pharyngo-laryngodysesthesias	Not metabolized by P450 enzymes	Low risk for QTc prolongation
Taxanes	Paclitaxel	Sensory peripheral neuropathy is not worse with continued treatment Rarely seizures and transient encephalopathy, and motor neuropathy Given with steroids	Metabolized by CYP 2C8 and CYP 3A4	Low risk for QTc prolongation
	Docetaxel	Like paclitaxel but with less neurotoxicity	Metabolized by CYP 3A4 and CYP 3A5	Low risk for QTc prolongation

(Continued)

TABLE 30.2
Possible Neuropsychiatric Side Effects of Cancer Drugs[a]—Cont'd

Chemotherapies

Class	Medication	Side Effects	Interactions With Psychiatric Medications	Cardiac Risk
Anthracyclines	Doxorubicin (Adriamycin)	Depression and anxiety, peripheral neuropathy, cognitive dysfunction, headache, dizziness, delirium, and seizures	Metabolized by CYP 3A4	High risk for QTc prolongation
	Daunorubicin	As above	Metabolized by CYP 3A4	High risk for QTc prolongation
	Epirubicin	Depression, mood swings, insomnia, peripheral neuropathy, delirium, cerebellar ataxia, seizures, stroke-like symptoms	Metabolized by CYP 3A4	High risk for QTc prolongation

Inhibitors of Kinase Signaling Enzymes

Class	Medication	Side Effects	Interactions With Psychiatric Medications	Cardiac Risk
Tyrosine Kinase Inhibitors (TKIs)	Imatinib	Most psychiatric reactions are mild, and include depression, insomnia, anxiety, and rarely delirium. It can cause fluid retention and fatigue, rarely low phosphate; confusion and papilledema	Potential increase risk of bleeding and bruising with SSRIs, increased risk of immune suppression with antipsychotics, rashes with mood stabilizers, and cardiovascular side effects with stimulants. All TKIs are metabolized by CYP 3A4, and imatinib is also metabolized by CYP 2D6, crizotinib is also metabolized by CYP 1A2, osimertinib and selpercatinib by CYP 2C9 and 2C19. Finally capmatinib, is a CYP 1A2 inhibitor/P-glycoprotein/ABCB1 inhibitor may increase concentration of certain psychiatric medications (e.g., duloxetine, olanzapine, ramelteon, risperidone)	Low risk for QTc prolongation
	Sunitinib	Rare reactions include depression, insomnia, delirium, headaches, also reports of psychosis and suicidal ideation. It can also lead to hypothyroidism; TSH should be checked every 3 months		Moderate risk for QTc prolongation
	Sorafenib	Like sunitinib. Also, fatigue and asthenia and rarely hypophosphatemia		Moderate risk for QTc prolongation
	Lapatinib	Depression, anxiety, irritability, agitation, hallucinations, delusions, suicidal thoughts of behaviors		Moderate risk risk for QTc prolongation
	Dasatinib	Fatigue and asthenia		High risk for QTc prolongation
	Nilotinib			Low risk for QTc prolongation
	Crizotinib	Fatigue, dizziness		Low risk for QTc prolongation
	Osimertinib			Low risk for QTc prolongation
	Selpercatinib			Low risk for QTc prolongation
	Capmatinib	Fatigue, weakness/asthenia		Low risk for QTc prolongation

Inhibitors of Kinase Signaling Enzymes

Class	Medication	Side Effects	Interactions With Psychiatric Medications	Cardiac Risk
Proteasome Inhibitors	Bortezomib	Postural hypotension and asthenia, confusion, psychosis, and suicidal thoughts have been reported	Metabolized by CYP 3A4 and CYP 2C19	Low risk for QTc prolongation
	Carfilzomib (Kyprolis)	Peripheral neuropathy, headache, dizziness, fatigue, insomnia, anxiety, depression, confusion, hallucinations, and seizures	Metabolized by CYP 3A4 and CYP 2D6	Moderate risk for QTc prolongation
	Ixazomib (Ninlaro)	Peripheral neuropathy, headache, dizziness, fatigue, insomnia, anxiety, depression, confusion, and hallucinations	Metabolized by CYP 3A4	Low risk for QTc prolongation

Targeted Therapies

Class	Medication	Side Effects	Interactions With Psychiatric Medications	Cardiac Risk
Poly-adenosine-diphosphate ribose poly-merase (PARP) Inhibitors	Olaparib	Fatigue, weakness/asthenia	CYP 3A4, CYP 2D6, CYP 2C9, CYP 2C19	Low risk for QTc prolongation
Bcl-2 Inhibitors	Venetoclax	Fatigue, confusion and seizure possible in the setting of tumor lysis syndrome	CYP 3A4, CYP 2C19. Use with 3A4 inhibitors during initiation phase can increase the risk for tumor lysis syndrome	Low risk for QTc prolongation
Anti-androgens	Enzalutamide	Posterior reversible encephalopathy syndrome (PRES) and seizures have been reported; strong CYP3 A4 inducer	CYP 3A4	Low risk for QTc prolongation
Androgen Synthesis Inhibitors	Abiraterone acetate	Insomnia, fatigue, hot flashes, adrenocortical insufficiency; moderate CYP 2D6 inhibitor	CYP 2D6, CYP 3A4	May prolong QTc interval particularly in the setting of drug-induced hypokalemia;
Proto-oncogene B-RAF (BRAF) Inhibitors	Encorafenib	Fatigue, dizziness, insomnia, intracranial hemorrhage	CYP 3A4, CYP 2C9, CYP 2C19	May prolong QTc when combined with binimetinib

Immunotherapies

Class	Medication	Side Effects	Interactions With Psychiatric Medications	Cardiac Risk
CAR T-cell Therapies	Idecabtagene vicleucel Axicabtagene ciloleucel Tisagenlecleucel	Risks of headache, confusion, anxiety, depression, and delirium/encephalopathy (immune effector cell–associated neurotoxicity syndrome [ICANS]), particularly associated with cytokine release syndrome (CRS)	No P450 metabolism reported	No evidence for QTc prolongation

(Continued)

TABLE 30.2

Possible Neuropsychiatric Side Effects of Cancer Drugs[a]—Cont'd

Immunotherapies

Class	Medication	Side Effects	Interactions With Psychiatric Medications	Cardiac Risk
Antibody-Drug Conjugates	Brentuximab vedotin	Depression and anxiety, headache, dizziness, dysgeusia, and somnolence. Less common but more serious include seizures, encephalopathy, posterior reversible encephalopathy syndrome, hallucinations, suicidal ideation, and suicide attempts	No P450 metabolism reported	Low risk for QTc prolongation
	Sacituzumab govitecan	Peripheral neuropathy, dizziness, fatigue, insomnia, delirium, and rarely seizures		Low risk for QTc prolongation
	Fam-trastuzumab deruxtecan-nxk	Peripheral neuropathy, headaches, delirium, more rarely seizures. Anxiety and depression are rare		Low risk for QTc prolongation
	Ado-trastuzumab emtansine	Peripheral neuropathy, headaches, anxiety, sleep disturbances, delirium, more rarely seizures		Low risk for QTc prolongation
Monoclonal Antibodies	Daratumumab	Peripheral neuropathy, confusion, dizziness, headache, and insomnia. Additionally, there have been rare reports of more serious neurological events such as PRES and acute encephalitis	No P450 metabolism reported	Low risk for QTc prolongation
	Bevacizumab	Fatigue and rarely causes PRES		Low risk for QTc prolongation
	Rituximab	Headache and dizziness		Low risk for QTc prolongation
	Trastuzumab	Headache, insomnia, and dizziness		Low risk for QTc prolongation
Immune Checkpoint Inhibitors	Pembrolizumab (anti-PD-1)	Fatigue, depression, confusion, rare class risk of immune-mediated encephalitis and meningitis	No reported drug-drug interactions; however, co-enzymes CYP 3A4 and CYP 2C9 are involved in the metabolism	No evidence for QTc prolongation
	Nivolumab (anti-PD-1)	Insomnia, dizziness, depression, confusion, rare class risk of immune-mediated encephalitis and meningitis	No P450 metabolism reported	No evidence for QTc prolongation
	Atezolizumab (anti-PD-L1)	Anxiety (up to 25%), insomnia, depression, dizziness, confusion, rare class risk of immune-mediated encephalitis and meningitis		Prolongs QTC interval (incidence 10%)
	Durvalumab (anti-PD-L1)	Fatigue, insomnia, depression, confusion, rare class risk of immune-mediated encephalitis and meningitis		No evidence for QTc prolongation
	Ipilimumab (anti-CTLA-4)	Fatigue, insomnia, headache, depression, confusion, rare class risk of immune-mediated encephalitis and meningitis		No evidence for QTc prolongation
	Cemiplimab (anti-PD-1)	Insomnia, headache, depression, confusion, rare class risk of immune-mediated encephalitis and meningitis, reports of aseptic meningitis		No evidence for QTc prolongation
	Avelumab (anti-PD-L1)	Fatigue, insomnia, headache, depression, confusion, rare class risk of immune-mediated encephalitis and meningitis		No evidence for QTc prolongation

[a]Based on data available in May 2023. Given novelty of many agents, this information is subject to change with increased clinical use and knowledge.
CNS, Central nervous system; CTLA-4, cytotoxic T lymphocyte-associated antigen 4; MAO, monoamine oxidase inhibitor; PD-1, programmed cell death receptor 1; PD-L1, programmed cell death ligand 1; SSRIs, selective serotonin reuptake inhibitors; TSH, thyroid-stimulating hormone.

throughout the continuum of cancer care to promote quality of life and survival for patients with a pre-existing mental illness and cancer.[3]

DISTRESS

Emotional distress is common in cancer, occurring on a spectrum of severity and at various points across the diagnostic and treatment trajectory. Roughly 25% of patients in outpatient cancer settings are very distressed, with estimates closer to 60% for those receiving palliative care.[4] The National Comprehensive Cancer Network (NCCN) defines distress as "a multifactorial unpleasant emotional experience of a psychological (cognitive, behavioral, emotional), social, and/or spiritual nature that may interfere with the ability to cope effectively with cancer, its physical symptoms and its treatment. Distress extends along a continuum, ranging from common and normal feelings of vulnerability, sadness, and fears to problems that can become disabling, such as depression, anxiety, panic, social isolation, and existential and spiritual crisis."[5] Greater cancer-related distress has been associated with a variety of risk factors (such as physical symptom burden, younger age, negative illness perception(s), poor social support, and financial burdens).[6]

Since 2015 cancer programs seeking accreditation from the American College of Surgeons Commission on Cancer have been required to screen patients for distress during their first course of treatment and to provide on-site psychosocial services or a referral to those who report moderate or severe distress. The widely used *distress thermometer*, a simple visual tool developed by the NCCN, serves as an initial single-question screen, identifying distress that arises from any source, even if it is unrelated to cancer.[7] Once distress is detected, a follow-up assessment is recommended to identify potential contributors. Tools such as the Patient Health Questionnaire-4 are sometimes used as screening measures for symptoms of depression and anxiety in cancer care settings.[8] Moreover, the experience of distress also extends to the family members and friends of those with cancer. As cancer care continues to shift more to the outpatient setting, caregivers are at risk for depression, anxiety, sleep difficulties, physical health conditions, and/or worsening of pre-existing mental health conditions.[9]

Psychosocial interventions during cancer care can improve patients' quality of life, alleviate symptoms (e.g., pain and fatigue), and significantly enhance medical outcomes.[10] Interventions that have garnered substantial empirical support for treating patient distress include supportive-expressive group psychotherapy, cognitive-behavioral therapy (CBT), and meaning-centered psychotherapy (MCP).[10] Studies have also explored the role of psychosocial interventions on cancer mortality rates, with some evidence to suggest an improvement in survival rates for those receiving psychosocial care.[11] The severity of cancer-related symptoms (such as fatigue and nausea) and the demanding schedules for cancer treatments may limit the ability of some patients to participate in traditional weekly 50-minute psychotherapy visits. Therefore psychotherapy visits should be flexible; they might be shorter, occur during chemotherapy treatments, and use telehealth services (i.e., phone or virtual visits). Interventions have also been developed and tested to address the psychosocial needs of family caregivers; these often involve psychoeducation, CBT, and MCP.[12]

ANXIETY

Anxiety is a common response to learning that one has cancer, and it fluctuates during the roller coaster ride of uncertainty and perceived threats that occur during the illness. Despite being understandable, symptoms of anxiety should neither be overlooked nor minimized, particularly when they are excessive and impair function. Clinically significant anxiety develops in roughly one-third of those with cancer, with 16% meeting the criteria for a formal anxiety disorder.[13] There is some evidence to suggest that certain cancers, such as cancer of the lung or brain, may be associated with more anxiety than those with other cancers.[13] A history of anxiety or trauma predisposes people to a re-activation of pre-morbid anxiety following a cancer diagnosis.[14] Medical issues (such as hypoglycemia, hypoxia, pulmonary edema, complex partial seizures), and side effects of medications (e.g., steroids, anti-emetics) may be misdiagnosed as primary anxiety and should first be ruled out and/or adequately addressed.

In the oncology setting, different domains of anxiety can arise, and patients may experience more than one type simultaneously. Situational anxiety develops as patients anticipate the results of laboratory tests and scans (sometimes informally called "scanxiety"), fear debilitating or embarrassing symptoms/side effects (e.g., hair loss, incontinence), and worry about upcoming procedures. Existential distress and/or death anxiety may develop, especially in those with advanced cancer.[15] Throughout the illness and even into remission/survivorship, certain physical symptoms may continue to ring the alarm of catastrophe. In addition, improving survival rates may come with a heightened or prolonged sense of uncertainty, as an individual learns to re-engage with their life after cancer.

Symptoms of a pre-existing anxiety disorder (e.g., generalized anxiety disorder, panic disorder, phobias, post-traumatic stress disorder [PTSD]) can also be activated by a cancer diagnosis and its treatment.[14,16] Having cancer provides ample opportunities for fearful rumination in patients who already struggle with excessive or impairing worry. Treatments and procedures may make a patient feel out of control; care should be provided when attending to patients' reactions, to minimize their anxiety. For example, claustrophobia becomes clinically important when a magnetic resonance imaging (MRI) scan is required or when a patient has limited mobility (e.g., following the repair of a leg riddled with osteogenic sarcoma, or weakness that is associated with a prolonged hospitalization). Needle phobia can be challenging in the context of frequent blood drawing and intravenous (IV) infusions. A trauma history might render the need for serial physical exams, invasive procedures, and overnight admissions in the hospital particularly challenging.

The management of anxiety in those with cancer often includes both pharmacologic and non-pharmacologic interventions. Symptom severity, patient preference, and resource availability all guide treatment planning. Selective serotonin reuptake inhibitors (SSRIs) can suppress a chronic state of alarm and reduce baseline anxiety. Benzodiazepines are best used for panic attacks and specific anxiety-provoking procedures or discussions. CBT and stress management techniques teach adaptive coping skills and address thoughts, feelings, and behaviors that can cause or exacerbate anxiety.[17] Further, mindfulness-based interventions,[18] Acceptance and Commitment Therapy (ACT),[19] and mobile CBT applications[20] have shown promise in treating anxious patients with cancer. A

trauma-informed approach to care may also be helpful for a patient with a history of trauma and/or PTSD.

NAUSEA AND VOMITING

Approximately one-half of patients with cancer develop nausea or vomiting during the course of their disease, either because of the cancer itself or because of its treatment.[21] Delayed nausea, which can come in the first days after chemotherapy (e.g., with platinum-based drugs), significantly compromises the quality of life even more than vomiting.[22] As a result of vomiting during or after chemotherapy, patients can develop conditioned nausea and anxiety linked with the smells and sights paired with treatment, sometimes even before arriving for treatment at the hospital. Anticipatory nausea is associated with psychological distress and many quality-of-life domains, such as emotional, role, cognitive, and social functioning.[23] Conditioned nausea can also morph into anticipatory anxiety, insomnia, and treatment aversion with potential downstream negative consequences for treatment adherence.

The primary approach to anticipatory nausea is to control chemotherapy-induced nausea and vomiting (CINV) at the start of treatment. The addition of a neurokinin-1 receptor antagonist, a 5-hydroxytryptamine-3 receptor antagonist, or a corticosteroid, markedly reduces the occurrence of CINV.[24] Olanzapine, a second-generation antipsychotic has significantly improved nausea prevention even when highly emetogenic chemotherapies are used and it may be useful for the prevention of both acute and delayed CINV.[25] When antipsychotics, steroids, and benzodiazepines are used to prevent or treat nausea, psychiatrists can offer valuable advice about side effects, drug-drug interactions, and safe dosing. Hypnosis, cognitive-behavioral techniques, relaxation strategies, systemic desensitization, and anti-anxiety agents (e.g., alprazolam or lorazepam) can reduce phobic responses, as well as anticipatory nausea and vomiting during and after chemotherapy.

SLEEP

Nearly half of all patients with cancer experience sleep problems that adversely affect function and quality of life. Insomnia in those with cancer has been associated with increased levels of pain and depression, a decreased quality of life, diminished immune function, impaired cognition, a worse overall survival rate, and even an increased risk of death.[26] Prominent worry during the initial evaluation or ahead of staging scans can lead to anxious rumination and insomnia. Physical symptoms (e.g., nausea, pain, hot flashes, urinary frequency), hospital environmental factors, and maladaptive sleep behaviors can make restful sleep elusive. Certain cancer treatments and medications, such as steroids, can lead to hyperarousal and disrupt sleep-wake cycles.

After addressing reversible causes of insomnia and ensuring adequate sleep hygiene, CBT for insomnia is considered a first-line treatment.[27] Relaxation techniques, meditation, yoga, exercise, and improving sleep hygiene may also be helpful. Pharmacotherapy may involve the use of antihistamines, sedative-hypnotics, sedating antidepressants (e.g., trazodone, doxepin, mirtazapine), and other medications, such as melatonin agonists and orexin antagonists. Benzodiazepines should be limited to short-term use, given their risk for delirium, tolerance, dependence, and rebound insomnia with chronic use. Drug-drug interactions of sleep aides and treatments for cancer (e.g., opioids) and other symptoms should be considered.

DEPRESSION

In patients with cancer, major depressive disorder (MDD) is associated with a diminished quality of life, worse adherence to treatment, longer hospital stays, a greater desire for hastened death, and an increased rate of suicide and death.[14] The prevalence of MDD in patients with cancer varies from 10% to 25%,[28] while nearly one-third (30%) of patients experience depressive symptoms.[13] Individuals with a history of depression are more likely to develop depressive symptoms after receiving a diagnosis of cancer,[14] but depressive symptoms can arise in those even without a history of depression.

As in individuals without cancer, the diagnosis of MDD is made using the *Diagnostic and Statistical Manual of Mental Disorders, Fifth Edition, Text Revision* (DSM-5-TR) criteria. However, the diagnosis can be complicated by symptoms that overlap with cancer and its treatment. To address this issue, alternative criteria have been proposed that recommend considering non-somatic symptoms (e.g., tearfulness, social withdrawal, guilt) rather than somatic symptoms (e.g., anorexia, insomnia, fatigue).[29] The Hospital Anxiety and Depression Scale is a valid instrument for the assessment of emotional distress in patients with cancer; it follows a similar approach.[30] Importantly, when making a diagnosis of MDD, an assessment for demoralization should also be conducted; this syndrome is conceptualized as clinically distinct from depression and it involves an inability to cope, subjective incompetence, helplessness, meaninglessness, and despair—usually without anhedonia (the loss of pleasure) and with intact emotional reactivity.[31]

In evaluating medically ill patients who appear depressed, potential medical contributions should also be considered when creating a differential diagnosis. Untreated pain, hypothyroidism, nutritional deficiencies, and medications (e.g., corticosteroids, chemotherapy) often contribute to depressed mood. Delirium, especially the hypoactive subtype, can frequently be mistaken for depression. Although mood symptoms occur as part of delirium, key features of delirium include impaired attention and cognition, waxing and waning symptoms, and a sleep-wake disturbance. Fatigue is a common cancer-related symptom that can be difficult to differentiate from MDD. Anhedonia may be the best distinguishing factor for MDD.[32] Apathy (e.g., that results from a lesion in the frontal lobes) can also be reminiscent of MDD. With apathy, there is a loss of interest, motivation, and spontaneous action or speech without the psychological anguish of depression.

The treatment of MDD in patients with cancer is like that of MDD treatment in the general population but with a closer eye on the medical and existential context within which they are being treated. While antidepressants are commonly used to treat MDD that is co-morbid with cancer, placebo-controlled trials of their efficacy in cancer are scarce. A meta-analysis focusing exclusively on pharmacological interventions reported that antidepressant treatment improved depressive symptoms more than placebo. Further, it was suggested that antidepressants may also improve subsyndromal depressive symptoms.[33] When using antidepressants, close attention should be paid to side effects, such as gastrointestinal (GI) upset and an increased risk of bleeding, as they can worsen or be worsened by pre-existing conditions.[14] Antidepressants are often chosen for their side-effect profile (e.g., sedation and increased appetite), which may be desirable in some cases. Some antidepressants (e.g., fluoxetine, duloxetine, paroxetine, bupropion) can affect the cytochrome P450 2D6 system and interfere with the metabolism of commonly used cancer medications. Monoamine oxidase inhibitors are largely avoided due to the risk of drug-drug interactions. Stimulants (e.g., methylphenidate) may also be beneficial for lifting mood, increasing appetite, and improving fatigue, but there is limited evidence to support this practice.[34] When the response to stimulants develops, it is usually seen within a week. Severe cases of MDD, especially those with wasting, may be treated with electroconvulsive therapy.

Although little research has been conducted on medications for MDD in people with cancer, many studies confirm the efficacy of psychosocial interventions.[28] The empirically supported therapies that treat depression among patients with cancer include CBT,[17] mindfulness-based interventions,[18] ACT,[35] MCP,[36] and dignity therapy.[37]

FATIGUE

Fatigue is a highly prevalent and troubling symptom in patients with cancer. Cancer-related fatigue is described as "*a distressing, pervasive sense of physical, emotional, and/or cognitive tiredness or exhaustion related to cancer or cancer treatment that is not proportional to recent activity and interferes with usual functioning.*"[38] Cancer-related fatigue can be severe and persistent, while also resistant to alleviation through deep rest or sleep.[39] Fatigue can arise before receiving a cancer diagnosis, during active cancer treatment, and into the survivorship years.

The diagnosis of cancer-related fatigue is made primarily by asking questions about its presence and severity. While there are validated instruments for measuring fatigue, administration of these questionnaires may not be feasible in busy clinical settings. The NCCN recommends screening for fatigue at office visits with a one-item, 0-to-10 scale, that is like the one used for the screening of pain, with 0 being "no fatigue" and 10 being "the most severe fatigue."[38] Scores ≥ 4 should prompt further evaluation. Clinicians should

explore potential modifiable causes of fatigue, including anemia, pain, sleep disturbance, depression, poor nutrition, and inactivity/deconditioning. Fatigue can also be a side effect of radiation therapy, medications, chemotherapies (e.g., gemcitabine, steroids, narcotics, anti-emetics, beta blockers), and other medical conditions (e.g., infection, hypothyroidism, hypogonadism, adrenal insufficiency, hypercalcemia, hepatic or heart failure). Psychiatrists can help distinguish between cancer-related fatigue and depression, given their frequent symptom overlap, although the two can co-exist.[38] Negative psychological features (e.g., guilt, hopelessness, and thoughts of suicide) are more likely to indicate a depressive episode.

The primary treatment for fatigue is modification of the contributing factors, which should be done in conjunction with the patients' other clinicians. Abundant evidence exists for exercise as a treatment of fatigue, with several studies demonstrating the benefits of exercise for fatigue in people with cancer.[38,39] Mental health clinicians can encourage exercise through motivational interviewing and recommending behavioral changes. Because patients can have serious physical conditions (e.g., bone metastases that could lead to fractures), consultation with an oncologist is recommended before initiating exercise. A physical therapist can assist in designing an exercise program that contains both strength and aerobic training and it is often appropriate for a person with physical limitations from cancer or its treatment. For patients with more medical complications, exercise might best be done in a cardiovascular or pulmonary rehabilitation center.

Behavioral interventions, such as CBT and energy conservation, may be beneficial as both primary and adjunctive treatments for fatigue in patients with cancer.[40] CBT emphasizes the management of fatigue rather than a cure for it. CBT can help address general coping with the experience of cancer, fear of recurrence, unhelpful thoughts and beliefs regarding fatigue, sleep challenges, activity dysregulation, and low social support.[39] Energy conservation is similar to CBT in some respects; it focuses on prioritizing activities and delegating, problem solving around difficulties caused by fatigue, as well as improving organizational skills.[39,40] In addition, psychoeducation around cancer-related fatigue for both patients and their caregivers, mindfulness-based stress reduction techniques, and yoga have also shown promise in addressing cancer-related fatigue.[38,39]

Pharmacologically, current evidence supports the use of psychostimulants to address cancer-related fatigue.[39] NCCN guidelines for patients in active treatment and post-treatment recommend trialing methylphenidate in concert with the treatment of other modifiable causes.[38] However, stimulants can raise blood pressure and heart rate, and they have been linked to arrhythmias. Methylphenidate and dextroamphetamine are not recommended for patients with some pre-existing cardiovascular conditions. Common side effects include constipation, insomnia, anxiety, and (at higher doses) anorexia. Modafinil has also been explored as a well-tolerated non-stimulant alternative, but it has shown mixed results in clinical trials.[41,42] If a depressive episode is present, the use of a more activating antidepressant, such as bupropion, might be helpful if it is not otherwise contraindicated.

NEUROPSYCHIATRIC SYMPTOMS IN CANCER

Delirium is highly prevalent in cancer. Its incidence ranges between 10% and 27% in early stages,[43] but it can increase to up to 44% in hospitalized patients[44] and to over 85% in those with a terminal illness.[45] Common causes include infection, hypoxia, metabolic abnormalities, pain, substance withdrawal, and side effects of treatment/medications (e.g., anticholinergic agents, opioids, hematopoietic stem cell transplantation, chimeric antigen receptor T-cell therapy [CAR-T]). In most patients with cancer, delirium is multi-factorial, with a median number of three precipitating factors per delirious episode.[46] The elderly and patients with structural brain disease, vascular disease, or lung, kidney, or liver impairment are predisposed to delirium.[47]

Specific cancer-related syndromes that may cause neuropsychiatric symptoms in those with cancer are listed below.

Hyponatremia

Hyponatremia can result from the syndrome of inappropriate antidiuretic hormone (SIADH) that occurs as a paraneoplastic syndrome (especially from small cell carcinomas, but also from non-small-cell lung cancer, mesothelioma, pancreatic cancer, duodenal cancer, lymphoma, endometrial cancer, and leukemia), lung infections, cerebral tumors, brain injury, and complications of many psychotropic medications (e.g., SSRIs, carbamazepine, and tricyclic antidepressants). Lethargy and confusion are attributable to cerebral edema caused by the movement of water across the osmotic gradient created by a reduction in the serum sodium[48]; chronic hyponatremia is associated with falls and inattention in the elderly.[49]

Cushing Syndrome

Cushing syndrome may cause delirium, psychosis, and muscle weakness in association with adrenocortical carcinoma or tumors with paraneoplastic adrenocorticotropic hormone (ACTH) production. Psychiatric symptoms are a common feature of the syndrome of ectopic ACTH production. Specific treatments for this syndrome include the use of steroidogenesis inhibitors or glucocorticoid receptor antagonists.

Brain Tumors

The incidence of primary brain tumors is 6.6 per 1,000,000, but the rate of metastatic brain tumors is higher (ranging from 8 to 11 per 100,000). Virtually any tumor can metastasize to the brain, the most common being non-small and small cell lung cancers, breast cancer, melanoma, and GI cancers.[50] In patients with small cell lung cancer, brain metastases are anticipated, and prophylactic whole-brain radiation is often recommended.[51] Isolated brain metastases from non-small cell lung cancer may be treated surgically, and modern radiation techniques target small brain areas.

Deterioration in consciousness develops in 33% to 85% of patients with space-occupying lesions and agitation and delirium arise in 15% to 19%.[52] Tumors (particularly of the frontal, temporal, and limbic lobes) that affect the hardwiring of motivation, attention, mood stability, and memory often come to psychiatric attention. Temporal lobe epilepsy can be associated with psychological symptoms (e.g., memory dysfunction, anxiety, hypergraphia, and viscosity). For these patients, neuropsychiatric consultation, testing, and cognitive rehabilitation may be critically important to define and treat the specific impairment. Multi-modal interventions may be appropriate for altered attention, memory, word retrieval, and problem-solving abilities.[53] Caregivers can understand more clearly the basis of some limitations, and patients can acknowledge their deficits and take whatever control is possible.

Leptomeningeal Disease

Leptomeningeal disease or carcinomatous meningitis (seen most often in breast cancer, lung cancer, melanoma, and non-Hodgkin lymphomas) can lead to a diffuse encephalopathy due to changes in brain metabolism or reductions in regional cerebral blood flow. If focal signs or findings are not seen on neuroimaging, the associated malaise may not be recognized as coming from cancer. In addition to mental changes, headaches, difficulty with walking, limb weakness, and seizures are common. Dizziness and sensorineural deafness have also been noted. Malignant cells in the cerebrospinal fluid (CSF) confirm the diagnosis but obtaining a large enough fluid sample improves the chance of making a diagnosis; from 50% to 70% of tests may be falsely negative. A brain MRI scan may be unremarkable in 20% but it is more likely to show hydrocephalus, brain metastases, or contrast enhancement of the sulci or cisterns.[54]

Toxic Leukoencephalopathy

White matter injury can be an early, temporary, or late consequence of cancer treatment. Whole-brain radiation and certain anti-cancer drugs can injure the projection fibers, association fibers, and commissural tracts that affect cognition and emotion. These drugs include methotrexate, carmustine, cisplatin, levamisole, fludarabine, thiotepa, ifosfamide, cytarabine, and fluorouracil. Acutely, confusion is related to patchy, reversible edema and later to widespread edema and demyelination. More severe delayed consequences result from loss of myelin and axons related to vascular necrosis and thrombosis. The risk of leukoencephalopathy is related to the patient's age, total radiation dose, fraction size, and timing of chemotherapy. Most cancer protocols have adjusted the doses and timing to minimize these adverse effects. However, sometimes patients with a vulnerable brain or delayed drug metabolism may be affected unexpectedly. Neurobehavioral sequelae occur acutely in 28% of patients and should also be considered in cancer survivors, even years out from treatment.[55] When seeing an adult patient who received chemotherapy or radiation to the brain during childhood, psychiatrists should consider white

matter injury as a cause of difficulties with learning or cognition.

The frontal lobes (the lobes with the greatest number of white matter tracts) are the ones most likely to be injured. Patients with a mild leukoencephalopathy may complain of difficulties with concentration and vigilance and of problems with attention. Apathy, anxiety, irritability, depression, or changes in personality may be seen with memory loss, slowed thinking, and failure of executive oversight. In more severe cases, dementia, abulia, stupor, and coma occur with necrotic areas and diffuse white matter hyperintensities that can be seen on MRI scans. This injury, unlike that seen in Alzheimer disease, spares language, praxis, perceptions, and procedural memory. The key bedside tests related to the mental status examination are the elements that test for attention (e.g., digit span, serial sevens, three-word delayed recall), visuospatial skills (clock drawing), and frontal lobe function (alternating motor sequences). The contribution of white matter injury should be documented on T_2-weighted MRI scans.[56]

This toxicity is seen in patients who have received high-dose methotrexate and radiation treatment for childhood acute lymphoblastic leukemia (ALL) or primary central nervous system (CNS) lymphoma. In the latter, a rapidly progressive subcortical dementia with psychomotor slowing, executive and memory dysfunction, behavioral changes, ataxia, and incontinence can be seen. Diffuse white matter disease and cortical-subcortical atrophy have also been noted.[57] Toxic effects of drugs or radiation may add to white matter damage of hydrocephalus, trauma, alcoholism, and hypertension. Patients with a history of psychosis or an affective disorder also tend to show more evidence of abnormal white matter on imaging.

Hematopoietic Stem Cell (Bone Marrow) Transplantation

The incidence of delirium among patients undergoing hematopoietic stem cell transplantation is high (43%–50%), with most cases developing within the first 2 weeks post-transplantation.[58,59] An engraftment syndrome may cause delirium with fever, headache, and rash. Usually, this syndrome occurs when the neutrophil count is >500/mm^3 and when there is a cytokine effect on the hematopoietic colony-stimulating factors.[60] In the transplant setting, immunosuppressive drugs (e.g., cyclosporine, tacrolimus, or the antifungal drug amphotericin B) can cause delirium. Risk factors include hypertension, use of steroids, uremia, and previous brain radiation.[61] Drug serum levels may facilitate diagnosis; tremor occurs in 40%, and paresthesia in 11%. Hypomagnesemia increases the risk of seizures. Immunosuppressants are rarely associated with a reversible posterior leukoencephalopathy syndrome that causes headaches, visual loss or blurring, visual hallucinations, and confusion.[62] Parkinsonism, ataxia, or dystonia can also occur. White matter edema is documented in the parieto-occipital area on fluid-attenuated inversion recovery (FLAIR) sequences. If this syndrome has occurred with one immunosuppressant, either tacrolimus or cyclosporine, the other agent may be used.[63]

Paraneoplastic Neurological Syndromes

Paraneoplastic neurological syndromes of the periphery or CNS are complications of cancer with immune-mediated pathogenesis, as supported by the identified presence of onconeural antibodies associated with certain tumors. They are a heterogeneous group of syndromes and can include sensory neuropathy, Lambert-Eaton myasthenic syndrome, rapidly progressive cerebellar syndrome, limbic encephalitis, diffuse encephalomyelitis, and others.[64] Affected patients may present with these clinical concerns before a cancer diagnosis is confirmed; identification of an antibody in the serum or the CSF can guide the subsequent search for an underlying tumor. Lung cancers (both small cell and non-small cell), breast cancer, ovarian cancer, and lymphomas are the most frequently associated cancers with paraneoplastic neurological syndromes.[64] While still considered rare, the syndrome is likely underdiagnosed and its frequency may increase as new antibodies are identified and immunotherapy use increases.[64,65]

Paraneoplastic limbic encephalitis (PLE) refers to a specific autoimmune syndrome involving limbic areas of the brain also associated with the presence of cancer. As with all paraneoplastic neurological syndromes, neurologic symptoms can present before the cancer diagnosis has been established. PLE can cause memory difficulties, anxiety, mood changes, agitation, disorientation, delusions, hallucinations, abnormal

movements, catatonia, and complex partial seizures. This syndrome has been most frequently associated with small cell lung cancer. Still, it also occurs with Hodgkin lymphoma, thymoma, and cancers of the testes, breasts, ovaries, stomach, uterus, kidney, thyroid, and colon.[66] Typical presentations involve progressive confusion and deficits in short-term memory. Less commonly, patients experience visual and auditory hallucinations, delusions, or frank paranoia.[66] Detection of antibodies directed against onconeural antigens in the serum or the CSF may assist in the diagnosis. MRI brain findings, if present, may involve an increased FLAIR signal in one or both medial temporal lobe(s) though MRI abnormalities are not always seen. Electroencephalogram (EEG) findings may include slowing or seizure activity in the temporal areas. Tumor removal is critical to the treatment of the syndrome; first-line immunotherapies (e.g., steroids, IV immunoglobulins, plasmapheresis) also minimize autoimmune responses and neural inflammation and can result in improvement in up to half of the cases. Second-line immunotherapies (e.g., rituximab, cyclophosphamide) are usually effective when first-line treatments fail.[67] Anticonvulsants and neuroleptics have also been used in the symptomatic treatment of psychiatric manifestations.[66]

Immune-Related Adverse Events

Cancer immunotherapy involves harnessing aspects of a patient's immune system to achieve remission from the disease. Current immunotherapies include immune checkpoint inhibitors (ICIs), bispecific T-cell engagers, and immune effector cell (IEC) therapies, such as chimeric antigen receptor (CAR) T-cell therapy. ICIs target cytotoxic T lymphocyte–associated antigen 4 (CTLA-4), programmed cell death receptor 1 (PD-1), and programmed cell death ligand 1(PD-L1). Immunotherapies have been associated with unique and potentially life-threatening toxicities.

Psychiatric adverse events related to ICIs occur in approximately 2% to 3% of patients and the proportion is slightly higher in patients receiving combination therapy (i.e., two ICIs in combination) than monotherapy. A recent review reported confusion/delirium, insomnia, anxiety, and depression as the five most common categories of psychiatric side effects related to ICIs.[68] Immune treatment is often associated with mild or moderate fatigue, which complicates the assessment of cancer-related fatigue or the neurovegetative symptoms of depression. Neurologic immune-related adverse events (irAEs) are uncommon but occasionally occur as myasthenia gravis or Guillain-Barre syndrome. Posterior reversible encephalopathy syndrome (PRES), aseptic meningitis, pancerebellitis, or autoimmune encephalitis may occur rarely.[69]

A variety of irAEs, like pneumonitis or colitis, arise; they are more common with blockers of CTLA-4 than PD-1 or PD-L1. Autoimmune endocrine conditions, like thyroiditis (hypothyroidism or hyperthyroidism), hypophysitis, and rarely adrenal insufficiency, may mimic the symptoms of depression or anxiety. Furthermore, corticosteroids used to treat these syndromes have their own dose-related psychiatric side effects (e.g., destabilized mood, insomnia, anxiety, and tearfulness). When steroids are stopped, the relative adrenal insufficiency at times of infection or iatrogenic adrenal insufficiency should be considered.

Immune Effector Cell–Associated Neurotoxicity Syndrome

Immunotherapy with CAR T-cell therapy is one of the most important advances in the treatment of cancer and, particularly, hematologic malignancies. CAR T-cell therapy can cause cytokine release syndrome (CRS), a supraphysiologic inflammatory state, associated with fever and shock.[70]

A distinct IEC-associated neurotoxicity syndrome (ICANS) can follow a CRS or develop alone. ICANS may be more common in younger patients or those with CRS, a pre-existing neurologic injury, ALL, a high disease burden, thrombocytopenia, lympho-depleting therapy with fludarabine and cyclophosphamide, or an elevated ferritin level in the 3 days after treatment.[71] The presentation may begin 3 to 10 days after CAR T-cell administration, often starting with attentional problems and language abnormalities. Without steroid treatment, symptoms can progress within hours to days, leading to confusion, behavioral changes, aphasia, focal motor weakness, seizures, and coma. Higher-grade presentations often require an intensive care unit level of care and may be fatal due to malignant cerebral edema. The grading of ICANS is based on the evaluation of consciousness, presence of seizures, motor findings, and signs of elevated intracranial pressure. Imaging can be normal. An EEG often shows diffuse slowing or evidence of seizures. CSF analysis following a lumbar puncture shows elevated protein concentrations and lymphocyte counts. Management includes supportive care, glucocorticoids to attenuate the inflammatory response and anticonvulsants for seizure prophylaxis or treatment. Antipsychotics, such as IV haloperidol, may be used to manage agitation, being mindful of the potential to further lower the seizure threshold. Tocilizumab, which is often given for concomitant CRS, should not be relied on for isolated ICANS as it does not cross the blood-brain barrier.[70]

HORMONAL THERAPY

Treatment of hormonal-sensitive tumors involves the use of medications aimed at reducing the availability of sex hormones that may drive tumor growth. Tamoxifen is a mixed agonist/antagonist of estrogen that is associated with hot flashes and insomnia. Aromatase inhibitors reduce estradiol to barely detectable concentrations. Both are indicated in the setting of hormone-sensitive breast cancer. These hormonal therapies are associated with side effects, such as hot flashes, mood swings, irritability, joint pain, and insomnia, which result in suboptimal adherence to the medication and, subsequently, an increased risk of recurrence.[72] Men receiving androgen ablation for prostate cancer experience hot flashes that are more frequent, severe, and longer lasting.[73] Venlafaxine and some SSRIs (e.g., paroxetine, citalopram, escitalopram) can reduce the frequency and severity of hot flashes and improve mood, sleep, anxiety, and quality of life in patients undergoing hormonal deprivation therapy for hormone-sensitive tumors.[73] Gabapentin and pregabalin have also been beneficial for decreasing hot flashes in patients with cancer.[74]

Notably, there has been concern regarding the concomitant use of tamoxifen with antidepressants known to inhibit CYP 2D6 due to concern that it would diminish tamoxifen's anti-cancer effects. More recent data suggest that tamoxifen's efficacy is mediated by other pathways than its CYP 2D6 conversion to a metabolite and that the use of tamoxifen and potent CYP 2D6-inhibiting SSRIs, rather than other SSRIs, was not associated with an increased risk of death. However, pragmatism and caution continue to dictate preferential avoidance of antidepressants known to strongly inhibit CYP 2D6 (e.g., fluoxetine, duloxetine, bupropion, paroxetine) in patients taking tamoxifen.[75]

Gonadotropin-releasing hormone agonists, such as leuprolide, have been associated with depression in populations without cancer; however, in patients with prostate cancer, clinical trials have shown diverse results and well-controlled prospective studies have suggested that even though depression occurs, fatigue is more prevalent and it may be mistaken for depression.[76] Leuprolide is now commonly used for breast cancer as well.

END-OF-LIFE CARE

Comprehensive end-of-life (EOL) care requires a team-based approach. A growing body of evidence over the last two decades has demonstrated that the early integration of palliative and oncologic care near the time of diagnosis of advanced solid tumors, such as metastatic lung cancer, leads to beneficial patient outcomes. Specifically, patients with advanced cancer who receive this model of care experience an improved quality of life, less severe depression symptoms, more accurate prognostic understanding, and longer lengths of stay in hospice, a key metric of higher quality EOL care. Moreover, studies show that these improved outcomes in quality of life and mood are accounted for by patients' use of adaptive coping strategies. Psychiatrists and other mental health clinicians, such as psychologists and social workers, play an essential role in the delivery of comprehensive EOL care for patients with advanced cancer, especially given their close alignment, if not integration, with palliative care teams. Specifically, mental health clinicians provide psychopharmacologic consultation for treating depression, anxiety, and delirium, which tend to worsen at the EOL and deliver evidence-based psychotherapies, such as CBT, meaning-centered psychotherapy, and dignity therapy, to enhance patients' use of adaptive coping skills and deepen the existential meaning and coherence before death.[77] They may also play an essential role in facilitating conversations about EOL goals and treatment preferences between the patient, their family caregivers, and the medical team.

SURVIVORSHIP IN CANCER

With the rapid advancement of cancer detection, treatments, and procedures, more and more patients are fortunately able to transition to a "survivorship" phase. Notably, "survivor" of cancer is a loaded term that many patients do not identify with and might find harmful.[78] Nonetheless, the post-treatment phase should not be overlooked, and psychiatrists and other mental health clinicians may play an important role in supporting this growing patient population. Although concerns vary, some of the most salient challenges that patients face in survivorship include coping with post-treatment side effects and adjusting to their changed bodies following surgical or other invasive treatment procedures, returning to work and financial toxicity, and handling concerns about ongoing cancer monitoring that may increase their anxiety (including the fear of cancer recurrence). Further, increased anxiety, depression, PTSD symptoms, and general adjustment distress are important psychological consequences following a cancer diagnosis and treatment.[79] Similarly to patients undergoing active treatment, patients in the survivorship phase often benefit from the use of psychotropics and psychotherapeutic interventions (e.g., psychoeducation, CBT, ACT, MCP, mindfulness, and relaxation training) as well as engagement in support groups with others being treated for cancer.[36,79,80] Lifestyle interventions that focus on enhancing health behaviors in survivorship (e.g., increasing physical activity, optimizing nutrition, reducing substance use) are important to mitigate the risk of recurrence and second primary tumors.

CONCLUSION

Psychiatrists can help patients cope with affective, behavioral, cognitive, and physical symptoms associated with cancer and its treatment, as well as with developmental losses, changes in relationships, and the effects of cancer on family systems and caregivers.

REFERENCES

1. Massie MJ. The role of the psychiatrist in the care of women with breast cancer. *BCO.* 2005;8(5):e26.
2. National Cancer Institute. *Understanding Cancer: Cancer Disparities.* Updated March 28, 2022. Available at: https://www.cancer.gov/about-cancer/understanding/disparities#contributing-factors. Accessed February 28, 2023.
3. Irwin KE, Henderson DC, Knight HP, Pirl WF. Cancer care for individuals with schizophrenia. *Cancer.* 2014;120(3):323–334.

4. Gao W, Bennett MI, Stark D, et al. Psychological distress in cancer from survivorship to end of life care: prevalence, associated factors and clinical implications. *Eur J Cancer Care.* 2010;46:2036–2044.

5. NCC Network. *NCCN Clinical Practice Guidelines in Oncology: Version 2. Distress Management*; 2023. Available at: https://www.nccn.org/login?ReturnURL=https://www.nccn.org/professionals/physician_gls/pdf/distress.pdf. Accessed January 21, 2023.

6. Liu JK, Kaji AH, Roth KG, et al. Determinants of psychosocial distress in breast cancer patients at a safety net hospital. *Clin Breast Cancer.* 2022;22(1):43–48.

7. Lo SB, Ianniello L, Sharma M, et al. Experience implementing distress screening using the National Comprehensive Cancer Network distress thermometer at an urban safety-net hospital. *Psychooncology.* 2016;25(9):1113–1115.

8. Pirl WF, Fann JR, Greer JA, et al. Recommendations for the implementation of distress screening programs in cancer centers: report from the American Psychosocial Oncology Society (APOS), Association of Oncology Social Work (AOSW), and Oncology Nursing Society (ONS) joint task force. *Cancer.* 2014;120(19):2946–2954.

9. Applebaum AJ, Kent EE, Lichenthal WG. Documentation of caregivers as a standard of care. *J Clin Oncol.* 2021;39(18):1955–1958.

10. Caruso R, Breitbart W. Mental health care in oncology. Contemporary perspective on the psychosocial burden of cancer and evidence-based interventions. *Epidemiol Psychiatr Sci.* 2020;29:e86.

11. Mustafa M, Carson-Stevens A, Gillespie D, et al. Psychological interventions for women with metastatic breast cancer. *Cochrane Database Syst Rev.* 2013(6): CD004253.

12. Sun V, Raz DJ, Kim JY. Caring for the informal cancer caregiver. *Curr Opin Support Palliat Care.* 2019;13(3):238.

13. Zeilinger EL, Oppenauer C, Knefel M, et al. Prevalence of anxiety and depression in people with different types of cancer or haematologic malignancies: a cross-sectional study. *Epidemiol Psychiatr Sci.* 2022;31:e74.

14. Pitman A, Suleman S, Hyde N, et al. Depression and anxiety in patients with cancer. *BMJ.* 2018;36:k1415.

15. Breitbart W, Pessin H, Rosenfeld B, et al. Individual meaning-centered psychotherapy for the treatment of psychological and existential distress: a randomized controlled trial in patients with advanced cancer. *Cancer.* 2018;124(15):3231–3239.

16. Cordova MJ, Riba MB, Spiegel D. Post-traumatic stress disorder and cancer. *Lancet Psychiatry.* 2017;4(4):330–338.

17. Traeger L, Greer JA, Fernandez-Robles C, et al. Evidence-based treatment of anxiety in patients with cancer. *J Clin Oncol.* 2012;30:1197–1205.

18. Oberoi S, Yang J, Woodgate RL, et al. Association of mindfulness-based interventions with anxiety severity in adults with cancer: a systematic review and meta-analysis. *JAMA Network Open.* 2020;3(8):e2012598.

19. Fishbein JN, Haslbeck J, Arch JJ. Network intervention analysis of anxiety-related outcomes and processes of acceptance and commitment therapy (ACT) for anxious cancer survivors. *Behav Res Ther.* 2023:104266.

20. Greer JA, Jacobs J, Pensak N, et al. Randomized trial of a tailored cognitive-behavioral therapy mobile application for anxiety in patients with incurable cancer. *Oncologist.* 2019;24(8):1111–1120.

21. Warr DG. Chemotherapy-and cancer-related nausea and vomiting. *Curr Oncol.* 2008;15(1):S4–S9.

22. Navari RM. Nausea and vomiting in advanced cancer. *Curr Treat Options Oncol.* 2020;21(2):14.

23. Akechi T, Okuyama T, Endo C, et al. Anticipatory nausea among ambulatory cancer patients undergoing chemotherapy: prevalence, associated factors, and impact on quality of life. *Cancer Science.* 2010;101(12):2596–2600.

24. Di Maio M, Bria E, Banna GL, et al. Prevention of chemotherapy-induced nausea and vomiting and the role of neurokinin 1 inhibitors: from guidelines to clinical practice in solid tumors. *Anticancer Drugs.* 2013;24:99–111.

25. Navari RM, Qin R, Ruddy KJ, et al. Olanzapine for the prevention of chemotherapy-induced nausea and vomiting. *N Engl J Med.* 2016;375(2):134–142.

26. Melton L. Cognitive behavioral therapy for sleep in cancer patients: research, techniques, and individual considerations. *J Adv Pract Oncol.* 2018;9(7):732–740.

27. Garland SN, Johnson JA, Savard J, et al. Sleeping well with cancer: a systematic review of cognitive behavioral therapy for insomnia in cancer patients. *Neuropsychiatr Dis Treat.* 2014;10:1113–1124.

28. Pirl WF. Evidence report on the occurrence, assessment, and treatment of depression in cancer patients. *JNCI Monograph.* 2004(32):32–39.

29. Saracino RM, Aytürk E, Cham H, et al. Are we accurately evaluating depression in patients with cancer? *Psych Assess.* 2020;32(1):98–107.

30. Annunziata MA, Muzzatti B, Bidoli E, et al. Hospital Anxiety and Depression Scale (HADS) accuracy in cancer patients. *Support Care Cancer.* 2020;28:3921–3926.

31. Kissane DW, Clarke DM, Street AF. Demoralization syndrome—a relevant psychiatric diagnosis for palliative care. *J Pall Care.* 2001;17(1):12–21.

32. Saracino RM, Rosenfeld B, Nelson CJ. Towards a new conceptualization of depression in older adult cancer patients: a review of the literature. *Aging Mental Health.* 2016;20(12):1230–1242.

33. Laoutidis ZG, Mathiak K. Antidepressants in the treatment of depression/depressive symptoms in cancer patients: a systematic review and meta-analysis. *BMC Psychiatry.* 2013;13:140.

34. Homsi J, Nelson KA, Sarhill N. A phase II study of methylphenidate for depression in advanced cancer. *Am J Hosp Palliat Care.* 2001;18:403–407.

35. Arch JJ, Fishbein JN, Ferris MC, et al. Acceptability, feasibility, and efficacy potential of a multimodal acceptance and commitment therapy intervention to address psychosocial and advance care planning needs among anxious and depressed adults with metastatic cancer. *J Palliat Med.* 2020;23(10):1380–1385.

36. van der Spek N, Vos J, van Uden-Kraan CF, et al. Efficacy of meaning-centered group psychotherapy for cancer survivors: a randomized controlled trial. *Psychol Med.* 2017;47(11):1990–2001.

37. Zhang Y, Li J, Hu X. The effectiveness of dignity therapy on hope, quality of life, anxiety, and depression in cancer patients:

a meta-analysis of randomized controlled trials. *Int J Nurs Stud.* 2022;132:104273.

38. NCC Network. *NCCN Clinical Practice Guidelines in Oncology: Version 2. Cancer-Related Fatigue*; 2023. Available at: https://www.nccn.org/professionals/physician_gls/pdf/fatigue.pdf.

39. Fabi A, Bhargava R, Fatigoni S, et al. Cancer-related fatigue: ESMO clinical practice guidelines for diagnosis and treatment. *Ann Oncol.* 2020;31(6):713–723.

40. Chapman EJ, Martino ED, Edwards Z, et al. Practice review: evidence-based and effective management of fatigue in patients with advanced cancer. *Palliat Med.* 2022;36(1):7–14.

41. Blackhall L, Petroni G, Shu J, et al. A pilot study evaluating the safety and efficacy of modafinil for cancer-related fatigue. *J Palliat Med.* 2009;12(5):433–439.

42. Spathis A, Fife K, Blackhall F, et al. Modafinil for the treatment of fatigue in lung cancer: results of a placebo-controlled, double-blind, randomized trial. *J Clin Oncol.* 2014;32(18):1882–1888.

43. Morrison C. Identification and management of delirium in the critically ill patient with cancer. *AACN Clin Issues.* 2003;14:92–111.

44. Centeno C, Sanz A, Bruera E. Delirium in advanced cancer patients. *Palliat Med.* 2004;18:184–194.

45. Massie MJ, Holland J, Glass E. Delirium in terminally cancer patients. *Am J Psychiatry.* 1983;140:1048–1050.

46. Lawlor PG, Gagnon B, Mancini IL, et al. Occurrence, causes, and outcome of delirium in patients with advanced cancer: a prospective study. *Arch Intern Med.* 2000;160:786–794.

47. Tuma R, DeAngelis LM. Altered mental status in patients with cancer. *Arch Neurol.* 2000;57:1727–1731.

48. Adrogué HJ, Madias NE. Hyponatremia. *N Engl J Med.* 2000;342:1581–1589.

49. Smith DM, Mckenna K, Thompson CJ. Hyponatraemia. *Clin Endocrinol.* 2000;52:667–678.

50. Nayak L, Lee EQ, Wen PY. Epidemiology of brain metastases. *Curr Oncol Rep.* 2012;14:48–54.

51. Auperin A, Arriagada R, Pignon J, et al. Prophylactic cranial irradiation for patients with small-cell lung cancer in complete remission. *N Engl J Med.* 1999;341:476–484.

52. Yamanaka R, Koga H, Yamamoto Y, et al. Characteristics of patients with brain metastases from lung cancer in a palliative care center. *Support Care Cancer.* 2011;19:467–473.

53. Cicerone KD, Dahlberg C, Kalmar K, et al. Evidence-based cognitive rehabilitation: recommendations for clinical practice. *Arch Phys Med Rehabil.* 2000;81:1596–1615.

54. DeAngelis LM. Current diagnosis and treatment of leptomeningeal metastasis. *J Neurooncol.* 1998;38:245–252.

55. Filley CM. Neurobehavioral aspects of cerebral white matter disorders. *Psychiatr Clin North Am.* 2005;28:685–700.

56. Crossen JR, Garwood D, Glatstein E, et al. Neurobehavioral sequelae of cranial irradiation in adults: a review of radiation-induced encephalopathy. *J Clin Oncol.* 1994;6:1215–1228.

57. Omuro AMP, Ben-Porat LS, Panageas KS, et al. Delayed neurotoxicity in primary central nervous system lymphoma. *Arch Neurol.* 2005;62:1595–1600.

58. Beglinger LJ, Duff K, Van Der Heiden S, et al. Incidence of delirium and associated mortality in hematopoietic stem cell transplantation patients. *Biol Blood Marrow Transplant.* 2006;12:928–935.

59. Fann JR, Roth-Roemer S, Burington BE, et al. Delirium in patients undergoing hematopoietic stem cell transplantation. *Cancer.* 2002;95:1971–1981.

60. Spitzer TR. Engraftment syndrome following hematopoietic stem cell transplantation. *Bone Marrow Transplant.* 2001;27:893–898.

61. Reece DE, Frei-Lahr DA, Shepherd JD, et al. Neurologic complications in allogeneic bone marrow transplant patients receiving cyclosporin. *Bone Marrow Transplant.* 1991;8:393–401.

62. Hinchey J, Chaves C, Appignani B, et al. A reversible posterior leukoencephalopathy syndrome. *N Engl J Med.* 1996;334:494–500.

63. Walter RW, Brochstein JA. Neurologic complications of immunosuppressive agents. *Neurol Clin.* 1988;6:261–278.

64. Graus F, Vogrig A, Muñiz-Castrillo S, et al. Updated diagnostic criteria for paraneoplastic neurologic syndromes. *Neurol Neuroimmunol Neuroinflamm.* 2021;8(4):e1014.

65. Vogrig A, Gigli GL, Segatti S, et al. Epidemiology of paraneoplastic neurological syndromes: a population-based study. *J Neurol.* 2020;267(1):26–35.

66. Foster AR, Caplan JP. Paraneoplastic limbic encephalitis. *Psychosomatics.* 2009;50:108–113.

67. Titulaer MJ, McCracken L, Gabilondo I, et al. Treatment and prognostic factors for long-term outcome in patients with anti-NMDA receptor encephalitis: an observational cohort study. *Lancet Neurol.* 2013;12:157–165.

68. Zhou C, Peng S, Lin A, et al. Psychiatric disorders associated with immune checkpoint inhibitors: a pharmacovigilance analysis of the FDA Adverse Event Reporting System (FAERS) database. *EClinicalMedicine.* 2023;59:101967.

69. Reynolds KL, Guidon AC. Diagnosis and management of immune checkpoint inhibitor-associated neurologic toxicity; illustrative case and review of the literature. *Oncologist.* 2019;24:435–443.

70. Reynolds KL, Cohen JV, Zubiri L, Stern TA, eds. *Facing Immunotherapy: A Guide for Patients and Their Families.* MGH Psychiatry Academy; 2020.

71. Schubert ML, Schmitt M, Wang L, et al. Side-effect management of chimeric antigen receptor (CAR) T-cell therapy. *Ann Oncol.* 2021;32:34–48.

72. Joffee H, Hall JE, Gruber S, et al. Estrogen therapy selectively enhances prefrontal cognitive processes: a randomized, double-blind, placebo-controlled study with functional magnetic resonance imaging in perimenopausal and recently postmenopausal women. *Menopause.* 2006;12:411–422.

73. Adelson KB, Loprinzi CL, Hershman DL. Treatment of hot flushes in breast and prostate cancer. *Expert Opin Pharmacother.* 2005;6:1095–1106.

74. Loprinzi CL, Qin R, Balcueva EP, et al. Phase III, randomized, double-blind, placebo-controlled evaluation of pregabalin for alleviating hot flashes, N07C1. *J Clin Oncol.* 2010;28:641–647.

75. Donneyong MM, Bykov K, Bosco-Levy P, et al. Risk of mortality with concomitant use of tamoxifen and selective serotonin reuptake inhibitors: multi-database cohort study. *BMJ.* 2016;354:i5014.

76. Pirl WF, Greer JA, Goode M, et al. Prospective study of depression and fatigue in men with advanced prostate

cancer receiving hormone therapy. *Psychooncology.* 2008;17: 148–153.

77. Greer JA, Applebaum AJ, Jacobsen JC, et al. Understanding and addressing the role of coping in palliative care for patients with advanced cancer. *J Clin Oncol.* 2020;38(9):915–925.

78. Berry LL, Davis SW, Godfrey Flynn A, et al. Is it time to reconsider the term "cancer survivor"? *J Psychosoc Oncol.* 2019;37(4):413–426.

79. Shapiro CL. Cancer survivorship. *N Engl J Med.* 2018;379(25): 2438–2450.

80. Cuthbert CA, Farragher JF, Hemmelgarn BR, et al. Self-management interventions for cancer survivors: a systematic review and evaluation of intervention content and theories. *Psychooncology.* 2019;28(11):2119–2140.

31

PULMONARY DISEASE

YELIZAVETA SHER, MD ■ EMMA M. TILLMAN, PHARMD,
PHD ■ SYLVIE·J. WEINSTEIN, BA ■ PRANGTHIP CHAROENPONG,
MD, MPH ■ ANNA M. GEORGIOPOULOS, MD

OVERVIEW

Psychiatrists in general hospitals may encounter children and adults with common pulmonary diseases (e.g., asthma, chronic obstructive pulmonary disease [COPD], non–cystic fibrosis bronchiectasis), as well as rare conditions (cystic fibrosis [CF], primary ciliary dyskinesia [PCD], pulmonary hypertension, interstitial lung disease [ILD]), and diseases associated with pulmonary conditions or complications (e.g., sleep disorders, neuromuscular disorders [NMDs]). Psychiatric disorders (such as anxiety, depression, neurocognitive impairment, and tobacco use disorders) occur more frequently in patients with pulmonary conditions than in the general population and are accompanied by a decreased quality of life, a lower adherence to care, and worse medical outcomes.[1-7] In addition, some pulmonary therapies are associated with neuropsychiatric side effects and psychological distress (Table 31.1).

Psychiatric Impact of Pulmonary Pharmacotherapies

Many common pulmonary therapies are associated with neuropsychiatric side effects. For example, bronchodilators and caffeine are associated with agitation, restlessness, anxiety, and insomnia. Steroids are associated with a bevy of psychiatric effects, ranging from mild changes in mood to severe symptoms that include, but are not limited to, euphoria, anger, agitation, anxiety, distractibility, fear, hunger, hypomania, indifference, insomnia, irritability, lethargy, labile mood, pressured speech,

restlessness, and tearfulness.[8] The adverse effects of steroids are dose related, with doses higher than 40 mg of prednisone equivalents being more likely to lead to neuropsychiatric side effects. CF transmembrane conductance regulator (CFTR) modulators have recently been linked to adverse neuropsychiatric effects (including anxiety, depression, insomnia, and brain fog) (Box 31.1).[9] Montelukast has been associated with psychiatric side effects, including thoughts of suicide and suicide attempts.[10] The immunosuppressive calcineurin inhibitors are also associated with adverse events, including mood changes, agitation, anxiety, insomnia, restlessness, psychosis, hallucinations, and posterior reversible encephalopathy syndrome (PRES).

Psychiatric Impact of Non-pharmacologic Pulmonary Therapies

Non-pharmacologic therapies for pulmonary conditions often become more intensive as pulmonary diseases progress. Moreover, complex psychological sequelae can accompany these interventions. For example, although long-term oxygen therapy (LTOT) is associated with improved survival, patients' quality of life may not improve,[10] and some individuals experience substantial distress.[11] Although oxygen therapy can improve independent functioning, it can be inconvenient and logistically challenging. LTOT may also represent a visible marker of progressive disease, leading patients to avoid participating in social activities or using the therapy. Therefore, it is important to recognize and address the psychological implications of LTOT, which can interfere with adherence and worsen

TABLE 31.1
Pulmonary Conditions and Therapies With Common Psychiatric Co-morbidities

Pulmonary Conditions	Pulmonary Therapies With Psychiatric Impact	Psychiatric Co-morbidities

■ Asthma
■ Cystic fibrosis (CF)
■ Non-CF bronchiectasis
■ Chronic obstructive pulmonary disease
■ Interstitial lung disease, including idiopathic pulmonary fibrosis
■ Neuromuscular disorders
■ Primary ciliary dyskinesia
■ Pulmonary hypertension
	Pharmacologic
	  ■ Bronchodilators
	  ■ Caffeine
	  ■ Calcineurin inhibitors (cyclosporine, tacrolimus)
	  ■ CF transmembrane conductance regulator modulators
	  ■ Montelukast
	  ■ Steroids
	Non-pharmacologic
	  ■ Extracorporeal membrane oxygenation
	  ■ Long-term oxygen therapy
	  ■ Lung transplantation
	  ■ Mechanical ventilation
	  ■ Non-invasive ventilation (Bilevel or continuous positive airway pressure)
	  ■ Tracheostomy
		■ Agitation
		■ Anxiety/panic
		■ Depression
		■ Delirium
		■ Neurocognitive impairment
		■ Post-traumatic stress disorder
		■ Sleep disturbance
		■ Substance use disorders (tobacco, cannabis, alcohol, opiates)

BOX 31.1
NEUROPSYCHIATRIC SIDE EFFECTS ASSOCIATED WITH CFTR MODULATORS

Case 2

Mr. A, a 19-year-old with advanced CF, heterozygous for F508del, was hospitalized for a pulmonary exacerbation after a period of relative stability. Over the prior 2 weeks, he noted a dramatic increase in coughing, dyspnea, and sputum production. Intravenous (IV) antibiotics were added to his outpatient regimen, and his respiratory symptoms improved; however, he engaged minimally in airway clearance and seemed uncharacteristically withdrawn. Psychiatry was consulted to evaluate his depressed mood.

Mr. A and his mother reported that as a child and adolescent, he had no psychiatric symptoms other than moderate anxiety related to medical procedures, although there was a family history of mood and anxiety disorders. His pulmonary health had improved substantially after he started the cystic fibrosis transmembrane conductance regulator (CFTR) modulator elexacaftor/tezacaftor/ivacaftor (ETI) 18 months earlier. However, his mother noted that he had become increasingly irritable since then, which she attributed to "the stress of being a teenager."

When he was interviewed alone, Mr. A reported having symptoms of depression and anxiety, including passive thoughts of suicide and insomnia. Recently, he read a blog post by a person with CF who said she had experienced mental health side effects from the same CFTR modulator that he takes, which resolved when she stopped the medication. As a result, he decided to stop the ETI, and he noticed an immediate improvement in his sleep and anxiety. His mood was also improving until his pulmonary symptoms worsened and he was admitted to the hospital, where the CFTR modulator was ordered by his inpatient team and he began taking it again. Now, he feels uncertain about whether he will continue to take the CFTR modulator, although given his rapid decline off the modulator, he also worries about the implications for his physical health without it. He agreed to share this dilemma with his healthcare team and family.

Mr. A, his mother, the hospitalist, his CF pulmonologist and social worker, and the consulting psychiatrist met to discuss his goals and preferences and to explore the risks and benefits of treatment approaches (including a referral for psychotherapy, starting a selective serotonin reuptake inhibitor (SSRI) for depression and anxiety as well as trazodone (as needed) for insomnia, and discontinuation of off-label dose reduction of ETI. Rather than discontinuing the modulator, he agreed to take a reduced dose while he was hospitalized, so that his response could be monitored closely by his medical team. He also agreed to meet with the psychiatrist as an inpatient and accepted a referral for outpatient psychiatric care at a hospital-associated clinic that had collaborated well with the CF team.

medical outcomes. On the other hand, some patients who are ready to be weaned off LTOT feel particularly anxious about removing this safety measure, which can impede the weaning process.

Patients who experience acute respiratory failure may require intubation and an intensive care unit (ICU) admission, both of which can be traumatic and associated with significant distress. Those who are intubated have a high prevalence of delirium (up to 80%) as well as higher rates of morbidity and mortality.[12] They experience significant pain, anxiety, loss of control and mobility, as well as a perceived loss of dignity that can be demoralizing. Despite their ventilatory needs being met, many patients often perceive dyspnea, which is further discussed in the dyspnea section. Moreover, approximately 20% of those who survive their ICU stay develop post-traumatic stress disorder (PTSD).[13]

In addition to intubation, some patients require extracorporeal membrane oxygenation (ECMO), a complicated, potentially life-saving, treatment that provides oxygenation and circulatory support for those with lung and/or heart failure. Psychiatrists are consulted frequently about patients who are intubated and/or who require ECMO, as they often experience significant distress as well as developing delirium and demoralization. Patients on ECMO acutely face their own mortality, which is typically stressful. Large catheters that protrude from their veins and arteries severely limit movement, even while in bed. These individuals are completely dependent on the assistance of others, and they understand the precariousness of their situation. Thus, it is not surprising that the symptoms of PTSD in long-term survivors have been reported in as many as 41% of such patients.[14] Triggers for PTSD include traumatic memories of their abrupt deterioration before the initiation of ECMO.[14] Moreover, ECMO circuits sequester medications, especially those that are highly protein bound or highly lipophilic.[15] Medication doses used for the treatment of delirium, anxiety, and agitation in patients on ECMO should be carefully titrated, based on their symptoms and scores of validated screening tools that assess delirium, agitation, and pain in sedated patients.[16]

Some patients with pulmonary problems eventually require lung transplantation, which is a treatment to prolong survival and improve their quality of life; however, transplantation does not provide a cure. It is important to appreciate how significant it is to contemplate lung transplantation, to undergo an evaluation, and to wait for approval and availability of donor lungs. While most evaluations for lung transplantation are accomplished in outpatient settings, in cases of emergencies, inpatients may also be evaluated. In such a case, the evaluation process is even more intense, and it requires rapid decision-making. A psychosocial evaluation, which is a regular component of any transplant evaluation, involves addressing psychosocial risk factors that are known to affect post-transplant outcomes (such as a patient's understanding of their illness, the transplant process, and their overall readiness; their support system; mental health issues; substance use disorders; and adherence to medical recommendations). Some of the most frequently used tools to facilitate such evaluations include the Psychosocial Assessment of Candidates for Transplantation,[17] the Stanford Integrated Psychosocial Evaluation for Transplantation (SIPAT),[18] and Transplant Evaluation Rating Scale.[17] Transplant social workers typically perform the initial psychosocial evaluation; if there are ongoing questions about an individual's psychosocial candidacy and/or particular psychiatric concerns, consultation psychiatrists are often consulted.

Undergoing a lung transplant evaluation requires an individual to face their mortality, and it is important for mental health professionals to address patients' fears and concerns. Although patients hope for a good outcome, they also prepare for dying. Referral to, and collaboration with, palliative care is also important. Furthermore, lung transplant recipients have some of the shortest survival times following solid organ transplantation, with a median survival time of approximately 5 years; as a result, these individuals often require support navigating the implications of this reality.[19] Patients can develop persistent anxiety after lung transplantation, which stems from adverse side effects of high-dose steroids and immunosuppressants, adjusting to new lungs while being weaned off of oxygen, and having ongoing existential concerns (including the realization that they have replaced one chronic disease with another). Lung transplant recipients frequently experience panic attacks; with 18% developing panic disorder within 2 years of their lung transplantation, as compared to a rate of 8% in a comparable surgical group, heart transplant recipients.[19] When lung transplant recipients are re-hospitalized for post-transplant complications, psychiatrists are frequently consulted for anxiety, demoralization, and depression.[20]

PRESENTATION AND TREATMENT OF PSYCHIATRIC DISORDERS ASSOCIATED WITH PULMONARY CONDITIONS

Disordered Sleep: Impact of Cough

Coughing is a protective mechanism that safeguards the airways against foreign particles and aids in the clearance of respiratory secretions. However, individuals with a chronic cough are particularly prone to coughing at night; approximately 50% of them report sleep disturbances attributed to their coughing.[21] Coughing can lead to difficulty falling asleep, frequent awakenings, sleep disruption, fragmented sleep, reduced sleep efficiency, and sleep deprivation. These disruptions can have detrimental effects on physical and mental health and interfere with an individual's overall quality of life.[22]

Managing a nocturnal cough involves addressing its underlying causes. For instance, smoking cessation is advised for smokers; proper adherence to inhalers is recommended for individuals with asthma or COPD; use of nasal steroids, antihistamines, and nasal saline irrigation can be beneficial for those with upper airway cough syndrome; and proton pump inhibitors and lifestyle modifications can reduce manifestations of gastroesophageal reflux disease.[23] While our understanding of how coughing adversely impacts sleep is still limited, recognizing and addressing nocturnal cough can contribute to improved sleep quality and overall well-being.[23]

Restless Legs Syndrome

Restless legs syndrome (RLS) is a neurological disorder characterized by an irresistible urge to move one or both legs that is often accompanied by uncomfortable sensations that occur during periods of inactivity and that are relieved by movement. RLS affects up to 15% of adults. Although its pathophysiology is incompletely understood, dysfunction of the dopamine pathway may play a role, and both genetic and environmental factors are believed to be relevant factors. Patients with other medical conditions, such as CF and iron deficiency anemia, are at an elevated risk for RLS.[24] Symptoms of RLS tend to worsen in the evening, which contributes to sleep-onset insomnia and nocturnal awakenings. Sleep disturbances caused by RLS can result in daytime sleepiness, fatigue, and impaired quality of life. Moreover, RLS increases the risk of depression, anxiety, suicide, and self-harm.[25,26]

Although RLS cannot be cured, treatment can alleviate its symptoms and enhance sleep. Making lifestyle adjustments (e.g., engaging in regular exercise, avoiding triggers such as caffeine and alcohol, and practicing good sleep hygiene) can offer relief. It is also advisable to assess and treat iron deficiency anemia. For individuals with persistent RLS, gabapentin analogs and dopamine agonists are treatment options. In cases where symptoms have been unresponsive to the above-mentioned treatments, the use of low-dose opioids can alleviate symptoms.[27] It is also important to consider that certain psychotropic medications, such as dopamine-blocking antipsychotics, can worsen the symptoms of RLS.

Obstructive Sleep Apnea

Obstructive sleep apnea (OSA) is the most prevalent sleep-related breathing disorder; it is characterized by recurring complete or partial collapse of the upper airway during sleep. This leads to apneic episodes, which cause hypoxia and awakenings from sleep. OSA affects approximately 14% of males and 5% of females.[28] Risk factors for OSA include obesity, male gender, advanced age, and abnormalities in the craniofacial structure and upper airway. Common symptoms of OSA include snoring or gasping during sleep, witnessed episodes of breathing cessation, excessive daytime sleepiness, difficulty concentrating, cognitive impairment, mood changes, and morning headaches. Individuals with OSA face an elevated risk of cardiovascular and cerebrovascular diseases (e.g., coronary artery disease, systemic hypertension, pulmonary hypertension, arrhythmias, heart failure, and stroke). In addition, OSA can increase the likelihood of neuropsychiatric disorders, such as depression and psychosis.[28] A systematic review[29] showed that the prevalence of OSA was 48% in patients with major depressive disorder, and 43% in those with post-traumatic stress disorder (PTSD), both rates that are significantly higher than in the general population. Central nervous system (CNS) changes, such as increased sympathetic activity, hyperarousal states, and disrupted sleep patterns associated with these disorders, can lead to instability in the upper airway, potentially contributing to the development of OSA.

The diagnosis of OSA relies on polysomnography, a comprehensive sleep study that measures various physiological parameters throughout sleep. The primary treatment for OSA is continuous positive airway pressure (CPAP), which helps to maintain an open upper airway during sleep, thereby reducing obstructive events.[30] Engaging in regular exercise and losing weight are crucial components of OSA management and these approaches should be combined with CPAP therapy. Patients with OSA should avoid the use of alcohol and sedative medications as they can act as CNS depressants, disrupt sleep architecture, and worsen OSA and daytime sleepiness.

Anxiety

Anxiety is common in patients with respiratory conditions, and it can further reduce one's quality of life. Anxiety disorders are characterized by feelings of worry and fear, ruminative thoughts (with distortion in danger appraisal), and anxious bodily sensations (e.g., shortness of breath, palpitations, nausea, trembling, shaking, butterflies, muscle tension).

Several studies have shown higher rates of psychiatric disorders in patients with pulmonary disorders. Patients with CF are two to three times more likely to have anxiety (22% of adolescents and 32% of adults).[2] In one study, 31% of children with non-CF bronchiectasis had an anxiety disorder.[31] In PCD, the prevalence of anxiety was 6% in adults and adolescents and 14% in children.[32] Up to 50% of patients with asthma are anxious. Patients with COPD are also more predisposed to anxiety, with a systematic review reporting rates of anxiety ranging from 10% to 55% among inpatients and 13% to 46% among outpatients.[33] Patients with pulmonary arterial hypertension have an increased burden of psychological disorders, with

19% to 51% experiencing anxiety and panic attacks.[34] In ILD, the prevalence of anxiety has been reported as being 21% to 60%.[35] In those with NMDs, one study found that anxiety was more common than in those in the general population, and was present in up to 30% of patients with amyotrophic lateral sclerosis.[36]

Multiple factors help to explain the co-morbidity among pulmonary conditions and anxiety. Some medications used to treat respiratory conditions, such as steroids or beta-agonists, can worsen anxiety. In addition, when pulmonary medications are started, medications that have been successfully addressing mental health conditions might become less effective due to drug-drug interactions. Not getting enough air to breathe is quite uncomfortable, and it can lead to acute anxiety, which can increase discomfort. Patients worry, understandably, about developing anxiety symptoms in triggering situations and developing avoidance behaviors that reinforce anxiety. Over the long term, existential distress can also contribute to anxiety, especially as pulmonary diseases progress.

Several hypotheses have been offered to explain the increased co-morbidity between respiratory conditions (such as COPD) and anxiety, especially panic attacks.[37] According to a physiologic model, patients with COPD who are predisposed to panic attacks are particularly sensitive to mild variations in carbon dioxide and pH levels. Increased carbon dioxide levels and a decreased pH activate the limbic system, which is involved in respiratory control as well as defensive anxious behaviors, such as panic attacks.[10] Hyperventilation can lead to reduced carbon dioxide levels and respiratory alkalosis, which precipitates dyspnea and panic attacks.[10] Finally, a cognitive-behavioral model suggests that traumatic COPD exacerbations might serve to sensitize predisposed individuals, leading them to misinterpret normal or near-normal bodily sensations and develop panic disorder.[10]

Selective serotonin reuptake inhibitors (SSRIs) are the mainstay of psychopharmacological treatment for anxiety disorders in the context of respiratory conditions. For example, international guidelines recommend sertraline, fluoxetine, citalopram, and escitalopram as first-line pharmacological interventions in adolescents and adults with CF who require pharmacotherapy for depression or anxiety.[2] SSRIs and nortriptyline (a tricyclic antidepressant [TCA]) have also been effective in the treatment of anxiety in COPD, according to small studies.[38] Mirtazapine, an alpha-2 antagonist with anti-histaminic properties, can also be used in those with anxiety who also have co-morbid disturbances of appetite or insomnia.[10] It can be particularly helpful acutely, for example, during a hospitalization and ICU stay, when anti-histaminic properties can provide immediate relief.

Caution is advised when using psychotropic medications (e.g., benzodiazepines, certain TCAs, sedating antipsychotics) that might promote carbon dioxide retention or decrease respiratory drive in patients with pulmonary conditions, especially when patients are decompensating. Sedating medications can worsen carbon dioxide retention and precipitate respiratory failure. Thus, if these medications are being prescribed, clinicians should start with a low dose and monitor the patient closely. Lorazepam and other shorter half-life benzodiazepines can be used on an as-needed basis, such as for anxiety associated with an acute intervention, and particularly for refractory symptoms, or care at the end of life.[39] Other as-needed medications for acute anxiety include hydroxyzine (an anti-histaminic medication) and gabapentin or pregabalin (calcium channel blockers).

Dyspnea

Dyspnea, the subjective experience of breathing discomfort, is a common symptom in people with respiratory conditions. While the proposed pathophysiology of dyspnea is complex, it can be divided into three mechanisms that underlie brain-lung connectivity facilitating breathing: cortico-brainstem connections leading to air hunger; chemoreceptor sensitivity leading to the perception of increased work of breathing; and stretch receptor sensitivity leading to the perception of chest tightness. When the brain's efforts to adjust ventilation fail to match the lungs' capability to do so, patients might report distinct types of dyspnea based on the affected mechanism.[40] This feeling is influenced by current medical factors, and by prior experiences, belief systems, and emotions.[41] Dyspnea occurs in outpatients and inpatients and is especially common among patients on ventilatory support and ECMO in the ICU. In a recent study of lung transplant recipients, 63% were found to be dyspneic according to provider reports.[42] Dyspnea, which relies on a patient's

self-report, is often underdiagnosed; moreover, it is even harder to identify in non-communicative ICU patients, which leads to an underestimation of patients' suffering by providers.

The first step in the management of dyspnea is to understand and treat any medical processes that can contribute to this sensation (e.g., pneumothorax, pneumonia, fever, anemia). Next, ventilatory settings should be addressed with ICU physicians and respiratory therapists. Finally, pharmacological and non-pharmacological interventions should be considered. While the only medication class that has been shown to reduce dyspnea is opiates, treatment of associated anxiety also improves quality of life.[43] Anxiety is almost 10 times more common in those who are experiencing dyspnea.[43] Medications that can be used to treat anxiety associated with dyspnea include SSRIs and mirtazapine when longer-term treatment of dyspnea is anticipated, but alpha-2 agonists (e.g., guanfacine), calcium channel blockers (e.g., pregabalin, gabapentin), and anti-histaminic medications (e.g., hydroxyzine, quetiapine) can be helpful more acutely. Care must be taken while mitigating dyspnea and anxiety to ensure that the patient does not become too sedated and develop respiratory depression. Non-pharmacological interventions include proper positioning of the patient, use of a fan if allowed by infection control, and relaxation techniques. Education and validation of the experience are important as well (Box 31.2).

Post-traumatic Stress

Many patients with progressive respiratory conditions grapple with their impending mortality and experience events that act as existential threats. Such events (e.g., hemoptysis) are common among people with CF, as are ICU stays, with invasive interventions (e.g., intubation, ECMO) that challenge one's sense of safety and thus may lead to PTSD. Predisposing factors for post-ICU PTSD include delirium, use of benzodiazepines, and prior psychopathology. ICU diaries, which can be created by family members, friends, or nurses to document the events of the hospital stay, can decrease post-ICU PTSD. They help patients integrate their memories with recorded events and make meaning out of their painful and distressing experiences.[44]

BOX 31.2
MANAGEMENT OF DYSPNEA AND ANXIETY

Case 2

Ms. B, a 62-year-old woman, underwent lung transplantation for ILD. Four days later, she was diagnosed with primary graft dysfunction, and slow weaning from the ventilator was required. With an expected prolonged hospital course, she had a tracheostomy. While she was supported with ventilation, the team had a difficult time decreasing her pressure support requirements. Whenever her pressure support was decreased, she felt like she was not getting enough air to breathe and became increasingly anxious. Although she maintained an oxygen saturation of 98% with a FiO_2 of 30%, her heart rate was 80 beats per minute, her blood pressure was 135/82 mm Hg, and her respiratory rate was 20 breaths per minute. Her medications included prednisone (20 mg twice per day) and a dexmedetomidine drip for anxiety. She received as-needed oxycodone for pain.

Psychiatry was consulted for anxiety that limited her weaning off the ventilator. While there were no acute processes that contributed to her presentation, her primary graft dysfunction was impeding her lung-brain communication, sending the signals to the brain that her lungs were unable to take full breaths. In addition, high doses of prednisone further worsened her anxiety, which was already provoked by dyspnea. Finally, she had existential concerns about her survival, which contributed to her overall anxiety. She was evaluated for delirium with a neurocognitive assessment and was found to be cognitively intact.

The consulting psychiatrist validated the patient's feelings, taught guided imagery to help reduce her acute anxiety, provided education about the interplay of dyspnea and anxiety in the context of her situation, and explained the importance of ongoing rehabilitation with slowly decreasing pressures. The psychiatrist recommended to the team to schedule oxycodone for pain and dyspnea. The psychiatrist also advised the team to use guanfacine to help taper the patient from dexmedetomidine and to help with anxiety, as well as pregabalin to help with pain and anxiety, and as-needed hydroxyzine.

Depression

Depression is characterized by low mood, a reduced ability to experience pleasure (anhedonia), and physical and emotional fatigue.[10] Demoralization, which is common in seriously ill individuals, is marked by feelings of disempowerment, helplessness, disappointment at having failed one's own or someone else's expectations, and viewing oneself as a burden; it can co-exist with depression.[10] Consequently, depressive symptomology can impair quality of life, adherence, and treatment outcomes.[10] Individuals with pulmonary disease who are facing disease progression may be at particular risk and should be screened for depression as part of a comprehensive needs assessment; this can be accomplished with a tool such as the Integrated Palliative Care Outcome Scale.[45]

Treatment of depression in those with pulmonary disease involves the use of tailored interventions. Antidepressants can be prescribed alongside psychotherapeutic strategies (such as cognitive re-structuring, providing religious and spiritual support, and exploring values and hopes in life).[10] If patients are approaching the end of their life, existential therapies, such as dignity therapy, can be particularly helpful.

Delirium

Delirium is a common neuropsychiatric condition that is characterized by impaired attention and other neuropsychological and behavioral symptoms. Inpatients with respiratory disorders are at an especially high risk for developing delirium due to risk factors that include older age, problems with oxygenation, and use of various pharmacologic agents (e.g., anticholinergic medications, steroids, sympathomimetics, opioids, antibiotics).[10] Patients undergoing lung transplantation have a 45% incidence of delirium within the week following transplantation.[10] Certain medications, such as benzodiazepines, while helpful for anxiety, can also increase the risk of delirium, and thus, if possible, they should be tapered and discontinued when patients undergo surgery. As stated above, delirium can also increase the risk of post-ICU PTSD, a fact that highlights the importance of preventing, detecting, and treating delirium.

Cognitive Impairment

Patients with progressive pulmonary conditions frequently experience a deterioration of their thinking, which is likely due to persistent hypoxia and hypercapnia, as well as to cardiovascular risk factors.

For example, patients with COPD have an increased prevalence of cognitive dysfunction, which correlates with illness severity.[10] A study of 46 patients with pulmonary arterial hypertension who had their cognitive function evaluated found that 58% had some impairment in verbal learning, verbal memory, and executive function.[46] Of patients awaiting lung transplantation, 47% have cognitive impairment.[10] This is important as cognitive dysfunction adversely affects the quality of life and independence, identifies more severe disease and the likely need for a caregiver, and is a risk factor for delirium.

Substance Use

The use of inhaled tobacco, electronic cigarettes (e-cigarettes), and inhaled cannabis is prevalent among those with pulmonary conditions, and it has serious implications regarding medical status and transplantation.[47,48] Exposure to secondhand smoke (SHS) also has detrimental effects on lung health, especially in children, and those with pre-existing pulmonary conditions (e.g., children with asthma and CF) are especially vulnerable. A 2015 meta-analysis found that SHS can trigger asthma exacerbations and children with asthma who were exposed to SHS were twice as likely to be hospitalized and significantly more likely to have lower pulmonary function test results.[49] A recent study of pediatric CF patients found that tobacco exposure may independently predict pulmonary decline and lower levels of lung function.[50] People with pulmonary disease and their families should be screened for tobacco use and exposure during hospitalizations. A variety of smoking cessation products are available (both over the counter and by prescription). Nicotine replacement product dosage forms include a topical patch, gum, lozenges, nasal spray, and inhalers. In addition, non-nicotine medications (such as varenicline and bupropion) can be prescribed.

Similarly, lung health is compromised by excessive alcohol use, which increases one's risk of pulmonary infections by suppressing immune responses.[51] Adverse effects on respiratory health have also been observed in people who use opiates, which affect central respiratory centers in the brain.[52] A survey of 1135 adults with CF determined that 77% drink alcohol and 54% of those who used alcohol met the criteria for an alcohol use disorder.[53] Adults with CF who misused substances (either alcohol or opiates) missed their outpatient CF visits more frequently, had more frequent "sick" visits, had more frequent and longer hospitalizations, and had a higher mortality rate than those who did not misuse these substances.[54] As noted above, substance misuse is a modifiable factor with implications for lung transplant eligibility.

CONSIDERATIONS FOR PRESCRIBING PSYCHOPHARMACOLOGIC AGENTS IN THE CONTEXT OF PULMONARY DISEASE

Pulmonary diseases can be treated with a bevy of medications. When considering treatment for psychiatric conditions in those with pulmonary disorders, potential drug-drug interactions should be considered. Common interactions involve the use of pulmonary and psychiatric drugs (Table 31.2).[55]

CONCLUSION

Patients with pulmonary diseases are frequently seen in general hospital settings, and they commonly experience anxiety, depression, PTSD, delirium, and cognitive symptoms. Exposure to tobacco smoke and substance misuse are associated with worse health outcomes and have implications for lung transplantation eligibility. Psychiatrists should be vigilant for existential concerns that accompany disease progression, as well as distress related to respiratory symptoms (e.g., dyspnea) and pulmonary therapies, such as the use of long-term oxygen and intubation. Neuropsychiatric effects can also be caused by pulmonary medications. Psychiatric symptoms in patients with pulmonary disease can generally be managed with usual treatments (e.g., antidepressants for depression/anxiety), by avoiding respiratory depression from sedating medications, and polypharmacy.

TABLE 31.2
Drug-Drug Interactions Specific to Pulmonary and Psychiatric Drugs[a]

Substrates

1A2	2B6	2C8	2C9	2C19	2D6	2E1	3A457
Amitriptyline	Bupropion	Olodaterol	Amitriptyline	Amitriptyline	Amitriptyline	Theophylline	Alprazolam
Clomipramine	Clobazam	Selexipag	Doxepin	Atomoxetine	Amphetamine		Amitriptyline
Clozapine			Fluoxetine	Citalopram	Aripiprazole		Aripiprazole
Doxepin			Fluvastatin	Clobazam	Brexipiprazole		Astemizole
Duloxetine			Olodaterol	Clomipramine	Cariprazine		Brexipiprazole
Fluvoxamine			Venlafaxine	Doxepin	Chlorpheniramine		Buspirone
Haloperidol			Zafirlukast	Escitalopram	Chlorpromazine		Caffeine
Imipramine				Hexobarbital	Citalopram		Cariprazine
Olanzapine				Imipramine	Clomipramine		Chlorpheniramine
Pirfenidone				Moclobemide	Desipramine		Citalopram
Riluzole				Venlafaxine	Dextromethorphan		Cyclosporine
Roflumilast				Vilazodone	Doxepin		Deflazacort
Theophylline					Duloxetine		Dexamethasone
Zileuton					Eliglustat		Dextromethorphan
					Escitalopram		Doxepin
					Fluoxetine		Elexacaftor
					Haloperidol		Eliglustat
					Imipramine		Escitalopram
					Methoxyamphatamine		Felodipine
					Minaprine		Haloperidol
					Nortriptyline		Hydrocortisone
					Paroxetine		Indacaterol
					Perphenazine		Ivacaftor
					Pimavanserin		Macitentan
					Risperidone		Pimavanserin
					Umeclidinium		Pimozide
					Venlafaxine		Quetiapine
					Vilazodone		Risperidone
					Zuclopenthixol		Roflumilast
							Salmeterol
							Selexipag
							Sildenafil
							Suvorexant
							Tacrolimus (FK506)
							Terfenadine
							Tezacaftor
							Trazodone
							Venlafaxine
							Vilazodone
							Ziprasidone
							Zolpidem

(Continued)

TABLE 31.2
Drug-Drug Interactions Specific to Pulmonary and Psychiatric Drugs[a]—Cont'd

Inhibitors

1A2	2B6	2C8	2C9	2C19	2D6	2E1	3A457
Citalopram		Montelukast	Fluvoxamine	Citalopram	Bupropion	Quercetin	Grapefruit juice
Fluvoxamine		Quercetin	Quercetin	Fluoxetine	Chlorpromazine		Ivacaftor
Furafylline			Zafirlukast	Fluvoxamine	Citalopram		Nefazodone
				Modafinil	Clemastine		Quercetin
				Quercetin	Clobazam		Star fruit
					Clomipramine		
					Diphenhydramine		
					Doxepin		
					Duloxetine		
					Escitalopram		
					Fluoxetine		
					Haloperidol		
					Hydroxyzine		
					Levomepromazine		
					Moclobemide		
					Paroxetine		
					Perphenazine		
					Sertraline		
					Tripelennamine		

Inducers

1A2	2B6	2C8	2C9	2C19	2D6	2E1	3A457
Beta-naphtoflavone	Lumacaftor	Lumacaftor	Lumacaftor	Lumacaftor		Ethanol	
Broccoli	Roflumilast		St. John's wort	Prednisone			Clobazam
Brussel sprouts				St. John's wort			Glucocorticoids
Char-grilled meat							Lumacaftor
Terifluomide							St. John's wort
Tobacco							

Inhibitor Key

Strong inhibitor	causes a ≥five-fold increase in the plasma area under the curve (AUC) values or >80% decrease in clearance
Moderate inhibitor	causes two-fold to five-fold increase in plasma AUC or a 50%–80% decrease in clearance
Weak inhibitor	causes a ≥1.25 but <two-fold increase in plasma AUC or a 20%–50% decrease in clearance
In vitro only	In vitro only inhibitor strength

[a]This table was adapted from the Flockhart table and includes select drugs that are commonly used for the treatment of pulmonary or psychiatric diseases.[55]

REFERENCES

1. Thomas M, Bruton A, Moffat M, et al. Asthma and psychological dysfunction. *Prim Care Respir J.* 2011;20(3):250–256. https://doi.org/10.4104/pcrj.2011.00058. PMID: 21674122; PMCID: PMC6549858.

2. Quittner AL, Abbott J, Georgiopoulos AM, International Committee on Mental Health, et al. International Committee on Mental Health in Cystic Fibrosis: Cystic Fibrosis Foundation and European Cystic Fibrosis Society consensus statements for screening and treating depression and anxiety. *Thorax.* 2016;71(1):26–34. https://doi.org/10.1136/thoraxjnl-2015-207488. Epub 2015 Oct 9. PMID: 26452630; PMCID: PMC4717439.

3. Balcells E, Gea J, Ferrer J, PAC-COPD Study Group., et al. Factors affecting the relationship between psychological status and quality of life in COPD patients. *Health Qual Life Outcomes.* 2010;8:108. https://doi.org/10.1186/1477-7525-8-108. PMID: 20875100; PMCID: PMC2957389.

4. Olsson KM, Meltendorf T, Fuge J, et al. Prevalence of mental disorders and impact on quality of life in patients with pulmonary arterial hypertension. *Front Psychiatry.* 2021;12:667602. https://doi.org/10.3389/fpsyt.2021.667602. PMID: 34135787; PMCID: PMC8200462.

5. van Groenestijn AC, Kruitwagen-van Reenen ET, Visser-Meily JM, et al. Associations between psychological factors and health-related quality of life and global quality of life in patients with ALS: a systematic review. *Health Qual Life Outcomes.* 2016;14(1):107. https://doi.org/10.1186/s12955-016-0507-6. PMID: 27439463; PMCID: PMC4955215.

6. Sher Y, Charoenpong P, Weinstein SJ, et al. Psychiatric care of patients with pulmonary disease. In: Stern TA, Wilens TE, Fava M, eds. *Massachusetts General Hospital Comprehensive Clinical Psychiatry.* 3rd ed. Elsevier; 2025:527–537.

7. Y Sher, AM Georgiopoulos, TA Stern. *Facing Cystic Fibrosis: a Guide for Patients and their Families.* Massachusetts General Hospital Psychiatry Academy; 2020.

8. Warrington TP, Bostwick JM. Psychiatric adverse effects of corticosteroids. *Mayo Clin Proc.* 2006;81(10):1361–1367. https://doi.org/10.4065/81.10.1361. PMID: 17036562.

9. Spoletini G, Gillgrass L, Pollard K, et al. Dose adjustments of Elexacaftor/Tezacaftor/Ivacaftor in response to mental health side effects in adults with cystic fibrosis. *J Cyst Fibros.* 2022;21(6):1061–1065. https://doi.org/10.1016/j.jcf.2022.05.001. Epub 2022 May 16. PMID: 35585012.

10. Sher Y. Psychiatric aspects of lung disease in critical care. *Crit Care Clin.* 2017;33(3):601–617. https://doi.org/10.1016/j.ccc.2017.03.014.

11. Goldbart J, Yohannes AM, Woolrych R, et al. 'It is not going to change his life but it has picked him up': a qualitative study of perspectives on long term oxygen therapy for people with chronic obstructive pulmonary disease. *Health Qual Life Outcomes.* 2013;11:124. Published 2013 Jul 25. https://doi.org/10.1186/1477-7525-11-124.

12. Ely EW, Shintani A, Truman B, et al. Delirium as a predictor of mortality in mechanically ventilated patients in the intensive care unit. *JAMA.* 2004;291(14):1753–1762. https://doi.org/10.1001/jama.291.14.1753.

13. Davydow DS, Gifford JM, Desai SV, et al. Posttraumatic stress disorder in general intensive care unit survivors: a systematic review. *Gen Hosp Psychiatry.* 2008;30(5):421–434. https://doi.org/10.1016/j.genhosppsych.2008.05.006. Epub 2008 Jul 30. PMID: 18774425; PMCID: PMC2572638.

14. Tramm R, Ilic D, Murphy K, et al. A qualitative exploration of acute care and psychological distress experiences of ECMO survivors. *Heart Lung.* 2016;45(3):220–226. https://doi.org/10.1016/j.hrtlng.2016.01.010.

15. Patel JS, Kooda K, Igneri LA. A narrative review of the impact of extracorporeal membrane oxygenation on the pharmacokinetics and pharmacodynamics of critical care therapies. *Ann Pharmacother.* 2023;57(6):706–726. https://doi.org/10.1177/10600280221126438. Epub 2022 Oct 15. PMID: 36250355.

16. Kusi-Appiah E, Karanikola M, Pant U, et al. Tools for assessment of acute psychological distress in critical illness: a scoping review. *Aust Crit Care.* 2021;34(5):460–472. https://doi.org/10.1016/j.aucc.2020.12.003. Epub 2021 Feb 27. PMID: 33648818.

17. Presberg BA, Levenson JL, Olbrisch ME, Best AM. Rating scales for the psychosocial evaluation of organ transplant candidates. Comparison of the PACT and TERS with bone marrow transplant patients. *Psychosomatics.* 1995;36(5):458–461. https://doi.org/10.1016/S0033-3182(95)71626-7.

18. Maldonado JR, Dubois HC, David EE, et al. The Stanford Integrated Psychosocial Assessment for Transplantation (SIPAT): a new tool for the psychosocial evaluation of pre-transplant candidates. *Psychosomatics.* 2012;53(2):123–132. https://doi.org/10.1016/j.psym.2011.12.012.

19. Bos S, Vos R, Van Raemdonck DE, et al. Survival in adult lung transplantation: where are we in 2020? *Curr Opin Organ Transplant.* 2020;25(3):268–273. https://doi.org/10.1097/MOT.0000000000000753. PMID: 32332197.

20. Dew MA, DiMartini AF, DeVito Dabbs AJ, et al. Onset and risk factors for anxiety and depression during the first 2 years after lung transplantation. *Gen Hosp Psychiatry.* 2012;34(2):127–138. https://doi.org/10.1016/j.genhosppsych.2011.11.009. Epub 2012 Jan 14. PMID: 22245165; PMCID: PMC3288337.

21. Lee KK, Birring SS. Cough and sleep. *Lung.* 2010;188(suppl 1):S91–94. https://doi.org/10.1007/s00408-009-9176-0. Epub 2009 Oct 13. PMID: 19823913.

22. Won HK, Lee JH, An J, et al. Impact of chronic cough on health-related quality of life in the Korean adult general population: the Korean National Health and Nutrition Examination Survey 2010-2016. *Allergy Asthma Immunol Res.* 2020;12(6):964–979. https://doi.org/10.4168/aair.2020.12.6.964. PMID: 32935489; PMCID: PMC7492512.

23. Singh DP, Jamil RT, Mahajan K. *Nocturnal Cough. StatPearls [Internet].* StatPearls Publishing; 2023. PMID: 30335306.

24. Jurisch P, Gall H, Richter MJ, et al. Increased frequency of the restless legs syndrome in adults with cystic fibrosis. *Respir Med.* 2019;151:8–10. https://doi.org/10.1016/j.rmed.2019.03.009. Epub 2019 Mar 23. PMID: 31047121.

25. Winkelmann J, Prager M, Lieb R, et al. "Anxietas tibiarum". Depression and anxiety disorders in patients with restless legs syndrome. *J Neurol.* 2005;252(1):67–71. https://doi.org/10.1007/s00415-005-0604-7. PMID: 15654556.

26. Zhuang S, Na M, Winkelman JW, et al. Association of restless legs syndrome with risk of suicide and self-harm. *JAMA Netw Open.* 2019;2(8):e199966. https://doi.org/10.1001/jamanetwork open.2019.9966. PMID: 31441941; PMCID: PMC6714009.

27. Silber MH, Buchfuhrer MJ, Earley CJ, Scientific and Medical Advisory Board of the Restless Legs Syndrome Foundation, et al. The management of restless legs syndrome: an updated algorithm. *Mayo Clin Proc.* 2021;96(7):1921–1937. https://doi. org/10.1016/j.mayocp.2020.12.026. PMID: 34218864.

28. Kapur VK, Auckley DH, Chowdhuri S, et al. Clinical practice guideline for diagnostic testing for adult obstructive sleep apnea: an American Academy of Sleep Medicine Clinical Practice Guideline. *J Clin Sleep Med.* 2017;13(3):479–504. https://doi.org/10.5664/jcsm.6506. PMID: 28162150; PMCID: PMC5337595.

29. Gupta MA, Simpson FC. Obstructive sleep apnea and psychiatric disorders: a systematic review. *J Clin Sleep Med.* 2015;11(2): 165–175. https://doi.org/10.5664/jcsm.4466. PMID: 25406268; PMCID: PMC4298774.

30. Epstein LJ, Kristo D, Strollo PJ Jr, Adult Obstructive Sleep Apnea Task Force of the American Academy of Sleep Medicine, et al. Clinical guideline for the evaluation, management and long-term care of obstructive sleep apnea in adults. *J Clin Sleep Med.* 2009;5(3):263–276. PMID: 19960649; PMCID: PMC2699173.

31. Ceyhan B, Bekir M, Kocakaya D, et al. The predictive role of psychological and disease severity indexes on quality of life among patients with non-CF bronchiectasis. *Turk Thorac J.* 2022;23(1): 17–24. https://doi.org/10.5152/TurkThoracJ.2021.21142. PMID: 35110196; PMCID: PMC9450191.

32. Verkleij M, Appelman I, Altenburg J, et al. Anxiety and depression in Dutch patients with primary ciliary dyskinesia and their caregivers: associations with health-related quality of life. *ERJ Open Res.* 2021;7(4):00274–2021. https://doi.org/10.1183/ 23120541.00274-2021. PMID: 34708110; PMCID: PMC8542938.

33. Willgross TG, Yohannes AM. Anxiety disorders in patients with COPD: a systematic review. *Respiratory Care.* 2013;58(5): 858–866. https://doi.org/10.4187/respcare.01862.

34. Bussotti M, Sommaruga M. Anxiety and depression in patients with pulmonary hypertension: impact and management challenges. *Vasc Health Risk Manag.* 2018;14:349–360.

35. Yohannes AM. Depression and anxiety in patients with interstitial lung disease. *Expert Rev Respir Med.* 2020;14(9): 859–862. https://doi.org/10.1080/17476348.2020.1776118. Epub 2020 Jun 12. PMID: 32460643.

36. Kurt A, Nijboer F, Matuz T, et al. Depression and anxiety in individuals with amyotrophic lateral sclerosis: epidemiology and management. *CNS Drugs.* 2007;21(4):279–291. https://doi. org/10.2165/00023210-200721040-00003. PMID: 17381183.

37. Pumar MI, Gray CR, Walsh JR, et al. Anxiety and depression-important psychological comorbidities of COPD. *J Thorac Dis.* 2014;6(11):1615–1631. https://doi.org/10.3978/j.issn.2072-1439. 2014.09.28. PMID: 25478202; PMCID: PMC4255157.

38. Tselebis A, Pachi A, Ilias I, et al. Strategies to improve anxiety and depression in patients with COPD: a mental health perspective. *Neuropsychiatr Dis Treat.* 2016;12:297–328. https:// doi.org/10.2147/NDT.S79354. Published 2016 Feb 9.

39. Kapnadak SG, Dimango E, Hadjiliadis D, et al. Cystic Fibrosis Foundation consensus guidelines for the care of individuals with advanced cystic fibrosis lung disease. *J Cyst Fibros.* 2020;19(3):344–354. https://doi.org/10.1016/j.jcf.2020.02.015. Epub 2020 Feb 27. PMID: 32115388.

40. Nishino T. Dyspnoea: underlying mechanisms and treatment. *Br J Anaesth.* 2011;106(4):463–474. https://doi.org/10.1093/bja/ aer040.

41. Schmidt M, Banzett RB, Raux M, et al. Unrecognized suffering in the ICU: addressing dyspnea in mechanically ventilated patients. *Intensive Care Med.* 2014;40(1):1–10. https://doi.org/ 10.1007/s00134-013-3117-3.

42. Sato T, Tanaka S, Akazawa C, et al. Provider-documented dyspnea in intensive care unit after lung transplantation. *Transplant Proc.* 2022;54(8):2337–2343. https://doi.org/10.1016/ j.transproceed.2022.08.034.

43. Jennings AL, Davies AN, Higgins JP, et al. A systematic review of the use of opioids in the management of dyspnoea. *Thorax.* 2002;57(11):939–944. https://doi.org/10.1136/thorax.57.11.939.

44. Jones C, Bäckman C, Capuzzo M, et al. Intensive care diaries reduce new onset post- traumatic stress disorder following critical illness: a randomised, controlled trial. *Crit Care.* 2010;14(5):R168. https://doi.org/10.1186/cc9260.

45. Kavalieratos D, Georgiopoulos AM, Dhingra L, et al. Models of palliative care delivery for individuals with cystic fibrosis: Cystic Fibrosis Foundation evidence-informed consensus guidelines. *J Palliat Med.* 2021;24(1):18–30. https://doi.org/10.1089/jpm. 2020.0311. Epub 2020 Sep 16. PMID: 32936045; PMCID: PMC77 57696.

46. White J, Hopkins RO, Glissmeyer EW, et al. Cognitive ECG. Cognitive, emotional, and quality of life outcomes in patients with pulmonary arterial hypertension. *Respir Res.* 2006;7(1):55.

47. Wills TA, Soneji SS, Choi K, et al. E-cigarette use and respiratory disorders: an integrative review of converging evidence from epidemiological and laboratory studies. *Eur Respir J.* 2021;57(1):1901815. https://doi.org/10.1183/13993003.01815- 2019. Published 2021 Jan 21.

48. Tashkin DP, Roth MD. Pulmonary effects of inhaled cannabis smoke. *Am J Drug Alcohol Abuse.* 2019;45(6):596–609. https:// doi.org/10.1080/00952990.2019.1627366.

49. Wang Z, May SM, Charoenlap S, et al. Effects of secondhand smoke exposure on asthma morbidity and health care utilization in children: a systematic review and meta-analysis. *Ann Allergy Asthma Immunol.* 2015;115(5):396–401.e2. https://doi. org/10.1016/j.anai.2015.08.005. Epub 2015 Sep 26. PMID: 26411971.

50. Oates GR, Baker E, Rowe SM, et al. Tobacco smoke exposure and socioeconomic factors are independent predictors of pulmonary decline in pediatric cystic fibrosis. *J Cyst Fibros.* 2020;19(5): 783–790. https://doi.org/10.1016/j.jcf.2020.02.004.

51. Mehta AJ, Guidot DM. Alcohol and the lung. *Alcohol Res.* 2017;38(2):243–254.

52. Dublin S, Walker RL, Jackson ML, et al. Use of opioids or benzodiazepines and risk of pneumonia in older adults: a population-based case-control study. *J Am Geriatr Soc.* 2011;59(10):1899–1907.

53. Lowery EM, Afshar M, West N, et al. Self-reported alcohol use in the cystic fibrosis community. *J Cyst Fibros.* 2020;19(1):84–90. https://doi.org/10.1016/j.jcf.2019.06.004. Epub 2019 Jul 11. PMID: 31303381; PMCID: PMC7351178.

54. Richards CJ, Friedman D, Pinsky H, et al. Alcohol and opiate misuse in adults with cystic fibrosis. *Pediatr Pulmonol.* 2023:9. https://doi.org/10.1002/ppul.26541. Epub ahead of print. PMID: 37294071.

55. Flockhart DA, Thacker D, McDonald C, et al. The Flockhart cytochrome P450 drug-drug interaction table. Division of Clinical Pharmacology, Indiana University School of Medicine (Updated 2021). https://drug-interactions.medicine.iu.edu.

32

BURNS, TRAUMA, AND INTENSIVE CARE UNIT TREATMENT

ASHIKA BAINS, MD ■ MLADEN NISAVIC, MD

OVERVIEW

Burns and traumatic injuries are a significant source of morbidity and mortality in the United States. Many afflicted individuals require psychiatric management that can be as challenging as their surgical care. Unrecognized and untreated underlying psychiatric conditions are associated with worse outcomes and increased morbidity and mortality in those with burns and other traumatic injuries. Moreover, caring for these patients can be painful for providers as they witness the distress of children and adults who have suffered from traumatic and, at times, life-threatening experiences. These feelings moderate as providers work to relieve pain, facilitate survival, and see improvement in disfiguring scars. Psychiatric education of providers around disasters and traumatic experiences is crucial to enhance resilience and increase preparedness.[1,2] Burn units and intensive care units (ICUs) bring together specialists from myriad disciplines to practice collaboratively.

HISTORY

The concept of a dedicated intensive care ward arose in 1953 when the anesthetist Bjorn Ibsen (who had suggested positive pressure ventilation for the treatment of patients during the Copenhagen polio epidemic) created the first ICU in Europe.[3] In that era, medical students were employed to hand ventilate the lungs of patients who required artificial ventilation through a tracheostomy.[3] Since then, critical care has grown as a specialty and developed into the multi-disciplinary field that it is today, with dedicated ICU physicians, nurses, physiotherapists,

pharmacists, dietitians, and technicians. Similarly, biomedical research and knowledge in burn care have flourished (e.g., recognizing the relationship between the size of a burn and mortality, the importance of burn surface area and skin grafting, and the use of antibiotics to prevent sepsis associated with severe burns).[4]

In 1943 Cobb and Lindemann,[5] early Massachusetts General Hospital psychiatrists, collaborated with other physicians and chronicled the deliria and post-traumatic reactions of the Cocoanut Grove fire survivors (a tragedy in which 491 people died). Lindemann,[6] in a classic paper (based in part on his work with 13 bereaved victims of the Cocoanut Grove fire and with relatives of those who served in the armed forces), reported for the first time on the symptoms and psychotherapeutic management of acute grief. These studies described the course of survivors, their children, and other relatives, and how their survivor guilt, traumatic grief, and post-traumatic stress disorder (PTSD) were treated.

BURN INJURIES

Epidemiology

An estimated 486,000 people are treated each year in the United States for burn-related injuries; roughly 40,000 of them are hospitalized for their burn-related injuries.[7] Currently, there are 128 designated burn treatment centers in the United States; the annual average number of admissions to each of these centers is approximately 200. Fortunately, statistics from 2005 to 2014 revealed an overall survival rate from burn injuries of 96.8%.[7] Demographically, roughly two-thirds (68%) of burn victims are males, and their mean age is 32 years. A bimodal age distribution for those who have sustained burn injuries has been observed, with most injuries occurring in children (aged 1–15.9 years) and adults (aged 20–59 years).[7,8] Most burns occur in the home (73%); the remainder of burn injuries occur at work (8%), on the street or the highway (5%), during recreational activities (5%), while 9% are designated as occurring in "other locations." Among those who require an inpatient admission, burns are most often related to flames (43%) and scald injuries (34%), while they occur less commonly from contact (9%), electrical (4%), chemical (3%), or other causes.[7]

Risk Factors

A combination of developmental and familial factors contributes to the risk of burns in children, including young age (<5 years old), male gender in younger children, non-White ethnicity, immigrant status, living in a single-parent family, having a low parental or guardian education level, unemployment in the parents, having poor living conditions, having a psychiatric diagnosis in childhood, and having a low socioeconomic status.[8–10] Most burns in pediatric patients occur due to contact with hot liquids (scald injuries) or hot objects (thermal injuries).[11,12] Burns in children most often involve the hands, legs, feet, and buttocks (Table 32.1).[11,12]

TABLE 32.1
Risk Factors for Burns in Children and Adolescents

Abuse/neglect

Immigrant status

Lack of employment among parents

Learning disabilities in child

Low parental/guardian education levels

Low socioeconomic status

Male gender in younger children

Non-White ethnicity

Psychiatric diagnosis in child (MDD, ODD, ADHD)[a]

Single-parent family

Unsafe housing

Young age (<5 years)

[a]Based on a representative sample in the United Kingdom.
ADHD, Attention-deficit hyperactivity disorder; *MDD,* major depressive disorder; *ODD,* oppositional defiant disorder.

Burns to children should not be labeled indiscriminately as a consequence of neglect or abuse, as they may result from a combination of developmental, environmental, and family variables. However, burns from neglect or abuse account for up to one-third of all pediatric burn injuries. Up to 45% of genital and perineal burns have been attributed to domestic violence. The age of maximum risk for abuse is 13 to 24 months, and scalds are the most common cause of burn injuries.[13] Factors that suggest abuse include an inconsistent history from the caregiver, a patient's history of repeated and similar injuries, a burn pattern with a clear shape from contact with a hot object, a pattern with a sharp stocking-and-glove demarcation (e.g., from forced immersion), sparing of flexed areas (protected), and other signs of violence (e.g., fractures) (Table 32.2).[12,13] If abuse or neglect is suspected, physicians must report (in most states) their concerns to the appropriate state agency.

Among adults, risk factors for burns include drug and alcohol intoxication and dependence, a major mental illness, an antisocial personality disorder, and exposure to occupational hazards (Table 32.3).[14–17] Nonintentional burn injuries occur more often in males than in females and are associated with low socioeconomic status, substance use and intoxication, and a low level of education.[11] The homeless and the elderly are more apt to suffer burns.[18,19] Homeless individuals have a higher rate of burn injuries due to assault (fourfold higher), self-inflicted injury (twofold higher), mental illness, and substance use.[20] Scald injuries are more common in elderly individuals with dementia and they typically occur during activities of daily living (ADLs).[21]

TABLE 32.2
Factors Suggestive of Abuse/Neglect in Burned Children

Inconsistent history from the caregiver

Patient history of recurrent similar injuries

Burn pattern with a clear shape from contact with a hot object (e.g., iron, cigarette)

Burn pattern of sharp stocking-and-glove demarcation (e.g., forced immersion)

Sparing of protected flexed areas

Other signs of violence (e.g., fractures)

Low socioeconomic status is a shared risk factor across all populations, regardless of age. Advancing age and the presence of an inhalation injury pose a significant risk of dying from a burn injury. For those under the age of 60 years, with a total body surface area (TBSA) burn between 0.1% and 19.9%, the presence of an inhalation injury increases the likelihood of death by nearly 24-fold. The most common complications of burn treatment are pneumonia, respiratory failure, cellulitis, septicemia, and wound infection; the risk of complications increases with the duration of the hospital stay. Risk factors for a higher mortality rate from burn injuries include the extent of the TBSA involved, older age, and the presence of an inhalation injury.[12] In those with severe burns (i.e., TBSA >70%): sepsis, thrombocytopenia ($<20,000/mm^3$), and ventilator dependency are independent risk factors for mortality.[22] Pre-existing frailty has also been associated with adverse outcomes among the elderly, as these individuals have a decreased level of organ perfusion and oxygenation in the acute phases of injury and are more susceptible to factors associated with increased mortality (e.g., infection, mental status changes, malnutrition).[8]

TYPES OF BURNS

Burns are classified by the depth of the injury (from first-degree to fourth-degree burns) with increasing depth being linked with an increased risk of complications. First-degree burns are characterized by an intact epithelium (i.e., the skin is pink, dry, and painful without blistering or scarring); these burns require no specific care. Second-degree burns are subdivided into superficial or deep. Superficial partial-thickness second-degree burns are painful, pink to red, and edematous; these may require dressing changes and wound care Deep partial-thickness second-degree burns indicate damage to the dermis; these injuries are less painful (due to injury of pain receptors), drier, and may require surgery. Laser Doppler imaging is a widely accepted method for early and accurate assessment of burn depth. Third-degree (full-thickness) burns of the dermis are leathery, dry, and lack sensation; these burns require surgical treatment. The most severe burns are fourth-degree burns; these extend through the subcutaneous tissue to the tendons, muscles, and bones, and they require complex surgical reconstruction (Table 32.4). A burn injury is designated as severe based on the percentage of the TBSA involvement and the patient's age (i.e., >10%

TABLE 32.3

Risk Factors for Burns in Adults

Alcohol use disorder

Antisocial personality disorder

Bipolar disorder

Chronic medical illness

Dementia

Depression

Homelessness

Low socioeconomic status

Occupational hazards

Older age

Poor education

Substance use disorder

Suicide attempts

Schizophrenia

TABLE 32.4

Classification of Burn Injuries

Degree	Dermal Involvement	Symptoms	Treatment
First degree	Intact epithelium	Pink, dry, painful	Symptomatic
Second degree: superficial partial thickness	Epidermis	Pink-red, painful, blisters	Wound care
Second degree: deep partial thickness	Dermis	Red, less painful, blisters	May require surgery
Third degree (full thickness)	Dermis	Leathery, dry, lack of sensation	Surgery
Fourth degree	Muscles, tendons, bones	Black or white color, lack of sensation	Surgery

TBSA in the elderly, >20% TBSA in adults, and >30% TBSA in children). Injuries to the skin and the underlying tissue can be accompanied by smoke inhalation or damage to other organs.

The operative treatment of burns includes wound debridement, escharotomy, and fasciotomy (release of burned skin and muscle, respectively), as well as grafting. Non-operative treatment involves daily wound care (performed several times each day), and systemic care and management of associated medical and surgical problems.[23]

PRE-BURN PSYCHOPATHOLOGY

Patients with a pre-existing psychiatric illness may be more apt to sustaining burn injuries, and the injury, its sequelae, and the duration of recovery can predispose patients to develop psychiatric disorders.

Numerous studies have noted psychiatric illnesses are common in those before their burn injuries. In a prospective series of 73 patients with burn injuries, Dyster-Aas and associates[24] found that two-thirds of the patients had at least one lifetime psychiatric diagnosis; most often this was major depression (41%), followed by alcohol use disorder (AUD) (32%), simple phobia (16%), and panic disorder (16%). Similarly, Wisely and co-workers[25] found that of 72 patients admitted to a burn unit over a 5-month period, 35% had a psychiatric diagnosis before the burn, most commonly depression, an alcohol/substance use disorder (SUD), a personality disorder, or a psychotic disorder. Hudson and colleagues[26] noted that burn patients with a pre-existing psychiatric diagnosis were more likely to have a co-morbid condition (e.g., cigarette smoking, hypertension, alcohol, and drug use), more severe burn characteristics (greater third-degree TBSA, inhalation injury), higher rates of treatment complications, and worse outcomes throughout their hospital course and on hospital discharge (e.g., placement issues).

Burn injuries are an uncommon method of self-harm and suicide in the United States; however, patients with a self-inflicted burn often have a high prevalence of mental illness (e.g., psychotic disorders, affective disorders, SUDs).[11] Psychosis and substance use are commonly identified as risk factors for suicide attempts by self-immolation. A review of 582 patients with self-inflicted burns found that 78% had a psychiatric history,[27] an increased likelihood of psychotic symptoms, an increased likelihood of being prescribed a psychotropic at the time of the burn, and an increased likelihood of being recently hospitalized psychiatrically.[28] A more recent systematic review of self-immolation reported that victims were often affected by psychiatric disorders (e.g., schizophrenia, depression, AUD, SUD) and had made one or more suicide attempts.[29] In the United States, self-immolation tends to occur in private (to minimize the unintended harm to others and to avoid being detected), while most who use this method are male. However, in other parts of the world, self-immolation is more common, and it is associated with different demographics. For example, in Iran and India, self-immolation occurs almost exclusively in females, often in those with little in the way of a pre-morbid psychiatric history (their most common diagnosis was adjustment disorder), and it is strongly associated with marital strife, isolation, and repressive gender politics.[30] These injuries often occur in public, to shame the immediate community of the victim.

A subset of patients inflicts burns on themselves without having suicidal intent. These patients are commonly females, younger, and may have comparatively higher rates of complex trauma and borderline personality disorder. These patients often apply heated objects to their skin and wish to feel numb or distracted from other intense emotions.[30]

INITIAL ASSESSMENT AND MANAGEMENT OF PATIENTS WITH BURN INJURIES

The role of the psychiatrist evolves during the recovery process. These patients may have a protracted hospital course that requires multiple surgical interventions. An initial psychiatric assessment focuses on safety and stabilization, then care transitions to diagnosis and treatment of any emerging affective or trauma responses, and eventually, the provider may target adjustment to chronic disability.

During the initial evaluation, psychiatrists should aim to obtain a history of the burn's circumstances, as well as information related to psychopathology, substance use, and social function. However, the initial assessment may be hampered by encephalopathy, acute intoxication, or severe injury that requires intubation and sedation. Thus the consulting psychiatrist often relies on medical records as well as pharmacy records, reports of emergency medical technicians (EMTs) and emergency services, surgical team notes, and input from the patient's friends and family to complete the assessment. While reviewing the record, the psychiatrist should pay attention to the mode of presentation (e.g., brought in by police and emergency medical service records) that describes the circumstances in which the patient was found, toxicology screens (with consideration given to drug or alcohol intoxication or withdrawal), and laboratory tests (e.g., that might indicate an increased risk of infection, organ injury, volume status changes). Special studies, including brain imaging (when there is a concern for a head injury, stroke, severe hypoxic insult, or a worsening mental status) and an electroencephalogram (when there is a concern for seizures or delirium) may be indicated. National controlled substance databases, pharmacy records, and electronic medical records may provide additional information about a patient's medical history, including their use of opioids and other sedatives (which may contribute to both pain control and withdrawal).

Pre-morbid psychiatric illness and medications may complicate acute pharmacological management of patients due to drug-drug interactions with agents required for sedation. Further, psychiatric medication drug doses may require adjustments due to changes in a patient's volume status or organ function. Even if certain drugs have been used safely before, the presence of multiple sedating agents in a burn patient may contribute to sedation and delirium, especially in older adults. These complexities can generate uncertainty in the primary team regarding the status or dosing of psychotropic medications in patients with burns. Consulting psychiatrists can educate their patients about the indications for psychotropics. The patient's condition (including their respiratory status and the presence of end-organ injury [e.g., renal, hepatic]), should be accounted for when considering whether to continue a pre-existing psychotropic. If they are continued, physicians should remain vigilant for potential drug-drug interactions or changes in the drug's pharmacokinetic/pharmacodynamic profile as a result of the active burn injury or its sequelae. It should be monitored and

re-assessed during the recovery process for eventual medication re-initiation.

Substance use (specifically alcohol intoxication and AUD) is a risk factor for burn injuries. Urine/blood toxicology screening for all patients with a burn injury is recommended, and regardless of test results, all patients should be engaged (in a supportive and non-stigmatizing manner) about the possibility of alcohol/drug use as a contributor to their injury. Patients with active alcohol use should be screened for their potential for developing alcohol withdrawal. For patients with milder burn injuries and mild/moderate AUD, symptom-triggered treatment with a benzodiazepine will usually suffice. The consulting physician should be aware of potential pain-related, inflammatory, and other metabolic contributors that may confound the assessment of withdrawal (e.g., by contributing to vital sign changes or encephalopathy). In our clinical experience, tremor is the most sensitive alcohol withdrawal syndrome (AWS) sign, and treatment is usually initiated once the patient displays tremor and at least one other sign of active withdrawal (e.g., severe tachycardia or hypertension unrelated to the underlying injury).

Subjective distress, anxiety, or agitation are preferentially managed with non-benzodiazepine agents (e.g., intravenous [IV] haloperidol or oral quetiapine), given the risk of worsening agitation or delirium associated with benzodiazepine use. For those with more severe burn injuries and/or a high risk for complications of alcohol withdrawal, or AWS-related complications, we typically use a phenobarbital-based withdrawal protocol (given its relative ease of administration and its favorable outcome/complication data in this patient population).[31]

DELIRIUM IN THE CONTEXT OF A BURN INJURY

A common early complication of a burn injury is delirium; it may contribute to an increased risk for morbidity (e.g., through unintended injuries, falls, pulling out IV lines) and mortality. The prevalence of delirium in burn patients ranges from about 13% to 80%, and delirium occurs at a rate that is roughly eight times higher on burn units than on general wards.[32] Risk factors associated with delirium include traumatic brain injury (TBI), advanced age, low cognitive reserve, pre-existing disease (e.g., diabetes, hypertension, heart disease), co-morbid dementia, and SUDs (including alcohol and tobacco). Many of these factors are also associated with an increased risk of sustaining a burn injury. Burn patients may be at increased risk for delirium due to carbon monoxide exposure and hypoxia due to inhalation injuries.[33] Higher burn severity (>30% TBSA) and the presence of complications, such as infections or electrolyte abnormalities, are also associated with delirium.[32] With more severe burns, patients are often initially anesthetized and intubated until their skin grafting is completed; thus acute delirium may be masked until later in the hospitalization. Iatrogenic factors, such as benzodiazepine use, IV opioid administration, use of anticholinergic agents, and an increased number and length of surgical procedures, are also associated with the development of delirium in burn patients.[32] Agarwal and associates[34] noted that benzodiazepine exposure independently predicted the development of delirium, while exposure to methadone and IV fentanyl (for pain control) was not associated with an increased delirium risk. Dexmedetomidine and propofol are less deliriogenic than benzodiazepines.[33]

Pharmacological treatment with antipsychotics may be useful in delirium-related agitation. Patients may be critically ill and should be monitored for adverse effects of medications (such as QT prolongation); anticholinergic side effects (e.g., tachycardia and constipation); antihistaminergic effects (e.g., sedation and weight gain); hypotension, bradycardia (secondary to alpha-agonism with agents such as dexmedetomidine); paradoxical worsening of agitation or respiratory depression (with benzodiazepine use); and akathisia, dystonia, tardive dyskinesia, or neuroleptic malignant syndrome (due to use of neuroleptics). Prompt evaluation, maintenance of safety (which may necessitate the use of restraints), treatment of the causative factors, institution of environmental changes, and provision of supportive contacts with staff and family are recommended. Treatment goals include adequate management of agitation, keeping in mind that inadequate pain control may contribute to the presentation.

Pain Management in Burn Patients

Burn-related injuries cause significant pain due to the irritation from adjacent damaged tissue in the injury itself and from multiple surgical procedures (e.g., debridement), dressing changes, repositioning, and physical therapy. Pain is often multi-modal, and patients often benefit from a multi-modal approach that involves the use of anti-inflammatory agents, conventional opioids, and finally, agents that target neuropathic pain. A summary of guidelines for pain management by the American Burn Association[35] is outlined in Table 32.5 and includes protocolizing pain assessments, utilizing acetaminophen in all patients if possible, individualizing therapy to the patient,

TABLE 32.5
Guidelines for Pain Management

- Pain assessments should be performed several times daily and be protocolized.
- Acetaminophen should be used for all burn patients, if possible.
- Therapy should be individualized for each patient and be adjusted frequently.
- The lowest amounts of opiate equivalents should be used to achieve the desired effect, and opioids should be used in conjunction with non-opioid and non-pharmacological measures.
- Decisions about the choice of opioid used should be based on the patient's physiology, pharmacology, and physician experience.
- Patients should be educated about the role of opioids and other pain medications in their recovery from burn injuries.
- NSAIDs should be considered in all patients, if not contra-indicated.
- Treatment of neuropathic pain (e.g., gabapentin or pregabalin) should be considered as an adjunct to opioids in patients with neuropathic pain or in those who are refractory to standard therapy.
- Ketamine can be considered for procedural sedation or as an adjunct to opioids, with appropriate training and monitoring.
- Dexmedetomidine and clonidine are recommended as adjuncts in patients with prominent anxiety.
- Patient should be offered non-pharmacological pain-control techniques, such as CBT, hypnosis, and virtual reality when available.

CBT, Cognitive-behavioral therapy; NSAIDs, non-steroidal anti-inflammatory drugs.

utilizing the lowest amounts of opiates in conjunction with non-opioid and non-pharmacological measures, and educating patients on the role of opioids and other pain medications during their recovery. Further consideration should be given to the use of non-steroidal anti-inflammatory drugs (NSAIDs) for all patients able to tolerate these medications and the use of adjunctive agents (e.g., gabapentin or pregabalin for neuropathic pain or refractory pain, low-dose ketamine during the post-operative period, and dexmedetomidine or clonidine for patients who show signs of withdrawal or prominent anxiety).

When considering an opioid agent for burn-related pain, clinicians should consider using agents for basal pain-control relief and additional agents for breakthrough pain and procedural pain. We often use methadone for baseline pain control (given its long half-life) and a short-acting agent (e.g., oxycodone, morphine, or hydromorphone) for breakthrough pain. Burn injuries often require extended hospitalizations and repeated interventions, thus generating catastrophic reactions to wound care, repositioning/mobilization, and other routine aspects of patient care. We commonly co-administer low-dose IV haloperidol with IV opioids 30 minutes before any such interventions to mitigate anticipatory fear and help improve a patient's engagement.[33] With prolonged hospitalizations, patients are also at risk of developing a dependence on opioids used chronically for pain management and they may benefit from a gradual taper to minimize the risk of developing a significant withdrawal reaction.

Patients with severe burn injuries may be unable to communicate effectively due to the extent and severity of their injuries or the presence of delirium. The American Burn Association[35] provides the following management guidelines: patients should be assessed repeatedly during different activities; assessments should be protocolized to ensure the use of consistent language; patient-reported scales should be used when possible; the Burn Specific Pain Anxiety Scale should be available; and Critical Care Pain Observation Tool can be used when a patient is unable to interact with his/her care providers.

Several studies have shown that about one-third of burn patients continue to have significant pain that results in functional impairment up to 9 years post-injury. In addition to pain, itching (particularly related to deep burns with hypertrophic scars) is a key longitudinal contributor to patient distress. Van Loey and colleagues[36] reported that itching is common following the initial injury (87% of patients at 3 months), and it diminishes over time (such that at 2 years, 21% of burn patients reported moderate/severe itching). Importantly, this study showed a correlation between the presence of early post-traumatic stress symptoms and itching following injury. Pharmacological treatment for burn-related itching (including naltrexone,[37] gabapentin, and doxepin[38]) is limited.

Pain Management in Patients With Chronic Opioid Use

Acute pain control in those with an opioid use disorder (OUD) and a burn injury can be challenging. Personality factors and pre-existing mood disorders, anxiety, and trauma-related illness may be accentuated soon after the burn injury and may heighten discomfort and reduce pain tolerance. In general, patients with chronic opioid use, whether illicit or iatrogenic, exhibit physiological tolerance to opioids and may show signs of opioid-related hyperalgesia. Therefore, these individuals frequently require higher-than-usual doses of opioids to achieve adequate pain control.[33] Patients who have been taking prescribed opioids for chronic pain, or taking methadone for an OUD, should not be taken off their medications, nor should it be assumed that their home regimen will provide them with sufficient pain control. For those receiving methadone, the treating clinician should communicate with their clinic (to avoid the risk of their being terminated from the clinic due to the lack of follow-up) and consider a dose increase for improved pain control. On discharge, close coordination among the patient, community prescribers, and family members (if available) can help to ensure appropriate pain control and minimize the risk for relapse and other complications (e.g., diversion, polypharmacy).[39] Patients on buprenorphine present an added dilemma, as the use of buprenorphine may limit the efficacy of conventional short-acting opioids. Typically, these patients have been managed by discontinuation of buprenorphine and initiation of methadone or another long-acting agent to mitigate buprenorphine withdrawal and enhance pain control. This approach often resulted in significant discomfort and anxiety, which contributed to patient-initiated discharges and the risk of relapse. A safer alternative is to reduce buprenorphine dosing to 8 mg/day (as a single daily dose or as a divided dose), which should be sufficient to prevent withdrawal and leave enough opioid receptors available for conventional agonists to achieve acute pain control.[40]

Post-Burn Psychopathology

Burn injuries can lead to long-term psychopathology, including major depressive disorder (MDD) and post-traumatic stress disorder (PTSD). Regarding depression, the prevalence has been estimated at up to 23%[41-43] with key risk factors including a history of MDD, female gender, and facial disfigurement.[41,44] The prevalence of post-burn acute stress disorder (ASD) ranges from 6% to 33%,[43] while rates of PTSD range from 24% to 40% at 6 months post-injury, up to 15% to 45% at 12 months post-injury[43] and as high as 58%.[44] Risk factors for PTSD include a history of psychiatric illness,[33] anxiety related to pain, visible burns,[41] younger age, a lack of social support, and avoidance-based or ambivalent coping strategies.[44] A retrospective review of adult burn survivors found that there were higher odds of developing symptoms of MDD and PTSD in association with female gender (two-fold), graft size (with a 2% increase for every 1% increase in graft size), a head/neck graft (2.5 times), a history of recent psychiatric treatment (2.2 times), electrical injury (four-fold), and having less than a high school education (0.53 times).[45] Finally, early treatment with a selective serotonin reuptake inhibitor (SSRI) for ASD had mixed results, even though they were generally considered to be first-line treatments for PTSD. Cognitive-behavioral therapy (CBT) has been an effective treatment for PTSD.[46,47] The efficacy of beta-blockers, e.g., propranolol, has been mixed. Benzodiazepines have consistently been shown to be ineffective, and they pose significant additional risks for delirium and may contribute to an increased risk of developing PTSD when used for ASD.

Longitudinal Assessment and Management of Patients with Burns

As the recovery process progresses, psychiatrists can shift their focus from stabilizing the patient to assessing the impact of the injury and evaluating emerging psychiatric illness. At this point, providers can differentiate an individual's ongoing distress, mourning the loss of physical health, demoralization, adjustment disorders, MDD, anxiety spectrum disorders, and/or trauma-related disorders. Many burn survivors with a changed physical appearance develop difficulties with psychological and social adaptation: Thombs and associates[48] found that at 1 year following a severe burn injury, body image satisfaction and distress were the most significant predictors of overall psychosocial function. Once the diagnosis of a primary psychiatric disorder has been established, pharmacological and psychotherapeutic interventions are indicated. The treatment for adjustment disorders typically includes targeting associated symptoms, such as insomnia and anxiety, and the use of psychotherapy to understand the person's strengths and coping style.

Even with appropriate community support and strong patient resilience, patients are at risk for body image disruption, and re-traumatization in the setting of repeated hospitalizations and surgical interventions. Watkins and colleagues[33] described key treatment interventions:

1. Educating the patient about their expected course of recovery.
2. Orienting the patient to what will occur during each aspect of their treatment (e.g., itching, nociceptive and neuropathic pain).
3. Working with patients to create a program for self-care and activities that help foster gradual and realistic progress toward recovery.
4. Focusing on developing abilities as opposed to remaining disabilities through continuous positive feedback.

TRAUMATIC INJURIES AND INTENSIVE CARE

Epidemiology

According to the Centers for Disease Control and Prevention Web-based Injury Statistics Query and Reporting System (WISQARS), from 2010 to 2020, the leading causes of non-fatal trauma-related emergency department (ED) visits were unintentional falls, unintentional strikes, and unintentional overexertion.[49] Most non-fatal injuries occurred in people 15 to 29 years of age. Assault was in the top 10 leading causes of non-fatal injury ED visits for those 10 years or older, and accounted for approximately 17 million injuries, while self-harm occurred in about 5 million individuals.[50]

Risk Factors

Traumatic injuries are more likely to affect males and younger people (between the ages of 10 and 24 years of age).[51] Risk factors for road-related injuries include increased vehicle speeds, alcohol use, fatigue, use of hand-held mobile telephones, inadequate visibility, traffic planning (e.g., schools located on busy roads, lack of median barriers), roadside hazards, and failure to use helmets (on two-wheeled vehicles) or seat belts.[52] Risk factors for falls included advanced age, low bone density, poor nutritional status, hypertension, diabetes, poor performance in ADLs, low levels of engagement in physical activity, poor cognitive function, impaired vision, a family history of hip fracture, a cluttered home environment, and alcohol consumption.[52,53] A review of injuries due to repeated assaults revealed that young age, low socioeconomic status, racialized groups, a history of mental illness or a SUD, and a history of incarceration were risk factors.[54]

In children, the most common unintentional injuries included fractures (15.8%), head injuries (4.3%), burns (2.3%), and poisoning (2.1%).[10]

Types of Trauma

The two main types of physical trauma are blunt force trauma (i.e., when an object or force strikes the body) and penetrating trauma (i.e., when an object pierces the skin or body). Depending on the location and the severity of the trauma, complications include concussions, TBIs, fractures, aspiration or pulmonary injuries, cardiac injuries, and splenic or abdominal injuries. Many trauma injuries require a surgical intervention, and they carry considerable risk for morbidity (e.g., loss of limb, chronic cognitive impairment) and mortality.

Traumatic Brain Injuries

Both penetrating and non-penetrating head trauma can result in a TBI (a disruption in normal cellular brain function through direct, rotational, or shear forces). TBI can occur in two phases: the primary injury, which is caused by an initial physical trauma

(with fractures, hematomas, contusions, or axonal injury); and a secondary injury that develops over time (with dysregulation of cellular pathways, demyelination, and altered permeability of cells or blood-brain barrier).[55,56] TBIs can produce vascular changes and parenchymal lesions that include diffuse axonal injury (DAI). Unlike acute bleeds and fractures associated with head trauma, DAI is commonly difficult to appreciate on a computerized tomography scan and may require a magnetic resonance imaging scan to make the diagnosis, unless it is severe. DAI, owing to diffuse neuronal network disruptions, can have a significant effect on a patient's quality of life[55] and lead to considerable morbidity and delayed recovery.

Following a head injury, patients may require acute interventions (e.g., a craniotomy or mechanical ventilation) and may require monitoring of intracranial pressure (ICP). Hypothermia or brief periods of hypocapnia may be utilized for a significantly elevated ICP.[55] The sequelae of moderate-to-severe TBIs include anterograde or retrograde amnesia, chronic pain, cognitive complaints, neurosensory deficits, seizures, neuroendocrine disorders, and hydrocephalus.[56-58] TBI is also associated with a range of behavioral disturbances (including MDD, PTSD, anxiety disorders, and psychosis) as well as neurocognitive deficits (e.g., memory impairment and executive and frontal deficits that include disinhibition and impulsivity). MDD is the most common psychiatric disorder associated with TBI, with generalized anxiety disorder being the second most common condition; thus it is appropriate to screen patients following a head injury for these symptoms and consider the use of an SSRI in an appropriate clinical setting.[56,57] Post-traumatic mania or hypomania is less common, with prevalence ranging from 1.7% to 9%.[57] Affect dysregulation, sleep disturbance, and impulsivity can be misattributed to mania in those with a TBI, and clinicians should assess for manic episodes and obtain a thorough history when the sequelae of injuries may contribute to dysregulation. In cases of post-traumatic mania or hypomania, valproic acid, and quetiapine are reasonable treatments.[57]

Paranoia in TBI is associated with post-trauma amnesia, although it can persist beyond the acute postoperative period; if it is observed, the use of atypical antipsychotics should be considered. Aggression and impulsivity often require a multi-modal approach, including behavioral and environmental strategies that focus on minimizing the unintentional risk of harm to the patient or their caretakers; likewise, many patients may benefit from medications that promote sleep and reduce aggression. Consensus expert opinions for non-pharmacological interventions for TBI-associated behavioral disorders include allowing time for processing information due to the potential of cognitive difficulties, providing structured and clear information (e.g., avoiding the use of jargon), respecting the patient's autonomy, providing information in forms that best address the patient's cognitive/sensory deficits, using a consistent approach among patient's providers, and utilizing professional/assistive services to limit feeling targeted by a patient's aggression.[59] A variety of pharmacologic agents (including beta-blockers, antipsychotics, SSRIs, anticonvulsants, and alpha-agonists) have been used to manage psychiatric symptoms in patients with TBI. Beta-blockers have the most consistent evidence for the treatment of DAI-associate impulsivity and agitation; although clinical evidence is often inconsistent, antipsychotics and sedating anticonvulsants (e.g., valproate) are commonly used to manage acute agitation, impulsivity, and insomnia. The use of antipsychotic agents comes with a word of caution about the risk of extrapyramidal symptoms and cognitive compromise.

Assessment and Management of Post-Trauma and Intensive Care Patients

When considering the initial psychiatric management of those who have sustained an acute trauma, the consulting psychiatrist should perform a thorough history and physical examination, paying close attention to the trauma's cause (e.g., self-inflicted or unintentional), the risk for developing delirium, pre-morbid substance use and risk for withdrawal emergence, and the utility (vs. risk) of continuing the patient's psychotropics. As with burn injuries, patients may not be able (due to injury or delirium) to provide an accurate history, and the consulting psychiatrist may need to rely on alternative sources of information (including family members, outside medical records, and prescription/pharmacy data). Acute pain management of those who have sustained a traumatic injury is like that of those who have received burns.

Longitudinal management includes the assessment of psychopathological responses and the initiation of appropriate pharmacological and psychological interventions. As with burn patients, survivors of trauma often experience symptoms of mood and anxiety disorders, as well as PTSD following their injury, especially as they face chronic challenges to their health. Trauma-focused care should be offered throughout the patient's recovery and there should be a low threshold for the involvement of psychiatry for diagnostic clarification and treatment recommendations. Patients with a TBI may experience sequelae that range from time-limited concussive symptoms to persistent motor and cognitive deficits; prompt recognition and treatment of these are key in ensuring a patient's ongoing recovery.

Management of Delirium in Surgical Trauma Patients

Marquetand and co-workers[60] reported delirium developed in 21.7% of their 2026 trauma patients. Delirium was associated with an increased risk of transiting to assisted living or a nursing home, the need for rehabilitation services, and patient mortality. Risk factors for delirium in surgical trauma patients include pre-existing neurocognitive conditions (e.g., dementia), polypharmacy, a significant underlying medical illness (e.g., cardiac insufficiency, brain edema, pneumonia, cerebral inflammation), the need for ICU management, and the use of mechanical ventilation. A systematic review reported a strong correlation of delirium with advancing patient age, a history of dementia, hypertension, mechanical ventilation, metabolic acidosis, coma, and multiple organ failure; this study found that the use of dexmedetomidine was associated with a lower delirium prevalence.[61] Proposals for the management of delirium in the ICU have included a so-called ABCDEF "bundle approach":

- A stands for assess, prevent, and manage pain
- B represents spontaneous awakening trials (SATs) for those on sedatives and spontaneous breathing trials (SBTs) if patients were on a mechanical ventilator
- C refers to choosing analgesics and sedatives that are less likely to contribute to delirium
- D denotes delirium monitoring or management (e.g., re-orientation, treating circadian rhythm dysregulation, improving vision and/or hearing if impaired)

- E stands for early exercise/mobility
- F refers to family engagement

Analysis for effectiveness of this approach revealed the potential to improve clinical outcomes. For example, early mobilization has improved delirium, and multiple studies have shown a reduction in patient mortality rates and length of stay following the implementation of the bundle approach.[62,63] The bundle approach was also effective in reducing the proportion of patient-days with coma and 28-day mortality.[63]

END-OF-LIFE CARE AND STAFF SUPPORT

Psychiatrists are uniquely positioned to identify and manage distress experienced by patients, families, and caregivers while facing potentially life-threatening illness and trauma. Through interactions with the members of the patient's health care team, the consulting psychiatrist can appreciate the complex (and often rapidly changing) clinical picture of the ICU patient, and pivot their assessment and treatment considerations to best assist the patient, their family, and the providers.

When critical illnesses do not respond to treatment or when life-sustaining interventions cannot meet the patient's goals, physicians should consider having discussions with the family about the patient's end-of-life goals. Psychiatrists are often consulted to assist in the care of dying patients and their families to minimize pain and suffering and to aid in decision-making at the end of life. It is essential to provide accurate explanations about the risk of death to families and patients. Advance directives, when available, can be used to guide medical decision-making. When directives are unavailable and the patient is unable to discuss goals of care meaningfully, family members may need to discuss the patient's wishes and a proxy will need to be involved in decision-making. Some patients and families, in collaboration with multi-disciplinary teams, may opt for palliative care, which aims to support the patient, minimize pain and anxiety, and promote death with dignity. The ICU experience is typically an emotionally and spiritually challenging process, and additional services (including spiritual care, legal counsel, ethics, and social work) may become involved in care.

Additional stress contributes to burnout in ICU staff; psychiatric skills may also benefit stress management. By providing interventions (such as education on responses to traumatic or difficult events and validating emotions for staff), psychiatrists can assist ICU colleagues who are managing stress and grief reactions.[2] The psychiatrist on the team typically encourages communication and reflection on the nuances of the medical and social circumstances for the patient.

REFERENCES

1. Stoddard FJ, Pandya A, Katz DL. *Disaster Psychiatry: Readiness, Evaluation and Treatment.* American Psychiatric Association Publishers; 2011.
2. Bains A. Liaison psychiatry during challenging times. *Acad Psychiatry.* 2021;45(5):647–648.
3. Kelly FE, Fong K, Hirsch N, et al. Intensive care medicine is 60 years old: the history and future of the intensive care unit. *Clin Med.* 2014;14(4):376.
4. Lee KC, Joory K, Moiemen NS. History of burns: the past, present and the future. *Burns Trauma.* 2014;2(4):2321–3868.
5. Cobb S, Lindemann E. Neuropsychiatric observations after the Cocoanut Grove fire. *Ann Surg.* 1943;117:814–824.
6. Lindemann E. Symptomatology and management of acute grief. *Am J Psychiatry.* 1994;101:141–148.
7. American Burn Association: Burn Incidence and Treatment in the United States: 2016. Available at: https://ameriburn.org/who-we-are/media/burn-incidence-fact-sheet/
8. Jeschke MG, van Baar ME, Choudhry MA, et al. Burn injury. *Nat Rev Dis Primers.* 2020;6(1):1–25.
9. Alnababtah K, Khan S, Ashford R. Socio-demographic factors and the prevalence of burns in children: an overview of the literature. *Paediatr Int Child Health.* 2016;36(1):45–51.
10. Rowe R, Maughan B, Goodman R. Childhood psychiatric disorder and unintentional injury: findings from a national cohort study. *J Pediatr Psychol.* 2004;29(2):119–130.
11. Peck MD. Epidemiology of burns throughout the World. Part II: intentional burns in adults. *Burns.* 2012;38(5):630–637.
12. Paul AR, Adamo MA. Non-accidental trauma in pediatric patients: a review of epidemiology, pathophysiology, diagnosis and treatment. *Transl Pediatr.* 2014;3(3):195–207.
13. Renz BM, Sherman R. Abusive scald burns in infants and children: a prospective study. *Am Surg.* 1993;59:329–334.
14. Anwar MU, Majumder S, Austin O, et al. Smoking, substance abuse, psychiatric history, and burns: trends in adult patients. *J Burn Care Rehabil.* 2005;26:493–501.
15. Rockwell E, Dimsdale JE, Carroll W, et al. Preexisting psychiatric disorders in burn patients. *J Burn Care Rehabil.* 1988;9:83–86.
16. Haum A, Perbix W, Hack AJ, et al. Alcohol and drug abuse in burn injuries. *Burns.* 1995;21:194–199.
17. Kolman PBR. Incidence of psychopathology in burned adult patients. *J Burn Care Rehabil.* 1984;4:430–436.

18. Kramer CB, Gibran NS, Heimbach DM, et al. Assault and substance abuse characterize burn injuries in homeless patients. *J Burn Care Res.* 2008;29:461–467.

19. Peck MD. Epidemiology of burns throughout the world. Part I: distribution and risk factors. *Burns.* 2011;37(7):1087–1100.

20. Vrouwe SQ, Johnson MB, Pham CH, et al. The homelessness crisis and burn injuries: a cohort study. *J Burn Care Res.* 2020;41(4):820–827.

21. Anwar MU, Majumder S, Austin O, et al. Smoking, substance abuse, psychiatric history, and burns: trends in adult patients. *J Burn Care Rehabil.* 2005;26:493–501.

22. Rex S. Burn injuries. *Curr Opinion Crit Care.* 2012;18(6):671–676.

23. Grunwald TB, Garner WL. Acute burns. *Plast Reconstr Surg.* 2008;121:311e–319e.

24. Dyster-Aas J, Willebrand M, Wikehult B, et al. Major depression and posttraumatic stress disorder symptoms following severe burn injury in relation to lifetime psychiatric morbidity. *J Trauma.* 2008;64:1349–1356.

25. Wisely FA, Hoyle E, Tarrier N, et al. Where to start? Attempting to meet the psychological needs of burned patients. *Burns.* 2007;33:736–746.

26. Hudson A, Al Youha S, Samargandi OA, et al. Pre-existing psychiatric disorder in the burn patient is associated with worse outcomes. *Burns.* 2017;43(5):973–982.

27. Geller JL. Self-incineration: a review of the psychopathology of setting oneself afire. *Int J Law Psychiatry.* 1997;20:355–372.

28. Mulholland R, Green L, Longstaff C, et al. Deliberate self-harm by burning: a retrospective case-controlled study. *J Burn Care Res.* 2008;29:644–649.

29. Simonit F, Da Broi U, Desinan L. The role of self-immolation in complex suicides: a neglected topic in current literature. *Forensic Sci Int.* 2020;306:110073–110080.

30. Nisavic M, Nejad SH, Beach SR. Intentional self-inflicted burn injuries: review of the literature. *Psychosomatics.* 2017;58(6):581–591.

31. Nejad S, Nisavic M, Larentzakis A, et al. Phenobarbital for acute alcohol withdrawal management in surgical trauma patients—a retrospective comparison study. *Psychosomatics.* 2020;61(4):327–335.

32. Ren Y, Zhang Y, Luo J, et al. Research progress on risk factors of delirium in burn patients: a narrative review. *Front Psychiatry.* 2022;13:1–10.

33. Nejad SH, Dobovsky A, Irwin K, et al. Burns. In: Fogel BA, Greenberg DB, eds. *Psychiatric Care of the Medical Patient.* 3rd ed. Oxford University Press; 2015.

34. Agarwal V, O'Neill PJ, Cotton BA, et al. Prevalence and risk factors for development of delirium in burn intensive care unit patients. *J Burn Care Res.* 2010;31:706–715.

35. Romanowski KS, Carson J, Pape K, et al. American Burn Association guidelines on the management of acute pain in the adult burn patient: a review of the literature, a compilation of expert opinion, and next steps. *J Burn Care Res.* 2020;41(6):1129–1151.

36. Van Loey NEE, Bremer M, Faber AW, et al. Itching following burns: epidemiology and predictors. *Br J Derm.* 2008;158(1):95–100.

37. Jung SI, Seo CH, Jang K, et al. Efficacy of naltrexone in the treatment of chronic refractory itching in burn patients: preliminary report of an open trial. *J Burn Care Res.* 2009;30:257–260.

38. Goutos I, Dziewulski P, Richardson PM. Pruritus in burns: review article. *J Burn Care Res.* 2009;30:221–228.

39. Ward EN, Quaye ANA, Wilens TE. Opioid use disorders: perioperative management of a special population. *Anesth Analg.* 2018;127(2):539–547.

40. Acampora GA, Nisavic M, Zhang Y. Perioperative buprenorphine continuous maintenance and administration simultaneous with full opioid agonist: patient priority at the interface between medical disciplines. *J Clin Psychiatry.* 2020;81(1):14112–14119.

41. Van Loey NE, Van Son MJ. Psychopathology and psychological problems in patients with burn scars. *Am J Clin Derm.* 2003;4(4):245–272.

42. Thombs BD, Bresnick MG, Magyar-Russell G. Depression in survivors of burn injury: a systematic review. *Gen Hosp Psychiatry.* 2006;28(6):494–502.

43. Wiechman S, Meyer W, Edelman L, et al. Psychological outcomes in American burn association consensus statements. *J Burn Care Res.* 2013;34(4):363–368.

44. Lodha P, Shah B, Karia S, et al. Post-traumatic stress disorder (PTSD) following burn injuries: a comprehensive clinical review. *Ann Burns Fire Disasters.* 2020;33(4):276–287.

45. Stockly OR, Wolfe AE, Goldstein R, et al. Predicting depression and posttraumatic stress symptoms following burn injury: a risk scoring system. *J Burn Care Res.* 2022;43(4):899–905.

46. Paggiaro AO, Paggiaro PBS, Fernandes RAQ, et al. Posttraumatic stress disorder in burn patient: a systematic review. *J Plast Reconstr Aesthet Surg.* 2022;75:1586–1595.

47. Chokshi SN, Powell CM, Gavrilova Y, et al. A narrative review of the history of burn-related depression and stress reactions. *Medicina.* 2022;58(10):1395–1412.

48. Thombs BD, Fauerbach JA, Lawrence JW, et al. Body image satisfaction in burn survivors: natural history across periods of wound healing, scar activity, and approaching scar maturity. *J Burn Care Rehab.* 2005;26:S56.

49. Centers for Disease Control and Prevention. *Web-based Injury Statistics Query and Reporting System: Leading Causes of Nonfatal Injury.* Available at: https://wisqars.cdc.gov/lcnf/?y1=2010&y2=2020&ct=5&cc=0&s=0&g=00&a=lcd1age&a1=0&a2=199&d=0

50. Centers for Disease Control and Prevention. Web-based Injury Statistics Query and Reporting System: Nonfatal Injuries. Available at: https://wisqars.cdc.gov/data/non-fatal/explore/selected-years?nf=eyJpbnRlbnRzIjpbIjAiXSwibWVjaHMiOlsiMzAwMCJdLCJ0cmFmZmljIjpbIjAiXSwiZGlzcCI6WyIxIiwiMiIsIjQiLCI1Il0sInNleCI6WyIxIiwiMiIsIjMiXSwiYWdlR3JvdXBzTWluIjpbIjAwLTA0Il0sImFnZUdyb3Vwc01heCI6WyIxOTkiXSwiY3VzdG9tQWdlc01pbiI6WyIwIl0sImN1c3RvbUFnZXNNYXgiOlsiMTk5Il0sImZyb21ZZWFyIjpbIjIwMTAiXSwidG9ZZWFyIjpbIjIwMjAiXSwiYWdlVnodG4iOiI1WXIiLCJncm91cl5MSI6IkFHRURQQIn0%3D

51. Norton R, Kobusingye O. Injuries. *N Engl J Med*. 2013; 368(18):1723–1730.

52. Norton R, Hyder AA, Bishai D, et al. Unintentional injuries. In: Jamison DT, Breman JG, Measham AR, et al., eds. *Disease Control Priorities in Developing Countries*. 2nd ed. Oxford University Press; 2006.

53. Peel NM. Epidemiology of falls in older age. *Can J Aging/La Revue Canadienne du Vieillissement*. 2011;30(1):7–19.

54. Strauss R, Menchetti I, Nantais J, et al. Repeat assault injuries: a scoping review of the incidence and associated risk factors. *Injury*. 2022;53(10):3078–3087.

55. Stocchetti N, Carbonara M, Citerio G, et al. Severe traumatic brain injury: targeted management in the intensive care unit. *Lancet Neurol*. 2017;16(6):452–464.

56. Capizzi A, Woo J, Verduzco-Gutierrez M. Traumatic brain injury: an overview of epidemiology, pathophysiology, and medical management. *Med Clinics*. 2020;104(2):213–238.

57. Polich G, Iaccarino AI, Zafonte R. Psychopharmacology of traumatic brain injury. In: Reus VI, Lindqvist D, eds. *Handbook of Clinical Neurology*, Vol 165. Elsevier; 2019.

58. O'Shanick GJ, Moses GT, Varney NR. Traumatic brain injury: evaluation and management for the psychiatric physician. In: Fogel BA, Greenberg DB, eds. *Psychiatric Care of the Medical Patient*. 3rd ed. Oxford University Press; 2015.

59. Wiart L, Luauté J, Stefan A, et al. Non pharmacological treatments for psychological and behavioural disorders following traumatic brain injury (TBI). A systematic literature review and expert opinion leading to recommendations. *Ann Phys Rehab Med*. 2016;59(1):31–41.

60. Marquetand J, Gehrke S, Bode L, et al. Delirium in trauma patients: a 1-year prospective cohort study of 2026 patients. *Eur J Trauma Emerg Surg*. 2022;48(2):1017–1024.

61. Zaal IJ, Devlin JW, Peelen LM, et al. A systematic review of risk factors for delirium in the ICU. *Crit Care Med*. 2015;43(1):40–47.

62. Trogrlić Z, van der Jagt M, Bakker J, et al. A systematic review of implementation strategies for assessment, prevention, and management of ICU delirium and their effect on clinical outcomes. *Crit Care*. 2015;19:1–17.

63. Zhang S, Han Y, Xiao Q, et al. Effectiveness of bundle interventions on ICU delirium: a meta-analysis. *Crit Care Med*. 2021;49(2):335–346.

33

PATIENTS WITH GENETIC SYNDROMES

TAMAR C. KATZ, MD, PHD ■ CHRISTINE T. FINN, MD ■ JOAN M. STOLER, MD

OVERVIEW

Genetic syndromes are disorders with a characteristic set of features that result from an underlying common genetic mechanism, either a specific genetic mutation or a chromosomal abnormality. This chapter provides a brief overview of the genetics of major psychiatric disorders, genetic syndromes, and inborn errors of metabolism that the general psychiatrist may encounter in the hospital or clinic setting. It emphasizes several characteristics of the genetics of major psychiatric disorders. First, psychiatric disorders have a substantial genetic component, and understanding the role of genetics is useful for understanding psychiatric disease physiology and treatment. Second, the environment plays a significant role in the expression of these disorders; interactions between the genetic background and the environment lead to disease expression. Third, this chapter explores several current approaches used to identify the genetic basis of psychiatric disorders and offers recent insights about psychiatric genetics. Finally, this chapter highlights the fact that psychiatric disorders, genetic syndromes, and metabolic diseases may each present with psychiatric symptoms as part of their observed presentation. Behavioral manifestations may be important clinical features for the identification of underlying genetic illnesses.

Knowing when to suspect that a genetic or metabolic issue may be contributing to the presenting condition of a patient is important in formulating a differential diagnosis. Proper identification of genetic and metabolic illness allows treatment or interventions to be directed at the primary process (e.g., correction of hyperammonemia in urea cycle disorders) rather than management of its downstream effects (e.g., delirium). For the most part, the disorders reviewed here may present in late childhood to adulthood; this chapter specifically excludes those disorders that are lethal in infancy or early childhood. When an underlying genetic syndrome or metabolic disease is suspected, a consultation by a geneticist can be highly beneficial and help direct clinical management.

Currently, there are no available treatments that can cure genetic syndromes or replace missing genetic material. For this reason, treatment is directed at symptomatic management, surveillance for associated medical conditions, and early developmental interventions. However, an improved understanding of the underlying genetic mechanisms of psychiatric illnesses vastly expands the potential for future targeted therapy, including targeted pharmacologic approaches, gene therapy, and pre-implantation genetic diagnosis, among others.

VARIED APPROACHES TO UNDERSTANDING PSYCHIATRIC GENETICS

Epidemiology of Psychiatric Disorders

Twin, family, and adoption studies can assess the magnitude of genetic versus environmental factors that give rise to a phenotype.[1,2] Family studies usually measure the lifetime prevalence of a disorder among first-degree relatives of the affected individual, known as the index case. Adoption studies can help further disentangle genetic and environmental influences by comparing rates of a disorder in biological family members with those in adoptive family members. In addition, comparing rates of a disorder in twins who were raised in the same household with twins reared in separate households can provide further evidence about the genetic and environmental influences that lead to the expression of the disorder. For example, comparing concordance rates in monozygotic twins raised apart (in different environments) can provide an estimation of the *heritability* of a disorder, as these individuals have near-identical DNA and differ primarily in their environment.

Heritability estimates the extent to which differences in the appearance of a trait *across a population* can be accounted for by genetic factors. Heritability is measured on an index from 0 to 1 and is an estimate of the additive sum of all the genetic influences on a trait in the population. A heritability index of 1 means that 100% of the variability between individuals in a population is due to genetic factors, with no environmental contribution. A helpful conceptualization of the heritability index is that all traits exist on a continuum from "genetic" to "environmental," with most traits receiving influence from both factors. Heritability is measured within a population and says nothing about the likelihood of a *given individual* inheriting a gene, the number of genes that are involved in a trait, or the effect size of a given gene. Thus, if the heritability of bipolar disorder (BPD) is 0.75, this indicates that 75% of the variability observed in those with BPD is due to

genetic causes, but it does *not* suggest that a specific individual has a 75% chance of developing BPD.

As Table 33.1 demonstrates, genes and environment both contribute substantially to the expression of psychiatric disorders, though the balance differs between disorders. For example, environment plays a more substantial role in the development of major depressive disorder (MDD)[3] or anxiety disorders[4] than schizophrenia or autism.[5] In all cases, the relationship between genetic and environmental influences is far more complicated than a simple linear relationship. Environmental factors that contribute to the expression of psychiatric disorders include early life events, stressors, early trauma, difficult family environments, exposure to toxins and infectious agents, and a dysregulated immune system.[6,7]

Gene-by-Environment Interactions

Gene-by-environment interaction is the tendency for environmental exposures to influence gene expression.[8] The primary theoretical framework used to model gene-by-environment interactions is termed the stress-diathesis model. This model suggests that individuals are born genetically vulnerable to psychiatric disorders, and diseases manifest only when the environment interacts with and exposes the underlying genetic vulnerability.[9-11] Thus, individuals with different genotypes differ in the impact of similar environmental exposure on their disease risk; conversely, two individuals with the same genotype, such as monozygotic (identical) twins, may differ in their

---

TABLE 33.1
Epidemiology of Common Psychiatric Disorders[3-15]

	Heritability	Monozygotic Concordance	Dizygotic Concordance	Lifetime Risk (General Population)	Increased Risk in Individuals With First-Degree Relatives
Bipolar disorder	60%–85%	45%	5%	1%	10-fold increased risk
MDD	40%	23%–49%	16%–42%	6.7%–17.1%	3-fold increased risk
Panic disorder	45%	24%	11%	4.7%	5-fold increased risk
Schizophrenia	70%–89%	50%	15%	1%	10-fold increased risk
Alcohol dependence	35%–60%	76%	61%	8%–10% females; 10%–15% males	6- to 10-fold increased risk
Autism	>90%	70%–90%	5%–10%	0.66%–1.5%	50- to 100-fold increased risk
ADHD	75%	82%	38%	8.1%	2- to 8-fold increased risk

ADHD, Attention-deficit hyperactivity disorder; *MDD*, major depressive disorder.

risk of developing a disease when exposed to different environments. This model previously addressed only adverse environmental exposures, but it has been updated to suggest that genetic variability may increase in response to both negative *and* positive environmental influences, known as the differential susceptibility model.[12,13]

The seminal example of a gene-by-environment interaction is the interaction of the serotonin transporter gene and stressful life events in the onset of episodes of MDD.[14] The serotonin transporter is the target of selective serotonin reuptake inhibitor antidepressants. There is a common polymorphism in the promoter of the serotonin transporter gene that leads to a "long" allele or a "short" allele lacking a 44 base-pair sequence. The short allele is associated with reduced expression of the serotonin transporter. The 2003 study by Caspi and colleagues[14] examined a birth cohort of 1037 children followed to age 26 years for evidence of a linkage between the short or long allele of the serotonin transporter gene, stressful life events, and MDD. Stressful life events included problems in employment, finances, housing, health, and relationships. In the absence of stressful life events, the presence of either the short or long allele of the serotonin transporter gene was not associated with depressive symptoms in these individuals. However, with an increasing number of stressful life events, individuals with the short allele of the serotonin transporter gene have an increasingly greater number of major depressive episodes, suicidal thoughts, and suicide attempts.[15] In addition, individuals with the short allele had an increased probability of adult major depressive episodes with increasing childhood maltreatment, whereas individuals with the long allele did not have more adult depression with childhood maltreatment. In both examples, individuals heterozygous for the short and long alleles had an intermediate phenotype compared with individuals homozygous for the short or long allele. These experiments show how an environmental factor, such as stressful life events, interacts with the genetic background of an individual, in this case, a functional polymorphism in the serotonin transporter gene, to lead to psychiatric disorders such as MDD.

A second study by Caspi and colleagues[16] highlights the effects of childhood trauma in the context of a functional polymorphism in the monoamine oxidase A (MAO_A) gene promoter. The MAO_A promoter has been shown to moderate the association between exposure to early childhood trauma and the development of antisocial or aggressive personality traits. Among children with low MAO_A levels, childhood abuse is associated with higher levels of aggression and antisocial traits, whereas high levels of MAO_A appear to be partially protective against the development of these traits even among childhood abuse victims.

While the concept of gene-environment interactions is a universally accepted phenomenon, specific findings have not always been easily replicated. Gene-by-environment research in psychiatry faces numerous challenges. Exposures to environmental stressors may differ across time and place, large sample sizes are required, and the complexity of psychiatric disorders often involves multiple loci with small effect sizes. To address these challenges, new research databases and algorithms, such as the Research Domain Criteria created in 2010, provide conceptual and statistical tools that integrate various types of information, including, but not limited to, genetics, circuits, behavior, and environment toward an integrated understanding of psychopathology and its mechanisms.[17]

Advances in Identification of Genetic Mutations That Underlie Psychiatric Disorders

A major current undertaking in psychiatric neurosciences is identifying genomic regions that influence psychiatric disorders and providing opportunities for diagnostic accuracy, mechanistic clarification, and treatment precision. While some disorders are due to single dominant genes, such as the role of the *methyl-CpG-binding protein 2*, which is implicated in 95% of Rett syndrome cases, a leading hypothesis for many psychiatric disorders is that multiple risk genes of small effect size interact with one another, and at times with environmental factors, to lead to the disease phenotype. Several approaches commonly used by scientists to identify genes linked to psychiatric disorders are elaborated here.

The *candidate gene approach* focuses on selecting one or a small group of genes believed to be implicated in a disease. This approach relies on the strong hypothesis that a gene's function is likely to be involved in a disease mechanism. For example, studies of the serotonin transporter gene and its role in MDD were derived from pre-existing knowledge that serotonergic function was implicated in depression. Targeted studies of this gene revealed that mutations in the serotonin transporter gene lead to higher rates of depression within the population. These studies focus on a small number of specific genes and as such, they are often faster and less expensive than whole genome studies (discussed below). However, this approach is often not effective for diseases without background knowledge, or those caused by the combined effect of multiple genes. Candidate gene approaches may utilize techniques such as *fluorescence in situ hybridization (FISH)*, a cytogenetic technique that uses fluorescent probes designed to bind complementarily to any gene of interest. These probes can localize where on the chromosome a gene is located and detect deletions and/or duplications within that gene. Similarly, sequencing is used for the identification of gene mutations other than deletions or duplications.

In contrast, in a *whole genome approach*, scientists sequence a nearly complete copy of an individual's genome to elucidate all mutations present in affected individuals as compared to healthy controls. This approach may identify unexpected genetic mutations anywhere in the genome that are implicated in disease pathology without requiring a priori knowledge of a specific gene's function. This higher identification rate is a mixed blessing; while it is more likely to identify the full spectrum of mutations involved in an illness it also yields more false positives or mutations of unclear clinical significance that may cloud treatment decisions.

Perhaps the most heavily utilized approach is *genome-wide association studies* (GWAS), in which hundreds or thousands of genomes are sequenced from individuals with and without disease and compared with one another to identify genomic variations among these populations.[18] Genomes may be compared among unrelated individuals, biological or adopted relatives, individuals of similar or different ethnicity, environment, or any number of parameters.

GWAS takes advantage of the fact that, while most genes are fixed within a population, some genes, known as *polymorphisms*, contain variants within a population. Most polymorphisms exist as single base-pair changes within the gene in which one of the four nucleotide bases is substituted for another. These variations, known as *single nucleotide polymorphisms (SNPs)*, occur approximately once every 300 base pairs, accounting for healthy genetic diversity within a population. Many versions of the same gene can exist that contain different SNPs and account for different versions of the gene. However, GWAS studies reveal that particular SNPs may be "associated," that is, more prevalent, in certain disease phenotypes.[18] The tendency of a particular SNP to be associated with an increased risk of a disease is known as *polygenic risk*, and it varies by disease—for example, the same individual may be at higher risk of developing obsessive-compulsive disorder (OCD) but at a lower risk of developing schizophrenia based on the *polygenic risk score* associated with each SNP contained within his/her genome. Recall that the simple presence of an SNP may or may not be sufficient to allow for the development of mental illness within an individual—due to gene-environment interactions some SNPs may increase *vulnerability* to a particular illness that may or may not give rise to a phenotype depending on whether the environment is protective. Understanding an individual's risk can help guide clinicians in practicing *precision medicine* to determine monitoring and interventions that are specific to a patient's needs.

Because SNPs occur normally within the population, GWAS requires thousands of patients to achieve statistical power to see an association and must consider factors such as race, sex, and geography to reduce false positives. GWAS have been instrumental in elucidating genes that are likely to be implicated in mental illness. For example, GWAS identified over 108 loci that meet genome-wide significance for schizophrenia with sample sizes in some studies exceeding 36,900 subjects.[19] Many of the identified genes are involved in regulatory functions that are impaired in patients with schizophrenia, including *DRD2* (D_2 dopamine receptor gene), *TCF4* (a transcription factor involved in neurogenesis), *NRGN* (a post-synaptic protein kinase substrate involved in learning and memory), and *ZNF804A* (a transcription factor involved in regulating neuronal connectivity). Multiple genes involved in glutamatergic neurotransmission and synaptic plasticity were also implicated.

In addition to studying SNPs, GWAS have identified over 1000 *copy number variants (CNVs)*, which are duplications or deletions of genomic segments ranging from 1 kilobase to several million bases that in some cases are enriched in patients with schizophrenia, autism, and BPD.[20] CNVs may be inherited from one or both parents, or may arise as new, or de novo, mutations in individuals. These CNVs may interrupt an implicated gene and may cause downshift mutations in later genes. A 2017 review recounted that novel CNVs were heavily enriched in individuals with schizophrenia as compared to healthy controls.[21] Most of the structural variants identified were different and rare, and these variants disrupted genes that are important for brain development. A large study of 3391 patients with schizophrenia found a 1.15-fold increased burden of CNVs in patients with schizophrenia relative to controls,[22–25] particularly rarer, single-occurrence CNVs. In addition, children with autism spectrum disorders have a significantly increased burden of de novo deletions and duplications.[26,27]

Cross-Disorder Approaches

Another advance of GWAS has been the identification of genes that are shared between psychiatric disorders that manifest similar behavioral traits.[28] For example, psychotic symptoms can occur in schizophrenia, BPD, trauma, or in some cases of affective psychosis associated with MDD.[29] A cross-disorder approach is based on the notion that current *Diagnostic and Statistical Manual of Mental Disorders* (DSM) diagnostic distinctions are arbitrary and that many psychiatric disorders exist on a continuum and involve a shared genetic underpinning, overlapping neurocircuitry, and neurotransmitter signaling.[1]

A compelling example of the overlapping genetic etiology of varying psychiatric disorders is the discovery of the gene called *Disrupted-in-Schizophrenia-1 (DISC-1)* in a large Scottish family with a high incidence of schizophrenia. This family had a balanced translocation between chromosomes 1 and 11, and *DISC-1* was discovered at the breakpoint of this translocation. *DISC-1* is involved in regulating brain development, neuronal migration, and a signaling pathway important for learning, memory, and mood.[30–33] The translocation in this large extended Scottish family is associated not only with schizophrenia but also with BPD and MDD.[33]

Genetic commonalities are increasingly found both within and between diagnostic families. For example, the cyclic AMP phosphodiesterase *PDE4B* is a second messenger that regulates many cellular responses to extracellular signals (such as hormones, light, and neurotransmitters). A 2019 GWAS of over 17,000 individuals found that altered activity of *PDE4* signaling is associated with many anxiety- and stress-related diagnoses, which share common anxiety-related features and fall within the continuum of anxiety-related disorders.[34] Similar studies have also identified genetic commonalities between distinct diagnostic families. In a study of over 18,000 individuals, multiple variants were identified that are shared between mood and anxiety disorders, presumably conferring a shared genetic risk to explain why mood and anxiety disorders are often co-morbid.[35]

The Psychiatric Genomics Consortium Cross-Disorder group conducted a large-scale GWAS meta-analysis of data from those with schizophrenia, BPD, MDD, attention-deficit hyperactivity disorder (ADHD), and autism in a sample of 33,332 cases and 27,888 controls.[36] They identified two SNPs in two different L-type voltage-gated calcium channel subunit genes (*CACNA1C* and *CACNB2*) which were broadly associated with an increased risk of each of these disorders, despite different diagnostic parameters of each diagnosis. This supports the notion, increasingly accepted, that many of our diagnostic distinctions may be arbitrary and fail to recognize a common continuum of symptom nuance and severity that extends beyond external DSM categorizations. However, while this study suggests an important advance about cross-disorder approaches, it also highlights the limitations of such studies; given the large sample size required, only two variants achieved statistical significance and both had relatively small odds ratios ranging from 1.07 to 1.13. Moreover, other studies, have highlighted similar limitations. Two recent studies[37,38] evaluated 8 to 11 different psychiatric disorders to determine whether genetic correlations among the disorders may explain the correlation in their behavioral traits. Despite the identification of multiple loci with a high genetic correlation across disorders, it was difficult to quantify the genetic risk associated with any specific variant. These findings underscore the complex and polygenic etiology of many psychiatric disorders and the current limitation of understanding how genetic susceptibility translates to phenotypic expression.

Once genetic loci of interest have been identified, *linkage studies* are used to generate a logarithm of the odds score (LOD score), which estimates whether two or more genetic loci are perturbed or inherited with a higher frequency in affected individuals than would be expected by random chance. An odds ratio of 1000:1 (corresponding to an LOD score of 3) is the typical threshold for linkage determination. These findings may be verified or determined by *multiple ligation-dependent probe amplification* (MLPA), which allows for the detection of differences in genetic copy numbers and can detect up to 50 different genes that differ by as little as one nucleotide.

An alternative approach is to determine the genetics of intermediate phenotypes or "endophenotypes," in which symptoms manifest at a low level that does not meet the criteria for an acute mental illness. For instance, the polymorphism in the serotonin transporter gene discussed previously has been associated with increased amygdala reactivity and reduced coupling of corticolimbic circuits seen by neuroimaging. Another intermediate phenotype that is studied is the inhibition of P50-evoked responses to repeated auditory stimuli in schizophrenia.[39]

Assessment of the Patient for Genetic Syndromes

Certain features of the medical history, family history, and physical examination may indicate the possibility of a genetic syndrome that underlies observed psychiatric symptoms. In addition to the comprehensive review of systems and medical history during the initial assessment of patients, the inclusion of questions about pregnancy and the perinatal period, birth defects, and surgeries in infancy or early childhood that may have been performed to correct congenital anomalies may provide valuable clues to an underlying genetic syndrome. In addition, a careful review of the developmental history (with special attention paid to early developmental milestones) may reveal the presence of specific developmental delays, intellectual disability, or learning disabilities. When inquiring about the family history, the clinician should ask specific questions about recurrent miscarriages; stillborn children; early infant deaths; and a family history of

intellectual disability, seizures, or congenital illness, which may help in uncovering an underlying genetic disease, especially when the pattern of illness appears to be Mendelian (e.g., dominant, recessive, or X-linked inheritance). Some standard assessment questions are summarized in Table 33.2. In addition, a careful physical examination may reveal abnormalities of growth, dysmorphic features, or involvement of various organ systems. Results of imaging studies may aid in the assessment of underlying malformations suggested by the physical examination (e.g., an echocardiogram to rule out structural heart defects when a murmur is appreciated, neuroimaging when neurological defects are detected).

Selected Genetic Disorders
Case 1

Ms. A, an 18-year-old female, presented to the psychiatric emergency room with auditory hallucinations and paranoid ideation. She had a history of ADHD and oppositional behavior. Her full-scale intelligence quotient (IQ) was 78, and her verbal IQ was 15 points greater than her performance IQ, characteristic of a non-verbal learning disorder. A review of systems revealed surgery in infancy for correction of a congenital heart defect and frequent episodes of sinusitis, otitis media, and pneumonia. On physical examination, she was short with a flat facial expression. Facial features included a high-arched palate, a small chin, and a nose with a broad, square nasal root. Ms. A was admitted to the inpatient psychiatric service and treated with atypical neuroleptics with a good result. Consultation with the genetics service for her dysmorphic facial features and congenital heart defect, along with her cognitive and psychiatric symptoms, resulted in a diagnosis of velocardiofacial syndrome.

Disorders Due to Chromosomal Abnormalities and Microdeletions

Velocardiofacial Syndrome/DiGeorge Syndrome. Velocardiofacial syndrome (VCFS) (including most patients previously diagnosed with DiGeorge syndrome), is due to a microdeletion on chromosome 22q11.2, resulting in the loss of up to 60 known and

TABLE 33.2
Additional History and Physical Examination Assessment for Genetic and Metabolic Illness

Prenatal History

Any complications with pregnancy?
Timing of complication(s)?
Maternal diabetes, systemic illness?
Maternal hypertension, eclampsia, or toxemia?
Maternal infection or high fevers?
Toxic exposures (medications, illicit substances, alcohol, radiation, chemicals)?
Any abnormalities on ultrasound?
Any indications for amniocentesis/chorionic villus sampling (CVS)?
Amniocentesis/CVS results?

Birth/Perinatal History

Mode of delivery (vaginal vs. cesarean section, natural vs. induced vs. emergent)?
Complications with delivery?
NICU or prolonged hospital stay in infancy?
Issues with feeding or growth?

Developmental History

Timing of major verbal and motor milestones?
History of speech, occupational or physical therapy?
Decline in school performance?
History of special education services, academic supports?

Family History

Ethnicity/race of parents?
History of consanguinity?
Patterns of illness in family members?
History of infertility, miscarriages?
History of infant/child deaths?
Family members with surgeries in childhood?

Multi-Organ Review of Systems

History of decompensation with illness?
Dietary history of food intolerances or unusual food preferences?
Episodic neurologic symptoms?
Problems with linear growth or weight gain?
HELLP (Hemolysis, Elevated Liver enzymes, Low Platelets)?

Physical Examination

Asymmetry of features?
Presence of dysmorphic features?
Signs of neurologic dysfunction?

Psychiatric Review of Systems

Non-specific behavioral problems (e.g., tantrums, violent behavior)?
History of developmental regression (outbursts, hyperactivity)?
Self-injurious behaviors?
Difficulties with sleep?

NICU, Neonatal intensive care unit.

TABLE 33.3
Selected Disorders With Associated Psychosis

Genetic Syndromes	Inborn Errors of Metabolism
Velocardiofacial syndrome/DiGeorge syndrome	Acute intermittent porphyria
	X-linked adrenoleukodystrophy
	Niemann-Pick disease, type C
Prader-Willi syndrome	Metachromatic leukodystrophy
Huntington disease	Tay-Sachs disease
	Wilson disease
	Mitochondrial disease

predicted contiguous genes.[40] VCFS has been called a "genetic subtype of schizophrenia," and it is estimated that as many as 2% of patients with schizophrenia may have this disorder and be undiagnosed.[41] This rate may be even higher among patients with childhood-onset schizophrenia. The spectrum of selected disorders with associated psychosis is summarized in Table 33.3. Psychiatric symptoms in those with VCFS and schizophrenia do not appear to differ from those without VCFS and schizophrenia. Roughly 60% to 75% of patients with VCFS have significant psychiatric morbidity, including mood disorders, ADHD, autism, substance abuse, anxiety disorders, and oppositional defiant disorder.[41-47] These behavioral difficulties can begin at an early age. The physical features of people with VCFS include a characteristic facial appearance (broad and squared nasal root, mid-face hypoplasia, short palpebral fissures, retruded chin), cleft palate, and/or velopharyngeal insufficiency (which may manifest as hypernasal speech, nasal regurgitation in infancy, or frequent ear infections); congenital heart defects, aplasia/hypoplasia of the thymus (leading to immune problems); problems with calcium homeostasis; low muscle tone; and scoliosis.[48] Facial hypotonia may result in a somewhat flat, expressionless appearance. Learning disabilities, especially non-verbal learning disorders, are common. However, patients can exhibit only some of these features, and the spectrum of findings may vary even within families. Diagnostic testing is available on a clinical basis and involves testing for microdeletion by FISH, chromosomal microarray (CMA), or MLPA.

Smith-Magenis Syndrome. Smith-Magenis syndrome is due to a microdeletion of chromosome 17p11.2 or a mutation in the gene RAI1.[49] In infancy, these patients may exhibit failure to thrive and hypotonia. Physical findings, which may change over time, include short stature, scoliosis, eye abnormalities, renal problems, heart defects, peripheral neuropathy, and hearing loss (both conductive and sensorineural). Characteristic facial features include a square face with a prominent forehead, deep-set and upslanting eyes, a broad nasal bridge with a short nose and fleshy nasal tip, full cheeks, and a "cupid's bow" tented upper lip. The jaw becomes more prominent with age. Although they may have hypersomnolence in infancy, a striking feature of this syndrome is marked sleep disturbance, with the absence of rapid eye movement sleep in some patients. In addition, abnormalities of circadian rhythms and melatonin secretion as well as cardiac defects have been documented.[49-51] Most patients have developmental delays, and their IQs may range from borderline intelligence to moderate intellectual disability. Patients have symptoms of ADHD, tantrums, impulsivity, and a variety of self-injurious behaviors, including onychotillomania (pulling out fingernails and toenails) and polyembolokoilamania (insertion of foreign bodies), head-banging, face-slapping, and skin-picking.[50-53] In addition, they may show stereotypies, most commonly a "self-hug" when happy.[54] The behavioral features may be seen as early as 18 months of age. Abnormalities of lipid profiles have been seen in these patients, with elevations of cholesterol, triglycerides, and low-density lipoprotein.[55] Diagnostic testing involves testing for the microdeletion with FISH, MLPA, and if negative, molecular testing of the RAI1 gene.[50,56]

Williams Syndrome.

A microdeletion on chromosome 7q11.23 results in Williams syndrome. The loss of different genes within the deletion contributes to the phenotype: the elastin gene is thought to be responsible for the supravalvular aortic or pulmonic stenosis and other connective tissue features, while the LIMK1 may be responsible for the visuospatial difficulties.[57] Patients with Williams syndrome are described as having an elfin facial appearance with a broad forehead that narrows at the temples, a short nose with a fleshy nasal tip, large and prominent ear lobes, a wide mouth with full lips, and a small jaw. The iris of the eye has a stellate or lacy appearance. Other characteristics include a hoarse voice and hyperacusis (hypersensitivity to sounds). Intellectual disability in the mild to severe range is usually present, with an average IQ of 56. Specific learning deficits in visual-spatial skills are in marked contrast to strengths in verbal and language domains and are important for the identification and care of these patients. Psychiatric symptoms and conditions include autism, ADHD, depression, and anxiety. Patients with this syndrome may show circumscribed interests or obsessions and may be somatically focused. Despite being socially disinhibited and overly friendly, they tend to have difficulty with peer relationships and may become socially isolated. Affected individuals are described as overly talkative, a feature that may be, in part, reflective of generalized anxiety. Diagnostic testing involves the detection of the microdeletion with FISH or MLPA techniques.[58-61]

Prader-Willi Syndrome.

Although several genetic mechanisms may result in Prader-Willi syndrome, the absence of a critical region of the paternally inherited chromosome 15q11–q13 is central to the disorder. This region of chromosome 15 undergoes the process of imprinting, by which genes are switched on or off depending on whether they are of maternal or paternal origin. In contrast to Prader-Willi syndrome, the absence of the maternally derived region results in Angelman syndrome (severe intellectual disability, seizures, ataxia, and characteristic behaviors). Patients with Prader-Willi syndrome may be hypotonic and show failure to thrive in infancy. Most have short stature and small hands, feet, and external genitalia; some have fair skin and hair coloring. A characteristic facial appearance with upslanting almond-shaped eyes and a thin upper lip is seen. The hallmark behavior of this disorder is hyperphagia, with resultant morbid obesity, which develops early in childhood. Behavioral interventions have been effective in controlling this behavior if started at an early age. Psychiatric symptoms and conditions include obsessional thoughts, compulsions, repetitive behaviors, mood disorders, anxiety, psychosis, ADHD, autism, skin-picking, and temper tantrums. Afflicted individuals may have a high pain threshold, and they rarely vomit. These patients may show decreased IQ and learning problems, although they also show areas of relative strength in visual-spatial skills (e.g., as with jigsaw puzzles). Diagnostic testing for Prader-Willi syndrome involves analysis of the critical region for methylation status (the process that determines whether genes are turned on or off) or the detection of the deletion by FISH, MLPA, or CMA.[62–65]

Down Syndrome. Most individuals with Down syndrome are diagnosed prenatally or soon after birth. This disorder is included in this chapter because of its known association with Alzheimer dementia, in which cognitive decline or changes in behavior in adults with Down syndrome may prompt psychiatric consultation. In 95% of cases, Down syndrome is due to an extra free copy of chromosome 21; the remainder of cases are due to unbalanced translocations or duplications involving the Down syndrome critical region on chromosome 21 or mosaicism. Down syndrome is the most common genetic cause of intellectual disability; an increased incidence is observed with older maternal age. Most clinicians recognize the characteristic Down syndrome face, which consists of eyes with upslanting palpebral fissures, epicanthal folds, Brushfield spots (white spots in the iris), a flat nasal bridge, low-set ears, and a protruding tongue. In addition, they have a short neck, short stature, and a single transverse palmar crease. These patients may also have a variety of congenital malformations, including heart defects, duodenal atresia, and high rates of hypothyroidism. Intellectual disability is seen in most individuals with Down syndrome, with an average IQ of 45 to 48 with a wide range. Social skills are usually more advanced than would be expected given the level of intellectual disability. Decline in cognition or changes in behavior in middle-aged adults with Down syndrome may indicate Alzheimer disease. The presence of an extra copy of the *amyloid precursor protein* gene (one of the causative genes in early-onset Alzheimer disease) on chromosome 21 is thought to contribute to increased rates of dementia in these patients. Non-specific behavioral symptoms, depression, and anxiety may also be seen. Diagnostic testing for Down syndrome involves karyotype analysis of chromosomes.[66–69]

Turner Syndrome. Approximately 50% of cases of Turner syndrome are due to the loss of an entire X chromosome, which is designated as 45,X. The other cases have other abnormalities of one of the X chromosomes or a mosaic karyotype with 45,X and another cell line. These patients are females, with physical characteristics of short stature, a webbed neck, and a flat, broad chest. Diagnosis may be delayed until adolescence when these girls fail to develop secondary sexual characteristics (as a result of gonadal dysgenesis). The use of hormonal therapy can help afflicted girls achieve pubertal changes but will not result in fertility. These patients may also have involvement in other organ systems, including congenital heart or kidney disease. Psychiatric symptoms and conditions include ADHD, depression, anxiety, and problems with social skills. Specific learning disabilities (especially visual-spatial deficits) have been reported. Diagnostic testing for Turner syndrome involves karyotype analysis of chromosomes.[70–72]

Klinefelter Syndrome. Klinefelter syndrome is due to the addition of an extra X chromosome, resulting in 47,XXY. These patients are male and usually described as tall, and they may be somewhat hypotonic and clumsy. They typically have a small penis and testes. Contrary to earlier descriptions, they have a male distribution of body fat and hair, although gynecomastia may be seen. They may be first diagnosed in adolescence, after they fail to enter puberty, or as part of an infertility work-up. The use of testosterone can help with the development of secondary sexual characteristics. An increased incidence of ADHD, immaturity, and depression has been reported in these patients. Cognitively, specific learning disabilities are seen. Diagnostic testing for Klinefelter syndrome involves karyotype analysis of chromosomes.[73]

47,XYY. Males with an extra copy of the Y chromosome have been of interest to the psychiatric profession for many years because of reported increased criminality and antisocial behaviors in these patients. Although early studies conducted on criminal populations were limited by ascertainment bias, more recent studies have continued to show small increases in these behaviors in 47,XYY males compared with controls. However, increased rates of antisocial or criminal behavior appear to be related to the cognitive deficits seen in some of these patients.[74] Physical findings may include accelerated linear growth in childhood and tall stature as adults. They may have a lower-than-average IQ or specific learning disabilities, especially in reading and language domains. Psychiatric conditions include ADHD and conduct disorders.[75] Overall, most of these patients never receive medical attention because they may lack any identifying features. Diagnostic testing for 47,XYY involves karyotype analysis of chromosomes.

Autosomal Dominant Single-Gene Disorders

Huntington Disease. Huntington disease is due to an increased number of CAG triplet repeats in the *HD* gene on chromosome 4p16. The normal number of CAG repeats ranges from 10 to 26 in unaffected individuals, whereas patients with Huntington disease have between 36 and 121 repeats. The number of repeats may expand from one generation to the next, and increased severity and earlier onset of illness (known as anticipation) may be seen in subsequent generations. Psychiatric symptoms are prominent in the early presentation of this disorder and may include changes in personality, depression, and apathy. Later, progressive cognitive decline and dementia occur. Mood lability and psychosis may also be seen. A high suicide rate is reported in these patients. Early physical findings include dysarthria and clumsiness with deterioration in both voluntary and involuntary movements and the development of chorea. The abnormal movements are often treated with high-potency neuroleptics, but no treatment stops the progressive neurologic decline in this disease. Characteristic atrophy of the caudate and putamen may be apparent on magnetic resonance imaging (MRI) or CT of the brain. Changes in the volume of these structures may be seen on MRI before the onset of symptoms.[76] Diagnostic testing involves molecular detection of an increased number of CAG repeats in the *HD* gene.[77-79]

Tuberous Sclerosis. Tuberous sclerosis is due to mutations in the *TSC1* (on chromosome 9q23) or *TSC2* (on chromosome 16p13.3) genes. Patients with tuberous sclerosis exhibit characteristic skin findings of flat hypopigmented macules (ash-leaf spots), shagreen patches (raised area with dimpled texture), and angiofibromas (red papular lesions). They may have small pits in their tooth enamel. Tumors occurring in different organ systems are seen, including central nervous system (CNS) tubers, retinal hamartomas, cardiac rhabdomyomas, and renal angiomyolipomas. Seizures are a common feature of this disorder. Patients with tuberous sclerosis have been reported to have symptoms of pervasive developmental disorder and ADHD. Intellectual disability may occur, depending on the extent of CNS involvement. The diagnosis is made using clinical diagnostic criteria and mutation analysis of the *TSC1* and *TSC2* genes.[80,81]

Neurofibromatosis Type I. Neurofibromatosis type I (NF1) is due to a mutation in the *NF1* gene on chromosome 17q11.2, which is believed to result in loss of tumor suppressor function. Abnormalities of skin pigmentation (*café au lait* spots, freckling in axilla or groin), Lisch nodules (small brown spots) on the iris, bony abnormalities, neurofibromas (cutaneous, subcutaneous, or plexiform), and macrocephaly are some of the physical findings in NF1. Complications may arise depending on the size or location of neurofibromas or because of the development of malignant tumors. Psychiatric symptoms may include learning disabilities and ADHD. Diagnosis is made using clinical criteria and mutation analysis of the *NF1* gene.[80,82,83]

X-Linked Dominant Disorders

Fragile X Syndrome. In contrast to Down syndrome, which is the most common *genetic* cause of intellectual disability, fragile X syndrome is the most common *inherited* (i.e., transmitted from a mother who carries the abnormal gene) cause of intellectual disability. Fragile X is the result of dysfunction of the *FMR1* gene at Xq27.3 caused by increased numbers of trinucleotide repeats. Normal alleles have approximately 5 to 44 repeats, and borderline alleles have approximately 45 to 58 repeats. Having greater than approximately 200 CGG repeats results in the full syndrome; a "premutation" allele with approximately 59 to 200 repeats may expand to the full syndrome when passed on from a mother to her children. The full syndrome is most often found in male subjects, but female subjects who carry a full-length mutation on one of their X chromosomes may have features of the disorder of variable severity. Approximately one-third of female subjects with a full-length mutation are thought to be normal, one-third are mildly affected, and the remaining one-third have findings like those of the full syndrome in males. In addition to intellectual disability in the moderate-to-severe range, physical features, such as large testes, connective tissue disease (loose joints), low muscle tone, and characteristic facial appearance (large head with prominent forehead and jaw, long face with large ears) may help identify males with this disorder. Of note, the facial features and testicular size may be more apparent after puberty. Psychiatric symptoms include autistic features, ADHD, oppositional defiant disorder, mood disorders, and avoidant personality disorder and traits. Premutation carriers (especially males) are at risk for fragile X tremor ataxia syndrome with progressive ataxia, intention tremor, deficits in executive function, and cognitive decline. Generalized anxiety disorders and phobias have also been noted in premutation carriers.[84,85] Diagnostic testing to determine the number of trinucleotide repeats in the *FMR1* gene is widely available.[86-88]

Rett Syndrome. Rett syndrome is due to a mutation in the *MECP2* gene on chromosome Xq28. This syndrome is described in girls who appear normal at birth and during the first several months or years of life. They then experience a progressive loss of developmental skills associated with acquired microcephaly. Additional features include impaired language, loss of purposeful hand movements (replaced by stereotyped hand movements), gait abnormalities, seizures, bruxism, and screaming spells. Girls with less dramatic regression, milder intellectual disability, and autistic-like features have been noted, referred to as variant Rett syndrome.[89] Mutations in the *MECP2* gene, once thought to be fatal in males, have been recognized as a cause of neonatal encephalopathy in males and also intellectual disability with manic-depressive psychosis and pyramidal signs in boys.[90] Diagnostic testing for analysis of the *MECP2* gene is available.[91,92]

METABOLIC DISEASE

Inborn errors of metabolism are a class of genetic disorders that result in dysfunction of the production, regulation, or function of enzymes or enzyme cofactors. The disruption of normal metabolic processes may lead to a buildup of pathway by-products or the production of alternate substances that cause toxicity. In addition, the absence of essential pathway end products may lead to disease states. Classically, disorders of metabolism have been described in children. However, presentation or recognition of disease may be delayed in patients with relative preservation of enzyme activity that is seen in milder forms of disease, and many disorders have later-onset forms. Metabolic disorders are most often classified based on the abnormal substances involved or by the cell location where the enzyme dysfunction occurs.

Testing for metabolic illness begins at birth by population screening for a variety of illnesses by state-mandated newborn screening programs. However, the number of diseases tested for varies widely by state, and even the most comprehensive testing has been available only for the past several years. Thus, it is unlikely that older children and adults would have benefited from these screening programs. Furthermore, even the most comprehensive state panels do not rule out all, or even most, genetic and metabolic diseases. For this reason, suspicion of a metabolic disease should be pursued vigorously. Early identification of metabolic illness is crucial to maximize good outcomes.

Assessment of the Patient for Metabolic Illness

Essential to the evaluation for possible metabolic illness is careful history taking. Questions about dietary history (e.g., food intolerances, unusual food preferences, colic or reflux), a history of decompensation associated with minor illness, or a history of transient neurologic symptoms (e.g., lethargy, encephalopathy, ataxia, confusion) may lead to detection of an underlying metabolic illness. In addition, a careful review of developmental history, especially a history of developmental regression, loss of skills, or decline in cognition, is important. Because many metabolic illnesses are inherited in an autosomal recessive fashion, a review of family history should include questions about consanguinity and ethnicity. In addition, a history of stillbirths or early infant deaths may prove informative. For example, it is thought that many children who died of Reye syndrome (manifested by vomiting, liver dysfunction with fatty infiltration, and hypoglycemia) may have had underlying problems with disorders of fatty acid oxidation.

Abnormal results of routine and specialized laboratory studies may be abnormal only during the period of acute illness or metabolic decompensation, thus, prompt collection of indicated specimens is crucial for diagnosis. Some general laboratory tests to consider when evaluating a patient for metabolic illness are listed in Table 33.4. Abnormal results on preliminary testing may direct a more specific assessment of certain metabolic pathways.[93] Thorough ophthalmologic examination may prove particularly helpful when evaluating metabolic illnesses because the retina provides a window through which to observe the metabolic processes in the brain.

Many metabolic illnesses affect the brain, either directly (e.g., via destruction of white matter in metachromatic leukodystrophy) or indirectly (e.g., as encephalopathy in urea cycle disorders). For this reason, neuropsychiatric symptoms associated with metabolic disease may vary widely. Conversely, many metabolic illnesses may have similar acute presentations (e.g., delirium). As is the case with genetic syndromes, some patients meet the full criteria for psychiatric disorders, whereas others may exhibit non-specific behavioral findings.

Treatment of psychiatric and behavioral symptoms related to inborn errors of metabolism is typically symptom focused and uses traditional psychotropic medications like treating symptoms in the general population. However, the ultimate treatment for some of these conditions may be prompt identification of the disorder and mitigation of disease progression via directly addressing the metabolic deficit. Further, the chance for a greater risk of side effects from psychotropic medication use, and the potential to directly impact the metabolic pathway (e.g., with porphyria below) must be considered.[94]

Selected Metabolic Disorders With Psychiatric Features
Case 2

Mr. B, a 57-year-old man, was admitted to the medical service due to a change in mental status. He was reported to have prominent mood lability, disorientation, and disorganized and racing thoughts. His medical history was significant for hypertension, dental surgery, and a history of hepatitis 6 months previously (attributed to alcohol intake and medication side effects). Mr. B had been consuming six beers at a time, several times a week. His family history was unremarkable. On evaluation, he appeared anxious and restless, and a tremor was noted. He had difficulty with speech and had abnormal facial movements. He exhibited mood lability and had difficulty completing cognitive tasks. Laboratory studies showed a mild elevation of liver transaminases, low serum ceruloplasmin, and a greatly increased urine copper excretion, which led to a diagnosis of Wilson disease.

Autosomal Dominant Disorders

Porphyrias and Acute Intermittent Porphyria. The porphyrias are a group of disorders with dysfunction of heme biosynthesis. One of the more common porphyrias is acute intermittent porphyria (AIP), which results from mutations in the *hydroxymethylbilane synthase* gene on chromosome 11q23.3 that cause decreased activity of porphobilinogen (PBG)

TABLE 33.4
Laboratory Studies to Evaluate Metabolic Illness

Laboratory Test	Metabolic State/Disorders Tested for
Electrolyte panel	Acidosis, calculation of anion gap
Liver function tests	Storage of abnormal substances in the liver
Blood gas	Determination of pH (acidosis vs. alkalosis)
Ammonia (NH_3)	Urea cycle disorders—primary elevation, organic acidemias, disorders of fatty acid oxidation—secondary elevation
Lactate, pyruvate	Disorders of energy metabolism
Plasma amino acids	Amino acid disorders (e.g., urea cycle defects, homocystinuria)
Urine organic acids	Organic acidemias
Acylcarnitine profile	Disorders of fatty acid oxidation, organic acidemias
Very long-chain fatty acids	Peroxisomal disorders
Urine mucopolysaccharides	Lysosomal storage disorders
Urine oligosaccharides	Lysosomal storage disorders

deaminase. AIP is inherited in an autosomal dominant manner. Episodic neurovisceral attacks are the predominant manifestations of AIP; they consist of recurrent abdominal pain, vomiting, generalized body pain, and weakness. Photosensitivity is not a feature of AIP as it is with some types of porphyria. Psychiatric symptoms and conditions, such as delirium, psychosis, depression, and anxiety, may accompany the acute attacks. Between attacks, constitutional and psychiatric symptoms resolve, although anecdotally these patients are often described as having a distinct personality with long-standing histrionic traits. Over time, indications of demyelination may develop. Of importance to the psychiatric consultant is that medications that upregulate heme biosynthesis may worsen attacks. For this reason, patients treated with medications that upregulate the cytochrome P450 system may make symptoms worse, because heme is an essential part of the cytochrome ring; these patients may be incorrectly labeled as treatment refractory. Offending agents include benzodiazepines, some tricyclic antidepressants, barbiturates, some anticonvulsants (valproate and carbamazepine), oral contraceptives, cocaine, and alcohol. Diagnostic testing focuses on the identification of by-products of heme synthesis in the urine or the measurement of PBG deaminase levels in the blood. Molecular testing may help to identify relatives of an affected patient who also are at risk for the disorder. Urine that is left standing may discolor, turning dark red or brown as a result of the presence of PBG and aminolevulinic acid. Treatment for AIP includes supportive care during attacks and the avoidance of offending agents. In addition, a high-carbohydrate diet, folic acid (a PBG diamine co-factor), intravenous heme, and the use of medications that suppress heme synthesis may be helpful.[95-98]

Autosomal Recessive Disorders

Homocystinuria. Classic homocystinuria is due to mutations of the *cystathionine β-synthase (CBS)* gene on chromosome 21q22.3 that result in decreased enzymatic activity of *CBS* and problems with conversion of homocystine to cystine and re-methylation of homocystine to methionine. Patients with preservation of some enzyme activity may respond to high dosages of pyridoxine (vitamin B_6), which acts as a co-factor for *CBS*. Deficiencies of other

enzyme co-factors (e.g., B_{12} and folate) may also lead to symptoms. Patients with homocystinuria usually have unremarkable early histories, with the development of symptoms in childhood. The patients tend to be tall and thin and are sometimes described as "marfanoid." They may have features of connective tissue disease, such as *pectus excavatum*, lens dislocation, scoliosis, and a high-arched palate. Unlike patients with Marfan syndrome, they may have restricted mobility in their joints. It is thought that high levels of homocysteine may interfere with collagen cross-linking, which results in connective tissue symptoms. In addition, abnormalities in collagen can lead to disruptions of the vascular endothelium and thrombotic events with disabling or fatal consequences. High levels of homocysteine or other factors are also thought to be neurotoxic and, when left untreated, lead to intellectual disability and learning disabilities. During the 1960s and 1970s, these patients were reported to have increased rates of schizophrenia, which was attributed to the hypothesized central role of methionine in both disorders. More recent studies have not supported an increased risk of schizophrenia or psychosis but have shown depression, OCD, personality disorders, and other behavioral disturbances. Urinary nitroprusside testing for disulfides and measurement of high levels of homocysteine and methionine (the precursor of homocysteine) in the blood help make the diagnosis. Newborn screening for homocystinuria has been available in some states for more than 30 years. Molecular testing is also available to detect biallelic pathogenic variants in *CBS*. Treatment focuses on providing a diet low in methionine and supplementation with vitamin co-factors and cystine (which becomes an essential amino acid in these patients). The use of the supplement betaine also aids in lowering homocysteine levels.[99,100]

Wilson Disease. Wilson disease is due to mutations in the *ATP7B* gene, located on chromosome 13q14.21, which lead to copper deposition in the CNS as a result of decreased levels of copper-transporting adenosine triphosphatase. Signs and symptoms of liver dysfunction (e.g., jaundice, hepatomegaly, cirrhosis, hepatitis) may be present, along with abnormal liver function tests. Of particular importance to psychiatrists are changes in personality, mood lability (including pseudobulbar palsy), cognitive decline, and other behavioral changes that may be among the earliest symptoms of Wilson disease.[101] A recent small study has also reported significantly higher rates of BPD and depression in patients with Wilson disease.[102] Neurologic symptoms are most often extrapyramidal and can include tremor, dysarthria, muscular rigidity, parkinsonism, dyskinesia, dystonia, and chorea. Seizures may also occur. The hallmark of this disorder is the Kayser-Fleischer ring, a yellow-brown ring (a consequence of copper deposition in the cornea) that is visible on slit-lamp ophthalmologic examination. Accumulations of copper in other organ systems may result in a variety of complications, including arthritis, renal tubular dysfunction, and cardiomyopathy. Confirmatory diagnostic testing includes measurement of reduced bound copper and ceruloplasmin in the serum and increased copper excretion in the urine, as well as testing to detect *ATP7B* mutations. Copper deposits may be seen on head MRI or in the liver by way of a liver biopsy. Treatment, in the form of chelation of copper (with medications such as D-penicillamine), treatment with zinc, and supplementation with antioxidants, is available. Avoidance of copper-rich foods (such as shellfish, liver, chocolate, and nuts) is recommended. Of note, patients with Wilson disease may be overly sensitive to the extrapyramidal effects of antipsychotic medications.[103] Unfortunately, liver damage may progress to liver failure and necessitate liver transplantation in some patients.[104]

Metachromatic Leukodystrophy. Metachromatic leukodystrophy is a lysosomal storage disorder with a deficiency of the enzyme arylsulfatase A and mutations in the *ARSA* gene located on chromosome 22q13.31. As a result, abnormal storage of galactosyl sulfatide (cerebroside sulfate) occurs in the white matter of the central and peripheral nervous systems. The disorder may occur in infancy, childhood, or adulthood. For the later-onset forms psychiatric symptoms may be an earlier manifestation of the disease, with a decline in cognition, personality changes, and psychotic features (including hallucinations and delusions). In some cases, psychosis may predate the onset of other symptoms by several years. Two adult-onset forms are associated with specific genetic changes, including homozygous *P426L* mutations and heterogeneous carriers of

I179S mutations. Neurologic symptoms may include ataxia and walking difficulties, dysarthria and dysphagia, and pyramidal signs. Vision loss may also occur. Brain MRI may show periventricular changes; eventually, white matter atrophy caused by the loss of myelin may be noted. In this disorder, the relationship between myelination deficits and psychosis may provide a better understanding of the role of connectivity in the development of schizophrenia. Diagnostic testing involves the measurement of elevated urine sulfatides and decreased levels of arylsulfatase A in the blood. Confirmatory molecular testing of the ARSA gene is available. No treatment is currently available, although bone marrow transplantation may delay the progression of symptoms and is most beneficial when done before symptom onset.[94,105–107]

Niemann-Pick Disease, Type C. Niemann-Pick disease, type C (NPC) is a condition that results in abnormal cholesterol esterification and lipid storage in lysosomes caused by mutations in the *NPC1* gene on chromosome 18q11–q12 or the *NPC2* gene on 14q24.3. The disorder may appear in childhood or adolescence (and rarely in adulthood) with early findings of ataxia, coordination problems, and dysarthria. Vertical supranuclear palsy is the hallmark of the disorder. Seizures and hepatosplenomegaly may be present. Psychiatric symptoms include progressive cognitive decline and dementia and may be presenting symptoms in late-onset disorders. In addition, several reports have documented the initial presentation of this disorder as psychosis or schizophrenia as well as BPD and OCD. Diagnosis is based on the demonstration of characteristic pathologic findings in the skin or bone marrow; abnormal cholesterol esterification in fibroblasts; and molecular analysis of the *NPC1* gene, which is positive in 95% of cases. Of note is that panels testing blood and urine specimens for lysosomal storage diseases will be normal in NPC, so diagnostic suspicion must direct a more comprehensive work-up.[108–111]

GM2 Gangliosidosis (Tay-Sachs Disease, Late-Onset Type). Tay-Sachs disease is another lysosomal storage disease, with the accumulation of GM2 gangliosides in neurons. Mutations in the *HEXA* gene on chromosome 15q23–q24, which encodes the alpha subunit of hexosaminidase A, lead to an enzyme deficiency.

Most clinicians are familiar with the infantile-onset form of the disorder but may not be aware of the later-onset forms that can occur with the preservation of some enzymatic activity. Patients may present with psychiatric symptoms of psychosis, mood lability, catatonia, and cognitive decline. Physical findings are those of progressive neurologic dysfunction and include early ataxia, coordination problems, dysarthria, and progressive neurologic dysfunction (e.g., with dystonia, spasticity, and seizures). Macular cherry-red spots, the hallmark of the early-onset form, are not present in the later-onset form. Diagnosis is based on analysis of enzyme levels in the blood or mutation analysis, which is especially helpful for prenatal genetic counseling. Tay-Sachs may occur in people of various ethnic and racial backgrounds, and prenatal screening is offered, especially to those of Ashkenazi Jewish descent, wherein the carrier rate is estimated to be 1:30, and to French Canadians, who have a carrier rate of 1:50. There is no treatment available for Tay-Sachs disease.[112,113]

X-Linked Disorders

X-Linked Adrenoleukodystrophy. X-Linked adreno-leukodystrophy is also a disorder of abnormal storage but in the peroxisome instead of the lysosome. In this disorder, deficiency of lignoceroyl-CoA ligase results from mutations in the *ABCD1* gene on Xq28 and leads to the accumulation of very long-chain fatty acids (VLCFAs) in the cerebral white matter and adrenal cortex. On account of its X-linked manner of inheritance, male subjects are described with the full syndrome. Female carriers, however, can also exhibit a spectrum of associated symptoms with varying degrees of severity, and they may be misdiagnosed with other disorders, including multiple sclerosis. Often, the first signs and symptoms of the disorder result in a diagnosis of ADHD for affected males. In the adult-onset form, high rates of mania and psychosis are reported. Other early signs may include difficulty with gait, handwriting, or speech. Progressive loss of motor skills, vision, and hearing, accompanied by continued decline in cognition, occurs over months to years. Accumulation of VLCFAs in the adrenal cortex may cause elevation of adrenocorticotropic hormone and other findings associated with adrenal dysfunction. These adrenal abnormalities, brain MRI findings, and elevated levels of VLCFAs in the blood can lead to the diagnosis. Confirmatory molecular testing for mutations in the *ABCD1* gene is available. Treatment for adrenal dysfunction is recommended, but there is no treatment available for the neurologic sequelae of this disease, insofar as the use of Lorenzo's oil has not proven to be effective. Bone marrow transplantation has been proposed but concerns about the high morbidity and mortality rate associated with the procedure have limited its use.[114-116]

Urea Cycle Defects—Ornithine Transcarbamylase Deficiency. Disorders of the urea cycle interfere with the normal urinary excretion of excess nitrogen via conversion to urea. Several enzymes make up the urea cycle, and deficiencies of these enzymes lead to variable failure to manage nitrogenous waste from protein. Ornithine transcarbamylase (OTC) deficiency is one of the more common urea cycle disorders, and it is inherited in an X-linked manner as a result of mutations in the *OTC* gene on Xp21.1. Although male subjects with this disorder usually present in the neonatal period with marked hyperammonemia and resultant sequelae, female carriers of the *OTC* gene may have a more variable course, owing to the lyonization of X chromosomes. Their presentations may occur at any age, and female carriers range from being asymptomatic to being as severely affected as their male counterparts. Psychiatric symptoms in affected female carriers may include intermittent episodes of delirium, ataxia, lethargy, and confusion.[117-122] Patients may report a history of self-restriction of protein in the diet or severe decompensations with vomiting illnesses or fasting (which may result in an endogenous protein load via catabolism of muscle). During symptomatic episodes elevations of ammonia, urine orotic acid, and liver function, accompanied by a characteristic pattern of plasma amino acids, aid in diagnosis. Confirmatory molecular diagnostic testing by mutation analysis, or enzymatic assay of liver tissue, is available. Treatment is focused on maintaining a low intake of dietary protein and providing supplemental essential amino acids and urea cycle intermediates. Acutely, medications that allow alternate excretion of nitrogen compounds may be used for high ammonia levels; in some cases, hemodialysis is required for rapid control of hyperammonemic episodes. Of note, the use of valproate has been reported to cause acute liver failure in patients with OTC and to precipitate a hyperammonemic crisis in female carriers. It is thought that valproate inhibits urea synthesis and can lead to hyperammonemia.[123,124] Hyperammonemic crisis has also been observed in female carriers on a high-protein diet.

Lesch-Nyhan Syndrome. Lesch-Nyhan syndrome is a disorder of purine metabolism owing to a deficiency of hypoxanthine-guanine phosphoribosyltransferase (HPRT), caused by mutations in the *HPRT1* gene at Xq26–27.2. Hyperuricemia and hyperuricuria occur and can result in the deposition of urate crystals in the joints, kidneys, and bladder. Affected males exhibit hallmark behaviors of self-injury and self-mutilation (including head-banging and biting of lips and fingers). Mutilation may be severe enough to warrant the removal of teeth or the use of restraints. Additional symptoms may include aggression, depression, anxiety, motor stereotypies, distractibility, and attentional deficits and seem to be more strongly related to deficiencies of guanine recycling. Intellectual disability may occur, although progressive loss of cognition does not. Diagnostic testing reveals increased uric acid production and excretion, decreased HPRT activity, and confirmatory molecular analysis of the *HPRT1* gene. Although allopurinol may control sequelae of high uric acid, it does not ameliorate the neurologic or psychiatric symptoms. There is some suggestion that dysfunction of dopamine metabolism may be related to the CNS pathology in this disorder.[125–128]

Mitochondrial Disorders

Disorders that involve dysfunction of the mitochondria are diverse and include disorders of fatty acid beta-oxidation or pyruvate metabolism and dysfunction of the Krebs cycle or oxidative phosphorylation by the electron transport chain. Commonly, they may be thought of as disorders of energy metabolism. Mitochondrial disorders are inherited from the mother, in the case of those coded for by genes located in the mitochondrial genome, or from either or both parents in those coded for by genes located in the nuclear genome. Mitochondrial syndromes may be characterized as specific disorders (e.g., mitochondrial encephalopathy with lactic acidosis and stroke-like episodes) or may

involve dysfunction of multiple organ systems (e.g., cardiomyopathy, diabetes, hearing loss). Body tissues with high energy demands, including the brain, may be preferentially affected. Psychiatric symptoms and conditions in mitochondrial disorders are largely uncharacterized but may include depression, delirium, dementia, and psychosis. Additionally, current thinking about the role of inflammation in contributing to the development of psychiatric disorders may indicate a pathway where deficiencies in energy production can lead to symptoms. Mitochondrial dysfunction may be suggested by elevations of lactate or pyruvate or by the presence of by-products of fatty acid oxidation or other mitochondrial pathways. Diagnosis by analysis of specific mutations is available for some disorders, whereas others require functional analysis of pathways using skin or muscle tissue. Dietary and vitamin supplementation, prevention of lactic acidosis with acute decompensations, and management of associated medical conditions are the mainstays of treatment for mitochondrial disorders.[129,130]

Teratogen Exposure

A variety of syndromes and characteristic features are associated with prenatal exposure to prescribed medications, alcohol and drugs of abuse, maternal illnesses (e.g., diabetes) and infectious agents, chemicals, radiation, and other toxins. Physical, cognitive, and psychiatric findings vary depending on the amount and timing of exposure. A detailed prenatal history should be obtained as part of a comprehensive patient evaluation.

Fetal Alcohol Spectrum Disorders. Alcohol is the major teratogen to which fetuses are exposed; it can result in a wide spectrum of cognitive, behavioral, and physical findings known as fetal alcohol spectrum disorder (FAS). The severity of symptoms appears to be dose related, although a critical threshold for alcohol intake has not been identified. High levels of blood alcohol (achieved by binge drinking) may result in more severe manifestations. Psychiatric symptoms and conditions include ADHD, depression, mood lability, anxiety, aggression, and oppositional defiant behaviors. Physical features include prenatal and postnatal growth deficiency and a characteristic facial appearance manifested by a small head, a flattened mid-face, the presence of epicanthic folds, a flat philtrum with a thin upper lip, and a small jaw. Learning disabilities and cognitive limitations are common. Diagnosis rests on clinical features with recognition of characteristic findings in the context of a known history of prenatal alcohol exposure. There is a spectrum of features seen encompassing full fetal alcohol syndrome on the most severe end to partial FAS (with some of the features) and/or alcohol-related neurodevelopmental disorder (where there may be no outward physical features). Exposure to multiple drugs in utero should also be considered in all patients evaluated for FAS. No confirmatory laboratory or imaging tests are available, although recent MRI studies have documented structural abnormalities of the brain with the absence or small size of the corpus callosum being reported in patients with FAS.[131–134]

CONCLUSION

Because the selected genetic and metabolic syndromes described in this chapter are frequently associated with psychiatric symptoms, an awareness of these disorders is important for the general psychiatrist. Given the surge in recent psychiatric genetic technologies, we anticipate that an understanding of the underlying genetics of psychiatric disorders will become increasingly important in the refinement of diagnostic and treatment criteria in the coming years.

REFERENCES

1. Smoller JW, Andreassen OA, Edenberg HJ, et al. Psychiatric genetics and the structure of psychopathology. *Mol Psychiatry.* 2019;24:409–420.
2. Kendler KS. What psychiatric genetics has taught us about the nature of psychiatric illness and what is left to learn. *Mol Psychiatry.* 2013;18(10):1058–1066.
3. Kupfer DJ, Frank E, Phillips ML. Major depressive disorder: new clinical, neurobiological, and treatment perspectives. *Lancet.* 2012;379:1045–1055.
4. Hettema JM, Prescott CA, Myers JM, et al. The structure of genetic and environmental risk factors for anxiety disorders in men and women. *Arch Gen Psychiatry.* 2005;62:182–189.
5. Jutla A, Foss-Feig J, Veenstra-VanderWeele J. Autism spectrum disorder and schizophrenia: an updated conceptual review. *Autism Res.* 2022;15:384–412.
6. Lund C, Brooke-Sumner C, Baingana F, et al. Social determinants of mental disorders and the sustainable development goals: a systematic review of reviews. *Lancet Psychiatry.* 2018;5:357–369.
7. Meyer HC, Lee FS. Translating developmental neuroscience to understand risk for psychiatric disorders. *Am J Psychiatry.* 2019;176:179–185.
8. Musci RJ, Augustinavicius JL, Volk H. Gene-environment interactions in psychiatry: recent evidence and clinical implications. *Curr Psychiatry Rep.* 2019;21:81.
9. Kessler RC, Berglund P, Demler O, et al. Lifetime prevalence and age-of-onset distributions of DSM-IV disorders in the National Comorbidity Survey replication. *Arch Gen Psychiatry.* 2005;62:593–602.
10. Hettema JM, Prescott CA, Myers JM, et al. The structure of genetic and environmental risk factors for anxiety disorders in men and women. *Arch Gen Psychiatry.* 2005;62:182–189.
11. Klengel T, Binder EB. Epigenetics of stress-related psychiatric disorders and gene x environment interactions. *Neuron.* 2015;86:1343–1357.
12. Musci RJ, Augustinavicius JL, Volk H. Gene-environment interactions in psychiatry: recent evidence and clinical implications. *Curr Psychiatry Rep.* 2019;21(9):81.
13. Albott CS, Forbes MK, Anker JJ. Association of childhood adversity with differential susceptibility of transdiagnostic psychopathology to environmental stress in adulthood. *JAMA Netw Open.* 2018;1e:185354.
14. Caspi A, Sugden K, Moffitt TE, et al. Influence of life stress on depression: moderation by a polymorphism in the 5-HTT gene. *Science.* 2003;301:386–389.
15. Pezawas L, Meyer-Lindenberg A, Drabant EM, et al. 5-HTTLPR polymorphism impacts human cingulate-amygdala interactions: a genetic susceptibility mechanism for depression. *Nat Neurosci.* 2005;8:828–834.
16. Caspi A, McClay J, Mofitt TE, et al. Role of genotype in the cycle of violence in maltreated children. *Science.* 2002;297:851–854.
17. Insel T, Cuthbert B, Garvey M, et al. Research domain criteria (RDoC): toward a new classification framework for research on mental disorders. *Am J Psychiatry.* 2010;167:748–751.
18. Lee SH, Ripke S, Neale BM, et al. Genetic relationship between five psychiatric disorders estimated from genome-wide SNPs. *Nat Genet.* 2013;45:984–994.
19. Ripke S, Neale BM, Corvin A. Biological insights from 108 schizophrenia-associated genetic loci. *Nature.* 2014;511:421–427.
20. Plomin R, Davis OS. The future of genetics in psychology and psychiatry: microarrays, genome-wide association, and non-coding RNA. *J Child Psychol Psychiatry.* 2009;50:63–71.
21. Zhuo C, Hou W, Lin C, et al. Potential value of genomic copy number variations in schizophrenia. *Front Mol Neurosci.* 2017;10:204.
22. Kirov G, Grozeva D, Norton N, et al. Support for the involvement of large CNVs in the pathogenesis of schizophrenia. *Hum Mol Genet.* 2009;18:1497–1503.
23. Stefansson H, Rujescu D, Cichon S, et al. Large recurrent microdeletions associated with schizophrenia. *Nature.* 2008;455:232–236.
24. Walsh T, McClellan JM, McCarthy SE, et al. Rare structural variants disrupt multiple genes in neurodevelopmental pathways in schizophrenia. *Science.* 2008;320:539–543.

25. Xu B, Roos JL, Levy S, et al. Strong association of de novo copy number mutations with sporadic schizophrenia. *Nat Genet.* 2008;40:880–885.

26. Grove J, et al. Identification of common genetic risk variants for autism spectrum disorder. *Nat Genet.* 2019;51:431–444.

27. Morrow EM, Yoo SY, Flavell SW, et al. Identifying autism loci and genes by tracing recent shared ancestry. *Science.* 2008;321:218–223.

28. Bulik-Sullivan BK, et al. LD Score regression distinguishes confounding from polygenicity in genome-wide association studies. *Nat Genet.* 2015;47:291–295.

29. Selzam S, Coleman JR, Caspi A, et al. A polygenic p factor for major psychiatric disorders. *Transl Psychiatry.* 2018;8:205.

30. Muir WJ, Pickard BS, Blackwood DH. Disrupted-in-schizophrenia-1. *Curr Psychiatry Rep.* 2008;10:140–147.

31. Ross CA, Margolis RL, Reading SA, et al. Neurobiology of schizophrenia. *Neuron.* 2006;52:139–153.

32. Mao Y, Ge X, Frank CL, et al. Disrupted in schizophrenia 1 regulates neuronal progenitor proliferation via modulation of GSK3beta/beta-catenin signaling. *Cell.* 2009;136:1017–1031.

33. Porteous D. Genetic causality in schizophrenia and bipolar disorder: out with the old and in with the new. *Curr Opin Genet Dev.* 2008;18:229–234.

34. Meier SM, Trontti K, Purves KL, et al. Genetic variants associated with anxiety and stress-related disorders: a genome-wide association study and mouse-model study. *JAMA Psychiatry.* 2019;76(9):924–932.

35. Otowa T, Hek K, Lee M, et al. Meta-analysis of genome-wide association studies of anxiety disorders. *Mol Psychiatry.* 2016;21:1485.

36. Cross Disorders Group of the Psychiatric Genomics Consortium. Identification of risk loci with shared effects on five major psychiatric disorders: a genome-wide analysis. *Lancet.* 2013;81:1371–1379. 3.

37. Lee PH, et al. Genomic relationships, novel loci, and pleiotropic mechanisms across eight psychiatric disorders. *Cell.* 2019;179:1469–1482.

38. Grotzinger AD, Mallard TT, Akingbuwa WA, et al. Genetic architecture of 11 major psychiatric disorders at biobehavioral, functional genomic and molecular genetic levels of analysis. *Nat Genet.* 2022;54:548–559.

39. Calkins ME, Dobie DJ, Cadenhead KS, et al. The Consortium on the Genetics of Endophenotypes in Schizophrenia: model recruitment, assessment, and endophenotyping methods for a multisite collaboration. *Schizophr Bull.* 2007;33:33–48.

40. Cleynen I, Engchuan W, Hestand MS, et al. Genetic contributors to risk of schizophrenia in the presence of a 22q11.2 deletion. *Mol Psychiatry.* 2021;26:4496–4510.

41. Bassett AS, Chow EW. Schizophrenia and 22q11.2 deletion syndrome. *Curr Psychiatry Rep.* 2008;10:148–157.

42. Arnold PD, Siegel-Bartelt J, Cytrynbaum C, et al. Velo-cardio-facial syndrome: implications of microdeletion 22q11 for schizophrenia and mood disorders. *Am J Med Genet.* 2001;105:354–362.

43. Murphy KC. Schizophrenia and velo-cardio-facial syndrome. *Lancet.* 2002;359:426–430.

44. Kraus C, Vanicek T, Weidenauer A, et al. DiGeorge syndrome: relevance of psychiatric symptoms in undiagnosed adult patients. *Wien Klin Wochenschr.* 2018;130:283–287.

45. Gothelf D, Schaer M, Eliez S. Genes, brain development and psychiatric phenotypes in velo-cardio-facial syndrome. *Dev Disabil Res Rev.* 2008;14:59–68.

46. Prasad SE, Howley S, Murphy KC. Candidate genes and the behavioral phenotype in 22q11.2 deletion syndrome. *Dev Disabil Res Rev.* 2008;14:26–34.

47. Shprintzen RJ. Velo-cardio-facial syndrome: 30 years of study. *Dev Disabil Res Rev.* 2008;14:3–10.

48. Biswas AG, Furniss F. Cognitive phenotype and psychiatric disorder in 22q11.2 deletion syndrome. A review. *Res Dev Disabil.* 2016:242–257. 53–54.

49. Onesimo R, Versacci P, Delogu AB, et al. Smith-Magenis syndrome: report of morphological and new functional cardiac findings with review of the literature. *Am J Med Genet A.* 2021;185:2003–2011.

50. Poisson A, Nicolas A, Bousquet I, et al. Smith-Magenis syndrome: molecular basis of a genetic-driven melatonin circadian secretion disorder. *Int J Mol Sci.* 2019;20:3533.

51. Gropman AL, Elsea S, Duncan WC Jr, et al. New developments in Smith-Magenis syndrome (del 17p11.2). *Curr Opin Neurol.* 2007;20:125–134.

52. Rinaldi B, Villa R, Sironi A, et al. Smith-Magenis syndrome-clinical review, biological background and related disorders. *Genes.* 2022;13:335.

53. Elsea SH, Girirajan S. Smith-Magenis syndrome. *Eur J Hum Genet.* 2008;16:412–421.

54. Finucane BM, Konar D, Haas-Givler B, et al. The spasmodic upper-body squeeze: a characteristic behavior in Smith-Magenis syndrome. *Dev Med Child Neurol.* 1994;36:78–83.

55. Smith AC, Gropman AL, Bailey-Wilson JE, et al. Hyper-cholesterolemia in children with Smith-Magenis syndrome: del (17)(p11.2p11.2). *Genet Med.* 2002;4:118–125.

56. Girirajan S, Elsas LJ, Devriendt K, et al. RAI1 variations in Smith-Magenis syndrome patients without 17p11.2 deletions. *J Med Genet.* 2005;42:820–828.

57. Hoogenraad CC, Akhmanova A, Galjart N, et al. LIMK1 and CLIP-115: linking cytoskeletal defects to Williams syndrome. *Bioessays.* 2004;26:141–150.

58. Meyer-Lindenberg A, Mervis CB, Berman KF. Neural mechanisms in Williams syndrome: a unique window to genetic influences on cognition and behaviour. *Nat Rev Neurosci.* 2006;7:380–393.

59. Paterson SJ, Schultz RT. Neurodevelopmental and behavioral issues in Williams syndrome. *Curr Psychiatry Rep.* 2007;9:165–171.

60. Royston R, Waite J, Howlin P. Williams syndrome: recent advances in our understanding of cognitive, social and psychological functioning. *Curr Opin Psychiatry.* 2019;32:60–66.

61. Mervis CB, Velleman SL. Children with Williams syndrome: Language, cognitive, and behavioral characteristics and their implications for intervention. *Perspect Lang Learn Educ.* 2011;18:98–107.

62. Angulo MA, Butler MG, Cataletto ME. Prader-Willi syndrome: a review of clinical, genetic, and endocrine findings. *J Endocrinol Invest.* 2015;38:1249–1263.

63. Schwartz L, Xaixas A, Dimitropoulos A, et al. Behavioral features in Prader-Willi syndrome (PWS): consensus paper from the International PWS Clinical Trial Consortium. *J Neurodev Dis.* 2021;13:25.

64. Cassidy SB, Driscoll DJ. Prader-Willi syndrome. *Eur J Hum Genet.* 2009;17:3–13.

65. Butler MG, Miller JL, Forster JL. Prader-Willi syndrome—clinical genetics, diagnosis and treatment approaches: an update. *Curr Pediatr Rev.* 2019;15:207–244.

66. MacLennan S. Down's syndrome. *InnovAiT.* 2020;13:47–52.

67. Plaiasu V. Down syndrome—genetics and cardiogenetics. *Maedica.* 2017;12:208–213.

68. Dykens EM. Psychiatric and behavioral disorders in persons with Down syndrome. *Ment Retard Dev Disabil Res Rev.* 2007; 13:272–278.

69. Asim A, Kumar A, Muthuswamy S, et al. Down syndrome: an insight of the disease. *J Biomed Sci.* 2015;22:41.

70. Kesler SR. Turner syndrome. *Child Adolesc Psychiatr Clin N Am.* 2007;16:709–722.

71. Cui X, Cui Y, Shi L, et al. A basic understanding of Turner syndrome: incidence, complications, diagnosis, and treatment. *Intractable Rare Dis Res.* 2018;7:223–228.

72. Gravholt CH, Viuff MH, Brun S, et al. Turner syndrome: mechanisms and management. *Nat Rev Endocrinol.* 2019;15:601–614.

73. Bonomi M, Rochira V, Pasquali D, et al. Klinefelter syndrome (KS): genetics, clinical phenotype and hypogonadism. *J Endocrinol Invest.* 2017;40:123–134.

74. Re L, Birkhoff JM. The 47,XYY syndrome, 50 years of certainties and doubts: a systematic review. *Aggress Violent Behav.* 2015; 22:9–17.

75. Ross JL, Roeltgen DP, Kushner H, et al. Behavioral and social phenotypes in boys with 47,XYY syndrome or 47,XXY Klinefelter syndrome. *Pediatrics.* 2012;129:769–778.

76. Aylward EH, Sparks BF, Field KM, et al. Onset and rate of striatal atrophy in preclinical Huntington disease. *Neurology.* 2004;63:66–72.

77. Rosenblatt A. Neuropsychiatry of Huntington disease. *Dialogues Clin Neurosci.* 2007;9:191–197.

78. Andhale R, Shrivastava D. Huntington's disease: a clinical review. *Cureus.* 2022 Aug 27;14(8):e28484.

79. McColgan P, Tabrizi SJ. Huntington's disease: a clinical review. *Eur J Neurol.* 2018;25:24–34.

80. Uysal SP, Şahin M. Tuberous sclerosis: a review of the past, present, and future. *Turk J Med Sci.* 2020;50:1665–1676.

81. Prather P, de Vries PJ. Behavioral and cognitive aspects of tuberous sclerosis complex. *J Child Neurol.* 2004;19:666–674.

82. Mautner VF, Kluwe L, Thakker SD, et al. Treatment of ADHD in neurofibromatosis type 1. *Dev Med Child Neurol.* 2002;44: 164–170.

83. Boyd KP, Korf BR, Theos A. Neurofibromatosis type 1. *J Am Acad Dermatol.* 2009;61:1–14.

84. Cordeiro L, Abucaja F, Hagerman R, et al. Anxiety disorders in fragile X permutation carriers: preliminary characterization of probands and non-probands. *Intractable Rare Dis.* 2015;4: 123–130.

85. Kalus S, King J, Lui E, et al. Fragile X-associated tremor/ataxia syndrome: an under-recognised cause of tremor and ataxia. *J Clin Neurosci.* 2016;23:162–164.

86. Lozano R, Azarang A, Wilaisakditipakorn T, et al. Fragile X syndrome: a review of clinical management. *Intractable Rare Dis Res.* 2016;5:145–157.

87. Reiss AL, Hall SS. Fragile X syndrome: assessment and treatment implications. *Child Adolesc Psychiatr Clin N Am.* 2007;16:663–675.

88. Bassell GJ, Warren ST. Fragile X syndrome: loss of local mRNA regulation alters synaptic development and function. *Neuron.* 2008;60:201–214.

89. Archer HL, Whatley SD, Evans JC, et al. Gross rearrangements of the MECP2 gene are found in both classical and atypical Rett syndrome patients. *J Med Genet.* 2006;43:451–456.

90. Moog U, Smeets EE, van Roozendaal KE, et al. Neurodevelopmental disorders in males related to the gene causing Rett syndrome in females (MECP2). *Eur J Paediatr Neurol.* 2003;7:5–12.

91. Fu C, Armstrong D, Marsh E, et al. Consensus guidelines on managing Rett syndrome across the lifespan. *BMJ Paediatr Open.* 2020;4:e000717.

92. Chahrour M, Zoghbi HY. The story of Rett syndrome: from clinic to neurobiology. *Neuron.* 2007;56:422–437.

93. Demily C, Sedel F. Psychiatric manifestations of treatable hereditary metabolic disorders in adults. *Ann Gen Psychiatry.* 2014;13:27.

94. Walterfang M, Bonnot O, Mocellin R, et al. The neuropsychiatry of inborn errors of metabolism. *J Inherit Metab Dis.* 2013;36:687–702.

95. Crimlisk HL. The little imitator—porphyria: a neuropsychiatric disorder. *J Neurol Neurosurg Psychiatry.* 1997;62:319–328.

96. Bissell DM, Anderson KE, Bonkovsky HL. Porphyria. *N Engl J Med.* 2017;377:862–872.

97. Duque-Serrano L, Patarroyo-Rodriguez L, Gotlib D, et al. Psychiatric aspects of acute porphyria: a comprehensive review. *Curr Psychiatry Rep.* 2018;20:5.

98. Bonkovsky HL, Maddukuri VC, Yazici C, et al. Acute porphyrias in the USA: features of 108 subjects from porphyrias consortium. *Am J Med.* 2014;127:1233–1241.

99. Di Lorenzo R, Amoretti A, Baldini S, et al. Homocysteine levels in schizophrenia patients newly admitted to an acute psychiatric ward. *Acta Neuropsychiatr.* 2015;27:336–344.

100. Almuqbil MA, Waisbren SE, Levy HL, et al. Revising the psychiatric phenotype of homocystinuria. *Genet Med.* 2019;21:1827–1831.

101. Kasztelan-Szczerbinska B, Cichoz-Lach H. Wilson's disease: an update on the diagnostic workup and management. *J Clin Med.* 2021;10:5097.

102. Carta MG, Sorbello O, Moro MF, et al. Bipolar disorders and Wilson's disease. *BMC Psychiatry.* 2012;30:12–52.

103. Zimbrean PC, Schilsky ML. The spectrum of psychiatric symptoms in Wilson's disease: treatment and prognostic considerations. *Am J Psychiatry*. 2015;172:1068–1072.

104. Ala A, Walker AP, Ashkan K, et al. Wilson's disease. *Lancet*. 2007;369:397–408.

105. Rauschka H, Colsch B, Baumann N, et al. Late-onset metachromatic leukodystrophy: genotype strongly influences phenotype. *Neurology*. 2006;67:859–863.

106. Shaimardanova AA, Chulpanova DS, Solovyeva VV, et al. Metachromatic leukodystrophy: diagnosis, modeling, and treatment approaches. *Front Med*. 2020;7:3389.

107. van Rappard DF, de Vries ALC, Oostrom KJ, et al. Slowly progressive psychiatric symptoms: think metachromatic leukodystrophy. *J Am Acad Child Adolesc Psychiatry*. 2018;57:74–76.

108. Sandu S, Jackowski-Dohrmann S, Ladner A, et al. Niemann-Pick disease type C1 presenting with psychosis in an adolescent male. *Eur Child Adolesc Psychiatry*. 2009;18:583–585.

109. Sevin M, Lesca G, Baumann N, et al. The adult form of Niemann-Pick disease type C. *Brain*. 2007;130:120–133.

110. Whitehouse C, Harris S, Heptinstall L. Niemann-Pick type C in adults. *J Inherit Metab Dis*. 2002;25:385–389.

111. Sullivan D, Walterfang M, Velakoulis D. Bipolar disorder and Niemann-Pick disease type C disease. *Am J Psychiatry*. 2005;162:1021.

112. Navon R, Argov Z, Frisch A. Hexosaminidase A deficiency in adults. *Am J Med Genet*. 1986;24:179–196.

113. MacQueen GM, Rosebush PI, Mazurek MF. Neuropsychiatric aspects of the adult variant of Tay-Sachs disease. *J Neuropsychiatry Clin Neurosci*. 1998;10:10–19.

114. Sedel F, Baumann N, Turpin JC, et al. Psychiatric manifestations revealing inborn errors of metabolism in adolescents and adults. *J Inherit Metab Dis*. 2007;30:631–641.

115. Garside S, Rosebush PI, Levinson AJ, et al. Late-onset adrenoleukodystrophy associated with long-standing psychiatric symptoms. *J Clin Psychiatry*. 1999;60:460–468.

116. Zhu J, Eichler F, Biffi A, et al. The changing face of adrenoleukodystrophy. *Endocrine Rev*. 2020;41:577–593.

117. Sloas 3rd HA, Ence TC, Mendez DR, et al. At the intersection of toxicology, psychiatry, and genetics: a diagnosis of ornithine transcarbamylase deficiency. *Am J Emerg Med*. 2013;31:1420.

118. Rowe PC, Newman SL, Brusilow SW. Natural history of symptomatic partial ornithine transcarbamylase deficiency. *N Engl J Med*. 1986;314:541–547.

119. Legras A, Labarthe F, Maillot F, et al. Late diagnosis of ornithine transcarbamylase defect in three related female patients: polymorphic presentations. *Crit Care Med*. 2002;30:241–244.

120. Honeycutt D, Callahan K, Rutledge L, et al. Heterozygote ornithine transcarbamylase deficiency presenting as symptomatic hyperammonemia during initiation of valproate therapy. *Neurology*. 1992;42:666–668.

121. Nassogne MC, Heron B, Touati G, et al. Urea cycle defects: management and outcome. *J Inherit Metab Dis*. 2005;28:407–414.

122. Gropman AL, Batshaw ML. Cognitive outcome in urea cycle disorders. *Mol Genet Metab*. 2004;81(suppl 1):S58S62.

123. Hjelm M, Oberholzer V, Seakins J, et al. Valproate-induced inhibition of urea synthesis and hyperammonaemia in healthy subjects. *Lancet*. 1986;2:859.

124. Kay JD, Hilton-Jones D, Hyman N. Valproate toxicity and ornithine carbamoyltransferase deficiency. *Lancet*. 1986;2:1283–1284.

125. Robey KL, Reck JF, Giacomini KD, et al. Modes and patterns of self-mutilation in persons with Lesch-Nyhan disease. *Dev Med Child Neurol*. 2003;45:167–171.

126. Bell S, Kolobova I, Crapper L, Ernst C. Lesch-Nyhan syndrome: models, theories, and therapies. *Mol Syndromol*. 2016;7:302–311.

127. Schretlen DJ, Ward J, Meyer SM, et al. Behavioral aspects of Lesch-Nyhan disease and its variants. *Dev Med Child Neurol*. 2005;47:673–677.

128. Schretlen DJ, Callon W, Ward RE, et al. Do clinical features of Lesch-Nyhan disease correlate more closely with hypoxanthine or guanine recycling? *J Inherit Metab Dis*. 2016;39:85–91.

129. McFarland R, Taylor RW, Turnbull DM. Mitochondrial disease—its impact, etiology, and pathology. *Curr Top Dev Biol*. 2007;77:113–155.

130. Taylor RW, Turnbull DM. Mitochondrial DNA mutations in human disease. *Nat Rev Genet*. 2005;6:389–402.

131. Riley EP, Infante MA, Warren KR. Fetal alcohol spectrum disorders: an overview. *Neuropsychol Rev*. 2011;21:73–80.

132. Mattson SN, Bernes GA, Doyle LR. Fetal alcohol spectrum disorders: a review of the neurobehavioral deficits associated with prenatal alcohol exposure. *Alcohol Clin Exp Res*. 2019;43:1046–1062.

133. Williams JF, Smith VC. The committee on substance abuse: fetal alcohol spectrum disorders. *Pediatrics*. 2015;136:3113.

134. Donald KA, Eastman E, Howells FM, et al. Neuroimaging effects of prenatal alcohol exposure on the developing human brain: a magnetic resonance imaging review. *Acta Neuropsychiatr*. 2015;27:251–269.

SUGGESTED READING

Gene Clinics. <http://www.Geneclinics.org>

Online Mendelian Inheritance in Man (OMIM). <http://www.ncbi.nlm.nih.gov/omim/>

POSSUM and software. <http://www.possum.net.au/>

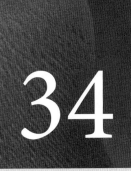

34

COPING WITH MEDICAL ILLNESS AND PSYCHOTHERAPY OF THE MEDICALLY ILL

STEVEN C. SCHLOZMAN, MD ■ JONAH N. COHEN, PHD ■ THEODORE A. STERN, MD

BACKGROUND

Coping with illness can be a serious problem for both the patient and the physician. Increasingly, clinicians and researchers have focused on the problems that coping presents for family and community members of those who are ill. Indeed, the irony of our increasing prowess in healing is our growing discomfort and our sense of impotence when a cure cannot be found, and when coping is the order of the day. This dilemma is both consciously realized and unconsciously experienced; patients, practitioners, and families feel the ripple effect.[1-4]

Psychiatrists are perhaps among those best suited to assist patients and their non-psychiatric providers and caregivers with the complexities of medical illness and to pay careful attention to the complex feelings that chronic suffering engenders (in inpatient consultative settings as well as in outpatient practices). In fact, there is a growing body of literature that focuses on the mechanisms by which patients cope with chronic conditions and the corresponding psychotherapeutic interventions for patients with chronic illness. This chapter addresses how patients and their families cope, as well as on the art of working psychotherapeutically with the medically ill.

HISTORY

At virtually every step of patient care, physicians and patients alike appraise their coping skills. Although this appraisal is not always conscious, it is clear that conclusions drawn about how a patient is processing his or her illness can have a significant bearing on

therapeutic decisions, on the psychological well-being of the patient, and on the overall course of the patient's illness.[1] However, achieving an accurate appraisal of coping skills is hampered by muddled definitions of coping, perhaps even more muddled definitions of resilience, competing standardized assessments, and a general lack of conscious consideration of how patients cope and whether their particular coping styles are effective or helpful.[5-8]

Early conceptualizations of coping centered around the "Transactional Model for Stress Management," put forth first by Lazarus and colleagues in the late 1960s.[9] This conceptualization emphasized the extent to which patients interact with their environment as a means of attempting to manage the stress of illness. These interactions involve assessment of the current medical condition, given the psychological and cultural overlay that varies from patient to patient. Although this definition of coping is useful, many believe that it is also too broad to allow for standardized assessments in patient populations. Thus, while multiple studies of patient coping exist, most clinicians favor a more open-ended evaluation of each patient, taking into consideration the unique backgrounds that the patient and the physician bring to the therapeutic setting.[6]

Coping is perhaps best defined as a problem-solving behavior that is intended to bring about relief, reward, quiescence, and equilibrium. Furthermore, the term "coping" is often used interchangeably with the term "resilience," and given that multiple definitions exist for each of these terms, general conclusions about how one best copes or remains resilient should be viewed with utilitarianism and caution.[7] We will address the different definitions of resilience later in this chapter. At this point, it is more important to remember that nothing in any of these definitions promises a permanent resolution of problems encountered. Both coping and resilience, however, *do* imply a combination of knowing what the problems are and how to go about embarking upon a path that will help achieve a more comfortable state.[1,6,9]

In ordinary language, the term *coping* is used to characterize a means of managing a problem, and it overlooks the intermediate processes of appraisal, performance, and correction that most problem-solving entails. Coping is not a simple judgment about how some difficulty worked out. It is an extensive, recursive process of self-exploration, self-instruction, self-correction, self-rehearsal, and guidance gathered from outside sources. Indeed, these assertions were central to Lazarus' initial conceptualizations.[9] More recent research has focused on the ways that different stages of development affect one's approach and ability toward effective coping.

CLINICAL AND RESEARCH CHALLENGES

Coping with illness and its ramifications is an inescapable part of medical practice. Therefore, the overall purpose of any intervention, physical or psychosocial, is to improve coping beyond the limits of the illness itself. Such interventions must account for both the problems to be solved and the individuals most closely affected by the difficulties. In fact, when one considers varied definitions of coping and resiliency, it becomes clear that despite the different conceptualizations of this complicated process, they all have in common the need that one adapt to the highest level of individual functioning.

How anyone copes depends on the nature of a problem, as well as on the mental, emotional, physical, and social resources that one has available for the coping process. It also depends on the developmental stage of the person doing the coping and of those who are engaged in the caretaking. In this sense, the hospital psychiatrist is well-positioned to evaluate how physical illness can interfere with the patient's life and to see how psychosocial stressors can impede the course of illness and recovery. This is accomplished largely by knowing which psychosocial problems are pertinent, which physical symptoms are most distressing, what the developmental meaning of the reasons for the hospitalization entails, and which interpersonal relations support or undermine coping.

Assessment of how anyone copes, especially in a clinical setting, requires an emphasis on the "here and now." This emphasis has been borne out by the growing momentum that practices, such as mindfulness, have brought to the bedside.[10] Furthermore, the recent global COVID-19 pandemic yielded important information about how, and in what circumstances, individuals and communities cope with an existentially threatening medical experience.[11] Issues such as the locus of control, positive versus negative religious interpretations of events, and openness with one's partner all play significant roles in successful coping.[12–14] Nevertheless, ongoing research is needed to assess best practices in this next frontier of treatment.

More traditional, long-range, forays into the medical, social, family, and psychiatric history are relevant only if such investigations are likely to shed light and understanding of the present predicament. In fact, clinicians are increasingly adopting a focused and problem-solving approach to therapy with medically ill patients. For example, supportive and behavioral therapies for medically ill children and adults in both group and individual settings have reduced psychiatric morbidity and led to measurable improvements related to the course of non-psychiatric illnesses.

Few of us always cope well. For each of us, sickness imposes a personal and social burden, with a risk to our well-being and happiness. Furthermore, these reactions are seldom proportional to the actual dangers of the primary disease. Therefore, effective copers may be individuals with a special skill or with personal traits that enable them to master many difficulties. Characteristics of good copers are presented in Box 34.1. No one always copes superbly, especially with problems that threaten one's sense of sense or survival. Notably, effective copers seem adept at selecting the kind of situation in which they are most likely to prosper and hold enough confidence to maintain resourcefulness. Finally, it is our impression that those individuals

BOX 34.1
CHARACTERISTICS OF GOOD COPERS

- They are optimistic about mastering problems and, despite setbacks, generally maintain a high level of morale.
- They tend to be practical and emphasize immediate problems, issues, and obstacles that must be conquered before even visualizing a remote or ideal resolution.
- They select from a wide range of potential strategies and tactics, and their policy is not to be at a loss for fallback methods. In this respect, they are resourceful.
- They heed various possible outcomes and improve coping by being aware of consequences.
- They are generally flexible and open to suggestions, but they do not give up the final say in decisions.
- They are quite composed and vigilant in avoiding emotional extremes that could impair judgment.

BOX 34.2
CHARACTERISTICS OF POOR COPERS

- They tend to be excessive in self-expectation, rigid in outlook, inflexible in standards, and reluctant to compromise or to ask for help.
- Their opinion of how people should behave is narrow and absolute; they allow little room for tolerance.
- Although prone to firm adherence to preconceptions, bad copers may show unexpected compliance or be suggestible on specious grounds, with little cause.
- They are inclined to excessive denial and elaborate rationalization; in addition, they are unable to focus on salient problems.
- Because they find it difficult to weigh feasible alternatives, bad copers tend to be more passive than usual and fail to initiate action on their own behalf.
- Their rigidity occasionally lapses, and bad copers subject themselves to impulsive judgments or atypical behavior that fails to be effective.

who cope effectively do not pretend to have knowledge that they do not have; they feel comfortable turning to experts whom they can trust. The clinician's tasks are to assess how patients and their families and friends cope and to pinpoint the traits that they seem to lack. The clinician then must focus on these missing traits to maximize the emotional equilibrium with existing medical challenges.[8]

It is too simplistic to indicate that bad copers have the opposite characteristics of effective copers. As was stressed earlier, each patient brings a unique set of cultural and psychological attributes to his or her coping capacity. Also, it is important to keep in mind that a bad coper is not a bad person. Instead, bad copers are those who face more challenges when coping with unusual, intense, and unexpected difficulties because of a variety of traits. Box 34.2 lists some characteristics of these individuals. Investigations into the psychiatric symptoms of the medically ill have yielded many of the attributes of those who do not cope well. Problems such as demoralization, anhedonia, anxiety, pain, and overwhelming grief have each been documented in medical patients for whom psychiatric attention has been indicated. Additionally, some individuals fare more poorly because of an absence of social and emotional support outside of the medical setting.[4]

The significance of religious or spiritual conviction for the medically ill deserves special mention. Virtually every psychiatrist works with patients as they wrestle with issues such as mortality, fate, justice, and fairness. Such topics often invoke religious considerations in patients and their physicians; moreover, there is a growing appreciation in the medical literature for the important role that these considerations can play.[15–17]

In some studies, being at peace with oneself and with one's sense of a higher power predicts physical and psychiatric recovery.[12] Other studies suggest that resentment toward God, fears of God's abandonment, and a willingness to invoke Satanic motivation for medical illness predict worsening health and an increased risk of death.[16,17]

Inasmuch as psychiatrists seek to identify and strengthen those attributes that are most likely to aid a patient's physical and emotional well-being, effective therapy for the medically ill can involve exploring the religious convictions of patients; fostering those elements is likely to be helpful. Although it is *never* the role of the physician to encourage religious conviction de novo, ignoring religious content risks omitting an important element of the psychotherapeutic armamentarium.

PRACTICAL POINTERS

Coping refers to how a patient responds to problems that relate to *disease, sickness,* and *vulnerability.* In approaching chronically ill patients, it is helpful to conceptualize the *disease* as the categorical reason for being sick, *sickness* as the individual style of illness and patienthood, and *vulnerability* as the tendency to be distressed and to develop emotional difficulties in the course of trying to cope.[1] One must also keep in mind the various definitions of resilience while approaching these clinical challenges. Some have defined resilience as the establishment of a stable trajectory after a highly adverse event. Others have noted that those who are resilient possess the ability to harness those aspects of their lives that will maintain well-being. In this sense, the hospital psychiatrist must forecast both for and with a patient how that individual will most efficiently and effectively obtain a trajectory that will ensure the maximum level of intended functioning. In other words, the work of the hospital psychiatrist in this setting involves something akin to a negotiation with the patient and those around the patient. What is the desired level of functioning? How long does this level of functioning take to obtain? And are these expectations reasonable?

Most importantly, the psychiatrist must ask *why now?* What has preceded the consultation request? How does the patient show his or her sense of futility and despair, or is there instead a desire to think about how best to remain optimistic? How did the present medical problems and their corresponding coping challenges, come about? Was there a time when such problems could have been thwarted? It is also worth noting that the treatment team can often be even more exasperated than the patient. In these instances, one must guard against the assumption that only the patient is troubled by the medical predicament.

In fact, if there is any doubt about the gap between how the medical staff and patients differ in their cultural bias and social expectations, just listen to the bedside conversation between the patient and the clinicians involved in his or her care. Good communication may not only reduce potential problems but also help patients to cope better. Good coping is a function of empathic connectedness between the patient and the physician regarding the risks and stresses in the current treatment. Psychiatrists are by no means alone in their professional concern about coping, but the unique skills and mandates of psychiatric care are ideally suited to address the vicissitudes of how patients cope. Many chronic conditions evoke existential issues. These are fundamental psychiatric considerations for which there is a bevy of educational resources that can empower patients and their family members, preparing them with knowledge, skills, and strategies that can enhance coping.[18–39]

It is important to remember that psychiatry does not arbitrarily introduce psychosocial problems. If, for example, a patient is found to have an unspoken but vivid fear of death or is noted to suffer from an unrecognized and unresolved bereavement, fear and grief already exist; they are not superfluous artifacts of the evaluation itself. Open discussion of these existential quandaries is likely to be therapeutic, and active denial of their existence is potentially detrimental, risking empathic failure and the poor adherence that accompanies the course of patients who feel misunderstood or unheard. These considerations were borne out in investigations of how individuals coped with contracting COVID-19.[11]

Being sick is, of course, much easier for some patients than it is for others, and for certain patients, it is preferred over trying to make it in the world outside of the medical domain. For some, there is too much anxiety, fear of failure, inadequacy, pathological shyness, expectation, frustration, and social hypochondriasis to make the struggle to holding one's own appealing. At key moments of life, sickness can be a solution. Although healthy people are expected to tolerate defeat and withstand disappointments, others legitimize their low self-esteem with a variety of excuses, denial, self-pity, and symptoms, long after other individuals are back to work. Such patients thrive in a complaining atmosphere and even blame their physicians. Although these are forms of coping, they pose significant challenges. They are also contrary to the collective similarities in definitions of resilience.[8,40]

These complexities complicate the role of psychiatrists. Clinicians must assess the motivation of staff and patients to ask for a psychiatric intervention. For example, the request for psychiatric consultation to treat depression and anxiety in a negativistic and passive-aggressive patient is inevitably more complicated than the simple recognition of certain psychiatric symptoms. Such patients (through primitive defenses such as denial and projection) can generate a profound sense of hopelessness and discomfort in their treaters.

It is often an unspoken and unconscious desire by physicians and ancillary staff that psychiatrists shift the focus of negativity and aggression onto themselves and away from the remainder of the treatment team. If the consulting psychiatrist is unaware of these subtleties, the intent of the consultation will be misinterpreted, and the psychiatrist's efforts will ultimately fall short.

Everyone needs, or at least deserves, a measure of support, sustenance, security, and self-esteem, even when they are not patients, but merely human beings encountered at a critical time.

In assessing problems and needs, psychiatrists can help by identifying potential pressure points (e.g., health and well-being, family responsibility, marital and sexual roles, jobs and money, community expectations and approval, religious and cultural demands, self-image and sense of inadequacy, and existential issues) where trouble might arise. In these circumstances, it is paramount that one pay close attention to the developmental stage of the patient. A young patient at the prime of her career will have different needs and concerns than a long-retired grandparent.[12]

Social support is not a hodgepodge of interventions designed to cheer up difficult patients. Self-image and self-esteem, for example, depend on the sense of confidence generated by various sources of social success and support. In a practical sense, social support reflects what society expects and demands regarding health and conduct. There is, in fact, a burgeoning literature that addresses the necessity of support at all levels of care for patients with chronic illness.

Social support is not a "sometime" thing, to be used only for the benefit of those who are too weak, needy, or troubled to get along by themselves. It requires a deliberate skill, which professionals can cultivate, to recognize, refine, and implement what any vulnerable individual needs to feel better and cope better. In this light, it is not an amorphous exercise in reassurance, but a combination of therapeutic strategies intended to normalize a patient's attitude and behavior. Techniques of support range from concrete assistance to extended counseling and family interventions.[4,41,42] Such techniques aim to help patients get along without professional support. Social support depends on an acceptable image of the patient, not one that invariably "pathologizes." If a

counselor only corrects mistakes or points out what is wrong, bad, or inadequate, insecurity increases, and self-esteem inevitably suffers.

Vulnerability is present in everyone, and it shows up at times of crisis, stress, calamity, and threats to well-being and identity.[43–51]

How does a patient visualize threat? What is most feared when approaching a surgical procedure? The diagnosis? Anesthesia? Possible invalidism? Failure, pain, or abandonment by the physician or family?

Coping and vulnerability have an inverse relationship in that the better one copes, the less distress he or she experiences as a function of acknowledged vulnerability. Another way of looking at this is by noting that resilient patients acknowledge and come to terms with the challenges of their predicament. In general, distress often derives directly from a sense of uncertainty about how well one will cope when called on to do so. This does not mean that those who deny or disavow problems and concerns are exceptional copers. The reverse may be true. Courage to cope requires that anxiety be confronted, with an accurate appraisal of how much control the patient has over his or her predicament.

Table 34.1 shows 13 common types of distress. Table 34.2 describes how to find out about salient problems, the strategy used for coping, and the degree of resolution attained.

Many interventions call on the consulting psychiatrist to ask patients to fill out forms that indicate their degree of anxiety, level of self-esteem, perceived illness, and so on. Although such queries often provide valuable information, these standardized inquiries are no substitute for careful and compassionate interviews. There is a strong element of social desirability present in any attempt to assess how a person adapts. How a patient deals with illness may not be the same as how he or she wishes to manage it. Vulnerability, except in extreme forms (such as depression, anger, or anxiety), can be difficult to characterize, so the astute clinician must rely upon a telling episode or metaphor that typifies a reaction.

Thus far, we have discussed the following: salient characteristics of effective and less effective copers; differing definitions of resiliency in medical settings, methods by which deficits in patients can be identified and how clinicians can intervene; potential pressure

TABLE 34.1	
Vulnerability	
Hopelessness	The patient believes that all is lost; effort is futile; there is no chance at all; there is a passive surrender to the inevitable.
Turmoil/perturbation	The patient is tense, agitated, restless, hyperalert to potential risks (real and imagined).
Frustration	The patient is angry about an inability to progress, recover, or get satisfactory answers or relief.
Despondency/ depression	The patient is dejected, withdrawn, apathetic, tearful, and often unable to interact verbally.
Helplessness/ powerlessness	The patient complains of being too weak to struggle anymore; cannot initiate action or make decisions that stick.
Anxiety/fear	The patient feels on the edge of dissolution, with dread and specific fears about impending doom and disaster.
Exhaustion/apathy	The patient feels too worn out and depleted to care; there is more indifference than sadness.
Worthlessness/ self-rebuke	The patient feels persistent self-blame and no good; he or she finds numerous causes for weakness, failure, and incompetence.
Painful isolation/ abandonment	The patient is lonely and feels ignored and alienated from significant others.
Denial/avoidance	The patient speaks or acts as if threatening aspects of illness are minimal, almost showing a jolly interpretation of related events, or else a serious disinclination to examine potential problems.
Truculence/ annoyance	The patient is embittered and not openly angry; feels mistreated, victimized, and duped by forces or people.
Repudiation of significant others	The patient rejects or antagonizes significant others, including family, friends, and professional sources of support.
Closed time perspective	The patient may show any or all of these symptoms, but in addition foresees an exceedingly limited future.

TABLE 34.2	
Coping (To Find Out How a Patient Copes)	
Problem	In your opinion, what has been the most difficult for you since your illness started? How has it troubled you?
Strategy	What did you do (or are doing) about the problem?
	Get more information (rational/intellectual approach).
	Talk it over with others to relieve distress (share concern).
	Try to laugh it off; make light of it (reverse affect).
	Put it out of your mind; try to forget (suppression/denial).
	Distract yourself by doing other things (displacement/dissipation).
	Take a positive step based on your present understanding (confrontation).
	Accept, but change the meaning to something easier to deal with (re-definition).
	Submit, yield, and surrender to the inevitable (passivity/fatalism).
	Do something, anything, reckless or impractical (acting out).
	Look for feasible alternatives to negotiate (if x, then y).
	Drink, eat, take drugs, and so on, to reduce tension (tension reduction).
	Withdraw, get away, and seek isolation (stimulus reduction).
	Blame someone or something (projection/ disowning/externalization).
	Go along with directives from authority figures (compliance).
	Blame oneself for faults; sacrifice or atone (undoing self-pity).
Resolution	How has it worked out so far?
	Not at all.
	Doubtful relief.
	Limited relief, but better.
	Much better; actual resolution.

Adapted from Weisman AD. *The Realization of Death: A Guide for the Psychological Autopsy.* Jason Aronson; 1974.

points that alert clinicians to different psychosocial difficulties; types of emotional vulnerabilities; and a format for listing different coping strategies, along with questions about resolution.

The **assessment and identification** of ways in which a patient copes or fails to cope with specific problems requires both a description by the patient and an evaluation by the psychiatrist. Even so, this may be inadequate. Details of importance may not be explicit or forthcoming. In these situations, clinicians must elucidate the specifics of each situation. If not, the result is only an approximation that generalizes where it should be precise. Indeed, clinicians should ask again and again about a topic that is unclear and re-phrase, without yielding to clichés and general impressions. This is where family, community, and members of the treatment team can be particularly helpful.[4]

Psychiatrists have been trained to leverage empathy and intuition. Although immediate insights and inferences can be pleasing to the examiner, sometimes these conclusions can be misleading and inaccurate. It is far more empathic to respect each patient's individuality and unique view of the world by making sure that the examiner accurately understands in detail how problems are confronted. To draw a quick inference without being sure about a private and idiosyncratic state of mind is distinctly non-empathic. Like most individuals, patients give themselves the benefit of the doubt and claim to resolve problems in a socially desirable and potentially effective way. It takes a little experience to realize that disavowal of any problem through pleasant distortions is itself a coping strategy, not necessarily an accurate description of how one has coped.

Patients who adamantly deny any difficulty tend to cope poorly. Sick patients have difficult lives, and the denial of adversity usually represents a relatively primitive defense that leaves such patients ill-prepared to accurately assess their options. Carefully timed and empathic discussions with patients that convey a genuine appraisal of their current condition can help them avoid this maladaptive approach and address their treatment more effectively.

On the other hand, patients may attempt to disavow any role in their current illness. By seeking credit for having suffered so much, such patients reject any implication that they might have prevented, deflected, or corrected what has befallen them (see Table 34.2). Helping these patients does not necessarily require that they acknowledge their role in their predicament. Instead, the empathic listener identifies and provides comfort around the implicit fear that these

patients harbor (i.e., that they somehow deserve their debilitation).

Suppression, isolation, and projection are common defenses. Effective copers seem to pinpoint problems clearly, whereas poor copers seem only to seek relief from further questions without attempting anything that suggests reflective analysis.

In learning how anyone copes, a measure of authentic skepticism is always appropriate, especially when it is combined with a willingness to correct it later. The key is to focus on points of ambiguity, anxiety, and ambivalence while tactfully preserving a patient's self-esteem. A tactful examiner might say, for example, "I'm really not clear about what exactly bothered you, and what you really did. …"

The purpose of focusing is to avoid premature formulation and closure that gloss over points of ambiguity. An overly rigid format while approaching an evaluation risks overlooking individual tactics that deny, avoid, dissemble, and blame others for difficulties. Patients, too, can be rigid, discouraging alliance, rebuffing collaboration, and preventing an effective physician-patient relationship.

Coping with illness is only one special area of human behavior. It is important to recognize that in evaluating how patients cope, examiners should learn more about their own coping styles and, in effect, learn from patients. Clearly, it is not enough to mean well, to have a warm heart, or to have a head filled with scientific information. Coping well requires open-ended communication and self-awareness. No technique for coping applies to everyone. In fact, the concept of technique may be antithetical to true understanding. A false objectivity obstructs appraisal and an exaggerated subjectivity only confuses what is being understood about whom.

Psychiatrists and patients can become better copers by cultivating the characteristics of effective copers. Coping is, after all, a skill that is useful in a variety of situations, although many modifications of basic principles are required. Confidence in being able to cope can be enhanced only through repeated attempts at self-appraisal, self-instruction, and self-correction. Coping well with illness—with any problem—does not predict success, but it does provide a foundation for becoming a better coper.

Access a list of MCQs for this chapter at https://expertconsult.inkling.com

REFERENCES

1. Schlozman SC, Groves JE, Gross AF, et al. Coping with illness and psychotherapy of the medically ill. In: Stern TA, Freudenreich O, Smith FA, eds. *Massachusetts General Hospital Handbook of General Hospital Psychiatry*. 7th ed. Elsevier; 2018.

2. Williams CM, Wilson CC, Olsen CH. Dying, death, and medical education: student voices. *J Palliative Med*. 2005;8(2):372–381.

3. Gordon GH. Care not cure: dialogues at the transition. *Patient Educ Couns*. 2003;50(1):95–98.

4. Ferraris G, Bei E, Coumoundouros C, et al. The interpersonal process model of intimacy, burden and communal motivation to care in a multinational group of informal caregivers. *J Soc Personal Relationships*. 2023;40(8):1–23.

5. Orbach I, Mikulincer M, Sirota P, et al. Mental pain: a multidimensional operationalization and definition. *Suicide Life Threat Behav*. 2003;33(3):219–230.

6. Coyne JC, Gottlieb BH. The mismeasure of coping by checklist. *J Pers*. 1996;64(4):959–991.

7. Southwick SM, Bonanno GA, Masten AS, et al. Resilience definitions, theory, and challenges: interdisciplinary perspectives. *Eur J Psychotraumatol*. 2014;5(1).

8. Bonanno GA, Westphal M, Mancini AD. Resilience to loss and potential trauma. *Annu Rev Clin Psychol*. 2011;7:511–535.

9. Lazarus RS. *Psychological stress and the coping process*. McGraw-Hill; 1966.

10. Dadzie HAN, Teye-Kwadjo E, Oppong Asante K, et al. Psychological factors associated with mental adjustment to breast cancer: a hospital-based observational study. *Illness Crisis & Loss*. 2023. https://doi.org/10.1177/10541373231176018.

11. Iles-Caven Y, Gregory S, Northstone K, et al. The beneficial role of personality in preserving well-being during the pandemic: a longitudinal population study. *J Affect Disord*. 2023;331:229–237.

12. Heyda A, Bieleń A, Wygoda A, et al. Walking through the valley of the shadow of death—The psychotherapy of the head and neck cancer patient expressing suicidal ideations and impulses. *J Clin Psychol*. 2023;79:1562–1571.

13. Koch EJ, Shepperd JA. Is self-complexity linked to better coping? A review of the literature. *J Pers*. 2004;72(4):727–760.

14. Vamos M. Psychotherapy in the medically ill: a commentary. *Aust N Z J Psychiatry*. 2006;40(4):295–309.

15. Gijsberts MJ, Echteld MA, van der Steen JT, et al. Spirituality at the end of life: conceptualization of measurable aspects—a systematic review. *J Palliat Med*. 2011;14(7):852–863.

16. Laubmeier KK, Zakowski SG, Bair JP. The role of spirituality in the psychological adjustment to cancer: a test of the transactional model of stress and coping. *Int J Behav Med*. 2004;11(1):48–55.

17. Pargament KI, Koenig HG, Tarakeshwar N, et al. Religious struggle as a predictor of mortality among medically ill patients: a 2-year longitudinal study. *Arch Intern Med*. 2001;161:1881–1885.

18. Stern TA, Sekeres MA. *Facing Cancer: A Complete Guide for People With Cancer, Their Families, and Caregivers*. McGraw-Hill; 2004.

19. Stern TA, Beach SR, Januzzi JL. *Facing Heart Disease: A Guide for Patients and Their Families*. MGH Psychiatry Academy; 2018.

20. Wexler DJ, Celano CM, Stern TA. *Facing Diabetes: A Guide for Patients and Their Families*. MGH Psychiatry Academy; 2018.

21. Stanford FC, Stevens JR, Stern TA. *Facing Overweight and Obesity: A Complete Guide for Children and Adults*. MGH Psychiatry Academy; 2018.

22. Bolster MB, Stern TA. *Facing Osteoporosis: A Guide for Patients and Their Families*. MGH Psychiatry Academy; 2020.

23. Bolster MB, Stern TA. *Facing Scleroderma: A Guide for Patients and Their Families*. MGH Psychiatry Academy; 2020.

24. Bolster MB, Stern TA. *Facing Lupus: A Guide for Patients and Their Families*. MGH Psychiatry Academy; 2020.

25. Bolster MB, Stern TA. *Facing Rheumatoid Arthritis: A Guide for Patients and Their Families*. MGH Psychiatry Academy; 2020.

26. Kourosh AS, Stern TA. *Facing Psoriasis: A Guide for Patients and Their Families*. MGH Psychiatry Academy; 2020.

27. Kourosh AS, Stern TA. *Facing Eczema: A Guide for Patients and Their Families*. MGH Psychiatry Academy; 2020.

28. Kourosh AS, Stern TA. *Facing Vitiligo: A Guide for Patients and Their Families*. MGH Psychiatry Academy; 2020.

29. Kourosh AS, Stern TA. *Facing Acne: A Guide for Patients and Their Families*. MGH Psychiatry Academy; 2020.

30. Kourosh AS, Friedstat J, Stern TA. *Facing Burns and Scars: A Guide for Patients and Their Families*. MGH Psychiatry Academy; 2020.

31. Sher Y, Georgiopoulos AM, Stern TA. *Facing Cystic Fibrosis: A Guide for Patients and Their Families*. MGH Psychiatry Academy; 2020.

32. Reynolds KL, Cohen JV, Zubiri L, Stern TA. *Facing Immunotherapy: A Guide for Patients and Their Families*. MGH Psychiatry Academy; 2020.

33. Sher Y, Stern TA. *Facing Transplantation: A Guide for Patients and their Families*. MGH Psychiatry Academy; 2020.

34. De EJB, Stern TA. *Facing Pelvic Pain: A Guide for Patients and Their Families*. MGH Psychiatry Academy; 2021.

35. Wang JP, Tannyhill RJ, Stern TA. *Facing Post-operative Pain: A Guide for Patients and Their Families*. MGH Psychiatry Academy; 2021.

36. Chemali Z, Stern TA. *Facing Memory Loss and Dementia: A Guide for Patients and Their Families*. MGH Psychiatry Academy; 2021.

37. Freudenreich O, Cather C, Stern TA. *Facing Serious Mental Illness: A Guide for Patients and Their Families*. MGH Psychiatry Academy; 2021.

38. Sher Y, Fishman J, Stern TA. *Facing COVID-19: A Guide for Patients and Their Families*. MGH Psychiatry Academy; 2021.

39. Williams WW, Ivkovic A, Stern TA. *Facing Chronic Kidney Disease: A Guide for Patients and Their Families*. MGH Psychiatry Academy; 2022.

40. Panter-Brick C, Leckman JF. Editorial Commentary: Resilience in child development – interconnected pathways to wellbeing. *J Child Psychol Psychiatry*. 2013;54:333–336.

41. Clarke DM, Mackinnon AJ, Smith GC, et al. Dimensions of psychopathology in the medically ill: a latent trait analysis. *Psychosomatics*. 2000;41:418–425.

42. Stern TA, Prager LM, Cremens MC. Autognosis rounds for medical housestaff. *Psychosomatics*. 1993;34(1):1–7.

43. Stauffer MH. A long-term psychotherapy group for children with chronic medical illness. *Bull Menninger Clin*. 1998;62:15–32.

44. Saravay SM. Psychiatric interventions in the medically ill: outcomes and effectiveness research. *Psychiatr Clin North Am*. 1996;19:467–480.

45. Bird B. *Talking With Patients*. 2nd ed. JB Lippincott; 1973.

46. Coelho G, Hamburg D, Adams J. *Coping and Adaptation*. Basic Books; 1974.

47. Jackson E. *Coping With Crises in Your Life*. Hawthorn Books; 1974.

48. Kessler R, Price R, Wortman C. Social factors in psychopathology: stress, social support, and coping processes. *Annu Rev Psychol*. 1985;36:531–572.

49. Moos R. *Human Adaptation: Coping With Life Crises*. DC Heath; 1976.

50. Murphy L, Moriarity A. *Vulnerability, Coping and Growth*. Yale University Press; 1976.

51. Weisman A. *The Coping Capacity: On the Nature of Being Mortal*. Human Sciences; 1984.

35

RESILIENCE, WELLNESS, AND COPING WITH THE RIGORS OF PSYCHIATRIC PRACTICE

ABIGAIL L. DONOVAN, MD ■ JENNIFER SHEETS, PSYD ■ FELIPE A. JAIN, MD ■ THEODORE A. STERN, MD

OVERVIEW

The practice of medicine is focused on disease, not health, and on treatment, not primary prevention. Therefore it should not be surprising that physicians and other clinicians have difficulty minimizing their own stress and preventing burnout in their own lives. Throughout medicine (and especially in psychiatry) clinicians confront suffering and despair more often than they see success and happiness. In addition, the same character traits that make physicians and other clinicians successful (e.g., perfectionism, an exaggerated sense of responsibility, and selflessness) also make them vulnerable to stress. *Stress*, defined as the condition that occurs in response to adverse external influences, can affect both physical and psychological health. *Resilience* is the adaptive capacity to respond to stressful events and withstand adversity. The daily stress of clinical work, when exceeding the capacity for resilience of the clinician, can progress over time to burnout. Burnout is a pathological syndrome in which prolonged occupational stress leads to emotional and physical depletion, and ultimately to the development of maladaptive behaviors (e.g., cynicism, depersonalization, hostility, and detachment). Clinicians can enhance their own resilience through a variety of coping skills, including mindfulness. Understanding the root causes of stress and burnout, exploring ways to reduce vulnerability to burnout, and learning skills to cope with stress are important factors in building and maintaining a successful career and establishing a fulfilling life.

EPIDEMIOLOGY

Despite their academic and vocational success, clinicians are immune to neither disease nor suffering. Rather, one can argue that clinicians are more likely to experience emotional distress and burnout, given the nature of their work. A seminal study completed in 2011 reported that 46% of physicians endorsed at least one symptom of burnout.[1] Burnout rates have only increased since that time; in 2014, 54% of physicians reported symptoms of burnout.[2] Furthermore, burnout rates may be rising even more dramatically among female physicians.[3] However, burnout is not limited to physicians; 21% to 67% of mental health clinicians report experiencing burnout,[4] which is strongly associated with decreased job satisfaction, emotional exhaustion, depersonalization, and a decreased sense of personal accomplishment.[5] Of significant concern is the finding that burnout is also associated with an increased risk of patient safety incidents.[5] In addition, studies have identified high rates of suicide among physicians. While physicians, as a group, have lower mortality rates from several diseases (e.g., chronic obstructive pulmonary disease, liver disease),[6] they have a higher rate of suicide than do other professionals and members of the general population[6,7] (Fig. 35.1); for male physicians, the relative risk ranges from 1.1 to 3.4, and for female physicians, the relative risk ranges from 2.5 to 5.7.[8] Physicians in the United States appear to be at elevated risk of suicide compared to physicians in other countries.[7] Psychiatrists, in particular, have higher suicide rates than those in other

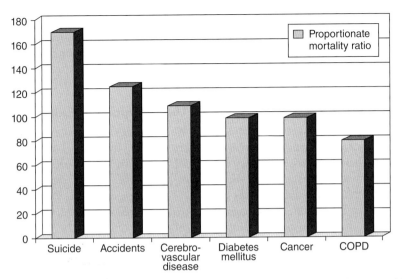

Fig. 35.1 ■ Proportionate mortality ratio for causes of death among White male physicians. The proportionate mortality ratio compares the proportion of deaths due to a specific cause in White male physicians with the proportion of that cause of death in all White male professionals.[6] *COPD,* Chronic obstructive pulmonary disease.

specialties.[9] In the general population, the suicide rate is four times higher for males than it is for females; in physicians, the rate of suicide for females is equal to or higher than that of males.[10]

ETIOLOGIES FOR STRESS AND BURNOUT

The current practice of psychiatry is both challenging and rewarding; however, it is also stressful and not without the potential for burnout. Although the classic image of a clinician with a cozy couch in an idyllic office may come to mind, clinicians often toil in busy outpatient settings, hospitals, inpatient and residential units, emergency departments (EDs), or are embedded within other medical practices. Several aspects of clinical work leave the clinician especially vulnerable to stress and, ultimately, to burnout (Fig. 35.2).

Frequent Encounters With Distress

Mental health clinicians encounter human suffering daily, witnessing countless stories of sadness, anger, and betrayal. While moments of joy and happiness can arise, to many clinicians they often seem few and far

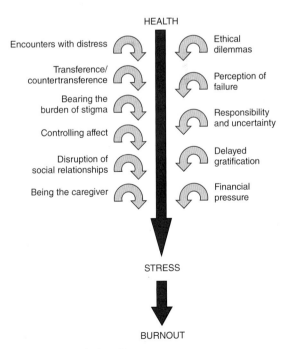

Fig. 35.2 ■ Etiologies of stress.

between. In addition, clinicians commonly provide behavioral health services in specialty clinics (managing chronic pain, grief, and complications of cancer and organ failure), where the nature of the work often entails working with patients whose outcome despite care will be death. The chronic and devastating nature of many psychiatric conditions, and the physical illnesses that accompany them, increases the emotional burden on clinicians. Since clinicians must remain emotionally available to their patients so that they can experience the empathy that is necessary for a therapeutic alliance, this emotional availability makes clinicians particularly vulnerable to suffering alongside their patients. Clinicians must consistently maintain enough distance to remain objective; a critical balance must be maintained, and a precise emotional distance must be preserved.

Ethical Dilemmas

The patient's reliance on their clinician for guidance can raise a host of ethical conflicts. Clinicians may find themselves in the position of watching their patients make unwise—and even dangerous—decisions and feel powerless to curtail this destructive behavior. Clinicians may have to enforce mandated treatment regimens, hospitalize patients against their will, or even physically restrain violent patients. There may even be times when a clinician must intentionally break a patient's confidentiality to ensure their patient's safety or that of others. None of these decisions is made lightly, and each requires a great deal of reflection and emotional energy.

Transference and Countertransference

The daily practice of psychiatry is filled with the management of transference and countertransference, which involve intense emotions in the patient and in the clinician. Furthermore, several psychiatric illnesses have, as core symptoms, difficulty with interpersonal interactions. Afflicted patients, including those with borderline and narcissistic personality disorders, are often challenging. Treatment may necessitate working through the patient's hostile, aggressive, or devaluing transferences; this process is often extremely difficult for the treater. This difficulty may be further compounded if the clinician cares for many such patients or if the negative transference is particularly long lived. In addition, clinicians, through the course of listening to, and empathizing with their patients, may also become the object of loving feelings or dependent attachments. Coping with intense transference, while monitoring one's own countertransference, can be exhausting.

The Perception of Failure

Mental health clinicians treat chronic illnesses, which are subject to relapse, and carry significant risks for morbidity and mortality; thus the very nature of psychiatric disease can lead clinicians to experience feelings of failure. Despite having knowledge of treatment-response rates, clinicians may believe that if they could only find the right medication or say the right words in therapy, their patient would be healed. Failure to respond to treatment can be, and frequently is, viewed as a failure of both the medical intervention and the treater.

Controlling Affect

Despite the intensely emotional nature of clinical work, clinicians must consistently control their emotions to do their jobs well. When patients are overwhelmed by sadness, despair, anger, or frustration, clinicians must keep their own reactions in check, sometimes bottled deep within. While this control of affect is necessary for the provision of high-quality clinical care, it can ultimately lead to the denial of emotions. If one denies the existence of one's affect (even after the patient has left the office), it can lead to increased stress and vulnerability to burnout. Instead, informal debriefings with colleagues, or formal supervision, may encourage the necessary expression of what is controlled during patient sessions.

Responsibility and Uncertainty

The practice of psychiatry is multi-dimensional, incorporating interpersonal and individual dynamics, sociology, biology, and pharmacology. The complex nature of psychiatry makes it an exhilarating, yet uncertain, field. Psychiatrists and other mental health clinicians frequently base their clinical decisions on biased, incomplete, or ambiguous data. While the breadth and depth of psychiatric research are growing exponentially, there is still a dearth of research to guide many clinical decisions. These challenges are further compounded by the added stress of answering to institutions, insurers, patients, and their families. Health insurance organizations often establish standards of care without clinician involvement, undermining the pride and self-determination of practitioners.

Disruption of Social Relationships

Mental health clinicians frequently work in isolation, leaving them alone to face the effects of psychopathology. Furthermore, rules regarding confidentiality preclude sharing the details of one's day with family and friends. Long work hours can limit the time available for socializing, and social engagements and family time can be interrupted (without warning) by emergencies. These factors can fracture social relationships, decrease social support, and increase the risk of burnout. Furthermore, vocational burnout is, in turn, associated with low satisfaction in relationships (with patients and with clinical staff).

Delayed Gratification

The ability to delay gratification is an important developmental milestone. The practice of medicine raises it to an art form. To successfully complete 4 years of medical school, 1 sleep-deprived year of internship and 3 grueling years of residency, physicians must be adept at delaying gratification. But this skill, when taken to an extreme, can lead to burnout. Clinicians may be tempted to put personal, non-work-related goals on hold, in the service of career success (e.g., "I can't get married, have children, or buy a house until I finish training, have a stable practice, or have enough money in the bank."). Such rationalizations can be extended indefinitely and may lead to a life lacking balance and devoid of non-vocational success.

Being the Caregiver

Clinicians, in general, have a strong need to be needed and to care for others. These traits are part of what initially draws clinicians to the practice of psychiatry. At the same time, the dependence some patients develop on their clinician can be overwhelming in its intensity. Furthermore, focusing intently on the needs of others can lead to denial of one's own need to be cared for.

Financial Stress

While the popular perception is that all clinicians make copious amounts of money, the reality is quite different.

The costs of medical education and attending graduate school can be astronomical and they continue to rise each year; however, the salaries of many clinicians do not enjoy the same growth, and the increases in earnings over time may not even match the rate of inflation. Many clinicians finish training with enormous debt, and with limited options for repayment and deferment of loans. Furthermore, the practical options for improving one's financial situation are limited to working longer hours or seeing more patients (for shorter periods of time). Either option is likely to increase, rather than decrease, vocational stress. This pressure may be especially intense for early career clinicians.

SPECIAL SITUATIONS IN PSYCHIATRY

Coping With Patient Suicide

A Profound and Enduring Effect

Half of all psychiatrists have had one (or more) of their patients commit suicide[11,12]; approximately one-third of those psychiatrists experienced such a loss while they were still in residency training.[11] Furthermore, one-fourth of psychiatrists who experienced patient suicide stated that it had "a profound and enduring effect" on them throughout their careers.[11] While the practice of most medical specialties entails dealing with death, suicide in the practice of psychiatry takes on additional meaning. Since one of the primary tools in psychiatry is the individual, when the treatment fails, it can feel as if the treater has failed. Furthermore, while death from cancer can be seen as inevitable, death from suicide can be viewed as a choice.[13] When coping with patient suicide, it is important to remember that "a patient suicide is neither a unique event nor a personal failure."[14]

Reactions to Suicide

Clinicians' reactions to a patient's suicide can be varied and intense.[15] In addition, clinicians must cope not only with their own reaction but also with the reactions of their patient's family and friends; this can evoke feelings of grief, guilt, inadequacy, anxiety, depression, shock, shame, betrayal, and anger. The experience of anger and hostility toward the patient who has committed suicide may further trigger self-blame. A sense of rejection may also be particularly poignant. While the clinician was working their hardest and trying all available therapies, they may feel that through suicide the patient has in effect said, "You just weren't good enough." Younger clinicians may be especially vulnerable to this intense distress.

Coping

To cope effectively with a patient's suicide, clinicians must give themselves permission to experience a variety of emotions.[16] While challenging, experiencing anger and hostility toward the patient is a necessary component of healing. Clinicians may also find themselves ruminating over treatment decisions, asking, "What if?" While it is important to review the treatment course to learn from the outcome, obsessive ruminations may diminish one's confidence in decision-making and impair coping with the tragedy. Shame and embarrassment, as well as a sense of personal failure, may prevent clinicians from reaching out to colleagues. However, several colleagues have likely had similar experiences, and all parties may benefit from sharing their experiences.

Treating Dying Patients

In extreme situations, clinicians may find themselves refusing to care for suicidal patients or wanting to leave clinical care altogether. These wishes defend against the fear of future traumatic experiences with at-risk patients. Yet, as a seasoned therapist once said about treating suicidal patients, "If we do not treat dying patients, our patients will die alone".

Coping With Boundary Crossings and Violations

Boundary Violations

The practice of psychiatry is filled with intense emotions. Furthermore, clinical care is composed of regular, frequent, and lengthy patient contact, all behind closed doors. These facts, in addition to disrupting a clinician's personal relationships, can set up boundary crossings and violations. *Boundary crossings* are considered harmless deviations from clinical practice or from the therapeutic frame; for example, allowing a few extra minutes of a session at a particularly challenging moment or taking a patient's arm if she/he stumbles. However, *boundary violations* are more serious deviations that are harmful and exploitive to the patient's emotional, financial, or sexual needs.

Decreasing Vulnerability

All clinicians must recognize that they are at risk for boundary violations; denial of this vulnerability prevents introspection and analysis of motives, as well as early consultation in dilemmas. Other factors (including crises at work, at home, or in individual physical or psychological health) may make a clinician particularly vulnerable to boundary violations. In such situations, the clinician may be tempted to convey their personal problems to the patient; such self-disclosure should serve as a serious warning sign. Other warning signs include: idealizing the patient, and thus believing that s/he is deserving of special treatment; holding sessions at the end of the day or even "after hours"; frequently allowing sessions to go on longer than the allotted time; engaging in repeated outside of-session phone calls; allowing the patient to maintain a large, unpaid bill[17]; and, most importantly, a reluctance to discuss the case with colleagues or supervisors. Any of these signs should immediately prompt the clinician to seek objective consultation to examine these issues in depth.

Coping With Malpractice Litigation

Practicing modern medicine leads many clinicians to fear litigation, regardless of actual negligence. This fear, when extreme, can be paralyzing and may lead to the desire to treat only "low-risk patients." Unfortunately, there are no reliable methods to predict which patients are going to be litigious. Thus it is the responsibility of the practitioner to cope effectively with the continuous risk of malpractice litigation.

Protecting Yourself

There are steps all practitioners can take to protect themselves against potential litigation. Appropriate documentation is critical. The most frequent malpractice claim occurs when a patient has committed suicide; thus regular documentation of both the risks and the protective factors, in addition to the rationalizations behind clinical decisions, is crucial. Perhaps the most protective factor is a strong alliance with the patient. Maintaining and enhancing the therapeutic alliance can be accomplished in several ways. Clinicians can use language that reflects a joint effort with the patient, such as "Our problem is." or "Our goal is." This language allows the clinician and the patient to speak of the therapy as a third entity in the room. It promotes a detachment from the illness and lets the patient know that s/he is not alone in the battle, but rather that s/he will fight right alongside the clinician. Similarly, it may be beneficial for the clinician to maintain an alliance with the patient's family, although adhering to principles of confidentiality may make this goal challenging. Even if the patient refuses contact, it may be helpful simply to convey one's desire to speak with the family, in the present or in the future. Building an allied and collaborative relationship with a patient is a key component of effective treatment, and it may offer some protection against future litigation.

Coping With a Lawsuit

How can a clinician cope when facing a lawsuit?[18] Unfortunately, the very same traits that constitute careful and competent clinicians (e.g., responsibility, perfectionism, high standards) also subject them to self-doubt and unearned guilt when confronted with a lawsuit. It may be of some solace to remember that only a small percentage of malpractice lawsuits go to trial, and those that do usually find in favor of the clinician. During the preparation, it may be helpful to work closely with your lawyer, restoring a sense of control and ownership over the future. It is also critically important to maintain personal interests and relationships outside of the workplace. Regardless of whether negligence occurred, it is normal to feel shame, guilt, and anger during (and even after) a lawsuit.

Coping With Residency Training

While the rigors of a psychiatric practice can be challenging, psychiatric residency training and clinical training in other programs are simply grueling. Several factors make training especially demanding: a lack of control, sleep deprivation, responsibility without authority, and balancing autonomy with dependence.[19] Trainees have little control over their daily schedules. Moreover, trainees have little-to-no control over which patients they treat, and they frequently treat the sickest, most disadvantaged, and most difficult patients. Long hours and regular calls mean that trainees are constantly sleep deprived. Trainees also have a tremendous amount of responsibility, but without complete authority over treatment decisions, and without the

credence that years of practice bring. Trainees must also negotiate a balance between autonomy and dependence. In training, there is a desire to appear strong and competent to both colleagues and supervisors; trainees may view asking for help as a sign of dependency or weakness. Yet, if trainees knew everything, they would not need to be trainees anymore. The low predictability, high meaning of work, and multiple role conflicts conspire to make trainees especially vulnerable to burnout.[20]

WHEN THE COBBLER'S CHILDREN HAVE NO SHOES

Ironically, the proverbial cobbler was so busy making shoes for everyone else that he neglected to make them for his own children. Similarly, it is easy, in days filled with caring for the needs of others, to put our own needs second, or to neglect them entirely. Yet, to be good clinicians, we must care for ourselves as well. Neglecting self-care can cause a further progression from stress to burnout. Several factors contribute to this type of self-neglect (Fig. 35.3).

Denial of Vulnerability

As clinicians, we treat ourselves as if we are superhuman. While it is necessary for others to sleep, eat regular meals, and take vacations, we frequently deny ourselves these basic needs. Moreover, mental health clinicians typically wish to see themselves as

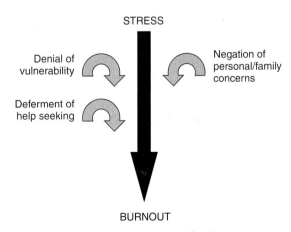

Fig. 35.3 ■ Factors contributing to self-neglect.

consummate copers, immune to emotional impairment. When placed under stress, it is common to work harder and longer, and withdraw from non-vocational activities, which ends up compounding the initial problem.

Negation of Personal and Familial Concerns

Personal and familial concerns can be misjudged as being less critical than relieving the pain and suffering of patients. It can seem easy, if not important, to spend 1 more hour at work to see a patient in crisis; however, this practice can rapidly expand, becoming a pattern of working longer and sacrificing personal time. After long and stressful days, clinicians may be too emotionally exhausted for empathic listening, even-handed conversation, or recreation. As a result, clinicians may turn inward, internalizing their concerns and cutting themselves off from family and friends. This behavior compromises the strength of family and social relationships and decreases the support available for the clinician.

Deferment of Seeking Help

It is common to view seeking help for personal problems as a sign of frailty or personal failure. While clinicians experience depression and other mental illnesses at similar rates to those in the general population, they are less likely to seek help,[21] perhaps because of the stigma of mental illness. In general, while clinicians may be more open to psychotherapy for themselves, the possibility of a formal diagnosis, breaches of confidentiality, or having to report a problem to a licensing board can make seeking help difficult. The intense pressure of clinicians' work can foster the creation of unachievable expectations. However, the clinician's well-being is only undermined by this intolerance for human vulnerability.

How to Recognize Stress in Oneself

As mental health clinicians, we are good at recognizing stress in others; however, recognizing stress in oneself requires a different skill set. Unrecognized and unmanaged stress can lead to anxiety or depression, and it can have long-lasting effects on clinicians, patients, and families. Signs of stress include exhaustion, chronic fatigue, apathy, anhedonia, irritability,

and despair, as well as somatic manifestations, including headaches and gastrointestinal disturbances. Further warning signs include disrupted sleep, conflict in family relationships, poor interactions with patients, reduced efficacy of personal coping skills, and changes in memory, concentration, and problem-solving ability. Perhaps the most important warning sign is the suggestion from friends, family, and colleagues that help is needed.

Stress can also affect attitudes toward patients. Stress and burnout may impair professional competence, reduce treatment efficacy, or increase the risk of harm to the patient. Clinicians may develop reactive misanthropy when they frequently encounter patients' pain and suffering, especially when expressed by the patient as hostility or devaluation. Clinicians may then find that warmth and concern are replaced with apathy, or even defensiveness and contempt. This emotional detachment can progress and carry over to all patients, so that the clinician is no longer able to appreciate fulfilling patient relationships.

Stress, when prolonged or unmanaged, can progress to burnout. Signs of burnout include detachment from the meaning of one's work, open hostility, deep-rooted cynicism, and overwhelming occupational dissatisfaction. In addition, reactive misanthropy can progress to malignant misanthropy in a burned-out clinician. In this malignant form, misanthropy extends to other relationships, including those with staff, colleagues, other health professionals, and even friends or family. The unfortunate result is then a conflict with one's social values and intentions, leading to self-punishment and feelings of guilt.

HEALING THE WOUNDED HEALER: PROMOTING RESILIENCE

Resilience is a psychological construct that assesses a person's ability to adapt to stressful life events (Table 35.1).[22] Early conceptualizations of resilience focused on a "rubber band" characteristic: the pre-existing capacity to experience a stressor and then return to a former homeostasis. More recent conceptualizations include the ability of the person to change, grow, and make meaning from a stressful life event. Some conceptualizations of resilience describe it as an active process instead of

TABLE 35.1
Varying Conceptualizations of Resilience

Resilience as a Capacity

Ability to experience adversity with brief symptoms and then return to stable functioning (homeostasis)

Faculty for moving forward insightfully and in an integrated manner, even if adversity causes severe symptoms

Capacity to adapt to disturbances that threaten development, function, or viability

Resilience as a Process

Process of harnessing resources to sustain well-being

Process of adapting well in the face of adversity, trauma, tragedy, threats, or significant sources of stress

Resilience as an Outcome

Absence of a mental disorder

Presence of positive functioning

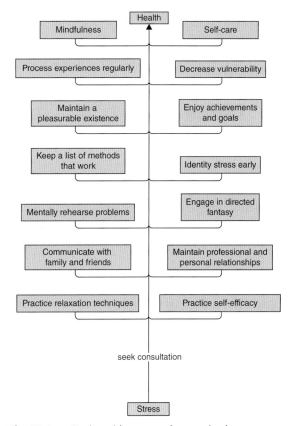

Fig. 35.4 ■ Coping with stress and preventing burnout.

a hard-wired personality trait, such as the process of adapting well in the face of adversity, trauma, or other significant sources of stress. In this view, resilience also may include the harnessing of external resources to sustain well-being when facing difficult situations. Resilience is critical to managing the numerous stressors inherent in the practice of psychiatry. Enhancing resilience can be accomplished through a variety of mechanisms described further below and in Fig. 35.4, beginning with mindfulness.

Mindfulness

Mindfulness is an ancient Buddhist practice that has been simplified and adapted for a Western audience and adopted within many psychological treatment settings. Within Buddhist traditions, mindfulness includes an approach to the cognitive processing of emotions and thoughts. The first successful adaptation of mindfulness to the clinical setting was achieved in the early 1980s by Jon Kabat-Zinn. Kabat-Zinn defined mindfulness as, "paying attention in a particular way: on purpose, in the present moment, and non-judgmentally."[23] This adaptation of mindfulness emphasized a mental focus on present-moment attention and non-judgment regarding experience. An important characteristic of both early Buddhist mindfulness and Kabat-Zinn's mindfulness adaptation is thought "decentering," or the ability to see thoughts or feelings as objective events in the mind

rather than personally identifying with them.[24] This decentering capacity, an aspect of meta-cognition, has been postulated as a key mechanism by which mindfulness exerts its effects.

Mindfulness and resilience are posited to be related based on a modified cognitive model of emotion. In the cognitive model, external events may result in transitory experiences of distress or pain, but the meaning and interpretation ascribed by the individual results in ongoing suffering and persistent psychological symptoms (Fig. 35.5). Even if the acute stressor results in distress or pain, the individual might exhibit resilience based on a hopeful or optimistic cognitive response, or the ability to reframe the experience. A mindful state of non-judging and non-reactivity to thoughts and emotions promotes resilience based on different mechanisms: decentering, lower rumination, and decreased

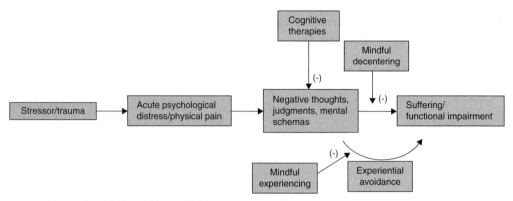

Fig. 35.5 ■ Hypothesized model by which mindfulness improves resilience in response to a stressor or trauma. The stressor or trauma causes acute psychological distress or physical pain, which leads to the development of negative thoughts, judgments, and mental schemas. Suffering and prolonged impairment are related to the degree of maladaptive cognitive processing. Mindfulness results in decentering, or the ability to see thoughts separate from reality.

experiential avoidance (Fig. 35.5). Through decentering, mindfulness changes the relationship between the person and their thoughts. By reducing the primacy of *thought as reality*, mindfulness decreases reactivity to judgments about experience, which can help reduce psychological symptoms of depression and anxiety.

Reduced rumination through mindful observation and acting with awareness may also be a mechanism that links mindfulness and resilience. Observing experience and acting with awareness imply a focus on the present without distracting mind wandering, thus diminishing rumination. Rumination has been linked to negative outcomes due to trauma, including higher rates of post-traumatic stress disorder and depression.[25] Thus engaging a mindful attitude might lead to resilience through lower rumination.

Finally, reducing experiential avoidance through mindfulness may improve resilience. By encouraging a focus on present-moment observation of experience, mindfulness might reduce a tendency toward dissociation or avoidance.[26] Mindfulness- and acceptance-based theories suggest that experiential avoidance and non-mindful behavior play a role in the development and maintenance of post-traumatic symptoms. Further, persistent (consistent) dissociation, or disruptions in consciousness, may be a risk factor for trauma-based symptomatology. To develop resilience to trauma, individuals must disengage from such mental states and engage in behaviors that allow for positive psychological adjustment post-trauma. Indeed, during

the COVID-19 pandemic, Götmann and Bechtoldt[27] reported that facets of dispositional mindfulness were associated with lower avoidance or disengagement coping, and with greater use of adaptive coping strategies, such as problem-solving. Mindfulness is thought to facilitate a state of non-judgmental experiencing and non-avoidance of a triggered emotion, which is hypothesized to lead to an immediate upregulation of autonomic reactivity during a stressor, followed by a more rapid and robust recovery post-stressor due to present-focused, non-judgmental awareness.

Mindfulness may be particularly important for healthcare workers. Longitudinal evidence suggests that mindfulness may be protective against the stressors that healthcare workers encounter on the job. In Switzerland, Westphal and colleagues[28] conducted a study that examined whether dispositional mindfulness in healthcare workers who were beginning work in an ED predicted depression, anxiety, and social impairment months later. One hundred and twenty-one participants, including residents, medical students, and nurses, completed measures of anxiety and depressive symptoms, perceived social support at work, social adjustment, and mindfulness soon after beginning work in the ED, and at least one follow-up within 6 months. After controlling for work-related stress, negative life events, and social support at work, higher mindfulness levels at study entry were associated with lower levels of depression, anxiety, and social impairment 6 months later. Furthermore, mindfulness moderated the relationship between poor social support at work and depressive symptoms: those with higher mindfulness exhibited fewer depressive symptoms than those with low mindfulness despite the same (poor) levels of social support.

Based on findings such as these, there has been increased interest in developing practices and strategies that may promote resiliency, reduce burnout, and improve mental health in healthcare personnel. Several new mindfulness programs have been recently developed and studied. In Ontario, Canada, an online mindfulness skill building program comprised of four weekly 30-minute sessions was developed for healthcare workers during the COVID-19 pandemic.[29] Researchers found that immediately post-intervention, resiliency significantly increased, and the effects were sustained after 1 month. A second group at the Ohio State University College of Medicine developed an 8-week mindfulness intervention.[30] The results indicated that from pre- to post-intervention, burnout and stress levels significantly decreased, while resilience and work engagement significantly increased.

Mindfulness is not the only technique to promote resilience. Additional skills are discussed further below and in Fig. 35.4.

Self-Care

Self-care is defined as the ability to care for oneself through awareness, self-control, and self-reliance to achieve, maintain, or promote optimal health and well-being.[31] Self-care can be individualized to suit one's own unique needs, availability, and interests, taking both a macro- and a microperspective. Macro self-care focuses on the big picture, often requiring more careful planning: organizing a schedule to achieve a particular routine, maintaining important connections with friends and family, and disconnecting by taking a vacation.[32] Micro self-care consists of the elements that complement daily life: listening to music, breathwork, time with a pet, exercising, spending time in nature, reading a book, prayer or other spiritual/religious practice (if important to the individual), or enjoying a conversation with a friend.[32] These small activities add value and can be completed before or after a workday, or perhaps between patients. It is important to implement these strategies proactively to enhance resilience.

Process Experiences Regularly

Talking with colleagues and supervisors regularly about difficult interactions or reserving the commute home as a time for processing the day's events can be invaluable. Many clinicians have found that supportive relationships with colleagues can buffer the demands of practicing medicine[33]; in mental health fields, support from colleagues has been identified as a resource to reduce the impact of work-related stress.[34] Coping with stress daily, and processing emotions before one arrives home, can decrease the risk that one may take the strain of the day out on family or friends. Furthermore, learning important lessons from difficult events may mitigate some of the distress that they cause.

Review Your Own History and Keep a List of Methods That Work

Clinicians can identify useful coping strategies from the past and eliminate maladaptive ones. Since it can be difficult to recall adaptive strategies during moments of extreme distress or duress, making a list of coping strategies that have previously helped can be beneficial. By engaging in constructive activities, such as athletics, one can discharge fury and anger, while exercise and yoga can relieve muscle tension. Even releasing emotion through tears can restore a psychic balance. It can also be helpful to identify prior manifestations of stress, so that one can recognize them early and intervene before they reach a caustic level.

Decrease Vulnerability to Stress

There are many aspects of clinical practice (such as long hours and copious amounts of record-keeping) over which clinicians have no control, but there are factors (e.g., treating physical illness, eating a balanced diet, exercising, getting enough sleep) that clinicians can control and that can reduce vulnerability to emotional stress.

Clinicians are frequently poor patients. Despite access to health care, many clinicians rarely visit their primary care physician, even when ill. But untreated illness only compounds the stress.

While hectic schedules sometimes necessitate taking meals on-the-go or taking no meals at all, nutrition is crucial for a healthy body and a healthy mind.

Exercise releases endorphins, and it can improve mood and energy. Furthermore, exercise is an excellent way to relieve stress and reduce tension. Regular physical exercise contributes to physical health and an overall sense of well-being.

Sleeping at least 8 hours every night has benefits; fatigue can leave one vulnerable to emotional stress and dysregulation.

Practice Self-Efficacy

Self-efficacy, the belief that one can achieve goals, is a skill that can be honed over time. Self-efficacy can be manifest in several ways, including having confidence that one can find solutions, communicating needs effectively, and utilizing coping strategies when faced with difficulties. These skills may be particularly useful in the workplace when needing to set limits with caseload expectations, when facing limited access to resources due to systemic barriers, and when unforeseen difficulties arise with a complex patient. Having confidence in one's ability to solve problems and achieve goals can combat uncertainty, rumination, and distress.

Mentally Rehearse Potential Problems

When a potentially difficult meeting or conversation is anticipated, it is helpful to rehearse statements and responses to questions. Having responses in mind before a crisis arises makes it more likely that one will remain calm in a tense situation. This technique also fosters a sense of control over the unexpected.

Engage in Directed Fantasy

One can imagine expressing intense feelings (e.g., anger, sadness, fear) as a means of decompression. One can also imagine affectively intense scenarios (e.g., hitting that frustrating patient with a flaming ax). The more outrageous these fantasies are, the more effective they will be at discharging emotion. The more unrealistic and outlandish, the easier it will be to distinguish between fantasy and a corresponding reality.

Cultivate and Maintain Professional and Personal Relationships

Healthy relationships are a key buffer against stress and burnout. Strong relationships with colleagues create a natural support network with whom one can share common challenges and stressors and serve to decrease feelings of professional isolation. Professional insight into complex patients, difficult situations, and general work management can be shared formally and informally. Personal relationships are essential to maintain the balance between work and life, and strong connections with family and friends place work issues in perspective. Personal relationships offer not only support and understanding but also provide rejuvenation and meaning to life outside of work.[35]

Communicate With Family and Friends About Anticipated Unavailability

This communication will help clinicians prepare for, and lessen, the likelihood that they will respond with anger and withdrawal. As one communicates about future work commitments, one can also plan social commitments. This action allows family and friends to know they are still held in high regard and it sets a framework for ongoing relationships. Above all else, open communication and a sense of togetherness should be maintained; hardship experienced as a team deepens intimacy and mutual respect.

Enjoy Your Achievements and Your Goals

Previous triumphs, both professional and personal, should be pondered and joyful moments recalled. Original goals should be remembered, the progress made toward achieving them noted, and new professional and personal goals set. Being mindful of the progress toward life goals instills a sense of pride and mastery. The strength gathered from memories of the high points of one's life facilitates coping with everyday stresses.

Learn and Practice Relaxation Techniques

Tension and overstimulation can make sleep difficult, and the fear of returning to work without rejuvenation only compounds this difficulty. While facing this pressure, one may be tempted to resort to using alcohol or sedatives. However, one can learn deep breathing techniques, progressive muscle relaxation, or self-hypnosis to promote tranquility and facilitate sleep. These exercises can also be used in the middle of a hectic day or during a stressful night on call to rejuvenate an exhausted mind and body.

Maintain a Pleasurable Existence

It can be helpful to commit yourself to taking a break from work each day to engage in a pleasurable experience. A pleasurable event can involve having a cup of tea, taking a short walk outside, reading a favorite poem, or speaking with a friend on the telephone. Keeping a balance between stress and pleasure day by day prevents burnout and promotes a positive mind-set.

Seek Consultation

Consultation offers an objective point of view; it can be the first step in seeking help for the overwhelmed clinician. Seeking consultation is not a sign of weakness; rather, it is the sign of a wise practitioner who recognizes that to help patients, one must first help oneself. Consultation should be considered for a variety of problems: symptoms of depression, disabling anxiety, self-prescribing, escalating use of alcohol or other substances, impulsive behavior, impaired clinical judgment, or inappropriate expressions of anger. Other signals that should prompt consultation include working longer hours, having trouble in significant relationships, and becoming socially isolated.

Obtain Professional Help

It may not be easy for a clinician to acknowledge that professional help is needed. It can be extremely difficult to surrender control when one is used to being in complete control. But it may also be a wise decision, especially to halt a downward spiral.

Psychotherapy

Psychotherapy provides the mental health clinician with the valuable opportunity to experience the other side of the therapeutic relationship. Psychotherapy can be a rich, life-enhancing experience, it can improve coping skills, and it provides much-needed support for the overwhelmed clinician.

Psychopharmacology

Many psychiatrists and mental health clinicians see the need for medication as a sign of weakness or failure. However, doctors would rarely fail to use chemotherapy to treat a cancer patient or insulin to treat a patient with diabetes. So too should medication be used to treat a biologically based psychiatric illness.

Couples Therapy

Strong family relationships are crucial for resilience. Ironically, family relationships are often among the first victims of vocational burnout. Couples therapy or family therapy can heal wounded relationships and restore lines of open communication, ultimately building protection against future stressors.

Group Therapy

Group therapy allows individuals to recognize that they are not alone in their suffering. Professional support groups can facilitate the sharing of common experiences and emotions and promote connections between people who have similar strengths and difficulties. More general groups promote understanding of the difficulties inherent to all lifestyles.

Autognosis Rounds

Autognosis literally means "self-knowledge." Autognosis rounds allow clinicians to share common experiences and identify individual reactions to clinical situations. This knowledge can then be used to inform diagnoses and to minimize potentially harmful reactions to patients (e.g., managing hostility toward a patient so that it will not interfere with treatment). Autognosis rounds have proven valuable for psychiatric resident groups at the Massachusetts General Hospital for the past four decades.[36]

CONCLUSION

The practice of psychiatry, with its inherent stresses, is an honor and a fulfilling calling. While the work is deeply gratifying, to hold a space that allows for healing, acceptance, loss, and growth, challenges remain. "When we find ways to cope with… conflicts, we move toward the equanimity that can enable us to serve our patients with greater effectiveness and compassion. We also progress toward greater satisfaction in this noble profession of medicine and in our personal lives as well…. I offer the suggestions in this [chapter] to my young and future colleagues with the hope that they will do no harm; that they will fortify and strengthen; and that they will contribute something to the glorious privilege that medical practice can be."[37]

ACKNOWLEDGMENTS

This chapter is dedicated to Dr. Edward Messner, whose commitment to resident well-being was unparalleled. He taught us not only how to heal our patients but also how to heal ourselves.

REFERENCES

1. Shanafelt TD, Boone S, Tan L, et al. Burnout and satisfaction with work life balance among US physicians relative to the general US population. *Arch Intern Med.* 2012;172:1377–1385.
2. Shanafelt TD, Hasan O, Dyrbye LN, et al. Changes in burnout and satisfaction with work-life balance in physicians and the general US working population between 2011 and 2014. *Mayo Clin Proc.* 2015;90(12):1600–1613.
3. Martinez KA, Sullivan AB, Linfield DT, et al. Change in physician burnout between 2013 and 2020 in a major health system. *South Med J.* 2022;115(8):645–650.
4. Simpson S, Simionato G, Smout M, et al. Burnout amongst clinical and counselling psychologist: the role of early maladaptive schemas and coping modes as vulnerability factors. *Clin Psychol Psychother.* 2019;26(1):35–46.
5. Hodkinson A, Zhou A, Johnson J, et al. Associations of physician burnout with career engagement and quality of patient care: systematic review and meta-analysis. *BMJ.* 2022;378:e070442.
6. Frank E, Biola H, Burnett CA. Mortality rates and causes among US physicians. *Am J Prev Med.* 2000;19:155–159.
7. Dutheil F, Aubert C, Pereira B, et al. Suicide among physicians and health-care workers: a systematic review and meta-analysis. *PLoS One.* 2019;14:e0226361.
8. Center C, Davis M, Detre T, et al. Confronting depression and suicide in physicians. *JAMA.* 2003;289:3161–3166.
9. Duarte D, El-Hagrassy MM, Couto TCE, et al. Male and female physician suicidality: a systematic review and meta-analysis. *JAMA Psychiatry.* 2020;77(6):587–597.
10. Silverman M. Physicians and suicide. In: Goldman LS, Myers M, Dickstein LI, eds. *The Handbook of Physician Health: Essential Guide to Understanding the Health Care Needs of Physicians.* American Medical Association; 2000.
11. Ruskin R, Sakinofsky I, Bagby RM, et al. Impact of patient suicide on psychiatrists and psychiatric trainees. *Acad Psychiatry.* 2004;28:104–110.
12. Chemtob CM, Hamada RS, Bauer G, et al. Patients' suicides: frequency and impact on psychiatrists. *Am J Psychiatry.* 1988;145:224–228.
13. Maltsberger JT. The implications of patient suicide for the surviving psychotherapist. In: Jacobs D, ed. *Suicide and Clinical Practice.* American Psychiatric Press; 1992.
14. Hendin H, Lipschitz A, Maltsberger JT, et al. Therapists' reactions to patients' suicides. *Am J Psychiatry.* 2000;157:2022–2027.
15. Hendin H, Haas AP, Maltsberger JT, et al. Factors contributing to therapists' distress after the suicide of a patient. *Am J Psychiatry.* 2004;161:1442–1446.
16. Lafayette JM, Stern TA. The impact of a patient's suicide on psychiatric trainees: a case study and review of the literature. *Harv Rev Psychiatry.* 2004;12(1):49–55.
17. Norris DM, Gutheil TG, Strasburger LH. This couldn't happen to me: boundary problems and sexual misconduct in the psychotherapy relationship. *Psychiatr Serv.* 2003;54:517–522.
18. Brazeau CM. Coping with the stress of being sued. *Fam Pract Manag.* 2011;8:41–44.
19. Thomas NK. Resident burnout. *JAMA.* 2004;292:2880–2889.
20. Borritz M, Bultmann U, Rogulies R, et al. Psychosocial work characteristics as predictors for burnout: findings from 3-year follow up of the PUMA study. *J Occup Environ Med.* 2005;47:1015–1025.
21. Elkbuli A, Sutherland M, Shepherd A, et al. Factors influencing US physician and surgeon suicide rates 2003 to 2017: analysis of the CDC-National Violent Death Reporting System. *Ann Surg.* 2022;276(5):e370–e376.
22. Southwick SM, Bonanno GA, Masten AS, et al. Resilience definitions, theory, and challenges: interdisciplinary perspectives. *Eur J Psychotraumatol.* 2014;5:25338.
23. Kabat-Zinn J. *Wherever You Go, There You Are: Mindfulness Meditation in Everyday Life.* Hyperion; 1994.
24. Segal ZV, Williams JMG, Teasdale JD. *Mindfulness-Based Cognitive Therapy for Depression.* 2. The Guilford Press; 2013:36–37..
25. Ehring T, Frank S, Ehlers A. The role of rumination and reduced concreteness in the maintenance of posttraumatic stress disorder and depression following trauma. *Cognit Ther Res.* 2008;32:488–506.
26. Thompson RW, Arnkoff DB, Glass CR. Conceptualizing mindfulness and acceptance as components of psychological resilience to trauma. *Trauma Violence Abuse.* 2011;12:220–235.
27. Götmann A, Bechtoldt MN. Coping with COVID-19 - Longitudinal analysis of coping strategies and the role of trait mindfulness in mental well-being. *Pers Individ Dif.* 2021:175.
28. Westphal M, Wall M, Corbeil T, et al. Mindfulness predicts less depression, anxiety, and social impairment in emergency care personnel: a longitudinal study. *PLoS One.* 2021:16.
29. Kim S, Crawford J, Hunter S. Role of an online skill-based mindfulness program for healthcare worker's resiliency during the COVID-19 pandemic: a mixed-method study. *Front Public Heal.* 2022;10:907528.
30. Klatt M, Bawa R, Gabram O, et al. Synchronous mindfulness in motion online: strong results, strong attendance at a critical time for health care professionals (HCPs) in the COVID era. *Front Psychol.* 2021:12.
31. Martínez N, Connelly CD, Pérez A, et al. (2021). Self-care: a concept analysis. *Int J Nurs Sci.* 2021;8(4):418–425.
32. Bush AD. *Simple Self-Care for Therapists: Restorative Practices to Weave Through Your Workday.* WW Norton & Company; 2015.

33. McKinley T. Toward useful interventions for burnout in Academic Medical Faculty: the case for unit-specific approaches. *J Contin Educ Health Prof.* 2022;42(1):e69–e74.

34. Rupert PA, Dorociak KE. Self-care, stress, and well-being among practicing psychologists. *Prof Psychol Res Pr.* 2019;50(5):343–350.

35. Zwack J, Schweitzer J. If every fifth physician is affected by burnout, what about the other four? Resilience strategies of experienced physicians. *Acad Med.* 2013;88:382–389.

36. Stern TA, Prager LM, Cremens MC. Autognosis rounds for medical house staff. *Psychosomatics.* 1993;34:1–7.

37. Messner E.*Resilience Enhancement for the Resident Physician.* Essential Medical Information Systems; 1993.

36

DEVICE NEUROMODULATION AND BRAIN STIMULATION THERAPIES

JAMES LUCCARELLI, MD, DPHIL ■ MICHAEL E. HENRY, MD ■ CARLOS G. FERNANDEZ-ROBLES, MD, MBA ■ CRISTINA CUSIN, MD ■ JOAN A. CAMPRODON, MD, MPH, PHD ■ DARIN D. DOUGHERTY, MD, MSc

OVERVIEW

Therapeutic options for patients with affective, behavioral, or cognitive disorders include psychotherapy, pharmacotherapy, and somatic therapies. This chapter focuses on the latter.

Somatic therapies, also known as *brain stimulation* or *neuromodulation*, are a group of device-based techniques that target specific structures of the nervous systems via surgical ablation or electrical modulation with the goal of therapeutically modifying pathological patterns of brain activity and circuit connectivity. Somatic therapies can be divided into two general groups: invasive and non-invasive modalities. Invasive treatments require the surgical implantation of stimulating electrodes (or surgical ablative disconnection of aberrant pathways) and include ablative limbic system surgeries, deep brain stimulation (DBS), and vagus nerve stimulation (VNS). Non-invasive techniques can modulate brain activity trans-cranially without surgical intervention and include transcranial magnetic stimulation (TMS) as its most paradigmatic modality. Electroconvulsive therapy (ECT), the oldest of all somatic therapies, occupies a space between the two categories, as it does not require surgical intervention but does require general anesthesia; it is generally considered minimally invasive.

Studies have demonstrated that only 30% to 40% of patients with major depressive disorder (MDD) treated with pharmacotherapy achieve full remission, and 10% to 15% experience no symptom improvement.[1] Thus, somatic therapies provide an important therapeutic option for patients who do not respond to initial pharmacotherapy. While invasive neuromodulation should be reserved for the most refractory patients, non-invasive techniques (including ECT) can be considered in earlier phases of the therapeutic process, given their efficacy and relatively benign safety profile (which can be significantly better than certain pharmacological options).

TRANSCRANIAL MAGNETIC STIMULATION

TMS is a non-invasive neuromodulation modality that uses powerful and rapidly changing magnetic fields applied over the surface of the skull to generate targeted electrical currents in the brain, painlessly and without the need for surgery, anesthesia, or the induction of seizures. In 2008 the US Food and Drug Administration (FDA) approved the use of high-frequency repetitive TMS (rTMS) over the left dorsolateral prefrontal cortex (DLPFC) for the treatment of MDD. Deep TMS H-coils were approved for MDD in 2013, with further approvals in 2018 for the treatment of obsessive-compulsive disorder (OCD), 2020 for smoking cessation, and 2021 for co-morbid anxiety symptoms in patients with depression.

One of the primary advantages of TMS is its non-invasive nature, which is made possible by the application of Faraday's principle of electromagnetic induction. Briefly (and overly simplified), this principle states that a changing electrical current flowing through a circular coil generates a magnetic field tangential to the plane of the coil. If this magnetic field contacts another conductive material (e.g., a pick-up coil), it will generate a secondary electrical current (Fig. 36.1). TMS systems use an electrical capacitor to generate a brief powerful current that flows through the TMS coil, which is a circular loop of wire connected to the capacitor and embedded in a protective plastic case. According to Faraday's principle, when the electrical current flows through the circular coil, a rapidly changing magnetic field is generated. If the TMS coil is placed on the surface of the skull, this magnetic field will travel towards the intra-cranial space unaltered by the structures it will cross (e.g., soft tissue, bone, cerebrospinal fluid), until it reaches the electrically conductive neurons of the cortex. These neurons will then act as an organic pick-up coil, and a secondary electrical current will be generated that can trigger action potentials and force brain cells to fire (see Fig. 36.1). As a result, the stimulation of neurons in TMS is electrical, not magnetic, and the term "magnetic stimulation" is a misnomer: the magnetic pulses are used only as a vehicle for the non-invasive transfer of electrical currents from the coil to the cortex.

Although the magnetic field is essentially unaltered by the various structures it encounters on its path to the cortex, the strength of the field weakens as it moves from its source in the TMS coil. As a result, the 1 to 2 Tesla magnetic pulse originated in the TMS coil becomes too weak to generate neuronal action potentials 2 to 4 cm away from its origin on the skull's surface. This sets a practical limitation to this technique, as only superficial cortical structures can be directly stimulated by TMS. Nevertheless, the effects of TMS are not only local but circuit-wide; once an action potential is generated in a cortical neuron, the volley of activation travels through its axon and stimulates the post-synaptic neuron, leading to a cascade of events through the entire neural circuit (including deep cortical, sub-cortical, and contralateral regions). This cascade of electrical events is specific to the brain circuit that the target region is connected to, and not generalized like the effects of ECT. Therefore, although it is true that TMS only directly modulates superficial cortical nodes, these nodes act as windows that provide modulatory access to an entire functional network of cortical and sub-cortical neurons.[2]

The effects of TMS are not only specific to the target of stimulation but also to the parameters used. This is important as we consider statements such as "TMS is (or is not) effective for a given condition," which lack meaning and are not informative. Alternatively, "TMS applied over a determined anatomical target at a specific frequency and dose for a particular condition" would be more clinically and scientifically meaningful. Since the effects of TMS are specific to the stimulated region and the parameters used, we should expect that stimulating prefrontal cortical areas that process working memory or spatial attention will have little effect on mood, anhedonia, or neurovegetative symptoms of depression. Similarly, inhibiting a pathologically hypoactive region will most likely worsen a patient's condition, though its activation may prove therapeutic. Last, applying 2 weeks of stimulation when 4 to 6 or more weeks are needed should have minimal or no therapeutic impact. This highlights the need to have a basic understanding of the TMS parameters that clinicians and scientists can manipulate: the location or target of stimulation, the focality and depth, the frequency, and

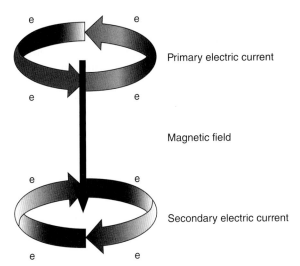

Primary electric current

Magnetic field

Secondary electric current

Fig.v 36.1 ■ This schematic illustrates the principle of electromagnetic induction, by which a primary electrical current (e, top) generates a perpendicular magnetic field that, when in contact with a conductive material, leads to a secondary electrical current in the same plane but opposite sense to the primary (e, bottom). Redrawn from Jalinous R. *A Guide to Magnetic Stimulation.* Magstim Company Ltd; 1998.

the dose of stimulation (which is a composite measure of stimulation intensity and duration) (Box 36.1).

As mentioned above, the choice of the anatomical site of stimulation is crucial, as this will grant us access to modulate a specific functional network of interest. Similarly, the focality of stimulation will be of relevance as the clinical impact and specificity will not be the same if one modulates a cortical area of 0.25 or 1 cm². Although the intensity of stimulation has an influence on the focality of its effects (the stronger the magnetic field, the deeper and less focal its effects),[3] focality is primarily controlled by the choice of TMS coil. Various types of coils are manufactured with differences in their internal architecture that allow varying degrees of focality and depth. The most common types are the circular coils (less focal), the figure-of-eight or butterfly coils (more focal), and the H-coils (deep).

TMS can either inhibit (down-regulate) or activate (up-regulate) populations of neurons depending on the frequency of stimulation. With parameters similar to the ones leading to long-term depression or long-term potentiation, low frequencies of 1 Hz are known to be inhibitory[4] while high frequencies of > 5 Hz (typically 10 or 20 Hz) are activating.[5] Newer TMS protocols with more complex patterns of stimulation (such as theta burst stimulation [TBS]) have been developed more recently, and allow for longer-lasting behavioral

---

BOX 36.1

TRANSCRANIAL MAGNETIC STIMULATION PARAMETERS

ANATOMICAL

1. Location (can be optimized with neuroimaging and neuro-navigation).
2. Focality (depends primarily on coil architecture, also on intensity).
3. Depth (also depends primarily on coil architecture and partially on intensity).

PHYSIOLOGICAL

1. Frequency (can facilitate or inhibit a target region).
2. Intensity of stimulation (usually expressed as a percentage of the motor threshold).
3. Number of pulses per session (will also determine the duration of the session).
4. Number of sessions (treatment protocols require multiple sessions over weeks).

---

effects despite a significantly shorter stimulation time (a traditional therapeutic protocol for MDD lasts 37.5 minutes, while TBS can be performed in 3 minutes). Once the target of stimulation and direction of modulation is set, the dose will be determined by deciding the strength of the magnetic field (pulse intensity) and the total number of pulses (duration). Duration also relates to the total number of sessions, typically daily sessions over weeks. Other more complex variables, such as the waveform of the electromagnetic current, are also relevant to define the dose.[6] As we improve our understanding of the mechanism of action of TMS, the parameter space available becomes more complex, granting greater control and specificity to clinicians and scientists.[7]

The safety profile of TMS is notoriously benign, given its non-invasive nature. The only contraindication considered to be absolute is the presence of metallic hardware in the area of stimulation, such as cochlear implants, brain stimulators, or medication pumps.[7] Still, the use of TMS on patients with DBS has been tested and considered relatively safe when the DBS system is off, although data are still very limited, and extreme caution (in addition to an accurate risk/benefit analysis) should be used in these cases.[8] The primary safety concern with TMS remains the induction of seizures with repetitive trains, even if this is a very rare phenomenon; approximately 20 seizures have been reported out of the estimated 300,000 sessions (clinical or research) since its development in the early 1980s.[7] Since the 2008 FDA approval of the NeuroStar TMS Therapy system (Neuronetics, Inc.), seven seizures have been reported in the United States from 250,000 treatment sessions in 8000 patients.[9] This represents 1 case in 35,000 patients, which is similar to or fewer than the seizure risk of most antidepressant medications. It should be noted that TMS may trigger a seizure but not cause epilepsy; seizures are always during (not after) rTMS and do not lead to spontaneous events afterward. Nevertheless, one should screen patients for a personal history of epilepsy and possible risk factors that increase their seizure risk (such as brain lesions or medications that lower the seizure threshold). Other less severe but more common side effects include headaches, local discomfort in the area of stimulation, facial twitching, tinnitus, anxiety, and vasovagal syncope.[7]

The evidence for the use of high-frequency rTMS to the left DLPFC, low-frequency rTMS to the right DLPFC, a combination of the two techniques (termed bilateral treatments), deep TMS over the left DLPFC, and TBS in the treatment of depression is supported by multiple clinical studies including over 4000 patients, demonstrating robust odds ratios of 2.54 to 4.66 for response relative to sham TMS.[10] Recent developments in image-guided TMS using neuro-navigation have proved to increase the anatomical specificity and clinical efficacy of TMS. One protocol involved functional MRI imaging to locate the region of the left DLPFC most functionally anti-correlated with the sub-genual anterior cingulate cortex, which is then targeted with 10 TMS sessions per day over 5 days. This accelerated protocol resulted in a 69% reduction in depression scores in 5 days, compared to 14% in those receiving sham treatment.[11] A device utilizing this protocol received FDA approval for the treatment of depression in 2022.

As TMS has entered clinical practice with more homogeneous protocols leading to greater effect sizes and decreased variability, researchers have explored what variables may predict the antidepressant response of TMS. Fregni and colleagues analyzed the pooled data for 195 patients from six independent studies.[12] They reported that age and the number of previously failed medication trials were negative predictors of response, that is, younger and less treatment-refractory patients had better outcomes. As the field moves towards identifying not only clinical or demographic variables but also biological markers that predict response to treatment, the hope is that the biomarkers linked to the therapeutics targets specifically modulated by the different treatment modalities will help stratify patients and individually select the most effective treatments.[13]

ELECTROCONVULSIVE THERAPY

ECT involves the delivery of an electrical current to the brain through the scalp and skull to induce a generalized seizure. ECT has been in use since 1938; it received FDA clearance in 2018 for the treatment of severe unipolar depression, bipolar depression, and catatonia in patients aged 13 and older. There is additional evidence for ECT as an effective treatment for both mania and schizophrenia, with recent treatment guidelines recommending ECT in patients with treatment-resistant disease refractory to clozapine. Compared with other antipsychotic augmentation strategies, it is evident that the effectiveness of ECT exceeds any other option and can accelerate the initial response by a few weeks. Furthermore, augmenting clozapine with ECT yields a response rate of 76% in patients with severe disease. In current practice, it remains a critical treatment for patients whose symptoms are unresponsive to drugs or who are intolerant of their side effects.[14] The neurobiological mechanism of ECT remains unknown and likely involves both neurohormonal effects resulting from the clinical seizure and changes in brain structure following treatment.[15]

Although most patients initially receive a medication trial regardless of their diagnosis, several groups of patients are appropriate for ECT as a primary treatment. These include patients who are severely malnourished, dehydrated, and exhausted due to protracted depressive or catatonic illnesses (however, they should be treated promptly after careful re-hydration); patients who have been unresponsive to medications during previous episodes (because they are often better served by proceeding directly to ECT); and, patients with catatonia who are showing signs of metabolic failure (as they respond promptly to ECT). In addition, due to its life-threatening nature, patients with significant suicidal ideation or a recent suicide attempt, especially in the context of psychotic illness, may be appropriate candidates for initial ECT treatment due to the speed of response.

To minimize the risks of injury from a generalized seizure, general anesthesia and muscle relaxant are given before ECT. Due to the numerous physical effects of ECT, careful patient selection and collaboration with an experienced anesthesia team are essential for the safe delivery of ECT. The routine pre-ECT work-up usually includes a thorough medical history and physical examination, along with an electrocardiogram, urinalysis, complete blood count, and serum electrolytes. Additional studies may be necessary at the clinician's discretion, particularly in the presence of baseline medical illness. As the technique for ECT delivery has improved, factors that were formerly considered near-absolute contraindications to ECT have become relative risk factors. The patient is best served by weighing the risk of treatment against the morbidity or lethality of remaining depressed. The prevailing view is that there are no longer any absolute contraindications to ECT, but several conditions (e.g., space-occupying lesions with increased intra-cranial pressure [ICP], recent cerebral infarction, and cardiac conditions) warrant careful work-up and management.

The brain is physiologically stressed during ECT, with cerebral oxygen consumption doubling during treatment and cerebral blood flow increasing several-fold. Increases in ICP and the permeability of the blood-brain barrier also develop. These acute changes may increase the risk of ECT in patients with a variety of neurological conditions.[16] Space-occupying brain lesions with associated increased ICP were previously considered essentially an absolute contraindication to ECT, however, more recent reports indicate that with careful management patients with a brain tumor or a chronic subdural hematoma may be safely treated. Recent cerebral infarction probably represents the most common intra-cranial risk factor. Case reports of ECT after recent cerebral infarction indicate that the complication rate is low,[16] and consequently ECT can be used for post-stroke depression, although clinical trials in this setting are lacking. Although one month is considered a standard amount of time for healing, the interval between infarction and the time of ECT should be determined by the urgency of treatment for depression. ECT is instrumental in treating severe depression during pregnancy, and its safety has been documented extensively. The most common risk to the mother is premature contractions and pre-term labor, which occur infrequently and are not caused by ECT; nonetheless, fetal monitoring is recommended before and after each ECT treatment.[17]

In addition to therapeutic brain effects, the electrical stimulus administered during ECT causes cardiac stimulation.[18] Cardiac work increases abruptly at the onset of the seizure initially because of sympathetic outflow from the diencephalon, through the spinal sympathetic tract, to the heart (Fig. 36.2). This outflow persists for the duration of the seizure and is augmented by a rise in circulating catecholamine levels that peak about 3 minutes after the onset of seizure activity (Fig. 36.3A).[19] After the seizure ends, the parasympathetic tone remains strong, often causing transient bradycardia and hypotension, with a return to baseline function in 5 to 10 minutes (see Fig. 36.3B).

The cardiac conditions that most often worsen under this autonomic stimulus are ischemic heart disease, hypertension, congestive heart failure (CHF), and cardiac arrhythmias. These conditions, if properly managed, have proved to be surprisingly tolerant to ECT. Vascular aneurysms should be repaired before ECT if possible, but in practice, they have proved surprisingly durable during treatment.[20] Critical aortic stenosis should be surgically corrected before ECT to avoid ventricular overload during the seizure. Patients with cardiac pacemakers generally tolerate ECT uneventfully, although proper pacer function should be ascertained before treatment. The 2020 American Society of Anesthesiologists Practice Advisory recommends "suspending the Implantable cardioverter defibrillator anti-tachycardia therapy with either a magnet or a programmer" before ECT.[21] Patients with compensated CHF generally tolerate ECT well, although a transient decompensation into pulmonary edema for 5 to 10 minutes may occur in patients with a baseline ejection fraction below 20%. It is unclear whether the underlying cause is a neurogenic stimulus to the lung parenchyma or a reduction in cardiac output because of increased heart rate and blood pressure.

Antidepressants are generally continued during ECT treatment. However, if the current antidepressant trial has been of adequate dose and duration, it is a good time to consider changing medications. As tolerated, anticonvulsants prescribed as mood stabilizers may be tapered before ECT to enhance seizure quality. Likewise, benzodiazepines should be reduced if possible, and withheld the night before treatment and the morning of ECT. When tapering, the anticonvulsant load, including benzodiazepines, should be reduced carefully as too aggressive a taper can increase the risk of severe post-treatment agitation. In the patient with a pre-existing seizure disorder, the anticonvulsant regimen should be continued for patient safety. The elevated seizure threshold can almost always be overridden with an ECT stimulus, and patients managed in this manner usually have the same clinical response as patients not taking anticonvulsants.[22]

The typical course of ECT treatment includes two phases: acute treatment, to rapidly improve symptoms, followed by continuation and maintenance treatment to prolong the time to symptom relapse. In the acute phase, treatments are generally given two to three

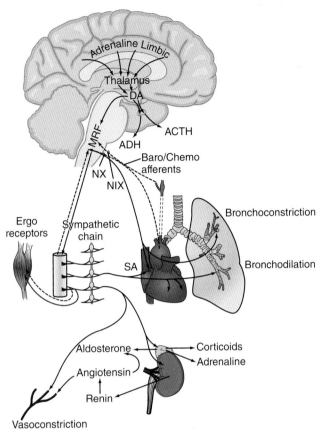

Fig. 36.2 ■ Schematic of sympathetic outflow from the diencephalon to the heart and other organs. *ACTH,* Adrenocorticotropic hormone; *ADH,* antidiuretic hormone; *DA,* defense area in hypothalamus; *SA,* sinoatrial node; *MRF,* medullary retiuclar formation; *NIX,* 9th cranial nerve; *NX,* 10th cranial nerve.

times per week and continued until symptom remission or a plateau in treatment response. In prospective trials, the median number of treatments required to reach remission is 7.3,[23,24] but in ordinary clinical practice longer courses are often required,[25] and for patients who continue to demonstrate clinical benefit there is no absolute number of acute course treatments that may be administered.

ECT is not a single technique, but rather a range of stimulation types. The ECT electrodes can be placed to stimulate both sides of the brain (bilateral) or just one hemisphere (typically the right) (Fig. 36.4A and B). Present evidence suggests equal efficacy of the two electrode placements in depression, with fewer cognitive effects of right unilateral treatment,[24] but optimal electrode placement for particular patients and disorders

remains an active area of research. Additionally, the width of the electrical stimulus is variable, with modern brief pulse and ultra-brief pulse retaining treatment efficacy while reducing cognitive side effects relative to earlier sine wave stimuli. The efficacy of acute course ECT in the treatment of depression is established by numerous clinical trials and meta-analyses, with demonstrated response rates of around 75% for both unipolar and bipolar depression.[26] The efficacy of ECT is higher than that of TMS and other non-surgical brain stimulation techniques, with similar tolerability.[27,28] Older age is associated with greater benefit from ECT treatment,[29] although efficacy remains high even in children and adolescents.[30]

Following successful treatment with ECT, without any continuation therapy, the risk of depressive relapse

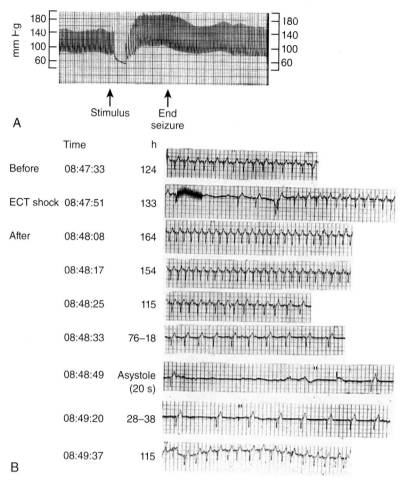

Fig. 36.3 ■ (A) Graphic of the impact of electroconvulsive therapy (ECT) on catecholamine levels and blood pressure following a seizure. (B) Graphic of the effects of ECT on cardiac rhythm.

is greater than 80% at 6 months.[31] As a result, ongoing treatment with pharmacotherapy and/or additional ECT is necessary. Ongoing treatment with ECT following symptom improvement is termed continuation or maintenance of ECT. In a recent comparison of pharmacotherapy alone versus ECT plus pharmacotherapy, relapse rates at 1 year were 61% with pharmacotherapy alone and 32% with pharmacotherapy plus maintenance ECT.[32] Continuation ECT alone (weekly for 4 weeks, biweekly for 8 weeks, and monthly for 3 months) lowers the relapse rate at 6 months to below 40%.[23] Large controlled trials of other antidepressant drugs after ECT have not yet been conducted. Although questions remain about the relative effectiveness of continuation

ECT and continuation pharmacotherapy, the cumulative evidence over the last decade indicates that continuation ECT is a valuable and effective strategy for most patients, with a cohort of 100 maintenance ECT patients maintaining benefit from 50 or more treatments over a median of 22 months.[33]

Pooled data indicate a mortality rate of ECT of 2.1 per 100,000 treatments, which is lower than the general anesthesia mortality rate of 3.4 per 100,000 in surgery procedures.[34] Although there is no evidence for structural brain damage as a result of ECT, there are important effects on cognition. Memory impairment varies greatly in severity and is associated with bilateral electrode placement, high stimulus intensity,

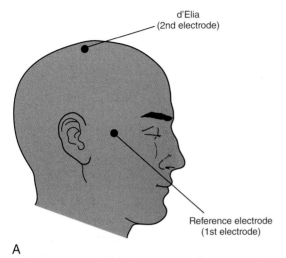

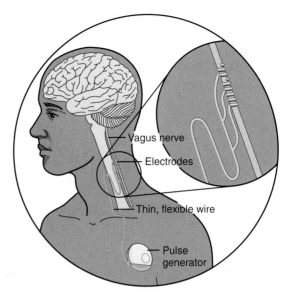

Fig. 36.5 ■ A schematic demonstrating the locations of the electrode lead on the left vagus nerve and the internal pulse generator following vagus nerve stimulation device implantation. (Redrawn from Cyberonics, Inc. *Physician's Manual for the VNS Therapy Pulse Model 102 generator and VNS Therapy Pulse Duo Model 102 R Generator*; 2003.)

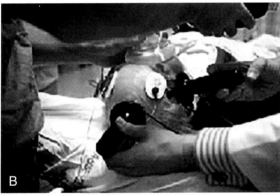

Fig. 36.4 ■ (A) Schematic of electrode placements during electroconvulsive therapy (ECT). (B) Photograph of electrodes being placed during ECT.

inadequate oxygenation, prolonged seizure activity, advanced age, alcohol abuse, and lower pre-morbid cognitive function. Difficulty recalling new information (anterograde amnesia) is usually experienced during the ECT series, but it normally resolves within a month after the last treatment. Difficulty remembering events before ECT (retrograde amnesia) is usually more severe for events closer to the time of treatment. A meta-analysis of cognitive function testing in 2981 patients in 84 studies found significant decreases in cognitive performance scores 0 to 3 days after completion of a series of ECT.[35] However, within 15 days of the last ECT treatment, almost all mean test scores were at or above pre-ECT levels. After 15 days, improvements compared to baseline were observed in processing speed, working memory, anterograde memory, and aspects of executive function.

VAGUS NERVE STIMULATION

VNS was approved for treatment-refractory MDD and bipolar disorder in 2005. The FDA-approved language states that VNS is an adjunctive treatment for treatment-resistant depression (TRD) and that it should be used in patients with severe, chronic, recurrent TRD who have failed at least four adequate antidepressant trials. Implantation of the VNS device involves surgical placement of electrodes around the left vagus nerve via an incision in the neck (only the left vagus nerve is used for VNS because the right vagus has a much higher percentage of parasympathetic branches to the heart) (Fig. 36.5.) A second incision is used to place an internal pulse generator (IPG) sub-cutaneously in the left sub-clavicular region, and the wire between the electrodes on the vagus nerve and the IPG is connected using sub-cutaneous tunneling between the two incision sites.

The interest in studying the efficacy of VNS for MDD arose from the clinical experience of treating over 40,000 patients with treatment-resistant epilepsy with VNS. Depression is more prevalent in patients with epilepsy than it is in the general population, and it was noted that many patients with treatment-resistant epilepsy being treated with VNS experienced improvement in symptoms of MDD.[36] The left vagus nerve enters the brain and first innervates the nucleus tractus solitarius (NTS). While the mechanism of action of VNS is not completely understood, the NTS communicates with the parabrachial nucleus (PBN), the cerebellum, the dorsal raphe, the periaqueductal gray, the locus coeruleus, and ascending projections to limbic, paralimbic, and cortical regions.[37] Functional neuroimaging studies of subjects receiving VNS show increased cerebral blood flow in many of these brain regions that are implicated in the pathophysiology of MDD.[38] For instance, the locus coeruleus and dorsal raphe nuclei contain the cell bodies of noradrenergic and serotonergic neurons that then project throughout the central nervous system. Last, the PBN communicates with other brain regions (including the hypothalamus, thalamus, amygdala, and nucleus of the stria terminalis) implicated in the pathophysiology of MDD.[37]

VNS is an adjunctive treatment for depression, therefore all patients who receive VNS should continue to receive pharmacotherapy, psychotherapy, or both (and even ECT, if necessary), referred to as *treatment as usual*. In an 8-week clinical trial of 112 patients in the active VNS treatment group and 110 patients in the sham VNS treatment group, active VNS failed to demonstrate statistically significant efficacy on the primary outcome measure, the Hamilton Depression Rating Scale (a clinician-administered scale), at 8 weeks.[39] However, step-wise increases in response and remission at 3, 6, 9, and 12 months were demonstrated during the subsequent open-label phase of the study and the FDA-approved VNS for TRD in 2005 based on these data. Better results have been demonstrated in longer-term studies. In a 5-year open-label study of 795 patients, 494 receiving VNS and 301 receiving treatment-as-usual, 5-year cumulative remission rates were 43.3% in the VNS arm compared to 25.7% in the treatment-as-usual arm.[40] Moreover the rate of suicide deaths and all-cause mortality in the VNS arm was less than half of that in the treatment-as-usual group.

Adjustment of the VNS stimulation parameters is performed by using a device that communicates transcutaneously with the IPG. The dose parameters used by the clinician for VNS therapy include the magnitude of the electrical charge delivered to the left vagus nerve, the stimulation frequency, the stimulation pulse width, and the duration of stimulation. Finally, decreasing the stimulation pulse width or stimulation frequency is often helpful for addressing potential side effects associated with VNS therapy.

Potential risks associated with VNS include standard risks associated with the surgical procedure itself. The most common side effects associated with active VNS therapy are likely due to stimulation of the laryngeal and pharyngeal branches of the left vagus nerve. The most common side effect is voice alteration during the active phase (seen in 54%–60% of patients). Other relatively common side effects include cough, neck pain, paresthesia, and dyspnea.[41] These side effects typically decrease or dissipate over time. Despite these side effects, the device is well tolerated, and patients also can turn off the device at any time by placing a magnet provided by the manufacturer over the IPG. The IPG will remain off (i.e., no stimulation will occur) while the magnet is in place. When the magnet is removed, the IPG returns to its previously set stimulation parameters.

DEEP BRAIN STIMULATION

DBS grew from the therapeutic tradition of ablative stereotaxic surgery and the technical developments that led to cardiac pacemakers.[42] It requires the surgical placement of stimulating electrodes in disease-specific deep brain structures via craniotomy and stereotaxic surgery. The intracranial electrodes are connected to an IPG, which consists of a battery and mini-processor that can generate electrical currents according to clinician-determined parameters. The IPG is surgically implanted in the pectoral region (although other sites are also possible) and connects to the intra-cranial electrodes via a wire that travels through the head and neck's subcutaneous tissue. Clinicians who employ DBS use devices that communicate transcutaneously with the IPG to control and interrogate the system. Clinicians can change the voltage, frequency, and pulse width of the electrical pulses according to safety and efficacy criteria. Most commercially available DBS systems have four contact positions in each stimulating electrode, which can be independently activated to provide positive or negative electrical charges, therefore changing the size and shape of the electric field. This flexibility allows clinicians a significant range of electrode combinations that increase the anatomical precision of stimulation, which can be individualized according to clinical response or biomarkers, such as MRI diffusion tractography.[43]

DBS is a surgical procedure and therefore invasive. Iatrogenic adverse events can be categorized into two primary groups: those related to surgical procedures and those related to the stimulation of brain regions. Surgical adverse events have an incidence rate of 1% to 4% and include seizures, infection, and hemorrhage.[44] Effects related to stimulation vary depending on the anatomical location of the electrodes and include worsening depression, (hypo)mania, acute anxiety, and gustatory or olfactory sensations. Unlike ablative interventions, permanent cognitive deficits have not been reported in DBS patients. Nevertheless, reversible cognitive effects (such as diminished concentration) have been described, though these are stimulation dependent and remit with re-adjustment of DBS parameters.

The primary indications for DBS are Parkinson disease and other movement disorders, such as dystonia and essential tremor. The therapeutic approach for these conditions requires the surgical modulation of key nodes in the motor circuitry: sub-thalamic nucleus for Parkinson disease, globus pallidus pars interna for Parkinson disease and dystonia, and ventral intermediate nucleus of the thalamus for essential tremor. As of 2019, more than 160,000 patients worldwide have been estimated to have been implanted with DBS devices.[45]

Basic and clinical research studies investigated the use of DBS for refractory OCD using various brain targets that included the anterior limb of the internal capsule, the ventral capsule/ventral striatum (VC/VS), the nucleus accumbens (NAcc), the sub-thalamic nucleus, and the inferior thalamic peduncle. It should be noted that the first three anatomical targets are very similar, if not practically the same. In 2009 the FDA approved the use of DBS to the VC/VS for the treatment of treatment-resistant OCD (under the humanitarian device exemption mechanism), thus approving

the first psychiatric indication and allowing DBS to enter clinical practice in psychiatry.[46]

Several open-label clinical trials have been published using DBS for the treatment of MDD stimulating three main regions: the VC/VS (the same as for OCD), the sub-genual cingulate gyrus or Brodmann area 25 (BA25/Cg25) and the NAcc. Response rates (from 50% to 60%) were similar for all regions.[47] Prospective randomized trials, however, have failed to demonstrate the benefit of DBS in depression. A prospective randomized sham-controlled trial of DBS at the VC/VS in 29 patients failed to demonstrate the superiority of active treatment compared to sham,[48] with a further study of 90 patients randomized to receive DBS to the subcallosal cingulate or sham treatment failing to demonstrate a difference between the two groups.[49] Other approaches for DBS including changes in intra-operative targeting are being explored, but overall the use of DBS for depression remains experimental.

In addition to OCD and MDD, DBS is also being investigated as a treatment for other conditions that result from physiological changes in the brain circuit and lead to pathological processing of affect, behavior, and cognition. A few examples under current active research include addiction, obesity, eating disorders, Tourette syndrome (TS), Alzheimer disease (AD), and schizophrenia. Structures (such as the ventral tegmental area and the NAcc) are targeted for addiction and schizophrenia and the hippocampal fornix is targeted for AD. As we improve our understanding of the mechanism of action of DBS and its effects on key targets, and we will be able to develop new technologies that increase its specificity, efficacy, and safety, DBS may become a more commonly used treatment for the most treatment-refractory patients.[45]

ABLATIVE LIMBIC SYSTEM SURGERY

Concerns regarding ablative neurosurgery for psychiatric indications are understandable given the indiscriminate use of crude procedures, such as frontal lobotomy, in the middle of the twentieth century. These procedures were associated with severe adverse events, including frontal lobe symptoms (e.g., apathy) or even death. In the latter half of the twentieth century, neurosurgeons began to use much smaller lesions in well-targeted and specific brain regions. As a result, the incidence of adverse events dropped precipitously.[42] Currently used procedures include anterior cingulotomy, sub-caudate tractotomy, limbic leucotomy (which is a combination of an anterior cingulotomy and a sub-caudate tractotomy), and anterior capsulotomy (Fig. 36.6). Each of these procedures uses craniotomy techniques. However, because of the small lesion volume required for anterior capsulotomy, a gamma knife (a technique that uses focused gamma rays to create ablative lesions) can be used to perform

this procedure. These procedures have been used in patients who suffer from intractable mood and anxiety disorders; response rates range from one-third to one-half, based on a meta-analysis of uncontrolled studies.[50] Because patients eligible for these procedures have failed all other available treatments, a significant positive response to these interventions can be life saving. While post-operative side effects may occur, they are almost always temporary. Among the side effects are headache, nausea, and edema; more serious adverse events include infections, urinary difficulties, weight

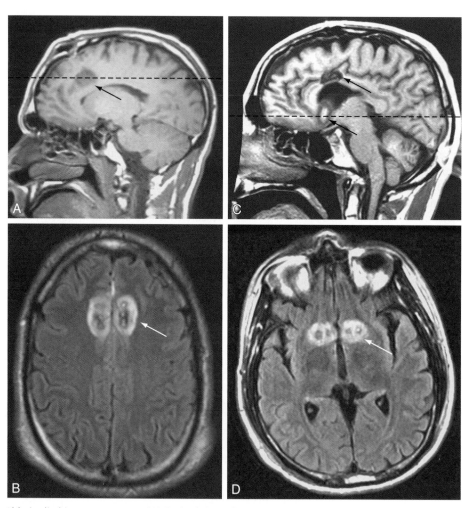

Fig. 36.6 ■ Ablative limbic system surgery. (A) Sagittal view of anterior cingulotomy lesions (*arrow*). (B) Axial view (at the level of the dotted line in panel A) of anterior cingulotomy lesions (*arrow*). (C) Sagittal view of anterior cingulotomy (*upper arrow*) and sub-caudate tractotomy (*lower arrow*) lesions. (D) Axial view (at the level of the dotted line in panel C) of sub-caudate tractotomy lesions (*arrow*).

gain, seizures, cerebral hemorrhage or infarction, and cognitive deficits, all of which are uncommon.

CONCLUSION

This chapter provided an overview of neurotherapeutic interventions for psychiatric disorders, which are currently available or being studied in clinical trials. Some of these treatments have been available for several decades (e.g., ECT and ablative limbic system surgery), and some (such as VNS, DBS, or TMS) have only been approved more recently by the FDA for psychiatric indications. Systems neuroscience and translational neuropsychiatry research are on the path to expanding our therapeutic armamentarium even further with new indications and protocols for these treatments and novel technologies.

REFERENCES

1. Fava M, Davidson KG. Definition and epidemiology of treatment-resistant depression. *Psychiatr Clin North Am.* 1996;19(2):179–200. https://doi.org/10.1016/s0193-953x(05)70283-5.

2. Strafella AP, Paus T, Barrett J, et al. Repetitive transcranial magnetic stimulation of the human prefrontal cortex induces dopamine release in the caudate nucleus. *J Neurosci Off J Soc Neurosci.* 2001;21(15). https://doi.org/10.1523/JNEUROSCI.21-15-j0003.2001.

3. Trillenberg P, Bremer S, Oung S, et al. Variation of stimulation intensity in transcranial magnetic stimulation with depth. *J Neurosci Methods.* 2012;211(2):185–190. https://doi.org/10.1016/j.jneumeth.2012.09.007.

4. Chen R, Classen J, Gerloff C, et al. Depression of motor cortex excitability by low-frequency transcranial magnetic stimulation. *Neurology.* 1997;48(5):1398–1403. https://doi.org/10.1212/wnl.48.5.1398.

5. Pascual-Leone A, Valls-Sole J, Wasserman EM, et al. Responses to rapid-rate transcranial magnetic stimulation of the human motor cortex. *Brain J Neurol.* 1994;117(Pt 4). https://doi.org/10.1093/brain/117.4.847.

6. Peterchev AV, Wagner TA, Miranda PC, et al. Fundamentals of transcranial electric and magnetic stimulation dose: definition, selection, and reporting practices. *Brain Stimul.* 2012;5(4):435–453. https://doi.org/10.1016/j.brs.2011.10.001.

7. Rossi S, Hallett M, Rossini PM, et al. Safety, ethical considerations, and application guidelines for the use of transcranial magnetic stimulation in clinical practice and research. *Clin Neurophysiol.* 2009;120(12):2008–2039. https://doi.org/10.1016/j.clinph.2009.08.016.

8. Deng ZD, Lisanby SH, Peterchev AV. Transcranial magnetic stimulation in the presence of deep brain stimulation implants: induced electrode currents. *Annu Int Conf IEEE Eng Med Biol Soc.* 2010;2010:6821–6824. https://doi.org/10.1109/IEMBS.2010.5625958

9. George MS, Taylor JJ, Short EB. The expanding evidence base for rTMS treatment of depression. *Curr Opin Psychiatry.* 2013;26(1):13–18. https://doi.org/10.1097/YCO.0b013e32835ab46d.

10. Brunoni AR, Chaimani A, Moffa AH, et al. Repetitive transcranial magnetic stimulation for the acute treatment of major depressive episodes: a systematic review with network meta-analysis. *JAMA Psychiatry.* 2017;74(2):143–152. https://doi.org/10.1001/jamapsychiatry.2016.3644.

11. Cole EJ, Phillips AL, Bentzley BS, et al. Stanford Neuromodulation Therapy (SNT): a double-blind randomized controlled trial. *Am J Psychiatry.* 2022;179(2):132–141. https://doi.org/10.1176/appi.ajp.2021.20101429.

12. Fregni F, Marcolin MA, Myczkowski M, et al. Predictors of antidepressant response in clinical trials of transcranial magnetic stimulation. *Int J Neuropsychopharmacol.* 2006;9(6):641–654. https://doi.org/10.1017/S1461145705006280.

13. Fidalgo TM, Morales-Quezada JL, Muzy GSC, et al. Biological markers in noninvasive brain stimulation trials in major depressive disorder: a systematic review. *J ECT.* 2014;30(1):47–61. https://doi.org/10.1097/YCT.0b013e31828b34d8.

14. Petrides G, Malur C, Braga RJ, et al. Electroconvulsive therapy augmentation in clozapine-resistant schizophrenia: a prospective, randomized study. *Am J Psychiatry.* 2015;172(1):52–58. https://doi.org/10.1176/appi.ajp.2014.13060787.

15. Espinoza RT, Kellner CH. Electroconvulsive therapy. *N Engl J Med.* 2022;386(7):667–672. https://doi.org/10.1056/NEJMra2034954.

16. Hsiao JK, Messenheimer JA, Evans DL. ECT and neurological disorders. *Convuls Ther.* 1987;3(2):121–136.

17. Ward HB, Fromson JA, Cooper JJ, et al. Recommendations for the use of ECT in pregnancy: literature review and proposed clinical protocol. *Arch Womens Ment Health.* 2018;21(6):715–722. https://doi.org/10.1007/s00737-018-0851-0.

18. Hermida AP, Mohsin M, Marques Pinheiro AP, et al. The cardiovascular side effects of electroconvulsive therapy and their management. *J ECT.* 2022;38(1):2–9. https://doi.org/10.1097/YCT.0000000000000802.

19. Liston EH, Salk JD. Hemodynamic responses to ECT after bilateral adrenalectomy. *Convuls Ther.* 1990;6(2):160–164.

20. Drop LJ, Viguera A, Welch CA. ECT in patients with intracranial aneurysm. *J ECT.* 2000;16(1):71–72.

21. Streckenbach SC, Benedetto WJ, Fitzsimons MG. Implantable cardioverter-defibrillator shock delivered during electroconvulsive therapy despite magnet application: a case report. *A A Pract.* 2020;14(11):e01284. https://doi.org/10.1213/XAA.0000000000001284.

22. Lunde ME, Lee EK, Rasmussen KG. Electroconvulsive therapy in patients with epilepsy. *Epilepsy Behav EB.* 2006;9(2):355–359. https://doi.org/10.1016/j.yebeh.2006.06.013.

23. Kellner CH, Knapp RG, Petrides G, et al. Continuation electroconvulsive therapy vs pharmacotherapy for relapse prevention in major depression: a multisite study from the Consortium for Research in Electroconvulsive Therapy (CORE). *Arch Gen Psychiatry.* 2006;63(12):1337–1344. https://doi.org/10.1001/archpsyc.63.12.1337.

24. Semkovska M, Landau S, Dunne R, et al. Bitemporal versus high-dose unilateral twice-weekly electroconvulsive therapy for depression (EFFECT-Dep): a pragmatic, randomized, non-inferiority trial. *Am J Psychiatry*. 2016;173(4):408–417. https://doi.org/10.1176/appi.ajp.2015.15030372.

25. Luccarelli J, McCoy TH, Shannon AP, et al. Rate of continuing acute course treatment using right unilateral ultrabrief pulse electroconvulsive therapy at a large academic medical center. *Eur Arch Psychiatry Clin Neurosci*. 2021;271(1):191–197. https://doi.org/10.1007/s00406-020-01202-2.

26. Bahji A, Hawken ER, Sepehry AA, et al. ECT beyond unipolar major depression: systematic review and meta-analysis of electroconvulsive therapy in bipolar depression. *Acta Psychiatr Scand*. 2019;139(3):214–226. https://doi.org/10.1111/acps.12994.

27. Mutz J, Vipulananthan V, Carter B, et al. Comparative efficacy and acceptability of non-surgical brain stimulation for the acute treatment of major depressive episodes in adults: systematic review and network meta-analysis. *BMJ*. 2019;364 https://doi.org/10.1136/bmj.l1079.

28. Ren J, Li H, Palaniyappan L, et al. Repetitive transcranial magnetic stimulation versus electroconvulsive therapy for major depression: a systematic review and meta-analysis. *Prog Neuropsychopharmacol Biol Psychiatry*. 2014;51:181–189. https://doi.org/10.1016/j.pnpbp.2014.02.004.

29. Luccarelli J, McCoy Jr TH, Seiner SJ, et al. Real-world evidence of age-independent electroconvulsive therapy efficacy: a retrospective cohort study. *Acta Psychiatr Scand*. 2022;145(1):100–108. https://doi.org/10.1111/acps.13378.

30. Luccarelli J, McCoy TH, Uchida M, et al. The efficacy and cognitive effects of acute course electroconvulsive therapy are equal in adolescents, transitional age youth, and young adults. *J Child Adolesc Psychopharmacol*. 2021;31(8):538–544. https://doi.org/10.1089/cap.2021.0064.

31. Sackeim HA, Haskett RF, Mulsant BH, et al. Continuation pharmacotherapy in the prevention of relapse following electroconvulsive therapy: a randomized controlled trial. *JAMA*. 2001;285(10):1299–1307. https://doi.org/10.1001/jama.285.10.1299.

32. Nordenskjöld A, von Knorring L, Ljung T, et al. Continuation electroconvulsive therapy with pharmacotherapy versus pharmacotherapy alone for prevention of relapse of depression: a randomized controlled trial. *J ECT*. 2013;29(2):86–92. https://doi.org/10.1097/YCT.0b013e318276591f.

33. Luccarelli J, McCoy TH, Seiner SJ, et al. Maintenance ECT is associated with sustained improvement in depression symptoms without adverse cognitive effects in a retrospective cohort of 100 patients each receiving 50 or more ECT treatments. *J Affect Disord*. 2020;271:109–114. https://doi.org/10.1016/j.jad.2020.03.152.

34. Tørring N, Sanghani SN, Petrides G, et al. The mortality rate of electroconvulsive therapy: a systematic review and pooled analysis. *Acta Psychiatr Scand*. 2017;135(5):388–397. https://doi.org/10.1111/acps.12721.

35. Semkovska M, McLoughlin DM. Objective cognitive performance associated with electroconvulsive therapy for depression: a systematic review and meta-analysis. *Biol Psychiatry*. 2010;68(6):568–577. https://doi.org/10.1016/j.biopsych.2010.06.009.

36. Elger G, Hoppe C, Falkai P, et al. Vagus nerve stimulation is associated with mood improvements in epilepsy patients. *Epilepsy Res*. 2000;42(2-3):203–210. https://doi.org/10.1016/s0920-1211(00)00181-9.

37. Nemeroff CB, Mayberg HS, Krahl SE, et al. VNS therapy in treatment-resistant depression: clinical evidence and putative neurobiological mechanisms. *Neuropsychopharmacol Off Publ Am Coll Neuropsychopharmacol*. 2006;31(7):1345–1355. https://doi.org/10.1038/sj.npp.1301082.

38. Kosel M, Brockmann H, Frick C, et al. Chronic vagus nerve stimulation for treatment-resistant depression increases regional cerebral blood flow in the dorsolateral prefrontal cortex. *Psychiatry Res*. 2011;191(3):153–159. https://doi.org/10.1016/j.pscychresns.2010.11.004.

39. Rush AJ, Marangell LB, Sackeim HA, et al. Vagus nerve stimulation for treatment-resistant depression: a randomized, controlled acute phase trial. *Biol Psychiatry*. 2005;58(5):347–354. https://doi.org/10.1016/j.biopsych.2005.05.025.

40. Aaronson ST, Sears P, Ruvuna F, et al. A 5-year observational study of patients with treatment-resistant depression treated with vagus nerve stimulation or treatment as usual: comparison of response, remission, and suicidality. *Am J Psychiatry*. 2017;174(7):640–648. https://doi.org/10.1176/appi.ajp.2017.16010034.

41. Rush AJ, Sackeim HA, Marangell LB, et al. Effects of 12 months of vagus nerve stimulation in treatment-resistant depression: a naturalistic study. *Biol Psychiatry*. 2005;58(5):355–363. https://doi.org/10.1016/j.biopsych.2005.05.024.

42. Schwalb JM, Hamani C. The history and future of deep brain stimulation. *Neurother J Am Soc Exp Neurother*. 2008;5(1):3–13. https://doi.org/10.1016/j.nurt.2007.11.003.

43. Lujan JL, Chaturvedi A, Choi KS, et al. Tractography-activation models applied to subcallosal cingulate deep brain stimulation. *Brain Stimulat*. 2013;6(5):737–739. https://doi.org/10.1016/j.brs.2013.03.008.

44. Hardesty DE, Sackeim HA. Deep brain stimulation in movement and psychiatric disorders. *Biol Psychiatry*. 2007;61(7):831–835. https://doi.org/10.1016/j.biopsych.2006.08.028.

45. Lozano AM, Lipsman N, Bergman H, et al. Deep brain stimulation: current challenges and future directions. *Nat Rev Neurol*. 2019;15(3):148–160. https://doi.org/10.1038/s41582-018-0128-2.

46. Mar-Barrutia L, Real E, Segalás C, et al. Deep brain stimulation for obsessive-compulsive disorder: a systematic review of worldwide experience after 20 years. *World J Psychiatry*. 2021;11(9):659–680. https://doi.org/10.5498/wjp.v11.i9.659.

47. Kaur N, Chou T, Corse AK, et al. Deep brain stimulation for treatment-resistant depression. *Psychiatr Ann*. 2013;43(8):358–365. https://doi.org/10.3928/00485713-20130806-04.

48. Dougherty DD, Rezai AR, Carpenter LL, et al. A randomized sham-controlled trial of deep brain stimulation of the ventral capsule/ventral striatum for chronic treatment-resistant depression. *Biol Psychiatry*. 2015;78(4):240–248. https://doi.org/10.1016/j.biopsych.2014.11.023.

49. Holtzheimer PE, Husain MM, Lisanby SH, et al. Subcallosal cingulate deep brain stimulation for treatment-resistant depression: a multisite, randomised, sham-controlled trial. *Lancet Psychiatry*. 2017;4(11):839–849. https://doi.org/10.1016/S2215-0366(17)30371-1.

50. Volpini M, Giacobbe P, Cosgrove GR, et al. The history and future of ablative neurosurgery for major depressive disorder. *Stereotact Funct Neurosurg*. 2017;95(4):216–228. https://doi.org/10.1159/000478025.

37 PSYCHOPHARMACOLOGY IN THE MEDICAL SETTING

JONATHAN E. ALPERT, MD, PHD ▪ DAVID MISCHOULON, MD, PHD ▪ MAURIZIO FAVA, MD ▪ THEODORE A. STERN, MD

OVERVIEW

Co-morbid medical disorders and concurrent medications often hinder the detection of psychiatric symptoms and alter the effectiveness, tolerability, and safety of psychopharmacological treatments. In today's complex medical environment, many patients receive a host of medications from different specialties.[1] As illustrated in the case below, communication among clinicians may not occur, particularly when care is provided in different healthcare systems using dissimilar information management platforms or on an emergency basis. Successful psychopharmacology in the medical setting involves (1) communication and collaboration with other treaters across disciplines; (2) knowing where, when, and how to use medicines safely and effectively considering intended therapeutic effects, optimal dosing, potential side effects, and drug interactions; and (3) recognizing when to change medicines, when to combine them with other medications or treatment approaches, and when to stop them.

As a guide to making informed decisions about the use of psychotropic medications in the medical setting, this chapter is divided into three sections. The first section focuses on principles of psychopharmacologic practice. The second portion reviews the expanding knowledge base regarding pharmacokinetics and drug-drug interactions. The final segment reviews some of the important psychiatric uses of non-psychiatric medications in clinical practice. This chapter aims to share what adept psychopharmacologists do to help patients achieve relief from their symptoms, avoid harm from potential drug-drug interactions, and ideally, achieve improved overall health outcomes and quality of life.

Case 1

Mr. C, a 75-year-old with schizophrenia, was well-managed on clozapine (300 mg/day) for 3 years. His medical problems included hypertension, a dilated cardiomyopathy, and a history of ventricular tachycardia (VT) for which he received an automatic implanted cardioverter defibrillator (AICD).

Four months after placement of his AICD, he was noted to be hypoxic during a routine outpatient AICD interrogation. Mr. C was sent to the emergency department (ED), where a transthoracic echocardiogram revealed a large circumferential pericardial effusion, without tamponade. A subxiphoid pericardial window was created and his AICD generator lead was removed as the suspected cause of his hemopericardium (via perforation of the right ventricle).

Within 48 hours of this procedure, however, Mr. C developed VT (with rates up to 200 beats per minute); a "code" was called. He received magnesium and intravenous (IV) amiodarone (150 mg), which resulted in a return to normal sinus rhythm within 10 minutes. Considering his AICD-related complication, Mr. C was loaded on amiodarone instead of replacing his AICD. Mr. C remained hemodynamically stable and was discharged on a regimen of amiodarone (400 mg/day) and his pre-admission dose of clozapine.

Mr. C returned to his group home. However, 2 days later, he developed dry mouth, dizziness, blurred vision with dilated pupils, sedation, and confusion.

A clozapine serum level revealed a concentration of 1580 ng/mL, which was significantly greater than his pre-hospital level (242 ng/mL). Staff at his group home confirmed that he had been adherent to his medication regimen. Mr. C's outpatient psychiatrist, suspicious that potent cytochrome P450 isoenzyme (CYP) inhibitors (e.g., amiodarone) could increase levels of relevant CYP substrates (e.g., clozapine), halved the dose of clozapine (to 150 mg/day). Two weeks later, Mr. C's serum clozapine level decreased (to 355 ng/mL) and his mental status returned to baseline.

PRINCIPLES OF PSYCHOPHARMACOLOGIC PRACTICE

The complicated clinical and psychosocial contexts in which psychotropic medications are often administered in the general hospital require a sound understanding of basic principles that underlie the practice of psychopharmacology and the interacting influence of medical illness.[2] When pharmacologic efforts fail to achieve their intended goals, a review of these principles often helps uncover potential explanations and re-direct treatment.

Initiating Treatment

The appropriate use of psychotropic medications starts with as precise a formulation of the diagnosis as possible. Antidepressant monotherapy for a depressed college student presenting to an ED might be appropriate if the diagnosis is a major depressive episode although seriously inadequate and possibly harmful if the primary diagnosis is first episode psychosis or bipolar disorder. The establishment of a psychiatric diagnosis often requires a longitudinal assessment of the course and treatment response. Symptoms of psychiatric disorders may be obscured by co-occurring medical conditions, substance use, or incomplete patient reports. In acute clinical situations, however, it is often not possible to defer the implementation of psychotropic medications until a diagnosis is fully clarified. In this context, it is crucial to document a differential diagnosis, the rationale for selecting a particular treatment over others, and the information that will be needed to achieve greater diagnostic certainty over time. When

a disorder appears in a form that fails to meet full diagnostic criteria, such as sub-syndromal depression or atypical panic symptoms, the rationale and goals for proceeding with psychopharmacologic treatment should be articulated clearly.

The identification of target symptoms plays an integral role in establishing a pre-treatment baseline and in monitoring the impact of treatment longitudinally. These symptoms might include insomnia, anhedonia, irritability, disorganized thinking, delusions of reference, or the frequency and intensity of suicidal longings. The identification of target symptoms serves to focus attention on the problems associated with the greatest danger, disability, and distress to the patient while also informing the patient about specific goals for which psychotropic medications have been recommended.

Despite the likely value of measurement-based psychiatric care and the wide availability of standardized scales for assessing symptoms and function, such scales remain grossly under-utilized in clinical psychopharmacological practice. Clinician-rated instruments, such as the Brief Psychiatric Rating Scale,[3] the Hamilton Rating Scale for Depression,[4] the Hamilton Rating Scale for Anxiety,[5] and the Young Mania Scale,[6] may enhance the serial assessment of relevant symptoms. Useful patient-rated scales that can be administered electronically or in paper form include the Patient Health Questionnaire-9[7] or Quick Inventory for Depressive Symptomatology—Self Rated[8] for depression and Generalized Anxiety Disorder-7[9] for anxiety. In addition, periodic collateral observations from significant others and other caregivers may be valuable as part of a comprehensive monitoring plan. In the case of episodic or complex presentations, the use of daily mood charts may reveal temporal patterns (e.g., rapid mood cycling) and associations (e.g., menstrual cycle, physical activity, sleep routine, or medication changes) that are difficult to discern cross-sectionally during office or bedside visits.

Along with the symptom assessment at baseline and during treatment, evaluation of functioning and quality of life has been increasingly appreciated as integral to good psychopharmacologic practice. Thus for an outpatient, the clinician might inquire about activities of daily living, work or school functions, family and other social relationships, and use of leisure time. For an inpatient, engagement in unit activities and progress in independent functioning can help confirm the adequacy of treatment while lack of improvement along these dimensions directs attention to residual symptoms or to problems not initially apparent.

The Global Assessment of Function scale, once part of the multi-axial diagnostic framework in psychiatry, was removed from The *Diagnostic and Statistical Manual of Mental Disorders, 5th edition* (DSM-5) and its subsequent text revision.[10] In its place, some clinicians use the Clinical Global Impression scale.[11] Widely used in clinical trials, this scale rates the severity of disease on a scale of 1 to 7 (from normal to most extreme) and improvement on a scale of 1 to 7 (from very much improved to worse) and provides a simple quantitative means to document overall treatment outcome. As a more specific scale, the DSM-5 TR Disability Study Group has recommended the World Health Organization Disability Assessment Schedule (WHODAS 2.0).[12] WHODAS 2.0 evaluates the patient's ability to perform activities in six domains of functioning—understanding and communicating, getting around, self-care, getting along with people, life activities, and participation in society—relevant to all individuals including those with mental health and other health conditions.[13]

The understanding that a patient's psychiatric condition is influenced by psychosocial factors does not imply that psychotropic medications should be withheld. Depression or anxiety evolving in the setting of job loss or a spouse's chronic illness may well be as severe and as responsive to pharmacologic treatment as similar conditions that develop in individuals without obvious precipitants. Vague encouragement to seek counseling does not constitute sufficient treatment under such circumstances and may be viewed by patients as amorphous and dismissive. If psychotherapy is recommended and pharmacotherapy deferred, the referral to psychotherapy—whether, for example, to individual cognitive-behavioral therapy, couples therapy, or a pain management group—must be viewed with the same deliberateness and precision as the prescription of medication, including a follow-up plan. If notable progress is not made within a clinically appropriate time frame (e.g., 6–12 weeks for major depressive disorder [MDD]), the potential role of medications should be re-visited. As an overarching principle, severity, disability, safety, chronicity,

and risk of recurrence are more relevant in determining the need for pharmacotherapy of psychiatric conditions than the presence or absence of aggravating life circumstances.

Reciprocally, the expanding range of safe and well-tolerated psychotropic agents, such as selective serotonin reuptake inhibitors (SSRIs) and serotonin-norepinephrine reuptake inhibitors (SNRIs) and other newer monoaminergic and non-monoaminergic antidepressants, does not alter the imperative to explore the use of non-medication interventions whenever medications are considered. An assessment of a patient for psychiatric medications should include an equally careful evaluation of other targeted interventions. In addition to the increasingly rich array of evidence-based psychotherapies, psychosocial supports that may be uniquely helpful include vocational assessment and rehabilitation; elder or child care resources; parenting skills groups; and in-person or online peer support groups for bereaved persons with medical disorders such as epilepsy or multiple sclerosis, or mental health conditions (e.g., as sponsored by Depression and Bipolar Support Alliance, National Alliance for Mental Illness, or Postpartum Support International) or substance use related problems (e.g., as sponsored by Alcoholics Anonymous, Narcotics Anonymous, and Al-Anon).

Patient education and informed consent are important legal and ethical imperatives that are also critical to the success of treatment with psychotropic medications. If the capacity of the patient to make his or her own decisions fluctuates or is questionable, the clinician should obtain the patient's permission to include significant others in important treatment decisions. When a patient cannot clearly make such decisions, formal legal mechanisms for substituted judgment should be used. Such mechanisms, however, in no way diminish the importance of sharing information with a patient to the extent possible. When presenting recommendations to a patient, information about diagnosis, target symptoms, treatment options, and anticipated means of follow-up should be included, as well as the medication name, class, and dosing instructions. Side effects that are common (e.g., dry mouth, nausea, tremor, drowsiness, sexual dysfunction, weight gain) should be reviewed together with side effects that are uncommon but require immediate attention, such as a dystonia due to an antipsychotic, painful, and prolonged erection on trazodone, or a rapidly progressing rash on lamotrigine. Potential clinically important longer-range risks (such as fetal malformations on valproic acid in patients of child-bearing potential or tardive dyskinesia on antipsychotics) should be discussed as should significant drug interactions that may require active monitoring or may alter drug effects such as the potential that certain psychotropic medications will reduce the efficacy of oral contraceptives. Patients should be cautioned specifically about the risks of abrupt discontinuation of psychotropic drugs. Dietary and drug restrictions must be clearly described and, particularly in the case of preventing a hypertensive crisis with monoamine oxidase inhibitors (MAOIs), should be provided in written form as well.

Prescribers have a duty to disclose to patients the information necessary for them to make informed decisions about their treatment.[14] Some prescribers are reluctant to disclose side effects, not wishing to promote undue anxiety or non-adherence. However, sharing of common side effects and uncommon but serious side effects often engenders trust between the prescriber and the patient while respecting patient autonomy and rights and mitigating against legal risk for the clinician. In the context of urgent, life-threatening conditions (such as acute mania), counseling about some potential adverse effects, particularly those not anticipated in the foreseeable future (e.g., tardive dyskinesia, metabolic syndrome, or perinatal risks), may need to be deferred until greater clinical stability is achieved when the risks and benefits of longer-term treatment can be meaningfully addressed.

Relevant information that should be imparted to the extent possible also includes the probable time course to notice a response (whether hours or weeks), anticipated length of treatment, availability of strategies to address side effects or lack of efficacy, reasonable alternative treatments, and the risks of withholding treatment.

Psychopharmacological decisions often possess special meaning to patients. Patients may view medicine as a magic bullet, a Band-Aid, or a toxin; they may view the act of prescribing as caring or dismissive; they may construe medication recommendations as evidence of a clinician's confidence that the patient's condition will improve or convey that they will not. Demonstrating curiosity about a patient's inner experience when considering medications advances the therapeutic alliance and guides future discussions. Exploring a patient's reluctance to initiate treatment often elicits myriad concerns, including the fear that medication will be stigmatizing; might engender physical or psychological dependence; might be "mind altering," creativity dampening, or personality transforming; might mask a problem rather than treat it; might consign them to life-long treatment; or reflects an overly narrow therapeutic philosophy on the part of the clinician. The faithfulness of a patient to a recommended course of treatment is invariably strengthened by a physician's dedicated efforts to frame realistic expectations while eliciting and addressing misgivings and potential misunderstandings. Referral to relevant, evidence-based websites and written materials on diagnosis and treatment is typically welcomed by, and empowering to, patients and family members in their efforts to get better informed, particularly when longer-term treatment is anticipated.

Selecting and Administering Medication

For many common psychiatric disorders, at least several agents are known to have roughly equivalent efficacy. Decisions regarding the choice of a particular medication should give considerable weight to a patient's previous treatment response and the current feasibility of the medication in terms of cost, tolerability, and complexity of dosing. Anticholinergic, hypotensive, and sedative effects of drugs must be considered carefully, particularly when prescribing medications to elderly patients or patients who are medically frail.

In some cases, knowledge of a patient's pharmacogenetic profile may be helpful. Although still at a nascent stage, pharmacogenetics, including pharmacogenomic testing, promises to become more impactful to clinical practice as more is learned about the genetics that underlie the mechanisms and metabolism of psychiatric medications Within psychiatry, studies have found genetic variations associated with altered treatment response and efficacy, as well as side effect risk. Genetic testing for such variations may help identify which patients are more likely to respond to psychotropics and which are likely to experience an increased side effect burden.[15] Further advances in pharmacogenomics are required, including in diverse real-world populations, to advance the goal of precision medicine in psychiatry.

Once a drug is chosen, the goal should be to achieve a full trial with adequate dosages and an adequate duration of treatment. Inadequate dosing and duration are among the principal factors that underlie treatment failure for patients with accurate diagnoses. In the service of decisions regarding a patient's future care weeks or months later, it is crucial to document whether a trial of medication succeeded, failed, or was abbreviated because of clinical deterioration, medication side effects, poor adherence to treatment, or problematic substance use. Suffering is unnecessarily prolonged, and resources are poorly used both when medications that were previously ineffective have been tried again because of inadequate documentation of failure and when medications that could have been effective are neglected because previous trials of those medications had not been flagged as having been incomplete.

Medication dosages should be adjusted to determine the lowest effective dosage and the simplest regimen. Due to significant variability among individual patients with respect to response, blood levels, the expression of side effects, and the development of toxicity, recommended dose ranges provide only a general guide. Documentation of a patient's response to a particular dosage becomes a meaningful reference point for future treatment. As a rule, elderly patients should be started on lower dosages than younger patients, and the interval between dosage changes should be longer because the time to achieve steady-state levels is often prolonged. In the elderly, often there is also prolonged storage of medication and active metabolites in body tissues. Nevertheless, the goal of reaching an effective dosage must be pursued with equal determination in the elderly as in younger patients.

For patients with chronic psychiatric conditions, exacerbation of symptoms might prompt increases in the dosages of medications or the addition of other medications. So too, for patients who present acutely with severe disorders, medication dosages may be escalated more rapidly than usual or combined with other psychotropic medications at an early point, such that the lowest effective dosage and simplest regimen are likely to be unclear. Under these circumstances, re-evaluation for cautious reduction of dosage when an appropriate interval of stability has followed should be routine. When a patient's care is likely to be transferred to another clinician or another setting, such as a chronic care facility or a community health center, such a plan must be communicated to the accepting clinical staff to avoid committing a patient to long-term treatment with dosages or regimens that are excessive.

The attentive management of side effects plays an important role in developing a therapeutic alliance and improving the quality of life for a patient who may be on psychopharmacologic treatment for months or years. Although some adverse events require immediate discontinuation of the drug (e.g., serotonin syndrome, neuroleptic malignant syndrome [NMS], a blistering rash on lamotrigine), most can be addressed initially with a dosage reduction, modification in the timing of doses or by dividing doses, taking the medication with or without food, a change in the preparation of medication (e.g., from tablet to liquid or shorter acting to longer acting), or guidance about sleep hygiene, exercise, or diet (e.g., use of caffeine, fluids, or fiber). When such measures prove unhelpful in addressing a side effect that is causing distress or that poses a safety risk, other measures must be considered, such as prescribing benztropine for extrapyramidal symptoms (EPS) on high-potency antipsychotic medicine or mirtazapine for nausea or insomnia while on SSRIs or replacing the offending medication with a more tolerable agent. For side effects that are likely to be transient and not dangerous, a patient's understanding that a variety of straightforward strategies are available in the case of persistence or worsening may be enough to help the patient endure the side effects until they subside.

Sometimes the most appropriate steps in psychopharmacology involve staying the course with careful re-assessment at regular intervals to avoid premature medication changes. When possible, it is best to avoid responding to short-term crises with long-term changes in medications. The decision to switch a previously effective antidepressant in the setting of despair and insomnia in the acute aftermath of a relationship break-up, for example, may offer the patient the prospect of benefit from the new medication weeks later but withdraw from the patient's active treatment known to have been helpful. Although it is often tempting to respond proportionally to a patient's marked distress with a fundamental change in established treatment, exacerbations that are thought likely to be transient are sometimes most reasonably addressed with interventions that are short term and focused if they are paired with close follow-up.

Approach to Treatment Failure

Lack of improvement, clinical worsening, or the emergence of unexpected symptoms require a concerted re-evaluation of diagnosis, dosage, drugs, and disruptions. Some patients require higher-than-usual doses of medicines or augmentation strategies that involve combined medication regimens.

Diagnosis

Among at least one-third of patients with most major psychiatric disorders, initial treatment fails to bring about significant improvement despite accurate diagnosis. Nevertheless, treatment failure should routinely motivate a careful review of history, initial presentation, and symptoms that seem incongruous with the provisional diagnosis (e.g., confusion in a patient with seemingly mild depression; olfactory hallucinations in a patient who presents with panic attacks). A patient with fatigue out of proportion to other depressive symptoms might have obstructive sleep apnea, hypothyroidism, anemia, or postural orthostatic tachycardia syndrome. A depressed and cachectic elderly patient who fails to improve despite a series of adequate courses of antidepressants might turn out to have psychotic depression, early dementia, or a frontal lobe tumor. A patient with obsessive-compulsive disorder who appears increasingly bizarre and erratic on an SSRI might have an undiagnosed bipolar disorder exacerbated by the antidepressant.

Dosage

Apparent treatment refractoriness is often the result of non-adherence or the prescribing of subtherapeutic dosages. When treatment fails, the onus is on the clinician to confirm the adequacy of the dosage and to confirm that the patient is taking the medication in the way the clinician believed it was recommended. In cases of uncertain adherence, blood levels of prescribed medications help establish whether a patient is taking the medications. Moreover, for medications with established dosage ranges (e.g., lithium, anticonvulsants, clozapine, and tricyclic antidepressants [TCAs], although not most antipsychotics or newer antidepressants), blood levels help ensure dosing within the therapeutic range. When adequate dosages of a drug prescribed to a conscientious patient fail to achieve consistent plasma concentrations or clinical response, the clinician must consider factors that affect drug metabolism, such as cigarette smoking, chronic alcohol use, food (e.g., with levothyroxine) or use of concurrent medications such as carbamazepine, oral contraceptives, or rifampin that result in lower levels of the drug. Less commonly, patients experience clinical deterioration after changes in their prescription brand, such as when generic preparations are substituted for brand name medications, causing variation in the bioavailability of the active agent.

Drugs

Many patients compartmentalize their use of medications and forget to mention as-needed or over-the-counter (OTC) medications or treatments prescribed by other clinicians. When psychopharmacologic treatments fail, a careful re-evaluation of the patient's current non-psychiatric medication use is warranted. Thus a patient whose panic disorder responds incompletely to full dosages of a high-potency benzodiazepine may be unaware that his or her condition is aggravated by the use of a β-agonist inhaler, a sympathomimetic decongestant, or caffeinated energy drinks. So, too, a patient with bipolar disorder, previously stabilized on lithium but now presenting with hypomania, might not have thought to mention that prednisone had been recently added for a flare of inflammatory bowel disease.

Herbal and other agents marketed as health supplements online and OTC can participate in clinically important drug interaction[16]; the possibility of such interactions may be easily missed, however, because the use of alternative and complementary therapies is typically reported by patients only on direct inquiry by their clinician. Details of alcohol and other substances and supplements must be carefully elicited as factors that can resemble or exacerbate other psychiatric disorders and can jeopardize the safety and efficacy of pharmacotherapy.

Disruptions

Although psychosocial stressors are not an excuse for psychopharmacologic nihilism, neither can they be meaningfully ignored as potential impediments to treatment. Incomplete remission of depressive symptoms in a patient living with a spouse who drinks alcohol excessively or of a psychotic exacerbation in a patient with schizophrenia whose residential treatment facility has closed should be met both with aggressive efforts to ensure the adequacy of pharmacologic treatment and with equally determined efforts to develop a plan to address the contextual factors that appear to be compromising a patient's recovery.

Combined Therapy

In clinical practice, many patients receive multiple medications, particularly older patients. Moreover, general medical co-morbidity is common among patients with a psychiatric disorder, elevating the likelihood of complex medication regimens and polypharmacy. As in other areas of medicine, polypharmacy has become an accepted approach in psychiatry for addressing difficult-to-treat disorders. The term *polypharmacy* may carry a pejorative connotation suggesting a thoughtless, irrational, or non-evidence-based approach to the prescribing of medicine. Indeed, haphazard polypharmacy puts patients at risk due to an increased likelihood of adverse medication reactions and drug-drug interactions. In contrast, "rational" or "strategic" combined psychopharmacologic approaches can be used positively for the treatment of psychiatric or medical co-morbidity, as augmentation for patients with an insufficient response to a single agent, and for the management of treatment-emergent adverse effects.[17]

Therefore, while a patient's use of multiple psychotropic medications ought to be scrutinized, it should not be viewed reflexively as in need of dismantling. One patient may accumulate multiple medications in a disjointed fashion across siloed treaters whereas another might arrive at a precisely adjusted, albeit complicated, regimen through a series of careful trials guided by an experienced clinician or clinical team. For the former patient, a directed plan to taper medications and perhaps even to "start from scratch" may be most helpful whereas for the latter even a modest dosage change may result in a severe relapse that threatens the patient's safety or livelihood. To the extent possible, obtaining further information about the background of a patient's complex regimen through medical records and conversations with treaters or significant others can be extraordinarily helpful in determining whether fine-tuning or major restricting is the best approach.

Discontinuing Medications

The discontinuation of psychotropic drugs must be carried out with as much care as their initiation. For patients on complicated regimens of psychotropic medications, periodic reviews for potential dosage reduction or discontinuation should be standard. Because data providing guidelines for drug discontinuation are scarce, the process is often empirical. Successful discontinuation, therefore relies heavily on a good knowledge of a patient's history, together with adequate follow-up.

Assessment of a patient for the discontinuation of a drug involves appreciating the short-term risks of rebound and withdrawal as well as the long-term risks of relapse and recurrence. Rebound effects are the transient return of symptoms for which medication has been prescribed (e.g., insomnia or anxiety), while withdrawal effects are the development of new symptoms characteristic of abrupt cessation of the medication, such as muscle spasms, delirium, or seizures following discontinuation of high-dosage benzodiazepine; nausea, muscle aches, or disconcerting, though not dangerous, shock-like sensations following discontinuation of an antidepressant.[18]

To make sound decisions regarding the re-instatement of medications, it is essential to distinguish rebound and withdrawal effects from relapse. *Relapse* is typically a persistent rather than self-limited state associated with a more delayed onset and the re-emergence of clinically significant symptoms of the underlying illness in the absence of (or sometimes despite the continuation of) active treatment. The return of daily panic attacks after a remission of several months and an exacerbation of psychosis requiring hospitalization after many years of stable outpatient treatment are examples of relapse.

For disorders that may occur episodically, such as MDD, the term *relapse* refers more precisely to the recrudescence of symptoms during an initial period of remission, whereas the additional term *recurrence* refers to the return of symptoms following a defined period of full remission (at least 4–6 months) on or off continued treatment. In the case of recurrence, the re-appearing symptoms are conceptualized as denoting a new episode rather than a continuation of the one previously treated.

In parallel with the concepts of relapse and recurrence, *continuation treatment* refers to the ongoing use of medication prescribed to consolidate a remission of symptoms brought about by an initial (acute) phase of treatment to prevent relapse. *Maintenance treatment* refers more precisely to a course of pharmacotherapy extended beyond the continuation phase to prevent recurrences. Maintenance treatment is typically reserved for patients with an illness characterized by chronicity, past recurrences, or high severity. For MDD, acute treatment is typically in the range of 6 to 12 weeks, whereas continuation treatment extends 4 to 6 months beyond that point, and maintenance treatment may extend a further 1 to 5 years or more depending on the clinical context. Although antidepressants appear to be more effective than placebo during long-term treatment and in routine practice, many patients remain on antidepressants for several or more years, the number of controlled antidepressant trials focusing on treatment of depression beyond the first year remains limited.[19]

A taper of medications over 48 to 72 hours is typically adequate to minimize the risk of serious acute rebound or withdrawal. With respect to mitigating against relapse or recurrence, however, patients at risk may well benefit from a more protracted, carefully monitored taper of medications. This allows rapid reinstatement of full-dosage treatment at the early signs of worsening to avert a more serious clinical deterioration. In addition, some but not all analyses of discontinuation of lithium[20] and antipsychotic agents[21] suggest that rapid cessation may increase the risk of relapse when compared with a more gradual taper. Findings such as these suggest that for elective discontinuation of psychotropic medications, a monitored taper lasting at least 2 to 4 weeks should be considered. Indeed, with patients for whom the consequences of relapse are likely to be severe (e.g., most patients with bipolar and psychotic disorders), an extended taper with dosage reductions of no more than 25% at intervals of no less than 4 to 6 weeks is likely to be a more prudent course. For patients who have anxiety disorders and are maintained on high-potency benzodiazepines, the introduction of a targeted course of therapy (e.g., a cognitive behavioral panic disorder group) in preparation for a drug taper is likely to further reduce the risks of relapse.[22]

Far from being an afterthought, decisions regarding the timing and pace of drug discontinuation and leverage of non-pharmacological supports should be regarded as an integral part of psychopharmacologic management and remain an important topic for further study.

PHARMACOKINETICS

Pharmacokinetic processes refer to absorption, distribution, metabolism, and excretion, factors that determine plasma levels of a drug and the local availability of a drug to biologically active sites—in short, what the body does to the drug.[23] Pharmacokinetics also refers to the mathematical analysis of these processes. Advances in analytic chemistry and computer methods of pharmacokinetic modeling and a growing understanding of the molecular pharmacology of the hepatic isoenzymes responsible for metabolizing most psychotropic medications have furnished increasingly sophisticated insights into the disposition and interaction of administered drugs.

Because the pharmacokinetics of medication are subject to myriad influences, including age, genes, gender, diet, disease states, and concurrently administered drugs, a working knowledge of pharmacokinetic principles is quite relevant to psychopharmacology in medical settings. Although pharmacokinetics refers to only one of the two broad mechanisms by which drugs interact (the other being pharmacodynamics), pharmacokinetic interactions involve all classes of psychotropic and non-psychotropic medications. An overview of pharmacokinetic processes is a helpful prelude to a discussion of specific drug-drug interactions by psychotropic class.

Absorption

Factors that influence drug absorption are generally of less importance in determining the pharmacokinetic properties of psychiatric medications than factors that influence subsequent drug disposition (e.g., drug metabolism). The term *absorption* refers to processes that generally pertain to orally (rather than parenterally) administered drugs, for which alterations in gastrointestinal (GI) drug absorption can affect the rate (time to reach maximum concentration) or the extent of absorption, or both. The extent or completeness of absorption, also known as *fractional absorption*, is measured as the area under the curve when plasma concentration is plotted against time. The bioavailability of an oral dose of a drug refers, in turn, to the fractional absorption of orally compared with intravenously (IV) administered drug. If an agent is reported to have a 90% bioavailability (e.g., lorazepam), this indicates that the extent of absorption of an orally administered dose is nearly that of an IV-administered dose, although the rate of absorption may well be slower for the oral dose.

Because the upper part of the small intestine is the primary site of drug absorption through passive membrane diffusion and filtration and both passive and active transport processes, factors that speed gastric emptying (e.g., metoclopramide) or diminish intestinal motility (e.g., opioids or cannabis) can facilitate greater contact with, and absorption from, the mucosal surface into the systemic circulation, potentially increasing plasma drug concentrations. Conversely, bulk laxatives, such as psyllium, magnesium-based antacids, lactulose, kaolin-pectin, and cholestyramine, can bind to drugs, forming complexes that pass unabsorbed through the GI lumen.

Changes in gastric pH associated with food or other drugs alter the non-polar, un-ionized fraction of the drug available for absorption. In the case of drugs that are very weak acids or bases, however, the extent of ionization is relatively invariant under physiologic conditions. Properties of the preparation administered (e.g., tablet, capsule, or liquid) can also influence the rate or extent of absorption and, for an increasing number of medications (e.g., bupropion, lithium, most stimulant medicines, quetiapine, and venlafaxine—to name a few), preparations intended for slow release are available.

The local action of enzymes in the GI tract (e.g., monoamine oxidase [MAO]; cytochrome P450, CYP 3A4) may be responsible for the metabolism of a drug before absorption. This is of critical relevance to the emergence of hypertensive crises that occur when excessive quantities of the dietary pressor tyramine are systemically absorbed in the setting of irreversible inhibition of the MAO isoenzymes for which tyramine is a substrate.

Following gut absorption, but before entry into the systemic circulation, many psychotropic drugs are subject to first-pass liver metabolism. Therefore conditions that affect the hepatic metabolism of a drug (e.g., primary liver disease) or conditions that impede portal circulation (e.g., congestive heart failure) are likely to increase the fraction of drug available for distribution for most psychotropic drugs, thereby contributing to clinically significant increases in plasma levels of drugs.

The drug transporter P-glycoprotein (Pgp) also plays a role in drug absorption.[24] While the tissue distribution of Pgp influences the effects and interactions of psychotropics, other medications, recreational drugs, and supplements at the interface between the bloodstream and central nervous system (CNS), Pgp is also found in other areas of the body, such as the intestines, which are a major site for drug absorption into the body. The Pgps found in the gut have not been as extensively studied; however, it is well known that the expression of Pgp in other tissues can be induced and inhibited by a range of medications and other substances. It is thought that some interactions, mainly seen with the antiepileptic drugs, previously assumed to reflect CYP 450 effects, instead may be mediated by the modulation of the Pgp activity. The capacity of St. Johns wort to lower blood levels of several critical medications (e.g., cyclosporine, indinavir), for example, is hypothesized to be related to an effect of the botanical agent on this transport system.

Distribution

Drugs are distributed to tissues through the systemic circulation. The amount of drug ultimately reaching receptor sites in tissues is determined by a variety of factors, including the concentration of free (unbound) drug in plasma, regional blood flow, and physiochemical properties of the drug (e.g., lipophilicity or structural characteristics). For entrance into the CNS, penetration across the blood-brain barrier is required. Fat-soluble drugs (e.g., benzodiazepines, antipsychotics, cyclic antidepressants) distribute more widely in the body than water-soluble drugs (e.g., lithium), which distribute through a smaller volume of distribution. Changes with age, typically including an increase in the ratio of body fat to lean body mass, therefore result in a net greater volume of lipophilic drug distribution and potentially greater accumulation of the drug in adipose tissue in older than in younger patients. A similar potential exists for female compared with male patients because of their generally higher ratio of adipose tissue to lean body mass.

In general, psychotropic drugs have relatively high affinities for plasma proteins (including albumin, α_1-acid glycoproteins, and lipoproteins). Most psychotropic drugs are more than 80% protein bound. A drug is considered highly protein bound if more than 90% exists in bound form in plasma. Fluoxetine, aripiprazole, and diazepam are examples of the many psychotropic drugs that are highly protein bound. In contrast, venlafaxine, lithium, topiramate, zonisamide, gabapentin, pregabalin, levomilnacipran, and memantine are examples of drugs with minimal protein binding and therefore a negligible risk of participating in drug-drug interactions related to protein binding.

A reversible equilibrium exists between bound and unbound drugs. Only the unbound fraction exerts pharmacologic effects. Competition by two or more drugs for protein-binding sites often results in the displacement of a previously bound drug, which, in the free state, becomes pharmacologically active. Similarly, reduced concentrations of plasma proteins in a severely malnourished patient or a patient with a disease that is associated with markedly lowered serum proteins (e.g., liver disease, the nephrotic syndrome) may be associated with an increase in the fraction of unbound drug potentially available for activity at relevant receptor sites. Under most circumstances, the net changes in plasma concentration of active drugs are, in fact, quite small because the unbound drug is available for redistribution to other tissues and metabolism and excretion, thereby offsetting the initial rise in plasma levels. It is important to be aware, however, that clinically significant consequences can develop when protein-binding interactions alter the unbound fraction of previously highly protein-bound drugs that have a low therapeutic index (e.g., warfarin). For these drugs, relatively small variations in plasma level may be associated with serious untoward effects.

Metabolism

Most drugs undergo several types of biotransformation, and many psychotropic drug interactions of clinical significance are based on interference with this process. *Metabolism* refers to the biotransformation of a drug to another form, a process that is usually enzyme-mediated and results in a metabolite that might or might not be pharmacologically active and might or might not be subject to further biotransformation before eventual excretion. A growing understanding of hepatic enzymes, and especially the rapidly emerging characterization of the CYP isoenzymes and other enzyme systems including the uridine-diphosphate glucuronosyltransferases and flavin-containing mono-oxygenases,[25] has significantly advanced a rational understanding and prediction of drug interactions and individual variation in drug responses.

Phase I reactions include oxidation (e.g., hydroxylation, dealkylation), reduction (e.g., nitro reduction), and hydrolysis, metabolic reactions typically resulting in intermediate metabolites, which themselves may have pharmacological activity and are then subject to phase II reactions, including conjugation (e.g., glucuronide, sulfate) and acetylation. Phase II reactions typically yield highly polar, water-soluble metabolites suitable for renal excretion. Most psychotropic drugs undergo both phase I and phase II metabolic reactions. Notable exceptions are lithium and gabapentin, which are not subject to hepatic metabolism, and a subset of the benzodiazepines (lorazepam, oxazepam, temazepam), which undergo only phase II reactions and are therefore especially appropriate when benzodiazepines are used in the context of concurrent medications, advanced age, or disease states in which alteration of hepatic metabolism is likely to be substantial and the extended presence of active metabolites is undesirable.

The synthesis or activity of hepatic microsomal enzymes is affected by metabolic inhibitors and inducers, as well as distinct genetic polymorphisms (stably inherited traits). Table 37.1 lists enzyme inducers and inhibitors common in clinical settings. These should serve as red flags that beckon further scrutiny for potential drug-drug interactions when they are found on a patient's medication list. These red flag substances are often drugs but they may be other substances, such as grapefruit juice and acute alcohol intake (inhibitors), or cruciferous vegetables, such as cabbage or Brussels sprouts, or chronic tobacco or alcohol use (inducers).

Inhibitors impede the metabolism of a concurrently administered drug, producing a rise in its plasma level, whereas inducers enhance the metabolism of another drug, resulting in a decline in its plasma levels. Although inhibition is usually immediate, induction, which requires enhanced synthesis of the metabolic enzyme, is typically a more gradual process. A fall in plasma levels of a substrate might not be apparent for days to weeks following the introduction of the inducer. This is particularly important to keep in mind when a patient's care is being transferred to another setting where clinical deterioration may be the first sign that drug levels have declined. Reciprocally, an elevation in plasma drug concentrations could reflect the previous discontinuation of an inducing factor (e.g., cigarette smoking, carbamazepine) just as it could reflect the introduction of an inhibitor (e.g., fluoxetine, valproic acid).

Although the CYP isoenzymes represent only one of the numerous enzyme systems responsible for drug metabolism, they are responsible for metabolizing, at least in part, more than 80% of all prescribed drugs. In the 1990s, recognition of the capacity of many of the newly introduced SSRIs to inhibit CYP isoenzymes kindled much interest in the pattern of interaction of psychotropic and other drugs with these enzymes in the understanding and prediction of drug-drug interactions in psychopharmacology. The CYP isoenzymes represent a family of more than 30 related heme-containing enzymes, largely located in the endoplasmic reticulum of hepatocytes (but also present elsewhere, including gut and brain), which mediate oxidative metabolism of a wide variety of drugs as well as endogenous substances, including prostaglandins, fatty acids, and steroids. Most antidepressant and antipsychotic drugs are metabolized by or inhibited by one or more of these isoenzymes. Table 37.2 summarizes the interactions of psychiatric and non-psychiatric drugs with a subset of isoenzymes that have been increasingly well characterized. In addition to reviews in which these interactions are cited,[26] several relevant websites for prescribers are regularly updated, including www.drugs.com/professionals.html. The relevance of these and other interactions is highlighted in a later section of this chapter, in which clinically important drug-drug interactions are described.

Within the group of CYP isoenzymes, there appears to be a polymodal distribution of metabolic activity in the population with respect to certain isoenzymes (including CYP 2C19 and 2D6). Most people are normal (extensive) metabolizers with respect to the activity of these isoenzymes. A smaller number are poor metabolizers, with deficient activity of the isoenzyme. Very much smaller numbers are ultra-rapid metabolizers, who have more than normal activity of the enzyme, and intermediate metabolizers, who fall between extensive and poor metabolizers. Persons who are poor metabolizers with respect to a particular CYP isoenzyme are expected to have higher plasma concentrations of a drug that is metabolized by that isoenzyme, thereby potentially being more sensitive to or requiring lower dosages of that drug than a patient with normal activity of that enzyme. These patients might also have higher-than-usual plasma levels of metabolites of the drug that are produced through other metabolic pathways that are not altered by the polymorphism, thereby potentially incurring

TABLE 37.1
Commonly Used Drugs and Substances That Inhibit or Induce Hepatic Metabolism of Other Medications

Inhibitors	Inducers
Amiodarone	Barbiturates (e.g., phenobarbital, secobarbital)
Antifungals (ketoconazole, miconazole, itraconazole)	Carbamazepine
Macrolide antibiotics (erythromycin, clarithromycin, triacetyloleandomycin)	Oxcarbazepine
	Phenytoin
Fluoroquinolones (e.g., ciprofloxacin)	Rifampin
	Primidone
Isoniazid	Cigarettes
Antiretrovirals	Ethanol (chronic)
Antimalarials (chloroquine)	Cruciferous vegetables
Selective serotonin reuptake inhibitors (fluoxetine, fluvoxamine, paroxetine, sertraline)	Charbroiled meats
	St. Johns wort
Duloxetine	Oral contraceptives
Bupropion	Prednisone
Nefazodone	
β-Blockers (lipophilic) (e.g., propranolol, metoprolol, pindolol)	
Quinidine	
Valproate	
Cimetidine	
Calcium channel blockers (e.g., diltiazem)	
Grapefruit juice	
Ethanol (acute)	

TABLE 37.2
Selected Cytochrome P450 Isoenzyme Substrates, Inhibitors, and Inducers

Isoenzyme	Substrates	Inhibitors	Inducers
1A2	Acetaminophen, alosetron, aminophylline, asenapine, caffeine, clomipramine, clozapine, cyclobenzaprine, estradiol, fluvoxamine, mirtazapine, melatonin, olanzapine, propranolol, ramelteon, riluzole, ropinirole, tacrine, tizanidine, theophylline, zolmitriptan	Amiodarone, artemisinin, cimetidine, ciprofloxacin, fluoroquinolones, fluvoxamine, ginkgo, grapefruit juice, methoxsalen, mexiletine, oral contraceptives, tranylcypromine, vemurafenib, zileuton	Armodafinil, carbamazepine, charbroiled meats, cruciferous vegetables, insulin, modafinil, montelukast, primidone, rifampin, ritonavir, smoking (tobacco, cannabis), St. Johns wort
2B6	Bupropion, methadone, selegiline	Desipramine, doxorubicin, paroxetine, sertraline, sorafenib, thiotepa	Carbamazepine, dexamethasone, efavirenz, modafinil, nilotinib, phenobarbital, phenytoin, primidone, rifampin
2C9	Celecoxib, diazepam, diclofenac, fluoxetine, glipizide, meloxicam, piroxicam, S-warfarin, THC	Amiodarone, delavirdine, efavirenz, fluconazole, gemfibrozil, ketoconazole, leflunomide, miconazole, omeprazole, sorafenib	Carbamazepine, dexamethasone, griseofulvin, phenytoin, primidone, rifampin, rifapentine, secobarbital
2C19	Amitriptyline, cannabidiol, carisoprodol, citalopram, clomipramine, diazepam, escitalopram, imipramine, venlafaxine	Chloramphenicol, esomeprazole, fluconazole, fluoxetine, fluvoxamine, gemfibrozil, modafinil, omeprazole, sertraline, ticlopidine, tranylcypromine, voriconazole	Aspirin, carbamazepine, norethindrone, phenytoin, prednisone, rifampin St. Johns wort
2D6	Amitriptyline, amoxapine, amphetamine, aripiprazole, atomoxetine, brexpiprazole, β-blockers (lipophilic), chlorpromazine, clomipramine, clozapine, codeine, desipramine, deutetrabenazine, dextromethorphan, diltiazem, donepezil, doxepin, duloxetine, encainide, escitalopram, flecainide, fluoxetine, fluvoxamine, galantamine, haloperidol, hydroxycodone, iloperidone, imipramine, lidocaine, metoclopramide, mCPP, mexiletine, mirtazapine, nifedipine, nortriptyline, ondansetron, olanzapine, phenothiazines (e.g., thioridazine, perphenazine), propafenone, risperidone, tamoxifen, tramadol, trazodone, valbenazine, venlafaxine, vortioxetine	Amiodarone, antimalarials, **bupropion,** cannabidiol, **chlorpromazine,** cimetidine, **cinacalcet,** citalopram, clomipramine, clozapine, desipramine, duloxetine, fluoxetine, haloperidol, ketoconazole, methadone, metoclopramide, paroxetine, phenothiazines, protease inhibitors (ritonavir), quinidine, sertraline, terbinafine, THC, ticlopidine, tipranavir, tranylcypromine, yohimbine	Dexamethasone, glutethimide, rifampin
3A4, 3A5	Alfentanil, alprazolam, amiodarone, amprenavir, apixaban, aripiprazole, armodafinil, brexpiprazole, bromocriptine, buprenorphine, buspirone, Cafergot, calcium channel blockers, caffeine, carbamazepine, cisapride, clonazepam, clozapine, cyclosporine, dapsone, delavirdine, diazepam, disopyramide, efavirenz, estradiol, eszopiclone, fentanyl, guanfacine, HMG-CoA reductase inhibitors (lovastatin, simvastatin), iloperidone, indinavir, ketamine, lidocaine, lemborexant, levomilnacipran, lopinavir, loratadine, lumateperone, lurasidone, methadone, midazolam, mirtazapine, nimodipine, pimozide, prednisone, progesterone, propafenone, ramelteon, quetiapine, quinidine, ritonavir, sildenafil, suvorexant, tacrolimus, testosterone, triazolam, valbenazine, vardenafil, vilazodone, vinblastine, warfarin, zaleplon, ziprasidone, zaleplon, zolpidem, zonisamide, zuranolone	Antifungals, boceprevir, calcium channel blockers, clarithromycin, cimetidine, conivaptan, delavirdine, efavirenz, erythromycin, fluconazole, fluvoxamine, grapefruit juice, indinavir, itraconazole, mibefradil, nefazodone, nelfinavir, ritonavir, saquinavir, telaprevir, telithromycin, verapamil, voriconazole	Armodafinil, bosentan, carbamazepine, glucocorticoids, modafinil, nevirapine, oxcarbazepine, phenobarbital, phenytoin, primidone, pioglitazone, rifabutin, rifampin, rifapentine, ritonavir, St. Johns wort, troglitazone

Bold indicates strong inhibitor/inducer.

HMG-CoA, Hydroxy-methylglutaryl co-enzyme A; *mCPP,* metachlorophenylpiperazine; *THC,* tetrahydrocannabinol.

pharmacologic activity or adverse effects related to these alternative metabolites.

Studies on genetic polymorphisms affecting the CYP system have suggested ethnic differences.[27] Approximately 15% to 20% of Asian Americans and African Americans appear to be poor metabolizers with respect to CYP 2C19 compared with 3% to 5% of the White population. Conversely, the proportion of frankly poor metabolizers with respect to CYP 2D6 appears to be higher among White people (approximately 5%–10%) than among Asian and African Americans (approximately 1%–3%). As our understanding of the clinical relevance of genetic polymorphisms in psychopharmacology expands, commercial genotyping tests for polymorphisms of potential relevance to drug metabolism will likely become commonplace. For the use of certain drugs, notably carbamazepine, the US Food and Drug Administration (FDA) recommends genotyping Asians for the *HLA B*1502* allele owing to data implicating the allele as a marker for carbamazepine-induced Stevens-Johnson syndrome and toxic epidermal necrolysis in Han Chinese.[28] Continued research of genetic polymorphisms and their relevance to drug response will undoubtedly lead to improved medication selection and dosing based in part on knowledge of pharmacodynamic and pharmacokinetic genetic variations.

Excretion

Because most antidepressant, anxiolytic, and antipsychotic medications are largely eliminated by hepatic metabolism, factors that affect renal excretion (glomerular filtration, tubular re-absorption, and active tubular secretion) are generally far less important to the pharmacokinetics of these drugs than to lithium, for which such factors can have clinically significant consequences. Conditions resulting in sodium deficiency (e.g., dehydration, sodium restriction, use of thiazide diuretics) are likely to result in increased proximal tubular re-absorption of lithium, resulting in increased lithium levels and potential toxicity. Lithium levels and clinical status must be monitored especially closely in the setting of vomiting, diarrhea, excessive evaporative losses, or polyuria. Factors, such as aging, that are associated with reduced renal blood flow and glomerular filtration rate (GFR) also reduce lithium excretion. For this reason, as well as for their reduced

volume of distribution for lithium because of the relative loss of total body water with aging, elderly patients typically require lower lithium dosages than younger patients, and a low starting dosage (i.e., 150–300 mg/day) is often prudent. Separate from pharmacokinetic effects, however, elderly patients may also be more sensitive to the neurotoxic effects of lithium even at low therapeutic levels. On the other hand, factors associated with an increased GFR, particularly pregnancy, can produce an increase in lithium clearance and a fall in lithium levels.

For other medications, renal excretion can sometimes be exploited in the treatment of a drug overdose. Acidification of the urine by ascorbic acid, ammonium chloride, or methenamine mandelate increases the rate of excretion of weak bases, such as amphetamines and phencyclidine. Therefore such measures may be important in the emergency management of a patient with severe phencyclidine or amphetamine intoxication. Conversely, alkalinization of the urine by administration of sodium bicarbonate or acetazolamide can hasten the excretion of weak acids including long-acting barbiturates, such as phenobarbital.

Mildly to moderately impaired renal function does not typically prompt routine changes in the dosage or dosing intervals of psychotropic medications other than lithium. In patients with severe impairment of kidney function, however, there may be an accumulation of metabolites and, to a lesser extent, of the parent compound across repeated doses. An increase in the dosing interval and possible reduction in drug dosage should therefore be considered in this setting, particularly in the case of chronically administered agents with active metabolites.

Renal excretion is only one contribution to the *elimination half-life*, a pharmacokinetic construct that refers to the time required for the plasma concentration of a drug to be reduced by one-half. The elimination phase (also referred to as the β-phase) reflects all processes that contribute to drug removal, including renal excretion, hepatic metabolism, and, to a much lesser extent, other factors (e.g., loss of drug in sweat or biliary secretions) potentially affecting drug clearance (the volume of blood or plasma cleared of drug per unit time). For most drugs, whose elimination follows first-order kinetics (i.e., their rate of elimination is proportional to the amount of drug in the body rather than equal to a constant amount), steady-state drug levels are reached in four to five elimination half-lives, whereas, on discontinuation, almost all drug are out of the body within five half-lives.

For drugs that are administered for their single-dose effects (e.g., an as-needed benzodiazepine or antipsychotic) rather than for long-term effects of repeated administration (e.g., antidepressants), the duration of action of the drug depends not only on the elimination half-life but also often more critically on the initial phase of drug redistribution from the systemic circulation to other tissues, such as muscle and fat.

DRUG INTERACTIONS

The scientific literature on psychotropic drug-drug interactions has grown immensely since first reviewed in the *Massachusetts General Hospital Handbook of General Hospital Psychiatry* in 1978.[29] Despite impressive advances in clinical and molecular pharmacology, much of the literature on drug-drug interactions remains a patchwork of case reports, post-marketing analyses, extrapolation from animal and in vitro studies, and inferences based on what is known about other drugs with similar properties. Fortunately well-designed studies of drug-drug interactions are an increasingly integral part of drug development while sophisticated mining of big data such as electronic health records is helping to clarify the practical relevance of drug-drug interactions in clinical settings.

Drug-drug interactions refer to alterations in drug levels or drug effects (or both) attributed to the administration of two or more prescribed, recreational, or OTC agents in close temporal proximity. Although many drug-drug interactions involve drugs administered within minutes to hours of each other, some drugs can participate in interactions days or even weeks after they are discontinued because of prolonged elimination half-lives (e.g., fluoxetine) or owing to their long-term impact on metabolic enzymes (e.g., carbamazepine). Some drug-drug interactions involving psychotropic medications are life threatening, such as those involving the co-administration of MAOIs and drugs with potent serotoninergic (e.g., meperidine) or sympathomimetic (e.g., phenylpropanolamine) effects.[30] These combinations are therefore absolutely contraindicated.

However, most drug-drug interactions in psychopharmacology manifest in subtler ways, often leading to poor medication tolerability and compliance due to adverse events (e.g., orthostatic hypotension, sedation, jitteriness), diminished medication efficacy, or puzzling manifestations, such as altered mental status or unexpectedly high or low drug levels. Drug combinations that can produce these often less-catastrophic drug-drug interactions are usually not contraindicated. Some of these combinations may, indeed, be valuable in the treatment of some patients though wreaking havoc for other patients. The capacity to anticipate and recognize both the major, but rare, and the subtler, but common, potential drug-drug interactions allow the practitioner to minimize the impact of these interactions as an obstacle to patient safety and therapeutic success.

It is crucial to be familiar with the small number of drug-drug interactions in psychopharmacology that, though uncommon, are associated with potentially catastrophic consequences. These include drugs associated with ventricular arrhythmias, hypertensive crisis, serotonin syndrome, Stevens-Johnson syndrome, seizures, and severe bone marrow suppression. In addition, drug-drug interactions are important to consider when a patient's drugs include those with a low therapeutic index (e.g., lithium, digoxin, warfarin) or a narrow therapeutic window (e.g., indinavir, nortriptyline, cyclosporine), such that relatively small alterations in pharmacokinetic or pharmacodynamic behavior can jeopardize a patient's well-being. In addition, it is worthwhile to consider potential drug-drug interactions whenever evaluating a patient whose drug levels are unexpectedly variable or extreme or a patient with a confusing clinical picture or with unexpected side effects. Finally, drug-drug interactions are likely to be clinically salient for a patient who is medically frail or elderly, owing to altered pharmacokinetics and vulnerability to side effects, as well as for a patient who is heavily using alcohol, cigarettes, or recreational drugs or who is being treated for a drug overdose.

Given the widespread use of combined pharmacotherapeutic regimens for many difficult-to-treat disorders, the vast literature of reported and potential drug-drug interactions, and the litigious society in which physicians practice, the physician today is faced with a dilemma when evaluating the significance of myriad potential drug-drug interactions. Fortunately, an increasing range of resources is available, including e-prescribing software that will automatically check for potential drug-drug interactions at the point of electronic prescription or filling prescriptions, as well as regularly updated drug interaction websites. Agreement on drug-drug interactions across websites and other resources is generally high for the most serious interactions that reflect absolute contraindications to co-prescribing though remains more modest for interactions that are classified as minor to major where the combined use of two medications may entail some risk but is not ruled out.[31]

Numerous factors contribute to inter-individual variability in drug response. These factors include treatment adherence, age, gender, nutritional status, disease states, and genetic polymorphisms that can influence the risk of adverse events or inadequate benefit.[32] Drug-drug interactions are an additional factor that influences how patients react to drugs. The importance of these interactions depends heavily on the clinical context. In many cases, the practical impact of drug-drug interactions may be small compared with other factors that affect treatment response, drug levels, and toxicity. It is reasonable therefore to focus special attention on commonly used classes of drugs and the contexts in which drug-drug interactions are most likely to be clinically problematic.

Antipsychotic Drugs

Antipsychotic drugs, used in the treatment of schizophrenia, schizoaffective disorder, organic psychoses, mood disorders, and an increasingly broad range of other psychiatric conditions, include phenothiazines (e.g., chlorpromazine, fluphenazine, perphenazine, thioridazine, trifluoperazine); butyrophenones (haloperidol); thioxanthenes (thiothixene); indolones (molindone); diphenylbutylpiperidines (pimozide); dibenzodiazepines (loxapine); and the second-generation, atypical agents (clozapine, risperidone, olanzapine, quetiapine, ziprasidone, aripiprazole, paliperidone, asenapine, lurasidone, iloperidone, brexpiprazole, cariprazine, and lumateperone). As a class, they are generally rapidly, if erratically, absorbed from the GI tract after oral administration (peak plasma concentrations ranging widely from about 30 minutes to 6 hours).

They are highly lipophilic and distribute rapidly to body tissues with a large apparent volume of distribution. Protein binding in the circulation ranges from approximately 90% to 98%, except for molindone, paliperidone, and quetiapine, which are only moderately protein bound.

The antipsychotics generally undergo substantial first-pass hepatic metabolism (primarily oxidation and conjugation reactions), reducing their systemic bioavailability when given orally compared with intramuscular (IM) administration, the fractional absorption of which nearly approximates IV administration. Most of the individual antipsychotics have several pharmacologically active metabolites (e.g., paliperidone is 9-hydroxyrisperidone, the primary active metabolite of risperidone).

Because of their propensity to sequester in body compartments, the elimination half-life of antipsychotics is quite variable, ranging from approximately 6 to 90 hours. For some antipsychotics, elimination pharmacokinetics appears to be especially complex, and the disappearance of the drug from the systemic circulation may take much longer, as it does for brexpiprazole whose half-life can exceed 90 hours.[33]

The lower-potency antipsychotics (including chlorpromazine, clozapine, and quetiapine) are generally the most sedating and have the greatest anticholinergic, antihistaminic, and α_1-adrenergic antagonistic effects. In contrast, the higher-potency antipsychotics (including risperidone and haloperidol) are comparatively more likely to be associated with an increased incidence of EPS, including akathisia, dystonia, and parkinsonism.

The atypical antipsychotics generally have multiple receptor affinities, including antagonism at dopamine D_1 to D_4 receptors, serotonin (5-HT) $5-HT_1$ and $5-HT_2$ receptors, α_1- and α_2-adrenergic receptors, histamine H_1 receptor, and cholinergic muscarinic receptors, with variations across agents that contribute to very different side-effect profiles. Thus for example, clozapine and olanzapine have notably greater affinity at the muscarinic receptors than the other agents, and aripiprazole, brexpiprazole, and cariprazine are examples of partial agonists at the D_2 receptor.

Although the more complex pharmacologic profile of second-generation, atypical agents, as well as the older low-potency antipsychotics, has generally been associated with a lower risk of EPS, the same broad range of receptor activity also poses a greater risk of *pharmacodynamic interactions.* Pharmacodynamic interactions refer to the pharmacologic effects that result from interactions at the same or interrelated biologically active (receptor) sites.

Lower-potency drugs, as well as some atypical antipsychotics (e.g., asenapine, risperidone, quetiapine), can produce significant hypotension, especially when combined with vasodilator or antihypertensive drugs related to α_1-adrenergic blockade (Table 37.3).[34,35] Severe hypotension has been reported when chlorpromazine has been administered with the angiotensin-converting enzyme (ACE) inhibitor captopril. Hypotension can develop when epinephrine is administered with low-potency antipsychotics. In this setting, the α-adrenergic stimulant effect of epinephrine, resulting in vasodilation, is unopposed by its usual pressor effect because α_1-adrenergic receptors are occupied by the antipsychotic. A similar effect can result if a low-potency antipsychotic is administered to a patient with pheochromocytoma. Finally, hypotension can develop when low-potency antipsychotics are used in combination with a variety of anesthetics, such as halothane, enflurane, and isoflurane.

In addition, the low-potency antipsychotics have quinidine-like effects on cardiac conduction and can prolong Q-T and P-R intervals.[36] Ziprasidone may also cause Q-T prolongation, although clinically significant prolongation (QTc > 500 ms) appears to be rare when administered to otherwise healthy individuals. Significant depression of cardiac conduction, heart block, and life-threatening ventricular dysrhythmias can result from co-administering low-potency antipsychotics or ziprasidone with class I antiarrhythmics (e.g., quinidine, procainamide, disopyramide); it can also result from the TCAs, which have quinidine-like activity on cardiac conduction, and when administered in the context of other aggravating factors including hypokalemia, hypomagnesemia, bradycardia, or congenital prolongation of the QTc. Pimozide also can depress cardiac conduction as a result of its calcium channel-blocking action, and the combination of pimozide with other calcium channel blockers (e.g., nifedipine, diltiazem, verapamil) is contraindicated.

Another clinically significant pharmacodynamic interaction arises when low-potency antipsychotics, particularly clozapine or olanzapine, are administered with other drugs that have anticholinergic effects, including TCAs, benztropine, and diphenhydramine. When these drugs are combined, there is a greater risk of urinary retention, constipation, blurred vision, cognitive memory, and, in the setting of narrow-angle glaucoma, increased intraocular pressure. With intentional or inadvertent overdoses, severe anticholinergic syndrome can develop, including delirium, paralytic ileus, tachycardia, and dysrhythmias. With a lower affinity for muscarinic cholinergic receptors, the high-potency agents and non-anticholinergic atypical agents (e.g., risperidone, aripiprazole) are indicated when anticholinergic effects need to be minimized.

The sedative effects of low-potency agents and atypical antidepressants are also often additive to those of the sedative-hypnotic medications and alcohol. In patients for whom sedative effects may be especially dangerous, including the elderly, starting with low and divided doses is often an appropriate first step if sedating medications need to be used.

Because dopamine receptor blockade is a property common to all antipsychotics, they are all likely to interfere, although with varying degrees, with the efficacy of levodopa in the treatment of Parkinson disease (PD). When antipsychotic treatment is necessary in this setting, the low-potency antipsychotics, clozapine and quetiapine, have been preferred.[37] The FDA approval in 2016 of pimavanserin for hallucinations and delusions in PD has allowed for prescription in this patient population of this atypical antipsychotic that has predominant 5-HT$_{2A}$ antagonist or inverse agonist effects, a property it shares with quetiapine and clozapine, though without blocking D2 receptors.[38] Reciprocally, antipsychotics are likely to be less effective in the treatment of psychosis in the setting of levodopa, stimulant use, and direct dopamine agonists (e.g., ropinirole) that facilitate dopamine transmission. Nevertheless, these agents have been combined with antipsychotics, in cautious sometimes modestly successful efforts, to treat the negative symptoms of schizophrenia (including blunted affect, paucity of thought and speech, and social withdrawal).

Elevated prolactin is common in patients on anti-psychotics, particularly the higher-potency agents (e.g., haloperidol, risperidone, paliperidone). It often manifests with irregular menses, galactorrhea, diminished libido, or hirsutism. Antipsychotic-induced prolactin elevations associated with clinical symptoms can be abated by reducing the dosage of the offending agent, switching to a prolactin-sparing agent (e.g., aripiprazole, brexpiprazole, clozapine, quetiapine, ziprasidone), adding adjunctive amantadine (200–300 mg/day) or a dopamine agonist, such as cabergoline (0.5–4 mg/week).[39]

The risk of agranulocytosis, which occurs rarely with low-potency antipsychotics, is much higher with clozapine, with an incidence as high as 1% to 3%. For this reason, the combination of clozapine with other medications associated with a risk of myelosuppression (e.g., carbamazepine) should be avoided. Similarly, because clozapine lowers the seizure threshold to a greater extent than other antipsychotics, co-administration with other medications that significantly lower the seizure threshold should be avoided or combined with an anticonvulsant.

Pharmacokinetic drug interactions are quite common among the antipsychotic drugs. Plasma levels of the antipsychotic drugs, however, can vary as much as 10-fold to 20-fold between patients even on mono-therapy, and, as a class, they have a relatively wide therapeutic index.[40] Therefore factors that alter antipsychotic drug metabolism might not have apparent clinical consequences. However, for patients maintained on antipsychotics carefully tapered to the lowest dose, a small decrease in antipsychotic levels, as can occur with the introduction of a metabolic inducer or an agent that interferes with absorption, can bring them below the threshold for efficacy, whereas for patients whose regimen is already producing just barely tolerable side effects, an increase in blood level, as may occur with introduction of another medication that inhibits metabolism of the antipsychotic, may lead to an unsustainable or unsafe side-effect burden.

Antipsychotic drug levels may be lowered by aluminum-containing or magnesium-containing antacids, which reduce their absorption and are best given separately. Mixing liquid preparations of phenothiazines with beverages, such as fruit juices, presents the risk of causing insoluble precipitates and inefficient GI absorption.

Carbamazepine, known to be a potent inducer of hepatic enzymes, has been associated with the reduction of steady-state antipsychotic drug plasma levels by as much as 50%. This effect is especially important to bear in mind as a potential explanation when an antipsychotic-treated patient appears to deteriorate in the weeks following the introduction of carbamazepine. Oxcarbazepine can also induce antipsychotic drug metabolism, as can a variety of other anticonvulsants, including phenobarbital and phenytoin.

Cigarette smoking has been widely associated with a reduction in drug levels of many common antipsychotic drugs through enzyme metabolism.[41] As inpatient units and community residential programs have widely become smoke free, there are often substantial differences in smoking frequency between inpatient and outpatient settings. Among patients who smoke heavily, consideration should be given to the impact of these changes in smoking habits on antipsychotic dosage requirements, particularly for those taking olanzapine and clozapine.

SSRIs and other antidepressants with inhibitory effects on CYP isoenzymes can also produce an increase in the plasma levels of a concurrently administered antipsychotic agent (Table 37.3). Thus, increases in clozapine, olanzapine, haloperidol, and asenapine plasma levels can occur when these drugs are co-administered with fluvoxamine. Increases in risperidone, aripiprazole, brexpiprazole, iloperidone, and first-generation antipsychotic levels can follow the initiation of fluoxetine, paroxetine, bupropion, duloxetine, and sertraline. Quetiapine, cariprazine, lumateperone, lurasidone, and ziprasidone levels can potentially rise following the addition of nefazodone, fluvoxamine, or fluoxetine.

Phenothiazine drug levels may be increased when co-administered with propranolol, another inhibitor of hepatic microenzymes. Because propranolol is often an effective symptomatic treatment for antipsychotic-associated akathisia, the combined use of the β-blocker with an antipsychotic drug is common. When interactions present a problem, the use of a water-soluble β-blocker, such as atenolol, which is not likely to interfere with hepatic metabolism, provides a reasonable alternative.

TABLE 37.3

Selected Drug Interactions With Antipsychotic Medications

Drug	Potential Interaction
Antacids (aluminum and magnesium containing)	Interference with absorption of antipsychotic agents; fruit juice
Carbamazepine	Decreased antipsychotic drug plasma levels; additive risk of myelosuppression with clozapine
Cigarettes	Decreased antipsychotic drug plasma levels; reduced extrapyramidal symptoms
Rifampin	Decreased antipsychotic drug plasma levels; reduced extrapyramidal symptoms
TCAs	Increased TCA and antipsychotic drug plasma levels; hypotension, depression of cardiac conduction (with low-potency antipsychotics)
SSRIs	Increased SSRI and antipsychotic drug plasma levels; arrhythmia risk with thioridazine and pimozide
Bupropion, duloxetine	Increased antipsychotic drug plasma levels; arrhythmia risk with thioridazine
Fluvoxamine, nefazodone	Increased antipsychotic drug plasma levels, arrhythmia risk with pimozide; seizure risk with clozapine
β-Blockers (lipophilic)	Increased antipsychotic drug plasma levels; improved akathisia
Anticholinergic drugs	Additive anticholinergic toxicity; reduced extrapyramidal symptoms
Antihypertensive, vasodilator drugs	Hypotension (with low-potency antipsychotics and risperidone)
Guanethidine, clonidine	Blockade of antihypertensive effect
Epinephrine	Hypotension (with low-potency antipsychotics)
Class I antiarrhythmics	Depression of cardiac conduction; ventricular arrhythmias (with low-potency antipsychotics, ziprasidone)
Calcium channel blockers	Depression of cardiac conduction; ventricular arrhythmias (with pimozide)
Lithium	Idiosyncratic neurotoxicity

SSRIs, Selective serotonin reuptake inhibitors; *TCAs,* tricyclic antidepressants.

Mood Stabilizers

Lithium

Lithium is absorbed completely from the GI tract; it achieves peak plasma concentrations after approximately 1.5 to 2 hours for standard preparations and 4 to 4.5 hours for slow-release preparations. It distributes throughout total body water and, in contrast to most psychotropic drugs, does not bind to plasma proteins and is not metabolized in the liver. It is filtered and re-absorbed by the kidneys, and 95% of it is excreted in the urine. Lithium elimination is highly dependent on total body sodium and fluid balance; it competes with sodium for re-absorption in the proximal tubules. To a lesser extent, lithium is re-absorbed also in the loop of Henle but, in contrast to sodium, is not re-absorbed in the distal tubules. Its elimination half-life is approximately 24 hours; clearance is generally 20% of creatinine clearance but is diminished in elderly patients and patients with kidney disease. The risk of toxicity is increased in these patients as well as in patients with cardiovascular disease, dehydration, or hypokalemia. The most common drug-drug interactions involving lithium are pharmacokinetic.[42] Because lithium has a low therapeutic index, such interactions are likely to be clinically significant and potentially serious (Table 37.4).

Among the best studied of these interactions are thiazide diuretics and drugs that are chemically distinct but share a similar mechanism of action (e.g., indapamide, metolazone, quinethazone). These agents decrease lithium clearance and thereby steeply increase the risk of lithium toxicity. Loop diuretics (e.g., furosemide) appear to interact to a lesser degree with lithium excretion, presumably because they block lithium re-absorption in the loop of Henle, potentially offsetting possible compensatory increases in re-absorption more proximally. The potassium-sparing diuretics (e.g., amiloride, spironolactone, triamterene) also appear to be less likely to cause an increase in lithium levels, but close monitoring is indicated when these drugs are introduced. The potential impact of thiazide diuretics on lithium levels does not contraindicate their combined use, which, indeed, has been valuable in the treatment of lithium-associated polyuria. Potassium-sparing diuretics have also been used for this purpose. When a thiazide diuretic is used, a lithium

TABLE 37.4
Selected Drug Interactions With Lithium

Drug	Potential Interaction
Aminophylline, theophylline, acetazolamide, mannitol, sodium bicarbonate, sodium chloride load	Decreased lithium levels
Thiazide diuretics	Increased lithium levels; reduction of lithium-associated polyuria
Non-steroidal anti-inflammatory drugs, COX-2 inhibitors, tetracycline, spectinomycin, metronidazole, angiotensin II receptor antagonists, angiotensin-converting enzyme inhibitors	Increased lithium levels
Neuromuscular blocking drugs (succinylcholine, pancuronium, decamethonium)	Prolonged muscle paralysis
Anti-thyroid drugs (propylthiouracil, thioamide, methimazole)	Enhanced anti-thyroid efficacy
Antidepressants	Enhanced antidepressant efficacy
Calcium channel blockers (verapamil, diltiazem)	Idiosyncratic neurotoxicity
Antipsychotic drugs	Idiosyncratic neurotoxicity, neuroleptic malignant syndrome risk

COX-2, Cyclo-oxygenase-2.

dosage reduction of 25% to 50% and close monitoring of lithium levels are required. Monitoring of serum electrolytes, particularly potassium, is also important when thiazides are introduced because hypokalemia enhances the toxicity of lithium. Although not contraindicated with lithium, ACE inhibitors (e.g., captopril) and angiotensin II receptor antagonists (e.g., losartan) can elevate lithium levels, and close monitoring of levels is required when these agents are introduced.

A probable pharmacodynamic interaction exists between lithium and agents used clinically to produce neuromuscular blockade (e.g., succinylcholine, pancuronium, decamethonium) during anesthesia. Muscle paralysis can be significantly prolonged when these agents are administered to the lithium-treated patient.[43] Although the mechanism is unknown, the possible inhibition by lithium of acetylcholine synthesis and release at the neuromuscular junction is a potential basis for synergism.

Lithium interferes with the production of thyroid hormones through several mechanisms, including interference with iodine uptake, tyrosine iodination, and release of triiodothyronine (T_3) and thyroxine (T_4) and is associated with hypothyroidism in some patients. Reciprocally, lithium can enhance the efficacy of anti-thyroid medications (e.g., propylthiouracil, thioamide, methimazole) and has also been used preoperatively to help prevent thyroid storm in the surgical treatment of Graves disease.[44]

There have been isolated reports of various forms of neurotoxicity, which is usually, but not always, reversible, when lithium has been combined with SSRIs and other serotoninergic agents, calcium channel blockers, antipsychotics, and anticonvulsants (e.g., carbamazepine).[45] In some cases, features of the serotonin syndrome or NMS have been present.[46] Although it is worthwhile to be aware of this idiosyncratic drug interaction when evaluating unexplained mental status changes in a lithium-treated patient, the combination of lithium with these classes of medication is neither unusual nor contraindicated.

Many of the non-steroidal anti-inflammatory drugs have been reported to increase serum lithium levels, potentially by as much as 50% to 60% when used at full prescription strength. This can occur by inhibition of renal clearance of lithium by interference with a prostaglandin-dependent mechanism in the renal tubule. The cyclo-oxygenase (COX)-2 inhibitors (e.g., celecoxib, rofecoxib), can also raise lithium levels. Limited data available suggest that sulindac, phenylbutazone, and aspirin are less likely to affect lithium levels. Several antimicrobials are associated with increased lithium levels, including tetracycline, metronidazole, and parenteral spectinomycin. If these agents are required, close monitoring of lithium levels and potential dosage adjustments are recommended.

Conversely, a variety of agents can produce decreases in lithium levels, thereby increasing the risk of psychiatric symptom breakthrough and relapse. The methylxanthines (e.g., aminophylline, theophylline) can cause a significant decrease in lithium levels by increasing renal clearance; close blood level monitoring with co-administration is necessary. A reduction in lithium levels can also result from alkalinization of urine (e.g., with acetazolamide use or with sodium bicarbonate), osmotic diuretics (e.g., urea, mannitol), or from ingestion of a sodium chloride load, which also increases lithium excretion.

Valproic Acid

Valproic acid is a simple branched-chain carboxylic acid that, like several other anticonvulsants, has mood-stabilizing properties. Valproic acid is 80% to 95% protein bound and is rapidly metabolized primarily by hepatic microsomal glucuronidation and oxidation. It has a short elimination half-life of approximately 8 hours.[47] Clearance is essentially unchanged in the elderly and in patients with kidney disease, whereas it is significantly reduced in patients with primary liver disease.

In contrast to some other major anticonvulsants (e.g., carbamazepine, phenobarbital), valproate does not induce hepatic microsomes. Rather, it can inhibit oxidation reactions, thereby potentially increasing levels of co-administered hepatically metabolized drugs, notably including lamotrigine, as well as some TCAs, such as clomipramine, amitriptyline, and nortriptyline (Table 37.5).[48,49] A complex pharmacokinetic interaction occurs when valproic acid and carbamazepine are administered concurrently. Valproic acid not only inhibits the metabolism of carbamazepine and its active metabolite, carbamazepine-10,11-epoxide, but it also displaces both entities from protein-binding sites. Although the effect on plasma carbamazepine levels is variable, the levels of the active unbound epoxide metabolite are usually increased, with a concomitant increased risk of carbamazepine neurotoxicity. Conversely, co-administration with carbamazepine results in a decrease in plasma valproic acid levels. Nevertheless, the combination of valproate and carbamazepine has been used successfully in the treatment of patients with bipolar disorder who were only partially responsive to either drug alone.[50] Oral contraceptives as well as carbapenem antibiotics have also been associated with decreases in plasma valproic acid levels; enhanced monitoring of levels and valproate dose adjustments are recommended when these agents are used.

Cimetidine, a potent inhibitor of hepatic microsomal enzymes, is associated with decreased clearance

TABLE 37.5

Selected Drug Interactions With Valproate and Carbamazepine

Drug	Interaction With Valproate
Carbamazepine	Decreased valproate plasma levels; increased plasma levels of the epoxide metabolite of carbamazepine; variable effects on plasma levels of carbamazepine
Phenytoin	Decreased valproate plasma levels; variable effects on phenytoin plasma levels
Phenobarbital	Decreased valproate plasma levels; increased phenobarbital plasma levels
Oral contraceptives	Decreased valproate plasma levels
Carbapenem antibiotics	Decreased valproate plasma levels
Lamotrigine	Increased lamotrigine levels; hypersensitivity reaction
Aspirin	Increased unbound (active) fraction of valproate
Cimetidine	Increased valproate plasma levels
Fluoxetine	Same as above
Clonazepam	Rare absence seizures

Drug	Interaction With Carbamazepine
Phenytoin	Decreased carbamazepine plasma levels
Phenobarbital	Same as above
Primidone	Same as above
Macrolide antibiotics	Increased carbamazepine plasma levels
Isoniazid	Same as above

Drug	Interaction With Carbamazepine
Fluoxetine	Increased carbamazepine plasma levels
Danazol	Same as above
Verapamil	Same as above
Diltiazem	Same as above
Propoxyphene	Same as above
Oral contraceptives	Induction of metabolism by carbamazepine

of valproic acid, resulting in increased levels. The dosage of valproic acid may need to be reduced in the patient starting cimetidine, but not other H_2-receptor antagonists.[51] Elevated levels of valproic acid have also been reported sporadically with fluoxetine and other SSRIs. Aspirin and other salicylates can displace the protein binding of valproic acid,[52] thereby increasing the unbound (free) fraction, which can increase the risk of toxicity from valproate even though total serum levels are unchanged.

Lamotrigine

Lamotrigine is a phenyltriazine derivative anticonvulsant that is moderately (50%–60%) protein bound and metabolized primarily by glucuronidation. Its most serious adverse effect is a life-threatening hypersensitivity reaction with rash, typically, but not always, occurring within the first 2 months of use.[53] The incidence among patients with bipolar disorder is estimated at 0.8 per 1000 among patients on lamotrigine monotherapy and 1.3 per 1000 among patients on lamotrigine in combination with other agents.

The risk of adverse effects including hypersensitivity reactions and tremor is increased when lamotrigine is combined with valproic acid. As much as a two-fold to threefold increase in lamotrigine levels occurs when valproic acid is added, related to the inhibition of glucuronidation of lamotrigine.[54] Accordingly, prescribing guidelines recommend more gradual dosage titration of lamotrigine and lower target dosages when introduced in a patient already taking valproate. When valproate is added to lamotrigine, the dosage of lamotrigine should typically be reduced by one-half to two-thirds.

Conversely, lamotrigine levels can be decreased by as much as 50% when administered with metabolic inducers, particularly other anticonvulsants (including carbamazepine, primidone, and phenobarbital). Therefore, guidelines have been developed for dosing lamotrigine in the presence of these metabolic-inducing anticonvulsants. Similar magnitude reductions in lamotrigine levels have been reported in patients on oral contraceptives, requiring an increase in the dosage of lamotrigine.[55] Lamotrigine levels and symptom status should be monitored closely when oral contraceptives or metabolic-inducing anticonvulsants are started.

Carbamazepine and Oxcarbazepine

Carbamazepine is an iminostilbene anticonvulsant structurally related to the TCA imipramine.

Carbamazepine is slowly and inconsistently absorbed from the GI tract; peak serum concentrations are achieved approximately 4 to 8 hours after oral administration. It is only moderately (60%–85%) protein bound. Carbamazepine, a potent inducer of hepatic metabolism, can also induce its metabolism, such that elimination half-life can fall from 18 to 55 hours to 5 to 20 hours over a matter of several weeks, generally reaching a plateau after 3 to 5 weeks.

Most drug-drug interactions with carbamazepine occur by pharmacokinetic mechanisms. Drugs whose metabolism is increased by carbamazepine include valproic acid, phenytoin, ethosuximide, lamotrigine, alprazolam, clonazepam, TCAs, antipsychotics, doxycycline, tetracycline, thyroid hormone, corticosteroids, oral contraceptives, methadone, theophylline, warfarin, and cyclosporine. The concurrent administration of carbamazepine with any of these drugs can cause significant reductions in plasma levels and can lead to therapeutic failure. Patients of child-bearing potential who are taking oral contraceptives must be advised to use an additional method of birth control.

Several drugs inhibit the metabolism of carbamazepine, including macrolide antibiotics (e.g., erythromycin, clarithromycin, triacetyloleandomycin), isoniazid, fluoxetine, valproic acid, danazol, propoxyphene, and the calcium channel blockers verapamil and diltiazem. Because of its low therapeutic index, the risk of developing carbamazepine toxicity is significantly increased when these drugs are administered concurrently. Conversely, co-administration of phenytoin or phenobarbital, both microsomal enzyme inducers, can increase the metabolism of carbamazepine, potentially resulting in sub-therapeutic plasma levels. Carbamazepine has also been associated with bone marrow suppression, and its combination with other agents that interfere with blood cell production (including clozapine) should generally be avoided. The combination of carbamazepine with thiazide diuretics or furosemide has been associated with severe symptomatic hyponatremia,[56] suggesting the need for close monitoring of electrolytes when these medications are used concurrently.

Oxcarbazepine, a structural derivative of carbamazepine, appears to be a less-potent metabolic inducer than its parent compound, although it still can render certain important agents (particularly CYP 3A4 substrates) less effective because of similar pharmacokinetic interactions. Individuals of child-bearing potential should therefore receive guidance about supplementing oral contraceptives with a second effective form of birth control, as with carbamazepine. As with carbamazepine, oxcarbazepine is also associated with risk of hyponatremia.

Other Anticonvulsants

Other anticonvulsants such as topiramate, zonisamide, gabapentin, and pregabalin, do not appear to have efficacy like that of valproic acid, lamotrigine, or carbamazepine for any phase of bipolar disorder, though they may have a role as an adjunctive treatment in some patients with mood and anxiety disorders and other conditions and for side-effect management.

Topiramate. Topiramate is a sulfamate-substituted monosaccharide, related to fructose, a rather unusual chemical structure for an anticonvulsant. Topiramate is used less commonly for its putative mood-stabilizing effects[57] than its weight-reducing effects[58] and utility in substance-abusing populations.[59,60]

Topiramate is quickly absorbed after oral use. Most of the drug (70%) is later excreted in the urine unchanged; therefore it requires dosage reduction in the setting of renal insufficiency. The remainder is extensively metabolized by hydroxylation, hydrolysis, and glucuronidation. Topiramate inhibits carbonic anhydrase; therefore the concomitant use of other carbonic anhydrase inhibitors (e.g., acetazolamide) can lead to an increased risk of forming kidney stones.[61]

In the presence of hepatic enzyme inducers (e.g., carbamazepine), the elimination of topiramate may be increased by up to 50%. Based on its properties as a weak inhibitor of CYP 2C19 and an inducer of CYP 3A4, topiramate can increase plasma levels of phenytoin but decrease plasma concentrations of estrogens in patients taking oral contraceptives or hormonal therapy.

Zonisamide. Zonisamide is a sulfonamide anticonvulsant used in patients with partial seizures.[62] As with topiramate, zonisamide has been prescribed off-label to mitigate against weight gain on psychiatric medications and it might have fewer adverse cognitive effects. Zonisamide has been associated with metabolic acidosis in some patients. Zonisamide is metabolized mostly by the CYP 3A4 isoenzyme; its levels are therefore susceptible to the impact of CYP 3A4 inhibitors and inducers.

Gabapentin and Pregabalin. The gabapentinoids, gabapentin and pregabalin, bind to the α2-delta subunit of voltage-gated calcium channels, which decreases the release of glutamate, norepinephrine, and substance P. Although developed as anti-seizure medications, they have been used in a variety of clinical contexts.[63] Gabapentin is indicated for post-herpetic neuralgia, adjunctive therapy in epilepsy, and restless leg syndrome. It has been used off-label with various levels of evidence for myriad conditions ranging from anxiety, insomnia, fibromyalgia, and neuropathic pain to neurogenic cough. Although it is not a salt, it resembles lithium in so far as it is not hepatically metabolized, is minimally protein bound, and is excreted by the kidney largely as an unchanged drug. As with lithium, therefore changes in renal function require re-evaluation of gabapentin dosing. Pregabalin is rapidly absorbed when administered on an empty stomach, undergoes negligible metabolism in humans, has very low protein binding, and is also eliminated unchanged from the systemic circulation primarily by renal excretion. Although in vivo studies have shown no significant pharmacokinetic interactions for pregabalin, it might have potential pharmacodynamic interactions with opioids (pregabalin is synergistic with opioids in lower dosages), benzodiazepines, barbiturates, alcohol, and other drugs that depress the CNS. The two gabapentinoids are associated with some potential for misuse and should be used thoughtfully in patients at risk for problem substance use.

Antidepressants

The antidepressant drugs include TCAs, MAOIs, SSRIs, atypical agents (bupropion, trazodone, nefazodone, and mirtazapine), the SNRIs (venlafaxine, duloxetine, milnacipran, desvenlafaxine, and levomilnacipran), miscellaneous serotonergic agents (vilazodone, vortioxetine) and newer, rapidly acting non-monoaminergic agents including esketamine, brexanolone, and zuranolone. Although the TCAs and MAOIs are used infrequently, they continue to serve a valuable role in the treatment of more severe, treatment-resistant depressive and anxiety disorders despite the wide range of drug-drug and food drug interactions they entail.

SSRIs and Other Newer Antidepressants

The SSRIs (fluoxetine, sertraline, paroxetine, fluvoxamine, citalopram, escitalopram) and related agents (vilazodone, vortioxetine) share similar pharmacologic actions, including minimal anticholinergic, antihistaminic, and α_1-adrenergic blocking effects and potent presynaptic inhibition of serotonin reuptake. Vilazodone and vortioxetine act as serotonin reuptake inhibitors and agonize/antagonize various serotonin receptors (i.e., vilazodone is a partial agonist at the 5-HT_{1A} receptor, vortioxetine acts as an agonist or antagonist at 5-HT_{1A}, 5-HT_{1B}, 5-HT_3, 5-HT_{1D}, and 5-HT_7). Important pharmacokinetic differences account for distinctions among them with respect to potential drug interactions (Table 37.6).

Nefazodone, like trazodone, is distinguished from classic SSRIs by its antagonism of the 5-HT_2 receptor and differs from trazodone in its lesser antagonism of the α_1-adrenergic receptor. It is rarely used due to rare but serious liver toxicity. Mirtazapine blocks the 5-HT_2 receptor, 5-HT_3 receptor, and the α_2-adrenergic receptors. Venlafaxine, desvenlafaxine, duloxetine, milnacipran, and levomilnacipran are like TCAs in their inhibition of serotonin and norepinephrine reuptake, but, in contrast to TCAs, they are relatively devoid of post-synaptic anticholinergic, antihistaminic, and α_1-adrenergic activity. Milnacipran is FDA approved only for fibromyalgia, while its enantiomer levomilnacipran is approved for MDD. Venlafaxine is predominantly serotoninergic at low to moderate dosages and has greater noradrenergic effects at higher doses whereas duloxetine and, especially, milnacipran and levomilnacipran are potent inhibitors of both the norepinephrine and serotonin transporters across their clinical dosage ranges.

Although not an approved antidepressant, the norepinephrine reuptake inhibitor atomoxetine is indicated for the treatment of attention deficit hyperactivity disorder (ADHD) and might have a role in depression pharmacotherapy as an adjunctive treatment. It is neither a significant inhibitor nor inducer of the CYP system, but owing to its adrenergic effects, the risk of palpitations or pressor effects is likely to be greater than with serotoninergic agents when combined with

TABLE 37.6

Potential Drug Interactions With Selective Serotonin Reuptake Inhibitors and Other Newer Antidepressants

Drug	Potential Interaction
MAOIs	Serotonin syndrome
Secondary amine TCAs	Increased TCA levels when co-administered with fluoxetine, paroxetine, sertraline, bupropion, duloxetine
Tertiary amine TCAs	Increased TCA levels with fluvoxamine, paroxetine, sertraline, bupropion, duloxetine
Antipsychotics (typical) and risperidone, aripiprazole	Increased antipsychotic levels with fluoxetine, sertraline, paroxetine, bupropion, duloxetine
Thioridazine	Arrhythmia risk with CYP 2D6-inhibitory antidepressants
Pimozide	Arrhythmia risk with CYP 3A4-inhibitory antidepressants (nefazodone, fluvoxamine)
Clozapine and olanzapine	Increased antipsychotic levels with fluvoxamine
Diazepam	Increased benzodiazepine levels with fluoxetine, fluvoxamine, sertraline
Triazolobenzodiazepines (midazolam, alprazolam, triazolam)	Increased benzodiazepine levels with fluvoxamine, nefazodone, sertraline
Carbamazepine	Increased carbamazepine levels with fluoxetine, fluvoxamine, nefazodone
Theophylline	Increased theophylline levels with fluvoxamine
Type 1 C antiarrhythmics (encainide, flecainide, propafenone)	Increased antiarrhythmic levels with fluoxetine, paroxetine, sertraline, bupropion, duloxetine
β-Blockers (lipophilic)	Increased β-blocker levels with fluoxetine, paroxetine, sertraline, bupropion, duloxetine
Calcium channel blockers	Increased levels with fluoxetine, fluvoxamine, nefazodone
Tizanidine	Increased tizanidine levels with fluvoxamine

CYP P450, Cytochrome P450; *MAOIs*, monoamine oxidase inhibitors; *TCAs*, tricyclic antidepressants.

prescribed and OTC sympathomimetics, and its use with MAOIs is contraindicated.

Each of the SSRIs (except for fluvoxamine [77%], citalopram [80%], and escitalopram [56%]) as well as nefazodone, is highly protein bound (95%–99%). Venlafaxine, desvenlafaxine, milnacipran, and levomilnacipran are minimally protein bound (15%–30%), whereas duloxetine is highly protein bound (90%). Each of the antidepressants is hepatically metabolized, and all of them except paroxetine and duloxetine have active metabolites. The major metabolites of sertraline, citalopram, and desvenlafaxine, however, appear to be minimally active. Elimination half-lives range from 5 hours for venlafaxine and 11 hours for its metabolite, O-desmethylvenlafaxine, to 2 to 3 days for fluoxetine and 7 to 14 days for its metabolite, norfluoxetine. Nefazodone, like venlafaxine, has a short half-life (2–5 hours), with fluvoxamine, sertraline, paroxetine, citalopram, and escitalopram in the intermediate range of 15 to 35 hours. Food can have variable effects on antidepressant bioavailability, including an increase in sertraline, a decrease in nefazodone, and no change in escitalopram.

The growing knowledge about the interaction of the newer antidepressants with the CYP isoenzymes has revealed differences among them in their pattern of enzyme inhibition that are likely to be critical to the understanding and prediction of drug-drug interactions.

Cytochrome P450 2D6. Fluoxetine, norfluoxetine, paroxetine, bupropion, duloxetine, sertraline (to a moderate degree), and citalopram and escitalopram (to a minimal degree) all inhibit CYP 2D6, which accounts for their potential inhibitory effect on TCA clearance and the metabolism of other CYP 2D6 substrates. Other drugs metabolized by CYP 2D6—and whose levels can rise in the setting of CYP 2D6 inhibition—include the type 1 C antiarrhythmics (e.g., encainide, flecainide, propafenone) as well as β-blockers (e.g., propranolol, timolol, metoprolol), antipsychotics (e.g., risperidone, haloperidol, aripiprazole, iloperidone, thioridazine, perphenazine), TCAs, and trazodone. CYP 2D6 converts codeine and tramadol into their active form; hence the efficacy of these analgesics may be diminished when concurrently administered with a P450 2D6 inhibitor. So too, as P450 2D6 converts

tamoxifen into its active N-desmethyl tamoxifen form for the treatment of neoplasms, the use of inhibitors of 2D6 should be carefully re-evaluated during tamoxifen treatment.

These observations underscore the need to exercise care and to closely monitor when prescribing these SSRIs, bupropion, or duloxetine in the setting of complex medical regimens. Plasma TCA levels do not routinely include levels of active or potentially toxic metabolites, which may be altered by shunting to other metabolic routes when CYP 2D6 is inhibited. Therefore, particularly in the case of patients at risk for conduction delay, electrocardiography, and blood level monitoring are recommended when combining TCAs with SSRIs, duloxetine, or bupropion.

Cytochrome P450 3A4. Fluoxetine's major metabolite (norfluoxetine), fluvoxamine, nefazodone, and, to a lesser extent, sertraline, desmethylsertraline, citalopram, and escitalopram inhibit CYP 3A4. Each of these agents therefore has the potential for elevating levels of pimozide and cisapride (arrhythmia risks), methadone, oxycodone, fentanyl (respiratory depression risks), calcium channel blockers, the statins, carbamazepine, midazolam, and many other important and commonly prescribed substrates of this widely recruited CYP enzyme.

Cytochrome P450 2 C. Serum concentrations of drugs metabolized by this sub-family may be increased by fluoxetine, sertraline, and fluvoxamine. Reported interactions include decreased clearance of diazepam on all three SSRIs, a small reduction in tolbutamide clearance on sertraline, and increased plasma phenytoin concentrations reflecting decreased clearance on fluoxetine. Warfarin is also metabolized by this sub-family, and levels may be increased by the inhibition of these enzymes. SSRIs can interact with warfarin by still other, probably pharmacodynamic mechanisms (such as depletion of platelet serotonin). Although the combination is common, increased monitoring is recommended when SSRIs are prescribed with warfarin.

Cytochrome P450 1 A. Among the SSRIs, only fluvoxamine appears to be a potent inhibitor of CYP

1A2. Accordingly, increased serum concentrations of theophylline, haloperidol, clozapine, olanzapine, and the tertiary amine TCAs (including clomipramine, amitriptyline, and imipramine) can occur. Because theophylline and TCAs have a relatively narrow therapeutic index and because the degree of elevation of antipsychotic blood levels appears to be substantial (e.g., up to fourfold increases in haloperidol concentrations), additional monitoring and consideration of dosage reductions are necessary when fluvoxamine is co-administered with these agents.

Additional Interactions. Mirtazapine, although neither a potent inhibitor nor inducer of the CYP isoenzymes, has numerous pharmacodynamic effects including antagonism of the histamine, α_2-adrenergic, 5-HT$_2$ and 5-HT$_3$, and muscarinic receptors, creating the possibility of myriad pharmacodynamic interactions (including blockade of clonidine's antihypertensive activity).[64] It also has the possible benefit of attenuating nausea and sexual dysfunction that can occur with SSRIs.[65]

The serotonin syndrome is a potentially life-threatening condition characterized by clonus, tremor, diaphoresis, agitation, hyperreflexia, hypertonia, confusion, and coma.[66,67] Although this syndrome can arise whenever an SSRI is combined with drugs with serotonergic properties (e.g., L-tryptophan, clomipramine, venlafaxine, dextromethorphan, meperidine), the greatest known risk with SSRIs is associated with their co-administration with an MAOI which is, therefore absolutely contraindicated. Because of the long elimination half-life of fluoxetine and norfluoxetine, at least 5 weeks must elapse after fluoxetine discontinuation before an MAOI can be safely introduced. With the other SSRIs, an interval of 2 weeks appears to be adequate.

The weak, reversible MAOI antimicrobial linezolid, used for the treatment of multi-drug-resistant gram-positive infections, has been implicated in a small number of post-marketing cases of serotonin syndrome in patients on serotoninergic antidepressants, typically patients on SSRIs, as well as other medications, including narcotics.[68] The co-administration of SSRIs with other serotoninergic agents is not contraindicated, but it should prompt immediate discontinuation in any patient on this combination of drugs who presents with mental status changes, fever, or hyperreflexia of unknown origin.

Non-Monoaminergic Antidepressants

Since 2019 the pharmacotherapy of depression has been notably expanded beyond the monoaminergic agents with the FDA approval of both esketamine,[69] the non-selective antagonist of the *N*-methyl-D-aspartate ionotropic glutamate receptor antagonist which is administered intranasally due to poor oral bioavailability, and the positive allosteric modulators of GABA-A receptors, including brexanolone, administered intravenously, and zuranolone, administered orally.[70] Unlike many psychotropics, esketamine is only moderately (~45%) protein bound. It is primarily metabolized by CYP 2B6 and by CYP 3A4 which means potential alteration in levels by inducers or inhibitors of those agents. Esketamine is associated with abuse liability as well as acute dissociative reactions and typically mild hypertensive effects (systolic and/or diastolic) both peaking within the first hour. Due to these risks, the FDA requires in-clinic administration and monitoring. Esketamine is currently indicated for treatment-resistant depression as well as depressive symptoms in adults with MDD and suicidal ideation or behavior. Due to its potential effects on blood pressure, it is contraindicated in individuals with aneurysmal vascular disease. Although there are no absolute contraindications for medication co-administration, the concurrent use of psychostimulants or MAOIs may increase the risk of acute hypertensive reactions. Although not definitive, some evidence suggests that high-dose benzodiazepines may reduce the efficacy of esketamine in some patients. Based largely on data related to chronic recreational use of ketamine, it is possible that long-term use of esketamine, particularly at higher than usual doses, may carry the risk of bladder problems including bladder ulceration or interstitial cystitis. The GABA-A receptor modulators are currently FDA indicated for the treatment of post-partum depression, though have also been investigated for other conditions including depression outside of a perinatal context. They are both highly protein bound. Brexanolone, a synthetic version of allopregnanolone, is associated with a low (3%–5%) but clinically significant rate of loss of consciousness and must be administered in a hospital setting by slow IV infusion with monitoring. Both brexanolone and zuranolone may be sedating and should be administered with care with other CNS depressants, such as benzodiazepines. In addition, both have some abuse liability. Finally, as zuranolone is metabolized through CYP 3A4 its levels may be altered by the co-administration of inhibitors and inducers of this isoenzyme.

Tricyclic Antidepressants

TCAs are thought to exert their pharmacologic action by inhibiting the pre-synaptic neuronal reuptake of norepinephrine and serotonin in the CNS with subsequent modulation of both pre-synaptic and post-synaptic α-adrenergic receptors. While clinically effective, TCAs have been replaced by SSRIs and newer antidepressants that cause fewer side effects. TCAs also have significant anticholinergic, antihistaminic, and α-adrenergic activity as well as quinidine-like effects on cardiac conditions, and in these respects, they resemble the low-potency antipsychotic drugs, which are structurally similar.

TCAs are well absorbed from the GI tract and subject to significant first-pass liver metabolism before entry into the systemic circulation, where they are largely protein bound, ranging from 85% (trimipramine) to 95% (amitriptyline). Peak plasma concentrations are reached approximately 2 to 6 hours after oral administration. They are highly lipophilic, with a large volume of distribution. TCAs are extensively metabolized by hepatic microsomal enzymes, and most have pharmacologically active metabolites. Additive anticholinergic effects can occur when the TCAs are co-administered with other drugs possessing anticholinergic properties (e.g., low-potency antipsychotics, antiparkinsonian drugs), potentially resulting in an anticholinergic syndrome. SSRIs, SNRIs, atypical antidepressants, and MAOIs are relatively devoid of anticholinergic activity, although MAOIs can indirectly potentiate the anticholinergic properties of atropine and scopolamine. Additive sedative effects are not uncommon when TCAs are combined with sedative-hypnotics, anxiolytics, or narcotics or alcohol (Table 37.7).

TCAs possess class 1 A antiarrhythmic activity and can lead to depression of cardiac conduction, potentially resulting in heart block or ventricular arrhythmias when combined with quinidine-like agents

TABLE 37.7
Selected Drug Interactions With Tricyclic Antidepressants

Drug	Potential Interaction
Carbamazepine	Decreased TCA plasma levels
Phenobarbital	Same as above
Rifampin	Same as above
Antipsychotics	Increased TCA plasma levels
Methylphenidate	Same as above
SSRIs, bupropion, duloxetine	Same as above
Quinidine	Same as above
Propafenone	Same as above
Antifungals	Same as above
Macrolide antibiotics	Same as above
Verapamil	Same as above
Diltiazem	Same as above
Cimetidine	Same as above
Class I antiarrhythmics	Depression of cardiac conduction; ventricular arrhythmias
Guanethidine	Interference with antihypertensive effect
Clonidine	Same as above
Sympathomimetic amines (e.g., epinephrine)	Arrhythmias, hypertension (e.g., isoproterenol, epinephrine)
Antihypertensives	Hypotension
Vasodilator drugs	Same as above
Low-potency antipsychotics	Same as above; additive anticholinergic effects and risk of ventricular arrhythmias
Anticholinergic drugs	Additive anticholinergic toxicity
MAOIs	Delirium, fever, convulsions
Sulfonylurea hypoglycemics	Hypoglycemia

MAOIs, Monoamine oxidase inhibitors; *SSRIs*, selective serotonin reuptake inhibitors; *TCA*, tricyclic antidepressant.

(including quinidine, procainamide, and disopyramide as well as the low-potency antipsychotics).[71] The antiarrhythmics quinidine and propafenone, inhibitors of CYP 2D6, can additionally produce clinically significant elevations of the TCAs, thus increasing the risk of cardiotoxicity through both pharmacodynamic and pharmacokinetic mechanisms. The arrhythmogenic risks of a TCA are enhanced in a patient with underlying coronary or valvular heart disease, a patient with a recent myocardial infarction or hypokalemia, and in a patient receiving sympathomimetic amines, such as amphetamine stimulants.

TCAs also interact with several antihypertensive drugs. TCAs can antagonize the antihypertensive effects of guanethidine, bethanidine, debrisoquine, or clonidine via interference with neuronal reuptake by noradrenergic neurons. Conversely, TCAs can cause varying degrees of postural hypotension when co-administered with vasodilator drugs, antihypertensives, or low-potency neuroleptics.

Hypoglycemia has been observed with secondary and tertiary TCAs, particularly in the presence of sulfonylurea hypoglycemic agents, suggesting the need for close monitoring.

Pharmacokinetic interactions involving the TCAs are often clinically important. Antipsychotic drugs (including haloperidol, chlorpromazine, thioridazine, and perphenazine) are known to increase TCA levels by 30% to 100%. Cimetidine and methylphenidate can also raise tertiary TCA levels, as predicted by microsomal enzyme inhibition. The antifungals (e.g., ketoconazole), macrolide antibiotics (e.g., erythromycin), and calcium channel blockers (e.g., verapamil and diltiazem) as inhibitors of CYP 3A4, can also impair the clearance of tertiary amine TCAs, thereby requiring a reduction in TCA dosage. SSRIs have been associated with clinically significant increases in TCA plasma levels, believed to be the result of inhibition primarily, but not exclusively, of CYP 2D6. Similar elevations of TCA levels would be expected with other potent CYP 2D6 inhibitor antidepressants (e.g., duloxetine, bupropion). Inducers of CYP enzymes can increase the metabolism of TCAs. Thus, plasma levels of TCAs may be significantly reduced when carbamazepine, phenobarbital, rifampin, or isoniazid are co-administered or in the setting of chronic alcohol or cigarette use.

Monoamine Oxidase Inhibitors

Monoamine oxidase is an enzyme located primarily on the outer mitochondrial membrane and is responsible for the intracellular catabolism of monoamines. It is found in high concentrations in the brain, liver, intestines, and lungs. In pre-synaptic nerve terminals, MAO metabolizes cytoplasmic monoamines. In the liver and gut, MAO catabolizes ingested bioactive amines, thus protecting against absorption into the systemic circulation of potentially vasoactive substances, particularly tyramine.

Two sub-types of MAO have been distinguished: intestinal MAO is predominantly MAO_A, whereas brain MAO is predominantly MAO_B. MAO_A preferentially metabolizes norepinephrine and serotonin. Phenylethylamine and benzylamine are the prototypic substrates for MAO_B. Both MAO sub-types metabolize dopamine and tyramine. Among the currently available MAOIs, phenelzine, tranylcypromine, and isocarboxazid are non-specific inhibitors of both MAO_A and MAO_B; selegiline, available orally or in transdermal form, is primarily an inhibitor of MAO_B, though it is a mixed MAO_A and MAO_B inhibitor at higher dosages.

When patients are using MAOIs, dietary and medication[72-74] restrictions must be closely followed to avoid serious interactions. The MAOIs are, therefore generally reserved for use in responsible and motivated patients, or in supervised settings, when adequate trials of other classes of antidepressants have failed. The two major types of MAOI drug-drug interaction are the serotonin syndrome and the hypertensive (also called *hyperadrenergic*) crisis.

Hypertensive Crisis. A hypertensive crisis is an emergency characterized by an abrupt elevation of blood pressure, severe headache, nausea, vomiting, and diaphoresis; intracranial hemorrhage or myocardial infarction can occur. Prompt intervention to reduce blood pressure with the α_1-adrenergic antagonist phentolamine or the combination of sodium nitroprusside and a β-blocker may be life saving. Potentially catastrophic hypertension appears to be due to the release of bound intraneuronal stores of norepinephrine and dopamine by indirect vasopressor substances. The reaction can therefore be precipitated by the concurrent administration of vasopressor amines, stimulants, anorexiants, and many OTC cough and cold preparations; these include L-dopa, dopamine, amphetamine, methylphenidate, phenylpropanolamine, phentermine, ephedrine, and pseudoephedrine. By contrast, direct sympathomimetic amines (e.g., norepinephrine, isoproterenol, epinephrine), which rely for their cardiovascular effects on direct stimulation of post-synaptic receptors, rather than on pre-synaptic release of stored catecholamines, appear to be somewhat safer when administered to patients on MAOIs (although they are also contraindicated).

Hypertensive crises may also be triggered by the ingestion of naturally occurring sympathomimetic amines (particularly tyramine), which are present in various food products, including aged cheeses (e.g., stilton, cheddar, blue cheese, or camembert, rather than cream cheese, ricotta cheese, or cottage cheese), yeast extracts, fava (broad) beans, over-ripe fruits (e.g., avocado), pickled herring, aged meats (e.g., salami, bologna, and many kinds of sausage), chicken liver, fermented bean curd, sauerkraut, many types of red wine and beer (particularly imported beer), and some white wines. Although gin, vodka, and whiskey appear to be free of tyramine, their use should be minimized during MAOI treatment, as with other antidepressants, because of the risk of exaggerated side effects and reduced antidepressant efficacy. Other, less stringent requirements include a moderate intake of caffeine, chocolate, yogurt, and soy sauce. Because MAO activity can remain diminished for nearly 2 to 3 weeks following the discontinuation of MAOIs, a tyramine-free diet and appropriate medication restrictions should be continued for at least 14 days after an MAOI has been discontinued.

The lowest dose available of transdermal selegiline (6 mg/24 hour) has been shown to have minimal risks of hypertensive crisis on a normal diet and therefore does not require the same level of restriction. Based on the more limited data available for the doses of 9 mg and 12 mg/24 hours, food effects cannot be ruled out; therefore the FDA has advised that patients receiving these doses follow dietary modifications that include the avoidance of tyramine-rich food and beverages during treatment and for up to 2 weeks after therapy has been completed or the dose has been reduced to 6 mg. No dose adjustment is necessary for patients with mild-to-moderate renal or hepatic impairment.

Serotonin Syndrome. The serotonin syndrome the other major drug-drug interaction involving MAOIs, occurs when MAOIs and serotoninergic agents are co-administered.[66,67] Potentially fatal reactions most closely resembling the serotonin syndrome can also occur with other drugs with less-selective serotoninergic activity, most notably meperidine and dextromethorphan, a widely available cough suppressant. Both medications, similar to the SSRIs, SNRIs, and clomipramine, are contraindicated when MAOIs are used. Other serotoninergic medications (e.g., buspirone and trazodone) are not contraindicated but should be used with care.

The 5-HT$_1$ agonist triptans, used in the treatment of migraine, have been implicated in serotonin syndrome when administered to patients on MAOIs. Other narcotic analgesics (e.g., propoxyphene, codeine, oxycodone, morphine, alfentanil, or morphine) appear to be safer alternatives to meperidine, but, in conjunction with MAOIs, their analgesic and CNS-depressant effects may be potentiated, and rare serotonin syndrome-like presentations have been reported. If opioid agents are necessary, they should be started at one-fifth to one-half of the standard dosages and gradually titrated upward, with monitoring for untoward hemodynamic or mental status changes.

St. Johns Wort

Although data supporting the efficacy of St. Johns wort for depression have been inconsistent, it is among the most carefully studied herbal preparation with respect to drug-drug interactions. Initial concerns about the potential MAOI activity of this botanical and the risk of serotonin syndrome when combined with serotoninergic agents were only partially borne out, with few cases of serotonin syndrome reported despite widespread concurrent use of St. Johns wort with serotoninergic antidepressants. However, a much more serious pharmacokinetic drug interaction was observed whereby some critical medications are rendered less effective in some patients concurrently taking St. Johns wort.[16] These medications include immunosuppressants (such as cyclosporine and tacrolimus), coumarin anticoagulants, antiretrovirals, theophylline, digoxin, amitriptyline, and oral contraceptives. Although the precise mechanisms and herbal constituents responsible for these effects are not fully elucidated, the primary focus has been on CYP 3A4 and P-glycoprotein. A paucity of systematic information exists concerning potential drug interactions and adverse effects of other herbal products, including the risk of increased bleeding in patients on *Ginkgo biloba* and warfarin and hepatotoxicity in patients on certain kava preparations.

Psychostimulants and Related Agents

Psychostimulants

Amphetamine and methylphenidate-based psychostimulants, approved for the treatment of ADHD, have provided sometimes rapidly effective treatment of depressive symptoms among elderly and medically frail patients, including those with cardiac disease, acquired immunodeficiency syndrome, or cancer, who would be at particular risk from anticholinergic, hypotensive, sedative, or quinidine-like effects of the TCAs.[75-78] Although the broader range of options presented by the newer antidepressants has limited the need for stimulants in these settings, stimulants continue to be recruited as monotherapy and adjunctive therapy to FDA-approved antidepressants. In addition, the very cautious combination of methylphenidate and dextroamphetamine with MAOIs, though generally contraindicated, has been reported to be effective in a subset of treatment-refractory depressed patients[79,80] and in efforts to treat particularly severe postural hypotension from the MAOIs. Because of the high risk of hypertensive crises, the addition of stimulants to MAOIs for antidepressant augmentation should remain an option only in exceptional cases in which other options (e.g., electroconvulsive therapy) have been carefully weighed.

In combination with other drugs, psychostimulants, such as methylphenidate, have been linked to increased plasma levels of TCAs and possibly other antidepressants; increased plasma levels of phenobarbital, primidone, and phenytoin; increased prothrombin time on anticoagulants; attenuation or reversal of the guanethidine antihypertensive effect; and increased pressor responses to vasopressor drugs. Methylphenidate has been implicated in putative drug interactions more often than dextroamphetamine or mixed amphetamine salts; however, decades of clinical experience with methylphenidate and other psychostimulants suggests these medicines may be safe and effective for appropriately screened patients, including those on more complex medical regimens.

Modafinil/Armodafinil

The relatively benign side-effect profile of modafinil (and its R-enantiomer, armodafinil), together with its stimulant-like properties but differing mechanism, have motivated efforts to define the potential role in psychiatry of this wakefulness-promoting agent currently approved for the treatment of narcolepsy. Its success as a treatment for fatigue in neurologic conditions (e.g., multiple sclerosis)[81] suggests the possibility of usefulness as a treatment for drowsiness related to other causes, including medications (e.g., antipsychotic-induced sedation). In addition, it is used off-label, like the psychostimulants, for treating depression co-morbid with medical illness[82] and as an antidepressant adjunct in refractory depression.[83] Several studies have suggested efficacy for ADHD,[84-86] although the use of modafinil and armodafinil for this purpose remains off-label. Both medications are associated with risk of misuse although they have been explored as potentially less-problematic agents for potential treatment of cocaine and psychostimulant use disorders.

Modafinil and armodafinil are minimal to moderate inducers of CYP 3A4 and inhibitors of the CYP 2C isoforms.[87] Modafinil and armodafinil can thereby engage in drug-drug interactions with common substrates, including oral contraceptives (the levels of which can decrease) and β-blockers and warfarin (the levels of which can increase), thereby monitoring and patient education. It is important to advise the use of a second non-hormonal form of contraception in modafinil and armodafinil-treated patients on oral contraceptives. Like St. Johns wort, modafinil has also been implicated as a factor in lowered cyclosporine levels, presumably through P450 3A4 induction, and both modafinil and armodafinil should be used with extreme care in patients on immunosuppressants that rely on this enzyme for metabolism.

Benzodiazepines

The benzodiazepines are a class of widely prescribed psychotropic drugs that have anxiolytic, sedative, muscle-relaxant, and anticonvulsant properties. Their rate of onset of action, duration of action, presence of active metabolites, and tendency to accumulate in the body vary considerably and can influence both side effects and the success of treatment. Most benzodiazepines are well absorbed on an empty stomach, with peak plasma levels achieved generally between 1 and 3 hours, although with more rapid onset of some (e.g., diazepam, clorazepate) than others (e.g., oxazepam).

Duration of action of a single dose of benzodiazepine generally depends more on distribution from systemic circulation to tissue than on subsequent elimination (e.g., more rapid for diazepam than lorazepam). With repeated doses, however, the volume of distribution is saturated, and elimination half-life becomes the more important parameter in determining the duration of action (e.g., more rapid for lorazepam than diazepam). A benzodiazepine that is comparatively short acting on acute administration can therefore become relatively long acting on long-term dosing. Benzodiazepines are highly lipophilic and distribute readily to the CNS and tissues. Plasma protein binding ranges from approximately 70% (alprazolam) to 99% (diazepam).

Unlike most benzodiazepines, lorazepam, oxazepam, and temazepam are not subject to phase I metabolism. Because phase II metabolism (glucuronide conjugation) does not produce active metabolites and is less affected than phase I metabolism by primary liver disease, aging, and concurrently used inducers or inhibitors of hepatic microsomal enzymes, the 3-hydroxy substituted benzodiazepines are much preferred over other benzodiazepines such as diazepam in older patients and patients with liver disease. The most common and clinically significant interactions involving benzodiazepines are the additive CNS-depressant effects, which can occur when a benzodiazepine is administered concurrently with barbiturates, narcotics, or ethanol. These interactions can be serious because of their potential to cause excessive sedation, cognitive and psychomotor impairment, and, at higher dosages, potentially fatal respiratory depression. The specific benzodiazepine antagonist, flumazenil, may be used in the management of a severe benzodiazepine overdose.

Pharmacokinetic interactions include a decreased rate of absorption, but not the extent of absorption, of benzodiazepines in the presence of antacids or food. This is more likely to be a factor in determining the subjective effects accompanying the onset of benzodiazepine action for single-dose rather than repeated-dose administration. Carbamazepine, phenobarbital, and rifampin can induce metabolism, lowering levels of benzodiazepines that are oxidatively metabolized. In contrast, potential inhibitors of CYP 3A4 (including macrolide antibiotics, antifungals [such as ketoconazole and itraconazole], nefazodone, fluvoxamine, and cimetidine) have been associated with

decreased clearance and therefore increased levels of the triazolobenzodiazepines. A similar reaction occurs with several non-benzodiazepine sedative-hypnotics (e.g., zolpidem, zaleplon, eszopiclone), which are also metabolized through this pathway. The metabolism of diazepam depends in part on CYP 2C19. Decreased diazepam clearance may therefore occur in the setting of concurrent administration of a variety of agents including fluoxetine, sertraline, propranolol, metoprolol, omeprazole, disulfiram, low-dose estrogen-containing oral contraceptives, and isoniazid.

PSYCHIATRIC USES OF NON-PSYCHIATRIC MEDICATIONS

In the general hospital, consideration of the psychiatric complications of non-psychiatric medications is an integral part of the evaluation of alterations in mood, behavior, or mental status. Nevertheless, whether by extrapolation from known in vitro mechanisms or through serendipity, non-psychiatric drugs have also been found to be useful in the treatment of psychiatric illness. These include medications that ameliorate the side effects of psychotropic drugs, as well as medications that may have direct benefits for the treatment of neuropsychiatric disorders.

Medications for Psychotropic Drug Side Effects

The importance of attentive management of psychotropic drug side effects for reducing distress and risk, supporting the therapeutic alliance, and increasing treatment adherence continues to fuel the search for effective pharmacologic strategies when more conservative measures fail to reduce dangerous or difficult-to-tolerate side effects.[17] Anticholinergic agents (benztropine 1–2 mg twice a day; biperiden 1–3 mg twice a day; and trihexyphenidyl 1–3 mg twice a day) and, less often, anticholinergic antihistamines (diphenhydramine 25–50 mg twice a day) and amantadine (100 mg two to three times a day) are widely used for managing the parkinsonian side effects of antipsychotics. Benztropine (2 mg) and diphenhydramine (50 mg) are also used IM or IV for the acute management of dystonia. Anticholinergic side effects are not uncommon, however, and a combination of these drugs with other highly anticholinergic agents (e.g., tertiary amine TCAs) invites the risk of frank toxicity. In this regard, IV physostigmine has been used in the emergency management of anticholinergic syndrome, which includes delirium and tachyarrhythmias.

β-Blockers (including propranolol starting at 10–20 mg one to two times a day or the less centrally active atenolol [approximately 50 mg/day]) have been useful for akathisia from antipsychotics and antidepressants, for lithium-associated tremor, and, less commonly, for jitteriness on antidepressants.

Diuretics, including amiloride (5–10 mg one to three times a day) and hydrochlorothiazide (50–100 mg/day), have been successful in treating disruptive polyuria on lithium, albeit typically requiring reduction of lithium dosage and close monitoring of lithium levels and serum potassium. Anticholinergic side effects, including urinary retention, constipation, blurred vision, and dry mouth, may be treated with bethanechol (10–25 mg one to three times a day); dry mouth and blurred vision can also be treated with 1% pilocarpine ophthalmic solution. Excessive sweating on antidepressants is infrequently treated with the α_1-adrenergic agent terazosin (1 mg for every hour of sleep) and doxazosin (1–2 mg for every hour of sleep), as well as with anticholinergic agents, such as benztropine (0.5–1.0 mg once or twice daily) or glycopyrrolate (1–2 mg once daily to three times a day).

Pharmacologic attempts to reduce orthostatic hypotension on antidepressants have included caffeine or cautious introduction of T_3 (25–50 μg/day); T_4 (50–200 μg/day); the mineralocorticoid fludrocortisone (0.05–0.5 mg/day); salt tablets (600–1800 mg/day); methylphenidate, or dextroamphetamine (5–20 mg/day). These measures tend to be used after other measures have failed, including efforts to maximize hydration and to improve venous return from the lower extremities by calf muscle exercises or surgical support stockings.

Nausea or indigestion that is not responsive to a change in dosing strategy or a change in preparation has been successfully treated with nizatidine (150–300 mg/day), famotidine (20–40 mg/day), or metoclopramide (5–10 mg one to two times a day). Metoclopramide, a cholinergic agonist and dopamine antagonist, has been associated rarely with extrapyramidal and dyskinetic effects, akathisia, and a case

of mania, and because it increases gastric motility, it can potentially affect the absorption of co-administered medications. With respect to the H_2 antagonists, although all can produce mood and cognitive changes, including delirium, cimetidine, which has been most closely associated with these effects, is also a potent inhibitor of CYP metabolism, rendering it least preferable among these agents for use in patients on multiple psychotropic medications. Similarly, omeprazole, an inhibitor of the gastric proton pump, appears to be an inducer of CYP 1A2 and an inhibitor of CYP 2C, and its potential impact on the metabolism of concurrent medications should therefore be considered when it is prescribed. Agents that block 5-HT_3 receptors also may help reduce nausea related to serotoninergic agents. Although ondansetron is an option, a less expensive, albeit less selective, alternative for appropriate candidates is mirtazapine.

Diarrhea not responsive to changes in preparation or dosing is often responsive to standard agents, such as loperamide or diphenoxylate. Acidophilus (1 capsule/meal) and cyproheptadine (2–4 mg one to three times a day) have also been used as anti-diarrheal strategies.

Weight gain on psychotropic medications is common, distressing, and associated with the risk of diabetes and hyperlipidemia. In addition to behavioral strategies for weight reduction, attention has also been directed toward pharmacologic strategies. The recent approval of a combination agent containing the antipsychotic, olanzapine, and the μ-opioid receptor antagonist, samidorphan, reflects one such effort to counteract weight gain on psychotropic medications. Off-label approaches to weight gain on psychotropics, including antipsychotics and antidepressants, include metformin, topiramate, zonisamide, naltrexone, and the recent glucagon-like peptide 1 (GLP-1) agonists such as semaglutide and liraglutide. Whenever possible, coordination of the prescription of agents such as the GLP-1 agonists with other members of the treatment team, such as primary care clinicians or endocrinologists, is likely to contribute to optimal monitoring and outcomes. In all cases, proactive psychoeducation as well as lifestyle modifications and nutritional counseling are integral to the mitigation of weight gain through pharmacotherapy.

Sexual dysfunction has proved to be a particularly common and troublesome side effect of antidepressants, especially the serotonergic agents, including diminished libido, erectile dysfunction, ejaculatory delay, and anorgasmia. As an alternative to switching medications (e.g., to bupropion, mirtazapine, vilazodone, vortioxetine), a variety of partly effective strategies have been marshaled for when dosage reductions or drug holidays have not been feasible. These include sildenafil (25–100 mg/day) or other phosphodiesterase 5 inhibitors; yohimbine (2.7–5.4 mg as needed up to three times a day); cyproheptadine (4–16 mg/day); amantadine (100 mg two to three times a day), buspirone (5–20 mg up to three times a day), ropinirole (0.25–4 mg/day), and bupropion (75–300 mg/day). Improvement may be limited not only by the somewhat modest ability of these agents to offset the direct effects of serotonergic agents but also by the impact of depressive or other psychiatric illness on sexual interest and by the influence of other potential psychosocial factors (e.g., self-esteem; relationship conflict).

The management of tardive dyskinesia (TD) has been advanced substantially in recent years with the introduction of vesicular monoamine transporter type II (VMAT2) inhibitors which reduce the availability of dopamine in the pre-synaptic cleft.[88] Although the first of these agents was tetrabenazine, FDA approved for chorea in Huntington disease, valbenazine and deutetrabenazine, two similar agents differing primarily in half-life, are the VMAT2 inhibitors explicitly FDA approved for the treatment of TD. As valbenazine is metabolized through CYP 3A4 and CYP 2D6 dose adjustments need to be considered when co-administered with inhibitors of either isoenzyme. By increasing valbenazine blood levels, CYP 2D6 inhibitors may enhance drowsiness on this drug as well as increase the risk of QTc prolongation, which can be clinically significant at very high doses. In contrast, potent CYP 3A4 inhibitors may reduce levels and therefore effectiveness of valbenazine. Unlike valbenazine, deutratetrabenazine is not a CYP 3A4 substrate. However, like valbenazine, it is a CYP 2D6 substrate and can also prolong QTc interval at high blood doses.

α₁-Adrenergic Antagonists

Prazosin, the α₁-adrenergic receptor antagonist antihypertensive, has been demonstrated in some but not all controlled trials to offer benefit at dosages between 1 and 10 mg for core symptoms of post-traumatic stress disorder (PTSD), particularly nightmares, insomnia, and hyperarousal.[89] Although less well studied in this context, trazodone has shown similar effects in PTSD at low to moderate doses, presumably related to its shared α₁-adrenergic receptor antagonism. Side effects of prazosin include orthostatic blood pressure changes and dizziness, with possible syncope; caution is needed when administered concurrently with other agents with α₁-adrenergic blocking properties, including low-potency antipsychotics, as well as diuretics and other agents that may cause additive hypotension. Like trazodone, prazosin has been associated with rare priapism.

α₂-Adrenergic Agonists

The antihypertensive clonidine is highly lipophilic and readily crosses the blood-brain barrier, where it stimulates α₂-adrenergic receptors, thereby inhibiting norepinephrine release. Diminution of norepinephrine results in decreases in peripheral resistance, renal vascular resistance, heart rate, and blood pressure. Introduced as a treatment for hypertension in adults, clonidine has had a broad range of psychiatric uses, including oppositional defiant disorder, sleep disturbances, substance-induced withdrawal (particularly withdrawal from opioids), Tourette syndrome, chronic headaches, and hyperactive/impulsive behaviors in patients with autism spectrum disorders, and ADHD for which its longer acting forms are FDA approved as monotherapy or adjunctive therapy with stimulants.[90-93] Guanfacine, another α₂-adrenergic receptor agonist antihypertensive drug, appears to be useful for many of the same indications as clonidine and with the potential advantages of a longer half-life and generally less sedation. The α₂-adrenergic agents can potentiate the hypotensive as well as CNS depressive effects of other agents. In addition, they have been associated with bradycardia in patients receiving agents that affect sinus node function or atrioventricular node conduction (e.g., digitalis or calcium channel blockers). Both clonidine and guanfacine can cause rebound hypertension when stopped, particularly after long-term use of moderate to high doses. Gradual taper rather than abrupt discontinuation should be considered in these settings.

β-Blockers

In addition to their role in the treatment of akathisia and tremor, the non-selective β-adrenergic receptor antagonists, which block the β_1-adrenergic receptors in the heart and brain and β_2-adrenergic receptors in the lung, blood vessels, and brain (including glial cells), have been among the first-line treatments for neurologically based aggressive behavior.[94,95]

β-Blockers (e.g., propranolol 10–40 mg or the equivalent) have been used widely to reduce symptoms associated with performance anxiety and are not uncommonly used for this purpose by musicians and public speakers. β-Blockers have had limited use for the treatment of autonomic arousal associated with other anxiety states, including social phobia, PTSD, generalized anxiety disorder, and panic disorder.[95] Although a putative association between beta blockers and depression is often cited, studies on this topic largely refute a clinically meaningful link.[96,97]

The prescription of β-blockers is potentially hazardous in a variety of common clinical conditions, including bronchospastic pulmonary diseases, insulin-dependent diabetes, hyperthyroidism, significant peripheral vascular disease, and congestive heart failure. In addition, β-blockers entirely or primarily eliminated by the liver (e.g., propranolol, metoprolol, and pindolol) may be inhibitors of, as well as substrates for, hepatic microsomal enzymes and are therefore more likely to be subject to pharmacokinetic drug interactions than β-blockers primarily cleared by the kidney (e.g., atenolol, nadolol, and sotalol).

REFERENCES

1. Delara M, Murray L, Jafari B, et al. Prevalence and factors associated with polypharmacy: a systematic review and Meta-analysis. *BMC Geriatr.* 2022;22(1):601–613.
2. Levenson JL, Ferrando SJ, eds. *Clinical Manual of Psychopharmacology in the Medically Ill.* 3rd ed. American Psychiatric Press; 2024.
3. Overall J, Gorham D. The brief psychiatric rating scale. *Psychol Rep.* 1962;10:799–812.
4. Hamilton M. Development of a rating scale for primary depressive illness. *Br J Soc Clin Psychol.* 1967;6:278–296.
5. Hamilton M. Diagnosis and rating of anxiety. *Br J Psychiatry.* 1969;3:76–79.
6. Young R, Biggs J, Ziegler V, et al. A rating scale for mania: reliability, validity and sensitivity. *Br J Psychiatry.* 1978;133:429–435.
7. Kroenke K, Spitzer RL. The PHQ-9: a new depression diagnostic and severity measure. *Psychiatr Ann.* 2002;32:509–515.
8. Rush A, Trivedi M, Ibrahim H. The 16-item quick inventory of depressive symptomatology (QIDS), clinician rating (QIDS-C), and self-report (QIDS-SR): a psychometric evaluation in patients with chronic major depression. *Biol Psychiatry.* 2003;54:573–583.
9. Spitzer RL, Kroenke K, Williams JBW, et al. A brief measure for assessing generalized anxiety disorder—the GAD-7. *Arch Intern Med.* 2006;166:1092–1097.
10. American Psychiatric Association. *Diagnostic and Statistical Manual of Mental Disorders.* 5th ed. American Psychiatric Association Publishing; 2022.
11. Guy W, ed. *Early Clinical Drug Evaluation Unit Assessment Manual for Psychopharmacology.* Department of Health, Education and Welfare Publ. No. ADM-76-338, Washington, DC, 1976. U.S. Government Printing Office.
12. Konecky B, Meyer EC, Marx BP, et al. Using the WHODAS 2.0 to assess functional disability associated with DSM-5 mental disorders. *Am J Psychiatry.* 2014;171:818–820.
13. Üstün TB, Kostanjsek N, Chatterji S, et al. *Measuring Health and Disability: Manual for WHO Disability Assessment Schedule (WHODAS 2.0).* World Health Organization; 2010.
14. Stevens JR, Jarrahzadeh T, Brendel RW, et al. Strategies for the prescription of psychotropic drugs with black box warnings. *Psychosomatics.* 2014;55:123–133.
15. Bousman CA, Bengesser SA, Aitchison KJ, et al. Review and consensus on pharmacogenomic testing in psychiatry. *Pharmacopsychiatry.* 2021;54(1):5–17.
16. Le TT, McGrath SR, Fasinu PS. Herb-drug interactions in neuropsychiatric pharmacotherapy—a review of clinically relevant findings. *Curr Neuropharmacol.* 2022;20(9):1736–1751.
17. Goldberg JF, Stahl S, eds. *Practical Psychopharmacology.* Cambridge University Press; 2021.
18. Cosci F, Chouinard G. Acute and persistent withdrawal syndromes following discontinuation of psychotropic medications. *Psychother Psychosom.* 2020;89(5):283–306.
19. Kishi T, Ikuta T, Sakuma K, et al. Antidepressants for the treatment of adults with major depressive disorder in the maintenance phase: a systematic review and network meta-analysis. *Mol Psychiatry.* 2023;28(1):402–409.
20. Tondo L, Baldessarini RJ. Discontinuing psychotropic drug treatment. *Br J Psych Open.* 2020;6(2):e24. https://doi.org/10.1192/bjo.2020.6.
21. Patchan KM, Richardson C, Vyas G, et al. The risk of suicide after clozapine discontinuation: cause for concern. *Ann Clin Psychiatry.* 2015;27:253–256.
22. Otto MW, McHugh RK, Simon NM, et al. Efficacy of CBT for benzodiazepine discontinuation in patients with panic disorder: Further evaluation. *Behav Res Ther.* 2010;48:720–727.
23. Buston ILO. Pharmacokinetics: the dynamics of drug absorption, distribution, and elimination. In: Brunton LL, Knollmann BC, eds. *Goodman and Gilman's the Pharmacological Basis of Therapeutics.* 14th ed. McGraw-Hill; 2023.
24. Sandson N. Important drug-drug interactions for the addiction psychiatrist. *Psychiatr Clin North Am.* 2022 Sep;45(3):431–450.

25. Gonzalez FJ, Coughtrie M. Drug metabolism. In: Brunton LL, Knollmann BC, eds. *Goodman and Gilman's the Pharmacological Basis of Therapeutics*. 14th ed. McGraw-Hill; 2023.

26. Alpert JE, Mischoulon D. Drug interactions in psychopharmacology. In: Stern TA, Wilens TE, Fava M, eds. *Comprehensive Clinical Psychiatry*. 3rd ed. Elsevier; 2024.

27. Ono C, Kikkawa H, Suzuki A, et al. Clinical impact of genetic variants of drug transporters in different ethnic groups within and across regions. *Pharmacogenomics*. 2013;14:1745–1764.

28. Tangamornsuksan W, Chaiyakunapruk N, Somkrua R, et al. Relationship between the HLA-B*1502 allele and carbamazepine-induced Stevens-Johnson syndrome and toxic epidermal necrolysis: a systematic review and meta-analysis. *JAMA Dermatol*. 2013;149:1025–1032.

29. Bernstein J. Medical–psychiatric drug interactions. In: Hackett T, Cassem N, eds. *Massachusetts General Hospital Handbook of General Hospital Psychiatry*. Mosby; 1978:483–507.

30. Stahl S, Felker A. Monoamine oxidase inhibitors: a modern guide to an unrequited class of antidepressants. *CNS Spectr*. 2008;13:855–870.

31. Monteith S, Glenn T. Comparison of potential psychiatric drug interactions in six drug interaction database programs: a replication study after 2 years of updates. *Hum Psychopharmacol*. 2021;36(6):e2802. https://doi.org/10.1002/hup.2802.

32. Wilkinson G. Drug metabolism and variability among patients in drug response. *N Engl J Med*. 2005;52:2211–2221.

33. Greig SL. Brexpiprazole: first global approval. *Drugs*. 2015;75:1687–1697.

34. Freudenreich O, Goff D. Antipsychotics. In: Ciraulo A, Shader R, Greenblatt D, et al., eds. *Drug Interactions in Psychiatry*. 3rd ed. Williams & Wilkins; 2005.

35. Spina E, de Leon J. Metabolic drug interactions with newer antipsychotics: a comparative review. *Basic Clin Pharmacol Toxicol*. 2007;100:4–22.

36. Beach S, Celano C, Noseworthy P, et al. QTc prolongation, torsades de pointes, and psychotropic medications. *Psychosomatics*. 2013;54:1–13.

37. Zahodne LB, Fernandez HH. Pathophysiology and treatment of psychosis in Parkinson's disease: a review. *Drugs Aging*. 2008;25:665–682.

38. Weintraub D, Aarsland D, Biundo R, et al. Management of psychiatric and cognitive complications in Parkinson's disease. *BMJ*. 2022;379:e068718. https://doi.org/10.1136/bmj-2021-068718.

39. Kalkavoura CS, Michopoulos I, Arvanitakis P, et al. Effects of cabergoline on hyperprolactinemia, psychopathology, and sexual functioning in schizophrenic patients. *Exp Clin Psychopharmacol*. 2013;21:332–341.

40. Kennedy WK, Jann MW, Kutscher EC. Clinically significant drug interactions with atypical antipsychotics. *CNS Drugs*. 2013;27:1021–1048.

41. Desai H, Seabolt J, Jann M. Smoking in patients receiving psychotropic medications: a pharmacokinetic perspective. *CNS Drugs*. 2001;15:469–494.

42. Finley PR. Drug interactions with lithium: an update. *Clin Pharmacokinet*. 2016;55:925–941.

43. De Baerdemaeker L, Audenaert K, Peremans K. Anaesthesia for patients with mood disorders. *Curr Opin Anaesthesiol*. 2005;18:333–338.

44. Takami H. Lithium in the preoperative preparation of Graves' disease. *Int Surg*. 1994;79:89–90.

45. Shah VC, Kayathi P, Singh G, et al. Enhance your understanding of lithium neurotoxicity. *Prim Care Companion CNS Disord*. 2015;17(3).

46. Keck P, Arnold L. The serotonin syndrome. *Psychiatr Ann*. 2000;30:333–343.

47. DeVane C. Pharmacokinetics, drug interactions, and tolerability of valproate. *Psychopharmacol Bull*. 2003;37:25–42.

48. Fleming J, Chetty M. Psychotropic drug interactions with valproate. *Clin Neuropharmacol*. 2005;28:96–101.

49. Circaulo D, Pacheco M, Slattery M. Anticonvulsants. In: Ciraulo DA, Shader RI, Greenblatt DJ, eds. *Drug Interactions in Psychiatry*. 3rd ed. Williams & Wilkins; 2005:293–376.

50. Tohen M, Castillo J, Pope H, et al. Concomitant use of valproate and carbamazepine in bipolar and schizoaffective disorders. *J Clin Psychopharmacol*. 1994;14:67–70.

51. Webster L, Mihaly G, Jones D, et al. Effect of cimetidine and ranitidine on carbamazepine and sodium valproate pharmacokinetics. *Eur J Clin Pharmacol*. 1984;27:341–343.

52. Patsalos P, Froscher W, Pisani F, et al. The importance of drug interactions in epilepsy therapy. *Epilepsia*. 2002;43:365–385.

53. Wang XQ, Lv B, Wang HF, et al. Lamotrigine-induced severe cutaneous adverse reaction: update data from 1999–2014. *J Clin Neurosci*. 2015;22:1005–1011.

54. Kavitha S, Anbuchelvan T, Mahalakshmi V, et al. Stevens-Johnson syndrome induced by a combination of lamotrigine and valproic acid. *J Pharm Bioallied Sci*. 2015;7:S756–S758.

55. Sabers I, Ohman J, Christensen J, et al. Oral contraceptives reduce lamotrigine plasma levels. *Neurology*. 2000;361:570–571.

56. Yassa R, Nastase C, Camille Y, et al. Carbamazepine, diuretics, and hyponatremia: a possible interaction. *J Clin Psychiatry*. 1987;48:281–283.

57. Barzman D, Delbello M. Topiramate for co-occurring bipolar disorder and disruptive behavior disorders. *Am J Psychiatry*. 2006;163:1451–1452.

58. McElroy S, Frye M, Altshuler L, et al. A 24-week, randomized, controlled trial of adjunctive sibutramine versus topiramate in the treatment of weight gain in overweight or obese patients with bipolar disorders. *Bipolar Disord*. 2007;9:426–434.

59. Guglielmo R, Martinotti G, Quatrale M, et al. Topiramate in alcohol use disorders: review and update. *CNS Drugs*. 2015;29:383–395.

60. Kampman KM, Pettinati HM, Lynch KG, et al. A double-blind, placebo-controlled trial of topiramate for the treatment of comorbid cocaine and alcohol dependence. *Drug Alcohol Depend*. 2013;133:94–99.

61. Pearl NZ, Babin CP, Catalano NT, et al. Narrative review of topiramate: clinical uses and pharmacological considerations. *Adv Ther*. 2023 Jun 27 https://doi.org/10.1007/s12325-023-02586-y.

62. Leppik I. Zonisamide: chemistry, mechanism of action, and pharmacokinetics. *Seizure*. 2004;13:S5–S9.

63. Calandre EP, Rico-Villademoros F, Slim M. Alpha$_2$delta ligands, gabapentin, pregabalin and mirogabalin: a review of their clinical pharmacology and therapeutic use. *Expert Rev Neurother.* 2016;16(11):1263–1277.

64. Abo-Zena R, Bobek M, Dweik R. Hypertensive urgency induced by an interaction of mirtazapine and clonidine. *Pharmacotherapy.* 2000;20:476–478.

65. Kinrys G, Simon N, Farach F, et al. Management of antidepressant-induced side effects. In: Alpert J, Fava M, eds. *Handbook of Chronic Depression.* Marcel Dekker; 2003:348–352.

66. Boyer E, Shannon M. Current concepts: the serotonin syndrome. *N Engl J Med.* 2005;352:1112–1120.

67. Mikkelsen N, Damkier P, Pedersen SA. Serotonin syndrome-a focused review. *Basic Clin Pharmacol Toxicol.* 2023 Aug;133(2):124–129.

68. Lorenz R, Vandenberg A, Canepa E. Serotonergic antidepressants and linezolid: a retrospective chart review and presentation of cases. *Int J Psychiatry Med.* 2008;38:81–90.

69. Vasiliu O. Esketamine for treatment-resistant depression: a review of clinical evidence (review). *Exp Ther Med.* 2023;25(3):111.

70. Walkery A, Leader LD, Cooke E, et al. Review of allopregnanolone agonist therapy for the treatment of depressive disorders. *Drug Des Devel Ther.* 2021;15:3017–3026.

71. Teply RM, Packard KA, White ND, et al. Treatment of depression in patients with concomitant cardiac disease. *Prog Cardiovasc Dis.* 2016;58(5):514–528.

72. Gardner D, Shulman K, Walker S, et al. The making of a user-friendly MAOI diet. *J Clin Psychiatry.* 1996;57:99–104.

73. Rapaport MH. Dietary restrictions and drug interactions with monoamine oxidase inhibitors: the state of the art. *J Clin Psychiatry.* 2007;68:42–46.

74. Sarafidis PA, Georgianos PI, Malindretos P, et al. Pharmacological management of hypertensive emergencies and urgencies: focus on newer agents. *Expert Opin Investig Drugs.* 2012;21:1089–1106.

75. Kaufmann W, Murray G, Cassem N. Use of psychostimulants in medically ill depressed patients. *Psychosomatics.* 1982;23:817–819.

76. Masand P, Tesar G. Use of psychostimulants in the medically ill. *Psychiatr Clin North Am.* 1996;19:515–547.

77. Wallace A, Kofoed L. West A. Double-blind, placebo-controlled trial of methylphenidate in older, depressed medically ill patients. *Am J Psychiatry.* 2005;152:929–931.

78. Breitbart W, Rosenfeld B, Kaim M, et al. A randomized, double-blind, placebo-controlled trial of psychostimulants for the treatment of fatigue in ambulatory patients with human immunodeficiency virus disease. *Arch Intern Med.* 2001;161:411–420.

79. Fawcett J, Kravitz H, Zajecka J, et al. CNS stimulant potentiation of monoamine oxidase inhibitors in treatment-refractory depression. *J Clin Psychopharmacol.* 1991;11:127–132.

80. Thomas SJ, Shin M, McInnis MG, et al. Combination therapy with monoamine oxidase inhibitors and other antidepressants or stimulants: strategies for the management of treatment-resistant depression. *Pharmacotherapy.* 2015;35:433–449.

81. Rammohan K, Rosenberg J, Lynn D, et al. Efficacy and safety of modafinil (Provigil) for the treatment of fatigue in multiple sclerosis: a two centre phase 2 study. *J Neurol Neurosurg Psychiatry.* 2002;72:179–183.

82. Schwartz T, Leso L, Beale M, et al. Modafinil in the treatment of depression with severe comorbid medical illness. *Psychosomatics* 2002;43:336–337.

83. Menza M, Kaufman K, Castellanos A. Modafinil augmentation of antidepressant treatment in depression. *J Clin Psychiatry.* 2000;61:378–381.

84. Rugino T, Copley T. Effects of modafinil in children with attention-deficit/hyperactivity disorder: an open-label study. *J Am Acad Child Adolesc Psychiatry.* 2001;40:230–235.

85. Biederman J, Mick E, Faraone S, et al. Modafinil ADHD study group: a comparison of once-daily and divided doses of modafinil in children with attention-deficit/hyperactivity disorder: a randomized, double-blind, and placebo-controlled study. *J Clin Psychiatry.* 2006;67:727–735.

86. Taylor F, Russo J. Efficacy of modafinil compared to dextroamphetamine for the treatment of attention deficit hyperactivity disorder in adults. *J Child Adolesc Psychopharmacol.* 2000;10:311–320.

87. Robertson P, Hellriegel E. Clinical pharmacokinetic profile of modafinil. *Clin Pharmacokinet.* 2003;42:123–137.

88. Bashir HH, Jankovic J. Treatment of tardive dyskinesia. *Neurol Clin.* 2020;38(2):379–396.

89. Reist C, Streja E, Tang CC, et al. Prazosin for treatment of post-traumatic stress disorder: a systematic review and meta-analysis. *CNS Spectr.* 2021;26(4):338–344.

90. Newcorn JH, Krone B, Dittmann RW. Nonstimulant treatments for ADHD. *Child Adolesc Psychiatr Clin N Am.* 2022;31(3):417–435.

91. Pringsheim T, Hirsch L, Gardner D, et al. The pharmacological management of oppositional behaviour, conduct problems, and aggression in children and adolescents with attention-deficit hyperactivity disorder, oppositional defiant disorder, and conduct disorder: a systematic review and meta-analysis. Part 1: psychostimulants, alpha-2 agonists, and atomoxetine. *Can J Psychiatry.* 2015;60(2):42–51.

92. Kosten TR, Baxter LE. Review article: Effective management of opioid withdrawal symptoms: a gateway to opioid dependence treatment. *Am J Addict.* 2019.

93. Farhat LC, Behling E, Landeros-Weisenberger A, et al. Comparative efficacy, tolerability, and acceptability of pharmacological interventions for the treatment of children, adolescents, and young adults with Tourette's syndrome: a systematic review and network meta-analysis. *Lancet Child Adolesc Health.* 2023 Feb;7(2):112–126.

94. Ward F, Tharian P, Roy M, et al. Efficacy of beta blockers in the management of problem behaviours in people with intellectual disabilities: a systematic review. *Res Dev Disabil.* 2013;34:4293–4303.

95. Boyce TG, Ballone NT, Certa KM, et al. The use of β-adrenergic receptor antagonists in psychiatry: a review. *J Acad Consult Liaison Psychiatry.* 2021;62(4):404–412.

96. Riemer TG, Villagomez Fuentes LE, Algharably EAE, et al. Do β-blockers cause depression? Systematic review and meta-analysis of psychiatric adverse events during β-blocker therapy. *Hypertension.* 2021;77(5):1539–1548.

97. Molero Y, Kaddoura S, Kuja-Halkola R, et al. Associations between β-blockers and psychiatric and behavioural outcomes: a population-based cohort study of 1.4 million individuals in Sweden. *PLoS Med.* 2023;20(1):e1004164. https://doi.org/10.1371/journal.pmed.1004164.

38

PSYCHIATRIC CONSULTATION TO CHILDREN AND ADOLESCENTS

ROBYN P. THOM, MD ■ DAVID H. RUBIN, MD ■ ERIC P. HAZEN, MD ■ ANNAH N. ABRAMS, MD ■ KHADIJAH BOOTH WATKINS, MD, MPH ■ JEFFERSON B. PRINCE, MD

OVERVIEW

Pediatric psychiatry consults are requested to address a diverse set of issues and needs. Like the work that involves adult psychiatric consultations, child psychiatrists evaluate the patient, act as a liaison to the medical and nursing staff, manage the psychiatric needs of patients and their families, and help treatment teams unite around common goals of quality care. Additionally, pediatric consultants incorporate child development into their formulation, work closely with parents or caregivers, and interact with schools and social service agencies. This chapter reviews the pediatric consultation process and highlights its main differences from adult consultations. It focuses on important developmental and family-oriented concepts, common reasons for pediatric consultation, management of concerns surrounding child maltreatment, psychological issues related to chronic medical illness in both patients and their parents, ethical issues, pediatric considerations for psychopharmacology, and future directions in the field.

Early identification of children in need of consultation remains crucial. Bujoreanu and co-workers found that earlier psychiatric consultations during an inpatient admission led to shorter hospital stays and lower hospital charges.[1] One strategy to ensure early identification is to implement routine, automatic psychiatric consultations for specific diagnoses (such as cancer, diabetes, cystic fibrosis (CF), and failure to thrive), as well as for protracted or frequent hospital stays, non-adherence with treatment regimens, and psychosocial dysfunction.

The consultant needs to be attuned to the needs of the child and the family, as well as to the dynamics of the

pediatric unit.[2,3] Assessment of how the child's situation is experienced by the pediatric team requires an awareness of the patient mix on the unit, recent deaths or other traumas, and attitudes toward certain diseases and presentations that often evoke strong emotions among staff (e.g., irritation when caring for a patient whose problems are perceived as "self-induced," such as with an eating disorder or an intentional overdose). At times, the consultant may identify a psychologically vulnerable team member who needs a referral for additional support.

Case 1

An 11-year-old boy with autism spectrum disorder (ASD) was brought to the hospital by his parents due to a significant behavioral change and agitation over the previous 3 days. He was unable to communicate verbally and was dependent on his parents for toileting and other self-care needs. He was admitted to the pediatrics service for a medical work-up to determine if there was an organic etiology for his behavioral change. Child psychiatry was consulted to help with the management of his agitation.

In the hospital, he continued to be quite agitated. He tried repeatedly to leave his room, thrashed around in his bed, made loud yelling noises, and intermittently grabbed at members of the medical team. Hospital staff expressed frustration over not knowing how to calm him, especially when his parents were asleep or away from his bedside. His parents were understandably fatigued, stressed, and frustrated. Staff wanted more guidance from the family regarding what triggered his agitation and how best to soothe him, whereas his parents were looking to the staff for answers as to why their son was agitated and they expected the staff to provide the answers. As a result, his parents expressed significant anger towards the staff. One of the child psychiatry consultant's roles was to help validate the parent's concerns, while also supporting the staff and helping them understand the reasons behind the parents' behaviors.

The consulting child psychiatrist helped develop a behavioral plan to manage the patient's challenging behaviors. This was done in collaboration with the family, occupational therapy (OT), nursing staff, child-life specialists, and the pediatrics team. A developmental framework for this boy was particularly important, given his degree of developmental delay. History from the parents revealed that he enjoyed having a stuffed dog toy in his bed, preferred specific clothing, and enjoyed certain cartoons that were usually watched by younger children. He routinely listened to music at night before going to sleep. OT brought a large exercise ball for him to bounce on, as well as other soft toys to squeeze. A customized behavioral plan was printed out and placed on his door. This included potential triggers to avoid (such as having many strangers in the room at once) and effective behavioral techniques for calming him (such as playing soothing music or using sensory toys, e.g., a squeeze ball). Recommendations for possible medications to be used in the event of severe agitation were also made.

A medical work-up revealed severe constipation that likely caused his abdominal pain and contributed to his agitation. This was treated effectively by the pediatrics team. He received rewards, such as extra time watching a preferred cartoon, when he cooperated with his treatment regimen. As his constipation resolved, his agitation improved. The consulting child psychiatrist communicated with the patient's outpatient psychiatrist to coordinate care and ensure appropriate follow-up.

THE PEDIATRIC CONSULTATION PROCESS

Initial Steps

The first step in any consultation is to understand the consultation questions (e.g., Who initiated the consultation? What concerns underlie the question? What feedback does the consultee need to be satisfied, and within what time frame?). It can also be helpful to ask whether the patient and family have been notified about the consult. Once these questions are clarified, the consultant must gather the necessary history, including data provided by members of the medical team, the hospital record, observations from staff, and collateral information from social agencies or nonparental caretakers involved in a child's care, when appropriate.

Some pediatricians are very attuned to psychological concerns and have known the patient and the family for several years. In university-affiliated hospitals, the consultant often primarily interacts with house staff who work on monthly rotating schedules and therefore plays an important teaching role. A crucial function of ongoing consultation is the trusting relationship that should develop between the pediatrician, unit personnel, and the consultant. This trust creates an atmosphere in which the psychological needs of children are recognized, and the consultant's recommendations are carried out, even when they may take additional time and effort.

In the review of the medical record, it is especially important to note the observations of the nurses and child-life specialists. These individuals often have a wealth of information from sustained contact with the child and the family. They frequently have had considerable experience with other children of a similar age and with the same diagnosis, and thus can sense how this child is coping compared to a relevant peer group. The nurse usually takes a self-care and daily habit history on admission that emphasizes the child's pre-admission level of functioning. The nurse may also record the most careful observations of the child's level of anxiety, state of aggression, and temperamental characteristics. The role of the child-life specialist, trained in development, is to help children cope with the stress of hospitalization by organizing activities and providing coping strategies for challenges such as blood draws or other medical procedures. The child-life specialist often observes how children interact with peers and uses special hospital play materials.[4] Furthermore, many pediatric inpatient services have a social worker who reviews all or some of the admissions; this expanded social history may be helpful before the consultant meets the family and the child. Staff input is a critical component of the consultant's assessment and formulation, which is usually based on only one or two interviews.

Interview Techniques for Child Psychiatric Consultation

The child and family should be prepared for the consultation. The referring physician should discuss the reasons for the referral with both the child and the parents so that the child feels included and does not feel that information is being withheld.

The interview of young children (<3 years old) requires largely indirect expressions of feelings and concerns via play and observation rather than direct questioning. The consultant's interactive style should be active, interested, and playful. Toys could include finger puppets, stuffed animals, and dolls. First, one should carry out an unstructured observation, after which a gross developmental assessment is conducted. For children in this age group, observations of the parent-child dyad are crucial. One should note: What is the eye contact like between the parent and child? Does the parent respond to cues in the child and vice versa? Does the parent provide answers to questions for the child or encourage the child to speak for themselves? Are the parent and child "in sync"? Does the child look to the parent for reassurance and comfort? What is the child's temperament like, and how does the parent handle frustration? How do the child and parent handle separation? How does the child respond to strangers? Stranger anxiety in the very young is expected, and the lack of any stranger anxiety may be a sign of attachment difficulties.

The 3- to 6-year-old child may still require that a parent be present throughout the interview. That request should be respected, although, at some point in the interview, an attempt could be made to have the parent leave the room, depending on the clinical situation. Developmental assessment, including language, social interaction, and gross and fine motor coordination, is a mandatory part of the interview. Drawings become a more important tool for some children to express troubling thoughts and feelings. The psychiatrist should not expect to complete the evaluation in one visit. It may take several sessions and the sessions may be brief. The consultant may need to arrange visits to coincide with appropriate times for observing key behaviors, such as around mealtimes or dressing changes.

The latency-age child (age 7–12 years) can be a more verbal participant in the interview. The child should be questioned about current and previous school attendance, school behavior, school performance, after-school activities, friends, health (including mental health) of family members, family problems, and interaction of family members in response to traumatic events. The mental status examination should initially focus on the manner of relating. The child may be active and verbal or shy and inhibited. The consultant's approach should be flexible, depending on the child's interactive style. The active and verbal child can be approached with a more traditional interview. The shy child may be engaged through drawings or games, such as checkers or video games. These activities can prove helpful in facilitating an alliance and demonstrating organic or developmental deficits. The first few sessions may be necessary for the child to develop trust in the consultant and recognize that they will not be performing invasive or painful procedures. Many helpful observations of the child can occur in this initial phase, including assessment of pain, anorexia, insomnia, coping strategies, and supportive comments about ways to deal with symptoms and difficult feelings.

Interviewing an adolescent (ages 13–18 years) can be more challenging with regard to building an alliance. In general, it is best to take some time to interview adolescents without their parents or guardians present to provide a space to discuss uncomfortable or sensitive topics and to ensure that their voices are heard. Many adolescents wish to have a greater sense of agency in their treatment; giving them choices, when possible, can help provide this. One such commonly offered choice is to ask who the patient would prefer that the consultant speak with first: the patient or the parent.

Some adolescents are reluctant to talk, while others express their emotions more intensely. Some adolescents give an incomplete or distorted history, making collateral information from other family members essential. In general, it is helpful to approach the adolescent in an easy-going manner. The consultant can build an alliance by providing a structure to the encounter, such as: informing the patient how long the interview might last, providing a thorough explanation and reason for the referral, clarifying the limits and expectations of the interview, addressing confidentiality and its limits, and presenting the consultant as a member of the medical team who is here to help figure out more ways to help the patient. With the frameset, adolescents often feel more in control of the encounter, which may facilitate their engagement in the interview. The consultant should also clarify with the patient what he or she understands about their medical condition and allow the patient to provide explanations from his or her point of view.

Some adolescents are reluctant to engage and merely shrug their shoulders in response to questions. It is important to recognize that silence may represent anxiety and vulnerability, rather than disinterest. It may be helpful to initiate the interview by asking about some safe topics, such as a sporting event, a television show, or a question about a photo or other belongings in the hospital room. Making empathic statements that address common issues, such as anxiety and the shocking novelty of being sick in the hospital, may also help facilitate more sharing.

Liaison With the Medical Team

Child psychiatric consultation usually involves contact with more people than just the patient and the referring physician. Parents are inherently a part of the treatment, as they provide critical information and need to be actively involved in the implementation of treatment recommendations. In addition, nurses may assume some parental roles while the pediatric unit serves as the child's temporary home. Child and family behaviors can impact staff and evoke intense feelings. Lastly, patients with a chronic illness may return repeatedly to the same pediatric floor over a 5- to 10-year period. Thus many children become well known to the staff, and the depth of the staff's involvement grows year by year. Unavoidably, primary nurses often become intensely involved in the child's personal and family life; thus they have critical information and share the stress of the child's illness. Child psychiatric consultation includes an essential liaison role that is relevant to the care of patients and their families, inter-staff tensions, and the stress of individual staff members. The child psychiatrist can provide suggestions and supervision for dealing with difficult families or crises, review when a psychiatric referral is indicated,

and help in understanding the painful issues of chronic disease, suicide, and terminal illness.

For house staff, a common stressor is being relatively inexperienced and yet confronted by complex medical and psychological circumstances. This source of stress is clearest in the intensive care unit, where frustration mounts rapidly as children may not respond to treatment and can suffer lifelong physical and neurologic damage. The consequences of multiple stressors (e.g., frustration with the patient's course, lack of sleep, and feeling incompetent) may lead to depression, substance abuse, or bitter tensions among house staff or nurses.

Part of the child psychiatrist's liaison function is to attend rounds, be aware of difficult clinical and family situations, get to know nurses and house staff through teaching and informal discussion concerning patients, and be aware of the early signs of behaviors that are destructive to patient care and staff. With sufficient credibility, the child psychiatric consultant can organize family or multi-disciplinary staff meetings that have a beneficial impact on the unit's functioning and can relieve family or staff suffering.

DEVELOPMENTAL AND FAMILY-CENTERED APPROACHES TO CONSULTATION

In assessing a hospitalized child, the consultant must appreciate how the child's current presentation can be understood in the context of his or her baseline level of functioning and behavior, as well as relative to other children in the same developmental phase. The consultant uses a developmental perspective, informed by collateral data regarding temperament, pre-morbid personality, and the family's functioning to evaluate the child's behavior, emotional state, and defensive style.

Knowledge of psychological defense mechanisms provides insight into how children and their families cope with illness and hospitalization. Defenses (including denial, isolation of affect, and intellectualization) help with the modulation of anxiety.[5] For example, a teenager with CF may use isolation of affect and intellectualization when discussing what is needed for lung transplantation. An example of effective denial is the 10-year-old child with terminal cancer who is invested in completing his schoolwork and getting promoted to the fifth grade; this can maintain a sense of hope and future orientation, which can preserve day-to-day functioning. The use of an array of defenses that permits adherence to one's health care and facilitates investment in age-appropriate activities should be supported. However, when denial is used by a withdrawn child, it can mask psychopathology and prevent referral.[6]

Infancy

For the hospitalized infant, the key developmental challenge is to maintain the quality of the attachment between the parent and the child. The parental component of attachment begins while anticipating the infant's birth or adoption. An infant is a parent's most personal product, embodying the hopes that their child will ultimately possess the strengths and values the parent most values in himself or herself, and the wish that their child will have capacities that offset the parent's self-perceived deficiencies. No infant can meet each of the parents' conscious and unconscious expectations, yet most infants are accepted and loved when they enter the world. Parents adapt to the reality of the infant and embark on the lifelong process of attachment that enables the child and their parent to weather the stresses and strains of caretaking and growing up while remaining committed and connected.

Several parent and infant factors can affect attachment. The psychiatric consultant may be called on to differentiate between depression, character pathology, or anxious adjustment in the setting of inadequate parental attachment. Infants with medical conditions that interfere with feeding, limit access to holding and soothing, affect appearance, or cause irritability, present special challenges to the process of attachment. Ill infants require parents to be more mature because the unexpected circumstances they face may leave a parent feeling incompetent or unloved by the newborn. The medical staff can play a crucial role in successfully supporting new parents through this difficult early phase.

Infants and toddlers are largely non-verbal and rely on a small, consistent number of caretakers who know them well enough to be attuned to their non-verbal communications. Therefore the infant's experience of the stress of hospitalization is exacerbated by separations from the mother or primary caretaker. In response to the findings of short-term and long-term consequences of maternal separations, hospitals encourage mothers to stay overnight with children and to participate in their child's care. In addition, many nursing departments have instituted a primary nursing model to limit the number of nurses who care for each child.

Pre-School Age

Medical conditions in the pre-school phase (ages 3–6 years) are affected by three important aspects of the child's emotional and cognitive development: egocentricity, magical thinking, and body image anxiety. Egocentricity is the child's perception that all life events revolve around him or her. The child cannot imagine that others see the world from a vantage point different from his or her own. Magical thinking is the creative weaving of reality and fantasy to explain how things occur in the world. The combination of egocentricity and magical thinking may lead the pre-school-aged child to imagine that medical conditions are a punishment for the child's bad thoughts or deeds. For example, a 4-year-old with leukemia reported that he got his "bad cells" from eating too many cookies. The young child needs ongoing support from family and medical staff to understand that the medical condition is not punishment or due to some unrelated experience. Without this support, the child's anxiety is likely to be much greater and be expressed as inhibition and withdrawal, or as behavioral outbursts. One understanding of the cause of body image anxiety comes from the preschooler's cognitive development, which leads the child to envision the body as a shell (skin) filled with blood, food, and stool, which could ooze out of any hole in the skin. This concept of the body being like a tire or water balloon that can be punctured with dire results may explain the preoccupation with bandages at this age, as well as the fear of needle sticks and surgical procedures that seem to exceed what can be explained by painful experiences alone.

Some regression is to be expected in the stressed preschooler.[6] This may take the form of enuresis in a previously toilet-trained child, increased dependence on parents for help with dressing or eating, episodes of unwillingness to use words to express their wishes, or the return of "baby talk." Each of these regressed behaviors serves to engage parents and nursing staff in a style of caretaking that may be more commonly associated with a baby or a toddler.

Several treatment approaches can help the pre-schooler adjust to medical illnesses and interventions and that can minimize regression. Pain should be controlled or eliminated whenever possible, even when it is not the fastest way to proceed. Procedures should be explained in simple terms to the child. The child needs to hear in the most basic terms what will be done, why it is needed, and what parts will be uncomfortable or painful. They will want to know where their parents will be before, during, and after the procedure. Interventions should be performed in designated locations, such as treatment rooms, and there should be safety zones, usually the child's hospital room and the playroom, in which no procedures are done. Children of all ages must have safe places within the hospital setting so that they are not on "high alert" at all times. Similarly, warning children about impending procedures may lead to protest acutely, but over time allows children to relax and not be constantly anticipating an unpleasant "surprise attack."

School Age

School age (6–12 years), also referred to as latency age, is characterized by a host of new and developing skills in many arenas—academic, athletic, and artistic. The world outside the family becomes more important with the advent of best friends and status in friendship or interest groups. In the context of medical illness, the age-appropriate investment in mastery of skills may lead to improved coping with a better understanding of medical illnesses (although still rudimentary); pride in learning to anticipate regular treatments, medications, and procedures; better capacity to verbalize needs; and, establishment of relationships with nursing staff and physicians. Children with pre-morbid competencies may weather the stress of illness somewhat better than their less capable peers. The stress of medical conditions, however, routinely leads to regression in all age groups, so the improved coping skills associated with latency may not be observed in the hospital setting. Regression is common early in chronic illnesses, with the potential for developing better coping after there has been time for adjustment. The level of function fluctuates according to the individual stressors (e.g., mood, malaise, pain, procedures, and prognostic

changes) and family function. Offering age-appropriate activities (such as board games, video games, computers, puzzles, arts and crafts), and school tutors, helps children to function closer to their pre-morbid level and serves as a counterweight to the regressive pull of dependency, helplessness, and loss of control that often accompanies hospitalization. Later in a chronic illness, flexible denial can be a healthy component of coping. Flexible denial denotes the child's ability to suppress thoughts about the illness and to invest in an array of activities, without abandoning the appropriate measures necessary for the treatment of the illness.

It is common for latency-age children to have distorted or magical notions about the cause of the illness, which are typical of the thinking of younger children. It is helpful to invite all questions—by saying things like "I like to hear what children wonder about" or "There is no such thing as a silly question"—and invite fantasies about the medical condition by direct questions, such as "What do you think might have caused your cancer?" Creative outlets for expression, such as drawings or stories, can help to elucidate the fears that underlie the child's anxiety.

With chronic illnesses, the latency-age years offer a less conflicted opportunity to foster positive health-related behaviors. The child should be able to give a simple, accurate explanation of the illness. The child should be learning the names of medications, their purpose, and when they are to be taken. At this age, a partially independent relationship between the child and the treating physician can be developed. Psychiatric intervention is warranted if the child is resistant to learning about the illness, if the child is regressed, if parents are noted to be intrusive or over-involved in the healthcare regimen, or if non-adherence to the medical treatment plan has become a means of fighting between child and parent. Allowing these patterns to proceed into adolescence will likely increase the risk of dysfunction and make intervention more difficult.

Adolescence

Most adolescents, like adults, enter medical settings with the capacity to understand the meaning of an illness, including its possible ramifications. Developmentally, adolescents venture out with a more independent posture and leave behind their intense dependency on their parents, which is seen in younger children. This brings with it a particular sensitivity and vulnerability. The multiple demands of hospitalization (including deciphering the meaning of diagnoses and treatments while bearing the physical discomfort, limitations, pain, impact on appearance, and fears about the present and future) may overwhelm the adolescent's ability to exercise newly acquired independence in a developmentally appropriate way. The physical limitations imposed by illness may put adolescents at risk for major depression, especially when the illness interferes with activities that are key to the adolescent's emerging self-image.[7]

The assault on a teenager's autonomy may be particularly difficult to bear because it coincides with the strong developmental pull to individuate from parents and establish an independent identity. Often the illness occurs at a time when other tensions arise between the adolescent and their parent, making reliance on the parents uncomfortable or unacceptable. Faced with this emotionally complex dilemma, some teens become sullen, aggressive, non-adherent, or withdrawn, whereas others negotiate the discomfort of returning to a more dependent, supportive relationship with their parents.

Interview styles should respect the adolescent's wish for autonomy. One should engage the adolescent first before looking to the parents for their input. Sexual experiences or concerns and worries about parental coping or even death may not be voiced without privacy. The risks and benefits of treatments need to be presented to the adolescent with the recognition that his or her adherence is central to the success or failure of any treatment plan.

Family-Centered Care

The child cannot be understood separately from the family. Serious or chronic illness in a child is a family crisis. Parents must cope with uncertainty as well as the highs and lows associated with hospitalization. Abnormal laboratory results, adverse reactions, life-threatening crises, limitations on the child's future, and the specter of death suddenly become their reality. They observe their child in distress and they often feel fundamentally unable to protect the child. The hospital environment brings with it a host of medical professionals with as many personalities as there are consultants and caregivers; often, each seems to hold a crucial piece of the puzzle. Small nuances in the presentation of data or differing styles of optimism or pessimism among staff may radically shift the family's mood.

Parental anxiety negatively affects the child's capacity to cope; yet to expect a parent to be other than anxious is unthinkable.[8,9] Parents are the child's most trusted and valuable resource; therefore strategies to support parents are crucial. Most parents evoke staff empathy and appreciate the treatment team's skill and compassion. Certain parents are challenging to support because of a combination of personality characteristics and coping styles. Their distress, often fueled by a sense of helplessness, may be expressed either by devaluing staff or as an apparent insensitivity to the sick child's needs. The consultant helps the team of caregivers understand the psychological meaning of the parents' troubling behavior so that they can continue to provide optimal care.[10,11]

Siblings are often the forgotten sufferers in the context of chronic or life-threatening illness.[12,13] They worry about their sick sibling and often lose the support of their parents. The parents may be physically absent, spending time at the hospital with the ill child, and attempting to meet at least minimal work demands to support the family financially. They are often emotionally absent, depressed, or drained by the emotional demands of the sick child. Many parents feel angry at the good siblings for making any demands and for not selflessly understanding the seriousness of the ill child's predicament. This compounds the siblings' guilt in response to the predictable feelings of resentment and jealousy toward the ill child who is receiving so much attention. If the illness results in death, the feelings of guilt and responsibility may become overwhelming.

A carefully planned family meeting can begin to clarify distortions, reduce family turmoil, improve coping skills, and dispel conflict between family and staff. During the meeting, the staff or the psychiatrist should evaluate the family's psychological state, which includes an assessment of coping mechanisms, their anxiety level, available support, and ability to comprehend information.

REASONS FOR CONSULTATION REQUESTS

The child psychiatry consult practice pattern study by Shaw and associates[14] listed the most common reasons for consultation as: (1) conducting a suicide assessment (78.5% of survey responders indicated this as a common consult question), (2) creating a differential diagnosis for medically unexplained symptoms (72.3%), (3) facilitating adjustment to illness, including depression and anxiety (58.5% and 55.4%, respectively), (4) evaluating the need for psychotropic medications (49.2%), (5) diagnosing and managing delirium (29.2%), (6) treating non-adherence (24.6%), and (7) managing psychiatric patients who are boarding on medical floors (23.1%).[14] Consultants can also be called on to address behavioral difficulties that contribute to hospitalization, behavioral difficulties during the hospitalization that compromise optimal medical care, child maltreatment in the form of physical or sexual abuse or medical neglect, and children and families who must cope with a life-threatening or chronic illness.[14]

Primary Psychiatric Illnesses

Depression

Depression is a common condition in hospitalized children. It may be a response to having an acute or chronic illness, or it may be the primary diagnosis and present with somatic symptoms or behavioral problems. One of the obstacles to making a diagnosis of depression in the hospitalized child is the misconception that the child's dysphoric mood is appropriate to the stress of the situation, and it therefore does not deserve to be called depression. On the contrary, stress increases the likelihood that depression will occur; it does not invalidate the diagnosis.

Like adults, children and adolescents can develop a variety of depressive disorders (including major depressive disorder [MDD]; persistent depressive disorder; mood disturbances that are associated with medical conditions; substance-induced mood disorders; or an adjustment to psychosocial problems).

In medical settings, clinicians are challenged to differentiate transient symptoms of depression from true depressive disorders. Children and adolescents often manifest symptoms that resemble depression (including worry, hopelessness, sadness, anger, or withdrawal as a response to their medical illness or the stress of hospitalization). The consultant needs to distinguish between a depressive disorder and a reaction to illness or its treatment. If the symptoms occur only in certain contexts (such as in the hospital) or are associated with limited impairment, they are generally considered to be an adjustment disorder with a depressed or anxious mood. These patients usually respond to reassurance, environmental intervention, or interpersonal or cognitive-behavioral therapy.

Although the criteria for depression are the same for children and adults, there are some differences in how the symptoms manifest. For children younger than 6 years of age, the hallmarks of depression often include a poor appetite or a failure to grow and gain weight appropriately, a disturbance of sleep, hypoactivity, and an indifference to their surroundings and primary caretakers. Pre-pubertal children with an episode of MDD can present with separation anxiety, somatic complaints, irritability, or behavioral problems.[15] These children may not give an accurate self-assessment of sustained mood, so dysphoria must be observed by caretakers over a prolonged period. Making the diagnosis of depression can be difficult in children who are sick because many of the symptoms they exhibit (e.g., decreased energy or loss of appetite) may be attributed to their medical illness.[16] In addition, children who are sick often use denial as a coping mechanism and under-report their symptoms.[17]

Treatment of depression frequently involves psychotherapy, as well as consultation with a child-life and recreational therapist to support the child and family; sometimes, therapy is used in conjunction with an antidepressant medication. Unfortunately, the pharmacotherapy of youth with depression is less straightforward than it is with adults. Unlike in adults, tricyclic antidepressants are not an effective treatment for adolescents with depression. Fluoxetine, a selective serotonin reuptake inhibitor (SSRI), has seemed effective in meta-analyses[18] and randomized controlled trials.[19-21] Escitalopram, another SSRI, is

US Food and Drug Administration (FDA) approved for the treatment of adolescent depression, but the evidence is inconsistent for other antidepressants.

Update on Antidepressant-Associated Suicidality

In 2004 the FDA issued a black box warning describing the probable risk of increased suicidality in children and adolescents using antidepressant medications and suggested close monitoring for side effects and response in youth. The following year, antidepressant manufacturers were required to include a black box warning on antidepressant product labels.[22] Then, in 2007, the FDA updated the warning on antidepressants to include young adults (aged 18–24 years) during initial antidepressant treatment.

The FDA black box labeling of antidepressant medications for the pediatric population has had far-reaching consequences. Some authors[23] reported a 47% reduction in the use of antidepressants in the United States from 2002 to 2006 among patients aged 5 to 21 years, who had not previously been exposed to antidepressants. Interestingly, antidepressant rates remained the same in this age group for those who had been previously exposed to treatment.[23] Researchers[24] found a decrease in the use of all SSRIs in the pediatric population after the FDA issued its 2004 advisory; others[25] showed that fluoxetine prescriptions increased for those newly prescribed an antidepressant following the regulatory action. Moreover, after the FDA's warnings, prescribing clinicians reported that 14% to 22% of guardians and 9% of pediatric patients refused treatment with antidepressants.[24,26] The most serious and unintended effect of FDA advisories may have been on pediatric suicides. Gibbons and co-workers[27] provided a comparative study of suicide prevalence rates in the pediatric populations in the United States and the Netherlands, pre- and post-regulatory agency warnings. This study showed that, after 2003, antidepressant prescription rates in the United States decreased for all groups under the age of 60 years. The decrease in SSRI prescription rates in youth occurred at a time when the suicide rate *increased* by 14% from 2003 to 2004 among children and adolescents.[28]

Suicide risk in relation to antidepressant use remains controversial.[28,29] Several studies, including a meta-analysis, suggest a significant association with such risk,[29] especially in young people. Individuals younger than 25 years of age treated with antidepressants are more likely than older adults to develop thoughts about suicide. However, a large meta-analysis[30] showed that the benefits of such treatments still outweighed the risks (number needed to treat 10 vs. number needed to harm 143).

Suicide

Suicide is the second leading cause of death among adolescents and young adults aged 10 to 25 years in the United States, accounting for nearly 17% of all deaths in this age group; furthermore, the frequency of suicide in this age group appears to be on the rise.[31] In most cases, children who have made a suicide attempt must remain in the hospital or another secure facility until a thorough evaluation has been completed and an appropriate disposition has been decided. This may occur via admission to the pediatric service, in conjunction with crisis intervention services in the emergency department (ED), or in some cases, by direct transfer to a psychiatric facility.

During the assessment of a potentially suicidal child, one should:

1. Gather details of the suicide attempt, including access to potentially lethal means (e.g., firearms, pills, a rope).
2. Assess the risk of an attempt—What did the child imagine would happen? What was the likelihood of rescue?
3. Determine the child's mind-set at the time of the attempt—Was there a clear precipitant? Was it an impulsive or a planned act? What prompted the attempt on that specific day?
4. Obtain a history of any suicide attempts in the patient, family members, or peers.
5. Pursue the child's understanding of death and fantasy of what his or her death would elicit in the family or other significant person (such as a boyfriend or girlfriend).
6. Ask about the child's feelings of remorse about the attempt or regrets about having survived.
7. Assess whether the child expresses feelings of hopelessness, helplessness, or despair.
8. Assess whether sexual orientation and/or gender identity are relevant issues, including familial or

peer rejection, societal discrimination, bullying, or abuse.[32,33]

9. Assess how their racial or ethnic identity fits into the context of their community, and the extent of marginalization and vulnerability as a result of their minority status.
10. Assess whether the child is lonely or emotionally disconnected from others.
11. Determine whether the child used drugs or alcohol at the time of the attempt.
12. Determine whether the child is depressed, manic, or psychotic.
13. Determine whether the child identifies with someone who has committed suicide.
14. Assess the probability of physical or sexual maltreatment.
15. Conduct a family interview. Determine whether the parents are sad and frightened by the attempt or angry at the child for being manipulative.
16. Learn about therapeutic interventions that have been tried in the past. What is in place currently, and how good has adherence been with outpatient treatment?

The consultant is initially asked to decide on the appropriate safety management for the suicidal child. This may include one or more of the following: one-to-one supervision, restrictions on movements around the unit or hospital, restrictions on access to potentially harmful objects, such as sharp objects or ligatures (which may require a search of the belongings to which the patient has access in the hospital), and strategies for managing potential agitation. Ultimately the consultant needs to perform a thorough risk assessment and determine whether the child or adolescent should be psychiatrically hospitalized or managed as an outpatient (while either living at home or in another setting). Indications for psychiatric hospitalization include the serious risk of death through suicide; little wish to be rescued; psychosis; identification with someone who has committed suicide; co-morbid drug or alcohol abuse; intense feelings of hopelessness and helplessness; intense anger or severe depression; lack of support systems; history of inability to use help; and vulnerability to further losses. Appropriate outpatient or day treatment will be required if the patient is not transferred to a psychiatric facility. In this case, it is important to educate and engage the patient and his or her family in safety planning. This includes developing a plan for dealing with a crisis (such as contact information for treaters and access to hotlines), directing attention to limiting the availability of lethal means of suicide, such as guns and medications (including over-the-counter medications, such as acetaminophen), and emphasizing the need for vigilance about likely environmental contributors to suicidal behavior (such as substances and psychosocial stress).

Feeding and Eating Disorders

Anorexia nervosa (AN) is an illness characterized by significantly low weight in the context of a fear of gaining weight and/or a distorted perception of the thin body as fat. Amenorrhea is also a symptom of AN in post-menarche females; however, it is no longer a criterion for diagnosis in the DSM-5.[34] The onset of AN is typically in mid-to-late adolescence (14–18 years) and is predominantly seen in females[34]; onset may be associated with a stressful life event. Hospitalization of afflicted children is usually associated with severe weight loss, cardiovascular abnormalities (usually bradycardia), hypothermia, or electrolyte imbalance. Electrolyte disturbances may reflect binging or purging, which can include vomiting or the misuse of laxatives and/or diuretics. The goal of pediatric hospitalization is medical stabilization; additional interventions in the hospital are nutritional assessment and treatment, psychological assessment of the child and family, and recommendations for appropriate levels of psychiatric intervention after medical stabilization.[35] The assessment as to whether medical stabilization must be followed by an intensive day or inpatient psychiatric treatment includes determination of the adolescent's recognition that he or she has a problem with eating behaviors and self-image, the adolescent's motivation to participate in treatment (e.g., is he or she in denial about the eating disorder and resistant to eating the adequate nutrition presented in the hospital diet), and the parents' ability to support the adolescent and the need for treatment.

The DSM-5 introduced a new diagnosis related to disordered eating, Avoidant/Restrictive Food Intake Disorder (ARFID).[34] ARFID is characterized by an eating or feeding disturbance that leads to significant weight loss, nutritional deficiency, dependence on enteral feeding or oral nutritional supplements, and/ or a significant impact on psychosocial functioning. Unlike AN, ARFID is not associated with body image distortion. Clinically, ARFID is seen in children who have a fear of aversive consequences (e.g., choking, vomiting), lack of interest in food or eating, or severe food selectivity due to sensory sensitivities. It is important to note that ARFID is intended to describe patients who are malnourished. Children who are simply "picky eaters" but otherwise healthy and medically stable would not qualify for a diagnosis of ARFID.

The consultant will be called on to assist with the assessment and management of a child with eating issues as well as to give recommendations about disposition once the patient is medically stable. Placement is based on whether the child or adolescent can live at home safely while consuming adequate calories and attending outpatient treatment appointments (e.g., psychotherapy, nutrition, and pediatric visits) versus the need for a more intensive and structured program (such as a day treatment or residential eating disorder unit). Often, the consultant, in conjunction with the social worker, spends a significant amount of time helping the parents accept the plan for psychotherapeutic treatment, especially if the team recommends that the patient not return home.

Somatic Symptoms and Related Disorders

Some patients present to their pediatrician with intense somatic complaints (e.g., headaches, abdominal pain, constipation, dysmenorrhea, fatigue). In general, when cases are referred for psychiatric consultation, the pediatrician suspects that the intensity or the nature of the complaints is more likely to be an expression of emotional factors than a medical condition. Somatic symptoms and related disorders, as described in the DSM-5-TR, refer to a cluster of physical symptoms suggestive of a medical condition, but the severity of the symptoms or the level of functional impairment is not fully explained by the medical condition.[34] Although the DSM-5-TR lists specific disorders, including somatic symptom disorder, illness anxiety disorder, and functional neurological disorder/conversion disorder, the criteria for these conditions were established for adults. Often, children do not meet the full criteria for these specific

diagnoses. Recurrent somatic complaints are common in the pediatric population and are a frequent reason for psychiatric consultation. There may also be developmental considerations, with pre-pubertal children most often presenting with recurrent abdominal pain or headaches, while older children present with other types of pain and neurologic symptoms.[36]

The pediatrician's assessment that symptoms are psychological in origin, is often at odds with the patient's and the parents' assessment. With psychosomatic illnesses, the child and family may be highly invested in having a medical cause to explain the somatic complaints. They are not reassured by routine medical work-ups and they may pressure the physician to continue to search for a medical cause. Although the families of children who somatize have been found to have higher rates of anxiety and depression and to be more dysfunctional than other families,[37] they are often resistant to undergoing psychiatric assessment. Parents may view any suggestion of the important role of psychological factors as an insult and as an indication that the clinician does not believe that the symptoms are real. They often prefer that their children have more radiologic scans and procedures for the assessment of abdominal pain than further discussions about stressors (such as school difficulty, family loss or death, and parental discord) that might impact a child's presentation. Often the child and parents focus on minimally abnormal test results and pressure the physician to pursue these findings. They may connect a series of irrelevant bits of data to create a medical theory that is not endorsed by the pediatrician. Some families seek multiple specialists in an attempt to find someone who will support their medical theory. Unfortunately, if the parents search long enough, they will find a specialist who will ignore the psychological factors and validate the parents' perspective or a more junior clinician who lacks the clinical experience to stop the "rule-out approach." If the psychological issues are not attended to, the condition is likely to become chronic and result in significant morbidity. The presenting somatic symptoms serve as a solution, albeit a maladaptive one, to an emotional dilemma.

The psychiatric consultant is well-positioned to advocate for a balanced view of attention to medical and psychological factors when a somatic symptom disorder is on the list of possible diagnoses. This includes keeping in mind that it is not necessary to come to a conclusive diagnosis immediately, despite the wishes of the family. The consultant can assist the team in limiting the pursuit of equivocal organic findings without sacrificing a complete and appropriate medical work-up. It is often helpful to focus on improving function, such as returning to school and activities and gaining mobility, rather than on emphasizing the importance of a final, definitive diagnosis.

Campo and Fritz[38] proposed a method for assessing and managing pediatric somatization that includes the key elements in the assessment: acknowledgment of patient suffering and family concerns; exploration of prior assessments and treatment; investigation of patient and family fears provoked by the symptoms; maintenance of alertness to the possibility that unrecognized physical disease and communications are at play; avoidance of unnecessary tests and procedures; avoidance of diagnosis by exclusion; and, exploration of symptom timing, context, and characteristics. Mainstays of management include honesty, reassurance, emphasis on the rehabilitative approach (as opposed to the curative approach) to symptoms, and consideration of family and group interventions in addition to individual management and consolidation of care.

Therapeutic interventions for patients who somatize include a medical-psychiatric team approach that emphasizes a consistent relationship among clinicians, the child, and the family. It is important to foster the continued presence of the pediatrician, because there may be a tendency for the pediatrician to withdraw after a psychiatric referral has been made. If the family believes the presence of the psychiatrist leads to diminished access to the pediatrician, there may be escalating anxiety about physical symptoms, and it may become difficult for the psychiatrist to maintain a critical alliance with the family. Pediatric re-examination without re-testing helps calm the family's medical anxiety and reduces the likelihood of continued doctor shopping. Ongoing psychoeducation from team members can help the family re-frame the medical symptoms and enhance communication with caregivers. Inpatient pediatric rehabilitation may sometimes be necessary to address the physical components of the presentation and allow the child to regain strength and function in a supportive environment.

Often the child and family need different forms of psychotherapy to allow the child to let go of somatic symptoms and to move on to a healthy role. The child's medical symptoms frequently serve to stabilize the family system; therefore family therapy may be required to change patterns of interactions. Couples therapy may also be used to help parents strengthen their adult relationship, so the child's illness is not needed to hold the couple together or to distract them from their discord. A child's therapy helps to build self-esteem and allows the child to engage in developmentally appropriate activities that can increase his or her sense of agency or mastery, which leads to greater confidence and less of a need to rely on the sick role. Co-morbid psychiatric disorders in the child or family members must also be identified and treated appropriately, with the use of pharmacological agents as needed.

Psychiatric Factors That Affect Medical Illness

Medical illness and psychiatric illness are frequently co-morbid. Studies have shown higher rates of mental health problems in youth with a variety of chronic medical illnesses,[38,39] such as asthma,[40–42] diabetes,[43,44] epilepsy,[45–47] and inflammatory bowel disease.[48–50] In addition to the impact of illness-related symptoms and impairments on psychological function, complex interactions can arise among psychiatric factors and the symptoms, severity, complications, and even treatment of a medical illness. Patients and families who have experienced fear and helplessness in the course of life-threatening pediatric illness and treatment may develop post-traumatic symptoms of intrusive thoughts, hyperarousal, and avoidance.[51] Future medical care can then be complicated by post-traumatic symptoms that have been triggered by the medical setting.

Pediatricians typically rely on parental reports of young children and self-reports in older children to assess the need for intervention in many chronic conditions. When anxiety, dysphoria, emotional lability, or apathy arise, this increased distress often leads to a greater degree of medical interventions. In a study of patients with asthma, steroid prescription was correlated with patients' expressed anxiety about an exacerbation and not with the degree of change on pulmonary function tests.[52] Follow-up studies have categorized this expressed anxiety as "dysfunctional breathing," and cautioned medical providers to distinguish between the two.[53,54] Apathy or dysphoria in a patient with severe lung disease (e.g., CF), can lead to less therapeutic coughing and significant pulmonary compromise. Apathy (e.g., due to frustration or helplessness in a child undergoing rehabilitation) may interfere with physical therapy. Motivation is often a function of mood, and it is an essential feature of the sense of mastery and agency that is associated with striving toward maximal health. To help children become invested in their own best level of function, it is necessary to understand the emotional issues that impede the health-seeking process.

To understand the psychiatric factors involved in coping one should:

1. Ask the child what aspects of the illness and treatments are most difficult or frightening for him or her.
2. Invite the child to describe his or her own treatment goals and any disappointments experienced while reaching those goals.
3. Pursue the child's experience of how the illness and treatment affect his or her life outside of the hospital.
4. Learn whether the child feels that someone understands what it is like to be him or her.
5. Find out whether there is someone the child is particularly disappointed in for not understanding. Has the child felt deceived by anyone?
6. Determine whether the child knows someone with this condition, how that person's condition has evolved, and why.
7. Know the condition and its evolution.
8. Learn about the worst thing that could happen from the patient's point of view.

The physicians' goals are sometimes at odds with the child's goals. For example, a teenage girl who suffered a stroke but did not want to walk "like an old lady" with a cane, was sullen in rehabilitation because she did not want to give up her crutches. The many disappointments during hospitalization and unexpected re-hospitalizations are compounded when a patient feels that his opinion was not sought or that her best efforts still resulted in setbacks, leading to anger, frustration, mistrust, anxiety, or apathy.[55,56] Engaging the child in voicing his or her experience may be therapeutic in and of itself. There may be ways of altering the hospital protocols to suit the child or adapting the child's treatment program to accommodate home-life priorities. The consultant is asked to assist the child during the hospital stay and to determine whether outpatient psychotherapy is warranted. Knowing how time is spent outside of the hospital and what the content of the frustrations covers informs this decision. Psychopharmacologic interventions may also be helpful, depending on the symptoms and the psychiatric diagnoses.

Behavioral Factors That Affect Health Outcomes

Accidents and non-adherence with medical regimens are the two major categories of behavioral difficulties that lead to the hospitalization of children.

Accidents

Unintentional injury remains the number one cause of death among all children and young adults.[31] All children experience accidents, but they are more likely to occur in children who are reckless, active, impulsive, or inadequately supervised. It is necessary to entertain the possibility that an accidental injury could be the result of maltreatment, an act of intentional self-injury, a suicide attempt, or related to a medical/psychiatric condition (e.g., attention deficit hyperactivity disorder [ADHD], fetal alcohol syndrome, lead exposure). When a child presents with an accidental injury, an assessment must be made as to whether the supervision has been adequate for the child's age; this usually involves an assessment of the parents or other caretakers. Supervision, particularly in younger children, plays a significant role in maintaining child safety. Adolescents tend to view themselves as invulnerable; therefore they may be prone to greater risk-taking and accidents. The following information about the patient's behavior before the accident can clarify whether there is a medical or psychiatric etiology related to the accident:

1. Has the child had behavioral difficulty in school, at home, or with peers?
2. Has there been a change in the child's mood?
3. Is there evidence of a thought disorder?

4. Have there been problems leading to legal interventions?

5. Are these worrisome behaviors new or are they longstanding?

Non-adherence

Non-adherence may be secondary to an inadequate understanding of, or capacity to implement, the intended medical regimen. Often non-adherence is not an active decision to defy treatment recommendations. Instead, it may result from the patient being overwhelmed by a medical regimen or being tired of its chronicity. Some children leave the hospital on numerous medications that are to be administered several times each day. Simplifying medication regimens as much as possible and having honest dialogues with parents and children about what is realistic at home is recommended. Highlighting critical medications and the consequences of not taking them engages the child and family as educated and informed collaborators in the child's health care.

Patients and families who are refractory to simple educational interventions to improve adherence may benefit from a more intensive intervention to address the issue, and the medical team may seek the consultant's input. Kahana and co-workers'[57] meta-analyses evaluated how effective psychological interventions were in promoting adherence to pediatric chronic illness. They concluded that adherence was most likely to be improved by interventions that emphasized applied behavioral methods (such as problem solving or parent training), or multi-component interventions, usually incorporating combined behavioral and educational treatments. Notably, education-only interventions did not lead to improved adherence.[57] As one might expect, these psychological interventions led to brief improvements and effects that were lost over time; this suggests that adherence-focused interventions likely need to be carried out over the long term.[57]

There can be many socioeconomic, emotional, and psychodynamic issues that lead children or parents to actively or passively disregard medical recommendations. For example, socioeconomic factors (such as low maternal education, low income, and households where mothers are not full-time caregivers) have been associated with decreased adherence in the pediatric cancer population.[58] Common emotional and psychodynamic issues that contribute to non-adherence include denial (on the part of parents and children) and anger. With regards to denial, the child or caretaker has the conscious or unconscious notion that if the prescribed medication or prescribed restrictions are ignored, it is as if the illness does not exist. The clinician may hear from the child, "Taking my pills makes me feel like I am sick," or from the parent, "I cannot make myself bring him in for his doctor's appointments because sitting in the clinic reminds me that he has a bad liver." Suppressing thoughts about illness can be a healthy defense, allowing medically ill children and their families to cope with the stress of the illness, but denial leading to non-adherence is maladaptive and warrants a psychotherapeutic intervention to minimize serious medical consequences. Non-adherence may also be an expression of anger. When the child is angry at the parents, non-adherence is guaranteed to elicit parental distress, which can be emotionally satisfying for the child. Psychotherapy serves the function of allying with the healthy part of the child and helping the child or adolescent appreciate that this style of acting out anger and frustration with parents is self-injurious. Similarly, when the anger being acted out is against the illness or the physician, the psychotherapeutic goal is to ally with the healthy part of the child, helping the child articulate the frustration with words rather than by acting them out in a self-destructive way. The consultant is called on to assess what aspect of this goal can be achieved during the hospital stay and when outpatient psychotherapy is warranted. The non-adherent child may be resistant to the idea of outpatient psychotherapy. Hospitalization offers the consultant a valuable opportunity for alliance building by letting the child experience how talking (therapy) can be helpful.

Behavioral Difficulties During Hospitalization

Some children are referred for psychiatric consultation for the management of specific behavioral symptoms that interfere with medical care or physical safety. Symptoms may include excessive activity, agitation, verbal or physical threats to staff and other children, and temper tantrums. Assessment should include medical, developmental, and social history from the child and family, a neurologic examination, nursing and child-life observations, and school reports, as needed.

Behavioral plans, especially for younger children, may be instrumental in reducing treatment-interfering behaviors. The guiding principle underlying behavioral plans is to identify the key behaviors that are most problematic and provide incentives for the child to behave in positive ways. In younger children, sticker charts for swallowing pills and allowing blood draw without a temper tantrum are examples of common behavioral interventions. Younger children may receive stickers as the full reward, or after receiving a pre-determined number of stickers, a child may earn a toy. Older children may work toward special privileges (such as a trip to the gift shop, time outside with the child-life specialist, or a favorite meal brought in from outside the hospital). Other incentives (such as tickets to a hockey game), may be provided by the family. In addition to behavioral plans, children benefit from having a schedule for the day. An unstructured day increases uncertainty, boredom, and anxiety. Scheduling activity times, mealtimes, rest times, and procedure times can help provide the child with an increased sense of control over the hospital milieu.

Parent interactions often play a major role in the child's behavior in the hospital. Some behavioral outbursts may reflect the child's anxious response to the parent's escalating anxiety and inability to help the child feel safer in the hospital setting. Some parents may find it difficult to set limits on their child, considering the sadness the parent feels regarding the child's medical condition. The child's behavior may represent an unconscious need to re-engage the parent in what had been the usual style of parenting. A parent's lack of limit setting often feels to the child-like emotional abandonment. In conjunction with the social worker doing family work or parent guidance, the consultant needs to help the parent feel competent to be active again.

Children with behavioral difficulties invariably arouse negative feelings in the staff. There may be disagreements between staff members about how best to respond to certain behaviors, and the inconsistencies may foster further behavioral disturbances. Team meetings to develop a consistent plan and to facilitate good communication are essential. These team meetings are a good opportunity for the consultant to share his or her understanding of the psychological meaning of the behavior in a way that helps the staff feel more empathic with the child and the family.

Psychopharmacologic interventions may also be appropriate in some situations. The child with generalized anxiety or separation anxiety may benefit from a trial of a long-acting benzodiazepine (e.g., clonazepam) and/or an antidepressant.[59] Children with anxiety in association with particular procedures may benefit from pre-medication with a shorter-acting benzodiazepine (e.g., lorazepam). Anticipatory anxiety can be managed with behavioral interventions (e.g., relaxation and visualization techniques, breathing exercises, distraction, combined cognitive-behavioral interventions), as well as with psychotropics.[59,60] When ADHD (present in 3%–10% of school-aged children[61]) is diagnosed, the child may respond quite dramatically to the addition of a stimulant medication. Occasionally an underlying psychosis may be discerned, and an appropriate antipsychotic agent should be instituted. Currently, atypical antipsychotics are first-line agents in the pharmacotherapy of psychosis in children and adolescents. Aripiprazole, olanzapine, quetiapine, and risperidone are FDA-approved to treat chronic psychosis (e.g., schizophrenia) in youth aged 13 years and older. In clinical practice, atypical antipsychotics are initiated at low doses and gradually titrated to achieve efficacy. Risperidone, for example, may be started at 0.25 mg twice a day and can be increased every day or two under close observation of the medical setting. In patients treated over the long term with risperidone, clinicians should monitor weight, vital signs, and laboratory results (e.g., levels of triglycerides, cholesterol, prolactin).[62,63] Olanzapine and quetiapine are generally more sedating and are initiated at 2.5 to 5 mg/day and 25 to 50 mg/day, respectively.[64] Agitation associated with delirium may also require the use of antipsychotics to maintain a child's safety while the underlying cause is being addressed.

Emergency Interventions: Treatment of Acute Agitation or Aggression

Typically, the request for the emergency use of psychotropics deals with the initial management of acutely assaultive or self-injurious behaviors. The use of emergency psychotropics should be conducted in concert with behavioral interventions and aimed at addressing the crisis, its causes, and its psychosocial impact.[65] If reduced stimulation and general calming measures are ineffective, pharmacotherapy should be considered. Low doses of a short-acting benzodiazepine (e.g., lorazepam 0.5–1 mg), a sedating antihistamine (e.g., diphenhydramine 25–50 mg), or a sedating alpha agonist (e.g., clonidine 0.05–1 mg) can be used to reduce acute anxiety, agitation, and insomnia with few side effects. These agents can be administered orally, intravenously (IV), or intramuscularly (IM). Behavioral disinhibition can occur among children and should be monitored. In severe or agitated psychotic states, low-to-medium doses of a sedating antipsychotic (e.g., chlorpromazine 25–150 mg, olanzapine 2.5–10 mg, or quetiapine 25–300 mg) may be very effective in reducing concomitant anxiety, agitation, or psychosis. For children with active hallucinations or severe disturbances of reality, a higher-potency antipsychotic (e.g., risperidone at 0.25–3 mg orally or haloperidol 2.5–10 mg orally, IV, or IM) may be necessary. Often a combination of a benzodiazepine and an antipsychotic may be necessary for severe agitation. Extra caution is advised when co-administering IM lorazepam and olanzapine due to an elevated risk of cardiorespiratory depression. Medications used for crisis management should not be continued indefinitely unless they are indicated for the treatment of a co-existing psychiatric disorder.

Delirium

Delirium is a transient derangement of cerebral function with global impairment of cognition and attention. It is frequently accompanied by disturbances of the sleep-wake cycle and changes in psychomotor activity. Delirium may be a harbinger of a deteriorating medical condition, a toxic insult, or a brain injury, and may be accompanied by self-injurious behaviors, such as pulling out IV lines. In adolescents, clinicians should consider substance intoxication and drug interactions (between prescribed medications and illicit substances, such as marijuana) in the differential.

Treatment is usually directed at both the cause and the symptoms. Correction of metabolic abnormalities, removal of agents that may be exacerbating the symptoms, or treatment of the underlying injury or infection is generally followed by reversal in the delirium. After attempting to re-orient and decrease the sensory input, the practitioner may need to implement a pharmacologic intervention. In general, antipsychotics are useful if hallucinations or delusions are present. Risperidone, olanzapine, quetiapine, or haloperidol can be used, with the dose repeated every 6 hours, if needed. Psychotropic medications should be withdrawn with the resolution of the delirium.

Autism Spectrum Disorder

There are several important considerations when children with autism spectrum disorder (ASD) are hospitalized.[66] Behavioral plans can be especially helpful for children with ASD. At baseline, children with ASD have high rates of social anxiety and sensory difficulties and often rely on familiar routines for comfort. In the hospital, their usual routines are disrupted, and many new people and interventions are introduced, which may be overwhelming. Most children with ASD have communication impairments that can interfere with their ability to express their distress or to understand their need for certain medical interventions. Behavioral outbursts, including aggression or self-injury, and anxiety are not uncommon in the hospital setting and can cause significant distress for the patient, family, other patients, and staff.

Patients with ASD can benefit from specific, individualized, behavioral plans that are developed collaboratively with the family and are easily accessible to staff (e.g., posted on the patient's door). Parents can provide information to the team about preferred methods of communication, known triggers, individual signs of distress or escalation, and soothing strategies that work. OT can help provide sensory-based interventions to help reduce agitation and distress. The use of visually-oriented materials (such as storyboards or visual schedules) can facilitate communication and help the patient understand what is happening and prepare for procedures or other interventions. Coordination and communication with outpatient providers can be helpful, as they have a longer-standing history and relationship with the patient and family. Ideally an effective behavioral plan will decrease behavioral outbursts, provide uniform care, and avoid the use of unnecessary medications or use of restraints.

CHILD MALTREATMENT

Child maltreatment is defined as any act or series of acts of commission or omission by a parent or other caregiver that results in harm, the potential for harm, or the threat of harm to a child.[67] Acts of commission constitute child abuse, in the form of physical abuse, sexual abuse, or psychological abuse. Acts of omission constitute child neglect, including a failure to provide (e.g., physical neglect, emotional neglect, medical neglect, or educational neglect) or a failure to supervise (e.g., inadequate supervision or exposure to violent environments). [67] In general, data collected from agencies such as the National Child Abuse and Neglect Data System, Administration for Children and Families, and Centers for Disease Control, all overseen by the US Department of Health and Human Services, have shown a trend from 1990 to 2021 toward a significant decline in the rate of overall child maltreatment. Neglect remains the most common form of maltreatment and it continues to gradually increase in proportion to other types of maltreatment.[68] Child maltreatment rates are higher among younger children and are the highest from the ages of less than 1 to 11 years. [68]

Maltreatment may occur in the setting of multigenerational inadequate parenting, parental stress, substance use, and multiple family stressors (including domestic violence, a disrupted family unit, and cognitively limited or psychiatrically ill parents).[69] Low family income[70] is a risk factor, particularly among single-parent families,[71] as well as having a child with a disability.[72] Risk factors notwithstanding, maltreatment occurs in all socioeconomic and demographic environments, demanding constant vigilance in those who work with children.

The consequences of child maltreatment, including mental health problems, can be far-reaching.[73,74] Psychiatry may be consulted in cases where maltreatment is suspected. In some healthcare settings, a specialized child protection team may also be available to provide consultation and coordinate care. All physicians are mandated reporters of maltreatment, but only suspicion is required; it is not necessary to prove maltreatment to file with the appropriate state child welfare agency.

Physical Abuse and Neglect

Physical abuse is defined as the intentional use of physical force against a child that results in, or has the potential to result in, physical injury. Acts constituting physical abuse can include hitting, kicking, punching, beating, stabbing, biting, pushing, shoving, throwing, pulling, dragging, dropping, shaking, strangling/choking, smothering, burning, scalding, and poisoning. Children with disabilities are at increased risk for violence,[75] and having an emotional, psychological, or learning disability is associated with more abuse.[76]

Neglect, by comparison, is the failure of a caregiver to meet a child's basic physical, emotional, medical, or educational needs. These children may present with failure to thrive or other consequences of inadequate nutrition, the occurrence of preventable accidents, dermatologic conditions related to poor hygiene, lack of routine and specialized medical appointments, and school absences.

Abuse and neglect must be suspected before they can be diagnosed. Certain types and locations of injuries are suspicious. Bruises that resemble finger or handprints, and those that appear on body surfaces that normally do not bear the brunt of an accidental fall (such as welts on the back as opposed to anterior shin bruises), should raise suspicion. Multiple bruises in various stages of healing are suggestive of ongoing abuse. Clinicians should be suspicious when bruises, broken bones, and accidents have occurred that are inconsistent with the caretaker's explanation, when the caretaker admits and then recants culpability, or admits having observed the abuse being perpetrated and then recants the story. The caretaker may blame the injury on the child, suggesting it was self-inflicted, or blame a sibling for an injury that appears beyond the developmental capability of the child. There may have been an inexplicable delay in seeking medical attention, or the person bringing the child for medical assistance may be vague or report having not been with the child during the injury and not knowing how it happened.

When physical maltreatment is suspected, the child at risk should be kept in a safe facility until the child welfare agency has determined the safety of the child's disposition. A full physical examination should be performed and well documented, checking the whole child for evidence of bruising or injury in various stages of healing. This is important both to ensure the child's safety and because there may be subsequent legal proceedings. A radiological bone series may be indicated to look for evidence of old and new fractures. A retinal examination should be performed for evidence of traumatic shaking of a young child. Siblings of a child suspected of having been abused must be assessed immediately because they are also at high risk for abuse.

Sexual Abuse

Sexual abuse is defined as any completed or attempted sexual act, sexual contact with, or exploitation (i.e., non-contact sexual interaction) of a child by a caregiver. This involves the exposure of a child to a sexual experience that is inappropriate for his or her emotional and developmental level and that is coercive.[77] It is important to note that sexual abuse is significantly under-reported due to reasons like shame and fear, as well as differences in definitions and screening tools.[78] Incest is present when sexual contact occurs between a child and a family member, including step-family members or members of a surrogate (foster) family.

Although there are no universal screening standards for sexual abuse, it is important to be aware of potential signs and symptoms.[78] Reported symptoms may include nightmares, difficulty sleeping alone, sudden or worsening fear of the dark, bedwetting in otherwise toilet-trained children, anger outbursts, irritability, sadness, and physical symptoms, such as headaches and stomachaches.[78] Observable signs may include caregiver separation anxiety, refusal to get undressed, unwillingness to be examined, using sexual language, sharing sexual knowledge that is not age appropriate, or being engaged in inappropriate sexual behaviors.[78]

In cases where there is an unmistakable traumatic injury, a sexually transmitted infection, or testimony that sexual abuse has occurred in the context of no physical evidence, assessment and documentation of the sexual abuse and disclosure must be approached with the assumption that legal proceedings are likely to follow. In these cases, there is ample information to make mandated reporting of the suspicion of abuse a requirement. The fewest number of people should question the child to minimize further trauma to

the child and to decrease distortions. Ideally a single interview of the child should be conducted by a mental health professional with expertise in child sexual abuse and the appropriate police agency representative. The child psychiatry consultant's role is to support the child in the pediatric unit, without being involved in the sexual abuse examination.

Providers may also face scenarios where there are physical or behavioral symptoms suggestive of sexual abuse but there is no disclosure or implication of a perpetrator. In such cases, the child may present with medical symptoms, such as a urinary tract infection or vaginitis, or behavioral changes, such as sleep problems or depression.[77] These findings may arouse suspicion and should be followed up with a psychological assessment by the designated professional with expertise in child sexual abuse. Such an individual may assess a preschooler through play therapy, looking for themes of abuse in the fantasy play. During the play, the young child may reveal new information about sexual experiences. In the latency-aged child, additional information may be gleaned from the child's drawings, especially self-portraits or pictures of the family. Children and teenagers may be invited to disclose sexual abuse to the evaluator with questions such as, "Has anyone touched you in ways that made you feel uncomfortable or scared?" A follow-up question might be, "Would you tell me if they had?" and "Who could you tell, if someone was touching you or making you uncomfortable?" Even if a child is not yet ready to disclose, one hopes that it is therapeutic to assist a child in conceptualizing a plan for disclosing when he or she does feel ready.

If abuse is entertained, a family assessment is essential. There is no single personality profile of a sexual abuse perpetrator. Perpetrators may come from within or outside of the family. The task of the psychiatric consultant is to sensitively explore the meaning of general symptoms that may be indicative of sexual abuse without suggesting that non-specific symptoms are pathognomonic of sexual abuse.

Medical Child Abuse

Medical child abuse is a caregiver pathology where as a result of the caregiver's reports of fabricated symptoms, the child can be a victim of physical abuse, psychological maltreatment, multiple unnecessary procedures, and potentially harmful medical care.[79,80] It was previously referred to as Münchausen syndrome by proxy and was first described as a pair of case reports in 1977.[81] It carries a DSM-5-TR diagnosis as "factitious disorder imposed on another" and has similar names such as "pediatric symptom falsification" and "caregiver fabricated illness" in the pediatrics literature.[79,80] Although rare overall, one common presentation is when a parent, usually a mother,[81] consciously distorts her description of her child's symptoms or does things to the child to fabricate a picture of medical illness; she then seeks hospitalizations and medical interventions for the child. One American Academy of Pediatrics review reported that the most common presentations included bleeding, seizures, central nervous system depression, apnea, diarrhea, vomiting, fever, and rash.[80] The parent may also starve a child due to inaccurate beliefs of multiple allergies,[79] or cause life-threatening illness by injecting the child with medication, blood, or feces to ensure that a medical work-up continues.

Some of the caregivers with this syndrome have had medical training in a health-related profession, such as nursing,[82,83] and they use their medical knowledge to create "illness" in their child. The mother is usually at the infant's or young child's bedside. She tries to establish friendships with the nursing staff and is content as long as continued hospitalization and medical procedures are being scheduled and performed. She may become angry and agitated if she receives a report that her child is well and should be discharged home. Often, she appears earnest and less anxious when serious diagnoses of the child are being entertained. If discharged, she may return within hours or days to the ED with an escalation of symptoms. The psychological understanding of this syndrome is that the mother needs the child to be sick to maintain her role as a "nurturant" mother in the protected, supported environment of the pediatric ward. She may gain a "curious sense of purpose and safety in the midst of the disasters which [she herself has] created."[82] She perceives the nurses to be her friends and the male physicians as caretaking men in her life. She lacks the empathy to be troubled by the pain and suffering she is inflicting on her child.

Medical child abuse is a difficult diagnosis to make without observing the caregiver doing something to the child. It may be suspected when a child's medical condition does not follow the expected course and the symptoms are persistently inconsistent. The symptoms may be observed only by the caregiver or may occur in conjunction with the caregiver's presence and may be consistent with an intentional action. Undertaking the investigation of this diagnosis and seeking concrete evidence of risk to the child at the hands of a parent may require input from hospital legal counsel and administration.

The American Academy of Pediatrics (AAP) Committee on Child Abuse and Neglect published an approach to recognizing and addressing medical child abuse.[79] They suggest that before making a diagnosis of medical child abuse, the physician must ask: (1) Are the history, signs, and symptoms of the disease credible?; (2) Is the child receiving unnecessary and harmful or potentially harmful medical care?; (3) And if so, who is instigating the evaluations and treatment? They propose that medical child abuse is when medical care is harming the child as a result of the caregiver who is driving it.[79] The diagnosis is a pediatric diagnosis focused on what is happening to the child and does not factor in the caregiver's motivations.[79]

It is crucial to protect the child's safety if this diagnosis is suspected as it is associated with high mortality rates and significant morbidity.[79] The AAP suggests following these clinical principles in medical child abuse cases: (1) consult a pediatrician with child abuse experience, (2) carefully review records from all sources and have all involved physicians collaborate closely, (3) work with a multi-disciplinary child protection team, (4) allow treatment to occur in the least restrictive setting possible, but if necessary, do not hesitate to involve social agencies, and (5) involve the whole family in treatment.[79] The hospital legal department and child protective services should be notified of this diagnosis to protect the best interest of the child. If the parent thinks that she is being suspected of having harmed her child, she may become angry and leave against medical advice (sometimes going straight to another hospital under the same or an assumed name). Perpetrators of medical child abuse are difficult to treat due to their psychological difficulties, persistent denial, and capacity for deception; recidivism is common.[84]

LIVING WITH CHRONIC ILLNESS

Most children with chronic illnesses cope well. They are not defined by their illnesses but rather by their individual strengths, personalities, and age-appropriate developmental issues. However, children with chronic illnesses are more likely than their peers to have a psychiatric disorder.[84] No one personality coincides with certain illnesses, but each chronic illness, such as asthma, diabetes, rheumatoid arthritis, CF, and sickle cell anemia, presents with particular challenges. These challenges present in terms of coping with (1) the symptoms (such as pain or shortness of breath), (2) the timing of diagnosis (at birth, childhood, or adolescence), and (3) the requisite healthcare regimen (such as inhalers, IV antibiotics, or dietary restrictions). The meaning of the illness to the patient evolves according to relevant developmental issues throughout the individual's life. The consultant's task is to understand the meaning of the illness to the individual patient and family at this moment in development. The earlier section on development provides some general principles for understanding the effect of chronic illness throughout childhood, but the consultant must assess the unique experience of the child and family.[85-88]

The consultant needs to ask many questions to elucidate the patient's subjective experience of living with the chronic illness. Diagnostic instruments used in physically healthy children may not be useful in children with chronic illnesses. Some useful questions include what the worst or hardest thing is about the illness and if there is anything good about the illness. Similarly, what is the child's personal experience of the healthcare regimen? How has the child's experience of the disease changed as the child has grown older, or what events in the future are of concern? What are the child's peer relationships like, and how, if at all, does the illness affect these relationships? Who does the child tell about his or her illness, and when does the child do so in the course of the relationship? How does the child explain the illness to others, and how can he or she explain it to the consultant? What is the child's perception of the parental concerns about the illness? What are the areas of conflict between parent and child and between child and pediatrician or sub-specialist?

Chronic illness requires adjustment on the part of the child, the family, and sometimes the school.

The child's personal strengths (such as music, sports, or academics) are assets in maintaining self-esteem and building important peer support. Some children enjoy peer group opportunities, such as specialized camps for children who share a particular illness. Temperament and interpersonal capacities are also factors in the ease of a child's adjustment. Parental attitude toward the illness is crucial in setting the stage for the child's attitude. This may raise difficulties because feeling worried, burdened, and isolated is a common experience among parents of children with a chronic illness.[88] Excessive parental anxiety, anger, sadness, and guilt, however, are likely to impede the child's adjustment.[88,89]

The extent to which an illness interferes with age-appropriate activities, especially school, is an important factor in adjustment. Multiple hospitalizations are associated with greater emotional morbidity than is seen in an individual hospital stay.[90] Structuring the admissions to provide the child with protected times and protected places for play and dialogue, appropriate to the child's age, decreases the stress of the hospital environment. In-hospital tutoring for prolonged hospital stays and continued contact with friends in person, by phone, or online, can assist the child's comfort in returning to school.

CARE AT THE END OF LIFE

In recent years, the emerging sub-specialty of pediatric palliative care has helped focus the attention of clinicians who participate in end-of-life care on the complex challenges of providing the best possible care to these children and their families.[91-93] In some treatment settings, there may be specialized clinical services dedicated to pediatric palliative care, and the psychiatric consultant may work closely with these services to address psychosocial needs.[94] In circumstances where these services are not available, the psychiatric consultant may be called on to aid the patient, family, and medical team in a variety of ways.

A consultation request may stem from issues related to problem solving and decision-making in the context of a life-limiting illness.[95] This may include initiating a dialogue between the medical team and the patient and family of the patient with a life-threatening illness, clarifying the goals and hopes of treatment, and assisting in the evaluation of pros and cons related to specific treatments or treatment settings, including end-of-life care outside of the hospital[96] and planning for the location of death.[97] Because these issues may be frequently accompanied by emotional distress on the part of patients, families, and caregivers, psychiatric expertise may be sought. The psychiatric consultant may help to facilitate emotionally intense discussions and to help anticipate and interpret the reactions of children to issues around death and dying in the relevant developmental context.

In children, a mature conception of death can be viewed in components that may not be acquired simultaneously.[98] Key components include, in approximate order of typical acquisition,[99] concepts of universality, irreversibility, non-functionality (i.e., that the functions of life cease with death),[100] and causality. It should not be assumed that children either do not understand the concept of death or are too fragile to talk about it. The child's parents and the medical team may need education about whether and how to talk with the child about death and to involve the child in the plan of care.[101-103]

In addition, helping the seriously ill child to communicate his or her preferences (such as being called a nickname rather than a formal name or whether to wake him or her for optional events or social activities) can create a greater sense of agency and help stave off helplessness. Facilitating peer interactions in the hospital playroom for the child and encouraging both formal and informal support groups for children and their parents can be invaluable. Many parents and children feel that the enormity of the child's illness has so changed their lives that old friends feel inadequate. The worries of the well world can feel alienating and out of touch with the child and the family's new reality. This experience can be isolating. Sharing pleasures and frustrations with other families facing cancer, a terminal neurologic syndrome, or a metabolic disease can be an antidote to isolation. Many family friendships that begin on the ward survive long after a child dies.

Adolescents may desire to be more involved in their end-of-life planning, and consultants can help facilitate discussions in a developmentally appropriate manner. Wiener and associates highlighted how adolescents at the end of life value providing their input and thoughts on (1) what medical treatment they want or do not want, (2) how they would like to be cared for, (3) information for their family and friends to know, and (4) how they would like to be remembered.[104] The authors took these findings and created a new clinical tool, Voicing My CHOICES, which encompasses the above principles and can be a useful way of introducing and discussing these topics with adolescent and young adult patients.

The consultant may also have a role in helping with the treatment of symptoms at the end of life, which may be under-recognized or under-treated. Studies of children who died of cancer have found that symptoms of pain, fatigue, and dyspnea occur in many patients, resulting in significant suffering, and persist despite attempts to treat them.[105-108] In children with life-limiting illnesses of all kinds, the consultant may have a role in assisting with the treatment of pain,[109-112] fatigue,[112] dyspnea,[112] agitation,[113] anxiety, delirium, and depression.[114] Although the psychopharmacologic treatment of seriously ill or dying children is complicated, compassion dictates considering the use of psychiatric medications in this population if they may help relieve suffering.[115]

Families also need varying amounts of assistance to cope with the impending loss of a child, ranging from sympathy for their grief to guidance on how to make end-of-life decisions that reflect their values, preserve dignity, and minimize suffering. In a retrospective study of parents who lost children to cancer, the presence of unrelieved pain and a difficult moment of death were the most significant factors still affecting parents 4 to 9 years after the loss.[116] The same study also demonstrated that most parents had worked through their grief "a lot," and that factors which were associated with working through grief were sharing their problems with others during the child's illness, having access to psychological support during the last month of the child's life, and counseling being offered by healthcare staff within the last month of life.[117] Those parents who reported that they had not worked through their grief reported more physical and psychological health problems, increased sick leave, and increased utilization of healthcare services.[118] Parents who felt that health care given to their children was inadequate, that anxiety or pain had gone unrelieved, or that the parents' own needs (such as support and communication) were not met reported more feelings of guilt in the year following the death of the child.[119] Although support for grieving families at their time of loss can be beneficial, it is important to remember that grieving for the death of a child is a life-long process, and community resources for bereaved families may help to work through grief and find meaning in a tremendous loss.

The child's care team may also struggle with the loss of a patient. Commonly, feelings of sadness and helplessness can surface, and it may feel difficult to maintain empathy for patients and families whose circumstances appear trivial by comparison or whose disorders seem "less real" or self-inflicted. Even when these factors are not present, continuous compassion directed at those in crisis can create emotional exhaustion, which is termed "compassion fatigue."[120] The intensity of relationships formed in the course of providing care to children at the end of life may contribute to this phenomenon. The consultant may assist by educating members of the team about this phenomenon and dispelling stigma, and helping develop personal, professional, and organizational strategies to prevent and manage compassion fatigue.[121]

SUPPORT FOR PARENTS WITH SERIOUS ILLNESS

The Parenting at a Challenging Time (PACT) Model

Millions of children in the United States grow up in families in which a parent is medically ill. The psychiatric consultant may be asked to help facilitate communication about how parental illness can affect children, provide specific parent guidance, and share relevant community resources. Table 38.1 shows brief examples of parenting tips, with relevance to the child's developmental stage. Table 38.2 provides a list of various resources that parents could access to help with their own coping, their family's coping, events, and other relevant resources. There is a real clinical need for consultation in this capacity, as seen at the Massachusetts General Hospital Parenting at a Challenging Time (PACT) program. More clinical attention to, and research about, these issues is needed.

FUTURE CONSIDERATIONS

The long-term benefits of psychiatric intervention must be assessed through outcome studies that examine the

TABLE 38.1		
Key Points and Parenting Tips by Developmental Stage		
Developmental Stage	**Key Points**	**Parenting Tips**
Infancy (birth to 2.5 years)	Concern with attachment and self-regulation	Maintain familiar routines
		Keep number of caretakers to a minimum
Pre-school years (ages 3–6 years)	Egocentricity + magical thinking = "I am to blame"	Maintain routines and love limit setting
	Death is temporary and reversible	Repeatedly remind the child that the illness is not his or her fault
Latency (ages 7–12 years)	Mastery of skills	Protect family time by limiting visitors and turning off the phone at mealtimes
	Rules and fairness; simple cause-and-effect logic	
	Peer focused and image conscious	Set regular times for the child to show the ill parent the accomplishments of the week; attend to the details
	Intellectualization of death	
Adolescence (ages 13–18 years)	Abstract thinking and behavior are not on the same plane	Be cautious about assigning teens a parenting role with younger siblings
	Separation is developmental task but complicated by vulnerability of the parent	Support relationships with trustworthy non-parental adults
		Foster safer independent behavior
Young adults (19–23 years)	Living away from home	Provide enough information to allow for decision-making
	Serious relationship formation	
	Longer time frame with regard to decision-making	Encourage a balance between pursuing new life experiences and putting these on hold to spend precious time with the ill parent

TABLE 38.2
Resources for Patients

Resources for Cancer Patients

People Living with Cancer, from the American Society For Clinical Oncology (ASCO)
Offers educational information for patients and families (www.plwc.org)

American Psychosocial Oncology Society (APOS)
Provides a free helpline to connect patients and families with local counseling services, as well as webcasts for professionals on topics such as "Cancer 101 for Mental Health Professionals" and "Psychosocial Aspects of Cancer Survivorship" (co-sponsored by the Lance Armstrong Foundation) (www.apos-society.org)

American Cancer Society (ACS)
Provides information on talking to children about cancer, as well as numerous other cancer-related topics (www.cancer.org)

The Wellness Community
A national, non-profit organization that provides free online and in-person support and information to people living with cancer and their families (www.thewellnesscommunity.org)

Living Beyond Breast Cancer
A national education and support organization with the goal of improving quality of life and helping patients take an active role in ongoing recovery or management of the disease (www.lbbc.org)

Young Survival Coalition
Through action, advocacy, and awareness, this non-profit seeks to educate the medical, research, breast cancer, and legislative communities and to persuade them to address breast cancer in females of ages 40 and younger—and serves as a point of contact for young females living with breast cancer (www.youngsurvival.org)

BreastCancer.org
Offers medical information about current treatments and research in breast cancer care and survivorship (www.breastcancer.org)

Hurricane Voices Breast Cancer Foundation
Among other breast cancer–related resources, this organization offers a family reading list of books and stories for children of all ages dealing with cancer, in particular with breast cancer (www.hurricanevoices.org) (link is not active)

CancerCare
The mission of this national non-profit resource is to provide free professional help to people with all cancers through counseling, education, information, and referral and direct financial assistance. They offer online, telephone, and face-to-face support groups to those affected by cancer (www.cancercare.org)

Livestrong Foundation
Livestrong offers information and services to cancer survivors and the professionals who care for them (www.livestrong.org)

The Life Institute
This organization's online publication "Conversations from the Heart" provides an annotated list of resources for parents and professionals who want to learn more about how to have developmentally appropriate conversations with children about serious illness and death (www.thelifeinstitute.org)

Resources for other illnesses
American Heart Association (www.americanheart.org)
American Diabetes Association (www.diabetes.org)
ALS Association (www.alsa.org)
Brain Injury Association of America (www.biausa.org)
Colitis Foundation (www.colitisfoundation.org)
Cystic Fibrosis Foundation (www.cff.org/home)
Epilepsy Foundation (www.epilepsyfoundation.org)
National Multiple Sclerosis Society (www.nmss.org)
National Neurofibromatosis Foundation (www.nfnetwork.org)
Pulmonary Fibrosis Foundation (www.pulmonaryfibrosis.org)

impact of consultation on the quality of life of patients and families, on health outcomes, and the cost of care. Professionals who work with children are called on to advocate for the special needs of the young because they are not yet able to do so for themselves. Interventions that improve the psychological well-being of children maximize their productivity long into the future, and interventions that support families strengthen the community. As managed care, critical pathways, and advances in care decrease lengths of stay, increasingly consultation work will bridge to or be centered in outpatient settings and schools.[122] Being accessible, responsive, and communicative with primary care pediatricians will continue to be essential. Sustained improvement in pediatric mental health services will require continuing and expanding collaboration between medical and child and adolescent psychiatric providers.

Efforts to reduce the distance between pediatrics and child psychiatry have led to enhanced integration of behavioral care within the pediatric medical home, whether it is through an on-site embedded psychiatrist or other accessible consultation (such as phone consultations). For primary care settings, the Bureau of Child and Maternal Health of the Public Health Service and the American Academy of Pediatrics have collaborated on projects that emphasize the psychosocial needs of children. *Bright Futures* integrates psychosocial issues into every recommended primary care visit.[122] Many pediatric practices are assessing mental health needs by using screening tools such as a Pediatric Symptom Checklist.[123] Some sub-specialty clinics, including those treating CF, cancer, diabetes, and endocrine disorders, have become more open to consultation at the time of medical diagnosis, at key points in the illness, and for non-adherence. In pediatric oncology, this has led to the development of psychosocial standards of care.[124] More work is needed to develop psychosocial standards of care for other illnesses. Research is needed to evaluate how integration and early involvement of psychiatry can save costs, reduce medical burden, and lead to better outcomes overall.

REFERENCES

1. Bujoreanu S, White MT, Gerber B, et al. Effect of timing of psychiatry consultation on length of pediatric hospitalization and hospital charges. *Hosp Pediatr.* 2015;5:269–275.
2. Jellinek MS. Recognition and management of discord within house staff teams. *JAMA.* 1986;256:754–755.
3. Jellinek MS, Todres DI, Catlin EA, et al. Pediatric intensive care training: confronting the dark side. *Crit Care Med.* 1993;21:775–779.
4. American Academy of Pediatrics: Committee on Hospital Care Child life services. *Pediatrics.* 2000;106:1156–1159.
5. Knapp P, Harris E. Consultation-liaison in child psychiatry: a review of the past ten years. *J Am Acad Child Adolesc Psychiatry.* 1998;37:139–146.
6. Prugh DG, Staub EM, Sands H, et al. A study of the emotional reactions of children and families to hospitalization and illness. *Am J Orthopsychiatry.* 1953;23:70–106.
7. Aarons GA, Monn AR, Leslie LK, et al. Association between mental and physical health problems in high-risk adolescents: a longitudinal study. *J Adolesc Health.* 2008;43:260–267.
8. Rosenberg AR, Bradford MC, Junkins CC, et al. Effect of the promoting resilience in stress management intervention for parents of children with cancer (PRISM-P): a randomized clinical trial. *JAMA Netw Open.* 2009;4(2):e1911578.
9. Wakefield CE, McLoone JK, Butow P, et al. Parental adjustment to the completion of their child's cancer treatment. *Pediatr Blood Cancer.* 2010;56:524–531.
10. Harper FW, Eggly S, Crider B, et al. Patient- and family-centered care as an approach to reducing disparities in asthma outcomes in urban African American children: a review of the literature. *J Natl Med Assoc.* 2015;107:4–17.
11. Whitaker T. *Dealing with Difficult Parents.* Routledge; 2015.
12. Sharpe D, Rossiter L. Siblings of children with a chronic illness: a meta-analysis. *J Pediatr Psychol.* 2002;27:699–710.
13. O'Brien I, Duffy A, Nicholl H. Impact of childhood chronic illnesses on siblings: a literature review. *Br J Nurs.* 2009;18:1358–1365.
14. Shaw RJ, Pao M, Holland JE, et al. Practice patterns revisited in pediatric psychosomatic medicine. *Psychosomatics.* 2016;57:576–585.
15. Birmaher B, Ryan ND, Williamson DE, et al. Child and adolescent depression: a review of the past 10 years: I. *J Am Acad Child Adolesc Psychiatry.* 1996;35:1427–1439.
16. Kashani JH, Breedlove L. Depression in the medically ill. In: Reynolds WM, Johnston HF, eds. *Handbook of Depression in Children and Adolescents.* Springer-Verlag; 2013:427.
17. Canning EH, Canning RD, Boyce WT. Depressive symptoms and adaptive style in children with cancer. *J Am Acad Child Adolesc Psychiatry.* 1992;31:1120–1124.
18. Thapar A, Collishaw S, Pine DS, et al. Depression in adolescence. *Lancet.* 2012;379(9280):1056–1067.
19. March J, Silva S, Petrycki S, et al. Treatment for Adolescents with Depression Study (TADS) team. Fluoxetine, cognitive-behavioral therapy, and their combination for adolescents with depression: treatment for adolescents with depression study (TADS) randomized controlled trial. *JAMA.* 2004;292:807–820.
20. Goodyer I, Dubicka B, Wilkinson P, et al. Selective serotonin reuptake inhibitors (SSRIs) and routine specialist care with and without cognitive behaviour therapy in adolescents with major depression: randomized controlled trial. *BMJ.* 2007;335:142.
21. Goodyer IM, Dubicka B, Wilkinson P, et al. A randomized controlled trial of cognitive behaviour therapy in adolescents with major depression treated by selective serotonin reuptake inhibitors. The ADAPT Trial. *Health Technol Assess.* 2008;12:iii–iv, ix–60.

22. FDA Public Health Advisory: Reports of suicidality in pediatric patients being treated with antidepressant medications for major depressive disorder; 2003. Available at: http://www.fda.gov/drugs/drugsafety/postmarketdrugsafetyinformationforpatientsandproviders/ucm168828.htm.

23. Bhatia SK, Rezac AJ, Vitiello B, et al. Antidepressant prescribing practices for the treatment of children and adolescents. *J Child Adolesc Psychopharmacol*. 2008;18(1):70–80.

24. Pamer CA, Hammad TA, Wu YT, et al. Changes in US antidepressant and antipsychotic prescription patterns during a period of FDA actions. *Pharmacoepidemiol Drug Saf*. 2010;19(2):158–174.

25. Kurian BT, Ray WA, Arbogast PG, et al. Effect of regulatory warnings on antidepressant prescribing for children and adolescents. *Arch Pediatr Adolesc Med*. 2007;161(7):690–696.

26. Singh T, Prakash A, Rais T, et al. Decreased use of antidepressants in youth after US Food and Drug Administration black box warning. *Psychiatry (Edgmont)*. 2009;6(10):30–34.

27. Gibbons RD, Brown CH, Hur K, et al. Early evidence on the effects of regulators' suicidality warnings on SSRI prescriptions and suicide in children and adolescents. *Am J Psychiatry*. 2007;164(9):1356–1363.

28. Hetrick S, Merry S, McKenzie J, et al. Selective serotonin reuptake inhibitors (SSRIs) for depressive disorders in children and adolescents. *Cochrane Database Syst Rev*. 2007(3): CD004851.

29. Bridge JA, Yengar S, Salary CB, et al. Clinical response and risk for reported suicidal ideation and suicide attempts in pediatric antidepressant treatment: a meta-analysis of randomized controlled trials. *JAMA*. 2007;63:332–339.

30. Cozza KL, Armstrong SC, Oesterheld JR. *Concise Guide to Drug Interaction Principles for Medical Practice*. American Psychiatric Press; 2003.

31. Center for Disease Control: Injury Prevention and Control: Division of Violence Prevention. National Suicide Statistics. WISQARS. Available at: http://www.cdc.gov/violenceprevention/suicide/statistics/index.html (last updated 28.03.16).

32. Russell ST, Joyner K. Adolescent sexual orientation and suicide risk: evidence from a national study. *Am J Public Health*. 2001;91:1276–1281.

33. Grossman AH, D'Augelli AR. Transgender youth and life-threatening behaviors. *Suicide Life Threat Behav*. 2007;37: 527–537.

34. American Psychiatric Association. *Diagnostic and Statistical Manual of Mental Disorders*. 5th ed. American Psychiatric Association Publishing; 2013.

35. Anderson A, Bowers W, Evans K. Inpatient treatment of anorexia nervosa. In: Garner DM, Garfinkel PE, eds. *Handbook of Treatment for Eating Disorders*. 2nd ed. Guilford Press; 1997:327–353.

36. Postilnik I, Eisman HD, Price R, et al. An algorithm for defining somatization in children. *J Can Acad Child Adolesc Psychiatry*. 2006;15:64–74.

37. DeMaso DR, Martini DR, Cahen LA. Practice parameter for the psychiatric assessment and management of physically ill children and adolescents. *J Am Acad Child Adolesc Psychiatry*. 2009;48:213–233.

38. Campo JV, Fritz GK. A management model for pediatric somatization. *Psychosomatics*. 2001;42:467–476.

39. Wallander JL, Thompson RJ, Alriksson-Schmidt A. Psychosocial adjustment of children with chronic physical conditions. In: Roberts MC, ed. *Handbook of Pediatric Psychology*. 3rd ed. Guilford Press; 2003:141–158.

40. Peters TE, Fritz GK. Psychological considerations of the child with asthma. *Child Adolesc Psychiatr Clin N Am*. 2010;19:319–334.

41. Goodwin RD, Robinson M, Sly PD, et al. Severity and persistence of asthma and mental health: a birth cohort study. *Psychol Med*. 2013;43:1313–1322.

42. Blackman JA, Gurka MJ. Developmental and behavioral comorbidities of asthma in children. *J Dev Behav Pediatr*. 2007;28:92–99.

43. Butwicka A, Frisén L, Almqvist C, et al. Erratum. Risks of psychiatric disorders and suicide attempts in children and adolescents with type 1 diabetes: a population-based cohort study. *Diabetes Care*. 2015;38:453–459.

44. Zenlea IS, Mednick L, Rein J, et al. Routine behavioral and mental health screening in young children with type 1 diabetes mellitus. *Pediatr Diabetes*. 2013;15:384–388.

45. Ott D, Caplan R, Guthrie D, et al. Measures of psychopathology in children with complex partial seizures and primary generalized epilepsy with absence. *J Am Acad Child Adolesc Psychiatry*. 2001;40:907–914.

46. Sigita P, Dunn D, Caplan R. 10-year research update review: psychiatric problems in children with epilepsy. *J Am Acad Child Adolesc Psychiatry*. 2007;46:1389–1402.

47. Vega C, Guo J, Killory B, et al. Symptoms of anxiety and depression in childhood absence epilepsy. *Epilepsia*. 2011;52:74–78.

48. Szigethy E, Craig AE, Iobst EA, et al. Profile of depression in adolescents with inflammatory bowel disease: implications for treatment. *Inflamm Bowel Dis*. 2009;15:69–74.

49. Szigethy E, Levy-Warren A, Whitton S, et al. Depressive symptoms and inflammatory bowel disease in children and adolescents: a cross-sectional study. *J Pediatr Gastroenterol Nutr*. 2004;39:395–403.

50. Szigethy EM, Youk AO, Benhayon D, et al. Depression subtypes in pediatric inflammatory bowel disease. *J Pediatr Gastroenterol Nutr*. 2014;58:574–581.

51. Kazak AE, Kassam-Adams N, Schneider S, et al. An integrative model of pediatric medical traumatic stress. *J Pediatr Psychol*. 2006;31:343–355.

52. Hyland ME, Kenyon CA, Taylor M, et al. Steroid prescribing for asthmatics: relationship with Asthma Symptom Checklist and Living with Asthma Questionnaire. *Br J Clin Psychol*. 1993;32:505–511.

53. Hagman C, Janson C, Emtner M. A comparison between patients with dysfunctional breathing and patients with asthma. *Clin Respir J*. 2007;2:86–91.

54. Prys-Picard CO, Niven R. Dysfunctional breathing in patients with asthma. *Thorax*. 2008;63:568.

55. Bonn M. The effects of hospitalization on children: a review. *Curationis*. 1994;17:20–24.

56. Rennick JE, Dougherty G, Chambers C, et al. Children's psychological and behavioral responses following pediatric intensive care unit hospitalization: the caring intensively study. *BMC Pediatr*. 2014;14:276.

57. Kahana S, Drotar D, Frazier T. Meta-analysis of psychological interventions to promote adherence to treatment in pediatric chronic health conditions. *J Pediatr Psychol*. 2008;33:590–611.

58. Bhatia S, Landier W, Hageman L, et al. 6MP adherence in a multiracial cohort of children with acute lymphoblastic leukemia: a children's oncology group study. *Blood*. 2014;124:2345–2353.

59. Katzman MA, Bleau P, Blier P, et al. Canadian clinical practice guidelines for the management of anxiety, posttraumatic stress and obsessive-compulsive disorders. *BMC Psychiatry*. 2014;14:S1.

60. American Academy of Pediatrics: Committee on Quality Improvement SoA-DHD: diagnosis and evaluation of the child with attention-deficit/hyperactivity disorder. *Pediatrics*. 2000;105:1158–1170.

61. Martin A, L'Ecuyer S. Triglyceride, cholesterol and weight changes among risperidone-treated youths: a retrospective study. *Eur Child Adolesc Psychiatry*. 2002;11:129–133.

62. Martin A, Landau J, Leebens P, et al. Risperidone-associated weight gain in children and adolescents: a retrospective chart review. *J Child Adolesc Psychopharmacol*. 2000;10:259–268.

63. Bryden KE, Carrey NJ, Kutcher SP. Update and recommendations for the use of antipsychotics in early-onset psychoses. *J Child Adolesc Psychopharmacol*. 2001;11:113–130.

64. Steiner H, Saxena K, Chang K. Psychopharmacologic strategies for the treatment of aggression in juveniles. *CNS Spectr*. 2003;8:298–308.

65. Thom RP, McDougle CJ, Hazen EP. Challenges in the medical care of patients with autism spectrum disorder: the role of the consultation-liaison psychiatrist. *Psychosomatics*. 2019;60(5):435–443.

66. Leeb RT, Paulozzi L, Melanson C, et al. *Child Maltreatment Surveillance: Uniform Definitions for Public Health and Recommended Data Elements, Version 1.0*. Centers for Disease Control and Prevention, National Center for Injury Prevention and Control; 2008.

67. U.S. Department of Health & Human Services, Administration for Children and Families, Administration on Children, Youth and Families, Children's Bureau. *Child Maltreatment 2021*. Available from: https://www.acf.hhs.gov/cb/data-research/child-maltreatment; 20203.

68. Berkout OV, Kolko DJ. Understanding child directed caregiver aggression: an examination of characteristics and predictors associated with perpetration. *Child Abuse Negl*. 2016;56:44–53.

69. Hussey JM, Cheng JJ, Kotch JB. Child maltreatment in the United States: prevalence, risk factors, and adolescent health consequences. *Pediatrics*. 2006;118:933–942.

70. Berger LM. Income, family characteristics, and physical violence toward children. *Child Abuse Negl*. 2005;29:107–133.

71. Jones L, Bellis MA, Wood S, et al. Prevalence and risk of violence against children with disabilities: a systematic review and meta-analysis of observational studies. *Lancet*. 2012;380:899–907.

72. Gilbert R, Widom CS, Browne K, et al. Burden and consequences of child maltreatment in high-income countries. *Lancet*. 2009;373:68–81.

73. Shapero BG, Black SK, Liu RT, et al. Stressful life events and depression symptoms: the effect of childhood emotional abuse on stress reactivity. *J Clin Psychol*. 2013;70:209–223.

74. Jones L, Bellis MA, Wood S, et al. Prevalence and risk of violence against children with disabilities: a systematic review and meta-analysis of observational studies. *Lancet*. 2012;380:899–907.

75. Govindshenoy M, Spencer N. Abuse of the disabled child: a systematic review of population-based studies. *Child Care Health Dev*. 2007;33:552–558.

76. Britton H, Hensen K. Sexual abuse. *Clin Obstet Gynecol*. 1997;40:226–240.

77. Hanson RF, Adams CS. Childhood sexual abuse: identification, screening, and treatment recommendations in primary care settings. *Primary Care*. 2016;43:313–326.

78. Stirling J. Beyond Munchausen syndrome by proxy: identification and treatment of child abuse in a medical setting. *Pediatrics*. 2007;119:1026–1030.

79. Flaherty EG, MacMillan HL. Caregiver-fabricated illness in a child: a manifestation of child maltreatment. *Pediatrics*. 2013;132:590–597.

80. Meadow R. Munchausen syndrome by proxy: the hinterland of child abuse. *Lancet*. 1977;2:343–345.

81. Rosenberg DA. Web of deceit: a literature review of Munchausen syndrome by proxy. *Child Abuse Negl*. 1987;11:547–563.

82. Sheridan MS. The deceit continues: an updated literature review of Munchausen syndrome by proxy. *Child Abuse Negl*. 2003;27:431–451.

83. Shaw RJ, Dayal S, Hartman JK, et al. Factitious disorder by proxy: pediatric condition falsification. *Harv Rev Psychiatry*. 2008;16:215–224.

84. LeBlanc LA, Goldsmith T, Patel DR. Behavioral aspects of chronic illness in children and adolescents. *Pediatr Clin North Am*. 2003;50:859–878.

85. Sawyer M, Antoniou G, Toogood I, et al. Childhood cancer: a 4-year prospective study of the psychological adjustment of children and parents. *J Pediatr Hematol Oncol*. 2000;22:214–220.

86. Meijer SA, Sinnema G, Bijstra JO, et al. Social functioning in children with a chronic illness. *J Child Psychol Psychiatry*. 2000;41:309–317.

87. Hoekstra-Webbers J, Jaspers J, Kamps W, et al. Risk factors for psychological maladjustment of parents of children with cancer. *J Am Acad Child Adolesc Psychiatry*. 1999;38:1526–1535.

88. Trivedi D. Cochrane review summary: psychological interventions for parents of children and adolescents with chronic illness. *Prim Health Care Res Dev*. 2013;14:224–228.

89. Coffey JS. Parenting a child with chronic illness: a metasynthesis. *Pediatr Nurs*. 2006;32:51–59.

90. Himelstein BP, Hilden JM, Boldt AM, et al. Pediatric palliative care. *N Engl J Med.* 2004;350:1752–1762.

91. Liben S, Papadatou D, Wolfe J. Paediatric palliative care: challenges and emerging ideas. *Lancet.* 2008;371:852–864.

92. Zhukovsky DS, Herzog CE, Kaur G, et al. The impact of palliative care consultation on symptom assessment, communication needs, and palliative interventions in pediatric patients with cancer. *J Palliat Med.* 2009;12:343–349.

93. McSherry M, Kehoe K, Carroll JM, et al. Psychosocial and spiritual needs of children living with a life-limiting illness. *Pediatr Clin North Am.* 2007;54:609–629.

94. Feudtner C. Pediatric palliative care: a foundation for problem-solving and decision-making. *Pediatr Clin North Am.* 2007;54:583–607.

95. Carroll JM, Torkildson C, Winsness JS. Issues related to providing quality pediatric palliative care in the community. *Pediatr Clin North Am.* 2007;54:813–827.

96. Dussel V, Kreicbergs U, Hilden JM, et al. Looking beyond where children die: determinants and effects of planning a child's location of death. *J Pain Symptom Manage.* 2009;37:33–43.

97. Kane B. Children's concepts of death. *J Genet Psychol.* 1979; 134:141–153.

98. Kenyon BL. Current research in children's conceptions of death: a critical review. *Omega (Westport).* 2001;43:63–91.

99. Speece MW, Brent SB. Children's understanding of death: a review of three components of a death concept. *Child Dev.* 1984;55:1671–1686.

100. Beale EA, Baile WF, Aaron J. Silence is not golden: communicating with children dying from cancer. *J Clin Oncol.* 2005;23:3629–3631.

101. Kreicbergs U, Valdimarsdottir U, Onelov E, et al. Talking about death with children who have severe malignant disease. *N Engl J Med.* 2004;351:1175–1186.

102. Hinds PS, Drew D, Oakes LL, et al. End-of-life care preferences of pediatric patients with cancer. *J Clin Oncol.* 2005;23:9146–9154.

103. Wiener L, Zadeh S, Battles H, et al. Allowing adolescents and young adults to plan their end-of-life care. *Pediatrics.* 2012;130:897–905.

104. Wolfe J, Grier HE, Klar N, et al. Symptoms and suffering at the end of life in children with cancer. *N Engl J Med.* 2000;342:326–333.

105. Jalmsell L, Kreicbergs U, Onelov E, et al. Symptoms affecting children with malignancies during the last month of life: a nationwide follow-up. *Pediatrics.* 2006;117:1314–1320.

106. Theunissen JMJ, Hoogerbrugge PM, van Achterberg T, et al. Symptoms in the palliative phase of children with cancer. *Pediatr Blood Cancer.* 2007;49:160–165.

107. Pritchard M, Burghen E, Srivastava DK, et al. Cancer-related symptoms most concerning to parents during the last week and last day of their child's life. *Pediatrics.* 2008;121:e1301–e1309.

108. Monteiro Caran EM, Dias CG, Seber A, et al. Clinical aspects and treatment of pain in children and adolescents with cancer. *Pediatr Blood Cancer.* 2005;45:925–932.

109. Friedrichsdorf SJ, Kang TI. The management of pain in children with life-limiting illnesses. *Pediatr Clin North Am.* 2007;54:645–672.

110. Zernikow B, Michel E, Craig F, et al. Pediatric palliative care: use of opioids for the management of pain. *Paediatr Drugs.* 2009;11:129–151.

111. Ullrich CK, Mayer OH. Assessment and management of fatigue and dyspnea in pediatric palliative care. *Pediatr Clin North Am.* 2007;54:735–756.

112. Wusthoff CJ, Shellhaas RA, Licht DJ. Management of common neurologic symptoms in pediatric palliative care: seizures, agitation, and spasticity. *Pediatr Clin North Am.* 2007;54:709–733.

113. Kersun LS, Shemesh E. Depression and anxiety in children at the end of life. *Pediatr Clin North Am.* 2007;54:691–708.

114. Stoddard FJ, Usher CT, Abrams AN. Psychopharmacology in pediatric critical care. *Child Adolesc Psychiatr Clin N Am.* 2006;15:611–655.

115. Kreicbergs U, Valdimarsdottir U, Onelov E, et al. Care-related distress: a nationwide study of parents who lost their child to cancer. *J Clin Oncol.* 2005;23:9162–9171.

116. Kreicbergs UC, Lannen P, Onelov E, et al. Parental grief after losing a child to cancer: impact of professional and social support on long-term outcomes. *J Clin Oncol.* 2007;25:3307–3312.

117. Lannen PK, Wolfe J, Prigerson HG, et al. Unresolved grief in a national sample of bereaved parents: impaired mental and physical health 4 to 9 years later. *J Clin Oncol.* 2008;26:5870–5876.

118. Surkan PJ, Kreicbergs U, Valdimarsdottir U, et al. Perceptions of inadequate health care and feelings of guilt in parents after the death of a child to a malignancy: a population-based long-term follow-up. *J Palliat Med.* 2006;9:317–331.

119. Figley CR. *Compassion Fatigue: Coping with Secondary Traumatic Stress Disorder in Those Who Treat the Traumatized.* Brunner/Mazel; 1995.

120. Rourke MT. Compassion fatigue in pediatric palliative care providers. *Pediatr Clin North Am.* 2007;54:631–644.

121. Kearney MK, Weininger RB, Vachon MLS, et al. Self-care of physicians caring for patients at the end of life: "Being connected … a key to my survival". *JAMA.* 2009;301:1155–1164.

122. Green M, ed. *Bright Futures: Guidelines for Health Supervision of Infants, Children and Adolescents.* National Center for Education in Maternal and Child Health; 1994.

123. Jellinek MS, Little M, Murphy JM, et al. The pediatric symptom checklist: support for a role in a managed care environment. *Arch Pediatr Adolesc Med.* 1995;149:740–746.

124. Wiener L, Kazak A, Noll R, et al. Standards for the psychosocial care of children with cancer and their families: an introduction to the special issue. *Pediatr Blood Cancer.* 2015;62:S419–S424.

39

CHRONIC DISEASE AND UNHEALTHY LIFESTYLE BEHAVIORS: BEHAVIORAL MANAGEMENT

ELIZABETH PEGG FRATES, MD ■ ELYSE R. PARK, PHD, MPH ■
A. EDEN EVINS, MD, MPH ■ GREGORY L. FRICCHIONE, MD

OVERVIEW

Lifestyle behaviors (such as having an unhealthy diet, physical inactivity, inadequate sleep, chronic stress, a lack of social connectedness, and use of risky substances) are associated with the development of chronic non-communicable diseases (NCDs). Centuries ago, Hippocrates emphasized the power of exercise and nutrition; he noted, "If we could give every individual the right amount of nourishment and exercise, not too little and not too much, we would have found the safest way to health." Over the past few decades, a bevy of research papers have supported this ancient wisdom. Among these was a 1993 study on the identification of non-genetic factors that contribute to death in the United States.[1] McGinnis and Foege[1] examined the literature from 1977 to 1993 and determined that 19% of all deaths were attributable to tobacco use, 14% were attributable to poor diet and physical inactivity, and 5% were attributable to alcohol consumption. Eleven years later, Mokdad and colleagues[2] reported on statistics from the United States from the year 2000. They pointed out that the main chronic diseases causing death in the United States were cardiac disease, cancer, stroke, and chronic respiratory diseases. In addition, they highlighted the root causes of those diseases and thus, the actual causes of death; among these were behaviors (e.g., tobacco use, which accounted for approximately 19% of deaths; poor diet and physical inactivity, which accounted for approximately 17% of deaths; and alcohol consumption, which accounted for approximately 4% of deaths).[2] These studies and others helped to connect addictions and lifestyle behaviors

to the development of NCDs. To address these notable behaviors, *Healthy People 2030* created goals to: increase the proportion of adults who meet current guidelines for aerobic physical activity and muscle-strengthening activity; decrease the prevalence of smoking in adults to 6.1%; enhance restorative sleep (only 72.3% of adults get sufficient sleep, defined as ≥8 hours for those aged 18 to 21 years and ≥7 hours for those aged 22 years and older, on average, during 24 hours); and decrease the proportion of adults who are obese from 41.8% to 36.0%.[3]

According to the American Psychological Association, stress levels have been and remain high during and following the COVID-19 pandemic.[4] Roughly one-fourth (27%) of American adults said that on most days they felt so stressed that they could not function. Specifically, for those under the age of 35, nearly half (46%) felt that consequence of stress. However, only 4% of those aged >65 years felt that level of stress. In terms of race and ethnicity, 56% of Black adults aged <35 years felt so stressed they could not function, while less than half of White, Asian, or Latino/adults aged <35 years reported that level of stress.[4] Stress impacts health in many ways, especially related to lifestyle behaviors. The American Psychological Association estimates that nearly three-fourths (72%) of adults have negative health outcomes due to this stress, including feeling overwhelmed (33%), worrying constantly (30%), having difficulty sleeping (32%), and using alcohol, cigarettes, or drugs to relax (15%).[4]

NCDs (cardiovascular diseases, chronic respiratory diseases, cancer, diabetes, arthritis, and neuropsychiatric diseases) take an enormous toll, not only in terms of mortality but also in terms of disability and the ballooning of healthcare costs. For this reason, the NCDs represent the most important global health challenge of the 21st century.[5] Lifestyle is crucial in the etiology of NCDs, and healthcare professionals need to work with patients to reduce these important risk factors.[5]

The idea that Americans have some control over their chances of acquiring a chronic condition is becoming more mainstream. The five healthy habits index is commonly used in research. These five habits include: not smoking; maintaining a body mass index (BMI) <25; eating a healthy diet with a high intake of fiber, low levels of refined carbohydrates, a high ratio of polyunsaturated fat compared with saturated fat, and low intake of trans-fats; drinking alcohol in moderation (two drinks or less a day for males and one drink or less a day for females); and exercising regularly (at least 20 minutes three times a week of aerobic exercise).[6] Gradually, the public awareness of these healthy indices has increased. Unfortunately, over the past 20 years, changes in adherence rates to healthy habits in the United States have not changed for the better.[7] For example, obesity levels in the United States rose from 28% to 36%; the percentage of people engaging in regular physical activity dropped from 53% to 43%; the percentage of people eating ≥5 servings of fruits and vegetables in a day decreased from 42% to 26%; adherence to all five healthy indices went down from 15.2% to 8.5%; and, adherence rates to healthy habits were not more likely in people with chronic disease (e.g., cardiac disease, high blood pressure, high cholesterol, and diabetes).

Increased awareness of healthy lifestyles does not necessarily translate into increased adoption of healthy lifestyles. As Sir Francis Bacon stated in the 17th century, "Knowledge is power." However, knowledge alone is not powerful enough to instill lasting behavioral change. Environmental factors also influence lifestyle behaviors and patterns. The socioecological model of change reviews the layers that surround an individual (and includes relationships, community, and society). Although working to help people adopt and sustain healthy lifestyle patterns is important (to help them with their knowledge, skills, and attitudes), it is not enough. It is also essential to evaluate the individual's home environment, work environment, relationships in those places, their neighborhood, local grocery stores, green spaces, safe walking spaces, societal laws (especially those related to lifestyle factors like smoking, trans-fats in foods, driving under the influence punishments, and others).

To fully address an individual's lifestyle behaviors, the social determinants of health need to be factored into counseling sessions and treatment plans. The social determinants of health include economic stability, educational access and quality, healthcare access and quality, neighborhood and built environment, and the social and community context.[3] These social determinants of health were emphasized in *Healthy People 2030*. One update to the discussion of healthy behaviors is to take the focus away from choices and habits that put primary responsibility on the individual and neglect the environment that surrounds them. Instead of using the term lifestyle choices or habits, healthcare professionals can discuss lifestyle options and patterns that develop as a result of multiple factors, including what is available to the individual (e.g., fresh produce in grocery stores, food from a backyard garden, safe walking spaces, greenery and nature close to home, bike paths, and a quiet location at nighttime essential to sound sleep).

HEALTHY LIFESTYLES AND DISEASE PREVENTION AND MANAGEMENT

Lifestyle intervention studies have demonstrated that adopting healthy lifestyles reduces the morbidity and mortality of disease. Without question, obesity is a growing health concern. Therefore, losing weight and maintaining a healthy weight (i.e., ≤BMI) is a goal for many people in the United States. However, simply adding healthy lifestyle patterns, even if they do not alter someone's weight or BMI, is also beneficial. Matheson and colleagues[8] examined healthy lifestyle factors (e.g., being a non-smoker, consuming more than five servings of fruit and vegetables a day, engaging in physical activity >12 times a month, and drinking alcohol in moderation) in people in different weight categories (normal weight, overweight, and obese). Their results demonstrated that adding healthy behaviors to people's lifestyles resulted in a significant decrease in mortality, regardless of their baseline BMI. This was especially beneficial for those who were in the obese category by BMI.[8]

Research has shown that practicing healthy habits can reduce mortality and help people prevent chronic disease. For example, Ford and colleagues[9] found that by adhering to four healthy lifestyle factors: never smoking, maintaining a BMI <30, being physically active for ≥3.5 hours per week, and adhering to a healthy diet (with a high intake of fruits, vegetables, whole-grain bread, and low meat consumption) approximately 80% of chronic diseases could be prevented. Several years later, Akesson and colleagues[10] in Sweden, conducted a population-based prospective cohort study in Swedish males who were followed for 11 years. They concluded that by not smoking; consuming only moderate amounts of alcohol; following a healthy diet; walking/bicycling for >40 minutes each day; exercising for at least 1 hour a week; and maintaining a waist circumference <95 cm, 79% of myocardial infarctions could be avoided.

Collectively, current interventions target multiple risk factors (MRFs)—as a lifestyle change—rather than individual behaviors. Indeed, in 1982 the Multiple Risk Factor Intervention Trial, a randomized trial of a multi-factorial intervention program on mortality from coronary heart disease among high-risk males, consisted of treatment for hypertension, counseling for cigarette smoking, and dietary advice for lowering blood cholesterol levels.[11]

Lifestyle medicine is the medical specialty that encourages and prescribes healthy lifestyle behaviors (e.g., regular exercise, healthy eating patterns, sound sleep, positive social connections, stress management, and avoidance of risky substances to treat, reverse, and prevent disease). A landmark study published in the *New England Journal of Medicine* randomized overweight, pre-diabetic patients into three groups: placebo, metformin, and a lifestyle intervention. The lifestyle intervention targeted losing 7% of body weight by following a diet low in calories and low in fat, as well as aiming to accumulate 150 minutes of physical activity in a week. A 16-hour curriculum covering diet, exercise, and behavior modification was also part of the lifestyle intervention. These sessions, taught by case managers, were flexible and individualized. The participants also had monthly individual group sessions that reinforced the lessons. Subjects were followed for 4 years and then evaluated to see how many of them, who were all pre-diabetic, went on to develop diabetes. Compared with the placebo group, the cumulative incidence of diabetes in the metformin group was 31% less, and the cumulative incidence of diabetes in the lifestyle intervention group was 58% less than the placebo group. The lifestyle medicine intervention was more effective in helping pre-diabetic patients avoid the diagnosis of diabetes than both placebo and metformin.[12]

Our lifestyles affect our ability to manage, treat, and prevent disease through different mechanisms. One of those involves gene expression changes. Ornish and colleagues[13] demonstrated that a 3-month intensive lifestyle intervention with a focus on exercise, stress management, and nutrition could modulate gene expression in patients with prostate cancer. This epigenetics research encourages healthcare practitioners to prioritize counseling patients on behavioral change.

The effect of one component alone, specifically exercise, on health has been the subject of much research. A recent meta-analysis that examined the efficacy of exercise, compared with drug interventions, on the mortality rate of people suffering from specific chronic diseases (including heart disease, chronic heart failure, stroke, and diabetes), revealed that in many cases, exercise can be as effective as medicine.[14] Investigating the effects of exercise on mood and anxiety has also become a topic of interest in the medical literature. Several studies support the use of exercise as an adjunctive treatment for depression and anxiety.[15-20] In one study, researchers demonstrated that state anxiety was reduced after even one 50-minute session of aerobic or resistance training exercise at a level of 70% to 80% of one's maximum heart rate, in subjects with elevated anxiety levels.[21] These studies did not recommend using exercise instead of medicine, but rather in conjunction with medications. Exercise can be prescribed in a safe and effective way.[22] Moreover, providers who exercise are more likely to counsel their patients on exercise, and specifically, providers counsel patients on exercises that they perform, such as aerobic training or strength training.[23]

The evidence shows that adopting healthy lifestyles helps patients prevent and manage chronic disease. However, starting on, counseling in, and sustaining healthy behaviors is a challenge for patients and clinicians. Specific skills and tools (such as the use of the Transtheoretical Model of Change, the 5 As, motivational interviewing [MI], positive psychology, appreciative inquiry [AI], and goal setting) can be developed by practitioners to empower patients to adopt healthy lifestyles. There is a five-step cycle that incorporates each of these strategies and techniques and serves as a guide for providers counseling patients on lifestyle changes.

Patients often need support when seeking to stop an unhealthy behavior and start a new health-promoting behavior.

TRANSTHEORETICAL MODEL OF CHANGE

The Transtheoretical Model of Change was developed by James Prochaska, PhD, after working for 20 years with patients who suffer from addictions. It is useful, not only as a tool for treating addictions, often in conjunction with medication, but for increasing exercise, adopting a healthy diet, and changing other behaviors. This model separates patients into categories of readiness for change, including pre-contemplation (not willing or wanting to change), contemplation (considering changing), preparation (getting ready to make a change), action, and maintenance.[24] Recognizing the stage of change that a patient is in is the first step. Then, counseling follows according to their stage of change. This model allows providers to tailor their counseling to the needs of the patient based on their stage of change.

Pre-contemplation

Those individuals who are pre-contemplative say they cannot and are not ready to change. By raising their awareness of the importance of the problem, providers increase the chances that their patients will address the issue. For example, if an obese patient is eating "fast foods," reporting that he has no time to cook, no money to buy healthy foods, and states that since he has never been successful at losing weight he will not even try, then asking the patient about his understanding of the risks of being over-weight is a good place to start. "What is your understanding about the risks of being over-weight?" is an open-ended question that will allow a patient to share his knowledge and beliefs. Building on his response to this question, other risks can be added. This will raise his awareness. Sharing the story of a patient who lost weight and kept it off

might be another effective strategy for someone who is pre-contemplative. In this stage, the goal is for them to consider learning more about their behavior and the effects of their behavior.

For patients who are not motivated to change, the "5 Rs" can be used:

- Relevance—Make it relevant to the patient's current health and health goals
- Risks—Elicit the patient's perceptions of short- and long-term health risks of their behavior (e.g., obesity's impact on shortness of breath, long-term cardiac risk)
- Rewards—Encourage the patient to think about possible rewards for future changes in health behavior
- Roadblocks—Identify barriers to making a behavioral change (e.g., other smokers at work, friends who drink excessively)
- Repetition—Repeat these discussions each time you see the patient.

Contemplation

Contemplators say they may or might change. For contemplators, using experiential techniques, including raising awareness and dramatic relief, is effective. In this stage, a provider can also use self-re-evaluation by encouraging the patient to identify with a healthy role model. In addition, the use of imagery is helpful for contemplators. In so doing, the patient can begin to create a vision of who they might become. Asking the patient to consider what life would be like if they were enjoying healthy meals throughout the day and avoiding fast foods is one way to encourage the use of imagery. This allows the patient to ponder the possibilities of changing behavior and then to put those possibilities in their own words. By reviewing and emphasizing the pros of change and the cons of staying the same, the patient will start to realize the importance of change and the possible rewards that will come with change. When treating a contemplator, the goal is for him/her to think deeply about the reasons/causes that underlie their behaviors and consider evaluating different options.

Preparation

People who are in the preparation phase about their potential plans for modifying the target behavior have already convinced themselves that change is worth the effort. The focus is on making a commitment to change, using social support from family and friends, and finding healthy substitutes that can be used in place of unhealthy habits. For a patient looking to lose weight by consuming less fast food, the healthcare provider might brainstorm about quick healthy meals, starting with breakfast, to help the person in preparation move to action. Identifying a friend, co-worker, neighbor, or family member who can be a buddy in the process, or a supporter, will help the patient make progress. Creating a start date, or for smoking—a "quit date"—and making it public (e.g., by writing it down, posting it on social media, or sharing it with the healthcare provider, friends, or family) will help the person in preparation get ready for action. Making this commitment is called self-liberation. When treating someone in preparation, the goal is action, specifically, creating a plan to change behaviors and initiating medication if that is part of the plan.

Action

When treating someone in preparation, the goal is one of action, specifically, carrying out action-oriented plans. The people in the action phase have been practicing the new healthy behavior for at least a month, but less than 6 months, and they still need behavioral counseling and may still need medication treatment. Encouraging healthy substitutions and fostering relationships with people who support the healthy behavior pattern are also important. In addition to these strategies, focusing on the types of rewards the patient is experiencing and receiving from the newly adopted healthy behavior is key. Checking labs and pointing out a change in cholesterol or hemoglobin A1C can serve to encourage the patient to sustain the behavior. If the patient has experienced positive changes in their BMI or body composition, these can act as powerful rewards. The patient may notice improved mood or decreased stress. It is important to ask the patient what they noticed since adopting the healthy behavior.

Maintenance

People in the maintenance phase have been practicing healthy behavior for over 6 months, but they also need ongoing encouragement and support and may need to continue to take medication to sustain this behavior.

Using similar techniques to those in the action phase will work. Those patients in maintenance often respond well to the idea of becoming a mentor to someone new to the process of change. This can be a useful way for them to stay on track and to help another person who is struggling with a similar issue.

BEHAVIORAL MODIFICATION COUNSELING: THE "5 AS"

The 5 As of behavioral change counseling are: Assess, Advise, Agree, Assist, and Arrange. Following the 5 As of behavioral change, counseling is useful as it helps engage the patient, put a plan in motion, and track progress with the plan.[25]

Assess

First, assess the patient's risk factors, signs and symptoms, social history, past medical history, laboratory results, physical examination, exercise history, dietary patterns, stress levels, sleep quality and quantity, substance use, and level of social connection. Assessing the patient's current level of interest in change and the stage of change according to the Transtheoretical Model of Change is also part of the assessment phase of counseling.

Advise

After asking questions and gathering information during the initial assessment phase of the counseling, the provider moves to the second A: advising. The provider can then target the information on behavioral change to address the patient's current disease state, risk factors, and unhealthy behaviors. Meeting the patient's stage of change and tailoring the advice to the stage will save time and increase the chances that the advice is heard, understood, and followed. An understanding of the Transtheoretical Model of Change is essential for behavioral change counseling, especially when crafting advice that will be accepted and utilized by the patient.

Agree

After crafting advice that targets the patient's stage of change, disease state, symptoms, complaints, needs, desires, and hopes for the future, the next step is to check in with the patient. The third A stands for agree.

It is important to acknowledge the patient's autonomy and agreement with the plans for the change process. Instead of just telling the patient what to do without asking for feedback, this strategy ensures that the patient agrees with the plan. If the patient does not agree, a dialogue about the best way forward will unfold. This step creates a partnership between the patient and the provider.

Assist

Assist is the fourth A. In this phase, the provider assists the patient in making the change plan a reality. This could involve writing prescriptions for exercise or a healthy eating pattern, encouraging participation in a stress management program, or requesting a referral to a nutritionist, sleep laboratory, or physical therapist. The provider works closely with the patient to find support systems and community resources near the patient's home that can assist the patient in following through with the plan and achieving the stated goals.

Arrange

The fifth and final A represents arranging follow-up. This last phase is critical because it puts accountability into the change plan. The patient knows that there will be another visit during which the provider will follow-up on the topics and strategies discussed in the session. The provider needs to ask about the plan, which has been recorded in the medical record, during the follow-up visit. Focusing on all five steps of behavioral change counseling helps providers cultivate a supportive environment and conduct sessions that foster movement toward the targeted healthy behaviors.

A FIVE-STEP CYCLE FOR COACHING PATIENTS TO ADOPT AND SUSTAIN HEALTHY BEHAVIORS

The collaboration embodied in the "5 As" of behavioral change counseling helps propel patients forward on their behavior change journeys.[26] With collaboration, the expertise of the provider in disease management, health goals, behavioral change, and national guidelines are combined with the expert knowledge of that patient in their own life: needs, desires, fears, past successes, strengths, weaknesses, previous failed attempts to change, and potential supportive friends and family

that might help the patient achieve their goals. Both the provider and the patient provide essential information in the partnership. The provider refrains from telling the patient exactly what to do and realizes that the patient can have their own effective solutions to problems that arise during the process of behavioral change. Threatening, convincing, arguing, demanding, and cajoling are all ineffective tactics when counseling patients on behavioral change. An example of a threat is: "If you don't exercise regularly, you will keep gaining weight and suffer a heart attack." A more collaborative approach to motivate someone to begin an exercise program is to ask, "How would your life be different if you were exercising regularly?" Eliciting information from patients and building on their statements helps them feel heard, understood, and validated.

When collaborating with a patient to help start a new healthy behavior, there is a five-step cycle that can help providers conduct coaching conversations that are motivating, inspiring, and in line with the 5 As of behavioral counseling.[27] The five steps are as follows: (1) express empathy, (2) align motivation, (3) build confidence and self-efficacy, (4) co-create SMART goals, and (5) set accountability. Then, the cycle starts again with expressing empathy. The five-step cycle of collaboration is compatible with the 5 As. They are used in concert (Fig. 39.1).

Expressing empathy is the first step of the five-step cycle. Research demonstrates there is a correlation between physicians' self-reported empathy and instant feedback on patient-provider satisfaction by the patient, with higher empathy scores correlating to higher satisfaction scores.[28] Making sure to be fully present and mindful during the behavioral change counseling session is critical. This might require a provider to elicit their relaxation response by taking a few deep breaths before the session or by entering a mindful state through opening awareness in a non-judgmental way and finding a sense of calm before the session. With an open and quiet mind, the provider can listen fully to the patient's story and provide useful, individualized advice after thoughtful questioning. Fully understanding the patient's situation is important to increase the patient's trust in the provider. After listening carefully to the sentences, words, tone of voice, body language, cadence, and facial expressions of the patient, the provider can respond with reflections that demonstrate to

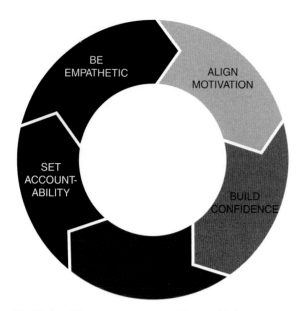

Fig. 39.1 ■ Five-step cycle as a coaching model. (From Frates EP, Moore MA, Lopez CN, et al. Coaching for behavior change in physiatry. *Am J Phys Med Rehabil*. 2011;90(12):1074–1082. Reprinted with permission.)

the patient that he or she was listening, that he or she followed the patient's story and train of thought and that he or she understood the patient's emotional state. As Theodore Roosevelt said, "No one cares what you have to say until they know how much you care." This first step in expressing empathy is the basis for creating a meaningful connection and for forming a therapeutic partnership for behavioral change.

The second step is to align motivation. In this step, the provider uses MI to help a patient discover and declare their own motivation for change.[29] Step 1 of the cycle emphasizes empathy and fully understanding the patient while taking a non-judgmental approach. In Step 2, the patient is encouraged to express their *change talk*. Change talk is the language that provides the pros for change, the cons for remaining the same, the desire for change, the ability to change, the reasons for change, and the need for change. One of the main goals of MI is to evoke change talk.

Through MI, a clinician can elicit a patient's reasons for change. The clinician's role is then, through questioning and listening, to illustrate the discrepancy between a patient's current behavior and their health goals. MI is influenced by the Stage of Change Theory,

Rogerian patient-centered therapy, and cognitive-behavioral therapy (CBT). Yet, distinct from CBT, MI conceptualizes motivation as a constantly changing state. Distinct from Rogerian therapy in its patient-centered approach, it differs in that it is directive. MI is also goal-directed, through negotiations between the clinician and the patient. During times of elevated motivation, CBT skills may be integrated with MI, to apply action goals, such as cutting back on the number of cigarettes per day, or to target barriers to achieving smoking cessation goals, such as using stress management practices to alleviate stress-related smoking triggers.

Underlying MI are the beliefs that motivation is a fluctuating state, in which ambivalence is a welcome and important part of change, and every patient has a potential for change. MI goals include: (1) building a patient's intrinsic motivation to change (e.g., beginning with an exercise routine or quitting smoking) and (2) resolving ambivalence about change (e.g., creating and amplifying the discrepancy between the patient's current behavior and their expressed goals). As an example of ambivalence, a patient says that they want to get 8 hours of sleep a night, to feel well rested, but consistently goes to bed 6 hours before their alarm rings. Finally, four MI principles are as follows: (1) express empathy (through skillful reflective listening), (2) develop discrepancy (ask evocative questions to enable the patients to express reasons for change), (3) roll with resistance (avoid arguing for change), and (4) support self-efficacy (the patient's belief, perceived confidence in their ability to change). A 2020 systematic review of 12 randomized controlled trials supported the effectiveness of brief intervention and MI to quit tobacco use.[30]

Some basic skills used in MI can be recalled through the mnemonic "OARS": asking Open-ended questions, stating Affirmations, using Reflections, and giving Summaries. MI involves establishing a connection and exploring the patient's feelings, beliefs (e.g., hopelessness), and values (e.g., importance of longevity) to help them work through ambivalence or ever-changing motivations. This includes addressing their reasons for their behaviors; understanding the relation of behaviors to their values and goals; and building their confidence.[29] Another technique used in MI is to elicit-provide-elicit. The provider elicits what information the patient would like to hear or what topics interest them. In this way, the provider checks in with the patient on how much the patient already knows; this diminishes wasting time by supplying the patient with information that he or she already has. With this method, the provider then provides that requested information. After imparting knowledge, the provider asks what the patient learned. This ensures a collaborative relationship in which the patient is an active member. It also makes sure that the provider was successful in explaining the concepts and checks in on what the patient was able to comprehend and recall. MI is an effective skill that can empower patients. It helps patients align their motivation for change. MI has been studied in weight loss and stroke and has shown promise in many other areas (including human immunodeficiency virus care, dental outcomes, alcohol use, tobacco use, and physical inactivity).[31-33]

Step 3 builds confidence and self-efficacy. Confidence is the feeling of strength that comes from a belief in one's abilities. Self-efficacy is the belief that one can complete a task successfully. In general, being confident and believing in one's self help patients persist in their process of behavioral change. Feeling assured that one can do a certain activity or conquer a specific challenge (such as taking a walk at lunchtime), is more specific and requires focused work on that task. To build self-efficacy, the patient needs to feel comfortable with the difficulty of the specific activity and to feel strong enough, mentally and physically, to meet that challenge. By practicing, patients build self-efficacy. By recalling times when they performed the target activity, the patient can also build self-efficacy. This step invites the provider to use positive psychology, a strengths-based approach, and AI to help the patient move forward on their behavioral change journey. Seligman,[34] considered one of the founders of the field of positive psychology, promotes the process of bringing out the patient's strengths. By identifying their strengths, the patient acknowledges the power inside him or her, and this helps to build confidence.[34] Finding ways to use these signature strengths in the pursuit of health goals and the behavioral change process can be an effective and rewarding technique to propel patients forward.

By asking questions that elicit a positive emotion, the provider is setting the stage for creative thinking and brainstorming, which are both important in a behavioral change counseling session. Positive emotions include love, joy, gratitude, serenity, interest, hope, pride, amusement, inspiration, and awe.[35] Frederickson's[36] broaden-and-build model highlights the fact that positive emotions can help people stimulate new ideas, gain new perspectives, as well as appreciate the broad picture in a situation. Thus positive emotions can help people build enduring personal resources.[36] Asking a question that explores a positive experience, such as "What was the highlight of your week?," "When was a time that you reached a goal? Tell me about that," or "What is going really well in your life right now?," will serve to bring out the positive core, and corresponding emotions, in a person.

Accentuating the positive core is a key concept in AI, an interviewing style that uses positive experiences in the present to create positive experiences in the future. In this method of interviewing, the idea is that appreciating and acknowledging the positive aspects of a person, situation, or organization brings forward more positive experiences.[37] This work has been used in the healthcare setting, and on an organizational and individual level with success. With AI, the provider works to build confidence by defining the focus or goal in the behavioral change process, then discovering the best of what is, after that, dreaming about what might be, then designing a plan, and finally, experiencing destiny by learning from and adjusting to what unfolds. The goal is to define, discover, dream, design, and deliver. A study using AI with patients suffering from dementia demonstrated positive results[38] and a recent review of the medical literature revealed that AI was effective in multiple domains, including caring for patients with dementia, elderly patients at the time of discharge from the hospital, and use within medical practices.[39] Building confidence and self-efficacy is an important step in the cycle and there are many different ways to accomplish this.

Step 4 is to co-create SMART goals. SMART goals are specific, measurable, action oriented, realistic, and time sensitive.

S = Specific: Goals should be straightforward and emphasize what you want to happen. Specific is the "What, Why, and How" of the SMART model.

M = Measurable: Goals with measurable outcomes should be selected, so that you can see the results of change. How will you know when you reach your goal?

A = Action oriented: Identify action goals and specify what you will do.

R = Realistic: The goal needs to be something you can strive toward and achieve.

T = Time sensitive: Set a time frame for the goal—initially very short term (i.e., this week).

Co-creation is used here to remind the provider to make sure the patient agrees with the goal. A provider can check to see if a goal is SMART by asking five questions: Is this a goal that is detailed and explicitly stated? How will the patient measure the outcome of the goal? Will the patient be doing something specific to achieve the goal? How likely is it that the patient can reach the goal in the stated time frame? What is the timeline for meeting the goal? To answer these questions, the provider must be connecting, communicating, and collaborating with the patient, as the patient is the only one who can determine if the goal is realistic. Working toward a goal provides a major source of motivation to reach the goal, which in turn, improves performance.[40] In addition, the Theory of Adult Learning, *andragogy*, states that adult learners are autonomous and self-directed, full of life experience and knowledge, goal-oriented, relevancy-oriented, and practical.[41] Keeping andragogy in mind when co-creating goals helps the provider treat the patient like an adult learner and a partner. It also facilitates the co-creation of compelling goals. Research demonstrates that when patients set health goals that match their life goals, they are more likely to reach their health goals.[42] Setting goals helps patients to focus on the behavioral change process and to prioritize it.

Step 5 in the cycle is setting accountability. This step ensures that patients are working on their goals. In the 5 As, this is consistent with the fifth A, for arranging follow-up. The patient needs to feel that this is important enough to the provider that he or she will check in on the goals the next time they meet. Before the next follow-up visit, a provider can check in by e-mail, by phone, or by postcard. This can be accomplished with the help of administrative staff at the office. Helping the patient identify a buddy for the behavioral change will allow for accountability between visits. A family member or friend can serve as the behavioral change buddy. If the buddy has similar goals and can take walks with the patient or start consuming more vegetables at the same time as the patient, it adds another level of importance to the goals for the patient and the buddy. Using a tracking system, such as a pedometer or wearable device, can be a useful method of providing feedback and thus setting accountability. A written log can be as effective as a method that uses the latest technology. The method must match the patient's preferences. Thus setting accountability is an important part of the five-step cycle.

After setting accountability, the cycle starts again with empathy. Empathy propels the cycle forward. When the patient returns for the follow-up visit, the provider needs to be open, non-judgmental, and supportive, regardless of the success or lack of success the patient experienced. If there is a failure, then the goal is to learn from the failure and move forward. Approaching the process with a growth mindset allows patients to take risks, try new things, and challenge themselves without the fear of shame, blame, and guilt, which often comes with failure. With a growth mindset, failures or mis-steps are opportunities to learn and grow.[43] Each week, there are usually moments of success or positivity, and asking about these in the follow-up appointment is important. "What went well this week?" is a great way to start a follow-up session. The patients usually report on their failures right away and often neglect the small successes. Expressing empathy after listening to the successes and setbacks that the patient experienced when trying to achieve the goal is a priority for follow-up sessions with a patient seeking to change behavior. Empathy is key when counseling on behavioral change.

Behavioral change is not a quick fix, and it is not easy. It takes collaboration, connection, time, patience, understanding, and an organized approach that will help patients stay engaged in their behavioral change plan.

Case 1

Mrs. M, a 57-year-old overweight female with a history of depression was recently informed by her primary care doctor that she has pre-diabetes. She is divorced and has two adult children in college. Mrs. M quit smoking 15 years ago. Over the past 10 years, her weight has been increasing, although she occasionally goes on a diet and loses 15 pounds but regains the weight within 3 months. She comes to the office today because she is anxious about her new diagnosis of pre-diabetes. Since she watched her uncle suffer from diabetes for years, she is afraid of having her lower leg amputated like her uncle did.

After listening attentively, the provider expressed empathy by reflecting on what she heard. "It sounds like you are anxious because you are afraid that the diagnosis of pre-diabetes means you are on your way to a below-the-knee amputation, and with that, your life will change dramatically." After that, the patient nods her head sheepishly. Then, the provider asks her an open-ended question, "What could you do to control your blood sugars?" She answers by reporting, "My primary care doctor said that if I lose weight, I could reverse the pre-diabetes and avoid the diagnosis of diabetes altogether, but I have tried to lose weight for 10 years, and I am afraid that I will never succeed." The provider notes that the patient is in the contemplative stage of change. She keeps listening attentively, and the patient continues, "If I could stick with eating more vegetables and fewer sweets and if I could find an exercise that I like, I might be able to lose weight and keep it off." Then, the provider uses another reflection. "If you can eat healthy foods in healthy portions and start exercising regularly, then you might be able to control your weight and stop worrying about getting an amputation, which is pretty powerful motivation to stick with a healthy lifestyle." Mrs. M. then reflects and says, "I have never had such a powerful motivator before. I really don't want an amputation. I wish I could find a plan that worked for me to lose weight. I want to do it. I just don't think I can." By reminding Mrs. M that she successfully quit smoking, the provider points out that the patient has been successful with behavioral change in the past. She admits that it took several attempts for her to be successful at quitting smoking and it was not until she had a powerful motivator, which was her teenager starting to smoke her cigarettes, that she was able to quit. She says that the fear of amputation is equally as powerful so she thinks this time maybe she can be successful with her weight loss attempts. The provider reviews the past successes and failures of the weight loss attempts

and highlights the importance of learning from the failed attempts. The provider also asks if she wants to hear about research on pre-diabetes and lifestyle interventions. Because the patient expresses an interest, the provider shares some data and statistics with her. After checking in with the patient to see how much of the discussion resonated with the patient, the provider learned that the patient is very interested in exercise, specifically. She had used walking with friends to help her quit smoking. With that cue, the provider asks if the patient wants to learn about some research on exercise and its ability to reduce anxiety levels. The patient is eager to hear about that topic and can demonstrate a clear understanding of how exercise could help her blood glucose as well as help reduce her anxiety level, which was the reason for her visit.

Together, the patient and provider create a SMART goal for the week. Originally, Mrs. M says she wants to walk for 1 hour for 7 days this coming week, because she read that people need to be active for 60 minutes each day to lose weight. The provider asks her how realistic this goal is, given her work schedule. Then, the patient remembers that she stopped walking because her old sneakers were bothering her bunions and her feet were hurting with each step. So, they co-created a SMART goal for this week, which is for Mrs. M. to buy sneakers with a wide-toe box and feel good when she walks. After purchasing appropriate sneakers, Mrs. B is to walk for one 20-minute session on Wednesday, which is her day off. They set accountability by making the follow-up appointment. At the end of the appointment, Mrs. M says her anxiety seems better already, since she has a doable plan to control her weight, and she is hopeful that she will be successful this time.

At the follow-up visit, Mrs. M proudly wears her new sneakers, and the provider congratulates her on making the time to go to the store and buy the sneakers. Although she was only able to walk for 10 minutes, because she said it started to rain, the provider recognizes her effort to meet her goal and reinforces the fact that walking for 10 minutes is better than not walking at all. She asks Mrs. M how it felt when she was walking, and Mrs. M reports that she liked walking outside and being in nature on a trail near her house.

Mrs. M gradually increases her walking to 5 days a week for 1 hour each session. She starts noticing that her clothes are feeling baggy. Also, she starts changing her diet to add more vegetables, to cut down on desserts, and to monitor the glycemic index of her foods. After 3 months, she has lost 15 pounds, and she is slowly losing more weight. She takes a cooking class at the local community center and starts eating healthy meals at home, while enjoying the preparation and creation of delicious food, following a Mediterranean dietary pattern of eating, with plenty of vegetables, nuts, seeds, healthy protein, and whole grains. After a year, her blood sugars are consistently in the normal range, and her BMI is normal.

SMOKING PREVALENCE AND CHARACTERISTICS OF SMOKERS

In 2021, 28.3 million adults in the US smoked cigarettes (i.e., 11.5% of adults).[44] The prevalence of smoking differs by gender and race/ethnicity and even by socioeconomic status; specifically, individuals who have lower incomes and fewer years of education and those with a mental illness have the highest rates of smoking. Individuals who smoke have higher rates of depression and mental illness; 36.5% across psychiatric disorders,[45] and smoking rates are estimated at 53% among individuals with serious mental illness. While counseling is effective, use of first-line medications in conjunction with counseling can increase abstinence rates by 200% to 300% over counseling alone.[46] In considering smoking patterns, the issue of electronic cigarettes (known as e-cigs) is also important. E-cigs are electronic devices that deliver nicotine vapor. Rates of e-cig use are increasing; the most common reasons for the use of e-cigs are to try to cut down/quit smoking or for use in places where combustible cigarettes are not allowed. The impact of e-cigs on mental health especially in the youth is concerning. Systematic reviews in the literature suggest that e-cigs and vaping are associated with depression, suicidality, attention-deficit hyperactivity disorder, and conduct disorder. [47] Using e-cigs to quit smoking creates a new problem to tackle quitting e-cigs. More research is needed to understand the long-term effects of e-cigs.

Quitting Cigarette Smoking

Most smokers begin by the age of 18, and most smokers want to quit. Each year, two-thirds of adult smokers try to quit,[48] but only 6% will become non-smokers, if unassisted.[49] Quitting is indeed a process. There are a variety of ways that a smoker can engage in quitting; individuals can quit by going "cold turkey" or by cutting back and tapering. Smokers cut back/taper by smoking only in certain places (e.g., no smoking in the car, or certain rooms in the home), only during certain times (e.g., only after work hours), or only a certain number of cigarettes smoked by day. Many individuals find it helpful to record one's smoking, to better understand their smoking behavior and associated patterns, and to set up a cutting back/tapering schedule. Daily monitoring of one's cigarette intake can be a great tool to facilitate a quit. Negative emotions (e.g., depression, anxiety, stress) complicate smoking cessation attempts. Individuals often use smoking to help regulate these emotions; in turn, quitting attempts with withdrawal symptoms can exacerbate these negative emotions. However, smoking cessation has been shown in many studies to improve anxiety, depression, negative affect, and stress.[50]

Smoking Cessation Behavioral Treatments

The US Public Health Service guidelines recommend that all smokers receive a brief clinician-delivered model (the 5 As: Ask, Advise, Assess, Assist, and Arrange follow-up).[51] The 5 As increase the likelihood of smoking cessation. Studies report that clinician-delivered rates of assistance (recommending and/or providing counseling or prescriptions) are low, which is unfortunate because these are the most impactful for patients.[52–55]

Smokers may obtain treatment in individual or group settings and treatment can be delivered via an in-person counselor, or with other modalities, such as stand-alone or adjunctive treatment, including telephone-based counseling, text messaging, web-based programs, and phone apps. Here, we discuss CBT and mindfulness approaches to smoking cessation.

Cognitive-Behavioral Therapy Approaches

Cognitive-behavioral treatments focus on building an awareness of and adaptation to negative thinking patterns and associated emotions and behaviors. CBT strategies for cessation include:

- Tracking daily intake
- Identifying and managing triggers, including withdrawal symptoms. A simple strategy for this is ACE, Avoid, Change, and Escape, in anticipating or coping with a trigger. Avoid: "How can you avoid triggers?"; Change: "What can you do to change a situation to lessen your chances of being around smoking?"; Escape: "How do you get away from a situation in which you are being exposed to smoking?"
- Engaging in social support (enhancing one's emotional and smoking-specific support)
- Engaging in emotional regulation (focusing on the role of mood changes, in relation to smoking and quitting attempts)
- Participating in stress management and relaxation training (using strategies such as meditation and deep breathing)
- Engaging in environmental modification (creating smoke-free environments or decreasing exposure to smokers and cigarette smoking)
- Coping with cravings. Many smokers experience physical and psychological urges to smoke, especially in the earlier stages of quitting. Stress management and mind-body strategies (e.g., diaphragmatic breathing, guided imagery, body scanning, yoga progressive muscle relaxation, a brief meditation, or mindful walking) can be used to deal with these urges. The "4 Ds" can also be helpful to remember and use: Delay—take a moment; Drink (water); Distraction—focus on or do something else; and Deep—breathing.

Mind-Body Approaches or Mindfulness

Mindfulness involves paying purposeful attention and having a non-judgmental awareness of present experiences.[56] Mindfulness exercises (e.g., mindful meditation, body scan, mindful walking) can increase awareness and acceptance of smoking cues, which, in turn, helps smokers tolerate smoking triggers and choose behaviors/responses other than smoking as a response to smoking cues. Focusing on this experience, a smoker may learn that an urge became fleeting. Mindfulness programs help smokers use mindfulness skills to manage negative emotions and thoughts about cues and be efficacious in helping smokers quit.[57,58]

Smoking Cessation Medications

The most effective way to quit smoking is to combine counseling treatment with US Food and Drug Administration (FDA)–approved smoking cessation medications. A careful psychiatric and medical intake, as well as a review of previous medication use, will determine the most effective medication and dose. Smoking cessation medications can be used for smokers with varying levels of quit motivation[59] during the process of quitting. Specifically, using this combination of evidence-based behavioral treatment and medication approximately doubles abstinence rates.[60] Currently, there are eight first-line medications for smoking cessation: five types of nicotine therapy (i.e., patch, lozenge, gum, inhaler, and spray), two forms of bupropion (Zyban, Wellbutrin), and varenicline. Nicotine-replacement therapy (NRT) involves using "clean" nicotine substitutes that target withdrawal symptoms. Bupropion SR (Zyban, Wellbutrin SR) is an antidepressant that inhibits the reuptake of dopamine and norepinephrine, reducing cravings for tobacco. Varenicline (Chantix) is a non-nicotine medication that interferes with nicotine receptors; it has both agonist and antagonist functions—blocking pleasure in conjunction with withdrawal symptoms. In 2009 the FDA published a public health advisory on the neuropsychiatric side effects of varenicline and bupropion, but research suggested that these fears may have been overstated, prompting an FDA review.[46] A recent Cochrane Database review found that varenicline and combination NRT were superior to mono-NRT or bupropion.[61] In the largest smoking cessation study to date, with over 8000 smokers randomized, and the first head-to-head comparison of all first-line smoking cessation aids in smokers with and without mental illness, varenicline, bupropion, and a nicotine patch were each more effective than placebo with varenicline more effective than bupropion and N RT; none had greater neuropsychiatric safety signal than placebo in either cohort. Quitting rates are consistently significantly higher for smokers who use varenicline than for other monotherapies.[46,62–65]

REFERENCES

1. McGinnis JM, Foege WH. Actual causes of death in the United States. *JAMA*. 1993;270(18):2207–2212.
2. Mokdad AH, Marks JS, Stroup DF, et al. Actual causes of death in the United States, 2000. *JAMA*. 2004;291(10):1238–1245.

3. Office of Disease and Prevention and Health Promotion. *Health People*. Available at: <https://www.apa.org/news/press/releases/stress/2014/stress-report.pdf>; 2030.

4. APA. *Stress in America 2022: Concerned for the Future, Beset by Inflation*. Available at: <https://www.apa.org/news/press/releases/stress/2022/concerned-future-inflation>; 2022.

5. Narayan KM, Ali MK, Koplan JP. Global noncommunicable diseases—where worlds meet. *N Engl J Med*. 2010;363(13):1196–1198.

6. Reis JP, Loria CM, Sorlie PD, et al. Lifestyle factors and risk for new-onset diabetes: a population-based cohort study. *Ann Intern Med*. 2011;155(5):292–299.

7. King DE, Mainous 3rd AG, Camemolla M, et al. Adherence to healthy lifestyle habits in US adults, 1988–2006. *Am J Med*. 2009;122(6):528–534.

8. Matheson EM, King DE, Everett CJ. Healthy lifestyle habits and mortality in overweight and obese individuals. *J Am Board Fam Med*. 2012;25(1):9–15.

9. Ford ES, Bergmann MM, Kroger J, et al. Healthy living is the best revenge: findings from the European Prospective Investigation into Cancer and Nutrition – Potsdam study. *Arch Intern Med*. 2009;169(15):1355–1362.

10. Akesson A, Larsson SC, Discacciati A, et al. Low-risk diet and lifestyle habits in primary prevention of myocardial infarction in men: a population-based prospective cohort study. *J Am Coll Card*. 2014;64(13):1299–1306.

11. Multiple Factor Intervention Trial Research Group Risk factor changes and mortality results. Multiple risk factor intervention trial. *JAMA*. 1982;248(12):1465–1477.

12. Knowler WC, Barrett-Connor E, Fowler SE, et al. Diabetes prevention program research group: reduction in the incidence of type 2 diabetes with lifestyle intervention or metformin. *N Engl J Med*. 2002;346(6):393–403.

13. Ornish D, Magbanua MJ, Weinberg V, et al. Changes in prostate gene expression in men undergoing an intensive nutrition and lifestyle intervention. *Proc Natl Acad Sci USA*. 2008;105(24):8369–8374.

14. Naci H, Ioannidis JP. Comparative effectiveness of exercise and drug interventions on mortality outcomes: meta-epidemiological study. *BMJ*. 2013;347:f5577.

15. Lee YC. A study of the relationship between depression symptom and physical performance in elderly women. *J Exerc Rehabil*. 2015;11(6):367–371.

16. Ross CE, Hayes D. Exercise and psychologic well-being in the community. *Am J Epidemiol*. 1988;127(4):762–771.

17. Stephens T. Physical activity and mental health in the United States and Canada: evidence from our population surveys. *Prev Med*. 1988;17(1):35–47.

18. Galper DI, Trivedi MH, Barlow CE, et al. Inverse association between physical inactivity and mental health in men and women. *Med Sci Sports Exerc*. 2006;38(1):173–178.

19. Ann HRM, Collins KA, Fitterling HL. Physical exercise and depression. *Mt Sinai J Med*. 2009;76(2):204–214.

20. Breus MJ, O'Connor PJ. Exercise-induced anxiolysis: a test of the "time out" hypothesis in high anxious females. *Med Sci Sports Exerc*. 1998;30(7):107–112.

21. Hare BS, Raglin JS. State anxiety responses to acute resistance training and step aerobic exercise across eight weeks of training. *J Sports Med Phys Fitness*. 2002;42(1):108–112.

22. Frates EP, McBride Y, Bonnet J. Its fun: a practical algorithm for counseling on the exercise prescriptions: a method to mitigate the symptoms of depression, anxiety, and stress-related illness. *Clin Exp Psychol*. 2016;2:116.

23. Abramson S, Stein J, Schaufele M, et al. Personal exercise habits and counseling practices of primary care physicians: a national survey. *Clin J Sport Med*. 2000;10(1):40–48.

24. Prochaska JO, Norcross JC, DiClemente CC. *Changing for Good: The Revolutionary Program that Explains the Six Stages of Change and Teaches You How to Free Yourself From Bad Habits*. New York: William Morrow; 1994.

25. Dosh SA, Holtrop JS, Torres T, et al. Changing organizational constructs into functional tools: an assessment of the 5 A's in primary care practices. *Ann Fam Med*. 2005;3(suppl 2):s50–s52.

26. Frates EP, Bonnet J. Collaboration and negotiation: the key to therapeutic lifestyle change. *Am J Lifestyle Med*. 2016;10(5):302–312.

27. Frates EP, Moore MA, Lopez CN, et al. Coaching for behavior change in physiatry. *Am J Phys Med Rehabil*. 2011;90(12):1074–1082.

28. Wang H, Kline JA, Jackson BE, et al. Association between emergency physician self-reported empathy and patient satisfaction. *PLoS One*. 2018;13(9):e0204113.

29. Miller WR, Rollnick S. *Motivational Interviewing: Helping People for Change*. 3rd ed. Guilford Press; 2013.

30. Kumar R, Sahu M, Rodney T. Efficacy of motivational interviewing and brief interventions on tobacco use among healthy adults: a systematic review of randomized controlled trials. *Invest Educ Enferm*. 2022;40(3):e03.

31. Lundahl B, Moleni T, Burke BL, et al. Motivational interviewing in medical care settings: a systematic review and meta-analysis of randomized controlled trials. *Patient Educ Couns*. 2013;93(2):157–168.

32. Watkins CL, Wathan JV, Leathley MJ, et al. The 12-month effects of early motivational interviewing after acute stroke: a randomized controlled trial. *Stroke*. 2011;42(7):1956–1961.

33. Pollack KI, Alexander SC, Coffman CJ, et al. Physician communication techniques and weight loss in adults: project CHAT. *Am J Prev Med*. 2010;39(4):321–328.

34. Seligman MEP. *Authentic Happiness: Using the New Positive Psychology to Realize Your Potential for Lasting Fulfillment*. Atria Books; 2004.

35. Frederickson BL. *Love 2.0: Finding Happiness and Health in Moments of Connection*. Plume; 2013.

36. Fredrickson BL. The role of positive emotions in positive psychology. The broaden-and-build theory of positive emotions. *Am Psychol*. 2001;56(3):218–226.

37. Cooperrider DL, Whitney D. *Appreciative Inquiry: A Positive Revolution*. Berrett-Koehler Publishers; 2005.

38. McCarthy B. Appreciative inquiry: an alternative to behaviour management. *Dementia*. 2016;16(2). https://doi.org/10.1177/1471301216634921.

39. Trajkovski S, Schmied V, Vickers M, et al. Implementing the 4D cycle of appreciative inquiry in health care: a methodological review. *J Adv Nurs*. 2013;69(6):1224–1234.

40. Lock EA. Motivation through conscious goal setting. *Appl Prev Psychol.* 1996;5:117–124.

41. Knowles MS. *The Adult Learner: A Neglected Species.* 4th ed. Gulf Publishing; 1990.

42. Zhang KM, Dindoff K, Arnold JMO, et al. What matters to patients with heart failure? The influence of non-health-related goals on patient adherence to self-care management. *Patient Educ Couns.* 2015;98(8):927–934.

43. Dweck C. *Mindset. The New Psychology of Success.* Ballantine Books; 2007.

44. Center for Disease Control and Prevention. *Smoking and Tobacco Use Fast Facts and Fac Sheets.* Available at: <https://www.cdc.gov/tobacco/data_statistics/fact_sheets/fast_facts/index.htm>.

45. Centers for Disease Control and Prevention (CDC). *Tobacco Use Among Adults with Mental Illness and Substance Use Disorders.* Available at: <http://www.cdc.gov/tobacco/disparities/mental-illness-substance-use/index.htm>.

46. Anthenelli RM, Benowitz NL, West R, et al. Neuropsychiatric safety and efficacy of varenicline, bupropion, and nicotine patch in smokers with and without psychiatric disorders (EAGLES): a double-blind, randomised, placebo-controlled clinical trial. *Lancet.* 2016;387:2507–2520.

47. Becker TD, Rice TR. Youth vaping: a review and update on global epidemiology, physical and behavioral health risks, and clinical considerations. *Eur J Pediatr.* 2022;181(2):453–462.

48. Centers for Disease Control and Prevention (CDC). Quitting smoking among adults–United States, 2001–2013. *MMWR Morb Mortal Wkly Rep.* 2015;64(40):1129–1135.

49. Centers for Disease Control and Prevention (CDC). Quitting smoking among adults—United States, 2001–2010. *MMWR Morb Mortal Wkly Rep.* 2001;60(44):1513–1519.

50. Taylor G, McNeill A, Girling A, et al. Change in mental health after smoking cessation: systematic review and meta-analysis. *BMJ.* 2014;348:g1151.

51. Tobacco Use and Dependence Guideline Panel. *Treating Tobacco Use and Dependence: 2008 Update.* US Department of Health and Human Services; 2008.

52. Quinn VP, Stevens VJ, Hollis JF, et al. Tobacco-cessation services and patient satisfaction in nine nonprofit HMOs. *Am J Prev Med.* 2005;29(2):77–84.

53. Ferketich AK, Khan Y, Wewers ME. Are physicians asking about tobacco use and assisting with cessation? Results from the 2001–2004 National Ambulatory Medical Care Survey (NAMCS). *Prev Med.* 2006;43(6):472–476.

54. Thorndike AN, Tegan S, Rigotti NA. The treatment of smoking by US physicians during ambulatory visits: 1994–2003. *Am J Public Health.* 2007;97(10):1878–1883.

55. Park ER, Gareen IF, Japuntich S, et al. Primary care provider-delivered smoking cessation interventions and smoking cessation among participants in the National Lung Screening Trial. *JAMA Intern Med.* 2015;175(9):1509–1516.

56. Kabat-Zinn J. An outpatient program in behavioral medicine for chronic pain patients based on the practice of mindfulness meditation: theoretical considerations and preliminary results. *Gen Hosp Psychiatry.* 1982;4(1):33–47.

57. Spears CA, Hedeker D, Li L, et al. Mechanisms underlying mindfulness-based addiction treatment versus cognitive behavioral therapy and usual care for smoking cessation. *J Consult Clin Psychol.* 2017;85(11):1029–1040.

58. Davis JM, Mills DM, Stankevitz KA, et al. Pilot randomized trial on mindfulness training for smokers in young adult binge drinkers. *BMC Complement Altern Med.* 2013;13:215.

59. Jardin BF, Cropsey KL, Wahlquist AE, et al. Evaluating the effect of access to free medication to quit smoking: a clinical trial testing the role of motivation. *Nicotine Tob Res.* 2014;16(7):992–999.

60. Fiore MC, Jaen C, Baker T, et al. *Treating Tobacco Use and Dependence: 2008 Update. Clinical Practice Guideline.* US Department of Health and Human Services. Public Health Service; 2008.

61. Cahill K, Stevens S, Perera R, et al. Pharmacological interventions for smoking cessation: an overview and network meta-analysis. *Cochrane Database Syst Rev.* 2013;5:CD009329.

62. Cahill K, Stead LF, Lancaster T. Nicotine receptor partial agonists for smoking cessation. *Cochrane Database Syst Rev.* 2012;4:CD006103.

63. Hughes JR, Stead LF, Lancaster T. Antidepressants for smoking cessation. *Cochrane Database Syst Rev.* 2007;1:CD000031.

64. Stead LF, Lancaster T. Behavioural interventions as adjuncts to pharmacotherapy for smoking cessation. *Cochrane Database Syst Rev.* 2012;12:CD009670.

65. Stead LF, Lancaster T. Combined pharmacotherapy and behavioural interventions for smoking cessation. *Cochrane Database Syst Rev.* 2012;10:CD008286.

40

COMPLEMENTARY MEDICINE AND NATURAL MEDICATIONS

ANA IVKOVIC, MD ■ FELICIA A. SMITH, MD ■
DAVID MISCHOULON, MD, PHD

OVERVIEW

Complementary and alternative medical therapies constitute a diverse spectrum of practices that often overlap with current medical practice. Typically, the descriptor, "alternative" medicine, is reserved for situations in which a non-mainstream approach is used in place of conventional medicine, whereas "complementary" or "integrative" medicine are the preferred terms when non-mainstream approaches are used alongside traditional medicine.[1] The National Center for Complementary and Integrative Health is the federal government's lead agency responsible for scientific research on complementary and integrative medicine. This chapter will focus on natural medications derived from natural products and not approved by the US Food and Drug Administration (FDA) for their proposed indication.[2] Natural medications include various products, such as hormones, vitamins, plants, herbs, fatty acids, amino acid derivatives, and homeopathic preparations. While natural medications have been used for thousands of years, their use in the United States has been much more recent, with a considerable increase over the past three decades. Surveys suggest that about 40% of the US population uses some sort of complementary therapy.[3] Ethnic considerations also impact usage, with African Americans being the group least likely in the United States to try natural remedies and Hispanics being the most prone to their use.[4] Given the considerable portion of the US population trying natural remedies, it is increasingly important for clinicians to be knowledgeable about these

medications so that they can provide comprehensive patient care. This chapter provides an overview of natural medications used for psychiatric indications. General safety and efficacy are discussed first, followed by an examination of natural remedies used for disorders of mood, anxiety, and sleep, as well as menstrual disorders and dementia.

EFFICACY AND SAFETY

Despite the increase in both government and industry sponsorship of clinical research involving natural medications, data regarding efficacy remain limited due to the paucity of systematic studies. Since the FDA does not regulate natural medications, questions of safety remain unaddressed. Another significant problem lies in the limited information regarding the safety and efficacy of combining natural medications with more conventional ones. This poses a particular challenge to the consultation psychiatrist because of the high prevalence of polypharmacy seen in inpatient medical settings. Notably, patients frequently do not disclose the use of integrative therapies to their physicians.[4] Asking specific questions about the use of both prescribed and over-the-counter medications may improve disclosures. Finally, preparations of natural medications often vary in purity, quality, potency, and efficacy and have myriad side effects. The remaining chapter outlines our current understanding of several primary natural medications and their potential psychiatric indications.

MOOD DISORDERS

Numerous natural medications have been used to treat mood disorders, including omega-3 fatty acids, St. Johns wort (SJW), S-adenosylmethionine (SAMe), folic acid, vitamin B_{12}, inositol, and N-acetyl cysteine (NAC) (Table 40.1). The efficacy, possible mechanisms of action, dosing, adverse effects, and drug interactions of each of these medications are discussed in the following section.

Omega-3 Fatty Acids

Omega-3 fatty acids are polyunsaturated lipids derived from fish oil, algae, and certain land-based plants (e.g., flax). Omega-3 fatty acids have been shown to have benefits in numerous medical conditions, including rheumatoid arthritis, inflammatory bowel disease, psoriasis, immunoglobulin A nephropathy, systemic lupus erythematosus, multiple sclerosis, and migraine headache, among others.[5] Cardioprotective benefits have been demonstrated, although one recent systematic review is less supportive of their role as preventive agents for cardiovascular disease.[6] From a psychiatric standpoint, omega-3 fatty acids may have a role in the treatment of unipolar depression, post-partum depression, bipolar disorder, schizophrenia, and attention-deficit/hyperactivity disorder (ADHD).[7] The most promising data are for the treatment of both unipolar and bipolar depression, yet recent meta-analyses have been more reserved in their enthusiasm about the antidepressant efficacy of omega-3s.[8] In countries with higher fish consumption, lower rates of depression and bipolar disorder provide a clue that omega-3 fatty acids may play a protective role in these disorders. Although there are three main omega-3 fatty acids, eicosapentaenoic acid (EPA) and docosahexaenoic acid (DHA) are the two primarily studied for psychiatric indications. The third omega-3 fatty acid, alpha-linolenic acid, is also thought to have neurotropic and other health-promoting effects. While their mechanisms of action are not completely clear, several have been proposed. These run the gamut from effects on membrane-bound receptors and enzymes that regulate neurotransmitter signaling to the regulation of calcium ion influx through calcium channels to the lowering of plasma norepinephrine levels, or possibly to anti-inflammatory effects leading to decreased

corticosteroid release from the adrenal gland.[9] Omega-3 fatty acids may be consumed from a variety of sources, including fatty fish, algae, various seeds and nuts, and enriched eggs. Commercially available preparations of omega-3 fatty acids vary in composition; the suggested ratio of EPA:DHA is at least 3:2 in favor of EPA.[8] Psychotropically active doses are generally thought to be at least 1 to 2 g/day, although higher doses may also be effective. Dose-related gastrointestinal (GI) distress is the major side effect. There is also a theoretical risk of increased bleeding, so concomitant use with high-dose non-steroidal anti-inflammatory drugs or anticoagulants is not recommended. Thus far, there are no known interactions with other mood stabilizers or antidepressants.

In sum, the use of omega-3 fatty acids is promising, particularly given the range of potential benefits and the relatively low toxicity observed thus far. However, larger and more definitive studies are still needed.

St. Johns Wort

SJW (Hypericum perforatum) is one of the biggest-selling natural medications on the market. It has been shown to be more effective than a placebo in the treatment of mild-to-moderate depression.[10] Studies have further suggested that SJW is as effective as low-dose tricyclic antidepressants (TCAs). When compared with selective serotonin reuptake inhibitors (SSRIs), the efficacy of SJW has been comparable to placebo.[11] Hypericum is thought to be the main antidepressant ingredient in SJW, while polycyclic phenols, pseudohypericin, and hyperforin are also thought to be active ingredients. Several theories regarding the mechanism of action of SJW have been proposed. These include the inhibition of cytokines, a decrease in serotonin (5-hydroxytryptamine [5-HT]) receptor density, a decrease in reuptake of neurotransmitters, and monoamine oxidase inhibitor (MAOI) activity.[9] Since SJW has MAOI activity, it should not be combined with SSRIs because of the risk of serotonin syndrome. Suggested doses range from 900 to 1800 mg/day. Adverse effects include dry mouth, dizziness, constipation, and phototoxicity. Care should be taken in patients with bipolar disorder due to the possibility of a switch to mania. Finally, there are several notable drug-drug interactions with SJW. Hyperforin is metabolized through the liver and induces CYP-3A4

TABLE 40.1

Natural Medications for Mood Disorders

Medication	Active Components	Possible Indications	Possible Mechanisms of Action	Suggested Doses	Adverse Events
Folic acid	Vitamin	Depression, dementia	Neurotransmitter synthesis	400–800 mcg/day; 15 mg/day 5-MTHF (Deplin)	Masking of B_{12} deficiency, lowers the seizure threshold in high doses, and adverse interactions with other drugs
Inositol	Six-carbon ring natural isomer of glucose	Depression, panic, OCD, and possibly bipolar disorder	Second messenger synthesis	12–18 g/day	Mild GI upset, headache, dizziness, sedation, and insomnia
NAC	Biological compound functioning as a mitochondrial modulator, involved in glutathione synthesis	Depression, bipolar disorder (including in children), OCD spectrum disorders, schizophrenia, substance use disorders, PTSD	Increases glutathione synthesis, reduces oxidative stress in the mitochondrial electron transport chain, protects brain cells, and may function similarly to lithium and valproate	600–3600 mg/day	Dry mouth, nausea, vomiting, diarrhea
Omega-3 fatty acids	Essential fatty acids (primarily EPA and DHA)	Depression, bipolar disorder, schizophrenia, ADHD	Effects on neurotransmitter signaling receptors; inhibition of inflammatory cytokines; lowering plasma norepinephrine (noradrenaline)	1000–4000 mg/day	Fishy taste and odor, GI upset, theoretical risk of bleeding
SAMe	Biological compound involved in methylation reactions	Depression	Neurotransmitter synthesis	300–3200 mg/day	Mild anxiety, agitation, insomnia, dry mouth, GI disturbance; also possible switch to mania and serotonin syndrome
St. Johns wort (Hypericum perforatum L.)	Hypericin, hyperforin, polycyclic phenols, pseudohypericin	Depression	Inhibition of cytokines, decreased serotonin receptor density, decreased neurotransmitter reuptake, MAOI activity	900–1800 mg/day	Dry mouth, dizziness, GI disturbance, and phototoxicity; also possible serotonin syndrome when taken with SSRIs and adverse interactions with other drugs
Vitamin B_{12}	Vitamin	Depression	Neurotransmitter synthesis	500–1000 mcg/day	None

ADHD, Attention-deficit/hyperactivity disorder; DHA, docosahexaenoic acid; EPA, eicosapentaenoic acid; GI, gastrointestinal; MAOI, monoamine oxidase inhibitor; NAC, N-acetyl cysteine; OCD, obsessive-compulsive disorder; PTSD, post-traumatic stress disorder; SAMe, S-adenosylmethionine; SSRI, selective serotonin reuptake inhibitor.
Adapted from Mischoulon D, Nierenberg AA. Natural medications in psychiatry. In: Stern TA, Herman JB, Rubin DH, eds. Psychiatry Update and Board Preparation, 4th ed. Massachusetts General Hospital Psychiatry Academy; 2018.

expression, which may reduce the activity of several common medications, including warfarin, calcineurin inhibitors, oral contraceptives, theophylline, digoxin, and indinavir.[12] Transplant recipients should avoid SJW; transplant rejections have been reported as a result of interactions between SJW, cyclosporine, and tacrolimus. Individuals with human immunodeficiency virus infection on protease inhibitors also should avoid taking SJW because of drug interactions.

In sum, SJW appears to be better than placebo and equivalent to low-dose TCAs for the treatment of mild depression. Emerging data indicate that SJW also compares favorably to SSRIs for mild depression. On the other hand, studies suggest that SJW may not be effective for more severe forms of depression. Drug-drug interactions should also be considered, as noted above.

S-Adenosylmethionine

SAMe, a compound found in all living cells, is involved in essential methyl group transfers and is the principal methyl donor in the one-carbon cycle. Levels of SAMe are dependent on folate and vitamin B_{12} sufficiency (Fig. 40.1). SAMe is involved in the methylation of neurotransmitters, nucleic acids, proteins, hormones, and phospholipids—its role in the production of

norepinephrine, serotonin, and dopamine may explain SAMe's antidepressant properties.[13] SAMe has been shown to elevate mood in depressed patients when doses of 300 to 3200 mg/day are used. Studies support the antidepressant efficacy of SAMe both when compared with placebo and TCAs (i.e., as monotherapy) and when used to augment SSRI- and serotonin-norepinephrine reuptake inhibitor-partial response. Oral preparations of SAMe are somewhat unstable, making high doses required for adequate bioavailability. Since the medication is relatively expensive (and not covered by most insurance plans), its high cost may be prohibitive for many individuals. Potential adverse effects are relatively minor; these include anxiety, agitation, insomnia, dry mouth, bowel changes, and anorexia. Sweating, dizziness, palpitations, and headaches have also been reported. Psychiatrists should monitor for a potential switch to mania. Finally, significant drug-drug interactions or hepatoxicity have not yet been reported with SAMe.

In sum, SAMe is a natural medication that appears to be relatively safe and shows promise as an antidepressant. Further study will help clarify its efficacy and safety.

Folate and Vitamin B_{12}

Folate and vitamin B_{12} are dietary vitamins that play a key role in one-carbon metabolism in which SAMe is formed[14] (see Fig. 40.1). SAMe donates methyl groups that are crucial for neurological function and play important roles in the synthesis of neurotransmitters. Deficiency of vitamin B_{12} may cause or contribute to a variety of neuropsychiatric and general medical conditions (e.g., macrocytic anemia, neuropathy, cognitive dysfunction/dementia, depression). Folate deficiency has several potential etiologies (e.g., inadequate dietary intake, malabsorption, inborn errors of metabolism, increased demand [e.g., as seen with pregnancy, infancy, bacterial overgrowth, rapid cellular turnover]). Drugs (e.g., anticonvulsants, oral contraceptives, sulfasalazine, methotrexate, triamterene, trimethoprim, pyrimethamine, and alcohol) may also contribute to folate deficiency. Like folate deficiency, vitamin B_{12} deficiency may also be caused by inadequate intake, malabsorption, impaired utilization, and interactions with certain drugs (e.g., colchicine, H_2 blockers, metformin, nicotine, oral contraceptive pills,

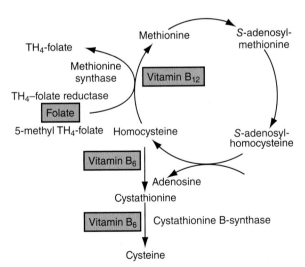

Fig. 40.1 ■ One-carbon cycle with SAMe, tetrahydrofolate (TH4), and vitamin B_{12}. *SAMe*, S-adenosylmethionine. (Redrawn from Dinavahi R, Bonita Falkner B. Relationship of homocysteine with cardiovascular disease and blood pressure. *J Clin Hypertens.* 2004;6:495. © 2004 Le Jacq Communications, Inc.)

cholestyramine, K-Dur, and zidovudine). From a psychiatric standpoint, deficiency of both folate and vitamin B_{12} has been linked with depression, although the association with folate seems to be greater.[15] Low folate levels have been associated with delayed and diminished clinical improvement of depression. Additionally, folate supplementation may be a beneficial adjunct for the treatment of SSRI-refractory depression. The folate form 5-methyl tetrahydrofolate (5-MTHF; Deplin) crosses the blood-brain barrier directly, without requiring enzymatic inter-conversion, and may deliver more active product to the brain. As such, this form may be particularly effective as augmentation therapy for the treatment of depression. Metabolically significant vitamin B_{12} deficiency, in turn, has been associated with a greater risk of depression, (including psychotic depression) and poor cognitive status, especially in the elderly.[16] Recent reviews support B-vitamin supplementation for mood disorders.[17] Adequate levels of each of these are thought to optimize neurotransmitter synthesis, which may aid in reversing depression. One caveat is that supplementation with folate alone may "mask" vitamin B_{12} deficiency by correcting macrocytic anemia while neuropathy persists; therefore vitamin B_{12} levels should be measured routinely when high doses of folate are given. Folate may also reduce the efficacy of other medications (e.g., phenytoin, methotrexate, and phenobarbital) and has been reported to lower the seizure threshold since high doses disrupt the blood-brain barrier.

In summary, correction of folate deficiency (and perhaps vitamin B_{12} deficiency) may improve depression or at least augment therapy with other medications. Folate (and possibly B_{12}) supplementation may also shorten the latency of response and enhance the treatment response for depressed patients, even when blood levels of these vitamins are normal. While overall data are inconclusive, psychiatrists should be vigilant for vitamin deficiency states by checking serum levels in individuals at risk for vitamin deficiencies and in those who have not responded to antidepressant treatment.

Inositol

Inositol is a natural isomer of glucose that is present in many foods. Myo-inositol is the isomer most common in the central nervous system of mammals; it is thought to modulate interactions between neurotransmitters,

receptors, cell-signaling proteins, and drugs through its activity in the cell-signaling pathway, and it is the putative target of the mood-stabilizing drug lithium.[18] Inositol has been effective in several small treatment studies of depression, panic disorder, obsessive-compulsive disorder, and bipolar depression.[19,20] While promising findings have been noted, negative monotherapy trials with inositol have been conducted in a variety of psychiatric illnesses, including schizophrenia, dementia, ADHD, premenstrual dysphoric disorder, autism, and electroconvulsive therapy-induced cognitive impairment. Effective doses are thought to be in the range of 12 to 18 g/day. Adverse effects are generally mild and include GI upset, headache, dizziness, sedation, and insomnia. At present, toxicity and drug interactions are absent.

In summary, treatment with inositol for psychiatric conditions treated with SSRIs and mood stabilizers appears to be safe and promising.

N-Acetyl Cysteine

NAC is a naturally occurring "mitochondrial modulator" with increasing applications in psychiatry. It appears to function by increasing glutathione synthesis, which in turn reduces oxidative stress in the mitochondrial electron transport chain. This may give NAC a protective effect on metabolically active brain cells, like the neuroprotective effects of lithium and valproate. A recent review by Bradlow and colleagues[21] reported promising data in various conditions, including major depressive disorder (2 trials), bipolar disorder (8 trials, including one in children ages 5–17), obsessive-compulsive spectrum disorders (10 trials), schizophrenia (8 trials), substance use disorders (15 trials covering tobacco, methamphetamine, gambling, cannabis, and cocaine, and including one study with co-morbid post-traumatic stress disorder [PTSD]). Overall, the data are promising. Typical doses range from 600 to 3000 mg/day. Safety and tolerability are reported as very good, with dry mouth, nausea, vomiting, and diarrhea as the main side effects.

ANXIETY AND INSOMNIA

Valerian

Valerian (*Valeriana officinalis*) is a flowering plant extract that has been used to promote sleep and reduce anxiety for over 2000 years. Typical preparations include capsules, liquid extracts, and teas made from roots and underground stems.[22] Valerian is thought to promote natural sleep after several weeks of use by decreasing sleep latency and improving overall sleep quality; however, methodological problems in most studies limit making firm conclusions in this area. A recent systematic review and meta-analysis[23] covering 60 studies found inconsistent outcomes regarding insomnia and anxiety, although safety and tolerability were deemed good, even in the elderly. A proposed mechanism involves decreasing gamma (γ)-aminobutyric acid (GABA) breakdown. Sedative effects are dose related within the usual dose range of 450 to 600 mg, administered about 2 hours before bedtime. Dependence and daytime drowsiness have not been problematic. Adverse effects, including blurry vision, GI symptoms, and headache, seem to be uncommon. Although data are limited, valerian should probably be avoided in those with liver dysfunction (due to potential hepatic toxicity).[22] Major drug interactions have not been reported.

In summary, valerian has been used as a hypnotic for centuries with relatively few reported adverse effects.

Melatonin

Melatonin is a hormone made in the pineal gland that has helped travelers avoid jet lag and decrease sleep latency for those suffering from insomnia. It may be particularly beneficial for night-shift workers. Melatonin is derived from serotonin (Fig. 40.2) and is thought to play a role in the organization of circadian rhythms via interaction with the suprachiasmatic nucleus.[24] Low-dose melatonin treatment has increased circulating melatonin levels to those normally observed at night and thus facilitates sleep onset and sleep maintenance without changing sleep architecture. Melatonin generally facilitates falling asleep within one hour, independent of when it is taken. While several studies have supported the use of melatonin as an effective hypnotic, a recent review, and meta-analysis suggested limited efficacy in adults, but greater efficacy in children and adolescents, with co-morbid and non-co-morbid chronic insomnia.[25] Optimal doses are thought to be in the range of 0.25 to 0.30 mg/day. Nevertheless, many preparations contain as much as 5 to 10 mg of melatonin.[24] Higher doses can cause daytime sleepiness and confusion; other adverse effects include decreased sex drive, retinal damage, hypothermia, and fertility problems. Melatonin is contraindicated in pregnancy and in those who are immunocompromised.[24] There are few reports of drug-drug interactions.

Melatonin seems to be a relatively safe hypnotic when taken in appropriate doses by appropriate populations.

Kava

Kava (*Piper methysticum*) is derived from a root originating in the Polynesian Islands, where it is used as a social and ceremonial herb.[22] Although it is thought to have mild anxiolytic and hypnotic effects, study results have been mixed, and recent reviews suggest that kava use leads to limited benefits.[10,26] The mechanism of action is attributed to kavapyrones, which are central muscle relaxants thought to be involved in blockade of voltage-gated sodium ion channels, enhanced binding to $GABA_A$ receptors, diminished excitatory neurotransmitter release, reduced reuptake of norepinephrine, and reversible inhibition of MAO_B. The suggested dose is 60 to 120 mg/day. Major side effects include GI upset, headaches, and dizziness. Toxic reactions, including ataxia, hair loss, respiratory problems, yellowing of the skin, and vision problems, have been seen at high doses or with prolonged use.[22] In the early 2000s, numerous reports of severe hepatotoxicity worldwide were published, including some cases that required liver transplantation.[22,26] For this reason, several countries withdrew kava from the market. Recent investigations suggest that kava is safe to use with proper precautions.[27]

While kava appears to be somewhat efficacious in the treatment of mild anxiety, safety concerns reduce our enthusiasm about its use, particularly for long-term treatment. If used, it should be done under medical supervision and with regular monitoring of liver function tests.

Lavender

Lavender (*Lavandula angustifolia*) is an aromatic plant long recognized anecdotally for its calming properties. Lavender essential oil can be taken by mouth or inhalation (i.e., as aromatherapy), or topically. Its

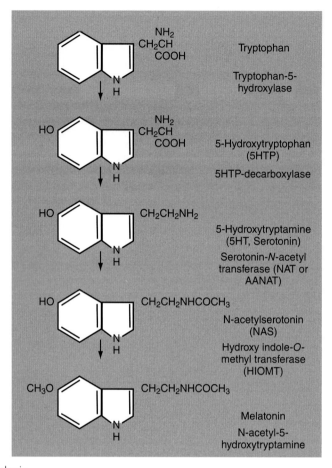

Fig. 40.2 ■ Melatonin synthesis.

anxiolytic effect is thought to occur through inhibition of voltage-gated calcium channels, reduction of 5-HT_{1A} receptor activity, and increased parasympathetic nervous system activation. Most studies on lavender have examined its anxiolytic effect when administered as aromatherapy. Silexan is a standardized, pharmaceutical-quality capsule form containing 80 mg of lavender essential oil per capsule. In a 10-week study of 539 adults with generalized anxiety disorder, Silexan outperformed placebo and paroxetine (determined by reduction of Hamilton Anxiety Scale scores) and was better tolerated than paroxetine (and it did not differ from placebo in terms of adverse effects).[28] Silexan and other forms of lavender are generally well tolerated and do not appear to cause dependency or withdrawal. Lavender's efficacy for insomnia is mixed.

Table 40.2 summarizes the natural medications discussed above for the treatment of insomnia and anxiety.

Cannabidiol

Cannabidiol (CBD), the cannabinoid constituent of cannabis, has been growing in popularity in the United States and worldwide given its increasing legalization and availability. It is often supplied as an oil containing only CBD (no tetrahydrocannabinol [THC]), a full-plant CBD-dominant hemp extract oil, capsules, dried cannabis, or liquid solution.[29] CBD is approved for multiple sclerosis-related pain in Canada and Sweden, and in the United States for certain childhood epilepsy disorders.[29] CBD is thought to work via multiple mechanisms, including serotonergic and anti-oxidant

TABLE 40.2

Natural Medications for Anxiety and Insomnia

Medication	Active Components	Possible Indications	Possible Mechanisms of Action	Suggested Doses	Adverse Events
CBD	Cannabidiol	Social anxiety, schizophrenia, insomnia PTSD, ADHD, MS-related pain, childhood seizure disorders	Serotonergic; antioxidant	Varies, depending on preparation and condition	Sleepiness, decreased appetite, diarrhea, fatigue, malaise, weakness, insomnia
Kava (*Piper methysticum*)	Kavapyrones	Anxiety	Central muscle relaxant, enhanced $GABA_A$ receptor binding, reversible inhibition of MAO_B	60–120 mg/day	Gastrointestinal disturbance, headaches, dizziness, ataxia, hair loss, visual problems, respiratory problems, rash, severe liver toxicity
Lavender (*Lavandula angustifolia*)	Terpenoids linalool and linalyl acetate	Generalized anxiety disorder, anxiety-related restlessness	Inhibition of voltage-gated calcium channels; decreased $5\text{-}HT_{1A}$ receptor activity; enhanced vagal tone	Silexan 80–160 mg/day	Nausea, dyspepsia (oral form); dermatitis (topical)
Melatonin	Hormone made in the pineal gland	Insomnia	Regulates circadian rhythm in the suprachiasmatic nucleus	0.25–0.3 mg/day (may increase up to 5 mg/day if needed)	Sedation, confusion, hypothermia, retinal damage, decreased sex drive, infertility
Valerian (*Valeriana officinalis*)	Valepotriates (from roots and underground stems)	Insomnia	Decrease GABA breakdown	450–600 mg/day	Blurry vision, headache, and possible hepatotoxicity

$5\text{-}HT_{1A}$, 5-Hydroxytryptamine 1A receptor; *ADHD*, attention-deficit/hyperactivity disorder; *CBD*, cannabidiol; *GABA*, γ-aminobutyric acid; *MAO*, monoamine oxidase; *MS*, multiple sclerosis; *PTSD*, post-traumatic stress disorder.
Adapted from Mischoulon D, Nierenberg AA. Natural medications in psychiatry. In: Stern TA, Herman JB, Rubin DH, eds. *Psychiatry Update and Board Preparation.* 4th ed. Massachusetts General Hospital Psychiatry Academy; 2018.

activity.[29] Potential clinical applications are broad. A recent review by Sarris and colleagues[30] found possible reductions of social anxiety, mixed (but mainly positive) evidence for adjunctive use in schizophrenia, and limited evidence in insomnia and PTSD. There was no apparent benefit for depression from high THC therapeutics or mania from CBD, but some potential efficacy for an oral cannabinoid/terpene combination in ADHD. Side effects have included sleepiness, decreased appetite, diarrhea, fatigue, malaise, weakness, and insomnia, but not significant intoxicating effects. Dosages and dosing strategies vary depending on the formulation used, but slow titration is recommended. Caution is recommended with its use in younger individuals as well as in individuals with anxious or psychotic disorders. Likewise, individuals with cardiovascular or respiratory disorders should use CBD cautiously, and CBD should probably be avoided during pregnancy and breast-feeding.[30] Occupational safety should also be considered with this yet-unproven treatment.

PREMENSTRUAL AND MENOPAUSAL SYMPTOMS

Black Cohosh

Black cohosh (Cimicifuga racemosa) is a member of the buttercup family native to the northeastern United States. The available natural supplement, derived from the root of the plant, at a dose of 40 mg/day or higher has reduced physical and psychological menopausal symptoms, as well as dysmennorhea.[31,32] Active ingredients are thought to be triterpenoids, isoflavones, and aglycones, which may participate in the suppression of luteinizing hormone in the pituitary gland, although studies in humans have shown mixed results. Anticancer effects are also inconsistent.[32] Headache, dizziness, GI upset, and weight gain are among its generally mild side effects. Limited data have not revealed specific toxicity or drug interactions. Black cohosh is not recommended for individuals who are pregnant or breast-feeding or who have heart disease or hypertension. Those with adverse reactions to aspirin should also avoid black cohosh since it contains salicylates.

Chaste Tree Berry

Chaste tree berry (Vitex agnus castus) is derived from the dried fruit of the chaste tree; ancient Greeks used it to help alleviate female reproductive complaints.[33,34] Its name comes from its historical use to help monks keep their vow of chastity by decreasing their sexual drive. The mechanism in both instances is thought to be via prolactin inhibition by binding dopamine receptors in the anterior pituitary, although this remains under investigation. It is most commonly used to alleviate premenstrual syndrome in doses of 200 to 400 mg/day.[33,34] Side effects such as nausea, headaches, GI disturbances, menstrual disturbance, acne, pruritus, and rashes seem to be minor.[35] While there are no clear drug-drug interactions, there is a theoretical risk of decreased efficacy of birth control due to its prolactin-inhibiting and ovulation-stimulating effects. Since it is thought to be a dopamine agonist, there may also be interactions with other dopamine agonists or antagonists.[35] A summary of the natural medications discussed here for premenstrual and menopausal symptoms is found in Table 40.3.

COGNITION AND DEMENTIA

Ginkgo Biloba

Ginkgo biloba has been used in Chinese medicine for thousands of years. This natural medication comes from the seed of the ginkgo tree, and it has generally been used for the treatment of impaired cognition and affective symptoms in dementias[36]; however, a possible new role has also emerged in the management of antidepressant-induced sexual dysfunction.[37] Target symptoms in those with dementia include memory and abstract thinking. Studies have shown modest but significant improvements in cognitive performance and

TABLE 40.3
Natural Medications for Premenstrual and Menopausal Symptoms

Medication	Active Components	Possible Indications	Possible Mechanisms of Action	Suggested Doses	Adverse Events
Black cohosh (Cimicifuga racemosa)	Triterpenoids, isoflavones, aglycones	Menopausal and premenstrual symptoms	Suppression of luteinizing hormone (LH) in the pituitary gland	40 mg/day	GI upset, headache, weight gain, and dizziness, unclear effects on breast cancer proliferation
Chaste tree berry (Vitex agnus castus)	Unknown	Premenstrual symptoms	Prolactin inhibition by binding to dopaminergic receptors in the anterior pituitary	200–400 mg/day	Minor GI disturbance, increased acne, increased menstrual flow, possible decreased efficacy of birth control

GI, Gastrointestinal.

Adapted from Mischoulon D, Nierenberg AA. Natural medications in psychiatry. In: Stern TA, Herman JB, Rubin DH, eds. Psychiatry Update and Board Preparation. 4th ed. Massachusetts General Hospital Psychiatry Academy, 2018.

TABLE 40.4
Natural Medications for Cognition and Dementia

Medication	Active Components	Possible Indications	Possible Mechanisms of Action	Suggested Doses	Adverse Events
Ginkgo biloba	Flavonoids, terpene lactones	Dementia and sexual dysfunction	Nerve cell stimulation and protection and free radical scavenging	120–240 mg/day	Mild GI disturbance, headache, irritability, dizziness, seizures in epileptics

GI, Gastrointestinal.
Adapted from Mischoulon D, Nierenberg AA. Natural medications in psychiatry. In: Stern TA, Herman JB, Rubin DH, eds. *Psychiatry Update and Board Preparation,* 4th ed. Massachusetts General Hospital Psychiatry Academy; 2018.

social function with doses of 120 mg/day.[36] Evidence suggests that progression of cognitive dysfunction may be delayed by 6 to 12 months; patients with mild dementia show the greatest improvement, while those with more severe disease may stabilize. Recent studies have suggested that ginkgo may be effective in combination with registered nootropic agents, the cholinesterase inhibitors.[38–40] Studies of healthy young volunteers taking *Ginkgo biloba* have shown mixed results regarding cognitive enhancement.[41–43] Flavonoids and terpene lactones are thought to be the active components, which may work by stimulating still-functional nerve cells. They may also play a role in protecting cells from pathological effects (such as hypoxia and ischemia). Ginkgo has been shown to inhibit platelet-activating factor, which suggests an increased bleeding risk, but a recent meta-analysis does not bear this out[44]; nonetheless, it should probably be avoided in those at high risk of bleeding until further data are available. Other noted side effects include headache, GI distress, seizures in epileptics, and dizziness. The suggested dose of *Ginkgo biloba* is 120 to 240 mg/day, with a minimum 8-week course of treatment; however, it may take up to a year to appreciate its full benefit.

Ginkgo biloba appears to be a safe and efficacious cognition-enhancing medication. It may have an additional role in reducing antidepressant-induced sexual dysfunction. Further studies are needed to fully understand its complete and long-term effects. Information about ginkgo biloba is summarized in Table 40.4.

CONCLUSION

Complementary and integrative medical therapies are increasingly popular in the United States and worldwide. The spectrum of such therapies is quite diverse and often significantly overlaps with more traditional medical practice. Lack of scientific research in this area historically has contributed to deficiencies in knowledge of the safety and efficacy of many of the natural remedies on the market today. The past three decades have generated new randomized clinical trials, meta-analyses, and systematic reviews that have allowed for more specific recommendations. For example, the Canadian Network for Mood and Anxiety Treatments recently published a series of guidelines for the use of complementary therapies in depressive disorders.[45] SJW, omega-3 fatty acids, and SAMe were the most highly recommended, including a first-line recommendation for SJW for mild-to-moderate depression. Folic acid received a second-line indication, and inositol was not recommended due to limited evidence. Many of the therapies discussed in this section may prove to be valuable additions to the psychopharmacologic armamentarium of psychiatrists. However, caution is needed regarding their potential drug-drug interactions and side effects. A general knowledge of these therapies and routine questioning about their use are essential parts of comprehensive care by psychiatrists.

REFERENCES

1. National Center for Complementary and Integrative Health. *Complementary, Alternative, or Integrative Health: What's in a Name?* Available from: <https://www.nccih.nih.gov/health/complementary-alternative-or-integrative-health-whats-in-a-name>; April 2021.
2. Mischoulon D, Nierenberg AA. Natural medications in psychiatry. In: Stern TA, Herman JB, Rubin DH, eds. *Psychiatry Update and Board Preparation.* 4th ed. Massachusetts General Hospital Psychiatry Academy; 2018.
3. Hassen G, Belete G, Carrera KG, et al. Clinical implications of herbal supplements in conventional medical practice: a US Perspective. *Cureus.* 2022;14:e26893.

4. Kelly JP, Kaufman DW, Kelley K, et al. Use of herbal/natural supplements according to racial/ethnic group. *J Altern Complement Med.* 2006;12:555–561.

5. Simopoulos AP. Omega-3 fatty acids in inflammation and autoimmune diseases. *J Am Coll Nutr.* 2002;21:495–505.

6. Ferrari R, Censi S, Cimaglia P. The journey of omega-3 fatty acids in cardiovascular medicine. *Eur Heart J Suppl.* 2020;22(suppl J):J49–J53.

7. Mischoulon D, Freeman MP. Omega-3 fatty acids in psychiatry. *Psychiatr Clin North Am.* 2013;36:15–23.

8. Appleton KM, Voyias PD, Sallis HM, et al. Omega-3 fatty acids for depression in adults. *Cochrane Database Syst Rev.* 2021(11):CD004692.

9. Mischoulon D. Update and critique of natural remedies as antidepressant treatments. *Psychiatr Clin North Am.* 2007;30:51–68.

10. Sarris J, Marx W, Ashton MM, et al. Plant-based medicines (Phytoceuticals) in the treatment of psychiatric disorders: a meta-review of meta-analyses of randomized controlled trials. *Can J Psychiatry.* 2021;66:849–862.

11. Haller H, Anheyer D, Cramer H, Dobos G. Complementary therapies for clinical depression: an overview of systematic reviews. *BMJ Open.* 2019;9:e028527.

12. Lippert A, Renner B. Herb-drug interaction in inflammatory diseases: review of phytomedicine and herbal supplements. *J Clin Med.* 2022;11:1567.

13. Sharma A, Gerbarg P, Bottiglieri T, et al. S-Adenosylmethionine (SAMe) for neuropsychiatric disorders: a clinician-oriented review of research. *J Clin Psychiatry.* 2017;78:e656–e667.

14. Maruf AA, Poweleit EA, Brown LC, et al. Systematic review and meta-analysis of l-methylfolate augmentation in depressive disorders. *Pharmacopsychiatry.* 2022;55:139–147.

15. Papakostas GI, Petersen T, Mischoulon D. et al. Serum folate, vitamin B_{12}, and homocysteine in major depressive disorder, part 1: predictors of clinical response in fluoxetine-resistant depression. *J Clin Psychiatry.* 2004;65:1090–1095.

16. Reynolds EH. Folic acid, ageing, depression, and dementia. *BMJ.* 2002;324:1512–1515.

17. Borges-Vieira JG, Cardoso CKS. Efficacy of B-vitamins and vitamin D therapy in improving depressive and anxiety disorders: a systematic review of randomized controlled trials. *Nutr Neurosci.* 2023;26(3):187–207.

18. Williams RS, Cheng L, Mudge AW, et al. A common mechanism of action for three mood-stabilizing drugs. *Nature.* 2002;417:292–295.

19. Belmaker RH, Levine J. Inositol in the treatment of psychiatric disorders. In: Mischoulon D, Rosenbaum J, eds. *Natural Medications for Psychiatric Disorders: Considering the Alternatives.* 2nd ed. Lippincott Williams & Wilkins; 2008.

20. Mukai T, Kishi T, Matsuda Y, Iwata N. A meta-analysis of inositol for depression and anxiety disorders. *Hum Psychopharmacol.* 2014;29:55–63.

21. Bradlow RCJ, Berk M, Kalivas PW, et al. The potential of N-acetyl-L-cysteine (NAC) in the treatment of psychiatric disorders. *CNS Drugs.* 2022;36:451–482.

22. Mischoulon D. Herbal remedies for anxiety and insomnia: kava and valerian. In: Mischoulon D, Rosenbaum J, eds. *Natural Medications for Psychiatric Disorders: Considering the Alternatives.* 2nd ed. Lippincott Williams & Wilkins; 2008.

23. Shinjyo N, Waddell G, Green J. Valerian root in treating sleep problems and associated disorders—a systematic review and meta-analysis. *J Evid Based Integr Med.* 2020;25:2515690X20967323.

24. Zhdanova V, Friedman L. Melatonin for treatment of sleep and mood disorders. In: Mischoulon D, Rosenbaum J, eds. *Natural Medications for Psychiatric Disorders: Considering the Alternatives.* 2nd ed. Lippincott Williams & Wilkins; 2008.

25. Choi K, Lee YJ, Park S. Efficacy of melatonin for chronic insomnia: systematic reviews and meta-analyses. *Sleep Med Rev.* 2022;66:101692.

26. Soares RB, Dinis-Oliveira RJ, Oliveira NG. An updated review on the psychoactive, toxic and anticancer properties of kava. *J Clin Med.* 2022;11:4039.

27. Thomsen M, Schmidt M. Health policy versus kava (Piper methysticum): anxiolytic efficacy may be instrumental in restoring the reputation of a major South Pacific crop. *J Ethnopharmacol.* 2021;268:113582.

28. Kasper S, Gastpar M, Müller WE, et al. Lavender oil preparation Silexan is effective in generalized anxiety disorder—a randomized, double-blind comparison to placebo and paroxetine. *Int J Neuropsychopharmacol.* 2014;17:859–869.

29. Levine MT, Gao J, Satyanarayanan SK, et al. S-adenosyl-l-methionine (SAMe), cannabidiol (CBD), and kratom in psychiatric disorders: clinical and mechanistic considerations. *Brain Behav Immun.* 2020;85:152–161.

30. Sarris J, Sinclair J, Karamacoska D, et al. Medicinal cannabis for psychiatric disorders: a clinically-focused systematic review. *BMC Psychiatry.* 2020;20:24.

31. McKenna DJ, Jones K, Humphrey S, et al. Black cohosh: efficacy, safety, and use in clinical and preclinical applications. *Altern Ther Health Med.* 2001;7:93–100.

32. Mohapatra S, Iqubal A, Ansari MJ, et al. Benefits of Black Cohosh (Cimicifuga racemosa) for women's health: an up-close and in-depth review. *Pharmaceuticals (Basel).* 2022;15:278.

33. Tesch BJ. Herbs commonly used by women: an evidence-based review. *Am J Obstet Gynecol.* 2002;188(5 suppl):S44–S55.

34. van Die MD, Burger HG, Teede HJ, Bone KM. Vitex agnus-castus (Chaste-Tree/Berry) in the treatment of menopause-related complaints. *J Altern Complement Med.* 2009;15:853–862.

35. Daniele C, Thompson Coon J, et al. Vitex agnus castus: a systematic review of adverse events. *Drug Saf.* 2005;28:319–332.

36. Tomino C, Ilari S, Solfrizzi V, et al. Mild cognitive impairment and mild dementia: the role of Ginkgo biloba (Egb 761*). *Pharmaceuticals (Basel).* 2021;14:305.

37. Niazi Mashhadi Z, Irani M, Kiyani Mask M, Methie C. A systematic review of clinical trials on Ginkgo (Ginkgo biloba) effectiveness on sexual function and its safety. *Avicenna J Phytomed.* 2021;11:324–331.

38. Yancheva S, Ihl R, Nikolova G, et al. GINDON Study Group Ginkgo biloba extract Egb 761*, donepezil or both combined in the treatment of Alzheimer's disease with neuropsychiatric features: a randomized, double-blind, exploratory trial. *Aging Ment Health.* 2009;13:183–190.

39. Cornelli U. Treatment of Alzheimer's disease with a cholinesterase inhibitor combined with antioxidants. *Neurodegener Dis.* 2010;7:193–202.

40. Canevelli M, Adali N, Kelaiditi E, et al. Effects of Gingko biloba supplementation in Alzheimer's disease patients receiving cholinesterase inhibitors: data from the ICTUS study. *Phytomedicine.* 2014;21:888–892.

41. Stough C, Clarke J, Lloyd J, et al. Neuropsychological changes after 30-day *Ginkgo biloba* administration in healthy participants. *Int J Neuropsychopharmacol.* 2001;4:131–134.

42. Elsabagh S, Hartley DE, Ali O, et al. Differential cognitive effects of Ginkgo biloba after acute and chronic treatment in healthy young volunteers. *Psychopharmacology (Berl).* 2005;179:437–446.

43. Kennedy DO, Jackson PA, Haskell CF, Scholey AB. Modulation of cognitive performance following single doses of 120 mg Ginkgo biloba extract administered to healthy young volunteers. *Hum Psychopharmacol.* 2007;22:559–566.

44. Kellermann AJ, Kloft C. Is there a risk of bleeding associated with standardized Ginkgo biloba extract therapy? A systematic review and meta-analysis. *Pharmacotherapy.* 2011;31:490–502.

45. Ravindran AV, Balneaves LG, Faulkner G, et al. Canadian Network for Mood and Anxiety Treatments (CANMAT) 2016 clinical guidelines for the management of adults with major depressive disorder: section 5. Complementary and alternative medicine treatments. *Can J Psychiatry.* 2016;61:576–587.

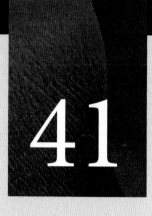

41 DIFFICULT PATIENTS

FRANKLIN KING IV, MD ■ JAMES E. GROVES, MD

OVERVIEW

The medical equivalent of war is the care of a difficult patient. Doctors soldier steadily on through all kinds of clinical chores, arduous schedules, and "administrivia," but when they get to the types of patients variously called "obnoxious," "needy," "crocky," "malignant," and even "hateful,"[1] they fight the worst battles of their careers, become prone to clinical blunders, mess up their personal lives, violate boundaries, and get sued. The good news is that—almost without exception—caring for the "difficult patient" makes the consulting psychiatrist more useful to treating physicians and patients alike than in any other medical encounter. Harrowing though such situations may temporarily be, it is just these kinds of consultations that earn the trust and respect of physician consultees and generate more consultation requests later on (and there are few better ways for a psychiatrist starting to build a practice than by becoming a specialist in the care of difficult patients). Before turning to management strategies, it is worth reviewing the presentations of difficult patients.

Case 1

Ms. A, a 38-year-old woman with a history reported in the chart as being significant for obesity, lower back pain, systemic lupus erythematosus, chronic tinnitus, fibromyalgia, and bipolar disorder, was admitted to the hospital for a fever and cough. Pneumonia was initially diagnosed, and her medical symptoms had been improving with antibiotics. However, care had been increasingly complicated by her escalating demands and seemingly endless physical complaints: she had been complaining of back pain "because of my lupus flare" (despite any objective evidence of autoimmune exacerbation), with repeated requests for oxycodone as the only medication that would help; urinary symptoms, despite a normal exam and laboratory findings; and insomnia and anxiety. In addition, Ms. A continued to leave the confines of the hospital to smoke cigarettes, at times, left the unit for hours at a time and lashed out at the medical team when they told her that she needed to be in her room during their morning rounds. Conflict erupted among staff; some nurses had excellent rapport with her and viewed her as a sympathetic character, who was at the mercy of a cold and indifferent attending physician and senior resident, as well as their apparently heartless colleagues on the night shift—who just did not seem to understand how much Ms. A was suffering. On her first night-float shift on this service, the junior resident prescribed lorazepam for insomnia, despite the daytime team's instructions to withhold benzodiazepines. This error was corrected the following night, but the next morning, Ms. A told the junior resident, "I need to sleep because of my bipolar disorder. If you don't give me my lorazepam, I'm gonna kill myself." An argument ensued between the patient and the junior resident, which escalated and resulted in a loud verbal conflict between the resident, the nurse, and the charge nurse. By the time the consultant received the consult request (delivered in an indignant, angry tone by the rotating subintern), the entire staff was in an uproar.

TYPES OF DIFFICULT PATIENTS

Delirious patients may be assaultive. Guilty, bereaved spouses can be litigious. Patients with temporal lobe epilepsy are often clingy and viscous. Those with mania are emotional cyclones. Celebrities often generate anxiety in their caregivers. Individuals with schizophrenia can be non-adherent to medical regimens. Anyone when ill can regress and become angry, dependent, and hypochondriacal—yet none of these problematic conditions necessarily produces "difficult patient" scenarios.

Difficult patients are often people with a personality disorder, or at least those who, in the face of medical illness, severe psychosocial stress, and alcohol and substance use disorders (SUDs), regressively display the maladaptive traits so characteristic of a patient with personality disorder. This highlights the importance of differentiating state versus trait: true personality disorders lie closer to trait because they are relatively durable over time, while SUDs and eating disorders lie closer to state because change, when it occurs, can be dramatic. In the *Diagnostic and Statistical Manual of Mental Disorders, 5th edition* (DSM-5),[2] personality disorders are defined by clusters of traits, while SUDs are associated with maladaptive behaviors that the substance gives rise to. However, the consultant will do well to remember that patients encountered on inpatient units are often at their worst—and as personality disorders are diagnosed based on traits observed over time, the patient with "borderline traits" may not meet the criteria for a *personality disorder* despite seeming to exhibit evidence during an acute medical illness. Despite their reputation of being intractable and chronic conditions, even the stability of full-fledged personality disorders over time has come under scrutiny in recent years, as prognosis, change, and recovery now appear perhaps more favorable for some disorders than previously thought.[3]

Not all patients with a personality disorder are difficult patients or necessitate psychiatric consultation. Looking at pure types through the lens of DSM-5, those not necessarily belonging to the difficult patient paradigm are paranoid, schizoid, and schizotypal personality disorders (cluster A), as well as avoidant, dependent, and obsessive-compulsive personality disorders (cluster C). Patients with a paranoid personality disorder deserve a brief mention, however, as their nearly boundless suspiciousness, hostility towards others, and extreme employment of projection often render them problematic to the primary clinical team when they must—always reluctantly—seek medical care.

Nonetheless, although some of these may be difficult patients, it is really when we scrutinize cluster B disorders that anxiety heightens: antisocial, borderline, and narcissistic (for the sake of this discussion, histrionic patients are grouped with borderline patients because, as difficult patients, they are almost indistinguishable). With these three diagnoses, comprising the dramatic-emotional-erratic cluster, there is almost a complete overlap between difficult patients and those with personality disorders. DSM-5 defines them as the following:

- Antisocial personality disorder involves a pattern of disregard for, and violation of, the rights of others.
- A borderline personality disorder is characterized by a pattern of instability in interpersonal relationships, poor self-image, labile and dysphoric affects, and marked impulsivity.
- Narcissistic personality disorder is embodied by a pattern of grandiosity, a need for admiration, and a lack of empathy.

The key word here is *pattern*. Personality traits lead to a personality disorder when they are "inflexible and pervasive across a broad range of personal and social situations," leading to significant distress or impairment in multiple domains of functioning.[4] These traits are enduring for most of the life span and deviate markedly from the expectations of the patient's culture. Finally, they do not result from another mental or physical disorder, such as depression or head trauma.

Antisocial and Narcissistic Personality Disorders

Patients with an antisocial personality disorder display the defining trait of disregard for the rights of others. The disorder satisfies the general criteria for the other personality disorders and consistently manifests at least three of the following traits:[2] rule-breaking; deceitfulness (e.g., lying, conning others); impulsivity or poor planning (resulting in a parasitic lifestyle that is sustained by manipulating others); aggressiveness (with repeated assaults and fights); irresponsibility (failing to sustain a job or uphold financial obligations); and a lack of conscience, remorse, or empathy.

Narcissistic personality disorder[2] is defined by the grandiosity and lack of empathy shown by at least five of the following traits: arrogance; a preoccupation with fantasies of power, beauty, love, brilliance, or money; convictions of "specialness"; a hunger for admiration; entitlement; exploitation and manipulativeness; stunted empathy (an inability to "feel into" the other person); envy; and displays of contemptuousness.

Antisocial personality disorder and narcissistic personality disorder are similar in terms of selfishness but different in terms of social destructiveness. One could think of the difference between criminality and shabby ethics. Whether these two entities differ more in degree or kind is a question perhaps better left to religion or philosophy, yet in psychiatry one view has been that personality disorders manifest similar ego defects (except in degree) and similar underlying psychic organizations or even a common *borderline personality organization*.[5] If it is true that a change in social context (e.g., incarceration) brings out a borderline personality in people who otherwise look antisocial, as some have claimed, there may be some utility to the notion of a core personality disorder called *borderline with several variant presentations*. At any rate, the management strategies discussed subsequently work for those with borderline and other personality disorders, given a rigorous application and a sufficiently strong social structure.

The concept of an underlying or core borderline personality organization is a metaphor that has considerable utility in the discussion of the difficult patient. The idea is that the underlying good-bad split or fragmented borderline personality organization is held together by the self-promoting program of the antisocial person and the grandiosity of the narcissist. Antisocial and narcissistic patients who believe their physicians' interests parallel their own are unctuous and un-difficult ("prison sincerity"). When the psychopathy and grandiosity are punctured by illness or injury and thwarted by medical treatment, the underlying fragmented, rageful, splitting, and attacking behavior comes out. In the discussion that follows,

therefore, *borderline personality* is the referent paradigm of difficulty, to be discussed more at length and used interchangeably with *difficult patient*.

Borderline Personality Disorder

"Borderline personality" was originally named because it seemed to psychoanalysts to lie between the psychoses (in which the patient is chaotic or irrational) and the neuroses (in which the patient desperately clings to others to feel real). Patients with borderline personality are dreaded for their impulsivity, swings from love to hate, and maddening irrationality. They split the world into exaggerated dichotomies of good and evil. An interpersonal middle ground does not exist. These patients, by some combination of innate rage and inept parenting, cannot find a moderate position in any aspect of mental life.

Those with a borderline personality have a multifaceted disorder that goes beyond the repeated self-injurious behavior for which the disorder is well known, with characteristics grouped into four broad domains of affective, interpersonal, behavioral, and cognitive features.[6] Such patients exhibit five or more of the following traits: frantic efforts to avoid or prevent (usually perceived) abandonment, a pattern of intense interpersonal relationships characterized by unstable alternations between idealization and devaluation; an unstable sense of self or identity; impulsive behaviors that may be self-damaging; recurrent thoughts of, attempts at, or threats of suicide, or self-mutilation; marked mood reactivity and affective instability; inappropriate, intense anger and poor self-control of anger; chronic feelings of emptiness, and transient paranoid ideation and dissociative symptoms.[2]

In the past, borderline personality was sometimes held to be a sub-set of a biological depressive illness or a variant of traditional diagnoses, such as hysteria, sociopathy, or alcoholism. This likely reflects the high rates of co-morbid psychiatric disorders found in this population: one of the more rigorously conducted studies to date followed 290 patients with a borderline personality, and found that even at 6-year follow-up, 75% of these patients met criteria for a mood disorder (61% for major depression), 35% for post-traumatic stress disorder (PTSD), 34% for an eating disorder, 29% for panic disorder, and 19% for an SUD.[7] More striking is the fact that this represented a decline from initial surveys and that even in patients whose borderline personality remitted, psychiatric co-morbidity remained high. Rates of remission of symptoms of both borderline personality and affective disorders have similarly been shown to reciprocally delay the time to recovery of each other, suggesting an interplay of related, but separate, etiologies.[8] Unfortunately, borderline personality disorder remains both under-diagnosed[9] as well as misdiagnosed (often as bipolar disorder).[10] The consultant would therefore do well to thoroughly review the diagnostic criteria and differential diagnosis of this disorder.

Regardless of sub-type or co-morbid diagnosis, however, patients with a borderline personality can abruptly flee treatment or develop psychotic transference and delusions about their caregivers. Short, circumscribed episodes of delusional thinking in unstructured situations and when under stress are almost pathognomonic.[11] Those with a borderline personality display a signature trait, a poor observing ego,[12] which is a dense denial of vital aspects of reality and irrationality to a degree that must be seen to be believed. Although the relationship between borderline personality and schizophrenia was long debated, it is likely that if there is a "border" with a biological illness, it is closer to affective illness without being completely tangential to it.

In borderline personality, the boundaries between the self and others are blurred, so that closeness seems to threaten fusion. Sexuality and dependency are confused with aggression. Needs are experienced as rage. Long-term relationships disintegrate because of an inability to find optimal interpersonal distance. Because of inadequate ego mechanisms of defense, there is little ability to master painful feelings or to channel needs or aggression into creative outlets. Ambivalence is poorly tolerated. Impulse control is impaired. The patient has a fragmented mental picture of the self and views others as all bad and simultaneously all potent, a chaotic mixture of shameful and grandiose images.[2]

In addition to the literature on inadequate parenting, borderline personality is linked with parental neglect and abuse, particularly severe sexual abuse.[13] The analytically based theory put forth is that the child victim of sexual abuse (especially chronic abuse[14]) used dissociation[15] as a defense against massive psychic trauma, and the dissociation became habitual,

undermining ego integration. This association with abuse is seen as variously explaining phenomena ranging from a propensity toward dissociative psychotic-like episodes, rage, sexual disorders, psychotic-erotic transferences in psychotherapy, and self-mutilation. The literature on abuse has the important effect of spotlighting the relationship between borderline phenomena and dissociation, something the older literature under-emphasized. Although the exact role that abuse plays in the development of borderline personality is still being worked out, it is clear that a significant number of patients with a borderline personality, when asked to give a history of such abuse, do so; this has to be taken into account in management.

Borderline personality occurs in perhaps 2% of the population.[16] Despite its small size, the borderline cohort stands out in the general hospital because of its florid presentation, notoriety for frequent utilization of both psychiatric and medical services, and because of the feelings of anger and helplessness stirred up in the caregivers.[17-19]

These patients often make themselves medical outcasts because they ruthlessly destroy the care they crave. However, because of this, the diagnosis of borderline personality has unfortunately attracted a considerable amount of bad press, both within the lay public, the medical community at large, and even among psychiatrists and other mental health clinicians.[20-22] This fact begs the question of how this affects psychiatric, medical, and nursing care, as clinicians who seek to avoid the difficult patient may overlook important clinical signs and under-diagnose disease in an unconscious effort to limit patient interactions. Medical co-morbidity in those with a borderline personality is significant, at least partly due to its association with obesity[23]; a 10-year longitudinal study found that comparing ever-recovered to never-recovered patients with a borderline personality, the latter had significantly higher rates of chronic health conditions—notably obesity, diabetes, urinary incontinence, and osteoarthritis—as well as poorly defined illnesses, such as chronic fatigue syndrome and fibromyalgia.[24] They also had higher rates of poor health-related lifestyle choices, financial burdens related to medical illness, and higher rates of utilization of costly medical services. Appropriate medical care is thus sorely lacking in this population, shunned as it is by the medical community—and thus adroit management of the inpatient medical team is of paramount importance in effecting sound patient care.

DIFFICULT BEHAVIOR AND THE CONSULTEE

The previous discussion about the DSM-5 diagnoses of difficult patients must be leavened with a simple fact: it is not the diagnosis of these patients that makes them difficult for the consultee—it is their behavior. The relationship of the behavior to other aspects of mental life is schematized in Fig. 41.1.

Such patients have abnormally intense affects and are poorer-than-average neutralizers of affect, or both. In any case, raw rage, naked dependency, and ontologic shame are present and are often found on the surface. The cognitive structures that ordinarily temper intense affects are distorted and primitive. The ego weakness of the patient is shown by the absence of higher-level

defenses and by the primitive nature of the ones that are present.[25]

Under the pressure of intense affect (rage, terror, shame), the patient uses dissociation to a greater or lesser extent and enters the dream-like state that persons ordinarily enter only in extreme emergencies. In this dissociated state (which is probably present much of the time to some degree), the patient is distracted, numb, and difficult to reach. The pervasiveness of dissociation is one feature of borderline personality that is insufficiently discussed in the literature; however, it can contribute drastically to the pathologic cognitions of patients with a borderline personality and place a distorting lens of unreality between them and the real world.

Besides dissociation, such patients use denial of major aspects of reality to cope. This mythification of the external, threatening world is displayed in defenses called *primitive idealization, omnipotence,* and *devaluation.* As the names imply, these are metaphors for the

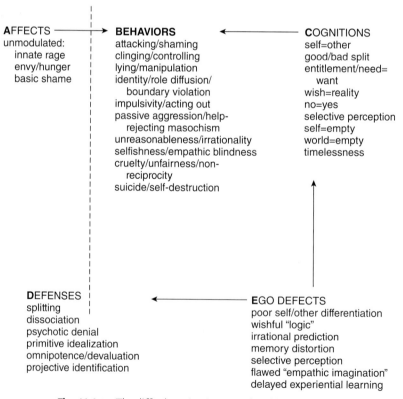

Fig. 41.1 ■ The difficult patient's types of problem behavior.

dreamy, wishful, mythified world the patient inhabits, a world of black and white and good and evil. These maladaptive defenses may be all too visible in the medical setting, but even more troubling are two others with which such patients unsuccessfully try to manage their extreme negative affects: splitting and projective identification.[25]

Splitting, by definition, involves a rigid separation of positive and negative thoughts or feelings. Normal persons are ambivalent and can experience two simultaneous contradictory feeling states; the individuals with a borderline personality characteristically shift back and forth, entirely unaware of one feeling state while in another. Sometimes one state is rigidly held while its opposite is projected onto the environment. Splitting may protect the patient from the anxiety of reconciling contradictory extremes (at the expense of the already unstable personality). In social systems, such patients can split the staff into warring "good" and "bad" factions that unwittingly act out the patient's internal world.

Projective identification[26] is said to consist of taking an unwanted aspect of the self, such as cruelty or envy, and wholly ascribing it to ("projecting it into") another. The patient then unconsciously pressures that person to own the projected attribute. Unaware that a self-fulfilling prophecy is being established, the recipient complies with the projection and acts it out. These two mechanisms can complement each other, with projective identification being used to "confirm" one side of a polarized, split view of the world.

Although the long-term psychotherapy of the patient with a borderline personality can involve therapeutic undoing of these defenses,[5] it is inadvisable—even dangerous—to confront such defenses in brief encounters in the medical setting. It is crucial, however, to be aware of their presence. For example, awareness of borderline splitting prepares the consultant to deal with the division of the medical staff into "good ones" and "bad ones." Recognition of the patient's idealization, of a physician for instance, can help the consultant prepare for the furious devaluing that is to follow.

Helping the Consultee

The medical setting is a social system with its own history, boundaries, hierarchy, customs, and taboos.

The introduction of a difficult patient into this culture sometimes places such stress on the system as to cause malfunctions in caregiving or outright extrusion of the patient, a situation that active psychiatric consultation can prevent. Difficult patients are exquisitely vulnerable to caregivers' ordinary imperfections in communication and consistency, and they are often remarkably attuned to their caregivers' normal negative feelings of anxiety, shame, anger, and depression. Such patients are especially vulnerable to feelings of rejection by caregivers, and their shaky defenses are even more compromised than usual by the stresses of illness and treatment.

After the initial diagnosis and treatment of the patient, the consultant's next priority should be to gauge the amount of distress the staff is facing. A psychologically naive medical staff can regress to a helpless or vengeful position in response to the patient's ingratitude, intractability, impulsivity, manipulativeness, dependency, entitlement, and rage. Regression in any social system can emerge as disagreement among staff; it can take the form of inappropriate confrontation with the patient, or it can manifest itself as a deterioration in the patient's behavior. Regression seems to occur when a large disparity exists between what is expected and what is found. Troublesome dissonance of this sort between the patient and the staff generally occurs in any or all of three dimensions: perception of reality, values governing control and aggression, and rules about interpersonal closeness (Table 41.1).

The earliest clue to the nature of the dissonance lies in the consultation request.[27] Its tone, covert messages, intensity, timing, and route by which it reaches the consultant all can reflect the dissonance between the expectations of the patient and the staff. Consultation is sought when the patient is out of touch with the staff's reality. In this case, dissonance can range from mild (when the patient is from a different culture) to severe (when the patient is psychotic). When the patient is docile, the request is matter-of-fact; when the patient manifests grotesquely sexual or aggressive behavior, the consultant might receive a shrill, disorganized call for help.

Consultation is sought when the patient's behavior violates staff expectations. The staff expects to be in control of the patient, who is expected to be grateful, compliant, and non-destructive. Dissonance in this

TABLE 41.1

Consultation Management of Staff and Difficult Patient Dissonance in the Medical Setting

Type of Dissonance: Consultation Request	Patient's Problem Behaviors	Consultant's Work With the Consultee	Consultant's Work With the Patient
Dissonant reality: vague, confusing request for help; puzzled tone	Inappropriate to realities of illness or hospital; denial and demandingness	Explains patient's reality to staff; models "reality testing"	Diagnosis of any cognitive disorders; gives medication and reality-testing request
Aggressive dissonance: request to control or remove patient; fearful or angry tone	Menacing, self-destructive, or suicidal	Recommends social, chemical, or physical restraints necessary for safety	Evaluates potential violence; search for source of the patient's panic
Staff and patient dissonance regarding interpersonal distance: request consultant to take over care of the patient; depressed, guilty tone to the consultation request	Dependent rejecting	Permission to say "no" to patient's unrealistic, excessive demands	Clarifies for patient that some, but not all, needs can be realistically met
		Diminishes guilt and depression by stating the impossibility of entirely satisfying patient	Allows patient some distance; repeatedly appeals to patient's "entitlement" and autonomous side
	Manipulative (dependent and rejecting)	Serves as a forum for hatred toward the patient; voices hateful feelings but behaves non-sadistically	Bargains; sets firm, non-interpretive limits on manipulation; clarifies patient's self-interest

dimension can range from mild, when the patient sulks, to severe, when the patient is violent or self-destructive. The tone of such a consultation request ranges from irritation to anger or outright fear, depending on the kind of aggression the patient displays.

Consultation is sought when the patient's need for closeness differs from what the staff deems appropriate. The staff expects the patient to be involved with the caregivers but to keep a certain distance. When the patient asks for repeated reassurances or when the patient makes inexhaustible or contradictory demands, a depressed, guilty request often ensues. Arrogant, peremptory consultation requests often herald a hostile, dependent, manipulative patient; depressed, tired requests can foretell an empty, clinging patient.

The primitive defenses[28] of the difficult patient can stimulate staff disagreement (Table 41.2). To cope with deep feelings of self-loathing, the patient might see the staff as loathsome—otherwise, why would they care (projective identification)? Or the patient may see the staff as magically all good, to keep all the badness in the world away (primitive idealization). To make sense of a world in which people are both good and bad, such a patient might choose some people on the staff to be "all good" and some to be "all bad" (splitting).

This "explains" for the patient "why" things always go wrong: the patient is caught between good and bad forces outside the self and therefore they are not the fault of the self. When the patient views the staff through the defense of splitting, the staff might eventually behave as if it were so. The patient will tell an "all good" staff member what terrible things an "all bad" staff member has done, said, or thought and then swear the "good" one to secrecy. As less and less communication takes place and the patient escalates demands, the "good" staff and "bad" staff begin to disagree about the care of the patient because the borderline patient may be "good" with "good" staff and vice versa. The remedy for this depends on re-establishing open staff communication, even if it is hostile, to enable staff to get a well-rounded view of the patient. A firm, non-punitive limit setting (Table 41.3) is crucial for inpatient treatment because it must be made clear that the patient cannot destroy the caregiving system or be destroyed by it, no matter how intense the wishes or fears may be.

It is a natural human instinct to confront such patients angrily, but caregivers should exercise precautions during confrontations. Avoiding a confrontation of narcissistic entitlement is as important as it is difficult.[28] Such patients exude an offensive sense

TABLE 41.2

Manifestations of Primitive Ego Defenses: The Difficult Patient in the Medical Setting

Splitting: Keeping completely apart two opposite ideas and their associated feelings. Staff are divided into "good ones" and "bad ones," reflecting the patient's incapacity to achieve ambivalence enough to see that caregivers have human limits, with "good" and "bad" qualities at the same time.

Projective identification: The tendency to see some staff as "bad" as the patient feels. This gets translated into behavior based on the following kind of "logic": "I'm bad and you take care of me, which means you're as rotten as I am, otherwise you wouldn't care for me." This perception is so powerfully held that the staff receiving it tend to act it out unconsciously.

Primitive denial: The alternating expungement from consciousness of first one and then another perception of opposite quality (which is called *splitting*) or a wish so powerful that it obliterates crucial aspects of reality contradicting that wish. For instance, fear might cause the patient to deny a serious condition and flee the hospital where it could be treated.

Primitive idealization: The tendency to see some staff as totally "good" to protect the patient from "bad" staff or from the patient's medical condition.

Omnipotence and devaluation: A shift (splitting) between the need to establish a relationship with a magical, powerful staff (primitive idealization) versus the conviction of omnipotence in the self that makes all others impotent by comparison (primitive idealization of the self). Omnipotent caregivers are supposed to deliver to the patient perfect care to protect against disease, and when this does not happen, the staff is seen as impotent and hateful. (Splitting makes the perception shift dramatically, whereas projective identification causes the staff to buy into the patient's primitive projections, making them come true).

Adapted from Groves JE. Management of the borderline patient on a medical or surgical ward: the psychiatric consultant's role. *Int J Psychiatry Med.* 1975;6:337–348.

TABLE 41.3

Rules for Confronting the Difficult Patient

- Acknowledge the real stresses in the patient's situation.
- Avoid breaking down needed defenses.
- Avoid overstimulating the patient's wish for closeness.
- Avoid overstimulating the patient's rage.
- Avoid confronting narcissistic entitlement.

Adapted from Adler G, Buie DH. The misuses of confrontation with borderline patients. *Int J Psychoanal Psychother.* 1972;1:109–120.

of deservedness that is always tempting for an overworked staff to confront angrily and suddenly. Often the difficult patient has only this sense of entitlement to keep a fragmented personality together during the stresses of hospitalization. Entitlement for the narcissist is what hope and faith are to normal persons. Preserving it requires a deliberate effort. Taken together, what Tables 41.2 and 41.3 show is that such behavior of the difficult patient (e.g., manipulativeness and entitled demanding)—obnoxious though they may be—sometimes function as defenses at a relatively high level for that patient. Stripping them away makes the patient fall back on even lower-level defenses, such as psychotic denial and dissociation, or—worse—to be defenseless, panic, or explode.

Setting limits, avoiding confrontation, and avoiding over-stimulation of the desire for closeness and rage are difficult to arrange in the fast-paced medical milieu. Prevention of staff splitting is especially difficult because of the various sub-cultures in medicine. If, for instance, the patient chooses the nurses to be "all bad" and the physicians to be "all good," the nurses may displace anger to the physicians but be unable to express it directly because of role-induced sanctions, and the physicians may see the nurses as incompetent and unable to comprehend their treatment plan for the patient. Such situations are fertile ground for the splitter and require concerted effort toward open communication.

Pathologic dependency manifests in one of its extremes as manipulativeness: an intense, covert, contradictory, self-defeating attempt to get needs met.[28] It is the behavioral manifestation of a need by the patient to get close but at the same time, maintain a safe distance from sources of emotional support. Some patients feel so empty that, paradoxically, getting their needs met threatens them with engulfment; they are so famished that closeness can make them feel merged with someone else and therefore not alive. Such patients seem to have a deathly fear of what they crave most.

In limit-setting confrontations with manipulative and entitled patients, the consultant might have to model for the staff firmness, repetition, and an appeal to the patient's sense of entitlement (rather than an assault on it): "You deserve the best medical care we can give, and that's why we're recommending X, Y, and Z." The consultant must keep the uppermost in mind the appeal to the entitlement and not get drawn into logical or illogical arguments. Moreover, it is important to avoid interpreting the resistance to cooperation as a fear of dependency, a tactic that would at best leave the patient somewhat bewildered. Repetition is crucial. Encounters to engage compliance often must be repeated two or three times at varying intervals before the patient agrees, for instance, to take medication.

Dependent, manipulative patients stir up sadism in caregivers, which inhibits the setting of effective limits. The consultant supports the staff's self-esteem and performance by reinforcing strengths rather than by pointing out weaknesses, by teaching, by lending a conceptual framework to mitigate anxiety, by modeling interactions, and, most of all, by matter-of-factly stating that such patients stir up hatred even in the best of caregivers. Whenever the staff brings even a hint of negative reference to the patient, the consultant can say something like, "Yeah, these patients are manipulative and irritating as hell!" or, "Everybody hates this kind of patient." This personalization, juxtaposed with the consultant's own non-sadistic behavior toward the patient, legitimizes hostility toward the patient, but shares it among staff rather than inflicting it on the patient.

In general, the earlier in the hospitalization the consultant is called, the more overt the reason for the consultation and the more effective will be the intervention because the difficult patient has had less time to project into the staff the intense, seemingly inborn shame such patients possess in great abundance. Late in the hospitalization, the consultant may be called urgently to see the patient for vague reasons and arrive to find the situation in shambles, the patient in restraints, the staff ashamed and in bitter conflict—and nobody either willing or able to say what has been happening.

Consultant's Role

The consultant's role in the management of the difficult patient consists of a specialized type of consultee-oriented approach, in which countertransference hatred and fear are drawn away from the patient and strategically metabolized within the relationship between staff and consultant. The consultant should actively promote a behavioral management practicum[28] placed in the medical chart for reference and as a symbol of the psychiatrist's helping presence. This "recipe" discusses communicating clearly with the patient and among staff; understanding the patient's need for constant interaction with personnel; dealing with entitlement without confronting needed defenses; and setting firm limits on dependency, manipulativeness, rage, and self-destructive behavior.

Generally, the consultant's approach should first lead directly to the consultee. The request should be elicited in person or at least over the phone because the written record never reveals the entirety of the problems in the management of the difficult patient. Then, the consultant goes to the nursing staff to obtain a history of the patient's responses to hospital routines. Next, the consultant reads the chart and compares medication orders with the records of medications administered. The consultant will have generated some hypotheses and is now ready to test them in the examination of the patient. As the consultant proceeds through these steps, an orderly plan emerges (Table 41.4).

One helpful approach is the consultee-oriented model of consultation,[29] which involves thinking of the patient and staff as a single entity and dealing as

---

TABLE 41.4

Order of Priorities for the Difficult Patient Consultation in the Medical Setting

1. Rapidly evaluate the most pressing psychiatric problems, beginning with physical or social restraints if the patient appears to lose control of violent or self-destructive impulses.
2. Create a differential diagnosis of the difficult patient, with an explicit biopsychosocial formulation of the predominant conflicts and stressors.
3. Identify dissonance between staff and patient and formulate a plan of action to reduce it (Table 41.1).
4. Provide treatment recommendations—psychological and pharmacologic (Table 41.1), short-term and long-term—accounting for the ongoing medical regimen and implicitly addressing dissonance between staff and patient while explicitly addressing the patient's conflicts.
5. Educate the consultee and staff to reduce dissonance and to lend a conceptual framework for dealing with future difficult patients.
6. Actively participate without grandstanding or taking over all of the patient's psychological care.
7. Follow-up and be involved in disposition planning for the medical and psychiatric needs of the patient.

much as possible with the strong, healthy part. The entity consists of two parts. One part, the difficult patient, has problems with object relations, pathologic behavior exacerbated under stress, and several self-defeating and infuriating defenses, especially splitting. To prevent being split, the consultant should try to deal mainly with the healthy part, the staff. Because the staff is often closely linked in an unwilling, hateful, and guilty alliance with the patient and its collective self-esteem is already damaged by encounters with the patient, the consultant should not damage it further by interpreting the staff's pathology.

The attempt to ally with staff rather than with the patient is destined to encounter several kinds of resistance at the outset. First, the patient is eager to engage the consultant to find out whether the consultant is "all good" or "all bad." Second, the staff, needing distance from its sense of failure, wants the consultant to take over the patient's care completely. Third, neither the staff nor the patient has the energy to understand what is going on; they are in pain and want relief now, preferably by the patient's removal.

The alliance with the staff depends to a large extent on previous experience with the consultant, how long it takes to answer the consultation request, and how much sense the advice makes. The alliance with the difficult patient is dramatically less important in terms of outcome than the alliance with the staff. Such patients are incapable of forming a real alliance, and their "alliances" are mostly primitive idealizations. Ideally, the patient should be seen only briefly if there are enough data from other sources, and the staff is told that the consultant will work mainly with staff and see the patient infrequently.

Visiting the patient should be reserved in the early stages for the specific purpose of the consultant's alliance with the staff. Following the initial patient interview, the consultant goes to see the patient when a magical gesture of "taking over" is needed to comfort a desperate staff, when staff members feel that the consultant does not know how much they are suffering, and when the staff needs a specific model for carrying out recommendations on limit setting or reality testing.

The consultant's note, by its tone, specific information, and description of the patient in a way the staff can immediately recognize, remains in a medical record day and night as a tangible symbol of the consultant's helping presence. It outlines the request, history, mental status at the hour of the examination, and psychiatric history. It is explicit about medications, and the potential for suicide and violence. It includes specific, concrete management recommendations.

Case 2

This was the conclusion of a consultation note for a difficult patient who had been spitting into her central line.

Impression: Ms. B is thought to have a borderline personality disorder, a chronic, severe personality disorder, meaning that her moods can fluctuate rapidly and severely, and she has only marginal social adjustment. These chronic traits have likely worsened as a result of the stress of her current medical condition.

Recommendations: Have brief, daily staff conferences to compare notes and reach a consensus about her surgical treatment plan. Try to have the same staff members work with Ms. B each day; bear in mind that she tends to panic at each change of shift. Set firm limits on her multiple and contradictory demands. She is quick to rage when her demands are not met and may threaten suicide. Do not imply that Ms. B does not deserve the things she demands, but rather say repeatedly that you understand what she is asking, but because you feel she deserves the best possible care, you are going to continue to recommend the course dictated by your experience and judgment. If she continues spitting into her central line, assure her that physical restraints may be needed. Initiate suicide precautions (and search her luggage). Medication recommendations are delineated as shown below.

The consultant addresses dissonance arising from the patient's version of reality; tendency to act out; and demandingness, neediness, and rage. The consultant gives a mandate for open communication and daily staff conferences to prevent staff splitting and to provide a supportive environment. Firm limits, without challenging the patient's entitlement, are set forth explicitly. The task now becomes one of seeing that the recommendations are carried out. There is nothing more frustrating than laboring to devise a treatment plan only to find that it is not enacted. When this happens, the consultant often finds that the source of resistance is a still-unresolved dissonance between the staff and the patient (Table 41.1).

Nowhere in the previous discussion is the unconscious motivation of the patient or the staff brought to the attention of either. This is what is meant by a *non-interpretive intervention*. Psychoanalytic interpretations foster a temporary regression and have no place in the consultation with the disruptive medical-surgical patient.[28] Instead, the consultant analyzes and reduces dissonance by speaking of its behavioral roots and consequences while resisting the temptation to illuminate interesting unconscious processes.

Medication

The psychopharmacologic management of those with a borderline personality disorder (the referent paradigm for difficult patients) is complex: despite the high exposure of this group to psychiatric polypharmacy,[30] robust evidence supporting the use of medications remains limited, and, as of 2023, there remains no US Food and Drug Administration–approved medication for the treatment of borderline personality. However, the general consensus among experts is that, although the role of medications in the long-term care of borderline personality remains to be determined and should never be the sole or first-line treatment modality, medications—especially for short-term use—nonetheless can help reduce specific symptoms within the borderline personality.[31] It is important to add that medications may also serve as transitional objects and vehicles for the patient's projection,[32] especially during times of dysregulation, such as may occur during admission to a general hospital. Thus, the inexperienced clinician may be easily deceived into attributing changes in symptoms to pharmacologic interventions—and fall into the trap of "symptom chasing" while ignoring the often context-specific manifestation of borderline personality symptoms (e.g., rapid improvement of "depression" on hospital admission or "relapse" of self-injurious behavior prior to, or just after, discharge). When prescribing medications, the consultant would do well to not "over-sell" the role of medications to the patient and the consultee, but to also provide the hopeful attitude that medications can

indeed play a role—albeit a partial one—in improving specific symptoms.

Given the present state of knowledge, it seems appropriate for the consultant to remember that mind and body are not separate, and that many seemingly insoluble problems respond to a search for an aggressive treatment of co-morbid psychiatric conditions, especially affective illnesses and SUDs. Common and uncommon medical conditions may mimic personality disorders (e.g., three random instances in the literature are narcolepsy, Wolfram syndrome, and Addison disease[33–35]). Also, over the lifetime of any given patient, the relationship with a supportive physician is as healing as any drug.

THE PSYCHIATRIST'S WORK WITH THE PATIENT

Although the design and promotion of the behavioral management protocol and a consultation with the staff are the initial work of the consultant, the psychiatrist performs the following tasks with the patient directly:

- Examination of the psychiatric mental status, creation of a differential diagnosis, and formulation (including the use of observations of transference and countertransference)
- Assessment of the patient's potential for suicide
- Assessment of the present need for the control of violence (as opposed to making a prediction about dangerousness)
- Assessment of, and recommendations for, co-morbid psychiatric disorders and maladaptive behaviors
- Rarely, a highly focused brief (one- or two-session) tactical psychotherapeutic intervention.

Differential Diagnosis

When the consulting psychiatrist does not provide them, there will not be a good mental status examination, psychiatric history, or biopsychosocial formulation in the medical record. However skilled or willing other specialists may be, only the psychiatrist has an understanding of the minute-to-minute fluctuations of transference and countertransference that occur early, even in a single interview (countertransference is so important as to be almost a diagnostic discriminator of borderline personality).[36] Also, there is a level of rigor and discipline that the experienced psycho-diagnostician brings to these situations: no one practitioners in the medical setting are, for instance, going to perform a Mini-Mental State Examination, ask about earliest memories, a history of sexual abuse, the content of dreams and fantasies, sexual worries, religious and spiritual concerns, disordered thoughts, and suicidal ideation—all in one interview—and then collate them into a differential diagnosis and formulation.

Differential diagnosis is crucial because co-morbidity is almost a hallmark of the difficult patient, and it is surprising (if not impossible) to encounter a patient with "cluster B" traits who does not also have at least one of the following diagnoses: another personality disorder, an SUD, an affective disorder, an anxiety disorder (especially panic or a phobia), an eating disorder, obsessive-compulsive disorder, PTSD, adult attention-deficit/hyperactivity disorder, an impulse control disorder, or another disorder.

Suicide Assessment

Patients with borderline personality disorder are at increased risk for suicide; specific risk factors described within this population include higher levels of impulsivity, hostility, low levels of harm-avoidance, high levels of novelty-seeking, co-morbid substance, and affective disorders, a personal connection to suicide (e.g., of a family member or caregiver), and poor psychosocial functioning.[37] Suicide risk assessment is discussed in detail in Chapter 42. However, it bears mentioning here, given that difficult patients on the inpatient medical unit—due to the interplay of personality factors, active psychiatric co-morbidity, and, often, psychological stressors and regression in the face of acute medical illness—are often at increased risk of suicide. For the difficult patient, in addition to the usual risk factors, recent worsening in the medical condition along with perceived rejection by caregivers[38] adds considerably to the risk of suicide. Suicide and suicide attempts in medical and surgical settings correlate highly with primary psychiatric disorders, but hopelessness related to severe medical illness and anger over the loss of social support have also been found to be significant.[38,39] Many suicide attempts occur in a clinical setting, in which the patient's experience is of being abandoned: during failing treatment, at times of imminent discharge, in conjunction with disputes with the staff, or during staff holidays. Negative countertransference itself may also be a poor predictor.[40] That the characteristics and demographics of suicides in non-psychiatric medical settings differ from those of patients in psychiatric settings,[41] coupled with the fact that patients with personality disorders may be at their most vulnerable during a medical admission, underscores the fact that a detailed and thorough consideration of the suicide risk is warranted for every difficult patient that the consultant encounters.

Assessment of the Potential for Violence

Problems that arise when the patient has difficulty controlling aggression are helped when the consultant defines for the staff the range of responses, from supporting the sulking patient or even giving in to a mildly over-controlling patient, to absolute limits on violence. The medical staff fears over-reacting, and the consultant reduces anxiety by defining the management of varying degrees of aggression. Disruptions are mostly born of self-protective or fearful impulses in the confused or delirious patient. Rarely, however, a patient becomes dangerous. In those instances, the most common warning is fear; someone becomes scared of the patient. Staff almost never fear delirious behavior, controllable anger, or senile pique, but they do tend to become wary, then edgy, and then frightened. This intuition in caregivers is often the only warning the consultant gets before an explosion. Ominous signs in the patient are rapidly increasing demandingness; more frequent and intense anger, especially with abusive language; and mounting agitation and paranoia. The general feeling in the medical setting of an implacable crescendo of menace surrounding the patient is another ominous sign.

Before any decision about physical restraint of the patient is made, hospital security guards should be standing by on the medical or surgical service. This is a first step in the decision-making process. Security can always be dismissed with thanks after standing by, but to delay summoning help until after such a decision is made risks panicking the patient, who may have an uncanny ability to sense an impending confrontation.

Such ideas refer to control of violent behavior in the immediate situation. Occasionally, however, the consultant is asked about the long-range "dangerousness" of the patient. This is an opinion that involves extrapolating from present behavior in a known, observed situation to a guess about the patient's interaction with a different milieu, one that might contain drugs, weapons, and situations beyond the psychiatrist's ken. Medicine is about healing, not social control. Dangerous persons (e.g., the person with an antisocial personality who commits rape) may in some sense be "difficult patients," but in these situations, they are not patients at all, but criminals.

Psychiatric opinions outside the medical purview violate an important boundary and feed the fallacy that all bad behavior is somehow psychiatric and that mentally ill persons have no personal responsibility for their behavior. What the psychiatrist can do, however, is document the medical history of the consenting patient about drugs, access to weapons, felony convictions, and the like. Surprisingly often, such a patient discloses useful information in the context of a skillfully elicited childhood history of enuresis, fire setting, and cruelty to animals. ("Were you ever accused of setting fires? Did anybody ever say you were mean to the neighbor's pets?") Such patients can be oddly eager to resurrect old denials and often are still indignant about them. Then, they sometimes continue to give themselves away and provide information needed to protect caregivers and other patients in the medical setting.

Substance Abuse

Substance use is one area in which the consultant can be most useful to patients with primitive personality problems. Substance use is such an issue for a significant proportion of difficult patients that excess alcohol can be thought of as a personality disorder in a bottle. A significant number of borderline patients—one-fifth in one study—abuse substances.[7] Of these, perhaps up to a fourth have such a good response to abstinence that they no longer meet diagnostic criteria for the disorder,[42] and the absence of an active SUD is the strongest single predictor of remission of borderline personality symptoms over time.[7]

Readers are referred to Chapter 13 for further information on the diagnosis and management of SUDs. However, it is important to note that patients with personality disorder can benefit from 12-step recovery programs, given that they have two ingredients known to help primitive character pathology:

an emphasis on taking responsibility for oneself (as opposed to cultivating the victim role) and a highly structured series of steps and methods. Moreover, there is a commonality between a central tenet of one of the most successful treatments for borderline personality, dialectical-behavioral therapy (DBT)—that of embracing both acceptance and change—and one of the philosophical underpinnings of 12-step programs, embodied in the Serenity Prayer. DBT itself can also be helpful for SUDs in patients with a borderline personality.[43] Not least in importance, there are myriads of such groups meeting at almost any hour of the day or night in every location in the urban United States.

Not surprisingly, it requires great skill to persuade a difficult patient to identify with one of the 12-step programs. First, there is almost always a dense denial of the abuse problem, along with a need to see the self as powerless and victimized. Patients who split and narcissists see themselves as "better than" persons in Alcoholics Anonymous, for example, and are so vulnerable to shame that they hesitate to take on another attribute that they see as shameful. Also, the general culture outside such programs has little real information about what they can accomplish, so the patient is not only ashamed but also usually ignorant of these resources.

There is an art to getting a difficult patient to consider that a problem with addiction, co-dependency, or the like may be the root of much of the suffering the patient endures. Practicing this art involves accumulating knowledge about such programs and having familiarity with some persons who have been helped by them. It involves the ability to discern when the patient might be receptive, first to acknowledging an addiction and second to considering such a program. It involves knowing how to elicit information in a non-shaming way ("Do you find yourself drinking more than you really want to be drinking?"), presenting the condition as a disease and "not the person's fault," and introducing the ideas gradually in a non-threatening manner ("Did your mom ever turn to Al-Anon for help with your father's drinking?" and "Did you ever get help from the Adult Children of Alcoholics program or something like that?").

No difficult patient is ever educated easily, and it usually requires multiple inputs from numerous sources over many months even to begin to get some of these options accepted by the patient. The consulting psychiatrist can introduce such ideas and, given the relapse rate of difficult patients, might get another opportunity with the same patient down the road. The consultant can, at the very least, start the educational process without making the patient feel ashamed.

Brief Tactical Psychotherapy

Psychotherapy is a risky proposition, and the consultant is wise to resist the temptation to do much on the medical-surgical unit. Rarely, however, the crisis of an illness provides a unique chance for a patient with a primitive personality for insight and growth. This lucid interval is incidentally produced when an illness and treatment cut through the veils of dissociation that surround such patients, their maladaptive projective defenses, and their habitual externalization of responsibility. In this context, sometimes the patient asks not only the superficial "Why me?" but also the deeper question, "Who am I that this is happening to?"

A study of changes in pathologic narcissism in a cohort of subjects followed for several years[44] found that most had improved significantly and that the improvement related to life achievements, new durable relationships, and disillusionment. These subjects displayed decreased grandiosity and a deeper empathy for others as evidenced by better relationships. The disillusionment related to these improvements, moreover, had occurred at a critical juncture in the person's development and was of a certain type—challenging but not devastating. The findings plausibly support the idea that certain painful constructive real-life experiences help people change their primitive pathology. (That brief therapeutic intervention can further this process, even in primitive patients, is shown in some of the therapies detailed by Malan, Budman, Strupp, Bloom, Horowitz, and especially Winnicott.)[45]

This is the rationale for a certain brief, tactical intervention by the psychiatric consultant who encounters a difficult patient during a medical or surgical crisis: how to keep the disillusionment from being completely devastating and help the patient make sense of it in terms of personal identity. (As Fig. 41.1 shows a vague sense of personal identity underlies much of the pathology of the difficult patient.) The patient is in the process of trying to adapt to the illness or injury, to work through it, to grieve losses, and to contain fears.

In this context, the psychiatrist's aim is not merely to help further this grieving or adjusting process, but to accomplish a deeper, more lasting goal: using the illness or injury process as a template or map for other life changes, using the crisis of the moment to help the patient learn new ways of thinking about the self, and coping with rage, terror, and shame.

The tactical brief therapy of the difficult patient falls into two types of maneuvers: *containment* and *intervention*. Containment involves control of uncontrolled affect, distorted cognition, and destructive behavior. Intervention consists of correcting the misdirection of the patient's trajectory, previously determined by pathologic affect, distorted cognition, and self-defeating behavior. Containment and intervention roughly correspond to the two parts of traditional psychotherapy: the frame (scheduling, vacations, fees, phone calls, limits on acting out, confidentiality) and the content (symptoms, history, development, associations, discourse, dreams, fantasies, defenses, adaptation, transference, countertransference, and other non-framework components of therapy). This "moment" of brief tactical psychotherapy assumes the patient in the medical situation is temporarily contained and already in a dialogue with the psychiatrist about the illness or injury that brought the patient to this place at this time.

The therapist's first task—and therapist is what the consultant becomes at this moment—is to listen to see whether the patient is asking for an intervention. The patient signals such readiness not only by addressing the impact of the illness or injury but also by mentioning the overall meaning of the patient's life, the patient's "story," the over-arching narrative that helps any human being make sense of the world. If the tactical intervention is to be helpful, the patient must be the one to push for it. The therapist's experience at this point is of being passively drawn into the patient's turbulent material, yet actively steering the discussion away from affects too intense on the one side and cognitions that are psychotically distorted on the other.

Up to this point, the therapist's job has been careful listening and containment. If the patient is ready, the patient will introduce these two themes: the overall story of the patient's life and its meaning, and the meaning of the illness or injury that is serving as the focus of the tactical psychotherapeutic moment. The patient will tend to see the medical crisis as thematically pertinent to the meaningful life story—for instance, just another in a long series of persecutions, a punishment for something bad the patient has done or is. The life story is generally a standard narrative of a search for perfect safety and love, a quest for power so the patient will never again be scared; there are seldom any major surprises at this point.

The therapist's first active step in the tactical intervention occurs now: labeling the life story; labeling the symbolic, adding metaphoric meaning of the illness or injury, and labeling the pain that is at the interface of the two. This is almost like offering a "title" for the story. ("All your life you've been a survivor; now you wonder if you can survive this terror.") The idea here is that, to survive, individuals must construct a meaningful narrative of the crisis. Under the pressure of converting experience into symbols and then into meaning, the primitive person may be forced to construct a more realistic life narrative (and hence a more coherent sense of personal identity).

If the patient continues to be receptive to a tactical intervention, two things happen at this point: first, production of deeper material in symbolic form (mention of a fantasy or recurrent dream, some external, cultural symbol or icon, a movie or a television character) and, second, a rather pointed question for the therapist about what to do (an acceptance by the patient of the therapist as a relatively separate, helpful person). This turning point requires careful listening because the key organizing theme of the patient's life (as the patient sees it) is presented in this one moment of symbol formation along with the rather concrete question that follows directly after.

Here the therapist does not answer the patient's question about what to do with the illness assaulting the meaning in the patient's life. The therapist labels the assault, points out the crisis in meaning, and thematically throws the question back to the patient. ("In a way you're asking how to cope with this thing, but in a deeper way you're saying that you're Scarlett O'Hara, since you just mentioned her. How would Scarlett handle what you're going through?")

What the patient says next reveals whether the tactical linking of the two meanings and two stories seemed useful to the patient. If so, the patient produces more details of the life story, again asking the therapist what to do about the illness or injury. Again,

the therapist throws responsibility back to the patient, labeling meaningfulness issues and the importance of the illness or injury to it. ("You just mentioned losing your husband—like Scarlett O'Hara—and now you're asking how to cope with your boyfriend's reaction to your mastectomy. Scarlett fell back on Tara and her own resources. What resources do you have to draw on?")

This working-through cycle of question and deflection continues if the therapist has the time and the patient has the strength to bear the rage, terror, or shame of the moment. Usually the patient fatigues and moves the subject back to some specific entitled demand, such as getting more pain medication. This signals that the therapy part of the encounter is now over and that the consultant is once again back to management of the difficult patient.

Although the brief tactical psychotherapy just described is probably the most useful first-line approach for the inpatient consultant, other psychotherapeutic methods have been designed for the treatment of borderline personality disorder and can be applied to other difficult patients as well.

Although full implementation of these therapies is not possible during a few consultation visits, familiarity with the theory and techniques they rely on can enhance the consultant's ability to make sense of, and employ, a therapeutic tool, in diverse situations. Indeed, as these very different forms of therapy have been found to produce similar results,[46] a set of common factors for any successful therapy of borderline patients has been proposed.[47]

Table 41.5 summarizes these treatments and provides examples of how they can be adapted to encounters with difficult patients.

TERMINATION

Preparation of the difficult patient for hospital discharge is fraught with hazards. The patient not only might intensify disruptive behavior to prolong the hospital stay but might also simultaneously try to leave prematurely. The patient might secretly infect dressings or intravenous lines with saliva or feces and develop a fever while threatening to leave the hospital against medical advice. Or the patient might increase suicidal gestures, such as wrist cutting, to manipulate

TABLE 41.5

Psychotherapies for Borderline Personality Disorder and Their Relevance to the Difficult Patient

Therapy	Developer	Relevant Theory[a]	Relevant Techniques	Example With the Difficult Patient
Dialectical-behavioral therapy	Marsha Linehan	The patient is more emotionally vulnerable and reactive and is therefore ill-suited to a normal social environment	Acknowledge and validate the patient's differences while also encouraging change	Consultant: "This ward is a difficult place for you. Everyone's too busy to give you the help you need, and this illness is one of the most distressing things that's ever happened to you. Your rage and fear make sense. That being said, the doctors and nurses here really are trying their best. They're at least meeting you a third of the way. Do you think you could cut them a little slack? Do you want me to communicate anything to them for you?"
Transference-focused psychotherapy	Otto Kernberg, John Clarkin	The patient is frozen in a state of immature emotional development where the self is split into multiple negative and positive parts experienced successively in time, each infused with maladaptively powerful affects. Personality therefore lacks consistency and cohesion	Interpret the patient's successive self-states to enhance the patient's awareness of the multiple roles she or he plays, which fosters a more integrated self	Consultant: "You say the doctors here are the best ever, but the nurses are all bitches. And at first, you told me I understood you like no one else. But now that I'm trying to enforce the rules to protect your safety, you're ready to throw me on the trash heap. So, it's almost like I experienced two different people: first, you were so warm and tender and the next minute you were like a warrior ready to cleave me in two. Aside from letting you take off your heart monitor leads, which you know is too dangerous right now, how can we help you feel better heard and cared for?"
Mentalization-based therapy	Peter Fonagy, Anthony Bateman	The patient cannot make sense of the actions of self and others based on intentional mental states, such as desires, feelings, and beliefs	Point out the patient's actions to help the patient draw a link between actions and what the patient is thinking and feeling; identify the patient's reactions to the therapist's words or actions and help them guess what you're feeling and thinking	Consultant: "Can you tell me what you were feeling and thinking while you were cutting yourself with that razor you brought in? Were you scared? Were you angry because we did something wrong?" Patient: "I told you to get the f*** out of here!!" Consultant: "I'm concerned about you and terrified when you scream like that. I know that scares other staff too. We'll need those restraints to keep you safe until we can understand you better and help you cope with this more safely."
Schema-focused therapy	Jeffrey Young; influenced by the work of Aaron Beck	The patient's inner world is characterized by five modes, or aspects of self, that interact in destructive ways: the abandoned and abused child, the angry and impulsive child, the detached protector, the punitive parent, and the healthy adult	Develop the "healthy adult" by "limited reparenting," emotion-focused work (e.g., imagery and dialogues), cognitive restructuring and education, and breaking behavioral patterns	Patient: "I don't take my heart pills or my insulin usually for the simple reason that I'm a dropout and a druggie and what's the point of someone like me continuing to take up space on this earth." Consultant: (who has already established that the patient is not depressed but rather personality disordered) "Multiple times already I've heard you be extremely hard on yourself. It would be useful to give that voice of yours a name. How about 'My Abusive Step-father?' When you hear yourself talking like that, try to remember that name. With outpatient therapy, you can learn how to tell that part of yourself to leave the rest of you alone and gradually he'll go away for good."

The patient = a borderline personality-disordered or difficult patient.

[a]With minor differences in emphasis, each of these theories assumes the same etiologic factors: innate temperamental difficulties or an abusive or neglectful (or poorly matched in terms of temperament) relationship with a caregiver in early life.

(get close to/stay distant from) the staff. Firm limits on sabotage and elopement should be discussed with the staff. Around termination, they should be more observant of the patient, as well as more visible, and firm. A specific discharge date should be firmly adhered to,[48] despite a predictable worsening in the patient's psychological status.

After the patient has left, it is preferable for the consultant to touch base with the staff and the consultee once more to review the treatment and to share some of the consultant's feelings. In this way, the consultant not only "terminates" with the staff but also paves the way for future work with the next difficult patient who comes to the general hospital.

REFERENCES

1. Groves JE. Taking care of the hateful patient. *N Engl J Med.* 1978; 298:883–887.
2. American Psychiatric Association. *Diagnostic and Statistical Manual of Mental Disorders.* 5th ed. American Psychiatric Association; 2013.
3. Gunderson JG, Stout RL, McGlashan TH, et al. Ten-year course of borderline personality disorder: psychopathology and function from the collaborative longitudinal personality disorders study. *Arch Gen Psychiatry.* 2011;68:827–837.
4. Hopwood CJ, Thomas KM. Paranoid and schizoid personality disorders. In: Widiger TA, ed. *The Oxford Handbook of Personality Disorders.* Oxford University Press; 2012.
5. Kernberg OF. Borderline Conditions and Pathological Narcissism. Jason Aronson; 1975.
6. Zanarini MC, Frankenburg FR, Vujanovic AA. Inter-rater and test-retest reliability of the revised diagnostic interview for borderlines. *J Pers Disord.* 2002;16:270–276.
7. Zanarini MC, Frankenburg FR, Hennen J, et al. Axis I comorbidity in patients with borderline personality disorder: 6-year follow-up and prediction of time to remission. *Am J Psychiatry.* 2004;161:2108–2114.
8. Gunderson JG, Stout RL, Shea MT, et al. Interactions of borderline personality disorder and mood disorders over 10 years. *J Clin Psychiatry.* 2014;75:829–834.
9. Paris J. Why psychiatrists are reluctant to diagnose: borderline personality disorder. *Psychiatry (Edgmont).* 2007;4:35–39.
10. Ruggero CJ, Zimmerman M, Chelminski I, et al. Borderline personality disorder and the misdiagnosis of bipolar disorder. *J Psychiatr Res.* 2010;44:405–408.
11. Chopra HD, Beatson JA. Psychotic symptoms in borderline personality disorder. *Am J Psychiatry.* 1986;143:1605–1607.
12. Sterba R. The dynamics of the dissolution of the transference resistance. *Psychoanal Q.* 1940;9:363–379.
13. Bandelow B, Krause J, Wedekind D, et al. Early traumatic life events, parental attitudes, family history, and birth risk factors in patients with borderline personality disorder and healthy controls. *Psychiatry Res.* 2005;134:169–179.
14. Silk KR, Lee S, Hill EM, et al. Borderline personality disorder symptoms and severity of sexual abuse. *Am J Psychiatry.* 1995;152:1059–1064.
15. Shearer SL. Dissociative phenomena in women with borderline personality disorder. *Am J Psychiatry.* 1994;151:1324–1328.
16. Cloninger CR, Dragan SM. Personality disorders. In: Kaplan HI, Sadock BJ, eds. *Comprehensive Textbook of Psychiatry.* 9th ed. Williams and Wilkins; 2009.
17. Adler G. Helplessness in the helpers. *Br J Med Psychol.* 1972; 45:315–326.
18. Bender DS, Dolan RT, Skodol AE, et al. Treatment utilization by patients with personality disorders. *Am J Psychiatry.* 2001;158:295–302.
19. Frankenburg FR, Zanarini MC. The association between borderline personality disorder and chronic medical illnesses, poor health-related lifestyle choices, and costly forms of health care utilization. *J Clin Psychiatry.* 2004;65:1660–1665.
20. Sheehan L, Nieweglowski K, Corrigan P. The stigma of personality disorders. *Curr Psychiatry Rep.* 2016;18:1–7.
21. Liebman RE, Burnette M. It's not you, it's me: an examination of clinician- and client-level influences on countertransference toward borderline personality disorder. *Am J Orthopsychiatry.* 2013;83:115–125.
22. Aviram RB, Brodsky BS, Stanley B. Borderline personality disorder, stigma, and treatment implications. *Harv Rev Psychiatry.* 2006;14:249–256.
23. Gerlach G, Loeber S, Herpertz S. Personality disorders and obesity: a systematic review. *Obes Rev.* 2016;17:691–723.
24. Keuroghlian AS, Frankenburg FR, Zanarini MC. The relationship of chronic medical illnesses, poor health-related lifestyle choices, and health care utilization to recovery status in borderline patients over a decade of prospective follow-up. *J Psychiatr Res.* 2013;47:1499–1506.
25. Zanarini MC, Frankeburg FR, Fitzmaurice G. Defense mechanisms reported by patients with borderline personality disorder and axis II comparison subjects over 16 years of prospective follow-up: description and prediction of recovery. *Am J Psychiatry.* 2013;170:111–120.
26. Ogden TH. On projective identification. *Int J Psychoanal.* 1979;60:357–373.
27. Kucharski A, Groves JE. The so-called "inappropriate" consultation request on a medical or surgical ward. *Int J Psychiatry Med.* 1976;7:209–220. 1977.
28. Groves JE. Management of the borderline patient on a medical or surgical ward: the psychiatric consultant's role. *Int J Psychiatry Med.* 1975;6:337–348.
29. Caplan G. *The Theory and Practice of Mental Health Consultation.* Basic Books; 1970.
30. Zanarini MC, Frankenburg FR, Harned AL, et al. Rates of psychotropic medication use reported by borderline patients and axis II comparison subjects over 16 years of prospective follow-up. *J Clin Psychopharmacol.* 2015;35:63–67.
31. National Health and Medical Research Council Clinical Practice Guidelines for the Management of Borderline Personality Disorder. National Health and Medical Research Council; 2012.

32. Adelman SA. Pills as transitional objects: a dynamic understanding of the use of medication in psychotherapy. *Psychiatry*. 1985;48: 246–253.

33. Aldrich MS. Narcolepsy. *N Engl J Med*. 1990;323:389–394.

34. Swift RG, Perkins DO, Chase CL, et al. Psychiatric disorders in 36 families with Wolfram syndrome. *Am J Psychiatry*. 1991;148:775–779.

35. Keljo DJ, Squires RH. Clinical problem-solving: just in time. *N Engl J Med*. 1996;334:46–48.

36. Zanarini MC, Gunderson JG, Frankenburg FR, et al. Discriminating borderline personality disorder from other axis II disorders. *Am J Psychiatry*. 1990;147:161–167.

37. McGirr A, Paris J, Lesage A, et al. Risk factors for suicide completion in borderline personality disorder: a case-control study of cluster B comorbidity and impulsive aggression. *J Clin Psychiatry*. 2007;68:721–729.

38. Reich P, Kelly MJ. Suicide attempts by hospitalized medical and surgical patients. *N Engl J Med*. 1976;294:298–301.

39. Roush JF, Guidry ET. Suicide risk among general hospital inpatients. *The Southwest Respiratory and Critical Care Chronicles*. 2015;3: 11–14.

40. Maltsberger JT, Buie DH. Countertransference hate in the treatment of suicidal patients. *Arch Gen Psychiatry*. 1974;30: 625–633.

41. Cheng IC, Hu FC, Tseng MC. Inpatient suicide in a general hospital. *Gen Hosp Psychiatry*. 2009;31:110–115.

42. Dulit RA, Fyer GL, Haas GL, et al. Substance use in borderline personality disorder. *Am J Psychiatry*. 1990;147:1002–1007.

43. Lee NK, Cameron J, Jenner L. A systematic review of interventions for co-occurring substance use and borderline personality disorders. *Drug Alcohol Rev*. 2015;34:663–672.

44. Ronningstam E, Gunderson J, Lyons M. Changes in pathological narcissism. *Am J Psychiatry*. 1995;152:253–257.

45. Groves JE, ed. *Essential Papers on Short-Term Dynamic Therapy*. New York University Press; 1996.

46. Clarkin JF, Levy KN, Lenzenweger MF, et al. Evaluating three treatments for borderline personality disorder: a multiwave study. *Am J Psychiatry*. 2007;164:922–928.

47. Weinberg I, Ronningstam E, Goldblatt MJ, et al. Common factors in empirically supported treatments of borderline personality disorder. *Curr Psychiatry Rep*. 2011;13:60–68.

48. Grunebaum HU, Klerman GL. Wrist slashing. *Am J Psychiatry*. 1967;124:527–534.

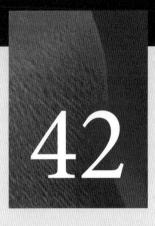

42

CARE OF THE PATIENT WITH THOUGHTS OF SUICIDE

KATHERINE A. KOH, MD, MSC ■ ABIGAIL L. DONOVAN, MD ■ SUZANNE A. BIRD, MD ■ THEODORE A. STERN, MD

OVERVIEW

Suicide, or intentional self-harm with the intent of causing death, is the 10th leading cause of death in the United States, accounting for nearly 45,000 deaths each year.[1] Non-lethal self-inflicted injuries are even more prevalent, accounting for more than 500,000 emergency department (ED) visits per year[1] and reflecting the high ratio of patients who present after a suicide attempt to those who have died by suicide. Psychiatric disorders are associated with more than 90% of deaths by suicide and with the most suicide attempts.[2] Therefore, psychiatrists must be familiar with the evaluation and treatment of patients who contemplate, threaten, or attempt suicide. Although guided by knowledge of epidemiological risk factors for suicide (Box 42.1), clinicians must rely on a detailed examination and clinical judgment in the evaluation of current suicide risk.

EPIDEMIOLOGY AND RISK FACTORS

Epidemiology

Suicide accounts for 1.3% of the total number of deaths in the United States each year.[1,3] For every person who dies by suicide, approximately 30 people attempt suicide.[4] Each year, ED visits for patients who have attempted suicide represent approximately 0.5% of all annual ED visits.[1]

The use of firearms is the most common method of ending one's life; for males in the United States, this method accounts for between 50% and 60% of suicides annually.[1] Suffocation, including hanging, is the second most common cause of suicide in the United States, and the second most common cause in males, accounting for more than 13,000 suicide deaths in 2019.[1] Poisoning, including drug ingestion, is the third most common cause of death by suicide in the United States and the most common cause in females between 1990 and 2020, accounting for approximately 5500 to 6500 deaths per year.[1] Historically, drug ingestion has accounted for most non-fatal suicide attempts.[5]

Suicide rates differ by age, sex, and race. Rates generally increase with age; people older than 65 years are 1.5 times more likely to take their life than are younger individuals, while White males over the age of 85 have an even higher rate of suicide.[5,6] The number of suicides among the elderly is disproportionately high; the elderly appear to make more serious attempts and are less apt to survive when medical complications from an attempt ensue—one out of four attempts in this group results in a suicide.[5,6] Although the elderly have the highest rate of suicide, suicide among young adults (between the ages of 15 and 24) rose three-fold between 1950 and 1990,[7] and as of 2022, suicide is the second-leading cause of death among people ages 15 to 24 in the United States. Males are three to four times more likely to take their own life than females, although the rate of non-fatal suicide attempts is comparable for females and males.[8,9] The reasons for these disparities have not been established clearly.

White and Native American people attempt and die from suicide more frequently than those of other races.[10] African Americans and Hispanic people have approximately half the suicide rate of White people.[10]

BOX 42.1
RISK FACTORS FOR SUICIDE

Psychiatric illness
- Major depression
- Bipolar disorder
- Alcohol and drug use disorders
- Schizophrenia
- Personality disorders
- Organic brain syndrome
- Panic disorder

Race (American Indian/Alaskan Native > White > Pacific Islander > Multi-racial > Black/Hispanic > Asian)
Marital status (widowed, divorced, or separated)
Living alone
Recent personal loss
Unemployment
Financial/legal difficulties
Co-morbid medical illness chronic illness, pain, or terminal illness
History of suicide attempts or threats
Male sex
Advancing age
Family history of suicide
Recent hospital discharge
Access to firearms
Hopelessness

TABLE 42.1
Percentage of Suicides With a Given Psychiatric Disorder

Condition	Percentage of Suicides
Affective illness	50
Drug or alcohol use disorders	25
Schizophrenia	10
Personality disorders	5
Secondary depression	5
Organic brain syndromes	2
None apparent	2

Psychiatric Risk Factors

Psychiatric illness is the most powerful risk factor for both dying from, and attempting, suicide. Psychiatric disorders are associated with more than 90% of deaths by suicide and with most suicide attempts.[2] Mood disorders, including major depressive disorder (MDD) and bipolar disorder (BPD), are responsible for approximately 50% of suicides, alcohol and drug use for 25%, psychosis for 10%, and personality disorders for 5%[11,12] (Table 42.1).

Up to 15% of patients with MDD or BPD die by suicide, almost always during depressive episodes[13]; this statistic represents a suicide risk 30 times greater than that of those in the general population.[14] The true lifetime risk may be somewhat lower, because these estimates (and those for the other diagnoses discussed later) typically derive from hospitalized patient samples.[11] The risk appears to be greater early in the course of a lifetime disorder, early on in a depressive episode,[15] in the first week following psychiatric hospitalization,[16] in the first month following hospital discharge,[16] and

in the early stages of recovery.[16] A 10-year follow-up study of almost 1000 patients found that those who died by suicide within the first year of follow-up were more likely to be suffering from global insomnia, severe anhedonia, impaired concentration, psychomotor agitation, alcohol abuse, anxiety, and panic attacks, whereas those who died by suicide after the first year of follow-up were more likely to be suffering from suicidal ideation, severe hopelessness, and had a history of suicide attempts.[17]

Approximately 15% to 25% of patients with an alcohol use disorder (AUD) or a substance use disorder (SUD) die by suicide, of which up to 84% suffer from both an AUD and a SUD.[18] The suicide risk appears to be greatest approximately 9 years after the onset of an AUD or a SUD.[19] Most patients with an AUD who die by suicide suffer from a co-morbid depressive disorder,[20] and as many as one-third have experienced the recent loss of a close relationship through separation or death.[21]

Nearly 20% of people who die by suicide are legally intoxicated at the time of their death.[22] Alcohol and drug use are associated with more pervasive suicidal ideation, more serious suicidal intent, more lethal suicide attempts, and a greater number of suicide attempts.[23] Use of alcohol and drugs may impair judgment and foster impulsivity.[16]

Approximately 10% of patients with schizophrenia die by suicide, mostly during periods of improvement after relapse or during periods of depression.[20] The risk for suicide appears to be greater among young males who are newly diagnosed,[24] who have a chronic course and numerous exacerbations, who are discharged from hospitals with significant psychopathology and functional impairment, and who have a realistic awareness and fear of further mental decline.[24] The risk may also be increased with akathisia and with the abrupt discontinuation of antipsychotic medications.[25] Patients who experience hallucinations (that instruct them to harm themselves) in association with schizophrenia, mania, or depression with psychotic features are probably at greater risk for self-harm.[26]

Between 4% and 10% of patients with borderline personality disorder and 5% of patients with antisocial personality disorder die by suicide.[27] The risk appears to be greater for those with co-morbid unipolar depression or AUD.[28] Patients with personality disorders often make impulsive suicidal attempts; these attempts may become progressively more lethal if they are not taken seriously. Even self-harming behaviors that are not associated with an intent to die can turn fatal.[26]

As many as 15% to 20% of patients with an anxiety disorder die by suicide,[29] and up to 20% of patients with panic disorder attempt suicide.[30] Although the risk of suicide in patients with anxiety and a panic disorder may be elevated secondary to co-morbid conditions (e.g., MDD, an AUD, a SUD), the suicide risk remains almost as high as that of MDD, even after co-existing conditions are accounted for.[31] The risk for suicide attempts may be elevated for females, with an early onset and with co-morbid alcohol or drug use.[30]

Medical Risk Factors

Medical illness, especially of a severe or chronic nature, is generally associated with an increased risk of suicide and is thus considered a risk factor for suicide even though there is most likely a multi-factorial relationship between medical illness and suicide.[32] Medical disorders are associated with as many as 35% to 40% of suicides and with as many as 70% of suicides in those older than age 60.[33] Acquired immunodeficiency syndrome (AIDS), cancer, head trauma, epilepsy, multiple sclerosis, Huntington chorea, organic brain syndromes, spinal cord injuries, hypertension, cardiopulmonary disease, peptic ulcer disease, chronic renal failure, Cushing disease, rheumatoid arthritis, and porphyria have each been reported to increase the risk of suicide. Notably, however, few investigations concerning the increased risk for suicide in these populations have controlled for the effects of age, sex, race, psychiatric disorders, other medical disorders, or use of medications.

Patients with AIDS appear to have a suicide risk that is greater than that of the general population, and previous estimates of the increased risk ranged from 7 to 66 times that of the general population.[11] Today, the risk of suicide in human immunodeficiency virus (HIV) infection has increased approximately threefold. Testing for antibodies to HIV has resulted in an immediate and substantial decrease in thoughts of suicide in those who turned out to be seronegative; no increase in suicidal ideation was detected in those who were seropositive.[34]

Patients with cancer have a suicide rate that is almost twice as great as that of the general population and seem to be at higher risk in the first 2 years after they are diagnosed.[33] Head and neck malignancies are associated with an 11 times greater risk of suicide compared with those in the general population, possibly due to increased rates of tobacco and alcohol use in this population and the resultant facial disfigurement and loss of voice.[33] In males, gastrointestinal cancers are associated with a greater risk of suicide, and in both sexes lung and upper airway malignancies are also associated with greater suicide risk.[33] Other factors, including poor prognosis, poor pain control, fatigue, depression, hopelessness, delirium, disinhibition, prior suicide attempts, recent losses, and a paucity of social supports, may place patients with cancer at greater risk.

Like those with cancer, individuals with head trauma, multiple sclerosis, and peptic ulcer disease have approximately twice the risk of suicide as those in the general population.[33] In patients with head injuries, the risk appears to be greater in those who suffer severe injuries and in those who develop dementia, psychosis, personality changes, or epilepsy.[35] In patients with multiple sclerosis, the risk may be higher for those diagnosed before age 40 and within the first 5 years after diagnosis.[36] In patients with peptic ulcer disease, the increased risk is hypothesized to be due to co-morbid psychiatric disorders and SUDs (especially AUD).[33]

Between the increased risk of suicide of approximately two-fold for cancer, head trauma, multiple sclerosis, and peptic ulcer disease, and the increased risk in patients with HIV/AIDS estimated to be at least nearly seven-fold, there are several medical illnesses with intermediate increases in suicide risk. These illnesses include epilepsy, systemic lupus erythematosus, spinal cord injuries, Huntington disease, organic brain syndromes, and chronic renal disease. Patients with end-stage renal disease on hemodialysis may have the highest relative risk of all subgroups.[33] As many as 5% of patients with chronic renal failure who receive hemodialysis take their own life; those who travel to medical centers for dialysis have a higher suicide rate than those who are dialyzed at home.[37]

Patients with epilepsy are five times more likely than those in the general population to die from, or attempt, suicide.[33] Sufferers of temporal lobe epilepsy, with concomitant psychosis or personality changes, may be at greater risk.[33]

Delirious and confused patients may suffer from agitation and destructive impulses and be unable to protect themselves from self-harm. For victims of spinal cord injury, the risk is greater for those with less severe injuries.[38]

Patients with hypertension and those with cardiopulmonary disease may also have a higher risk for suicide than those in the general population. Although previous reports suggested that beta-blockers could contribute to an increased risk by promoting depression,[39] evidence has since suggested that beta-blockers do not increase the risk of developing depression.[40] Finally, an association between suicide and very low cholesterol levels has been reported, but the connection is still under investigation.[11,32]

Familial and Genetic Risk Factors

A family history of suicide, a family history of psychiatric illness, and a tumultuous early family environment have each been found to have an important impact on the risk of suicide. A family history of suicide confers approximately a two-fold increase in risk for suicide even after controlling for a family psychiatric history.[41] This increased suicide risk may be mediated through a shared genetic predisposition for suicide, psychiatric disorders, or impulsive behavior, or through a shared family environment in which modeling and imitation are prominent.[26]

Genetic factors are supported by evidence that monozygotic twins have a higher concordance rate for suicide and suicide attempts than dizygotic twins

and by evidence that biological parents of adoptees who take their own lives have a higher rate of suicide than do biological parents of non-suicidal adoptees.[11] However, little is known about the specific genetic factors that confer this risk.[11] Studies have largely focused on serotonin neurotransmission, including genetic mutations in the rate-limiting enzyme in serotonin synthesis, L-tryptophan hydroxylase, serotonin receptors, and the serotonin transporter (SERT), but these investigations are still inconclusive.[41] While there is partial overlap with a vulnerability to depression, the predisposition to suicide is separate. Overall, it is estimated that one-third to one-half of the risk of suicide is genetically mediated.[41]

Recent evidence suggests that epigenetics, particularly alterations in promoter DNA methylation patterns, plays an important role in the neurobiology of suicide. Numerous familial environmental factors, which may be mediated through epigenetic changes, contribute to suicide risk.[42] A tumultuous early family environment (including factors of early parental death, parental separation, frequent moves, and emotional, physical, or sexual abuse) increases the risk for suicide.[43] Children's risk of future suicidal behavior may also be increased by suicidal behavior in important family members through modeling.[11]

Social Risk Factors

Widowed, divorced, or separated adults are at greater risk for suicide than are single adults, who are at greater risk than married adults.[44] Married adults with young children appear to carry the lowest risk.[16,26,45] Living alone substantially increases the risk of suicide, especially among adults who are widowed, divorced, or separated.[16] Social isolation from family, relatives, friends, neighbors, and co-workers also increases the risk of suicide.[45] Conversely, the presence of social support is protective against suicide.[41]

Significant personal losses (including diminution of self-esteem or status[33,45]) and interpersonal conflicts also place individuals, particularly young adults and adolescents, at greater risk for suicide.[46] Bereavement following the death of a loved one increases the risk of suicide over the next 4 or 5 years, particularly for people with a psychiatric history (including suicide attempts) and for people who receive little family support.[25] Unemployment, which may produce or exacerbate psychiatric illness or may result from psychiatric illness,[25] increases the likelihood of suicide and accounts for as many as one-third to one-half of deaths by suicide.[45] This risk may be particularly elevated among males.[16] Financial and legal difficulties also increase the risk of suicide.[16]

The presence of one or more firearms in the home appears to increase the risk of suicide independently for both sexes and all age groups, even when other risk factors, such as depression and alcohol use, are taken into account.[46] Therefore, it is important to ask about access to firearms during the suicide risk assessment and to take steps to limit access to firearms if indicated to mitigate the risk of suicide. Of note, adolescents with a gun in the household have suicide rates between 4 and 10 times higher than other adolescents.[47]

Recently, rates of suicide in the US military personnel have been increasing. Studies regarding rates of suicide in this population have historically drawn conflicting conclusions. Before the wars in Afghanistan and Iraq, rates of suicide in military personnel, when adjusted for age and sex, were consistently lower as compared to national rates from 1980 to 1992.[48] However, in 2008 the age- and sex-adjusted suicide rate in the Army was greater than the average suicide rate in the general population for the first time.[49] This trend continued and the US military reported that deaths from suicide surpassed deaths from combat from January to June 2012.[49] Veterans of Operations Enduring Freedom or Iraqi Freedom (OEF/OIF) as a whole trended toward having higher rates of suicide following deployment compared to those in the US general population.[49] OEF/OIF veterans who were in active duty units and therefore more likely exposed to combat trauma or those diagnosed with a mental disorder had statistically significantly higher rates of suicide than in the general population.[50] Clinicians treating this population should also screen for evidence of sleep disturbances as a warning sign for suicide, be aware of the parallel between increased prescribing and overuse of opioid analgesics in patients with post-traumatic stress disorder, and restrict access to firearms.[49]

Past and Present Suicidality

A history of suicide attempts is one of the most powerful risk factors for future attempts and death by suicide. While more than 50% of people who take their own life will do so on their first attempt, those who survive remain at elevated risk.[51] As many as 10% to 20% of people with prior suicide attempts die by suicide.[52] The risk for suicide following an attempted suicide is almost 100 times that of the general population in the year following the attempt; it then declines but remains elevated throughout the next 8 years.[25] People with prior suicide attempts are also at greater risk for subsequent attempts and account for approximately 50% of serious overdoses.[53] The clinical use of past suicide attempts as a predictive risk factor may be limited in the elderly because the elderly make fewer attempts for each fatal suicide.[5,6,45]

The lethality of past suicide attempts slightly increases the risk of dying by suicide,[25] especially among females with psychiatric illness.[54] The dangerousness of an attempt, however, may be more predictive of the risk for suicide in those individuals with significant intent to suicide and a realization of the potential lethality of their actions.[55]

The communication of present suicidal ideation and intent must be carefully evaluated as a risk factor for suicide and attempted suicide. As many as 80% of people who die by suicide communicate their intent either directly or indirectly.[52] Death or suicide may be discussed, new wills or life insurance policies may be written, valued possessions may be given away, or uncharacteristic and destructive behaviors may arise.[45]

People who intend to end their lives by suicide may, however, be less likely to communicate their intent to their healthcare providers than they are to close family and friends. Although 50% of people who die by suicide have consulted a physician the month before their death, only 60% of this group communicated some degree of suicidal ideation or intent to their physician.[56] In a study of 571 cases of suicide who had met with their healthcare professional within 4 weeks of their suicide,[57] only 22% discussed their suicidal intent. Many investigators believe that ideation and intent may be more readily discussed with psychiatrists than with other physicians.[57]

Hopelessness, or negative expectations about the future, is a stronger predictor of suicide risk than depression or suicidal ideation and may be both a short-term and long-term predictor of completed suicide in patients with MDD.[56]

Contact With Physicians

Nearly half of the people who die by suicide have had contact with their primary care provider (PCP) within 1 month of their death.[17,24,58] Approximately three-quarters of people who have taken their lives saw a PCP in the year before their suicide.[58] Many of these individuals sought treatment from their PCP for somatic rather than psychiatric complaints.[59] Rates of psychiatric encounters in the period before death by suicide are lower than those for primary care contacts.[59] In the month before taking their life, approximately one-fifth of those who took their own life obtained mental health services, and in the year before death by suicide, approximately one in three individuals who took their life had contact with a mental health professional.[59]

PATHOPHYSIOLOGY

Suicide is a behavioral outcome with many contributing factors, rather than a disease entity. Therefore, to understand the pathophysiology of suicidality, it is necessary to examine the differences between individuals with a given set of predisposing factors who do not attempt or die by suicide and those who do. Research has focused on a wide array of neurobiological and psychological topics to better understand the pathophysiology of suicide. Neurobiological inquiries have included neurotransmitter analyses, genetic studies, neuroendocrine studies, biological markers, and imaging studies.[34] Psychological aspects of suicide typically focus on psychodynamic and cognitive perspectives.

Neurobiology

Of all the neurotransmitters, the relationship of serotonin to suicidality has been most widely studied.[32] An association between decreased cerebrospinal fluid (CSF) levels of the serotonin metabolite 5-hydroxyindoleacetic acid (5-HIAA) and serious suicide attempts was first described in the 1970s. Since then, evidence of an association between the serotonergic system and suicidality has continued to grow, with most subsequent studies finding decreased CSF 5-HIAA levels in individuals who attempt suicide.[60] There have also been reports of a blunted prolactin response to the fenfluramine challenge, a marker for serotonergic dysfunction.[41,60] This finding is independent of an underlying psychiatric diagnosis; that is, it is consistent for those who attempt suicide with MDD, schizophrenia, and personality disorders compared to diagnosis-matched controls without a history of attempting suicide.[60] Low levels of 5-HIAA are associated with more serious attempts, and are negatively correlated with the degree of injury in the most recent suicide attempt or most serious past attempt[60]; that is, higher-lethality past attempts are associated with lower CSF 5-HIAA levels. Finally, low CSF 5-HIAA has also been shown to predict future suicide attempts and death by suicide.

Similarly, post-mortem brainstem analysis has shown a reduction in serotonin and its metabolite 5-HIAA in people who die by suicide.[11] This reduction in serotonin and 5-HIAA was similar for those with depression, schizophrenia, personality disorders, and AUDs, showing that decreased brainstem serotonin activity correlates with suicide irrespective of diagnosis.[61] Other brainstem abnormalities associated with those who took their own life include the presence of an increased number of serotonergic neurons compared to controls.[11,32]

Serotonin receptors, especially the SERT, have also been implicated in the neurophysiology of suicide. There is evidence for both pre-synaptic and post-synaptic changes in the prefrontal cortex of people who die by suicide, although not all studies have demonstrated these findings.[11] Specific findings in the prefrontal cortex of those who committed suicide include a decrease in pre-synaptic SERT binding on nerve terminals and increases in post-synaptic serotonin$_{1A}$ and serotonin$_{2A}$ receptors.[11,32] Changes in receptor expression and binding are also accompanied by changes in intracellular signaling.[60] Abnormalities include low protein kinase C activity in the prefrontal cortex, low cyclic adenosine monophosphate–mediated activity in the hippocampus and prefrontal cortex, and a decreased number of G-protein alpha subunits.[60]

Changes in norepinephrine (noradrenaline) transmission in suicide have also been investigated, but to a lesser degree than serotonergic changes. As a result, the implications of studies on the noradrenergic system remain comparatively preliminary. Post-mortem brainstem analysis of the locus coeruleus of suicide victims with MDD has revealed a decreased number of noradrenergic neurons.[62] However, this finding may be the result of illness, a stress-related phenomenon, or other factors.[60,61] Specifically, because of stress-related changes in the noradrenergic system during stress, the stress preceding suicide may be the cause of other observed changes in the brainstems of suicide victims, which include alterations in adrenergic receptor populations and tyrosine hydroxylase activity, the rate-limiting step in norepinephrine synthesis.[11,41,62] Overall, CSF studies have shown no significant difference in norepinephrine metabolites in people with suicidal behavior.[41]

Although some investigation into the role of dopamine in suicidal behavior and suicide has been done, overall, the data are relatively inconclusive. Postmortem studies are too few to determine whether there are changes in levels of dopamine and its metabolites in the brains of suicide victims.[62] CSF levels of dopamine metabolites have, in general, not been shown to differ in individuals with suicidal behavior compared to others.[41] Low levels of the dopamine metabolite homovanillic acid have been shown in individuals with MDD who attempted suicide.[62] However, it is unclear whether a relationship between dopamine and suicide exists independent of the known association of MDD and dopamine downregulation.[62]

The hypothalamic-pituitary-adrenal (HPA) axis has been implicated in the pathophysiology of suicide, although not all studies of the relationship between the HPA axis abnormalities and suicidal behavior have reached the same conclusions.[11,34,47] In general, heightened HPA axis activity, as evidenced by abnormal dexamethasone suppression test results, has been shown in MDD and is thought to be associated with suicidality.[11,32,41,60,62] However, while some studies of the relationship between HPA axis activity and suicidality have shown a relationship between dexamethasone non-suppression and suicidality, other recent investigations have not found a correlation.[41] Urinary cortisol production is elevated in suicidal behavior, and this finding has been replicated in CSF studies and postmortem brain analyses.[51] Elevated urinary cortisol and dexamethasone non-suppression have also been shown to correlate with future suicidality.[11,41,60,62]

Psychological, Psychodynamic, and Neuropsychological Perspectives

The psychodynamic and psychological understanding of suicide encompasses a vast literature; nonetheless,

according to one expert, "The psychological operation of this extraordinary phenomenon, whatever its neurochemical matrix may be, is far from obvious."[63] In conceptualizing the notion of murder turned against the self, Freud described confusion between the self and another person who is both loved and hated as central to suicide.[63] Suicide can, then, be conceptualized as anger turned on one's self or anger toward others directed at the self.[63,64] Suicide has also been seen as being motivated by three driving forces: the wish to die, the wish to kill, and the wish to be killed.[63] Deficits in ego functioning have also been postulated to predispose to suicide,[63] as having poor object relations.[64] Maltsberger has identified a core set of principles that are generally true in suicide; these include a central connection to object loss, mental anguish, confusion of parts of the self with others, the presence of fantasies of resurgence into a new life, and difficulty in self-regulation.[63]

Hopelessness is a central psychological correlate of suicide. Extensive studies on hopelessness have shown a stronger correlation among hopelessness, thoughts of suicide, and suicide than between hopelessness and depression, and depression and suicide.[47] Hopelessness may be the best overall predictor of suicide.[41] Shame, worthlessness, and poor self-esteem are also key concepts in the understanding of suicide; individuals with early traumatic relationships may be particularly vulnerable to narcissistic wounds.[64] Shneidman,[65] in setting forth his psychological approach to suicide, has argued that the psychology of suicide involves intense psychological pain, which he has termed *psychache*. This psyche occurs due to unmet psychological needs (specifically the vital needs individuals require when under duress).[65] He has identified five clusters of psychological pain that predispose to suicide: thwarted love; acceptance and belonging, fractured control, assaulted self-image, and avoidance of shame; ruptured key relationships; excessive rage and anger; and hostility.[65] Poor coping skills, antisocial traits, hostility, hopelessness, dependency, and self-consciousness have also been associated with suicide.[64] Other research has postulated correlations among observed neuroanatomic, neurotransmitter, and neuroendocrine findings in suicide and attendant cognitive traits of loser status, no escape, and no rescue as central to understanding suicidal behavior.[60]

CLINICAL FEATURES AND DIAGNOSIS

The patient at risk for suicide varies along a continuum (from an individual with private thoughts of wanting to be dead or to die by suicide, to a gravely ill individual who requires emergent medical attention as the result of a self-inflicted injury aimed at ending their life). Therefore, there is no single characteristic presentation of the suicidal patient. As a result, the evaluation of suicide risk depends on the clinical assessment of suicide risk in all patients and, on a detailed clinical examination of the patient who has contemplated, threatened, or attempted suicide. The thoughts and feelings of the individual must be elicited and placed in the context of known risk factors for suicide.

Although useful as a guide to general patient populations who may be more likely to attempt, or die, by suicide, risk factors alone are neither sensitive nor specific in the prediction of suicide. Their pervasive prevalence in comparison with the relatively low incidence of suicide in the general population may also lead to high false-positive rates. A multiple logistic regression model that used risk factors (such as age, sex, psychiatric diagnoses, medical diagnoses, marital status, family psychiatric history, prior suicide attempts, and thoughts of suicide) failed to identify any of the 46 patients who died by suicide over 14 years from a group of 1906 people with affective disorders.[66] Similarly, a multiple regression analysis aimed at predicting risk classification by treatment disposition of individuals after suicide attempts had only slightly more than a two-thirds concordance with the decisions made by the treating clinician.[67]

Screening for suicide risk should be completed for all patients with psychiatric illnesses seen in EDs and on hospital admission; in fact, as of 2020 it is a Joint Commission requirement that all patients 12 and older who are being seen in any treatment setting primarily for behavioral health conditions be screened for suicide using a validated screening tool. Moreover, a more extensive evaluation of suicide risk is indicated for all patients who have made a suicide attempt, who have voiced suicidal ideation or intent, who have admitted suicidal ideation or intent on questioning, or whose actions have suggested suicidal intent despite their protests to the contrary. All suicide attempts and thoughts of suicide should be taken seriously, regardless of their mode of expression, nature, or objective lethality. Critical features of a comprehensive assessment of patients with suicidal behaviors include a thorough psychiatric evaluation, a specific inquiry about suicidality, and an estimation of suicide risk.[64] The key facets of each of these components are detailed in Box 42.2.

The approach to the patient at potential risk for suicide should be non-judgmental, supportive, and empathic. The initial establishment of rapport may include an introduction, an effort to create some degree of privacy in the interview setting, and an attempt to maximize the physical comfort of the patient for the interview.[26] The patient who senses interest, concern, and compassion is more likely to trust the clinician and to provide a detailed and accurate history. Often ambivalent about their thoughts and plans, suicidal patients may derive significant relief and benefit from a thoughtful and caring clinician.[26]

The patient should be questioned about suicidal ideation and intent openly and directly. Patients with suicidal thoughts and plans are often relieved and not offended when they find someone with whom they

---

BOX 42.2
COMPONENTS OF THE SUICIDE EVALUATION

Conduct a thorough psychiatric examination
- Establish initial rapport
- Combine open-ended and direct questions
- Gather data from family, friends, and co-workers
- Conduct a mental status examination

Suicide assessment
- Ask specifically about thoughts of suicide and plans to die by suicide
- Examine the details of the suicide plan
- Determine the risk: rescue ratio
- Assess the level of planning and preparation
- Evaluate the degree of hopelessness
- Identify precipitants

Establish a differential diagnosis
- Obtain history
- Use data from a psychiatric examination
- Incorporate data from prior or current treaters

Estimate suicide risk
- Evaluate risk factors
- Evaluate available social supports

can speak about the unspeakable. Patients without suicidal ideation do not have the thoughts planted in their minds and do not develop a greater risk for suicide.[26] General questions concerning suicidal thoughts can be introduced gradually while obtaining the history of present illness. Questions such as "Has it ever seemed like things just aren't worth it?" or "Have you had thoughts that life is not worth living?"[26] may lead to a further discussion of depression and hopelessness. "Have you gotten so depressed that you've considered killing yourself?" or "Have you had thoughts of killing yourself?"[24] may open the door to a further evaluation of suicidal thoughts and plans.

Specific questions concerning potential suicide plans and preparations must follow any expression of suicidal ideation or intent. The patient should be asked when, where, and how an attempt would be made, and any potential means should be evaluated for feasibility and lethality. An organized and detailed plan involving an accessible and lethal method may place the patient at higher risk for suicide.[20] The seriousness of the wish or the intent to die must also be assessed. The patient who has begun to carry out the initial steps of a suicide plan, who wishes to be dead, and who has no hopes or plans may be at greater risk. The last-mentioned domain (plans) may be assessed by asking questions such as "What do you see yourself doing five years from now?" or "What things are you still looking forward to doing or seeing?"

Many clinicians have addressed the issues of lethality and intent using the risk:rescue ratio.[64] The greater the relative risk or lethality and the lesser the likelihood of rescue from a planned attempt, the more serious the potential for suicide. Although often useful, the risk:rescue ratio cannot be merely applied as a simple formula; instead, one must examine and interpret the beliefs of a specific patient. For example, a patient may plan an attempt with a low risk of potential harm but may sincerely wish to die and believe that the plan will be fatal; this patient may thus have a higher risk for suicide. Conversely, a patient may plan an attempt that carries a high probability of death, such as an acetaminophen overdose, but may have little desire to die and little understanding of the severity of the attempt; this patient may thus have a lower risk.[20,64]

The clinician must attempt to identify any possible precipitants for the present crisis to understand why the patient is suicidal. The patient who must face the same problems and stressors following the evaluation or who cannot or will not discuss potential precipitants may be at greater risk for suicide.[20] The clinician must also assess the social support in place for a given patient. A lack of outpatient care providers, family, or friends may elevate the potential risk.[45]

The clinician who interviews a patient after a suicide attempt needs to evaluate the details, risk:rescue ratio, and precipitants of the attempt. The patient who carries out a detailed plan, who perceives the attempt as lethal, who thinks that death will be certain, who is disappointed to be alive, and who must face unchanged stressors will be at a continued high risk for suicide. The patient who makes a calculated, premeditated attempt may also be at a higher risk for a repeat attempt than the patient who makes a hasty, impulsive attempt (out of anger, a desire for revenge, or a desire for attention), or the patient who is intoxicated.[26]

A thorough psychiatric, medical, social, and family history of the patient who may be at risk for suicide should be completed to evaluate the presence and significance of potential risk factors. Particular attention should be paid to the presence of MDD, alcohol or drug use, psychotic disorders, personality disorders, and anxiety disorders. The presence of multiple significant risk factors may confer an additive risk.

A careful mental status examination allows the clinician to detect psychiatric difficulties and assess cognitive capacities. Important aspects to evaluate in the examination include the level of consciousness, appearance, behavior, attention, mood, affect, language, orientation, memory, thought form, thought content, perception, insight, and judgment. A psychiatric review of systems aids in the detection of psychiatric disease.

The clinician should interview the family and friends of the patient at risk to corroborate the gathered information and to obtain new and pertinent data. The family may provide information that a patient is hesitant to provide and that may be essential to their care.[20,26] A patient who refuses to discuss an attempt or insists that the entire event was a mistake may speak openly and honestly only when confronted with reports from his or her family. The evaluation of suicidal risk and the protection of the patient at risk are emergent procedures, which may take precedence over the desire of the patient for privacy and the maintenance of confidentiality in the physician-patient relationship. Concern over a life-or-death situation may obviate obtaining formal consent from the patient before speaking to family and friends.[26]

TREATMENT OF SUICIDE RISK

The treatment of suicide risk begins with the stabilization of medical sequelae of suicidal behaviors. Attention to current or potential medical conditions must be prompt, and medical evaluations must be complete. The severity of the psychiatric presentation should not distract a clinician from his or her obligation to provide good medical care.[20] Once the patient is medically stable, or if the patient is suicidal but has not acted on suicidal impulses, the focus of treatment can shift to the initiation of treatment for the underlying causes of the desire for death. Components of the treatment of suicide risk include providing a safe environment for the patient, determining an appropriate treatment setting, developing a treatment plan involving appropriate somatic and psychotherapeutic interventions, and reassessing suicide risk, psychiatric status, and treatment response in an ongoing fashion[64] (Box 42.3).

Throughout the evaluation and treatment of the suicidal patient, safety must be ensured until the patient is no longer at imminent risk for suicide. Appropriate intervention and the passage of time may aid in the resolution of suicidal ideation and intent.[20,26] A patient who is at potential risk for suicide and who threatens to leave before an adequate evaluation is completed must be detained, in accordance with statutes in most states that permit the detention of individuals deemed dangerous to themselves or others. Patients who attempt

to leave nonetheless should be contained by locked environments or restraints.[20]

Potential means for self-harm should be removed from the reach of a patient at risk. Sharp objects (such as scissors, sutures, needles, glass bottles, and eating utensils) should be removed from the immediate area. Open windows, stairwells, and structures to which a noose could be attached must be blocked. Medications or other dangerous substances that patients may have in their possession must be secured by staff in a location outside of the patient's access.[20] Appropriate supervision should be provided at all times for a patient at risk for suicide. Frequent supervision, constant one-to-one supervision, physical restraints, and medications may be used alone or in combination to protect a patient at risk. The least restrictive means that ensure the safety of the patient should be used.

A decision about the appropriate level of care and treatment setting for the suicidal patient is critical. The patient's safety is paramount, and decisions about the level of care—from discharge home with outpatient follow-up to involuntary hospitalization—should be based on risk determinations and methods most likely to protect the patient from self-harm, even when the patient disagrees. Those who are at high risk for suicide, or who cannot control their suicidal urges, should be admitted to a locked psychiatric facility. A patient who is at high risk but who refuses hospitalization should be committed involuntarily.

A patient who requires hospitalization should be informed of the disposition decision in a clear, direct manner. Possible transfers should proceed as quickly and efficiently as possible because a patient may become quite tense and ambivalent about the decision to hospitalize. Those who agree to voluntary hospitalization and who cooperate with caregivers may have the highest likelihood of successful treatment.[26]

The clinician should always take a conservative approach to the treatment of suicidal risk and the maintenance of patient safety and err, if necessary, on the side of the more restrictive level of care. From a medico-legal standpoint, the clinician sued for involuntary commitment would be easier to defend than the clinician sued for negligence secondary to a death by suicide. Acting in accordance with good clinical judgment in the best interest of the patient brings little danger of liability.[26] Adequate documentation should

---

BOX 42.3
TREATMENT OF SUICIDE RISK

Stabilize the medical situation
Create a safe environment
- ■ Remove potential means for self-harm
- ■ Provide frequent supervision
- ■ Use restraints as needed
- ■ Detain involuntarily if necessary
Identify and treat underlying mental illness
Identify and modify other contributing factors

include the thought processes behind decisions to supervise, restrain, discharge, or hospitalize.[26]

Although managed care may place pressure on a clinician to avoid hospitalization through the use of less costly alternatives, there is no substitute for sound clinical judgment.[64] In particular, safety contracts or suicide prevention contracts, while intended to manage risk, are generally over-valued and of limited utility. Specifically, suicide contracts depend on the subjective beliefs of the psychiatrist and the patient and not on objective data; they have never been shown to be clinically efficacious.[64] In addition, many suicide attempters and completers had suicide contracts in place at the time of the suicidal act.[64] Finally, a suicide contract is not a legal contract and it has limited utility, if any, if litigation should ensue from a completed suicide.[64]

Somatic therapies to target underlying psychiatric illnesses are a mainstay of the treatment of suicidal patients. However, while psychiatric illness is a significant risk factor for suicide and treatment of underlying psychopathology is associated with decreased suicide risk, with few exceptions psychiatric medications have not independently been associated with a decrease in suicide. The two notable exceptions are long-term treatment with lithium (in affective illness) and clozapine (in schizophrenia). Because depression is the psychiatric diagnosis most associated with suicide, psychopharmacological treatment of depression is a central facet of the management of suicide risk. However, antidepressants have not been shown to decrease suicide risk.[64]

Controversy regarding the relationship between selective serotonin reuptake inhibitor (SSRI) antidepressant medications and suicide has now spanned three decades. In the early 1990s, reports of a possible increase in suicidal ideation and suicidal behavior in both adults and children on SSRIs emerged. In 2004 the US Food and Drug Administration (FDA) issued a "black box warning" for all antidepressant drugs related to the risk of suicide in pediatric patients, and more recent years extended this warning for individuals up to age 24. Nonetheless, controversy about SSRIs and suicide persists, in both adults and children. For example, in 2004 before the FDA advisory opinion, the American College of Neuropsychopharmacology's Task Force on SSRIs and Suicidal Behavior in Youth failed to find an association between SSRIs and increased suicidality in children.[68] Additionally, prescription fills for SSRIs decreased by 58% in the years following the 2004 FDA black box warning, with a significant spillover effect into the adult population with decreases in diagnosis and treatment of depression.[69] These decreases were associated with increases in rates of suicidality in pediatric patients.[70]

In adults, there has been similar controversy about a possible relationship between SSRIs and increased suicidality and self-harm. Multiple large studies that assessed the risk of suicide and self-harm have been conducted; they largely determined that SSRIs were not associated with a greater risk of suicide or violence.[64] However, debate has continued, and it is clear that more study is needed. Because SSRIs are prescribed for the treatment of an underlying illness characterized by anxiety, agitation, and suicidality, it is difficult to separate drug effect from the illness effect.[64] Despite there being an association between SSRIs and emergent suicidal ideation and behavior, treatment with antidepressants has not been demonstrated to increase suicide, and rates of suicide mortality have decreased as SSRI usage has increased. Notwithstanding the continuing controversy, SSRIs do have the obvious advantage over tricyclic antidepressants and monoamine oxidase inhibitors of being relatively safe in overdose. FDA warnings regarding the possible induction of suicidality have also been issued for antiepileptic drugs, varenicline, and tetrabenazine, but the clinical implications at this time are unclear. In general, physicians should be aware of the potential for SSRIs and other medications to be associated with suicidal thoughts and behaviors in a vulnerable subset of patients and therefore careful assessments, psychoeducation to patients and families, close monitoring, and follow-up care are indicated when initiating antidepressant treatment. However, the well-known beneficial effects of SSRIs need to be weighed against the risks. In addition, the anti-suicide effects of ketamine are promising.

Finally, because pharmacotherapy for depression typically requires several weeks for the onset of efficacy, electroconvulsive therapy (ECT) may be indicated in cases in which suicide risk remains high or antidepressants are contraindicated.[64] ECT is associated with a decrease in short-term suicidal ideation.[64] Its use is best established for depression, and it may also be recommended for pregnant patients and for patients who have not responded to pharmacological interventions for depression.[64]

Psychotherapeutic interventions are widely used to manage suicide risk, although few studies have addressed psychotherapy outcomes regarding the reduction of suicidality. Nonetheless, clinical practice and consensus support the use of psychotherapy and other psychosocial interventions, notwithstanding the need for further study.[64] There is emerging evidence of the efficacy of multiple psychotherapeutic modalities in the treatment of depression, borderline personality disorder, and suicide risk per se, including psychodynamic psychotherapy, cognitive-behavioral therapy, dialectical behavioral therapy, and interpersonal psychotherapy.[64]

DIFFICULTIES IN THE ASSESSMENT OF SUICIDE RISK

Clinicians may encounter obstacles with certain patients, or within themselves, during the evaluation of suicide risk. They must be adept in the examination of patients who are intoxicated, who threaten, or who are uncooperative, and they must be aware of personal feelings and attitudes (e.g., anxiety, anger, denial, intellectualization, or over-identification) to allow for better assessment and management of the patient at risk (Box 42.4).

A patient who is intoxicated may voice suicidal ideation or intent that is (frequently) retracted when sober. A brief initial evaluation while the patient is intoxicated and his or her psychological defenses are impaired may reveal the depth of suicidal ideation or

---

BOX 42.4
COMMON REACTIONS OF CLINICIANS TO SUICIDE

Anger
Anxiety
Depression
Denial
Helplessness
Indifference
Intellectualization
Over-identification
Rejection

---

the reasons behind a suicide attempt.[26] A more thorough examination when he or she is sober must also be completed and documented.[20,26]

A patient who is actively threatening harm toward themselves or others should be evaluated in the presence of security officers if necessary.[26] Patients who are at imminent risk of harm to themselves or others may require restraint and medication. Patients who are uncooperative or in distress may refuse to answer questions despite all attempts to establish rapport and create a supportive and empathic connection. Stating "I'd like to figure out how to be of help, but I can't do that without some information from you" in a calm but firm manner might be helpful. Patients should be informed that safety precautions will not be discontinued until the evaluation can be completed and that they will not be able to sign out against medical advice. Their capacity to refuse medical treatments should be carefully assessed.[26] A patient who refuses to cooperate until restraints are removed should be reminded of the importance of the evaluation and should be enlisted to cooperate to remove the restraints in mind. Statements such as "We both agree that the restraints should come off if you don't need them. I am very concerned about your safety, and I need you to answer some questions before I can decide if it's safe to remove the restraints" might be helpful.[26]

A clinician may experience personal feelings and attitudes toward a patient at risk for suicide; these must be recognized so that they do not interfere with appropriate patient care.[63] Clinicians may feel anxious because of the awareness that an error in judgment might have fatal consequences. They may feel angry at a patient with a history of multiple attempts or at a patient who has used trivial methods, potentially resulting in cursory evaluations and punitive interventions. Angry examiners may inappropriately transfer a patient with a low risk for suicide to a psychiatric facility or discharge a patient with a high risk to the home.[26]

Some clinicians are prone to experiencing denial as they evaluate and treat patients at risk for suicide. They may conspire with the patient or family in the stance that voiced suicidal ideation was "just talk" or that an attempt was "just an accident." Others may practice intellectualization and choose to believe that suicide is "an act of free will" and that patients should have the personal and legal right to kill themselves.[20]

Clinicians commonly over-identify with patients with whom they share personal characteristics. The thought "I would never end my own life" may become translated into the thought "This patient would never end their own life" and a serious risk may be missed.[26] The examiner may try to assure patients that they will be fine or may try to convince them that they do not feel suicidal. Patients may thus be unable to express themselves fully and may not receive proper evaluation and treatment.

A clinician who performs evaluations for patients who have made suicide attempts and who have been admitted to general hospital floors has to be aware of his or her own reactions to the patient, as well as to those of the staff. In addition, medical and surgical staff often develop strong feelings toward patients who have attempted suicide, and at times they wish that these patients were dead. The clinician must diffuse such charged situations, perhaps by holding group meetings for those involved to make them more aware of their negative feelings so that they are not acted out. Such intervention may prevent mismanagement and premature discharge.

CONCLUSION

All mental health clinicians will encounter patients with suicidal thoughts at some point in their careers. Therefore, clinicians must be knowledgeable about the risk and protective factors for suicide, as well as how to assess the individual patient who may be at risk. The patient's safety must be maintained while undergoing assessment and until suicide risk has decreased. Clinicians should also monitor their own counter-transference, which may be intense and varied with this vulnerable population.

REFERENCES

1. Centers for Disease Control and Prevention. *Web-Based Injury Statistics Query and Reporting System (WISQARS).* U.S. Department of Health and Human Services. https://www.cdc.gov/injury/wisqars/fatal.html.
2. Hirschfield RM, Russell JM. Assessment and treatment of suicidal patients. *N Eng J Med.* 1997;337(13):910.
3. Moscicki E. Epidemiology of suicide. In: Goldsmith S, ed. *Risk Factors for Suicide.* National Academy Press; 2001.
4. Han B, Kott PS, Hughes A, et al. Estimating the rates of deaths by suicide among adults who attempt suicide in the United States. *J Psychiatr Res.* 2016;77:125.

5. McIntosh JL. Suicide prevention in the elderly (age 65–99). *Suicide Life Threat Behav.* 1995;25:180–192.
6. O'Connell H, Chin A, Cunningham C, et al. Recent developments: suicide in older people. *BMJ.* 2004;329:895–899.
7. Kochanek KD, Kirmeyer SE, Martin JA, et al. Annual summary of vital statistics: 2009. *Pediatrics.* 2012;129(2):338.
8. Ivey-Stephenson AZ, Crosby AE, Jack SPD, et al. Suicide trends among and within urbanization levels by sex, race/ethnicity, age group, and mechanism of death—United States, 2001–2015. *MMWR Surveill Summ.* 2017;66(18):1.
9. Piscopo K, Lipari RN, Cooney J, et al. *Suicidal Thoughts and Behavior Among Adults: Results From the 2015 National Survey on Drug Use and Health. NSDUH Data Review.* Department of Health & Human Services; 2016.
10. Curtin SC, Warner M, Hedegaard H. Increase in suicide in the United States, 1999–2014. *NCHS Data Brief;* 2016.
11. Mann JJ. A current perspective of suicide and attempted suicide. *Ann Intern Med.* 2002;136:302–311.
12. Isometsa E, Henriksson M, Marttunen M, et al. Mental disorders in young and middle-aged men who commit suicide. *BMJ.* 1995;310:1366–1367.
13. Black DW, Winokur G. Suicide and psychiatric diagnosis. In: Blumenthal SJ, Kupfer DJ, eds. *Suicide Over the Life Cycle: Risk Factors, Assessment, and Treatment of Suicidal Patients.* American Psychiatric Press; 1990.
14. Jamison KR. Suicide and manic-depressive illness: an overview and personal account. In: Jacobs DG, ed. *The Harvard Medical School Guide to Suicide Assessment and Intervention.* Jossey-Bass; 1999.
15. Malone KM, Haas GL, Sweeney JA, et al. Major depression and the risk of attempted suicide. *J Affect Dis.* 1995;34:173–185.
16. Hirschfeld RMA. Algorithm for the evaluation and treatment of suicidal patients. *Prim Psychiatry.* 1996;3:26–29.
17. Black DW, Winokur G, Nasrallah A. Effect of psychosis on suicide risk in 1,593 patients with unipolar and bipolar affective disorders. *Am J Psychiatry.* 1988;145:849–852.
18. Miller NS, Giannini AJ, Gold MS. Suicide risk associated with drug and alcohol addiction. *Cleve Clin J Med.* 1992;59:535–538.
19. Fowler RC, Rich CL, Young D. San Diego suicide study: substance abuse in young cases. *Arch Gen Psychiatry.* 1986;43:962–965.
20. Buzan RD, Weissberg MP. Suicide: risk factors and prevention in medical practice. *Annu Rev Med.* 1992;43:37–46.
21. Murphy GE, Armstrong JW, Hermele SL, et al. Suicide and alcoholism: interpersonal loss confirmed as a predictor. *Arch Gen Psychiatry.* 1979;36:65–69.
22. Buzan RD, Weissberg MP. Suicide: risk factors and therapeutic considerations in the emergency department. *J Emerg Med.* 1992;10:335–343.
23. Crumley FE. Substance abuse and adolescent suicidal behavior. *JAMA.* 1990;263:3051–3056.
24. Tsuang MT, Fleming JA, Simpson JC. Suicide and schizophrenia. In: Jacobs DG, ed. *The Harvard Medical School Guide to Suicide Assessment and Intervention.* Jossey-Bass; 1999.
25. Hawton K. Assessment of suicide risk. *Br J Psychiatry.* 1987;150:145–153.

26. Shuster JL, Lagomasino IT, Okereke OI, et al. Suicide. In: Irwin RS, Rippe JM, eds. *Intensive Care Medicine*. 5th ed. Lippincott-Raven; 2003.

27. Goldsmith SJ, Fyer M, Frances A. Personality and suicide. In: Blumenthal SJ, Kupfer DJ, eds. *Suicide Over the Life Cycle: Risk Factors, Assessment, and Treatment of Suicidal Patients*. American Psychiatric Press; 1990.

28. McGlashan TH. Borderline personality disorder and unipolar affective disorder. *J Nerv Ment Dis*. 1987;175:467–473.

29. Noyes R. Suicide and panic disorder: a review. *J Affect Dis*. 1991;22:1–11.

30. Weissman MM, Klerman GL, Markowitz JS, et al. Suicidal ideation and suicide attempts in panic disorder and attacks. *N Engl J Med*. 1989;321:1209–1214.

31. Johnson J, Weissman MM, Klerman GL. Panic disorder, comorbidity and suicide attempts. *Arch Gen Psychiatry*. 1990;47:805–808.

32. Maris RW. Suicide. *Lancet*. 2001;360:319–326.

33. Conwell Y, Duberstein PR. Suicide among older people: a problem for primary care. *Prim Psychiatry*. 1996;3:41–44.

34. Perry S, Jacobsberg L, Fishman B. Suicidal ideation and HIV testing. *JAMA*. 1990;263:679–682.

35. Achte KA, Lonnquist J, Hillbom E. Suicides following war brain injuries. *Acta Psychiatr Scand Suppl*. 1971;225:3–94.

36. Stenager EN, Stenager E, Koch-Henriksen N. Multiple sclerosis and suicide: an epidemiological investigation. *J Neurol Neurosurg Psychiatry*. 1992;55:542–545.

37. Clayton PJ. Suicide. *Psychiatr Clin North Am*. 1985;8:203–214.

38. Geisler WO, Jousse AT, Wynne-Jones M, et al. Survival in traumatic spinal cord injury. *Paraplegia*. 1983;21:364–373.

39. MacKenzie TB, Popkin MK. Suicide in the medical patient. *Int J Psychiatry Med*. 1987;17:3–22.

40. Ko DT, Hebert PR, Coffey CS, et al. Beta-blocker therapy and symptoms of depression, fatigue, and sexual dysfunction. *JAMA*. 2002;288:351–357.

41. Joiner TE Jr, Brown JS, Wingate LR. The psychology and neurobiology of suicidal behavior. *Annu Rev Psychol*. 2005;56:287–314.

42. Labonte B, Suderman M, Maussion G, et al. Genome-wide methylation changes in the brains of suicide completers. *Am J Psychiatry*. 2013;170(5):511–520.

43. Lagomasino IT, Stern TA. The suicidal patient. In: Stern TA, Herman JB, Slavin PL, eds. *MGH Guide to Primary Care Psychiatry*. 2nd ed. McGraw-Hill; 2004.

44. Kyung-Sook W, SangSoo S, Sangjin S, et al. Marital status integration and suicide: A meta-analysis and meta-regression. *Soc Sci Med*. 2018;197:116.

45. Mans RW. Introduction. *Suicide Life Threat Behav*. 1991;21:1–17.

46. Brent DA, Perper JA, Allman CJ, et al. The presence and accessibility of firearms in the homes of adolescent suicides: a case-control study. *JAMA*. 1991;266:2989–2995.

47. Hirschfeld RMA, Russell JM. Current concepts: assessment and treatment of suicidal patients [review]. *N Engl J Med*. 1997;337:910–915.

48. Mahon MH, Tobin JP, Cusack DA, et al. Suicide among regular-duty military personnel: A retrospective case-control study of occupation-specific risk factors for workplace suicide. *Am J Psychiatry*. 2005;162:1688–1696.

49. Rozanov V, Carli V. Suicide among war veterans. *Int J Environ Res Public Health*. 2012;9:2504–2519.

50. LeardMann CA, Powell MS, Smith TC, et al. Risk factors associated with suicide in current and former US military personnel. *JAMA*. 2013;310(5):496–506.

51. Weissman MM. The epidemiology of suicide attempts, 1960–1971. *Arch Gen Psychiatry*. 1974;30:737–746.

52. Roy A. Risk factors for suicide in psychiatric patients. *Arch Gen Psychiatry*. 1982;39:1089–1095.

53. Stern TA, Mulley AG, Thibault GE. Life-threatening drug overdose: precipitants and prognosis. *JAMA*. 1984;251:1983–1985.

54. Appleby L. Suicide in psychiatric patients: risk and prevention. *Br J Psychiatry*. 1992;161:749–758.

55. Beck AT, Beck R, Kovacs M. Classification of suicidal behaviors: quantifying intent and medical lethality. *Am J Psychiatry*. 1975;132:285–287.

56. Fawcett J, Clark DC, Busch KA. Assessing and treating the patient at risk for suicide. *Psychiatry Ann*. 1983;23:244–255.

57. Isometsa ET, Heikkinen ME, Marttunen MJ, et al. The last appointment before suicide: is suicide intent communicated? *Am J Psychiatry*. 1995;152:919–922.

58. Luoma JB, Martin CE, Pearson JL. Contact with mental health and primary care providers before suicide: a review of the evidence. *Am J Psychiatry*. 2002;159:909–916.

59. Valente SM. Evaluating suicide risk in the medically ill patient. *Nurse Pract*. 1993;18:41–50.

60. Van Heeringen K. The neurobiology of suicide and suicidality. *Can J Psychiatry*. 2003;48:292–300.

61. Mann JJ, Arango V, Marzuk PM, et al. Evidence for the 5-HT hypothesis of suicide: a review of post mortem studies. *Br J Psychiatry*. 1989;155(Suppl. 8):7–14.

62. Mann JJ. Neurobiology of suicidal behavior. *Nature Rev Neurosci*. 2003;4:819–828.

63. Maltsberger JT. The psychodynamic understanding of suicide. In: Jacobs DG, ed. *The Harvard Medical School Guide to Suicide Assessment and Intervention*. Jossey-Bass; 1999.

64. American Psychiatric Association. Practice guideline for the assessment and treatment of patients with suicidal behaviors. *Am J Psychiatry*. 2003;160(11 Suppl):1–60.

65. Shneidman E. Perturbation and lethality: a psychological approach to assessment and intervention. In: Jacobs DG, ed. *The Harvard Medical School Guide to Suicide Assessment and Intervention*. Jossey-Bass; 1999.

66. Goldstein RB, Black DW, Nasrallah A, et al. The predication of suicide: sensitivity, specificity, and predictive value of a multivariate model applied to suicide among 1906 patients with affective disorders. *Arch Gen Psychiatry*. 1991;48:418–422.

67. Hepp U, Moergeli H, Trier S, et al. Attempted suicide: factors leading to hospitalization. *Can J Psychiatry*. 2004;49:736–742.

68. American College of Neuropsychopharmacology, Executive Summary. *Preliminary Report of the Task Force on SSRIs and Suicidal Behavior in Youth, 2004*.

69. Sussman N. FDA warnings and suicide rates: unintended consequences. *Prim Psychiatry*. 2008;15:22–232.

70. Gibbons RD, Brown CH, Hur K, et al. Early evidence on the effects of regulators' suicidality warnings on SSRI prescriptions and suicide in children and adolescents. *Am J Psychiatry*. 2007;164:1356–1363.

43

EMERGENCY PSYCHIATRY

ABIGAIL L. DONOVAN, MD ■ DIANA PUNKO, MD, MS ■ SUZANNE A. BIRD, MD ■ ANA IVKOVIC, MD ■ LAURA M. PRAGER, MD

INTRODUCTION

Over the past 30 years, emergency psychiatry has developed into an independent subspecialty practice within consultation-liaison psychiatry. Although there are no formal board certification requirements, all accredited United States (US) psychiatric residency training programs follow training guidelines for emergency psychiatry.[1] The evolution of emergency psychiatry as a specialized practice parallels the dramatic increase in patient volume in emergency care settings over recent years. Between 2009 and 2015 mental health–related emergency department (ED) visits in the United States increased by 40.8% for adults and 56.4% for children, while during the same period the number of non-mental health–related ED visits decreased.[2] Mental health problems are the fastest-growing component of emergency medical practice. The coronavirus disease 2019 (COVID-19) pandemic only intensified this challenge, resulting in even higher rates of mental health–related ED visits.[3]

Psychiatric emergencies encompass a range of clinical presentations. Typically, such patients seek or are brought to treatment in a crisis, unable to be contained by local support systems. Crises may arise from a variety of problems, including medical, psychological, substance-related, interpersonal, and social factors. Patients often present in significant distress, with impairment in functioning, and/or are viewed as increasingly dangerous to themselves or others. For example, patients may have thoughts of suicide or homicide, other violent thoughts, overwhelming depression or anxiety, psychosis, mania, or acute cognitive or behavioral changes. Substance use is also common and may play an exacerbating or causative role.

More recently, patients have used emergency services for non-emergent conditions.[4] An increasing number of patients seek treatment in EDs for urgent conditions, routine conditions, or outpatient referrals because they lack insurance coverage for routine outpatient care, there is a paucity of community healthcare resources, or they wish to avoid long waits to be seen by outpatient mental health providers. This volume increase, coupled with the dearth of available outpatient services, the limited number of inpatient psychiatric beds, and the demands of insurance companies for prior authorization for care, has led to longer lengths of stay for many psychiatric patients in EDs, a phenomenon known as "ED boarding."[5] These patients need psychiatric hospitalization, but unfortunately there is no available inpatient bed. ED boarding of psychiatric patients has added another layer of complexity to the practice of emergency psychiatry.

Psychiatrists who work in EDs typically require several core skills. In addition to being able to evaluate and treat a broad range of psychiatric conditions and substance use disorders (SUDs), emergency psychiatry practitioners must also evaluate and manage suicidal and homicidal thoughts and behaviors, violent behavior or agitation (often of unclear etiology), delirium, and substance intoxication and withdrawal. Medical co-morbidity is common; knowledge of the assessment and treatment of medical conditions with prominent psychiatric symptomatology is essential.

This chapter provides a foundation for the assessment and management of children, adolescents, and adults who present with psychiatric emergencies.

DEMOGRAPHICS

As noted in the introduction, mental health–related ED visits increased significantly between 2009 and 2015 and then even more dramatically during the early years of the COVID-19 pandemic. One cross-sectional study of almost 190 million ED visits reported that visit rates for mental health conditions, suicide attempts, all drug overdoses, intimate partner violence, and child abuse and neglect were higher in mid-March through October 2020, during the COVID-19 pandemic, compared with the same period in 2019.[3] Among emergency mental health visits, substance-related disorders (30%), mood disorders (23%), anxiety disorders (21%), psychosis (10%), and suicide attempts (7%) were the most common presentations.[4] Thoughts of suicide account for one-third to one-half of all patients who present with a psychiatric emergency.[6]

Although some patients self-refer to an ED when in crisis, others are referred by family, friends, general practitioners, medical specialists, community mental health providers, and employees of local and state agencies. Following several school shootings, teachers and school administrators have become a major source of ED referrals for the assessment of risk of violence or suicide. Police officers and representatives of the legal system also refer patients, as the ED often serves as a conduit between the psychiatric and judicial systems. The emergency psychiatric assessment of an individual in police custody helps police identify those individuals with an acute psychiatric illness who need immediate intervention and facilitate referral for appropriate care, while those without an acute psychiatric illness are returned to the judicial system.

TYPES OF DELIVERY MODELS

Two models are often used to deliver emergency psychiatric services. In one model, a dedicated psychiatric emergency service (PES) exists as an independent service, co-located with a general emergency medical service, or located separately in a stand-alone facility. In the other model, the PES functions as a consultation service for primary emergency medical services. Some institutions use a hybrid model. The specific model of services offered by healthcare systems is determined by the volume of emergency psychiatric patients seen and the financial and staffing resources available.

The primary benefit of providing emergency psychiatric services in an area that is separated from the chaos of a busy ED is safety; it provides a more secure and therapeutic environment (e.g., with limited access to sharp or dangerous objects, quiet surroundings to decrease stimulation, individual rooms for private interviews, and the ability to observe and rapidly initiate psychiatric treatment). The unit may also have on-site security staff who are trained to understand mental health issues and who help to maintain a safe environment. Many units have rooms designed specifically for patients who require restraint and seclusion.

Another benefit of a dedicated PES is the opportunity to staff the unit with specialized personnel who are trained in the delivery of emergency psychiatric care.[6] An interdisciplinary staff of psychiatrists, advanced practice providers, nurses, social workers, mental health technicians, and case managers can enhance the care of patients with acute psychiatric illnesses by coordinating medical evaluations with other ED colleagues, initiating psychopharmacologic treatment, focusing on therapeutic patient interactions, recognizing the need for immediate intervention, and using their specialized knowledge of local and regional psychiatric services to facilitate an appropriate disposition.

Some PESs also have access to "crisis beds" or units where patients can be observed for 24 to 72 hours and then be re-assessed. Observing patients whose mental state stabilizes after the initiation of psychotropic medications or following a period of enforced sobriety may obviate the need for inpatient hospitalization.[6]

THE MEDICAL EVALUATION

Regardless of the delivery model or the chief complaint, all ED visits for psychiatric concerns begin with a triage assessment. This assessment determines the likelihood that an emergency medical and/or psychiatric condition exists and what testing or interventions are indicated to stabilize the patient. Beginning in 2019 the Joint Commission (JC), the organization that accredits US healthcare organizations, mandated that all patients ≥12 years being evaluated for behavioral health conditions as their primary reason for care must be assessed for thoughts of suicide with a validated screening tool,[7] such as the Ask Suicide-Screening Questions (ASQ) Tool[8] or the Columbia-Suicide Severity Rating Scale (C-SSRS).[9] The results of this screening inform decisions about the level of monitoring and containment the patient requires during their ED visit.[7] Some EDs also screen patients for the risk of violence and agitation using standardized instruments, such as the Broset Violence Checklist[10] or the Aggressive Behavior Risk Assessment Tool.[11]

The initial medical work-up for patients with an acute psychiatric presentation is often referred to as "medical clearance." It is important to note that the division between "medical" and "psychiatric" diseases is a false dichotomy. Diseases primarily affecting thoughts, feelings, and behaviors for which there is not currently a fully elucidated pathophysiology (e.g., schizophrenia) are often considered "psychiatric," whereas diseases for which there is a fully elucidated pathophysiology (e.g., Parkinson disease) are often considered "medical" or "organic." Ultimately, all diseases that affect the human body (including psychiatric disorders) are medical, whether the pathophysiology leading to the disease is understood. A more accurate division may be based on which conditions are typically managed by psychiatrists or by non-psychiatrists, and those that are managed by several specialties simultaneously. Unfortunately, a widely accepted nomenclature that appropriately and succinctly describes these differences is lacking. Thus, this chapter will continue to use the terms "medical" and "psychiatric" when needed. "Medical clearance" generally denotes a medical evaluation aimed at ruling out underlying conditions that may cause or contribute to a psychiatric presentation as well as assessing patients' stability for transfer to a psychiatric setting. Despite many attempts to create consensus guidelines, there is no well-accepted standard for the medical evaluation of ED patients who present with an acute psychiatric complaint.[12] Non-geriatric patients who present in a fashion similar to their prior psychiatric presentations, without significant other medical conditions or active physical complaints, may be sufficiently evaluated by obtaining a history, a review of systems, a physical examination, and vital signs, without ordering additional laboratory testing. However, for any ED patient with a newly altered mental status (be it a change in cognition, emotional state, or behavior), it is crucial to rule out various medical conditions that might exacerbate or cause their symptoms. A change in mental state may indicate a primary psychiatric condition, a toxidrome secondary to substance use or ingestion, a substance- or medication-induced psychiatric disorder, a primary medical condition with psychiatric symptoms (e.g., delirium [an acute and reversible condition secondary to a medical illness], dementia [a chronic condition associated with long-term, irreversible brain pathology], or a wide range of other neuro-medical conditions, including but not limited to autoimmune, endocrine, epileptic, infectious, neoplastic, or nutritional disturbances). In addition, a medical work-up should be considered for the new onset of psychiatric symptomatology or any significant change or exacerbation of symptoms. It is important to consider medical etiologies for all psychiatric complaints because many psychiatric hospitals have limited resources to diagnose and treat non-psychiatric medical conditions. Indeed, the ED evaluation may be the most comprehensive physical assessment that the patient receives. A missed medical diagnosis because of an assumed psychiatric condition could result in dire consequences. In addition, failure to identify substance use or withdrawal as a potential cause or contributor to a patient's acute mental status changes may lead to inaccurate assignment of a psychiatric diagnosis and suboptimal decision-making about treatment.

One retrospective study of 212 consecutive patients (aged ≥ 16 years) who underwent a psychiatric evaluation in an ED demonstrated that among patients with a known psychiatric history and no physical complaints (38%), screening laboratories and radiographic results yielded no actionable additional information; those patients could have been appropriately referred for further psychiatric evaluation with the history, physical examination, and stable vital signs alone. Among the patients deemed to require further medical evaluation (62%), all had either reported physical complaints, or their medical histories suggested that further evaluation would be necessary.[13] Another study of ED patients with new-onset psychiatric symptoms demonstrated that two-thirds had a medical cause for their psychiatric symptoms.[12] These studies suggest that careful screening is important for patients with new-onset symptoms, but additional medical tests may be of little benefit among patients with known psychiatric disorders and without physical complaints or other active medical issues. However, an additional practical complication is that many psychiatric hospitals require screening laboratory and other testing (as a precaution) for all patients, regardless of a specific clinical indication.

The medical evaluation should involve a thorough medical history, a general review of systems, and measurement of vital signs, followed by a physical examination and/or laboratory tests as indicated.[14] Practitioners should also consider other factors that may put a patient at risk for a medical condition (e.g., lack of access to routine medical care, substance use,

and advancing age). The medical tests to consider in the ED are listed in Box 43.1.

THE PSYCHIATRIC INTERVIEW

Although a psychiatric assessment in the ED is often delayed until medical clearance has been completed, evaluation can begin at any point (assuming that the patient is awake and able to participate in an interview). The psychiatric emergency evaluation begins broadly; it becomes increasingly focused on guiding the diagnostic formulation (or differential diagnosis) and the safety assessment that will allow for the management of acute symptoms and disposition to the appropriate next level of care.

The cornerstone of the initial psychiatric evaluation is a careful history that focuses on the onset

---

BOX 43.1
TESTS TO CONSIDER IN THE MEDICAL EVALUATION OF PATIENTS WITH PSYCHIATRIC SYMPTOMS

- Complete blood count (to monitor for infection, anemia, or other dyscrasias)
- Electrolytes, blood urea nitrogen, creatinine (metabolic changes, hyponatremia or hypernatremia, abnormal kidney function, dehydration)
- Glucose (hypoglycemia or hyperglycemia)
- Liver function tests (liver dysfunction due to hepatitis or alcohol use disorder)
- Pregnancy test
- Serum toxicology screen (ingestion, intoxication, poisoning)
- Medication levels (medication toxicity, ingestions)
- Urine toxicology screen (to identify or confirm substance use)
- Calcium, magnesium, and phosphorus (hypoparathyroidism or hyperparathyroidism, eating disorders, poor nutrition)
- Folate, thiamine (alcohol use disorders, poor nutrition, depression)
- Vitamin B_{12} (cobalamin deficiency)
- Thyroid-stimulating hormone (hypothyroidism or hyperthyroidism)
- The following tests and imaging studies may also be considered in the medical work-up depending on the patient's presentation:
- Ammonia level (liver dysfunction)
- Antinuclear antibodies, erythrocyte sedimentation rate, C-reactive protein (autoimmune conditions)
- Methylmalonic acid and homocysteine (cobalamin deficiency)
- Rapid plasma reagin (neurosyphilis)
- Ceruloplasmin (Wilson disease)
- Heavy metal panel (toxicity)
- Lumbar puncture (infection, hemorrhage, limbic encephalitis)
- Electroencephalogram (seizure, changes due to ingestion of medications, delirium, dementia)
- Computed tomography (CT) (acute hemorrhage or trauma)
- Magnetic resonance imaging (higher resolution than CT for potential brain masses or lesions, posterior fossa pathology, or when radiation exposure is contraindicated)
- HIV (Human Immunodeficiency Virus)

Adapted from Alpay M, Park L. Laboratory tests and diagnostic procedures. In: Stern TA, Herman JB, eds. *Psychiatry Update and Board Preparation.* McGraw-Hill; 2000.

and development of symptoms, associated signs and symptoms, the level of distress and functional impairment, and possible precipitants. In addition, a history of physical illnesses, psychiatric diagnoses and treatment, use of prescription and over-the-counter (OTC) medications, allergies, adverse reactions to medications, patterns of substance use, a family history of psychiatric illness, and a psychosocial (including trauma) history, are also important. If available, past medical records should be reviewed. Box 43.2 describes the components of the evaluation, and Box 43.3 describes the special features of a substance use evaluation.

BOX 43.2
THE EMERGENCY PSYCHIATRIC INTERVIEW AND EVALUATION

- Chief complaint
- History of present illness, with a focus on symptoms and the context for these symptoms, includes a safety evaluation with an assessment of suicidal and homicidal ideation, plan or intent, and any associated risk factors
- Past medical history, with a focus on current problems
- Past psychiatric history, particularly symptoms or events similar to the current presentation, include diagnoses, previous hospitalizations, and suicide attempts
- Allergies and adverse reactions to medications
- Current medications, including an assessment of adherence
- Social history, particularly how it contributes to the context of the emergency visit
- Substance use history
- Family history, including symptoms or diagnoses similar to the patient's presentation
- Mental status examination
- Review of medical symptoms, particularly any medical symptoms that may account for the patient's presentation
- Vital signs
- Physical examination
- Laboratory studies and other tests, if indicated
- Assessment, including a summary statement, a statement about the patient's level of safety, and a rationale for disposition recommendations
- Diagnoses according to DSM-5-TR criteria
- Plan and disposition
- Document any significant interventions (such as medication administration) and the outcome

DSM-5-TR, Diagnostic and Statistical Manual of Mental Disorders, Fifth Edition, Text Revision

---

Practitioners should be familiar with all segments of the psychiatric interview, but they should focus on areas that are most relevant to the individual patient and their presenting complaint. For example, although the developmental history may not be a key part of the evaluation of an otherwise healthy-appearing adult patient with depression, it may be very important in the assessment of a young adult with obvious cognitive deficits. The interview is one part of a broader information-gathering mission, and the elements of the history as constructed from all sources should tell a story about the meaning and impact of current symptoms and provide support for the diagnosis (or diagnoses) and appropriate disposition.

The emergency evaluation always includes an assessment of the patient's living situation, social supports, and daily structure (e.g., at work, school, and/or in a day program). This assessment helps to define the patient's baseline level of function. In addition, a review of the patient's health insurance coverage is necessary because insurance often dictates the types of treatment programs that are available when the patient is released from the ED.

Often, PES presentations are complicated, and patients may be unable, or unwilling, to provide an accurate history. Therefore, information should be collected from multiple sources, including, but not limited

---

BOX 43.3
THE SUBSTANCE USE DISORDER INTERVIEW

For each substance used, assess the following:
- Age of first use
- Current amount and frequency of use
- Method of use (e.g., drinking, smoking, intranasal, intravenous)
- Time of last use and amount used
- Medical sequelae of use
- Social sequelae (relationship problems, school or work absences, legal problems)
- The longest period of sobriety
- Previous treatment (detoxification programs, outpatient programs, partial hospitalization)
- Methods of maintaining sobriety
- Participation in self-help programs (e.g., Alcoholics Anonymous, Narcotics Anonymous)
- Risk for withdrawal syndrome
- The patient's motivation to cut down or stop substance use
- The patient's need for assistance meeting goals to cut down or stop substance use

to, outside medical records, family, friends, treaters, police, emergency personnel, pharmacies, and/or statewide prescription monitoring programs. Ideally, patients will provide consent for contacting collateral sources. If a patient declines to give this permission, the importance of the type of information sought must be balanced against a violation of the patient's wishes and a potential violation of confidentiality. In addition, clinicians should be mindful to gather, but not release, information, particularly without a patient's consent. When data can be obtained and corroborated from several sources, psychiatrists can make more informed risk assessments and disposition decisions.

THE SAFETY EVALUATION

The safety evaluation is a critical component of every emergency evaluation; it assesses an individual's imminent risk of harm to themselves and others. Between 2000 and 2018 suicide rates in the United States increased by 30%.[15] Suicide was among the top 10 leading causes of death in 2020 for people aged 10 to 64.[15] Alarmingly, it was the second leading cause of death for youth aged 10 to 14 years and for adults aged 25 to 34.[15] More than 90% of patients who take their own lives have had at least one psychiatric diagnosis.[16] Patients aged 15 to 24 years and those over the age of 60 are in the highest-risk groups for suicide.[16]

The safety evaluation starts with screening for thoughts or plans for suicide (using a validated screening tool) for all patients who present with behavioral symptoms; this screening is a JC requirement for patients ≥12 years. Suicide screening should occur early during the ED visit, ideally as part of the triage evaluation. As noted earlier, there are several validated screening tools, including the ASQ Suicide Risk Screening Tool[8] and the C-SSRS,[9] described further in Table 43.1.[17–21] All patients who score positive on a screening tool require risk mitigation interventions, such as continuous observation and restriction of access to means of self-harm, until a full suicide risk assessment can be completed, ideally by a behavioral health provider.

There are also standardized instruments that can assist in risk stratification. For example, the ED-Safe Secondary Screener (ESS-6)[21] can be used after a positive screen for suicide risk to further stratify patients into low, medium, and high risk groups. The SAFE-T protocol, designed to be used with the C-SSRS, provides a five-step plan to identify risk and protective factors, conduct a suicide inquiry, and determine risk levels and potential interventions.[22]

The suicide risk assessment, whether guided by the structured SAFE-T protocol[22] or completed through the emergency psychiatric interview, must include direct questions about thoughts, plans, and intent to

TABLE 43.1
Validated Suicide Screening Tools

Tool	Validated Age Groups (Years of Age)	Psychometric Properties	Additional Notes[19]
Ask Suicide Screening Questions (ASQ)[8]	10–21	Sensitivity: 96.9% Specificity: 87.6%	Validated in children's hospitals only
Columbia-Suicide Severity Rating Scale (C-SSRS)[9]	≥11	Sensitivity: 93%–100% Specificity: 96%–100%	Validated in many settings, including the ED Can also be used to stratify suicide risk
Patient Health Questionnaire, 9 Item (PHQ-9)[17]	≥18	Sensitivity: 87.6% Specificity: 66.1%	
Patient Safety Screener-3 (PSS-3)[18]	≥18	Kappa: 0.94–0.95	Can be used with the ED-Safe Secondary Screener (ESS-6)[21] as a secondary tool to stratify suicide risk
Suicide Behaviors Questionnaire (SBQ)[20]	≥18	Chronbach's α: 0.75–0.8	SBQ-C has been adapted for <10 years

ED, Emergency department.

take one's life. This should be followed by more specific questions about access to the means of harm, including access to firearms. If a patient has a plan to take their own life or intends to die by suicide, the lethality of the plan, as well as the patient's perception of the risk, must be assessed. A medically low-risk plan may still coincide with a strong desire to die if the patient believes that the likelihood of lethality of the attempt is high. Similarly, the possibility that the patient could have been rescued if they had followed through on the plan should be evaluated (e.g., an impulsive ingestion of pills in front of a family member after an argument may convey less risk than a similar attempt while alone in a remote location). If a patient has attempted suicide previously, details of that attempt can facilitate an understanding of their current risk. In addition, the clinician should assess other risk factors for suicide (see Box 43.4), the strongest of which is a history of a suicide attempt. Clinicians may also want to distinguish between acute and chronic risk factors, as well as static and modifiable risk factors, the latter of which may suggest targets for intervention or treatment. Protective factors must also be assessed (see Box 43.4). The SAFE-T protocol (used by many EDs nationwide) is a structured method for obtaining this information.[22] In addition, obtaining collateral information is critical, especially for a higher-risk patient who is requesting to be discharged. In such situations, keeping a high-risk patient in the ED is often warranted until the requisite collateral information is obtained.

Assessment of violence includes asking the patient about thoughts of self-harm and about thoughts, plans, and/or intent to harm others. Observation of the patient's mental status, behavior, and impulsivity during the interview provides important information. In addition, because prior violence is the best predictor of future violence, it is important to learn about previous violent thoughts and behaviors, the triggers that led to those events, and any relationship to substance use. Collateral information is important; the risk assessment should include contact with others who know or who have recently observed the patient. Violent threats or homicidal ideation may or may not be directed toward a specific individual. If there is a likelihood of directed violence toward an identified person or persons, the ED psychiatrist may have a duty to warn or protect the identified target. The standards

---

BOX 43.4
SUICIDE RISK AND PROTECTIVE FACTORS

RISK FACTORS

Static Risk Factors

History of suicide attempts
Psychiatric illness (major depressive disorder, bipolar disorder, substance use disorders, schizophrenia, personality disorders)
Race
Marital status (widowed, divorced, or separated)
Co-morbid medical illness (chronic illness, pain, or terminal illness)
Male gender
Advancing age
Family history of suicide

MODIFIABLE OR ACUTE RISK FACTORS

Suicidal ideation
Active symptoms of psychiatric illness
Current symptoms of medical illness, especially pain
Recent personal loss (social, occupational, financial)
Recent psychiatric hospitalization
Substance use
Access to firearms or other lethal means
Unemployment
Financial or legal difficulties
Living alone

PROTECTIVE FACTORS

Married with young children
Social supports
Religion
Engaged in work or school
Therapeutic relationships with psychiatric providers
Future orientation

---

for the clinician's duty to protect the potential victim differ from state to state; however, most protocols are based on the original Tarasoff v. Regents case from the University of California in 1976.[23] Consultation with the hospital's legal counsel is recommended in situations involving the duty to warn.

Although civil commitment laws differ from state to state, most states have provisions for the time-limited containment of a patient who is deemed at risk for harm to oneself or others, or for the inability to care for oneself. In cases in which initial thoughts of suicide or homicide resolve during the ED visit, if a discharge is considered, a clear safety plan should be created that includes steps that the patient (and, ideally, an identified support person) understands and agrees to take if thoughts of suicide or homicide return. Most often, these plans involve contacting family members and treaters and a return to a psychiatric evaluation center or ED. For patients with access to lethal means, removing or restricting access to these must be seriously considered. Consultation with hospital legal counsel, hospital police or security, and/or local law enforcement is critical for any situation in which there is significant public safety concern.

PSYCHIATRIC SYMPTOMS AND PRESENTATIONS

Making a *Diagnostic and Statistical Manual of Mental Disorders, Fifth Edition, Text Revision* (DSM-5-TR)[24] diagnosis can be challenging in the PES since patients are seen at a single point in time, often in the worst crisis of their lives. Making a definitive diagnosis frequently requires a longitudinal assessment of symptoms. Although patients may not necessarily fit all diagnostic criteria, consideration of the most common disorders (e.g., mood disorders, psychotic disorders, anxiety disorders, SUDs, delirium) will help organize the assessment. The following sections will outline some of the most common psychiatric presentations and patient characteristics seen in the ED.

Depression

Depression is a common reason for seeking treatment at a PES. The severity of depression may vary from mild to extremely severe; it may occur with or without psychosis or suicidal ideation. Anhedonia, insomnia, and other neurovegetative symptoms of depression are frequent complaints. Anxiety or anger attacks are often co-morbid with depression. A history of mania must be assessed in every depressed patient to screen for bipolar disorder (BPD). The potential effects of substance use on mood must be considered. Alcohol use disorder (AUD) in particular can increase the frequency of depressive symptoms and the risk of suicide when co-morbid with depression. The potential role of medical conditions (including but not limited to hypothyroidism, sleep apnea, neurodegenerative disease, malignancy,

and/or chronic pain) should also be considered. The severity of symptoms and the ability to participate in work and other routines may contribute to disposition determination; in addition, the assessment of safety is essential for treatment planning.

Mania

Manic patients frequently present with pressured speech, grandiosity, irritability, flight of ideas, and psychomotor agitation. Such patients may be dressed or behave oddly or seductively, and they may have traveled impulsively across long distances. Paranoia, delusions, or hallucinations often arise in patients presenting with maniform psychosis, leading to a lack of insight and poor judgment. It is important to assess for various medical causes of mania, including autoimmune, infectious, neurologic, and toxicologic presentations (e.g., acute intoxication with cocaine, phencyclidine, methamphetamine, or other substances including prescribed or OTC stimulants). Steroids can contribute to manic symptoms, as can antidepressants in vulnerable patients. For patients with mania treated with lithium, valproic acid, carbamazepine, or lamotrigine, serum levels of these medications can clarify whether medication non-adherence is playing a role in the patients' presentation and can help to rule out medication toxicity in patients with BPD and an altered mental status.

Psychosis

Patients with psychosis can suffer from positive symptoms including disorganized thinking, hallucinations, delusions, or other forms of disordered thought (e.g., ideas of reference, thought broadcasting, or thought insertion), as well as negative symptoms including diminished emotional expression, a paucity of speech, and avolition. Patients with psychosis vary greatly in the severity and nature of their symptoms; they may be affected by paranoia that progressively interferes with work or relationships, or they may demonstrate overt disorganization in speech and behavior. Because some patients have lost touch with reality, they may be predisposed to dangerous and/or dysregulated behavior; the safety of staff and other patients must be maintained.

It is also important to rule out medical causes for symptoms, particularly among patients who lack a history of psychosis and in those whose age falls outside the usual range for the onset of psychosis without an identifiable medical cause (i.e., late teens to mid-20s). Auditory hallucinations are more common with primary psychiatric disorders, whereas visual hallucinations are more common in medical disorders (e.g., delirium) and substance use or withdrawal. A wide variety of neuro-medical conditions, including seizure disorders, metabolic changes, infection, ingestion, vitamin and mineral deficiencies, and substance intoxication or withdrawal, should be considered in the differential of new-onset psychosis. Among the elderly with new-onset hallucinations, conditions such as delirium, dementia, iatrogenic (i.e., medication related), and cortical-release phenomena (e.g., Charles Bonnet syndrome occurring in the context of sensory impairment) should be strongly considered.

Often, patients with a known psychotic illness are referred for an evaluation of worsening psychosis, which is frequently associated with medication nonadherence. Any new and/or atypical findings (e.g., cognitive impairment, catatonia, sensory changes) should prompt clinicians to consider new medical explanations for a patient's decompensation because patients with psychiatric illness are at increased risk for developing various medical co-morbidities, with new symptoms mistakenly attributed to their psychiatric diagnosis.[25]

Catatonia

Patients with catatonia require coordinated care between clinicians who specialize in emergency medicine and psychiatry. Rapid diagnosis and treatment are crucial since the condition may progress to life-threatening malignant catatonia. Because catatonia can be due to numerous underlying etiologies (e.g., seizures, infections, neoplasms, metabolic derangements, mood disorders, psychotic spectrum disorders), a thorough medical work-up of all potential etiologies is essential. While the underlying disorder will require specific treatment, treatment of catatonia should be initiated rapidly, typically with parenteral benzodiazepines. Antipsychotic medications should be avoided in the acute phase of catatonia. Malignant catatonia carries an increased risk of morbidity and mortality, and it is characterized by the triad of mental status change, rigidity, and fever. A full discussion of catatonia can be found in Chapter 21.

Anxiety

Although manifestations of anxiety often reflect a primary anxiety disorder, anxiety may also be a sign of other disorders. Patients with psychosis may first describe feeling anxious about people who might try to harm them; patients with depression may be anxious about financial or relationship difficulties. Psychomotor agitation, fidgeting, and pacing can co-exist with anxiety, but they may also be associated with psychosis, mania, alcohol withdrawal, or stimulant intoxication (due to caffeine, cocaine, or amphetamines). Medical problems (e.g., thyroid and parathyroid dysfunction, delirium, cardiac arrhythmia, mitral valve prolapse) and medication side effects (e.g., akathisia) may also be heralded by anxiety. Chest pain and shortness of breath from a panic attack may prompt frightened patients to seek help at an ED; these patients require a thorough physical evaluation in concert with a psychiatric assessment. Complex partial seizures should be considered for patients with recurrent panic, especially those at heightened risk for seizures (e.g., those with a history of head injury, another seizure disorder, cerebrovascular disease, or dementia).

Personality Disorders

Patients with borderline, narcissistic, and/or antisocial personality disorders often require a significant amount of time from PES staff to coordinate their care. Such patients may request services or accommodations that are outside of the normal ED routines. They may file complaints or even threaten to harm or kill themselves or others if staff are unwilling to provide their preferred treatment (i.e., they make contingent threats of harm). Often these threats are statements of acute distress, although each statement must be evaluated in the context of the patient's history and their current situation.

Problems often develop when the patient's psychopathology leads to splitting among staff members and disagreement over management approaches. The most important aspect of the treatment of these patients is for the PES team to provide clear boundaries and set limits regarding the scope of care available, the role of individual staff members, and the goals of the emergency intervention. Outside contacts who know the patient may be able to provide insights that can inform the safety assessment.

Trauma

Patients seen in the PES frequently have a history of trauma, even if it is not a presenting complaint. All patients should be asked whether they have been victims of violence or other trauma and whether they feel safe in their current living environment. Traumatized patients need not, and should not, be asked to review the details about past traumas lest the clinical interview unintentionally re-traumatize them. Indeed, the sights and sounds of the busy and acute ED can be overwhelming and triggering for patients with a trauma history. In addition, patients who have previously had negative interactions with the mental health field (including civil commitments or physical restraints) or with law enforcement may also find the psychiatric evaluation potentially re-traumatizing. Trauma-informed ED clinicians often provide explicit reassurance to the patient (that details around current or past trauma will not be explored, that safety is prioritized, and that boundaries will be maintained).

Intoxication or Withdrawal

Patients with substance intoxication or withdrawal often come to the attention of ED staff because of acute physical or cognitive symptoms (e.g., physical trauma, somnolence, difficulty breathing, confusion). However, they may also request referrals for detoxification services or other SUD treatment. SUDs are frequently co-morbid with other psychiatric conditions, and substance-induced disorders can be difficult to distinguish from non-substance–related psychiatric disorders when individuals initially present to the ED. The following sections will outline the substances most commonly encountered in ED presentations and key concepts in the assessment of SUDs.

Alcohol

Alcohol intoxication can cause disorientation, ataxia, and slurring of speech; when high blood alcohol levels (BALs) are present, respiratory depression, coma, and death may ensue. Chronic alcohol use leads to tolerance of a higher BAL (without symptoms of severe intoxication). For acute alcohol intoxication, treatment typically consists of observation, maintenance of the airway and physical safety, and administration of intravenous (IV) fluids, if indicated. Acutely intoxicated patients can be aggressive and require physical restraints and the use of intramuscular (IM) medications, generally with a high-potency antipsychotic, such as haloperidol. Patients with problematic alcohol use may also have thoughts of suicide while intoxicated. These patients should be observed until they are sober and then re-evaluated psychiatrically and for safety.

Alcohol withdrawal can be life threatening. In its mildest form, alcohol withdrawal leads to anxiety, irritability, tremor, and an elevated heart rate; more severe forms are associated with progressive autonomic instability (i.e., marked elevations of blood pressure, pulse, and temperature), and sometimes seizures. Patients with chronic alcohol use may experience withdrawal while they still have a measurable (or even a high) BAL because the measured level may be lower than what they require to prevent withdrawal. Treatment of alcohol withdrawal typically involves the use of oral or IV benzodiazepines (initially titrated to normalize vital signs and then tapered over several days), parenteral thiamine, folic acid, and fluid repletion. Phenobarbital may be an alternative treatment option.[26] A high-potency antipsychotic (e.g., haloperidol) can decrease psychomotor agitation associated with withdrawal. Prophylactic treatment with benzodiazepines and thiamine for patients at high risk of alcohol withdrawal can be beneficial. The severity of alcohol withdrawal symptoms can be monitored over time with the Clinical Institute Withdrawal Assessment for Alcohol—Revised protocol. All patients with AUDs, regardless of their withdrawal status, should be given thiamine prophylactically (to prevent and/or treat Wernicke encephalopathy), as well as folic acid, and a multi-vitamin. In situations where a patient with an active AUD has an altered mental status and an unclear dietary history (i.e., potentially subsisting on alcohol alone over several days), empiric niacin replacement (with nicotinamide 100 mg orally three times daily) should also be considered before laboratory confirmation given increased reports of pellagrous encephalopathy presenting as alcohol withdrawal delirium.[27]

In its most severe form, alcohol withdrawal can lead to delirium tremens (DTs), which consist of a change in mental status, disorientation, visual hallucinations, and severe autonomic instability. DTs is a medical emergency with a mortality rate of 5% to 10%;

it requires immediate medical care, including medical admission and intensive treatment with an IV gamma aminobutyric acid (GABA)-ergic medication, thiamine, and fluids.[28] High-potency antipsychotics are often required for the management of agitation and hallucinations.

Benzodiazepines and Barbiturates

Intoxication with benzodiazepines and barbiturates mimics intoxication with alcohol. Manifestations include slurred speech, confusion, ataxia, and respiratory depression. Withdrawal is similarly dangerous and life threatening; management is identical to that of alcohol withdrawal (including the use of oral or IV benzodiazepines or barbiturates).

Opioids

Patients who present to the ED with emergencies related to opioid use are most commonly using fentanyl, heroin, oxycodone, methadone, buprenorphine, or hydrocodone. Kratom is a legal plant product with opioid-like effects that is increasingly used given its accessibility via the internet. Opioid intoxication is characterized by drowsiness, decreased heart rate, and pupillary constriction. Patients often describe a sense of euphoria or calm. The greatest risk from an opioid overdose is respiratory depression. Frequently, accidental overdoses occur when individuals either miscalculate their dose after a period of abstinence (because of decreased tolerance), when the drug is more potent than expected, or when contaminants are present. Patients may also intentionally overdose on opioids as a suicide attempt and then characterize the overdose as a mistake or an attempt to "get high" when brought to medical attention. Careful evaluation for suicide risk, including an evaluation when the patient is no longer intoxicated, is critical. Opioid overdose can be treated emergently with the opioid antagonist naloxone. Drowsiness and respiratory depression may return as the naloxone wears off, given its short half-life. In addition, naloxone can cause an acute and uncomfortable withdrawal syndrome that often leads to agitation on awakening.

Opioid withdrawal is not life threatening but can be excruciatingly uncomfortable, prompting some patients to leave the ED if their discomfort is not adequately addressed. Early signs and symptoms include anxiety, yawning, diaphoresis, rhinorrhea, dilated pupils, muscle cramping, and chills. Elevations in blood pressure, pulse, and temperature, as well as nausea and vomiting, will follow. Bedside instruments, such as the Clinical Opiate Withdrawal Scale, can be helpful to quantify the severity of withdrawal. A urine drug screen can often confirm recent opioid use, although many opioids do not appear on standard toxicology screens. In the emergency setting, low-dose methadone can be given on an as-needed basis to treat withdrawal symptoms; however, initiating standing methadone treatment is not within the typical purview of the ED or PES. Medically stable patients who receive outpatient methadone maintenance treatment should receive their methadone dose in the ED after confirmation of the patient's dose and active enrollment in the patient's program. Alternatively, patients can be started on buprenorphine or another medication for opioid use disorder once they begin to exhibit withdrawal symptoms, with a referral to an outpatient prescriber as part of their discharge planning. Symptomatic treatment of opioid withdrawal consists of the use of clonidine for autonomic instability (which requires monitoring for hypotension), dicyclomine for abdominal cramps, and quinine sulfate for leg cramps (which should be limited to once per day due to the risk of cardiovascular and/or renal toxicity).

Cocaine

Patients with cocaine use disorders often present to the ED complaining of physical symptoms (e.g., chest pain), dysregulated mood, or psychotic symptoms. The symptoms and signs of cocaine intoxication include euphoria and grandiosity, irritability or agitation, insomnia, dilated pupils, and psychomotor restlessness (e.g., pacing, hand wringing, foot tapping, or choreiform movements). Patients may have elevations in blood pressure and temperature, tachycardia, palpitations, chest pain, or shortness of breath. Some patients develop hallucinations, paranoia, or agitation; benzodiazepines, as well as antipsychotic medications, are useful treatments in this setting. With very high doses of cocaine, some patients experience severe autonomic changes, seizures, cardiac arrhythmias (i.e., life-threatening ventricular fibrillation), and, ultimately, cardiac arrest and/or coma. Treatment is supportive. Serum toxicology screens for cocaine, if available, may confirm recent use of cocaine (within hours), whereas urine toxicology tests may confirm use within the last 48 hours. Identifying cocaine use is important, as those who regularly or excessively use cocaine may report symptoms and exhibit behavior that erroneously suggests a diagnosis of BPD.

Patients who are withdrawing after prolonged cocaine use often develop a strong urge to sleep, along with an increased appetite, fatigue, and a dysphoric mood.

Crystal Methamphetamine

Intoxication with crystal methamphetamine or other amphetamines (e.g., mixed amphetamine salts including prescribed or illicit use) may be recognized by mood lability or irritability, psychomotor agitation, confusion, and diaphoresis. More severe cases may include paranoia, hallucinations, cardiac abnormalities (e.g., arrhythmia, acute coronary syndrome, cardiomyopathy), seizures, renal injury, and fever. Treatment is primarily supportive, but benzodiazepines can be helpful with non-psychotic restlessness and mild agitation.[29] Antipsychotics can be added for the treatment of psychotic symptoms and more severe agitation. Similar to withdrawal from cocaine, withdrawal from amphetamines leads to irritability, sleep disturbance, psychomotor agitation, and depressed mood.

Cannabis and Synthetic Cannabinoids

Cannabis is an increasingly common drug used by patients treated in the PES. Synthetic cannabinoids (e.g., K2, Spice) are also frequently used, although they are not detectable on routine drug testing. Symptoms of intoxication include a relaxed or elevated mood, an alteration in the perception of time, tachycardia, and conjunctival injection. Patients may report paranoia or hallucinations, although in these cases, it is important to assess for other drug use and for underlying psychiatric disorders that may be exacerbated by cannabis use.

Substance Intoxication and the Safety Assessment

Even beyond these signs and symptoms, substance intoxication can impact the overall psychiatric assessment, especially the safety assessment. It is not unusual for intoxicated patients to report having thoughts of suicide or other safety concerns. While an initial assessment is important, a full safety assessment cannot be completed until the patient has been re-evaluated when sober (alert and oriented, able to speak clearly, and ambulate with a steady gait). Some patients may no longer feel suicidal when sober and may be appropriate for less restrictive levels of care. All patients should be informed that ongoing substance use is a risk factor for impulsive behavior, suicide, and violence toward others. Regardless of expressed safety concerns, no patient should be discharged from the ED while acutely impaired from intoxication. These patients frequently present management challenges to EDs and mental health providers alike.

Change in Mental Status

When evaluating a patient who presents with a significant change in mental status, the goal is to identify the underlying etiology. Frequently, changes in the mental status herald delirium due to a wide range of medical conditions, dementia with behavioral disturbances, or another neuropsychiatric condition. These conditions must be ruled out before psychiatric etiologies are considered. This is especially true for—but not limited to—geriatric patients without a psychiatric history. The Mini-Mental State Examination or Montreal Cognitive Assessment can both be useful screening tools for dementia and other cognitive impairments once the evaluator is confident that the patient is not delirious. Dementia, a chronic and progressive condition characterized by memory and other cognitive impairments, is discussed elsewhere in this textbook (see Chapter 10).

Delirium, also known as acute encephalopathy, is defined by the DSM-5-TR[24] as a fluctuating disturbance in attention and cognition accompanied by reduced awareness of the environment; it is caused by myriad medical conditions, substance intoxication or withdrawal, toxin exposure, or, frequently, a combination of multiple etiologies. Delirium typically has an acute onset (over hours or days), a fluctuating course, and it is usually reversible. Disturbance in consciousness, reduced awareness of the environment, attentional difficulties, disorientation, and an inability to think or speak coherently are common symptoms of delirium. Psychomotor agitation is also common, although psychomotor retardation can also occur. Symptoms typically associated with psychiatric diagnoses (e.g., auditory and visual hallucinations, acute changes in mood, and psychotic or disorganized thoughts) may be seen in delirious states. Indeed, delirium is often referred to as the "great imitator" given its protean manifestations. Hypoactive states, in particular, are frequently misdiagnosed as depression by non-psychiatric clinicians. Although certain medical conditions or their treatments are commonly associated with specific signs and symptoms that may provide clues to the etiology (or etiologies) of delirium for a particular patient (e.g., anxiety or agitation with pheochromocytoma, mania with the use of corticosteroids, and depression with interferon treatment), all possible medical conditions must be considered.

Delirium may be due to a serious or life-threatening condition. These conditions include Wernicke encephalopathy, hypoxia, hypoglycemia, hypertensive encephalopathy, intracerebral hemorrhage, meningitis/encephalitis, poisoning (exogenous or iatrogenic), and seizures. Their assessment and treatment are outlined in Table 43.2. Patients with other conditions, including subdural hematoma, septicemia, subacute bacterial endocarditis, hepatic or renal failure,

thyrotoxicosis or myxedema, DTs, anticholinergic toxicity, and complex partial status epilepticus, may also present with a change in mental status and require acute interventions. Elderly patients are particularly likely to present with signs and symptoms suggestive of delirium, especially those with multiple pre-morbid medical problems, including neurocognitive disorders. For such patients, even mild dehydration, constipation, or a urinary tract infection can be enough to precipitate an altered mental state.

Once acute and potentially life-threatening causes of delirium have been ruled out, other potential causes of delirium should be considered (see Chapter 9 for a more detailed discussion of delirium). Treatment of delirium involves immediate treatment of the underlying etiology; however, patients who are agitated, frightened, and/or psychotic from their delirious state may benefit from symptomatic treatment, typically starting with low-dose antipsychotics.

If delirium has been ruled out, particularly in the absence of catatonic features and potentially supported

TABLE 43.2
Potentially Life-Threatening Causes of Delirium

Condition	Diagnostics	Treatment
Wernicke encephalopathy	Classical clinical triad: change in mental status, gait instability, ophthalmoplegia	High-dose parenteral thiamine repletion (may see improvement over hours)
Hypoxia	Oxygen saturation/ABGs	Treat etiology
Hypoglycemia	Blood glucose	PO/IV administration of glucose, dextrose, sucrose, or fructose
Hypertensive encephalopathy	Blood pressure	Antihypertensive medication
Hyperthermia/hypothermia	Temperature	Cooling or warming interventions
Infectious process (e.g., sepsis, bacteremia, subacute bacterial endocarditis)	Infectious work-up	Treat infectious agent/site
Intracerebral hemorrhage	MRI/CT	Per hemorrhage type/location
Meningitis/encephalitis	LP, MRI	Antibiotic or antiviral medication, immunotherapy
Metabolic (e.g., chemical derangements, renal failure, hepatic failure, thyroid dysfunction)	Laboratory investigations	Per derangement
Poisoning/toxic reaction (e.g., environmental exposures, medications, alcohol, illicit substances)	Toxicology panel	Per toxin
Status epilepticus	EEG	Anticonvulsants or IV benzodiazepines (or both)

ABGs, Arterial blood gases; *CT*, computed tomography; *EEG*, electroencephalogram; *IM*, intramuscular; *IV*, intravenous; *LP*, lumbar puncture; *MRI*, magnetic resonance imaging; *PO*, oral (*per os*).

by a normal electroencephalogram (EEG) in particularly complex cases, a primary psychiatric diagnosis may also be considered (including the so-called pseudo-dementia of depression). A diagnosis of a primary mood or thought disorder can often be made based on symptomatology and history. Agitation or threatening behavior may also be representative of longer-standing problems with behavioral regulation, not due to a diagnosable disorder.

MANAGEMENT OF ACUTE SYMPTOMS

After ruling out contributory medical causes and identifying a working psychiatric diagnosis, the primary goal in emergency psychiatry is to manage acute crises. The intervention chosen will depend on the patient's needs, the severity of the illness, and the time and resources available. For some patients, the intervention may involve speaking to an understanding clinician who can ally, demonstrate empathy, and provide reassurance. Extremely agitated patients may require seclusion and/or chemical and/or physical restraints to protect them as well as staff and other patients. Between those extremes are various therapeutic interventions designed to decrease the acuity of the patient's situation, provide education about mental illness and treatment, and help the patient and family members make informed decisions. Staff must consider the following when making decisions about patient management: environmental factors, psychological techniques, and pharmacologic interventions.

Environmental Factors

The patient's attire and physical location while they wait for evaluation or management are important factors. Voluntary and cooperative patients without evidence of acute risk may be safe to wear street clothes and sit in a waiting room, while patients brought in by emergency medical services with an initial presentation suggestive of a serious condition should be changed into safe hospital attire (scrubs) and monitored in a secure area or single room. Patients may or may not be able to tolerate friends and family at the bedside; some patients are too labile or unpredictable (or have a known history of violence in healthcare settings) for a staff member to interview without security

being present. If possible, each interview should take place in a quiet, clean setting, where the patient and the clinician can both sit comfortably and not be overheard by strangers in the ED. Attending to patients' basic needs by providing tangible items, such as blankets, food, and an accessible restroom, is a vital part of every ED encounter.

Psychological Techniques

Forming an alliance during a brief interview in an emergency setting can be challenging. EDs and PESs are often busy, with long waits for evaluation and treatment. Using psychotherapeutic techniques (such as an empathic stance, acknowledgment or validation of the difficult circumstances, identification of mutual goals, and impartiality) can facilitate an alliance.

The psychiatric clinician should allow the patient a few minutes at the beginning of the interview to describe their situation. Starting with several open-ended questions will help the patient feel heard, allow for a brief assessment of the patient's mental status, and give the psychiatric clinician time to formulate a plan to guide the interview. Because of time constraints, the PES evaluation often involves more closed-ended screening questions (to rule out major symptoms or diagnoses) than occurs in other psychiatric arenas. Empathic comments demonstrate concern and allow the clinician to interject with appropriate questions to guide the interview. Some patients, particularly those who are brought to the ED against their will, may be unwilling to engage in an interview. For these patients, it may be possible to create an alliance around their distress over being held in the ED, potentially facilitating the development of rapport. At times, despite the best efforts of clinicians, it may be impossible to develop a therapeutic relationship with a patient.

For PES patients, psychological interventions may focus on education about psychiatric symptoms, treatments, or the mental health system. The clinician may help the patient gain insight into their problems and brainstorm solutions. Collaboration between the patient and the clinician can lead to a mutually agreeable treatment plan. The clinician may offer reassurance that a problem is not as overwhelming as it seems or that help is available. The simple act of validating a patient's feelings of being overwhelmed or providing a psychiatric diagnosis can help make sense of a patient's distressing symptoms and be therapeutic. The patient's and the family's unstated wishes or concerns should be identified and managed.

The patient should be encouraged to identify coping skills that have been helpful before. Although patients should be allowed to describe difficult feelings and release tension, providers should communicate the explicit expectation that the patient behave within the boundaries of what is safe and appropriate in a hospital environment (e.g., it is not appropriate to punch walls to demonstrate anger).

Another key to providing therapeutic care in an emergency setting is to understand provider reactions toward patients, and the role that conscious and unconscious bias plays in those reactions. Psychiatric emergency providers work in a chaotic, distracting, and fast-paced environment, often without comprehensive knowledge about patients whose acute presentations may elicit fear, anxiety, and frustration. This combination of factors can lead to clinical assessments and responses that are influenced by cultural stereotypes, as well as implicit and explicit biases. Maximizing cultural humility and structural competency amongst all staff contributes to more equitable and compassionate care for patients.

Amid the stress of the busy ED, staff members at every level can become overwhelmed, frustrated, anxious, or angry. However, clinicians must prevent these feelings from interfering with the treatment of patients, which could lead to unprofessional behavior, as well as compromised clinical care and safety. To mitigate this risk, for many years at Massachusetts General Hospital, psychiatric residents have participated in a weekly supervision session focused on recognizing provider reactions and enhancing resilience after long nights in the PES.[30] Awareness of stress among staff members and providing scheduled breaks (to eat meals and to relax during long shifts) are necessary for the provision of good care in an emergency service.

Pharmacologic Interventions

The power of medication in a psychiatric emergency should never be underestimated. For some patients, particularly those who are psychotic or acutely agitated, administering medication may be the primary intervention. Medication can decrease anxiety and paranoia, reduce disorganization, and help a manic patient to sleep. Benzodiazepines treat symptoms of alcohol withdrawal and can manage anxiety associated with a wide range of clinical presentations, including mitigating the stress of the ED encounter. Some patients who are overwhelmed initially can participate in the interview and psychological interventions only after medication has been administered. Medication should be considered early and often during an evaluation. Medication can also be offered before a psychiatric evaluation, when a patient first presents to the ED, to decrease the risk of subsequent agitation or to promote participation in the medical evaluation and subsequent psychiatric evaluation. Psychiatric clinicians can offer guidance to emergency medicine providers on appropriate early interventions. If the patient has used and tolerated a medication previously for similar symptoms, the same medication can be offered to avoid the potential side effects of new medications. If the patient has not tried medications, consideration of the symptoms, differential diagnosis, intended means of administration of the medication, and potential side effects will help narrow the options.[31]

Management of Agitation

In the emergency setting, evaluation and treatment may be complicated by agitation, defined as the physical manifestation of internal distress. The etiologies associated with agitation are numerous, including substance intoxication or withdrawal, delirium, dementia, pain, psychosis, mania, anxiety, and various personality disorders. Patients with intellectual disabilities or autism spectrum disorders may also be prone to agitation. Early signs of agitation include tapping of the fingers and feet, sighing, moaning, breathing heavily, fidgeting, staring intensely, and appearing distracted by internal stimuli. Changes in vital signs (e.g., elevations in blood pressure, pulse, or respiratory rate) may be noted. Pressured or loud speech, invasion of others' personal space, clenching of the jaw or hands, tension of other muscles, or pacing often indicate escalating agitation. Agitation often heralds a psychiatric emergency; it jeopardizes the safety of the patient as well as that of others in the treatment environment, and it impedes optimal evaluation and treatment.

Agitation is best managed by attempting to prevent or treat it as early as possible (see Case 1). If possible, the agitated patient should be enlisted in this task (i.e., to monitor their own internal state, report increases in anxiety or distress, and consider effective means for the reduction of distress to avert any behavioral dysregulation). Staff members should be well trained in de-escalation. Key components of de-escalation include the use of non-threatening body language, empathic listening to the patient's concerns, validation of the patient's position, respectfully stating expectations for behavior, and offering choices where possible to promote autonomy.[32] Staff should maintain an open, neutral stance, and speak calmly, in concise and simple language.

Modulation of the environment (by decreasing interpersonal interactions and auditory or visual stimulation) is an important initial step in management. A safe environment (without access to objects that could be used as weapons or ligatures and hang points that could be used for self-harm) is important to decrease the risk of harm. There should be adequate space for the patient and staff, including security staff, to interact safely. Paranoid or previously traumatized patients may be particularly sensitive to personal space. Attempts to make the environment more comfortable (e.g., by offering a warm blanket, a place to lie down, or food and drink) can go a long way to de-escalate patients.

As noted earlier, pharmacologic interventions are critical for the treatment of agitation. The goal of using medication is to calm patients so they can participate in the assessment and treatment planning. Potential medication regimens in the emergency setting include the use of benzodiazepines (particularly lorazepam [0.5–2 mg] oral or IM; a benzodiazepine should be the first choice if alcohol or other GABA-ergic withdrawal is suspected); second-generation antipsychotics (SGAs) (e.g., risperidone [0.5–2 mg] in oral tablet, liquid, or rapidly dissolving form; olanzapine [2.5–10 mg] in oral tablet, rapidly dissolving, or IM form; or quetiapine [25–100 mg] in an oral tablet form); and high-potency first-generation antipsychotics (FGAs) (e.g., haloperidol or fluphenazine) combined with a benzodiazepine (e.g., lorazepam) given as an IM injection for more severe agitation.[31] An alternative for moderately agitated patients who are willing to accept medication is oral risperidone combined with oral lorazepam. Newer parenteral formulations of SGAs for

the management of acute agitation are also available, including olanzapine 5 to 10 mg IM or 2.5 to 5 mg IV. Parenteral olanzapine should not be co-administered with parenteral benzodiazepines, given the risk of respiratory suppression.[33] Table 43.3 lists a range of medications used for adult patients. Elderly patients, patients with intellectual disabilities, and patients with a history of head injuries can be particularly sensitive to anticholinergic side effects or vulnerable to paradoxical reactions to medications, such as benzodiazepines. In these populations, it is better to use smaller initial doses of medication and to increase the dose gradually. A review of prior medication responses is particularly helpful in these populations.

Case 1

Mr. R, a 52-year-old man with a long history of schizophrenia (diagnosed in his early 20s after he became acutely paranoid and violently assaulted a stranger who he believed was going to harm him), had multiple psychiatric hospitalizations and was living at a shelter supported by the state's Department of Mental Health.

Over the past week, he stopped taking his medications (which included haloperidol and lorazepam) and he had become progressively more paranoid and disorganized. Police were called to his shelter after he threatened to harm several staff members, and he was brought to the local ED.

Upon arrival in the ED, he was extremely agitated. He was quickly escorted to a private room in the PES, where a psychiatrist, psychiatric nurse, and security staff attempted verbal de-escalation. Mr. R was quite upset that he was not allowed to smoke, but he accepted a nicotine patch. He was also offered, and accepted, haloperidol 5 mg and lorazepam 2 mg PO. He was given a dinner tray, at which point he asked to be left alone to eat. One hour later he was much calmer and participated in a complete assessment.

Restraint and Seclusion

Agitated or violent behavior should be managed with the least restrictive means possible; restraint (any method or device that immobilizes or restricts the patient's movement) and seclusion (involuntary

TABLE 43.3
Medications Frequently Used in the Psychiatric Emergency Service for Adult Patients

Medication	Starting Dose[a]	Formulation Available
BENZODIAZEPINES		
Clonazepam (Klonopin)	0.5–1 mg	PO
Chlordiazepoxide (Librium)	25–50 mg	PO/IM/IV
Diazepam (Valium)	5–10 mg	PO/IM/IV (oral solution available)
Lorazepam (Ativan)	0.5–2 mg	PO/IM/IV (oral solution available)
Oxazepam (Serax)	15–30 mg	PO
FIRST-GENERATION ANTIPSYCHOTICS		
Chlorpromazine (Thorazine)	25–50 mg	PO/IM (oral solution available)
Fluphenazine (Prolixin)	5–10 mg	PO/IM (oral solution available)
Haloperidol (Haldol)	5–10 mg	PO/IM/IV[b] (oral solution available)
Perphenazine (Trilafon)	4–8 mg	PO (oral solution available)
SECOND-GENERATION ANTIPSYCHOTICS		
Olanzapine (Zyprexa)	5–10 mg	PO[c]/IM/IV[b]
Quetiapine (Seroquel)	25–100 mg	PO
Risperidone (Risperdal)	0.5–2 mg	PO[c] (oral solution available)
OTHER AGENTS		
Benztropine (Cogentin)	0.5–1 mg	PO/IM/IV
Buspirone (BuSpar)	5–10 mg	PO
Clonidine (Catapres)	0.1 mg	PO
Diphenhydramine (Benadryl)	25–50 mg	PO/IM/IV (oral solution available)
Gabapentin (Neurontin)	100–200 mg	PO
Propranolol (Inderal)	20 mg	PO (oral solution available)
Trazodone (Desyrel)	25–50 mg	PO

[a]Starting doses are for healthy adult patients. Consider lower doses in patients who are pediatric, elderly, or have a history of head injury or neurodevelopmental disorder.

[b]Please note that haloperidol and olanzapine are not FDA-approved for IV use but can be administered off-label via this route.

[c]Also available in an orally disintegrating tablet.

FDA, US Food and Drug Administration; IM, intramuscular; IV, intravenous; PO, oral (per os).

confinement of a patient alone in a room or area) are interventions of last resort, used only when patients are at imminent risk of harming themselves or others and when other interventions have failed or have been refused. Restraint and seclusion can be associated with physical and psychological injuries to both patients and providers[34]; however, if verbal, environmental, and pharmacological interventions are unsuccessful, seclusion or restraint may be necessary to provide for patient safety and the safety of others. In such cases, the least restrictive intervention should be used; if patient safety permits, seclusion is preferable. For patients who remain at serious risk for harm, physical restraint may be required to maintain their safety and the safety of those around them. The use of restraints represents a true psychiatric emergency, and all members of the multi-disciplinary team should be involved in the decision to use restraints, although the ultimate responsibility lies with the physician.

The patient who has been placed in seclusion or restraints should be monitored at all times, in accordance with JC standards.[35] The time that the patient is permitted to remain in restraints is limited and determined by their age; however, attempts should always be made to remove the restraints as soon as possible. Almost every patient who requires restraint or seclusion will require medication to treat their agitation. For many acutely agitated patients, physical restraints may only be required briefly to allow for the safe administration of IM medication; restraints can and should be removed once the patient has calmed down. Debriefing after restraint is always recommended both with the patient when they are calm enough to participate and separately with involved staff. This process allows for a review of the events leading up to the restraint and a discussion of how similar events might be avoided in the future.

Disposition

The goals of the PES evaluation are to provide therapeutic interventions, arrive at a diagnostic and risk assessment, and determine the most appropriate disposition. The evaluator must account for the acuity of the patient's symptoms, complete a safety assessment, and assess the psychosocial support system and the availability of services to determine the appropriate level of care. Ideally, the patient, involved family, and any outpatient treaters should participate in the discussion regarding the next steps. In situations where there is no acute safety risk, the patient's willingness to engage in available treatment will ultimately be the deciding factor. Levels of care, ranging from most to least restrictive, include locked inpatient psychiatric units, unlocked crisis stabilization units, residential treatment services, detoxification units, partial hospitalization programs, and outpatient programs. The PES clinician must have a thorough knowledge of local mental health resources and the means to access them, supported by social workers who are ideally part of the emergency psychiatric team. The availability of outpatient treatment varies greatly by location. Some PESs offer prescriptions for medications on discharge and even provide follow-up while patients are awaiting referral to longer-term outpatient treatment. Other programs can refer patients to urgent psychiatry appointments or outpatient programs with short waitlists.

ED Boarding of Patients Awaiting Psychiatric Admission

Due to several complex factors, including a focus on de-institutionalization beginning in the 1960s and limitations in the availability of robust community-based psychiatric care, mental health–related ED visits have dramatically increased in recent years. Simultaneously, the number of psychiatric inpatient beds has decreased.[36] Furthermore, ED patients seeking psychiatric care have a longer length of stay than ED patients seeking other medical care (as much as 42% longer), and they are twice as likely to require hospital admission.[37] Thus, psychiatric patients are at significantly increased risk of boarding, defined by the JC as waiting more than 4 hours for an inpatient bed to become available after the decision to admit them has been made.[38] Several individual patient factors increase the risk for ED boarding, including a lack of insurance, having public government insurance (Medicare or Medicaid), being behaviorally dysregulated in the ED, or having a neurodevelopmental or neurocognitive disorder.[36,39]

ED boarding delays care for patients and creates significant challenges for ED staff. It contributes to overcrowding, disrupts ED throughput, and is associated with decreased staff morale and provider satisfaction.[36,39,40] ED boarding can exacerbate psychiatric symptoms due to a lack of appropriate psychiatric treatment and the overstimulating nature of the environment.[41]

While the ED is not equipped to provide the same level of care as an inpatient psychiatric unit, some measures can be taken to initiate critical psychiatric treatment in the ED. Typical emergency psychiatry practice operates on a shift basis, however boarding patients require active and ongoing longitudinal treatment during their ED stay. This treatment begins with the emergency psychiatry evaluation to determine the most likely underlying diagnosis or diagnoses. An ED psychiatric treatment plan should then be developed to stabilize these diagnoses. The individualized treatment plan may include starting, stopping, or adjusting psychiatric medications, adding as-needed medications that target decreasing distress and the risk of agitation, and monitoring for and treating substance withdrawal. Patients will benefit from a daily (or more frequently if indicated) evaluation with subsequent updates to their treatment plans. Patients with co-morbid medical problems should be treated with their home medications or started on appropriate medications after consultation with emergency medical colleagues. Particularly challenging or complex patients may need a specific behavioral plan created by the multi-disciplinary team (psychiatry, nursing, and security staff) that includes guidelines for privileges (e.g., phone, television, or electronic access), management of patient requests, frequency of nursing or provider contact, and behavioral expectations. Some EDs have hired mental health specialists and therapists to provide brief supportive interactions or therapy to patients boarding for psychiatric admission. While most boarding patients initially wait for inpatient care, treatment may be stabilizing enough that they can be discharged safely to a less restrictive level of care. For this reason, planning for possible outpatient disposition, including facilitating referrals to outpatient psychiatric care, is a core component of the ED treatment plan.

EMERGENCY ASSESSMENT OF CHILDREN

Demographics

Between 2009 and 2015, there was a 56.4% increase in the number of mental health–related pediatric ED visits[2]; however, during a similar period, pediatric ED visits for deliberate self-harm increased by 329%.[42] In 2015 pediatric mental health–related ED visits accounted for approximately 3.4% of all pediatric ED visits.[2] The most common diagnoses include anxiety, depression, SUDs, and conduct disorders.[43] Males and African American and Hispanic youth account for a higher frequency of mental health–related ED visits.[44]

The COVID-19 pandemic triggered a mental health crisis among youth. Youth experienced a multitude of stressors, including school closures and/or transitions to virtual schooling, physical and social isolation, the loss of family and friends due to COVID-19, family financial stress, and pervasive uncertainty. At the same time, typical avenues for stress relief and support, including visits to school counselors, peer relationships, family and social gatherings, religious services, school- and gym-based exercise, and sports, were curtailed or eliminated. As a result, global rates of depressive and anxiety symptoms nearly doubled in youth, rising to 25.2% and 20.5% prevalence, respectively.[45] As the prevalence of psychiatric symptoms increased, so did mental health–related ED visits. During the pandemic, the proportion of mental health–related ED visits increased by 24% for 5- to 11-year olds and by 31% for 12- to 17-year olds.[46] The acuity of ED visits

also increased during the pandemic; ED visits for suicide attempts increased by 50.6% for 12- to 17-year old girls.[47] Before the COVID-19 pandemic, youth were at increased risk of experiencing ED boarding while waiting for an inpatient placement, a problem that was only exacerbated during the pandemic. Factors associated with boarding include restraint use, agitation or aggression, co-morbid ASD or developmental delay, and prior psychiatric hospitalization.[48] As society gradually returns to a "new normal" state, it remains to be seen how the overall mental health of youth will adjust.

Basic Principles

Child psychiatric emergencies result from the complex interaction of psychosocial, biological, and system issues.

The primary goal is assessing and maintaining the safety of the child, and this principle must guide all subsequent treatment and disposition plans. Clinicians must always consider the possibility of abuse or neglect as the precipitant for a visit to the ED.

The evaluation itself is based on a developmental approach. Clinicians must choose age-appropriate techniques that facilitate the assessment, which must be based on a solid understanding of normative behavior within each developmental stage.

The emergency psychiatric assessment of a child is often more complicated and time-consuming than the evaluation of an adult. Clinicians must be familiar with resources for children and families within the community mental health system. Thorough evaluations and determination of appropriate disposition require gathering information from collateral sources (e.g., outside providers, including, but not limited to, pediatricians, school administrators, guidance counselors, and outpatient mental health professionals).

The Evaluation

The initial step in the assessment of a child in the PES is the identification of the child's legal guardian(s). In routine cases, the legal guardians are the biological parents who accompany the child to the hospital. In complex cases, the child's legal guardian may be court ordered to be only one parent, another relative, a foster parent, or a representative of the state agency responsible for the care and protection of children. Custody can be split into several parts, and one guardian can have legal (or decision-making) custody, while another guardian retains physical custody. Sometimes a child remains in the home of the biological parent, but a state agency assumes the responsibility for decisions regarding medical care. Clinicians should never assume that the adult who accompanies the child is the legal guardian or that a friend or neighbor can offer consent for the assessment. Except in rare, extenuating, circumstances, the legal guardian must come to the PES and participate in the evaluation, because that person must participate in the assessment and give permission to start medication (except for emergency situations when the patient or others are in danger) and will be a key factor in disposition.

Clinicians who evaluate children in an ED should base their method of assessment on the age of the child, although the interview may also include many standard elements of the psychiatric history as listed in Box 43.2. The *style* and *process* of the interview and mental status examination depend on the child's age.

Pre-schoolers (1- to 4-year olds) are generally unable to provide a coherent narrative of the events leading up to the ED visit. Clinicians must interview the parent or guardian to obtain the details of the history but should also pay careful attention to the interaction between the child and the caregiver, as well as to the child's hygiene. Mental status assessment should focus on the child's appearance, behavior, level of agitation, mood, affect, and ability to take direction and accept reassurance from the caregiver. Common precipitants for ED visits in this age group include impulsive or dangerous behaviors (e.g., running away from home or from a caregiver in a public place, fire setting, or hitting a younger sibling).

School-age children (5- to 11-year olds) can often provide a clear description of the precipitating event but usually lack the ability to place the specific event within a larger context. It is often helpful for clinicians to interview the parent or guardian before meeting with the child. The mental status assessment includes observations of the child's interaction with the caregiver, attention to speech and language, and direct questions about mood, affect, and risk for self-injurious behavior. Children who are younger than 6- or 7-year olds might retain their "magical thinking" and

thus not yet be able to distinguish fantasy from reality. The retention of magical thinking can make assessing suicidality (i.e., the wish to die) difficult, as children who are not yet able to distinguish fantasy from reality because of their developmental stage or a developmental delay may not recognize that death is a one-way street but instead, imagine it as a place to which one can go and return.

Adolescents (12- to 17-year olds) should ideally be interviewed alone before the clinician speaks with caregivers or other concerned adults. This approach reinforces and supports the adolescent's desire for autonomy and control. Mental status assessment involves the assessment of mood, affect, thought process and content, cognition, insight, and judgment, as well as thoughts of suicide and homicide.

Finally, the evaluation must include an assessment of the social situation. Being familiar with the local communities and school systems allows clinicians to better understand the patient's social context. An inner-city school with few resources is very different from an affluent suburban school with counselors and school nurses who can identify new problems and monitor medications; knowing this information will help clinicians make decisions about the treatment plan. It is also important to know the types of treatments that the child has participated in before. A child whose severe depression has failed to improve after several medication trials and participation in months of residential treatment programs is very different from one who seeks treatment for the first time with anxiety. The previous treatment history can inform the decision regarding the subsequent level of care.

Determining the health and safety of the child or adolescent is of paramount importance. As with adults, children and adolescents presenting with behavioral health problems should be screened for suicide risk with a validated instrument on arrival to the ED, which is a JC requirement for children 12 years and older (see Box 43.4). Children and adolescents who screen positive must have a full suicide risk assessment, which is typically done by a behavioral health clinician. The SAFE-T protocol provides a structure for this risk assessment[22]; it can assist in the determination of the disposition and be reviewed with the patient and guardian(s) so that everyone involved understands the rationale behind such decisions.

Management

The child or adolescent who presents with behavioral dysregulation requires rapid diagnostic assessment and management. The differential diagnosis should focus first on the medical causes of the behavior, including elevated lead levels (particularly for children under 5 years), seizure disorders, metabolic abnormalities, medication (prescription or OTC) ingestion or overdose, withdrawal from medication or recreational drugs, hypoxia, infection, and intoxication. Nutritional causes (e.g., deficiencies of iron, zinc, vitamin B_{12}, folate, thiamine, and vitamin C) should also be considered, particularly when the diet is limited, as is commonly seen with autistic, neglected, or eating-disordered children and adolescents.

If a medical etiology is suspected, vital signs and laboratory studies should be obtained immediately. Laboratory studies might include a complete blood count, serum electrolytes (including a blood glucose level), serum and urine toxicology screens, select nutritional markers, and, in patients with a female reproductive system, a pregnancy test. It is usually helpful to control the environment and to decrease stimulation by placing the child in a contained room, sometimes with one family member who can provide a reassuring and calming presence. It can also be helpful to offer food and drink, a warm blanket, or diversionary activities.

If the above measures are insufficient or ineffective, many medical centers employ behavioral response teams to de-escalate agitated patients. These are multi-disciplinary teams, usually consisting of nurses, milieu counselors, and security officers, who are specifically trained to manage behavioral emergencies in the ED and on inpatient medical floors. These teams also create treatment plans for the patients' ongoing management and are sometimes involved pro-actively with patients who are coming in for planned admissions for medical or surgical issues and who are known to struggle with behavioral dysregulation in times of stress.[49]

Sometimes, it is necessary to administer medication to control dysregulated or acutely intoxicated children, particularly if they are in danger of harming themselves or others. It is best to ask the parent or guardian which medications the child usually takes and administer either an additional dose of a standing medication or an existing as-needed (*pro re nata*) medication. Administration of oral medication is always preferable to an IM injection, but it is not always possible if the child is unable to respond to verbal direction or limit setting. If the child has never tried to swallow a pill before, oral medications that come in liquid formulations are best.

The choice of medication and route of administration depends on the etiology and severity of the dysregulation and the age of the child. Within the last few years, a national consortium of child and adolescent psychiatrists created guidelines for medication management of behavioral dysregulation in the emergency setting.[50] These guidelines highlight the notion that agitation can have multiple etiologies, and providers should consider both the etiology and the developmental stage of the child or adolescent when making medication recommendations. While there is insufficient evidence to support using a single medication or class of medications with all patients, diphenhydramine (if the child has not had a paradoxical reaction), benzodiazepines (although they may cause paradoxical excitation and disinhibition), and alpha-2 agonists are often helpful for mild or moderate agitation. More severe agitation will require FGAs or SGAs. See Table 43.4 for further details.

Physical restraints (e.g., locked Velcro restraints) are sometimes necessary and should be placed only by trained personnel following the physician's order and according to guidelines established by the JC.[35] Family members should leave the room during any form of restraint and be debriefed later about the course of events and the rationale for particular interventions.

LEGAL RESPONSIBILITIES OF THE EMERGENCY PSYCHIATRIC CLINICIAN

Emergency psychiatric clinicians are responsible for knowing the legal regulations and local standards of care related to involuntary containment of patients in the ED, capacity evaluations, confidentiality, release of information, civil commitment, and mandatory reporting for patients with psychiatric symptoms who are treated at the PES. Although specific standards may

TABLE 43.4

Medications Frequently Used in the Psychiatric Emergency Service for Pediatric Patients

Medication	Dose Range[a]	Formulation Available
Antihistamine		
Diphenhydramine (Benadryl)	12.5–50 mg 1 mg/kg/dose	PO/IM
Benzodiazepine		
Lorazepam (Ativan)	0.25–2 mg 0.05–0.1 mg/kg/dose	PO/IM/IV
Alpha-2 agonist		
Clonidine	0.05–0.1 mg	PO
First-Generation Antipsychotics		
Chlorpromazine (Thorazine)	12.5–60 mg 0.55 mg/kg/dose	PO/IM (oral solution available)
Haloperidol (Haldol)	0.5–5 mg 0.55 mg/kg/dose	PO/IM/IV[b] (oral solution available)
Second-Generation Antipsychotics		
Olanzapine (Zyprexa)	1.25–10 mg	PO/IM[c]
Risperidone (Risperdal)	0.25–1 mg 0.005–0.01 mg/kg/dose	PO[c] (oral solution available)
Quetiapine (Seroquel)	12.5–50 mg 1–1.5 mg/kg/dose (or divided)	PO

[a]Dose ranges are for healthy pediatric patients. Consider lower doses in patients who have significant medical co-morbidities or have a history of head injury or neurodevelopmental disorder.
[b]Please note that haloperidol is not FDA approved for IV use but can be administered off-label via this route.
[c]Also available in an orally disintegrating tablet.
FDA, US Food and Drug Administration; IM, intramuscular; IV, intravenous; PO, oral (per os).
Adapted from Gerson R, Malas N, Feuer V, et al. Best practices for evaluation and treatment of agitated children and adolescents (BETA) in the emergency department: consensus statement of the American Association for Emergency Psychiatry. *West J Emerg Med*. 2019 Mar;20(2):409–418.

differ, the following features may assist with understanding these general responsibilities. In all cases, careful documentation of decision-making is important. In complex cases, consultation with a forensic psychiatrist or legal counsel trained in mental health law may be helpful.

Capacity Evaluation

Capacity refers to the patient's ability to make an informed decision about a medical procedure or treatment. While any physician can determine capacity, psychiatrists may be called on to assist in challenging cases, especially when ED patients are refusing recommended treatment for acute medical problems. The determination of capacity is not based on legally determined criteria but rather on widely accepted clinical standards. In addition, a capacity evaluation applies to a single decision at a moment in time; when in question, the patient's ability to make global medical decisions is determined through a court-based competency hearing, which is outside the purview of the emergency psychiatric clinician. A patient is presumed to have the capacity to make medical decisions until proven otherwise. The key capacity evaluation components include the assessment of whether the patient can express a choice that is stable over time, understand the relevant information, appreciate the consequences of the decision, and logically manipulate all the data.[51] Furthermore, capacity exists on a sliding scale that incorporates a risk:benefit analysis of the particular treatment in question. A patient may have the capacity to decline a treatment with low benefit and high risk and at the same time lack the capacity to decline a treatment with high benefit and low risk. In many cases, the psychiatrist will find that the patient's ability to make a clear and rational decision is dependent on an opportunity to learn more about the specific medical procedure. Coordination with the medical or surgical team, involvement of trusted family members or outpatient providers, and further discussion with the patient may obviate the need for assessment of capacity.

Confidentiality and the Release of Information

It is often difficult to maintain privacy in the ED due to architectural design flaws (semi-private rooms, open bays, curtained alcoves) and high volume with overcrowding. Nevertheless, clinicians who take a psychiatric history should make every effort to preserve confidentiality.

The care of psychiatric patients requires a strong commitment to confidentiality; in the emergency setting, all attempts are made to gain permission for any collateral contact regarding the patient's condition. However, in the case of patients who present a potential risk of harm to themselves or others, it may be necessary to contact outpatient providers or family members without the patient's consent. There is a provision in the Health Insurance Portability and Accountability Act that allows for disclosure in emergencies as necessary to treat patients.[52] It is important to document in the medical record why the contact was made and to focus the contact on gaining information that will assist in the safety assessment. While the clinician may receive information necessary to perform the safety assessment, the clinician should limit the confidential information provided to the other party.

Another situation in which a breach of confidentiality may be justified is when a clinician learns that a patient intends to harm another individual.

Civil Commitment

Civil commitment refers to the state's ability to hospitalize an individual involuntarily because of the risk of harm or grave disability due to mental illness.[23] The commitment regulations and processes vary by state. Most regulations incorporate the risk of harm to self, risk of harm to others, and inability to care for self, all due to mental illness, as the basis for civil commitment. The safety evaluation described in this chapter provides clinicians with a basic outline of an assessment to determine risk and is an important component of the assessment that may lead to civil commitment.

Mandatory Reporting

Most states have regulations regarding mandatory reporting for suspected abuse or neglect of children, elders, and individuals with physical or mental disabilities. In most cases, mandatory reporters are obligated to report situations in which they suspect abuse or neglect, whether they have clear evidence; they are protected against claims of a breach of confidentiality under these conditions.[23] Mental health clinicians should be aware of when they are considered mandatory reporters in their state and how to contact the appropriate agencies.

CONCLUSION

Emergency psychiatry is a growing subspecialty within psychiatry, driven in part by rapidly increasing rates of ED visits related to mental illness and SUDs. The role of emergency clinicians is complex and includes rapid assessment, stabilization, and treatment planning for these complicated and acute patients. These clinicians must be experts not only in the assessment and care of a variety of acute psychiatric presentations, but also in medical illnesses with prominent psychiatric symptoms, management of agitation, local treatment resources, and legal issues in psychiatric care.

REFERENCES

1. Brasch J, Glick RL, Cobb TG, Richmond J. Residency training in emergency psychiatry: a model curriculum developed by the education committee of the American Association for Emergency Psychiatry. *Acad Psychiatry.* 2004;28(2):95–103. https://doi.org/10.1176/appi.ap.28.2.95.

2. Santillanes G, Axeen S, Lam CN, Menchine M. National trends in mental health-related emergency department visits by children and adults, 2009–2015. *Am J Emerg Med.* 2020;38(12):2536–2544. https://doi.org/10.1016/j.ajem.2019.12.035.

3. Holland KM, Jones C, Vivolo-Kantor AM, et al. Trends in US emergency department visits for mental health, overdose, and violence outcomes before and during the COVID-19 pandemic. *JAMA Psychiatry.* 2021;78(4):372. https://doi.org/10.1001/jama psychiatry.2020.4402.

4. Larkin GL, Claassen CA, Emond JA, et al. Trends in U.S. emergency department visits for mental health conditions, 1992 to 2001. *Psychiatric Services.* 2005;56(6):671–677. https://doi.org/10.1176/appi.ps.56.6.671.

5. Nordstrom K, Berlin J, Nash S, et al. Boarding of mentally ill patients in emergency departments: American Psychiatric Association resource document. *Western J Emerg Med.* 2019;20(5):690–695. https://doi.org/10.5811/westjem.2019.6.42422.

6. Allen MH. Definitive treatment in the psychiatric emergency service. *Psychiatric Quarterly.* 1996;67(3):247–262. https://doi.org/10.1007/BF02238956.

7. The Joint Commission. *R3 Report: National Patient Safety Goal for Suicide Prevention*; 2019.

8. Horowitz LM, Bridge JA, Teach SJ, et al. Ask suicide-screening questions (ASQ). *Arch Pediatr Adolesc Med.* 2012;166(12):1170. https://doi.org/10.1001/archpediatrics.2012.1276.

9. Posner K, Brown GK, Stanley B, et al. The Columbia–suicide severity rating scale: initial validity and internal consistency findings from three multisite studies with adolescents and adults. *Am J Psychiatry.* 2011;168(12):1266–1277. https://doi.org/10.1176/appi.ajp.2011.10111704.

10. Woods P, Almvik R. The Brøset violence checklist (BVC). *Acta Psychiatr Scand.* 2002;106:103–105. https://doi.org/10.1034/j.1600-0447.106.s412.22.x.

11. Kim SC, Berry B, Young L. Aggressive behaviour risk assessment tool for long-term care (ABRAT-L): validation study. *Geriatr Nurs.* 2019;40(3):284–289. https://doi.org/10.1016/j.gerinurse.2018.11.006.

12. Zun LS, Hernandez R, Thompson R, Downey L. Comparison of EPs' and psychiatrists' laboratory assessment of psychiatric

patients. *Am J Emerg Med.* 2004;22(3):175–180. https://doi.org/10.1016/j.ajem.2004.02.008.

13. Korn CS, Currier GW, Henderson SO. Medical clearance of psychiatric patients without medical complaints in the emergency department. *J Emerg Med.* 2000;18(2):173–176. https://doi.org/10.1016/S0736-4679(99)00191-2.

14. Henneman PL, Mendoza R, Lewis RJ. Prospective evaluation of emergency department medical clearance. *Ann Emerg Med.* 1994;24(4):672–677. https://doi.org/10.1016/S0196-0644(94)70277-2.

15. Ehlman DC, Yard E, Stone DM, et al. Changes in suicide rates—United States, 2019 and 2020. *MMWR Morb Mortal Wkly Rep.* 2022;71(8):306–312. https://doi.org/10.15585/mmwr.mm7108a5.

16. Hirschfeld RMA, Russell JM. Assessment and treatment of suicidal patients. *N Engl J Med.* 1997;337(13):910–915. https://doi.org/10.1056/NEJM199709253371307.

17. Na PJ, Yaramala SR, Kim JA, et al. The PHQ-9 Item 9 based screening for suicide risk: a validation study of the patient health questionnaire (PHQ)−9 item 9 with the Columbia Suicide Severity Rating Scale (C-SSRS). *J Affect Disord.* 2018;232:34–40. https://doi.org/10.1016/j.jad.2018.02.045.

18. Boudreaux ED, Jaques ML, Brady KM, et al. The patient safety screener: validation of a brief suicide risk screener for emergency department settings. *Arch Suicide Res.* 2017;21(1):52–61. https://doi.org/10.1080/13811118.2015.1040934.

19. Ambrose AJH, Prager LM. Suicide evaluation in the pediatric emergency setting. *Child Adolesc Psychiatr Clin N Am.* 2018;27(3):387–397. https://doi.org/10.1016/j.chc.2018.03.003.

20. Cotton CR, Peters DK, Range LM. Psychometric properties of the suicidal behaviors questionnaire. *Death Stud.* 1995;19(4):391–397. https://doi.org/10.1080/07481189508252740.

21. Boudreaux ED, Larkin C, Camargo CA, Miller IW. Validation of a secondary screener for suicide risk: results from the emergency department safety assessment and follow-up evaluation (ED-SAFE). *Jt Comm J Qual Patient Saf.* 2020;46(6):342–352. https://doi.org/10.1016/j.jcjq.2020.03.008.

22. Safe-T. *Suicide Assessment Five-Step Evaluation and Triage*; 2009.

23. Behnke S, Hilliard J. The Essentials of Massachusetts Mental Health Law: A Straightforward Guide for Clinicians of All Disciplines. WW Norton; 1998.

24. American Psychiatric Association. *Diagnostic and Statistical Manual of Mental Disorders, Fifth Edition, Text Revision.* American Psychiatric Association; 2022.

25. Hopkins SA, Moodley KK, Chan D. Autoimmune limbic encephalitis presenting as relapsing psychosis. *Case Reports.* 2013;2013. https://doi.org/10.1136/bcr-2013-010461.

26. Nisavic M, Nejad SH, Isenberg BM, et al. Use of phenobarbital in alcohol withdrawal management – a retrospective comparison study of phenobarbital and benzodiazepines for acute alcohol withdrawal management in general medical patients. *Psychosomatics.* 2019;60(5):458–467. https://doi.org/10.1016/j.psym.2019.02.002.

27. Oldham MA, Ivkovic A. Pellagrous encephalopathy presenting as alcohol withdrawal delirium: a case series and literature review. *Addict Sci Clin Pract.* 2012;7(1):12. https://doi.org/10.1186/1940-0640-7-12.

28. Schuckit MA. Recognition and management of withdrawal delirium (delirium tremens). *N Engl J Med.* 2014;371(22):2109–2113. https://doi.org/10.1056/NEJMra1407298.

29. Green AS. Stimulant use disorders and related emergencies. In: Donovan A, Bird S, eds. *Substance Use and the Acute Psychiatric Patient: Emergency Management.* Springer; 2019:51–68.

30. Messner E. *Resilience Enhancement for the Resident Physician.* Essential Medical Information Systems; 1993.

31. Wilson M, Pepper D, Currier G, et al. The psychopharmacology of agitation: consensus statement of the American Association for Emergency Psychiatry project BETA psychopharmacology workgroup. *Western J Emerg Med.* 2012;13(1):26–34. https://doi.org/10.5811/westjem.2011.9.6866.

32. Richmond J, Berlin J, Fishkind A, et al. Verbal de-escalation of the agitated patient: consensus statement of the American Association for Emergency Psychiatry project BETA de-escalation workgroup. *Western J Emerg Med.* 2012;13(1):17–25. https://doi.org/10.5811/westjem.2011.9.6864.

33. Marder SR, Sorsaburu S, Dunayevich E, et al. Case reports of postmarketing adverse event experiences with olanzapine intramuscular treatment in patients with agitation. *J Clin Psychiatry.* 2010;71(04):433–441. https://doi.org/10.4088/JCP.08m04411gry.

34. Knox D, Holloman G. Use and avoidance of seclusion and restraint: consensus statement of the American Association for Emergency Psychiatry project BETA seclusion and restraint workgroup. *Western J Emerg Med.* 2012;13(1):35–40. https://doi.org/10.5811/westjem.2011.9.6867.

35. The Joint Commission Edition. *The Joint Commission Comprehensive Accreditation and Certification Manual*; 2022.

36. Misek R, DeBarba A, Brill A. Predictors of psychiatric boarding in the emergency department. *Western J Emerg Med.* 2015;16(1):71–75. https://doi.org/10.5811/westjem.2014.10.23011.

37. Slade EP, Dixon LB, Semmel S. Trends in the duration of emergency department visits, 2001–2006. *Psychiatr Serv.* 2010;61(9):878–884. https://doi.org/10.1176/ps.2010.61.9.878.

38. Nolan JM, Fee C, Cooper BA, et al. Psychiatric boarding incidence, duration, and associated factors in United States emergency departments. *J Emerg Nurs.* 2015;41(1):57–64. https://doi.org/10.1016/j.jen.2014.05.004.

39. Kraft CM, Morea P, Teresi B, et al. Characteristics, clinical care, and disposition barriers for mental health patients boarding in the emergency department. *Am J Emerg Med.* 2021;46:550–555. https://doi.org/10.1016/j.ajem.2020.11.021.

40. Pearlmutter MD, Dwyer KH, Burke LG, et al. Analysis of emergency department length of stay for mental health patients at ten Massachusetts emergency departments. *Ann Emerg Med.* 2017;70(2):193–202.e16. https://doi.org/10.1016/j.annemergmed.2016.10.005.

41. Zeller SL. Treatment of psychiatric patients in emergency settings. *Prim Psychiatry.* 2010;17:35–41.

42. Lo CB, Bridge JA, Shi J, et al. Children's mental health emergency department visits: 2007–2016. *Pediatrics.* 2020;145(6). https://doi.org/10.1542/peds.2019-1536.

43. Hoge MA, Vanderploeg J, Paris M, et al. Emergency department use by children and youth with mental health conditions: a health

equity agenda. *Comm Ment Health J.* 2022;58(7):1225–1239. https://doi.org/10.1007/s10597-022-00937-7.

44. Kalb LG, Stapp EK, Ballard ED, et al. Trends in psychiatric emergency department visits among youth and young adults in the US. *Pediatrics.* 2019;143(4). https://doi.org/10.1542/peds.2018-2192.

45. Racine N, McArthur BA, Cooke JE, et al. Global prevalence of depressive and anxiety symptoms in children and adolescents during COVID-19. *JAMA Pediatr.* 2021;175(11):1142. https://doi.org/10.1001/jamapediatrics.2021.2482.

46. Leeb RT, Bitsko RH, Radhakrishnan L, et al. Mental health–related emergency department visits among children aged < 18 years during the COVID-19 pandemic—United States, January 1–October 17, 2020. *MMWR Morb Mortal Wkly Rep.* 2020;69(45):1675–1680. https://doi.org/10.15585/mmwr.mm6945a3.

47. Yard E, Radhakrishnan L, Ballesteros MF, et al. Emergency department visits for suspected suicide attempts among persons aged 12–25 years before and during the COVID-19 pandemic—United States, January 2019–May 2021. *MMWR Morb Mortal Wkly Rep.* 2021;70(24):888–894. https://doi.org/10.15585/mmwr.mm7024e1.

48. Hoffmann JA, Stack AM, Monuteaux MC, et al. Factors associated with boarding and length of stay for pediatric mental health emergency visits. *Am J Emerg Med.* 2019;37(10):1829–1835. https://doi.org/10.1016/j.ajem.2018.12.041.

49. Lelonek G, Crook D, Tully M, et al. Multidisciplinary approach to enhancing safety and care for pediatric behavioral health patients in acute medical settings. *Child Adolesc Psychiatr Clin N Am.* 2018;27(3):491–500. https://doi.org/10.1016/j.chc.2018.03.004.

50. Gerson R, Malas N, Feuer V, et al. Best practices for evaluation and treatment of agitated children and adolescents (BETA) in the emergency department: consensus statement of the American Association for Emergency Psychiatry. *Western J Emerg Med.* 2019;20(2):409–418. https://doi.org/10.5811/westjem.2019.1.41344.

51. Appelbaum PS. Assessment of patients' competence to consent to treatment. *N Engl J Med.* 2007;357(18):1834–1840. https://doi.org/10.1056/NEJMcp074045.

52. The Joint Commission Edition. *Health Insurance Portability and Accountability Act.* 104th Congress; 1996:1936–2103.

44 GERIATRIC PSYCHIATRY

M. CORNELIA CREMENS, MD, MPH

OVERVIEW

The population over the age of 65 years has increased dramatically over the past several years; this trend reflects improvements in health, nutrition, and access to medical care. This remarkable lengthening of the average life span in the United States, from 47 years in 1900 to more than 79 years now, will continue to increase along with improvements in medicine and the health consciousness of the baby boomers.[1] Equally noteworthy has been the increase in the number of those over the age of 85 years. Older adults continue to learn and contribute to society, despite the physiological changes associated with aging and the ever-present threat of illness and cognitive problems they face. Ongoing intellectual, social, and physical activity is important for the maintenance of mental health throughout the life cycle. Stressful life events (e.g., declining health; loss of independence; and the loss of a spouse or partner, family member, or friend) typically become more common with advancing age. However, major depressive disorder (MDD), anxiety disorders, memory loss, and unrelenting bereavement are not a part of normal aging; they should be treated when diagnosed. A host of effective interventions exist for most psychiatric disorders experienced by older adults and for many of the mental health problems associated with aging.

The prevalence of medical and psychiatric illness increases with advancing age in part due to stressful life events, the burden of co-morbid illness, and the various combinations of medications used.[2]

The reduction in hepatic, renal, and gastrointestinal function associated with aging impairs the ability to absorb and metabolize drugs; aging also interferes with the enzymes that degrade these medications (Table 44.1).[1]

Disability due to mental illness in the elderly will increasingly become a major public health problem. The elderly are more susceptible to disease and are more vulnerable to the side effects of prescribed drugs and other substances (be they illicit or over-the-counter substances).[3] Approximately 40% to 60% of medical and surgical inpatients are over the age of 65 years; moreover, they are at greater risk for functional decline while hospitalized than younger individuals.[4] Providing adequate treatment for older adults with psychiatric disorders facilitates their overall health by improving their interest and ability to care for themselves and to follow their primary care provider's (PCP's) directions and advice with regard to health promotion and medication adherence. Older individuals can also benefit from advances in psychotherapy, medications, and other treatment interventions for mental disorders when these interventions are modified for age and health status.

Barriers to access to appropriate mental health services exist in the organization and financing of elderly services. Unfortunately, numerous problems exist in the structure of Medicare, Medicaid, nursing homes, and managed care. PCPs are critical to the identification and treatment of mental disorders in older adults. Opportunities to improve mental health and medical outcomes are missed when mental illness is under-recognized and under-treated in primary care settings.

TABLE 44.1
Metabolic Changes Associated With Aging

Function	Impact	Domain
Hepatic function	Decreased	Blood flow
		Affects first-pass effect
	Decreased	Enzyme activity
		Demethylation
		Hydroxylation
Absorption	Decreased	Blood flow
		Acidity
		Motility
		Gastrointestinal surface area
Renal excretion	Decreased	Blood flow
		Can lead to lithium toxicity
		Glomerular filtration rate
		Hydroxymetabolites affected
		Tubular excretion
		Benzodiazepine clearance slowed
Distribution	Increased	Volume of distribution
		Especially for lipophilic drugs
	Increased	Fat stores
	Decreased	Water content
	Decreased	Muscle mass
	Decreased	Cardiac output and perfusion to organs
Protein binding	Decreased	Albumin levels (except alpha-1 glycoprotein)

General themes in geriatric psychiatry include the differentiating symptoms of normal aging from the symptoms of illness in later life; the modifiability of illness in later life; the modifiability of normal aging to improve function; the capacity to change; and distinguishing differences in the manifestations of early-onset and late-onset psychiatric disorders.

An understanding of geriatric mental health relies in part on an appreciation of neurochemistry. The neurochemistry of the aging human brain is closely correlated to an irreversible loss of function and a decline in global abilities. Fortunately, our brain has remarkable plasticity; this allows for the well-designed compensation for neuronal loss and functional decline that is linked with an age-related loss in neurons, dendrites, enzymes, and neurotransmitters.[5] Enzymes and neurotransmitters in the brain change as we age: for example, levels of monoamine oxidase increase while those of acetylcholine and dopamine decrease.[6] Some older adults by modifying their diet, increasing their exercise commensurate with their ability, and focusing on mental stimulation, age with better ability and enhanced clarity.

MENTAL HEALTH DISORDERS COMMON IN LATE LIFE

Late-Life Depression

Depression in late life lowers life expectancy. Depression and cognitive impairment affect approximately 25% of the elderly.[1] New research confirms that the risk for post-stroke depression increases especially in the "old-old" (i.e., those over 85 years of age).[7] According to Epidemiological Catchment Area (ECA) data, depression does not become more common with aging; however, making the diagnosis becomes more difficult. Depression is more common in older females than it is in older males; among those with a history of depression, there is a 50% chance of a second episode (either a recurrence or a relapse).[8] Use of medications for medical problems often generates adverse effects and complicates the diagnosis of depression; moreover, medical illness may mimic depression and depression may mimic medical illness. Depression (as occurs with a stroke, a fractured hip, arthritis, or cardiac illness) is common in disabled elderly. Depression is also associated with both acute and chronic medical illnesses and late-onset depression is closely associated with physical illness.[9] Of note, undiagnosed medical illness can manifest as depression. Grief and loss may also contribute to depression. As many as 60% of depressed patients have co-morbid anxiety and 40% of anxious patients have co-morbid depression.[10]

Neurological disorders also complicate the diagnosis of depression. The risk for depression in the post-stroke period is high, with 25% to 50% developing depression within 2 years of the event.[7] Alzheimer disease (AD) carries an increased risk of depression; approximately 20% to 30% (either before or at the time of diagnosis) are diagnosed with depression.

Delusions are also prominent in depression associated with dementia.[11] Recent research confirms the association of depression with the increased risk of developing late-onset AD.[12] Roughly half of patients with Parkinson disease develop depression or have a history of depression with anxiety, dysthymia, or frontal lobe dysfunction.[13] Degeneration of the sub-cortical nuclei (especially the raphe nuclei) is related to the development of depression in Parkinson disease.

Assessment of depression can be challenging. The Geriatric Depression Scale[14] is a helpful tool in this regard, and the information provided by caregivers is often crucial, as the elderly may not be forthcoming about their symptoms. However, the nine-item Patient Health Questionnaire (Table 44.2) used in primary care offices is easy to complete and therefore is used more readily.[15] The criteria for diagnosing depression in the elderly are the same as they are in the general population.

Treatment of late-life depression is challenging, in part, because there is a decline in one's biological ability to metabolize drugs and to bind proteins (because of reduced receptor sensitivity), as well as an increased sensitivity to medication side effects. To reduce the adverse effects of medications, drugs with the fewest side effects should be started (and be used in small doses); in addition, monotherapy should be attempted[16,17] (Tables 44.3 and 44.4). In more refractory cases or with psychotic symptoms, electroconvulsive therapy (ECT) should be considered early in treatment and as an adjunct to one or more drugs.[18,19] Recent developments in transcranial magnetic stimulation

TABLE 44.2
Patient Health Questionnaire (PHQ)-9

Nine-Symptom Checklist

Over the last 2 weeks, how often have you been bothered by any of the following problems?

	Not at all	Several days	More than half the days	Nearly every day
Little interest or pleasure in doing things	0	1	2	3
Feeling down, depressed, or hopeless	0	1	2	3
Trouble falling or staying asleep, or sleeping too much	0	1	2	3
Feeling tired or having little energy	0	1	2	3
Poor appetite or overeating	0	1	2	3
Feeling bad about yourself—or that you are a failure or have let yourself or your family down	0	1	2	3
Trouble concentrating on things, such as reading the newspaper or watching television	0	1	2	3
Moving or speaking so slowly that other people could have noticed? Or the opposite—being so fidgety or restless that you have been moving around a lot more than usual	0	1	2	3
Thoughts that you would be better off dead or hurting yourself in some way	0	1	2	3

(For office coding: Total Score _____ = ___ + ___ + ___)

If you checked off any problems, how difficult have these problems made it for you to do your work, take care of things at home, or get along with other people?

Not difficult at all	Somewhat difficult	Very difficult	Extremely difficult

From the Primary Care Evaluation of Mental Disorders Patient Health Questionnaire (PRIME-MD PHQ). The PHQ was developed by Drs. Robert L. Spitzer, Janet B.W. Williams, Kurt Kroenke, and colleagues. For research information, contact Dr. Spitzer at rls8@columbia.edu. PRIME-MD is a trademark of Pfizer Inc. Copyright© 1999 Pfizer Inc. All rights reserved, and Kroeke K, Spitzer RL. The PHQ-9: a new depression diagnostic and severity measure. *Psychiatr Ann.* 2002;32(9):1–7.

TABLE 44.3
Medications for Depression in the Elderly

Drugs	Dose Range	Comments
Tricyclic Antidepressants		
Nortriptyline	10–150 mg/day	Reliable blood levels, minimal orthostasis
Desipramine	10–250 mg/day	Mildly anticholinergic
Monoamine Oxidase Inhibitors		
Tranylcypromine	10–30 mg/day	Orthostasis (possibly delayed), pedal edema, weakly anticholinergic, requires dietary restrictions
Stimulants		
Dextroamphetamine	2.5–40 mg/day	Agitation, mild tachycardia
Methylphenidate	2.5–60 mg/day	
Modafinil	50–200 mg/day	
Selective Serotonin Reuptake Inhibitors		
Fluoxetine	5–60 mg/day	Akathisia, headache, agitation, gastrointestinal complaints, diarrhea/constipation
Sertraline	25–200 mg/day	
Paroxetine	5–40 mg/day	
Fluvoxamine	25–300 mg/day	
Citalopram	10–40 mg/day	
Escitalopram	2.5–20 mg/day	
Serotonin-Norepinephrine Reuptake Inhibitors		
Venlafaxine	25–300 mg/day	Increase in systolic blood pressure, confusion, light-headedness
Nefazodone	50–600 mg/day	Pedal edema, rash, hepatotoxicity (rare)
Duloxetine	20–60 mg/day	Diarrhea, dizziness
Alpha-2 Antagonist/Selective Serotonin		
Mirtazapine	15–45 mg/day	Sedation, weight gain
Atypical Antidepressants		
Trazodone	25–250 mg/day	Sedation, orthostasis, incontinence, hallucinations, priapism
	50–600 mg/day	Pedal edema, rash
Bupropion	75–450 mg/day	Seizures, less mania/cycling, headache, nausea

and ketamine infusions have been promising.[20,21] Individual psychotherapy or group therapy complements somatic treatments and often leads to a swift recovery.[22] Interpersonal therapy and cognitive-behavioral therapy are both well suited to this population as they are more focused and interactive treatments.[22]

Late-Life Depression and Suicide

Depression with psychotic features is associated with a higher risk of suicide. The rate of suicide in those greater than 65 years is twice that of the rate in the United States population, and those with the highest suicide rates of any age group are those aged 65 years and older.[23] In 2011 suicide ranked as the 10th leading cause of death among those aged 65; this group represented 12.5% of the population, but it accounted for 15.7% of all suicides. Suicide disproportionately affects the elderly; the suicide rate among those 65 to 69 years old was 13.1 per 100,000 (N.B.: all of the following rates are per 100,000 population), and the rates increased as age increased (i.e., it was 15.2 among those between 70 and 74, it was 17.6 among those between 75 and 79, it was 22.9 for those between 80 and 84 years, and it was 21.0 in people 85 or older). Firearms (71%), overdose (11%), and suffocation (11%) were the three most common methods of suicide used by those ≥65 years.

TABLE 44.4
Medications for Psychotic Symptoms in the Elderly

Drug	Dose Range	Sedation	Ach Potency	EPS/Comments
Atypical Antipsychotics				
Clozapine	12.5–100 mg	High	High	Very low
				Check WBC count weekly; excessive drooling, hypotension
Risperidone	0.25–3 mg	Low	Low	Low
				More EPS than initially reported
Olanzapine	2.5–10.0 mg	Moderate	Moderate	Low
Quetiapine	12.5–200 mg	High	Low	Low
Ziprasidone	20–80 mg BID	Moderate	Low	Low
Aripiprazole	15–30 mg	Low	Low	Moderate

Ach, Anticholinergic; *BID*, two times daily; *EPS*, extrapyramidal symptoms; *WBC*, white blood cell.

Firearms were the most common method of suicide by both males and females, accounting for 78% of males and 35% of females who committed suicide in that age group and cohort.[23,24]

Risk factors for suicide among the elderly differ from those among the young. In addition to a higher prevalence of depression, older persons are more socially isolated, and they more frequently use highly lethal methods. They also make fewer attempts per completed suicide, have a higher male-to-female ratio than other groups, have frequently visited a healthcare provider before their suicide, and have more physical illnesses. Approximately 20% of elderly (i.e., >65 years) persons who take their own life have visited a physician within 24 hours of their death, 41% visited with a physician within 1 week of their suicide, and 75% were seen by a physician within 1 month of their suicide. Of every 100,000 people aged >65 years, 14.3 take their own life. This figure is higher than the national average of 10.9 suicides per 100,000 people in the general population. White males ≥85 years had an even higher rate, with 17.8 suicide deaths per 100,000 people. Suicide rates among the elderly are highest for those who are divorced or widowed. Among males aged 75 years and older, the rate for divorced males was 3.4 times that for married males, and widowed males it was 2.6 times that for married males. In the same age group, the suicide rate for divorced females was 2.8 times that of married females, and for widowed females it was 1.9 times the rate among married

females. Several factors (including growth in the size of that population; health status; availability of, and access to, services; and attitudes about aging and suicide) relative to those over 65 years will play a role in future suicide rates among the elderly.

Suicide occurs early (often during the first 6 months) of an illness, but it can occur at any time, often in combination with other mental disorders. More than 90% of older people who take their own life have the following risk factors: depression or another mental disorder; a substance use disorder or a family history of such; stressful life events, in combination with other risk factors, such as depression; a prior suicide attempt or a family history of an attempt; family violence (including physical or sexual abuse); firearms in the home (the method used in more than half of suicides); incarceration; or exposure to the suicidal behavior of others, such as family members, peers, or media figures.[23,24] The rate of suicide is greater in this population than in any other age group; older adults account for 25% of all suicides. Older white males make up the highest-risk group, and rates are increasing. Isolation increases the risk of suicide, and alcoholism or substance abuse is a contributing factor to suicide in all populations, including older adults. Aggressive treatment with antidepressants is indicated for these individuals, and inpatient treatment is the safest venue for care.[25]

Most antidepressants are equally effective for the treatment of depression; however, drugs with anticholinergic effects and undue sedation should be avoided to reduce complications (such as falls, confusion, and poor adherence). However, matching the symptoms with the side effects is useful for a patient with significant weight loss and insomnia; a sedating medication that increases appetite may be beneficial. ECT early in the course of MDD should be considered strongly as an effective intervention for this high-risk population.

Alcoholism

Alcoholism is often overlooked; it may go unnoticed in the elderly despite a lifelong pattern of daily drinking. Even if the elderly drink only small amounts, they may become dependent on its use, and then, with a sudden or large decrease in the amount ingested, they can experience a significant and life-threatening withdrawal. Co-morbid illnesses (both psychiatric and medical) confound the diagnosis of both alcoholism and the medical or surgical diagnosis. Symptoms of problem drinking include insomnia, memory loss, confusion, anxiety, and depression, as well as somatic complaints that may mimic medical illness, further delaying an accurate diagnosis. Older adults who drink alcohol are at greater risk because they take more prescribed medications that can interact adversely with alcohol.[26]

The prevalence of alcoholism detected in the ECA study was 1.5% to 3.7%. Although cross-sectional studies suggested that the percentage of alcoholism declines after age 60, longitudinal studies proposed a stable pattern of lifelong alcohol abuse.[26,27] Females drink less than males at all ages, but older widowed females are at risk of increasing their intake. Studies note that the prevalence of alcohol use disorders (AUDs) in females is on the rise. Older adults with alcohol dependence also have a high prevalence of co-morbid nicotine dependence. Alcohol dependence can lead to liver damage, cancer, immune system disorders, and brain damage.

Depression is more common in those with alcoholism, as is grief, anxiety, psychosis, and dementia. Suicide risk is greater in the elderly who suffer from AUD; therefore obtaining a comprehensive history from family, friends, and caretakers is essential. Hospitalization is typically required for detoxification of the older patient.[25] Newer medications (such as naltrexone and acamprosate) and the familiar disulfiram (Antabuse) can be beneficial, but disulfiram may contribute to problematic side effects in older adults.[26,28]

Anxiety

Recently, anxiety (typically associated with normal aging and with medical, financial, and health-related hardships) has been increasingly recognized in the elderly. However, since anxiety is not a direct consequence of normal aging, the symptoms of anxiety should not be ignored. Among the most common categories of anxiety are simple phobias and generalized anxiety; if left untreated these conditions may lead to serious depression.[29] Anxiety may co-exist with many other psychiatric diagnoses (such as depression, bipolar disorder, alcoholism, and dementia). Diagnostic challenges often arise when anxiety (e.g., worry, fear, apprehension, concern, and foreboding), as well as somatic complaints (such as tachycardia, sweating, abdominal distress, dizziness, and vertigo) develop in the context of a medical illness (e.g., diabetes with hypoglycemia, hyperthyroidism, or cardiac disease with hypoxia) as it can be manifest by similar symptoms.[29] Worries, fears, and concerns are often related to finances, dependency issues, loneliness, and memory loss. Manifestations of medical illness can mimic psychiatric symptoms; certain substances or medications (e.g., caffeine, stimulants, ephedrine, and bronchodilators) produce anxiety-like symptoms. Withdrawal from a prescribed or illicit drug can precipitate severe anxiety and panic; life-threatening withdrawal can result from sudden abstinence from alcohol, benzodiazepines, or barbiturates.

Fortunately, anxiety in the elderly can be managed effectively, using medications, therapy, or a combination of the two.[30] Among the anxiolytics, benzodiazepines are the most frequently prescribed class of agents (especially by PCPs) for the elderly; however, significant side effects (such as confusion, falls, over-sedation, and paradoxical agitation) can arise.[30] Complications of long-term use include daytime somnolence, confusion, cognitive impairment, an unsteady stance or gait, paradoxical agitation, memory disturbance, depression, and respiratory depression.

Psychosis

Psychosis (manifest by hallucinations, delusions, disorganized speech, and disorganized or catatonic behavior) in the elderly has multiple etiologies (e.g., delirium, dementia, depression, mania, and schizophrenia). Not only is morbidity high with a diagnosis of delirium, but about 30% of those with delirium will die within 1 year of their illness.[31,32] The differential diagnosis of psychosis in the elderly includes various types of dementias (e.g., AD, Lewy body dementia [LBD], vascular dementia, frontal lobe dementia [Pick disease], and Parkinson disease), each of which can have psychotic symptoms at any point during the illness; delirium; delusional disorders; bipolar disorder; schizoaffective disorder; schizophrenia (either early onset or late onset); and MDD with psychotic features. Psychosis in dementia is common, and it can be episodic or persistent and can appear early or late during the disease.[33] Symptoms of psychosis (e.g., delusions, hallucinations, misconceptions, and misperceptions) are distressing to family members and to caregivers; they can be dangerous if the individual becomes frightened or energized by them. Alcoholism and substance abuse should also be considered as a possible etiology of psychosis.[27] The Charles Bonnet syndrome, with visual hallucinations beginning after a sudden loss of vision (as in macular degeneration), may be confused with a primary psychotic condition. Most individuals know that the hallucinations are not real, and they can adjust to them; however, when dementia or an anxiety disorder confounds the symptom, this may be problematic.[34]

Dementia

Many complaints of memory loss reflect the course of normal aging or the effects of a treatable condition (such as depression or delirium). Dementia is not usually diagnosed until its moderate to severe stages, as symptoms and a subtle decline in function (Box 44.1 and Box 44.2) develop over time. Factors worth considering during the evaluation of the geriatric patient with cognitive impairment are listed in Box 44.3.

The prevalence of dementia and cognitive impairment is higher in females than in males. While higher rates of AD are reported in females, higher rates of vascular dementia are reported in males.[35] AD typically affects 5% to 8% of those aged >65 years, 15% to 20% of those aged 75 years, and 25% to 50% of those aged >85 years; its course is that of a steady decline over approximately 8 to 10 years.[36,37]

BOX 44.1
ACTIVITIES OF DAILY LIVING

Feeding or eating
Bathing
Toileting
Dressing
Continence
Hygiene
Mobility or transferring

BOX 44.2
INSTRUMENTAL ACTIVITIES OF DAILY LIVING

Housework, light
Telephoning
Cooking and meal preparation
Grocery shopping
Using transportation
Managing medication
Managing finances

BOX 44.3
FACTORS TO CONSIDER DURING THE EVALUATION OF THE GERIATRIC PATIENT WITH COGNITIVE IMPAIRMENT (THE "5 MS")

Mobility
Medications
Mind
Multi-complexity
Matters most

The *ApoE-2* allele decreases the risk for AD (as it may have a protective effect), while patients with either sporadic or familial AD have a higher frequency of the *ApoE-4* allele than in the general population.[38]

The mechanisms by which these genetic markers confer increased risk are not completely known. Neurobiological changes associated with normal aging include lower levels of cortical acetylcholine, neuron and synaptic loss, decreased dendritic span, and decreased size and density of neurons (especially in the nucleus basalis of Meynert) and likely play a role in AD. AD is most accurately diagnosed by post-mortem examination of the brain (revealing a loss of neurons in the basal forebrain and cortical cholinergic areas, in addition to the depletion of choline acetyltransferase, the enzyme responsible for acetylcholine synthesis). The degree of this central cholinergic deficit is correlated with the severity of dementia; this has led to the "cholinergic hypothesis" of cognitive deficits in AD.[36] This hypothesis has led, in turn, to promising clinical interventions. Acetylcholine is probably not the only neurotransmitter involved in AD, and numerous medication trials are underway.[36]

Vascular dementia, the second most common cause of dementia, develops because of multiple ischemic events or strokes. Approximately 8% of patients develop vascular dementia after a stroke. Vascular dementia is generally manifested by an abrupt, stuttering, often stepwise, gradual decline; it commonly co-exists with AD.

Mixed dementia is a combination of AD and vascular dementia; it is common, and stroke can unmask an underlying AD.

In frontal lobe dementia, cognitive impairment may not be as noticeable as the behavioral and personality changes. In this condition, there is a loss of personal or social awareness, a lack of insight, indifference, inappropriate and stereotyped behaviors, aggression, distraction, a loss of inhibitions, apathy, or extroverted behavior.

Early or spontaneous parkinsonism, recurrent visual hallucinations, sensitivity to antipsychotics, fluctuating cognition, falls or syncope, and a transient loss of consciousness characterize LBD.

Mild cognitive impairment (MCI), formerly designated as age-associated memory impairment (or benign senescent forgetfulness) or age-related cognitive decline, is characterized by both subjective and objective cognitive impairment in the absence of dementia. Between 10% and 12% of persons with MCI develop AD; others remain with a stable impairment or a minimal decline or die from other causes.[39] MCI sub-classifications include an amnestic form (characterized by isolated memory impairments) one with multiple cognitive deficits and another with a single deficit.[39]

Behavioral and Psychological Symptoms of Dementia

More than 80% of patients with dementia exhibit a variety of psychological symptoms; most have delusions, as well as hallucinations, paranoia, anxiety, apathy, and misidentification syndromes. Behavioral symptoms include wandering, aggression, hostility, insomnia, inappropriate eating, and abnormal sexual behaviors.[40] The caregiver burden increases with behavioral and psychological symptoms of dementia (BPSD), and aggressive, hostile, and accusatory behaviors and psychotic symptoms often result in institutionalization. Caregivers are at risk for medical and psychiatric illness due to the stress associated with caring for such individuals. Therefore, providing treatment regimens or algorithms has the potential to improve the quality of life for both the patient and the caregiver. First-line treatment has involved non-pharmacological strategies that use environmental and behavioral interventions (such as regularly scheduled routines for meals, sleep, and bathing). Pharmacological interventions (that are not symptom driven) are less well established. Limited studies have shown the benefit of antipsychotics, but there are significant side effects from their use; these include a neurological risk of stroke, a cardiovascular risk for metabolic syndrome, and a propensity for anticholinergic symptoms.[41] Psychotic symptoms in the elderly are best treated with antipsychotics, while the atypical agents are of benefit due to their binding affinity to both dopamine and serotonin (Table 44.5). Agitated, hostile, and aggressive behaviors may respond to antipsychotics, anticonvulsants, or antidepressants. Patients with dementia may develop paradoxical agitation when given benzodiazepines, and these drugs should be administered with caution. Cholinesterase inhibitors have been used for the treatment of BPSD since cholinergic deficiency also appears to be involved in the development of BPSD, as well as AD.[42]

Schizophrenia

Although schizophrenia usually arises before the age of 30 years, late-onset schizophrenia is not rare. More

TABLE 44.5	
Medications for Alzheimer Disease and Other Dementias	
Donepezil	5–23 mg every day
Rivastigmine	1.5–6 mg twice a day
Galantamine	4–12 mg twice a day
Memantine	5–10 mg twice a day

Nausea, diarrhea, abdominal cramps, bradycardia, and fatigue may develop.

than 20% of cases are diagnosed after age 40, and at least 0.1% to 0.5% of the population >65 years has a diagnosis of schizophrenia that started late in life, with a prognosis that may be made worse by delay and avoidance of treatment.[43] Aggressive treatment of symptoms and supportive care for those with this diagnosis are imperative.

Approximately 85% of these individuals (mostly females) live in the community. Schizophrenia remains plastic into later life, with more negative symptoms than positive symptoms. Numerous confounding factors (including cognitive decline, dementia, depression, medical co-morbidity, and use of medications for medical conditions) occur with aging. Most older individuals with schizophrenia have been disabled for most of their life. The side effects of typical antipsychotics, such as tardive dyskinesia (TD) or extrapyramidal symptoms (EPS), may adversely affect independent living. Lowering the dose of these medications or switching to an atypical antipsychotic may be reasonable, noting the recent evidence that atypical agents are linked with an increased risk of stroke.[41] Caregiving and community support for these individuals is the key to maintaining health and stability.

Bipolar Disorder

Bipolar disorder (BPD) may be seen for the first time in late life, and it is not uncommon in older adults; its prevalence is 0.1% to 0.4%. For most elderly patients, the illness begins in middle age or late life and often has co-morbid neurological insults. Patients with co-morbid neurological diseases are more likely to have a significantly later age of onset and a family history of affective illness. In one study, roughly 25% of patients had mania after age 50, had a history of neurological disease before the onset of the mania, and had significantly lower genetic (familial) risk factors.[44] Several biological risk factors for BPD in the elderly, including genetic factors and medical illnesses, particularly vascular diseases.

Symptoms of mania or hypomania manifest differently in older patients, with more symptoms of anger or irritability and at times aggressive behavior, delusions, and paranoia; in addition less grandiosity and euphoria occur, episodes of mania are longer, and cycling may be more rapid. Treatment response is inconsistent, although lithium, anticonvulsants (e.g., divalproex sodium, carbamazepine, and lamotrigine),

atypical antipsychotics (e.g., olanzapine, quetiapine, and risperidone), and antidepressants have all been beneficial in the treatment of elderly patients with BPD. In the differential diagnosis of secondary mania, it is important to consider co-morbid illnesses. Many patients with dementia or delirium can present with a picture of mania secondary to their illness.[44,45] Although the treatment of the symptoms is similar in both cases, an accurate diagnosis is important.

Personality Disorders

Usually personality disorders in older adults have been lifelong and well articulated by family members. These disorders are distinguished from a change in personality resulting from an illness, dementia, delirium, depression, a disaster, or a catastrophic event. Neurological disorders (e.g., stroke, brain injury, trauma, frontal lobe syndrome, seizures, or Parkinson disease) are examples of conditions that may precipitate a personality change. In the differential diagnosis, although the patient may be paranoid, avoidant, or threatening, the personality change may be related to the underlying medical or neurological disorder and not classified as a personality disorder but a change in personality due to the specific diagnosis. MDD is commonly co-morbid with aging, ranging from 10% to 70%, most often associated with obsessive-compulsive personality disorder. Co-morbid depression and panic are also noted in older patients with somatic symptom disorder, specifically with illness anxiety disorder/hypochondriasis. The pattern of lifelong distress, social dysfunction, and exacerbation of prior symptoms or traits affirms the diagnosis of a personality disorder. The popular thought that modification of symptoms or traits and possibly adaptation may occur through prior psychotherapy, aging, or life experiences has not been demonstrated in the literature. Professionals working with older adults have noted that older adults are more vulnerable to illness, losses, and possibly forced dependency. These changes can be destabilizing and cause the emergence of otherwise controlled personality symptoms. Engaging patients and caregivers in communication to allay fears and engender trust and understanding, although not an easy task in those with cluster B personalities, is the entrée to stabilization. Medications may be of benefit, but their efficacy may be limited without concomitant therapy.

DISASTERS

Senior citizens comprise a sturdy and reliable generation that has proven over the years to have the ability to survive myriad disasters (e.g., the Great Depression, world wars, threats of nuclear holocaust, terrorist attacks, and hurricanes); yet they remain proud, tough, and resilient. Older adults are a generation of survivors.[46] However, when a disaster occurs, they often feel terrified, alone, and vulnerable. Older adults often need the most assistance but can mistakenly be overlooked during relief efforts. Feelings of helplessness can frighten the elderly, placing them at greater risk for both physical and mental health illnesses. It is important for older adults recovering from the after-effects of a disaster to talk about their feelings, to share their experiences with others, and to recognize that they are not alone. Symptoms of post-traumatic stress disorder (PTSD) can be triggered by war experiences or by recollections of childhood trauma. They should be encouraged to become involved in the disaster recovery process and to help others; this can be beneficial to their own recovery. Seeking assistance is a step toward recovery, and older adults should be encouraged to ask for any type of help needed (such as financial, emotional, and medical).[46]

CAREGIVER STRESS AND BURDEN

The health and well-being of the caregivers, family members, or employees of the patient need to be considered during the evaluation because they are at risk for depression.[47] Caring for the caregiver is as important as caring for the patient. The inordinate stress and burden can place the caregiver at risk for a medical and psychiatric crisis. Caregivers can become depressed or develop symptoms of depression related to burnout (i.e., fatigue, loss of social contacts, lack of interest in work, inability to perform at work, weight gain or loss, feeling helpless, and using alcohol or other substances).[48] Burnout may not present during the most stressful times of caring, instead it can emerge months later, somewhat like PTSD.

ELDER ABUSE

Each year thousands of elderly individuals, who are often frail and vulnerable, are abused, neglected, or exploited by family members, caregivers, friends, and others, on whom they depend to assist them with basic needs.[49] Elder abuse may be subtle and as simple as not providing medications or being avoided. Family and caregivers may not intend to harm or exploit the patient but often are overwhelmed and overextended. Hotlines are available in every state for helpful information, guidance, or reporting.

REFERENCES

1. Steffins DC, Zdanys K. *Textbook of Geriatric Psychiatry*. 6th ed. American Psychiatric Association Publishing; 2023.
2. Fogel BS, Greenberg DB, eds. *Psychiatric Care of the Medical Patient*. 3rd ed. Oxford University Press; 2015.
3. Gurwitz JH, Field TH, Harold LR, et al. Incidence and preventability of adverse drug events among older persons in the ambulatory setting. *JAMA*. 2003;289:1107–1116.
4. Lunney JR, Lynn J, Foley DJ, et al. Patterns of functional decline at the end of life. *JAMA*. 2003;289:2387–2392.
5. Marcantonio ER. Delirium. *N Engl J Med*. 2017;377:1456–1466.
6. Cummings JL, Mega SM. *Neuropsychiatry and Behavioral Neuroscience*. Oxford University Press; 2003.
7. Carota A, Berney A, Aybek S, et al. A prospective study of predictors of post stroke depression. *Neurology*. 2005;64: 428–433.
8. Dew MA, Whyte EM, Lenze EJ, et al. Recovery from major depression in older adults receiving augmentation of antidepressant pharmacotherapy. *Am J Psychiatry*. 2007;164:892–899.
9. Katon W, Lin EH, Kroenke K. The association of depression and anxiety with medical symptom burden in patients with chronic medical illness. *Gen Hosp Psychiatry*. 2007;29:147–155.
10. Lenze EJ, Mulsant BH, Shear MK, et al. Comorbid anxiety disorders in depressed elderly patients. *Am J Psychiatry*. 2000;157: 722–728.
11. Olin JT, Katz IR, Meyers BS, et al. Provisional diagnostic criteria for depression of Alzheimer disease. *Am J Geriatr Psychiatry*. 2002;10:129–141.
12. Vilalta-Franch J, Garre-Olmo J, López-Pousa S, et al. Comparison of different clinical diagnostic criteria for depression in Alzheimer disease. *Am J Geriatr Psychiatry*. 2006;14:589–597.
13. Ravina B, Camicioli R, Como PG, et al. The impact of depressive symptoms in early Parkinson disease. *Neurology*. 2007;69: 342–347.
14. Yesavage JA, Brink TL, Rose TL, et al. Development and validation of a geriatric depression rating scale: a preliminary report. *J Psychiatr Res*. 1983;17:27.
15. Richardson TM, He H, Podgorski C, et al. Screening depression aging services clients. *Am J Geriatr Psychiatry*. 2010;18: 1116–1123.
16. Cremens MC. Polypharmacy in the elderly. In: Ghaemi SN, ed. *Polypharmacy in Psychiatry*. Marcel Dekker; 2002.
17. Reynolds III CF, Dew MA, Pollock BG, et al. Maintenance treatment of major depression in old age. *N Engl J Med*. 2006;354: 1130–1138.

18. Greenberg RM, Kellner CH. Electroconvulsive therapy: a selected review. *Am J Geriatr Psychiatry*. 2005;13:268–281.

19. Kellner CH, Geduldig ET, Knapp RG, et al. More data on speed of remission with ECT in geriatric depression. *Br J Psychiatry*. 2015;206:167.

20. Lipsitz O, DiVincenzo JD, Rosenblat JD, et al. Safety, tolerability and real-world effectiveness of IV ketamine in older adults with treatment resistant depression. *Amer J Geriatr Psychiatry*. 2021;29:899–913.

21. Blumberger DM, Mulsant BH, Thorpe KE, et al. Effectiveness of standard bilateral repetitive transcranial magnetic stimulation vs bilateral theta burst stimulation in older adults with depression. *JAMA Psychiatry*. 2022;79:1065–1073.

22. Wei W, Sambamoorthi U, Olfson M, et al. Use of psychotherapy for depression in older adults. *Am J Psychiatry*. 2005;162:711–717.

23. Bruce ML, Ten Have TR, Reynolds CF, et al. Reducing suicidal ideation and depressive symptoms in depressed older primary care patients. *JAMA*. 2004;291:1081–1091.

24. Olin DW, Zubritsky C, Brown G, et al. Managing suicide risk in late life: access to firearms as a public health risk. *Am J Geriatr Psychiatry*. 2004;12:30–36.

25. Rowe JL, Conwell Y, Shulberg HC, et al. Social support and suicidal ideation in older adults using home healthcare services. *Am J Geriatr Psychiatry*. 2006;14:758–766.

26. Blow FC, Barry KL. Older patients with at-risk and problem drinking patterns: new developments and brief interventions. *J Geriatr Psychiatry Neurol*. 2000;13:134–140.

27. Alpert PT. Alcohol abuse in older adults: an invisible population. *Home Health Care Manag Pract*. 2014;26(4):269–272.

28. Olin DW. Late-life alcoholism: issues relevant to the geriatric psychiatrist. *Am J Geriatr Psychiatry*. 2004;12:571–583.

29. Lenze EJ, Rogers JC, Martire LM, et al. The association of late-life depression and anxiety with physical disability: a review of the literature and prospectus for future research. *Am J Geriatr Psychiatry*. 2001;9:113–135.

30. Pinquart M, Duberstein PR. Treatment of anxiety disorders in older adults: a meta-analytic comparison of behavioral and pharmacologic interventions. *Am J Geriatr Psychiatry*. 2007;15:639–651.

31. Inouye SK, Bogardus ST, Charpentier PA, et al. A multicomponent intervention to prevent delirium in hospitalized older patients. *N Engl J Med*. 1999;340:669–676.

32. Cole MG. Delirium in elderly patients. *Am J Geriatr Psychiatry*. 2004;12:7–21.

33. Leroi I, Voulgari A, Breitner JC, et al. The epidemiology of psychosis in dementia. *Am J Geriatr Psychiatry*. 2003:83–91.

34. Eperjesi N, Arkbarali S. Rehabilitation in the Charles Bonnet syndrome: a review of the treatment options. *Clin Exp Optom*. 2004;87:149–152.

35. Cremens MC, Okereke OI. Alzheimer's disease and dementia. In: Carlson KJ, Eisenstat SA, eds. *Primary Care of Women*. 2nd ed. Mosby; 2002.

36. Francis PT. Neuroanatomy/pathology and the interplay of neurotransmitters in moderate to severe Alzheimer disease. *Neurology*. 2005;65:S5–S9.

37. Cummings JL. Alzheimer's disease. *N Engl J Med*. 2004;351:56–67.

38. Palmer R, Berger AK, Monastero K, et al. Predictors of progression from mild cognitive impairment to Alzheimer's disease. *Neurology*. 2007;68:1596–1602.

39. Panza F, D'Introno A, Colacicco AM, et al. Current epidemiology of mild cognitive impairment and other pre-dementia syndromes. *Am J Geriatr Psychiatry*. 2005;13:633–644.

40. Ringman JM, Schneider L. Treatment options for agitation in dementia. *Curr Treat Options Neurol*. 2019;21:30.

41. Raivio MM, Laurila JV, Strandberg TE, et al. Neither atypical nor conventional antipsychotics increase mortality or hospital admissions among elderly patients with dementia: a two-year prospective study. *Am J Geriatr Psychiatry*. 2007;15:416–424.

42. Feldman H, Gauthier S, Hecker J, et al. Efficacy of donepezil on maintenance of activities of daily living in patients with moderate to severe Alzheimer's disease and the effect of caregiver burden. *Am J Geriatr Soc*. 2003;51:737–744.

43. Howard R, Rabins PV, Seeman MV, et al. Late-onset schizophrenia and very-late-onset schizophrenia-like psychosis: an international consensus. *Am J Psychiatry*. 2000;157:172–178.

44. Young RC, Mulsant BH, Sajatovic M, et al. GERI-BD: a randomized double-blind controlled trial of lithium and divalproex in the treatment of mania in older patients with bipolar disorder. *Am J Psychiatry*. 2017;174:1086–1093.

45. Brooks JO, Hoblyn JC. Secondary mania in older adults. *Am J Psychiatry*. 2005;162:2033–2038.

46. Rosenkoetter MM, Covan EK, Cobb BK, et al. Perceptions of older adults regarding evacuation in the event of a natural disaster. *Public Health Nurs*. 2007;24:160–168.

47. Borja B, Borja CS, Gade S. Psychiatric emergencies in the geriatric population. *Clin Geriatr Med*. 2007;23:391–400.

48. Steadman PL, Tremont G, Davis JD. Premorbid relationship satisfaction and caregiver burden in dementia caregivers. *J Geriatr Psychiatry Neurol*. 2007;20:115–119.

49. Lachs MS, Pillemer KA. Elder abuse. *N Engl J Med*. 2015;373:1947–1956.

45

CARE AT THE END OF LIFE

M. CORNELIA CREMENS, MD, MPH ■ ELLEN M. ROBINSON, RN, PHD HEC-C, FAAN

OVERVIEW

With more than 3.5 million deaths each year in the United States,[1] providing both competent and compassionate care for patients at the end of life is a crucial task for physicians. Caring for patients at the end of life often occurs amidst a complex background of medical, psychiatric, ethical, and legal concerns. The Institute of Medicine identified end-of-life care as one of the priority areas for improvement of quality of care, and it specifically identified pain control in advanced cancer and care of patients with advanced organ failure as areas of focus.[2]

Current concepts in ethics, as well as those at the interface of psychiatry and the law, surround this evolving area of medicine—where advances in medical technology and practice have extended the human life span and led to the emergence of novel ethical conflicts.[3] End-of-life care may create tension between two essential medical principles: to do no harm (primum non nocere) and to relieve suffering. For example, prescribing an opioid medication for pain relief may unintentionally hasten a patient's death via respiratory suppression.[4]

Caring for patients at the end of life occurs amid a complex background of medical, psychiatric, ethical, and legal concerns. Psychiatric co-morbidities, such as major depressive disorder (MDD), anxiety, delirium, and substance use disorders (SUDs) are common conditions encountered in the treatment of dying medically ill patients; psychiatric care often includes the patient and their family and friends who are also coping with the diagnosis, care, and treatment of patients at the end of life. In addition, with the recent emergence of physician-assisted suicide (alternatively called, medical aid in dying) and legal cases that surround the withdrawal of life-sustaining treatments, conflicts have emerged.

This chapter provides an overview of the central principles of care, diagnosis, and treatment of patients at the end of life from the psychiatric perspective. It also examines current concepts in ethics and legal precedents that surround this evolving area of medicine, where advances in medical technology and practice have extended the human life span and led to the emergence of both opportunities and conflicts at the end of life and the emergence of novel ethical conflicts.

GOALS OF TREATMENT

Psychiatrists face multiple challenges when caring for dying patients, encompassing issues of diagnosis and treatment as well as larger ethical and legal considerations. Psychiatrists may be uniquely qualified to help dying patients by optimizing palliative care and assisting patients and their families during the dying process. An important first step in this process is for the psychiatrist and the patient to define treatment goals. According to Saunders,[5] the primary aim of care is to help patients "feel like themselves" for as long as possible. Care at the end of life also offers an important opportunity, according to Kübler-Ross, to address and complete "unfinished business."[6] Common themes that arise include facilitating reconciliation with estranged friends or family and the pursuit of remaining hopes. Additionally, according to Kübler-Ross,[6] patients who are dying go through a transformational process (which includes stages of denial, anger, bargaining, guilt/depression, and eventual acceptance). These stages may occur in a unique order, may occur simultaneously, and may last for variable amounts of time. Psychiatrists, palliative care physicians, and other professionals may assist dying patients in the transition through these stages toward acceptance.

Hackett and Weisman[7] developed five goals for "appropriate death" that have helped to focus therapeutic efforts for the treatment of dying patients. These goals include freedom from pain, optimal function within the constraints of disability, satisfaction of remaining wishes, recognition and resolution of residual conflicts, and yielding control to trusted individuals. Perhaps the most important principle in the treatment of dying patients is that the treatment be tailored to the individual's circumstances. That is, within these general goals and paradigms, each patient's unique characteristics will necessitate careful tailoring of clinical interventions. This case-by-case approach can be accomplished only by getting to know the patient, responding to his or her needs and interests, proceeding at his or her pace, and allowing him or her to shape how those in attendance behave. There is no one best way to die. Everyone dies, but the goal for everyone is to have a good life to the end. In that spirit, a good death often means respecting the patient's wishes while caring for the patient, their family, and caregivers.

The recent surge of discussions regarding end-of-life care comes at a time when the aging population is burgeoning; people increasingly want their preferences to be respected, and they are invested in making their preferences known. Gawande[8] noted that the goals for palliative care and end-of-life wishes be established early in the course of illness and documented for the medical record, not merely at the end of life.[9]

Hospice care provides an important function for dying patients by incorporating spiritual and family support, pain management, respite services, and a multi-disciplinary approach to medical and nursing care. When St. Christopher's Hospice opened in 1967 with Saunders as its medical director, it was dedicated to enabling a patient, according to Saunders: "to live to the limit of his or her potential in physical strength, mental and emotional capacity, and social relationships."[5] Saunders viewed hospices as an "alternative to the negative and socially dangerous suggestion that a patient with an incurable disease likely to cause suffering should have the legal option of actively hastened death, that is, euthanasia."[5]

Currently, hospice care provides home nursing, family support, spiritual counseling, pain treatment, medications, medical care, and inpatient care for the terminally ill. In 1994[9] approximately 340,000 terminally ill individuals received hospice care in the United States, and by 2020 approximately 1.72 million patients had received hospice services.[10] Since Congress enacted the Medicare hospice benefit in 1982, most hospice services have been paid for by Medicare. To qualify for hospice benefits, recipients of hospice care must be terminally ill, and their physician and the hospice medical director must certify that the patient will be expected to live for ≤6 months if their illness runs its normal course.[9]

Just as hospice care has grown outside of hospital settings, palliative medicine has developed as a discipline within general hospitals to address the "care and management of the physical, psychological, emotional, and spiritual needs of patients and their families with chronic, debilitating, or life threatening illness."[11] This includes creating goals of care, addressing symptoms (especially pain and respiratory distress), working with patients' families, and educating medical teams about the unique needs of the dying. More than a decade ago, the average patient was enrolled in hospice only one month before their death, and most such patients had cancer.[8]

Higher hospice utilization rates were found for those with diseases that impose a higher burden on caregivers or with diseases with a higher prognostic accuracy.[8] The three conditions with the highest hospice utilization rates were malignancies, dementia, and heart disease. Females have used hospice services more often than males, Whites more than Blacks, and, overall, close to one in four older Americans have used hospice services.[11] The average length of stay (LOS) of Medicare patients enrolled in hospice has increased; in 2013 the LOS was 72.6 days, whereas in 2018 the LOS rose to 89.6 days.[10] The number of palliative care programs has also grown rapidly; moreover, outpatient palliative care programs now provide transitions in care and continuity of care.

ROLE OF THE PSYCHIATRIST

Psychiatrists play a crucial role in the management of patients at the end of life because of their appreciation of the medical aspects of the disease, their understanding of the highly subjective and individual factors that contribute to the personal significance of illness, their understanding of personality styles and traits, and their engagement with patients to modulate maladaptive responses to illness. To this end, psychiatrists may serve many functions, including facilitating medical treatment as well as augmenting communication among the patient, the family, and the caregivers.

Above all, the psychiatrist's primary goals are the diagnosis and management of psychiatric symptoms and illnesses. As with other patients, factors that contribute to psychiatric suffering include biological illnesses, psychological style, psychosocial factors, and functional capacity. Studies indicate that psychiatric morbidity in the setting of terminal illness is very high.[11-15] The most common issues that lead to psychiatric interventions for dying patients include MDD, anxiety, personality disorders, delirium, refractory pain, SUDs, cognitive impairment, and difficulties surrounding bereavement.[12,13]

Depression

As people become more seriously ill, it is more likely for them to develop MDD—the prevalence rates of clinically significant depression in the terminally ill range from 20% to 70%.[11,12,15] Risk factors associated with the development of depression in people with cancer include a high disease burden, lower functionality, insecure attachments, low self-esteem, and younger age.[11,12] Ganzini and colleagues[14] reported that severely depressed patients made more restricted advance directives when depressed, and then changed them once their depression remitted.

Aggressive treatment of depression is a cornerstone of care, as it dramatically decreases suffering and improves quality of life.[15] In terms of specific treatments, psychiatrists may consider the use of treatments that target specific symptoms, including antidepressants (e.g., selective serotonin reuptake inhibitors) as well as more rapidly acting agents (e.g., psychostimulants) that target decreased energy and appetite.[16] Advantages of psychostimulants include a rapid onset of improved mood and the potentiation of co-administered narcotics with less sedation.

Thoughts of suicide should not be thought of as an "understandable" response but rather as a condition that warrants immediate investigation and treatment.[17]

Desire to Hasten Death

It is also important to differentiate thoughts of suicide from a desire for hastened death. In one study (based on those with chronic kidney disease on dialysis), suicide was distinguished from life-ending acts and end-of-life decisions.[17] The desire to hasten death was also identified in a minority of older females with terminal illnesses.[18] Although the desire to hasten death is frequently associated with depression, other factors (e.g., pain, existential concerns, loss of function, and social circumstances) also play a critical role.

Anxiety

Anxiety frequently occurs at the end of life and requires psychiatric attention.[19] Impending death can generate severe anxiety in people facing death, as well as in their family members, friends, and caregivers. The patient who experiences anxiety surrounding death may not necessarily be able to articulate his or her fears, which may be expressed as anger, isolative behavior, or worry. Common fears associated with death include helplessness or loss of control, feelings of guilt and punishment, physical pain or injury, and abandonment.[13] Psychiatrists can be helpful by addressing these fears and by exploring issues related to isolation, abandonment, and suffering. Mindfulness-based techniques to reduce stress and anxiety are effective. Appropriate attention should also be directed toward psychopharmacologic management of anxiety symptoms.[20]

Personality Traits and Disorders

The terminally ill patient with a personality disorder (such as narcissistic or borderline personality disorder) or with problematic coping (e.g., associated with a history of trauma or post-traumatic stress disorder) can be challenging for healthcare providers.

Such patients can find it difficult, if not impossible, to accept help and trust their caregivers. This interferes with a patient's ability to accept offers of comfort from others.[21] For these patients, much of their situation is out of their immediate control; this elicits regression and the use of more primitive defenses (such as splitting). This may manifest as poor communication with treaters, inadequate pain control, and difficulty with the resolution of interpersonal conflicts.[22] Psychiatrists may find it useful to call upon their psychodynamically informed diagnostic and treatment skills to assist patients in accepting palliative care. Symptom-focused psychotherapeutic management can limit patient aggression and self-destructiveness, as well as enhance staff empathy while working with the patient.[23] Working closely with the family and friends of the patient, as well as with the medical team, is important in these situations.

Delirium and Cognitive Changes

As terminal illness progresses, medical complications (such as delirium and other cognitive changes) can arise. These complications often manifest as confusion, psychosis, agitation, or a multitude of other symptoms, and they are caused by the medical illness, its treatment, or both. The medical and pharmacologic treatments for delirium are essential. Palliative care interventions should also be considered earlier in the course of a deteriorating dementia that is often accompanied by worsening delirium.[24] Effective management of changes in affect, behavior, and cognition that result from delirium or dementia is critical, as cognitive impairment can indicate worsening of medical illness and can adversely affect the quality of life, dignity, and time spent with friends, family, and caretakers.[24]

Pain

Pain management can be complex and requires extensive expertise. Freedom from pain is basic to every care plan, and it should be achievable in most cases.[25] For a multitude of reasons, pain is often undertreated by medical staff.[26] Pain management is challenging for patients with a history of SUD, and patients with a history of addiction are more likely to be inadequately treated for their pain than patients without a history of SUD or dependence.[27] The reasons for this include concerns about higher-than-expected (and possibly escalating) doses of opiates, potential misuse or diversion of these drugs, and fears of the legal consequences of prescribing narcotics to a patient with a SUD.[27,28] Evidence of abuse may include unexpectedly positive results on a toxicology screen, frequent requests for higher drug doses, recurrent reports of lost

prescriptions, and multiple visits to various providers or emergency departments for prescription refills.

Physicians who prescribe to patients with SUDs have conflicting opinions regarding the treatment of SUDs in terminally ill patients. Some physicians carefully monitor the use of opiates in terminally ill patients, while others actively treat the patient's SUD. Physicians frequently need to separate the management of pain from the management of addiction, and then treat both.

A uniform set of practices for the care of such patients is essential for the avoidance of patient and staff distress.[27] Specifically, careful monitoring of a patient's narcotic use, creation of a multi-disciplinary team, limitation of prescribing to a single provider, and utilizing screening tests (e.g., urine toxicology) may all be useful in the management of a terminally ill person with substance dependence.[29]

Psychosocial Considerations

Optimal end-of-life care requires an understanding of the major areas of psychosocial concern (such as family, work, religion, faith, ethnicity, and culture). Family involvement is crucial to help patients resolve long-standing conflicts and to provide a context for honoring and remembering the patient. Psychiatrists and other mental health professionals can facilitate this by encouraging the sharing of feelings among family members and by helping to create specific plans for the family (such as the compilation of commemorative items). At the same time, understanding the complexities of family interactions (both positive and negative) helps prevent harm to a potentially fragile family system. For example, a randomized clinical trial of family-focused grief therapy found that it could help prevent pathologic grief in family members; however, it had the potential to increase conflict in families where the level of hostility was high.[30] As with family relationships, a sense of vocational identity can create meaning for a patient at the end of life.

Some patients feel less valued when their work ceases or retirement arrives; the presence of former and current colleagues can be quite supportive.

Similarly, thoughtful discussion about a patient's beliefs and faith can provide an opportunity for a patient to further their sense of meaning and thoughts about an afterlife.[31] Many patients are grateful for the opportunity to express thoughts about their faith. The patient's own religious leader, if available, can often provide invaluable information and insights about the patient and family and help smooth the course before death.

Last, patients from underserved communities or minority populations in the United States may have needs that go unmet by the current healthcare system.[32] Unfortunately, the same institutional, cultural, and individual factors that generate disparities in care for minority populations also affect care at the end of life.[33] These factors include lack of access to care, under-treatment of pain, and mistrust of the healthcare system. Furthermore, important differences between ethnic groups and cultures can be found in all segments of end-of-life care.[34] There are also important differences in terms of preferences for life-sustaining treatment. For example, in a study involving multiple ethnic groups, African Americans had the highest rate of preferring life-sustaining treatment, and European Americans had the lowest rates.

Culture may influence the decision-making process.[35] For example, family centered (rather than individual) decision-making is common in certain ethnic groups in the United States, which challenges the traditional Western model of the importance of individual autonomy. Studies have found a higher use of family-centered decision-making among Latino and Asian groups in the United States, which may include the decision to disclose (or not to disclose) the diagnosis of a terminal illness to an individual patient.[35] Thus, attention to cultural competency by psychiatrists plays a significant role in mediating end-of-life care for patients of all ethnicities and cultures.

CHALLENGES FOR CARE PROVIDERS

The emotional intensity associated with providing empathy and support for the dying patient during a time of need may challenge and tire caregivers (such as family and professional staff). A critical skill in end-of-life care is being able to hold end-of-life discussions[36] and to listen to the patient and their families, asking open-ended questions.[37] End-of-life discussions with physicians have been associated with fewer aggressive interventions, which, in turn, are associated with improved quality of life and caregiver bereavement adjustment. Structured, proactive, multi-disciplinary

communication systems that include an ethics consultation and palliative care teams have also been shown to improve communication during critical care and end-of-life care for patients and their families.[38-40] Barriers to patient–physician communication about end-of-life care include physicians' own perceptions that the patient is not ill enough or is not ready to have the conversation.[40] Special considerations should be given to pediatric populations.

Caregivers may also experience helplessness and despair in the face of their powerlessness over a patient's approaching death.[41] If left unaddressed, these feelings in caregivers can cause the caregiver to avoid the patient, retreat, or even convey to him or her how burdensome he or she is to caregivers. This could be devastating to the helpless patient, who looks to the caregiver for hope. Hence, among the greatest psychological requirements for caregivers is to learn to live with negative feelings and to resist the urge to avoid the patient—actions that convey to the patient that he or she no longer matters. Certain traits make these empathic difficulties hazardous for some caregivers. Dependent persons who expect patients to appreciate, thank, love, and nurture them are unconsciously prone to exhaust themselves regularly because they "can never do enough." This creates a pattern that may be sustainable for a patient with the capacity to nurture the caregiver, but it could have a disastrous outcome if the patient is depleted or intractably hostile. The harder the caregiver strives, the less rewarding the work becomes. Exhaustion and demoralization follow. Some caregivers want to please every physician they consult, and they come to a similar state of exhaustion because many of these patients cannot improve. For example, several studies have shown that African American patients, as well as older individuals from other ethnic backgrounds (such as Latino, Asian, or Native American), are somewhat less likely to have arranged for an advance directive as compared with Caucasian patients.

ETHICS AND END-OF-LIFE CARE

Principles

End-of-life care carries a host of ethical questions that psychiatrists are likely to encounter. A brief discussion of principles is not intended to supplant the need for concrete, individualized judgments for every patient. Principles provide anchor points from which clinical reasoning can proceed—specifically when the limitation of life-supporting treatment is proposed.

The primary obligation of physicians to their patients in traditional medical ethics has been expressed in both positive and negative terms. The negative goal, always referred to first, is not to harm the patient (*primum non nocere*). The positive obligation is to restore health, relieve suffering, or both. Our contemporary dilemma arose because we now have many situations in which these two aims come into conflict (i.e., the more aggressive the efforts to reverse an incurable illness, the more suffering is inflicted on the patient).

A related problem is the difficulty in distinguishing treatments administered to relieve pain and suffering from those intended to hasten death. The principle of double effect is commonly used to allow the administration of narcotics and sedatives with the intent to relieve the suffering of dying patients, even though such administration may hasten death.

Second, modern medicine respects patients' right to autonomy. This principle guarantees a competent patient the right to refuse any treatment, even a life-saving one. This was the emphasis of the medical ethics of the 1970s and 1980s, and it focused on refusing life-prolonging treatments, such as mechanical ventilation, and more recently, nutrition and hydration. Honoring such refusals presupposes that the patient is competent. It is important to remember that competent patients may make decisions that providers may view as irrational.[38] However, a patient cannot insist that the physician provide treatment that is considered futile.[39] Defining futility continues to be a goal of medical ethics as a balance is forged between the autonomy interest of patients to opt for aggressive treatment and concern by physicians that there is a duty not to offer or provide ineffective treatments.

Limitation of Life-Sustaining Treatment

One salient concept for psychiatrists to understand is the limitation of life-sustaining treatment. Whenever the risks or burdens of a treatment appear to outweigh the benefits, the use of that treatment should be questioned by both the physician and the patient. The limitation of life-prolonging treatment is generally reserved for three categories of patients. First, patients who have an irreversible illness, who are moribund, and who need to be protected from needlessly burdensome treatments may refuse life-sustaining treatment. This is widely accepted for patients who will die with or without treatment (those with advanced metastatic cancer). Second, because of the right to refuse treatment, competent patients who are not moribund but who have an irreversible illness have also been allowed to have life-sustaining treatments stopped. Third, competent patients with a reversible illness have the right to refuse any treatment, including life-saving treatments.

However, complications emerge when a patient is unable to make or voice a decision regarding his or her wishes. In the absence of this information, it is often up to a surrogate decision-maker to decide what the patient would have wanted in these circumstances. If no surrogate decision-maker is available, then the medical team (often in consultation with the hospital's legal counsel) will resort to the "reasonable person standard," that is, asking what a "reasonable person" would opt to do in that situation.

One example is that of Karen Ann Quinlan, a 21-year-old female who, in 1976, developed a vegetative state/unwakefulness syndrome (VS/UWS) while at a party. This case became a legal battleground between the rights of Quinlan's mother (who, as her guardian, wished to withdraw life-sustaining treatment from her daughter and allow her daughter to die) and the state's interest in preserving life. In the end, the Supreme Court of New Jersey decided that, if it was believed, to a reasonable degree, that the VS/UWS was irreversible, and life-sustaining treatment (e.g., with a respirator) could be removed.[42] The Quinlan case marked the beginning of the now well-established right to refuse life-sustaining treatment; a right that extends to the competent, once competent, and never competent person, enacted through their surrogate decision-maker.[43]

For patients in VS/UWS[44] (a state in which patients have a functioning brainstem but total loss of cortical function), a complicated scenario emerges.[45] The diagnosis of VS/UWS is made when a patient, by clinical examination, is unaware of himself or herself and his or her environment, and there is a diminishing prospect of any change in this state as time passes.[46] There have been several notable legal cases of patients in VS/UWS (formerly called a persistent vegetative state [PVS]) where there was conflict centered around whether they could be allowed to die (most notably the Nancy Cruzan case).[47] The complicated scenario of the VS/UWS was encountered in the Theresa Schiavo case. In this highly public and controversial case, Theresa Schiavo was deemed to be in a PVS in 1990. In 1998, her husband, who was her legal guardian, wished to withdraw her life-sustaining nutrition and hydration, in accordance with what he believed her wishes would have been. However, her parents opposed the removal of the life-sustaining measures because they believed Mrs. Schiavo to be conscious.[48] This case highlights the confusion and controversy that surrounds the withdrawal of medical care for patients with a VS/UWS.[45] The case revived public debate about the withdrawal of life-sustaining treatment at the end of life. Many states debated the level of proof required to establish that an incompetent patient, when competent, would have opted to have his or her life-sustaining care withdrawn.

In general, the legal cases regarding end-of-life decision-making explicitly give patients the right to exercise their autonomy regarding what care they receive at the end of life. Competent patients can make these wishes known through their use of advance directives, which take effect once future incapacity arises, to make or express decisions about their care. These directives may be instructional, may appoint a substitute decision-maker, or both. Instructional directives place limits on life-sustaining treatment; however, they may be difficult to interpret on clinical grounds. Advance directives that appoint a substitute decision-maker with whom the patient has discussed his or her wishes may be a more flexible way to enact a patient's wishes. Specifically, a substitute decision-maker can use his or her knowledge of the patient's prior expressed wishes in combination with the actual clinical scenario to effect (more reliably) the outcome that the patient would have wanted if they were competent.

Physician-Assisted Suicide, Medical Aid in Dying, and Euthanasia

One study of terminally ill patients with cancer found that attitudes toward euthanasia and assisted suicide were determined by psychosocial traits and beliefs, including religious beliefs and perceptions of the amount of burden on families, rather than on symptom intensity or disease severity. Euthanasia, even when requested by the patient, is illegal in all 50 states and all US districts and territories, but it is legal in the Netherlands, Belgium, Colombia, Luxembourg, Canada, New Zealand, Spain, and Australia. Physicians are prohibited from administering life-ending medication or directly causing death through affirmative action throughout the United States.[49]

Unlike euthanasia, the practice of physician-assisted suicide or medical aid in dying, allows physicians to help patients acquire the means to end their lives but does not permit the physician to administer those means. Medical aid in dying has begun to gain acceptance in the United States. Medical aid in dying provides the patient, after safeguards to protect against abuse, are established in each state, with lethal medication to aid in death with dignity. Medical aid in dying is currently legal in eleven states: Oregon, Washington, California, Colorado, Hawaii, Montana, New Jersey, New Mexico, Maine, Vermont, and the District of Columbia.

Under the Oregon Death with Dignity Act (DWDA),[50] physicians in Oregon are permitted to write prescriptions for lethal doses of medications to patients who request to die and meet the other requirements of the state law. The specific prevalence of psychiatric symptoms in individuals requesting physician-assisted suicide has not been extensively characterized. One study of 58 Oregon residents who had requested aid in dying from a physician or who had contacted an aid-in-dying advocacy organization found that 15 participants met the criteria for depression and 13 for anxiety.[50] Three of the 18 participants in the study who received a prescription for a lethal drug under the DWDA met the criteria for depression.

Although patients have broad rights of autonomy in expressing their wishes for end-of-life care, there are limits to a patient's ability to control his or her death. Specifically, a patient may express the wish to have a physician end his or her life (euthanasia). However, euthanasia, even when requested by the patient, is illegal in all 50 states and all US districts and territories.

CONCLUSION

End-of-life care aims to maximize the quality of life and minimize the suffering of terminally ill patients.

For many patients, the end of life marks an important opportunity to reflect, reconcile, and pursue their remaining hopes. Psychiatrists can play an important role in the diagnosis and treatment of psychiatric illness in this setting, as well as in facilitating treatment, enhancing communication, and modeling caregiver qualities for families. From a psychiatric perspective, MDD and anxiety are commonly seen; suicidality should not be considered "understandable" or "normal" in this setting. Delirium, pain, and difficulties with coping are also common reasons for consultation requests. As in all other forms of psychiatric evaluation and treatment, it is crucial to consider any medical contribution to psychiatric symptoms. Aggressive treatment of depression, anxiety, and other psychiatric symptoms is a crucial part of holistic management. Additionally, psychosocial factors may play an important (and, at times, complicating) role in the care of these patients. Psychiatrists also should be aware of, and be prepared to manage, many of the complex ethical and legal issues that arise in the care of these patients. Physicians have clear obligations in caring for their patients, and patients have right to autonomy in their decision-making.

The diagnosis, options for treatment in line with goals of care, and prognosis are best presented openly to guide the patients, family, and friends on a path to a peaceful, comfortable death with pain well controlled. Then, the conversations can continue toward acceptance, sadness, and an opportunity to say goodbye. Sound clinical and ethical practice requires that physicians assist terminally ill patients through the complex and often simultaneous processes of grieving and celebrating, reconciling conflicts, completing unfinished business, achieving last hopes, and accepting unrealized goals while alleviating suffering and maximizing autonomy and personhood until death.[51]

REFERENCES

1. Murphy S, Xu J, Kochanek K, et al. Deaths: final data for 2018. *Natl Vital Stat Rep.* 2021;69:1–82.
2. Institute of Medicine.. *Dying in America: Improving Quality and Honoring Individual Preferences Near the End of Life. Committee on Approaching Death: Addressing Key End of Life Issues.* Institute of Medicine, National Academies Press; 2015.
3. Qaseem A, Snow V, Shekelle P, et al. Evidence-based interventions to improve the palliative care of pain, dyspnea, and depression at the end of life: a clinical practice guideline from the American College of Physicians. *Ann Intern Med.* 2008;148:141–146.
4. Truog R, Cist A, Brackett A, et al. Recommendations for end-of-life care in the intensive care unit: the Ethics Committee of the Society of Critical Care Medicine. *Crit Care Med.* 2001;29:2332–2348.
5. Saunders C, ed.*The Management of Terminal Illness.* Year Book Medical;; 1978.
6. Kübler-Ross E.*On Death and Dying.* MacMillan; 1969.
7. Hackett T, Weisman A. The treatment of the dying. *Curr Psychiatr Ther.* 1962;2:121.
8. Gawande A. Quantity and quality of life: duties of care in life-limiting illness. *JAMA.* 2016;315(3):267–269.
9. Obermeyer Z, Makar M, Abujaber S. Association between the medicare hospice benefit and health care utilization and costs for the patient with poor prognosis. *JAMA.* 2014;312:1888–1896.
10. National Hospice and Palliative Care Organization. *Hospice Facts and Figures.* 2022
11. Blinderman CD, Billings JA. Comfort care for patients dying in the hospital. *N Engl J Med.* 2015;373(26):2549–2561.
12. Massie MJ. Prevalence of depression in patients with cancer. *J Natl Cancer Inst Monogr.* 2004(32):57–71.
13. Berens N, Kim SY. Rapid-response treatments for depression and requests for physician-assisted death: an ethical analysis. *Am J Geriatr Psychiatry.* 2022;30(11):1255–1262.
14. Ganzini L, Goy ER, Dobscha SK. Prevalence of depression and anxiety in patients requesting physicians' aid in dying: cross sectional survey. *BMJ.* 2008;337:a1682.
15. Rosenstein DL. Depression and end of life care for patients with cancer. *Dialogues in Clin Neurosci.* 2011;13:101–108.
16. Lee W, Chang S, DiGiacomo M, et al. Caring for depression in the dying is complex and challenging – survey of palliative physicians. *BMC Palliat Care.* 2022;21:11.
17. Bostwick J, Cohen L. Differentiating suicide from life-ending acts and end of life decisions: a model based on chronic kidney disease and dialysis. *Psychosomatics.* 2009;50:1–7.
18. Canetto SS, McIntosh JL. A comparison of physician-assisted/death-with-dignity-act death and suicide patterns in older adult women and men. *Am J Geriatr Psychiatry.* 2022;30:211–220.
19. Koslov E, Phongtankuel V, Prigerson H, et al. Prevalence, severity, and correlates of symptoms of anxiety and depression at the very end of life. *J Pain Symptom Manage.* 2019;58:80–85.
20. Szuhany KL, Simon NM. Anxiety disorders: a review. *JAMA.* 2022;328:2431–2445.
21. Hay JL, Passik SD. The cancer patient with borderline personality disorder: suggestions for symptom-focused management in the medical setting. *Psychooncology.* 2000;9:91–100.
22. Meyer F, Block S. Personality disorders in the oncology setting. *J Support Oncol.* 2011;9(2):44–51.
23. Terpstra TL, Williamson S. Palliative care for terminally ill individuals with borderline personality disorder. *J Psychosoc Nurs Ment Health Serv.* 2019;57(9):24–31.
24. Agar MR. Delirium at the end of life. *Age Ageing.* 2020;49:337–340.
25. Soares L, Chan V. The rationale for a multimodal approach in the management of breakthrough cancer pain: a review. *Am J Hosp Palliat Care.* 2007;24:430–439.
26. Ballantyne J, Mao J. Opioid therapy for chronic pain. *N Engl J Med.* 2003;349:1943–1953.

27. Gunnarsdottir S, Donovan HS, Ward S. Interventions to overcome clinician- and patient-related barriers to pain management. *Nurs Clin North Am*. 2003;38:419–434.

28. Kirsh KL, Passik SD. Palliative care of the terminally ill drug addict. *Cancer Invest*. 2006;24:425–431.

29. Renner JA, Ross JD, Gastfriend DR, et al. Drug-addicted patients. In: Stern TA, Fricchione GL, Cassem NH, eds. *Massachusetts General Hospital Handbook of General Hospital Psychiatry*. 6thed. Saunders; 2010.

30. Kissane DW, McKenzie M, Bloch S, et al. Family focused grief therapy: a randomized, controlled trial in palliative care and bereavement. *Am J Psychiatry*. 2006;163:1208–1218.

31. Rodin G, Mikulincer M, et al. Pathways to distress: the multiple determinants of depression, hopelessness, and the desire for hastened death in metastatic cancer patients. *Soc Sci Med*. 2009;68:562–569.

32. Krakauer EL, Crenner C, Fox K. Barriers to optimum end-of-life care for minority patients. *J Am Geriatr Soc*. 2002;50:182–190.

33. Siriwardena AN, Clark DH. End-of-life care for ethnic minority groups. *Clin Cornerstone*. 2006;6(1):43–48. discussion 49.

34. Perkins H, Geppert C, Gonzales A, et al. Cross-cultural similarities and differences in attitudes about advance care planning. *J Gen Intern Med*. 2002;17(1):48–57.

35. Kwak J, Haley W. Current research finding on end-of-life decision making among racially or ethnically diverse groups. *Gerontologist*. 2005;45(5):634–641.

36. Laury ER, MacKenzie-Greenle M, Meghani S. Advance care planning outcomes in African Americans: an empirical look at the trust variable. *J Palliat Med*. 2019;22(4):442–451.

37. Lo B. *Resolving Ethical Dilemmas*. 6th ed. Wolters Kluwer; 2020.

38. Brock DW, Wartman SA. When competent patients make irrational choices. *N Engl J Med*. 1990;322:1595–1599.

39. Luce J. Physicians do not have a responsibility to provide futile or unreasonable care if a patient or family insists. *Crit Care Med*. 1995;23(4):760–766.

40. Bernat JL. Medical futility: definition, determination, and disputes in critical care. *Neurocrit Care*. 2005;2(2):198–205.

41. Helft PR, Siegler M, Lantos J. The rise and fall of the futility movement. *N Engl J Med*. 2000;343:293–296.

42. Fine RL. From Quinlan to Schiavo: medical, ethical, and legal issues in severe brain injury. *Proc Bayl Univ Med Cent*. 2005;18:303–310.

43. Cantor NL. Twenty-five years after Quinlan: a review of the jurisprudence of death and dying. *J Law Med Ethics*. 2001;29(2):182–196.

44. Giacino JT, Katz DI, Schiff ND, et al. Practice guidelines update recommendations summary: disorders of consciousness. *Arch Physical Med Rehabil*. 2018;99:1699–1709.

45. Wade DT. Ethical issues in diagnosis and management of patients in the permanent vegetative state. *BMJ*. 2001;322:352–354.

46. Peterson A, Young MJ, Fins JJ, et al. Ethics and the 2018 practice guidelines on disorders of consciousness: a framework for responsible implementation. *Neurology*. 2022;98:712–718.

47. Annas GJ, Arnold B, Aroskar M, et al. Bioethicists' statement on the U.S. Supreme Court's Cruzan decision. *N Engl J Med*. 1990;323:686–688.

48. Perry JE, Churchill LR, Kirshner HS. The Terri Schiavo case: legal, ethical, and medical perspectives. *Ann Intern Med*. 2005;15(143):744–748.

49. Emanuel EJ, Onwuteaka-Philipsen BD, Urwin JW, Cohen J. Attitudes and practices of euthanasia and physician-assisted suicide in the United States. *JAMA*. 2016;316:79–90.

50. Ganzini L, Nelson H, Schmidt T, et al. Physicians' experiences with the Oregon Death with Dignity Act. *N Eng J Med*. 2000;342:557–563.

51. Kelley AS, Morrison RS. Palliative care for the seriously Ill. *N Engl J Med*. 2015;373:747–755.

46

PSYCHIATRIC ILLNESS DURING PREGNANCY AND THE POSTPARTUM PERIOD

CHARLOTTE S. HOGAN, MD ▪ BETTY WANG, MD ▪ MARLENE P. FREEMAN, MD ▪ RUTA NONACS, MD, PHD ▪ LEE S. COHEN, MD

OVERVIEW

Psychiatric consultation with obstetric patients typically involves evaluating and treating an array of psychopathology. Once thought to be a time of emotional well-being for women, studies now suggest that pregnancy does not protect women from the emergence or persistence of psychiatric disorders.[1,2] Because many psychiatric conditions are chronic or recurrent and have high prevalence rates in women during the reproductive years, many females become pregnant while receiving psychiatric treatment. Given the possibility of unplanned pregnancies, females of reproductive age should know the risks and benefits of their medications, even if they are not planning to become pregnant.

Optimally, a woman and her psychiatrist should plan for a pregnancy and assess the risks and benefits of treatment before conception. Ideally, this planning helps avoid abrupt cessation of medications because of fear of exposing the fetus to medication, which is important because rapid discontinuation of medication increases the risk of relapse of mood episodes during pregnancy.[3] Medications with relatively benign reproductive safety profiles should be used as first-line agents in females of reproductive potential. The risks of untreated psychiatric disorders during pregnancy include pre-term delivery, low birth weight, poor nutrition, poor prenatal care, substance use (such as cigarettes or alcohol), and termination of the pregnancy.[4] In addition, untreated psychiatric disorders during pregnancy have been associated with altered developmental trajectories in infancy and childhood.[5]

Depression during pregnancy is also a strong predictor of postpartum depression,[6] a condition that can have dire consequences for the mother, the baby, and the entire family. Therefore, it is critical to sustain maternal emotional well-being during pregnancy.

Pregnancy is an emotionally laden experience that evokes a spectrum of normal reactions, including heightened anxiety and increased mood reactivity. Psychiatric evaluation of pregnant females requires careful assessment of symptoms (e.g., anxiety or depression) and decisions about the nature of those symptoms, including normative or pathologic manifestations of a new-onset psychiatric disorder, and exacerbation of a previously diagnosed or undiagnosed psychiatric disorder. The American College of Obstetricians and Gynecologists and the US Preventive Services Task Force released formal recommendations calling for depression screening of all pregnant and postpartum women, with an emphasis placed on adequate systems to ensure treatment and follow-up after screening.[7] Screening for depression during pregnancy followed by thoughtful treatment can minimize maternal morbidity as well as the potential impact of an untreated psychiatric disorder on infant development and family functioning.

Treatment of psychiatric disorders during pregnancy involves a thoughtful weighing of the risks and benefits of proposed interventions (e.g., pharmacologic treatments) against the risks associated with untreated psychiatric disorders. In contrast to many other clinical conditions, treatment of psychiatric disorders during pregnancy is typically reserved for situations in which the disorder interferes in a significant fashion with maternal and fetal well-being; the threshold for treating psychiatric disorders during pregnancy tends to be higher than with other conditions. Women with similar illness histories often make different decisions about their care in collaboration with their physicians during pregnancy.

DIAGNOSIS AND TREATMENT OF MOOD DISORDERS DURING PREGNANCY

Studies suggest that rates of major and minor depression in gravid females (approximating 10% to 15%) are similar to those in non-gravid females.[8] Females with a history of major depressive disorder (MDD) appear to be at particularly high risk for recurrence of depression during pregnancy, especially when antidepressants have been discontinued.[3]

Making the diagnosis of depression during pregnancy can be difficult because disturbances in sleep and appetite, fatigue, and changes in libido do not always indicate an evolving affective illness. Clinical features that can support the diagnosis of MDD include anhedonia, feelings of guilt and hopelessness, poor self-esteem, and thoughts of suicide. In addition, symptoms that interfere with function signal a psychiatric condition that warrants treatment. Screening tools, such as the Edinburgh Postnatal Depression Scale (EPDS), a 10-item self-report questionnaire, validated for use during pregnancy and the postpartum period, exclude common constitutional symptoms of pregnancy. The EPDS may also be used to identify females with an anxiety disorder; however, screeners more specific to anxiety disorders, such as the Perinatal Anxiety Screening Scale, a 31-item self-report questionnaire, are also available. Suicidal ideation is not uncommon during pregnancy; however, the risk of clear-cut, self-injurious, or suicidal behavior appears to be relatively low in females who develop depression during pregnancy.[9]

Treatment for depression during pregnancy is determined by the severity of the underlying disorder, by a history of treatment responses, and by individual patient preferences. Neurovegetative symptoms that interfere with maternal well-being require treatment. Females with mild-to-moderate depressive symptoms may benefit from non-pharmacologic treatments that include supportive psychotherapy,[10] cognitive-behavioral therapy (CBT),[11] or interpersonal therapy (IPT),[12] each of which has been shown to ameliorate depressive symptoms during pregnancy.

Antidepressants

Selective serotonin reuptake inhibitors (SSRIs) are the first-line agents for the treatment of depression and anxiety and are the best-characterized antidepressants in pregnancy and lactation. The prevalence of antidepressant use is roughly 10% to 15% in reproductive-aged females and 7% in pregnant females.[13] As is the case with other medications, four types of risk are typically cited with respect to the potential use of antidepressants during pregnancy: risk of pregnancy loss or miscarriage, risk of organ malformation or teratogenesis, risk of neonatal toxicity or withdrawal syndromes during the acute neonatal period, and risk of long-term neuro-behavioral sequelae. In the past, a system established by the US Food and Drug Administration (FDA) that classified medications into five risk categories (A, B, C, D, and X), was used to inform physicians and patients about the reproductive safety of various prescription medications. In this system, medications in category A were designated safe for use during pregnancy, whereas category X drugs were contraindicated because of known risks to the fetus that outweighed any benefit to the mother. This system of classification had noteworthy limitations. First, categorization was often ambiguous and could lead to unwarranted conclusions. Second, the categorization was often assigned based on a small amount of animal data when human data were sparse or absent. Third, when larger and more rigorous studies became available on the reproductive safety profile of a medication, the category was rarely altered. Finally the categorization system failed to account for the risks of an untreated maternal psychiatric disorder for the female and her fetus. For these reasons, in June 2015 the FDA replaced this system with the Pregnancy and Lactation Labeling Rule, which requires descriptive safety information regarding pregnancy and lactation on the drug label. This includes a risk summary, clinical considerations, and data subsections for use in pregnancy, lactation, and treatment of patients with reproductive potential.[14] The letter classification system has been abolished and replaced by these more nuanced descriptions.

Randomized, placebo-controlled studies that examine the effects of medication use on pregnant patients are lacking and are largely considered unethical. Studies that have evaluated the reproductive safety of antidepressants have used a rigorous prospective design, or they have relied on large administrative databases or multi-center birth-defect surveillance programs. The following paragraphs provide an overview of currently available data on antidepressant use during pregnancy with regard to the risk of pregnancy loss or miscarriage, the risk of organ malformation or teratogenesis, the risk of neonatal toxicity or withdrawal syndromes during the acute neonatal period, and the risk of long-term neuro-behavioral sequelae.

Studies have not demonstrated a statistically increased risk of spontaneous miscarriage following prenatal exposure to antidepressants. When compared with females with depression, females on antidepressants do not experience a higher rate of miscarriage.[15]

Regarding teratogenic risk, SSRIs have been studied extensively for safety during pregnancy, although more limited data are available for less commonly prescribed SSRIs, such as fluvoxamine, and newer SSRIs, such as vortioxetine. Large studies are reassuring; as a group of medicines, SSRIs are not major teratogens and do not increase the risk of congenital malformation above the baseline incidence in any pregnancy.[16] Initial reports that suggested that paroxetine was associated with an increased risk of cardiac defects have not been duplicated in more recent studies, including independent, peer-reviewed, comprehensive meta-analyses of studies assessing paroxetine exposure during the first trimester.[17] Therefore, like other SSRIs, paroxetine may still be considered a first-line agent for females who have responded well to it before becoming pregnant.

More limited data is available on the use of serotonin-norepinephrine reuptake inhibitors (SNRIs), such as venlafaxine and duloxetine. Recent reports are reassuring, in that they have not demonstrated an increased risk of congenital malformations in infants exposed to duloxetine or venlafaxine above the background risk.[18,19]

Bupropion may be an attractive option for females who have not responded well to SSRIs or tricyclic antidepressants (TCAs). Most data thus far have not indicated an increased risk of malformations associated with bupropion use during pregnancy. However, several studies have observed a small increase in the risk of cardiovascular defects, specifically left ventricular outflow tract obstructions and ventricular septal defects. These studies have had several limitations, including potential confounding by indication, but it appears that the absolute risk is still relatively low (2.1–2.8 per 1000 births).[20]

Three prospective, and more than 10 retrospective, studies have examined the risk of organ malformation in over 400 cases of first-trimester exposure to TCAs. Both when evaluated on an individual basis and when pooled as a class, these studies have not found a significant association between fetal exposure to TCAs (except for clomipramine, which may increase the risk of cardiac defects) and the risk of any major congenital anomaly.[21] Among the TCAs, desipramine and nortriptyline are often preferred since they are less anticholinergic and are the least likely to exacerbate the orthostatic hypotension that may occur during pregnancy.

Limited information is available on other antidepressants, including mirtazapine, trazodone, vortioxetine, vilazodone, and esketamine. When possible, females taking these medications should, in general, switch to an antidepressant with a better-characterized reproductive safety profile. Scant information is available regarding the reproductive safety of monoamine oxidase inhibitors, and these agents are generally not used during pregnancy as they may produce a hypertensive crisis when combined with tocolytic medications, such as terbutaline.

Despite the growing literature that supports the relative safety of fetal exposure to SSRIs, some newborns who were exposed to SSRIs exhibit a transient period (limited to several days following delivery) of jitteriness, tachypnea, and tremulousness.[22] In general, this neonatal syndrome is a mild and benign syndrome that does not require any specific medical interventions.

Early reports raised a question about whether SSRI use later in pregnancy is associated with a serious but rare developmental lung condition, persistent pulmonary hypertension of the newborn (PPHN). More recent research has been reassuring, with multiple large studies showing that the risk is much lower than initially estimated, or even that there is no association between SSRI use and PPHN.[23] Importantly, PPHN is correlated with multiple risk factors, including cesarean section, race, body mass index, and other factors not associated with SSRI use.

Compared with the considerable data on the risk of congenital malformations with prenatal antidepressant exposure, reproductive safety data regarding the long-term effects of prenatal antidepressant exposure on the developing fetal brain are more limited. While previous studies yielded conflicting, albeit overall reassuring, findings, a recent study of over 145,500 exposed children did not find an increased risk of neurodevelopmental disorders (e.g., autism spectrum disorder, attention-deficit/hyperactivity disorder [ADHD], specific learning disorders, developmental speech/language disorder, developmental coordination disorder, intellectual disability, or behavioral disorders).[24]

Pharmacologic Treatment of Depression: Clinical Guidelines

Despite the growing number of reviews on the subject, the management of perinatal depression is still largely guided by experience, with few definitive data and no controlled treatment studies to inform management. The best treatment algorithms depend on the severity of the disorder, the patient's psychiatric history, her current symptoms, her attitude toward the use of psychiatric medications during pregnancy, and, ultimately, the patient's wishes. Clinicians must work collaboratively with the patient to arrive at the safest treatment plan that is based on currently available information.

In patients with mild depression, it is reasonable to consider discontinuation of pharmacologic therapy during pregnancy. Several psychotherapy modalities have reduced depressive symptoms during pregnancy.[25,26] Close monitoring of affective status is essential throughout pregnancy for females with a history of a mood disorder, regardless of whether their medication is continued or discontinued. Psychiatrically ill females are at high risk for relapse during pregnancy, and early detection and treatment of recurrent illness can significantly reduce the morbidity associated with having prenatal affective illness.

Many women who discontinue antidepressants during pregnancy experience recurrent depressive symptoms.[27] In one study, women who discontinued their medications were five times more likely to relapse (with a rate of relapse of 68%)[1] as compared to females

who maintained their antidepressants throughout their pregnancy. Thus, women with recurrent or refractory depressive illness may decide (in collaboration with their clinician) that the safest option is to continue pharmacologic treatment during pregnancy to minimize the risk of recurrent illness. In this setting, the clinician should attempt to select medications during pregnancy that have a well-characterized reproductive safety profile that might obviate switching to one with a better reproductive safety profile.

In an ideal world, switching to the best-studied medications would occur before becoming pregnant and would allow time for stabilization on a new medication. In other situations, one may decide to use a medication for which information regarding reproductive safety is sparse – for example, a woman with refractory depression who has responded only to one specific antidepressant for which data on reproductive safety are limited (e.g., mirtazapine). She may choose to continue this medication during pregnancy rather than risk relapse, which is associated with discontinuing the antidepressant or switching to another antidepressant for which the patient has no history of response.

Women can also experience a new onset of depressive symptoms during pregnancy. For females who present with minor depressive symptoms, non-pharmacologic treatments should be explored first. IPT or CBT may be beneficial for reducing the severity of depressive symptoms, and they can limit or obviate the need for medications. In general, pharmacologic treatment is pursued when non-pharmacologic strategies have failed or when it is felt that the risks associated with psychiatric illness during pregnancy outweigh the risks of fetal exposure to a specific medication.

In situations in which pharmacologic treatment is more clearly indicated, the clinician should select medications with the safest reproductive profile. SSRIs, with extensive data that support their reproductive safety, can be considered first-line choices. The TCAs and bupropion have also been relatively well characterized and can be considered reasonable treatment options during pregnancy.

When prescribing medications during pregnancy, an attempt should be made to simplify the medication regimen. For instance, one may select a more sedating antidepressant for a woman who presents with depression and sleep disturbance, instead of using a more activating antidepressant in combination with trazodone or a benzodiazepine.

In addition, the clinician must use an adequate dosage of medication to achieve or maintain remission. Often, the dosage of a medication is reduced during pregnancy to limit the risk to the fetus. However, this type of treatment modification might instead place the patient at greater risk for recurrent illness. During pregnancy, changes in plasma volume and increases in hepatic metabolism and renal clearance can significantly affect drug levels.[28] Several investigators have described a reduction (up to 65%) in serum levels of TCAs during pregnancy.[29] Sub-therapeutic levels may be associated with depressive relapse; therefore, an increase in daily antidepressant dosage may be required to obtain remission.

With multiple studies supporting the finding of transient neonatal jitteriness, tremulousness, and tachypnea associated with peripartum use of SSRIs,[30] some physicians have suggested discontinuing antidepressants just before delivery to minimize the risk of neonatal toxicity. Another potential rationale for discontinuing antidepressants before delivery is derived from the assumption that this would attenuate the risk of PPHN that has been associated with third-trimester exposure to SSRIs. However, this recommendation is not data driven and such a practice can carry significant risk because it withdraws treatment from a patient precisely as she is about to enter the postpartum period, a time of heightened risk for affective illness. In consideration of the well-characterized risks to the baby and siblings in the family of a woman with maternal depression, treatment goals should include having a woman approach the postpartum period in remission from depression. The strategy of discontinuing medication before delivery, however, would increase the risk of a patient entering the postpartum period with depression, and recovery could require substantial time.

Severely depressed patients who are acutely suicidal or psychotic require hospitalization and treatment; electroconvulsive therapy (ECT) is often selected as the treatment of choice. Reviews of ECT during pregnancy note the efficacy and safety of this procedure.[31] In a review of the 339 cases of ECT during pregnancy published since 1941, only 11 of the 25 fetal or neonatal complications, including two deaths, were likely the result of ECT.[31] Given its relative safety, ECT may also be considered an alternative to conventional pharmacotherapy for women who wish to avoid extended exposure to psychotropics during pregnancy or for females who fail to respond to standard antidepressants.[32]

BIPOLAR DISORDER

Case 1

Ms. A, a 31-year-old professional with a psychiatric history of bipolar disorder (BPD) type I, presents for consultation regarding pregnancy planning. She and her husband would like to conceive soon, and she seeks guidance on the safety of pregnancy given her psychiatric history and her medication regimen.

On interview, Ms. A was alert and engaged, presenting with a stable euthymic mood. She describes having had two manic episodes for which she was psychiatrically hospitalized. Since starting lithium monotherapy 3 years ago, her mood has remained stable.

After gathering a complete psychiatric, medical, gynecologic, family, and social history, the consulting psychiatrist engages Ms. A in a thoughtful discussion of the risks of mood disturbance during and after pregnancy, in addition to a discussion of the risks and benefits of various psychiatric treatments during and after pregnancy. Based on this discussion, Ms. A decided to plan for a pregnancy while continuing lithium monotherapy during pregnancy and the postpartum period. She and her psychiatrist plan for close follow-up and monitoring.

Historically, women with BPD have been counseled to defer pregnancy (given an apparent need for pharmacologic therapy with mood stabilizers) or to terminate pregnancies following prenatal exposure to drugs such as lithium or valproic acid. However, more recent and comprehensive data suggest that women can select treatment strategies that allow pregnancy with both the mother's and baby's safety in mind.

The risk of lithium exposure during pregnancy has been re-assessed and is considered far safer than it was decades ago. Concerns regarding fetal exposure to lithium, for example, have typically been based on early reports of higher rates of cardiovascular malformations (e.g., Ebstein anomaly) following prenatal exposure to this drug. While it is still thought to increase the risk of this rare condition, data suggest that the absolute risk of cardiovascular malformations following pre-natal exposure to lithium is quite low. In the general population, Ebstein anomaly occurs in 1/20,000 live births; with first-trimester lithium exposure, the risk is estimated as being at most 1/1000.[33] There appears to be a dose-response relationship between lithium and Ebstein anomaly. The risk of cardiac malformations at doses above 900 mg/day is three times higher than with doses below 600 mg/day, although not every women's illness may be effectively managed at such low doses.

Women may elect to proceed in various ways, given this risk. Potential options include continuing lithium, discontinuing lithium with the potential for re-intro-ducing lithium after the first trimester or at delivery, or switching to another mood-stabilizing agent. Prenatal screening with a high-resolution ultrasound and fetal echocardiography is recommended at about 16 to 18 weeks of gestation to screen for cardiac anomalies. A woman with BPD faced with a decision regarding the use of lithium during pregnancy may be appro-priately counseled about the very small risk of organ dysgenesis associated with prenatal exposure to this medicine. No clear consensus has been reached as to lithium blood level monitoring during pregnancy, although it should be noted that lithium levels decline during pregnancy. While some providers elect to adjust lithium only if symptoms emerge, others choose to follow levels closely and keep lithium levels within the therapeutic range.

Lamotrigine has emerged as a preferred agent for reproductive-aged women with BPD when clinically appropriate, although it has limited benefits in treating or preventing manic episodes. Well-studied by several preg-nancy registries, lamotrigine does not appear to increase the risk of major congenital malformations above that of the general population. Although early data raised concern for an increased risk of oral clefts following lamotrigine exposure, larger registries have not observed this association.[34] Dosing of lamotrigine must be care-fully considered as rising levels of estrogen in pregnancy decrease lamotrigine levels by up to 50%. Levels return to pre-pregnancy levels within 3 to 4 weeks following

delivery. Close monitoring of symptoms throughout pregnancy is essential, and dose changes may be made based on clinical indications.

Compared with lithium and lamotrigine, prenatal exposure to some anticonvulsants is associated with a far greater risk of organ malformation. Exposure to valproic acid in the first 2 months of gestation increases the risk of neural tube defects (with an adjusted odds ratio of 19.4), ventricular/atrial septal defects, pulmonary valve atresia, hypoplastic left heart syndrome, cleft palate, anorectal atresia, and hypospa-dias.[35] In addition, valproic acid has been associated with serious neurocognitive developmental anomalies, including a lower intelligence quotient and impaired cognition across several domains in children who were exposed in utero.[36] Valproic acid exposure before birth also appears to increase the risk of autism and attention-deficit disorders later in childhood.[36] Ideally, females of reproductive age should avoid treatment with valproate, and it should not be considered a first-line therapy in females with reproductive potential. No significant increase in neurodevelopmental disorders was found among children exposed to carbamazepine or lamotrigine. Information about the reproductive safety of other anticonvulsants sometimes used in patients with BPD (including gabapentin, oxcarbaze-pine, and topiramate) remains sparse.

Prenatal screening for congenital malformations following anticonvulsant exposure (including cardiac anomalies) with fetal ultrasound at 18 to 22 weeks' ges-tation is recommended. The possibility of fetal neural tube defects should be evaluated with maternal serum alpha-fetoprotein and ultrasonography. In addition, 4 mg a day of folic acid before conception and in the first trimester for females receiving anticonvulsants is often recommended. However, the supplemental use of folic acid to attenuate the risk of neural tube defects in the setting of anticonvulsant exposure has not been systematically evaluated.

Whereas the use of mood stabilizers (including lithium and some anticonvulsants) has become the mainstay of treatment for managing both acute mania and the maintenance phase of BPD, most patients with BPD are not treated with monotherapy. Rather, the use of adjunctive conventional and newer antipsychot-ics has become a common clinical practice for many patients with BPD.

To date, abundant data exist that support the reproductive safety of typical antipsychotics, and no definitive association between typical antipsychotic administration during pregnancy and the risk of congenital malformations has been identified.[37] There is growing, albeit more limited data, on the reproductive safety of the second-generation, "atypical" antipsychotic (SGA) medications. A recent review, including a meta-analysis, two large observational studies, and nearly 14,000 infants with prenatal SGA exposure, is reassuring. Thus far, no consistent increased risk for major congenital malformations has been observed. However, these studies included mostly exposures to risperidone, olanzapine, quetiapine, and aripiprazole; there is much less data on the newer, less commonly prescribed agents, such as lurasidone, asenapine, and cariprazine.[38] An atypical antipsychotic may be the optimal treatment for a pregnant female with BPD who has responded to that medication in the past.

Patients with a history of a single episode of mania and prompt full recovery, followed by sustained well-being, may tolerate discontinuation of a mood stabilizer before an attempt to conceive. Unfortunately, even among women with a history of prolonged well-being and sustained euthymia, discontinuation of prophylaxis for mania may be associated with subsequent relapse during pregnancy.

For women with BPD and a history of multiple and frequent recurrences of mania or bipolar depression, several options can be considered. Some patients may choose to discontinue a mood stabilizer before conception (as described earlier). An alternative strategy for this high-risk group is to continue treatment until pregnancy is verified and then taper off the mood stabilizer. Because uteroplacental circulation is not established until approximately 2 weeks after conception, the risk of fetal exposure is minimal. Home pregnancy tests are reliable and can document pregnancy as early as 10 days following conception, and with a home ovulation predictor kit, a patient may be able to time her treatment discontinuation accurately. This strategy minimizes fetal exposure to drugs and extends the protective treatment up to the time of conception, which may be particularly prudent for older patients because the time required for them to conceive may be longer than for younger patients. However, a significant potential problem with this strategy is that it can lead to relatively abrupt discontinuation of treatment, thereby placing the patient at increased risk for relapse. This strategy would require close clinical follow-up, so that patients could be monitored for early signs of relapse, and medications may be re-introduced as needed.

Another problem with the strategy of discontinuing mood stabilizers when the patient is being treated with valproic acid is that the teratogenic effect of valproic acid occurs early in gestation (between weeks 4 and 5), often before the patient knows she is pregnant. In such a scenario, any potential teratogenic insult from valproic acid may have already occurred by the time the patient documents the pregnancy.

For women who tolerate discontinuation of maintenance treatment, the decision of when to resume treatment is a matter of clinical judgment. Some patients and clinicians prefer to await the initial appearance of symptoms before re-starting medication; others prefer to limit their risk of a major recurrence by re-starting treatment after the first trimester of pregnancy since euthymia during pregnancy reduces the risk of postpartum mood episodes.

For women with particularly severe forms of BPD, such as with multiple severe episodes, and especially with psychosis and prominent thoughts of suicide, maintenance treatment with a mood stabilizer before and during pregnancy is strongly recommended. Many patients who are treated with sodium valproate or other anticonvulsants, such as gabapentin, for which there are particularly sparse reproductive safety data, never received a lithium trial before pregnancy. For such patients, a lithium trial before pregnancy may be a reasonable option.

Even if all psychotropics have been safely discontinued, pregnancy in a woman with BPD should be considered a high-risk pregnancy, because the risk of major psychiatric illness during pregnancy is increased in the absence of treatment with a mood-stabilizing medication, and it is even higher in the postpartum period. Extreme vigilance is required for the early detection of an impending relapse of illness, and rapid intervention can significantly reduce morbidity and improve the overall prognosis. Therefore, close monitoring with assessments of mood, sleep, and other symptoms is urged throughout pregnancy and during the immediate postpartum period.

The risk for relapse and chronicity following discontinuation of mood stabilizers is high; therefore, clinicians and women with BPD who are either pregnant or who wish to conceive must weigh the risks and benefits of medication carefully against the risks of symptom relapse and the consequences this has for both mother and fetus.

PSYCHOTIC DISORDERS

Acute psychosis during pregnancy is an obstetric and psychiatric emergency. Like other psychiatric symptoms of new onset, the first onset of psychosis during pregnancy requires a systematic evaluation. Psychosis during pregnancy may interfere with a woman's ability to care for herself, obtain appropriate and necessary prenatal care, and cooperate with caregivers during delivery. Psychosis during pregnancy is associated with adverse pregnancy outcomes, including a higher risk of operative delivery, ante/postpartum hemorrhage, placental abruption, pre-term delivery, premature rupture of membranes, poor fetal growth, fetal distress, and stillbirth.[39]

Treatment of psychosis during pregnancy may include the use of either typical or atypical antipsychotics. Regarding the typical antipsychotics, high-potency neuroleptics, such as haloperidol, are preferred because lower-potency antipsychotics have some historical data for possible increased risk of congenital malformations associated with prenatal exposure.[40] However, their use is not contraindicated. Atypical antipsychotics have recently been the subject of several large studies regarding reproductive safety data.[38] These are largely reassuring, and to date, do not identify any significant or consistent risk of major malformation with atypical antipsychotic exposure during pregnancy.

Psychiatric consultation may be requested to consider treatment options for mild or intermittent symptoms of psychosis or for pregnant females with chronic mental illness, such as schizophrenia, who have discontinued therapy with neuroleptics. Although as-needed neuroleptics are appropriate for treating milder symptoms of psychosis, introduction or re-introduction of maintenance antipsychotics should be considered in women with schizophrenia who have a new-onset illness or a recurrent disorder. This approach can limit overall exposure to these drugs by reducing the need for treatment with higher doses of drugs during relapse. Patients with florid psychosis during labor and delivery might benefit from intravenous (IV) haloperidol, which can facilitate the patient's cooperation with the obstetrician, thereby enhancing the overall safety of the delivery.

Decisions regarding the use of these agents and other psychotropics must be made on a case-by-case basis. Patients taking an antipsychotic drug may choose to discontinue their medication or switch to a better-characterized medication if they are taking a newer atypical antipsychotic. However, many women do not respond as well to the typical agents or have such severe illnesses that making any change in their regimen can place them at significant risk. Thus, women and their clinicians often choose to use whichever antipsychotic agent during pregnancy sustains function and prevents symptom relapse, while acknowledging that information regarding their reproductive safety remains incomplete.

ANXIETY DISORDERS

Although modest to moderate levels of anxiety during pregnancy is common, pathologic anxiety (including panic attacks) has been associated with a variety of poor obstetric outcomes, including increased rates of premature labor, low birth weight, low Apgar scores, and placental abruption.[41] Anxiety disorders are prevalent during pregnancy; however, specific prevalence estimates vary widely.[42] For females with pre-pregnancy diagnoses, there is considerable variability in the reported illness course, especially for obsessive-compulsive disorder (OCD) and panic disorder, with some studies suggesting improvement during pregnancy and others reporting worsening of symptoms.

Consultation requests regarding the appropriate management of anxiety symptoms during pregnancy are common. The use of non-pharmacologic treatments, such as CBT and other types of psychotherapy, may be of great value in attenuating symptoms of anxiety, and for most patients, it should be part of the treatment plan. For some patients, psychotherapy may be sufficient to manage anxiety disorders during pregnancy.

For other patients, especially those who experience panic attacks associated with new-onset or recurrent panic disorder or those with severe generalized anxiety, pharmacologic intervention may be necessary. Many patients respond well to antidepressants, whose risks and safety profiles were discussed earlier. While older studies of diazepam indicated an increased risk of oral clefts, newer data have not shown an association between benzodiazepines and an increased risk of congenital malformations.[43] Benzodiazepines, when used judiciously, may be a reasonable option for treating anxiety during pregnancy.

For patients with panic disorder who wish to conceive and who do not wish to remain on anxiolytic medication, a slow taper of the medication is recommended. Adjunctive CBT can help patients discontinue anti-panic agents, and it may increase the time to a relapse. Some patients conceive inadvertently on anxiolytics and present for an emergent consultation. Abrupt discontinuation of anxiolytic maintenance medication is not recommended given the risk of rebound panic symptoms or a potentially serious withdrawal syndrome. However, a gradual taper of a benzodiazepine (over more than 2 weeks) with adjunctive CBT may be pursued in an attempt to minimize fetal exposure to medication.

If the tapering of medication is unsuccessful or if symptoms recur during pregnancy, reinstitution of pharmacotherapy may be considered. For patients with severe panic disorder, maintenance medication may be a clinical necessity. TCAs or SSRIs, perhaps in addition to benzodiazepines, are reasonable options for managing panic disorder during pregnancy. Although some patients choose to avoid first-trimester exposure to benzodiazepines (given historical data suggesting a risk for cleft lip and palate), benzodiazepines may be used without significant risk and can offer some advantage over antidepressant treatments because they may be used on an as-needed basis. Pharmacotherapy for severe anxiety during pregnancy includes treatment with benzodiazepines, TCAs, SSRIs, or SNRIs in addition to CBT.

With respect to the peripartum use of benzodiazepines, there are reports of hypotonia, neonatal apnea, neonatal withdrawal syndromes, and temperature dysregulation.[44] These risks have prompted recommendations to taper and discontinue benzodiazepines at the time of parturition. This approach is risky given data that suggest a risk of puerperal worsening of anxiety

disorders in women with a history of panic disorder and OCD.[45,46] Discontinuation of a drug near the time of delivery places a woman at risk for postpartum worsening of these disorders, and low-dose benzodiazepines may be safely administered until delivery.

ELECTROCONVULSIVE THERAPY

Consideration of the use of ECT during pregnancy typically generates anxiety among clinicians and patients. However, its safety record has been well documented since the 1940s,[47] particularly when instituted in collaboration with a multi-disciplinary treatment team, including an anesthesiologist, a psychiatrist, and an obstetrician. Requests for psychiatric consultation for pregnant patients who require ECT tend to be emergent and dramatic. For example, expeditious treatment is imperative in instances of mania during pregnancy or psychotic depression with suicidal thoughts and disorganized thinking. Such clinical situations are associated with a danger of impulsivity or self-harm. A limited course of treatment may be sufficient, followed by the institution of treatment with one or a combination of agents (such as antidepressants, neuroleptics, benzodiazepines, or mood stabilizers). An additional option to consider for treatment-resistant depression (TRD) (or for a pregnant female with depression who does not want to take medications) would be transcranial magnetic stimulation (TMS), which appears to be safe during pregnancy and may be less likely than ECT to cause side effects. At least one study has demonstrated the efficacy of TMS for the treatment of depression during pregnancy,[48] but no studies have assessed its effectiveness in treating severe depression, and it is not clear how TMS compares to antidepressants for the treatment of depression during pregnancy. For severe depression during pregnancy, pharmacotherapy and/or ECT remain the preferred treatment.

ECT during pregnancy tends to be under-used because of concerns that the treatment will harm the fetus. Despite one report of placental abruption associated with the use of ECT during pregnancy,[49] considerable experience supports its safe use in severely ill gravid females. Thus, it becomes the task of the psychiatric consultant to facilitate the most clinically appropriate intervention in the face of partially informed concerns or objections.

Attention-Deficit Hyperactivity Disorder and Pregnancy

An increasing number of women seek consultation to better understand the reproductive safety data of psychostimulants used for the management of ADHD, as well as for adjunctive treatment of mood disorders. Several recent studies have evaluated the reproductive safety profile of psychostimulants when taken as prescribed. Two studies have demonstrated a small increase in the risk of ventricular septal defects with the use of methylphenidate in pregnancy. In contrast, with over 5500 exposures, amphetamines have not demonstrated such a risk.[50,51] In a fashion consistent with the risk posed outside of pregnancy, stimulant use has been associated with gestational hypertension.[52] No other obstetric complications during pregnancy, such as pre-term delivery or low birth weight, have thus far been identified as having an increased risk with either stimulant class.

There is a paucity of data evaluating the longitudinal course of ADHD throughout pregnancy. Presently, untreated ADHD does not appear to pose a risk to pregnancy; however, secondary effects of untreated ADHD might. For example, females with ADHD may experience a higher risk of physical accidents or injuries due to inattention, with special concern for the risk of motor vehicle collisions. Inattention may also result in profound impairment in functioning at work, school, and/or at home, which may result in adverse financial, occupational, academic, and relational outcomes, in turn causing or worsening mood and anxiety symptoms. Finally the indication for stimulant use extends outside of ADHD, and this must be factored into any decision regarding continued stimulant use in pregnancy, as the medication might be used for TRD or may be conferring benefits from a mood standpoint.

If their use is non-essential, these medications would ideally be discontinued during pregnancy. Optimizing non-pharmacological interventions, such as workplace or school accommodations, executive coaching, and utilization of public transportation, may be appropriate. If medication continuation is considered essential, the lowest effective dose of shorter-acting formulations is recommended, with potential drug holidays on days when use is non-essential.

BREAST-FEEDING AND PSYCHOTROPIC DRUG USE

The emotional and medical benefits of breast-feeding to mother and infant are clear. However, for some women, establishing breast-feeding can be difficult and can contribute to extreme sleep deprivation that can worsen the postpartum course of illness. It is important to consider the benefits and risks of breast-feeding given each woman's situation.

Given the prevalence of psychiatric illness during the postpartum period, a significant number of females might require pharmacologic treatment while nursing. The appropriate concern is raised, however, regarding the safety of psychotropic drug use in females who choose to breast-feed while using these medications. Efforts to quantify psychotropic drugs and their metabolites in the breast milk of mothers have been reported. The serum of infants can also be assayed to assess more accurately neonatal exposure to medications. The data indicate that all psychotropic drugs, including antidepressants, antipsychotic agents, lithium carbonate, and benzodiazepines, are secreted into breast milk. However, concentrations of these agents in breast milk vary considerably.

The amount of medication to which an infant is exposed depends on several factors: the maternal dosage of medication, the frequency of dosing, the rate of maternal drug metabolism, and characteristics of the drug itself (e.g., molecular weight, protein binding, lipid solubility). Typically, peak concentrations in the breast milk are attained approximately 6 to 8 hours after the medication is ingested. Thus the frequency of feedings and the timing of the feedings can influence the amount of drug to which the nursing infant is exposed. By restricting breast-feeding to times during which breast milk drug concentrations would be at their lowest (either shortly before or immediately after dosing medication) exposure may be reduced; however, this approach might not be practical for newborns, who typically feed every 2 to 3 hours.

The nursing infant's chances of experiencing toxicity depend not only on the amount of medication ingested but also on how well the ingested medication is metabolized. Most psychotropics are metabolized by the liver. During the first few weeks of a full-term infant's life, there is a lower capacity for hepatic drug metabolism, which is about one-third to one-fifth of the adult's capacity. Over the next few months, the capacity for hepatic metabolism increases significantly, and by about 2 to 3 months of age, it surpasses that of adults. In premature infants or infants with signs of compromised hepatic metabolism (e.g., hyperbilirubinemia), breast-feeding may be deferred because these infants are less able to metabolize drugs and are thus more likely to experience toxicity.

Consultation surrounding the safety of psychotropic use in breast-feeding should include a discussion of the known physical and psychological benefits of breast-feeding, the potential risks of breast-feeding (such as sleep interruption), the risks of untreated maternal mental illness, the known safety of the individual medication in lactation, the limitations of data, and the infant's status (e.g., age, weight, behaviors, stability).

The available data, particularly on SSRIs during breast-feeding, have been encouraging and suggest that the amounts of drug to which the nursing infant is exposed are low and that significant complications related to neonatal exposure to psychotropic drugs in breast milk are rare.[53–55] Typically very low or nearly undetectable levels of the drug have been identified in the infant's serum; exposure to an SSRI during nursing does not appear to result in clinically significant blockade of serotonin (5-HT) reuptake in infants. Although less information is available on other antidepressants, serious adverse events related to exposure to these medications have not been reported.

Anxiety is prevalent during the postpartum period, and anxiolytics are often used in this setting. Data regarding the use of benzodiazepines while nursing indicate that the amounts of medication to which the nursing infant is exposed are generally low.[56] The risk of adverse events in nursing infants exposed to benzodiazepines is very low; rare reports of sedation, particularly in infants exposed to other sedating drugs in addition to benzodiazepines, lead to a recommendation to monitor for sedation.[57] Benzodiazepines should be considered a reasonable treatment option for breast-feeding women with anxiety.

For females with BPD, breast-feeding can pose more significant challenges. First, on-demand breast-feeding can significantly disrupt the mother's sleep and thus can increase her vulnerability to relapse during the acute postpartum period. Second, there have been reports of toxicity in nursing infants related to exposure to some mood stabilizers in breast milk. Lithium is excreted at high levels in the mother's milk, and infants' serum levels are relatively high, about one-fourth that of the mother's serum levels, thereby increasing the risk of neonatal toxicity (which includes cyanosis, hypotonia, and hypothermia).[58] Although breast-feeding typically is avoided in females taking lithium, the lowest possible effective dosage should be used, and both maternal and infant serum lithium levels should be followed in mothers who breast-feed. In collaboration with the pediatrician, the child should be monitored closely for signs of lithium toxicity, and levels of lithium, thyroid-stimulating hormone, blood urea nitrogen, and creatinine should be monitored every 6 to 8 weeks while the child is nursing.

Several studies have suggested that lamotrigine reaches infants through breast milk in relatively high doses, ranging from 20% to 50% of the mother's serum concentrations; this may be explained by poor neonatal metabolism of lamotrigine.[59] In addition, maternal serum levels of lamotrigine increase significantly after delivery unless the dose is adjusted, contributing to high levels found in nursing infants.[60] One worry shared by clinicians and new mothers is the risk for Stevens-Johnson syndrome, a severe, potentially life-threatening rash, most commonly resulting from a hypersensitivity reaction to a medication, that occurs in about 0.1% of patients who have BPD and are treated with lamotrigine.[61] Thus far, there have been no reports of Stevens-Johnson syndrome in infants exposed to lamotrigine.

Similarly, concerns have arisen regarding the use of carbamazepine and valproic acid. Each of these mood stabilizers has been associated in adults with abnormalities in liver function and with fatal hepatotoxicity. Hepatic dysfunction associated with carbamazepine exposure in breast milk has been reported several times.[62,63] The risk for hepatotoxicity appears to be greatest in children younger than 2 years; thus, nursing infants exposed to these agents may be particularly vulnerable to adverse events. Although the American Academy of Pediatrics has deemed carbamazepine and valproic acid to be appropriate for use in breast-feeding mothers, few studies have assessed the impact of these agents on fetal well-being, particularly in mothers who are not taking them for the treatment of epilepsy. In females who choose to use valproic acid or carbamazepine while nursing, monitoring of drug levels and liver function testing is recommended. In this setting, ongoing collaboration with the child's pediatrician is crucial.

Consultation about the safety of breast-feeding among women treated with psychotropics should include a discussion of the known benefits of breast-feeding to mothers and infants and the possibility that exposure to medications in breast milk can occur. Although routine assay of infants' serum drug levels was recommended in earlier treatment guidelines, this procedure is probably not warranted; in most instances, infants have low or non-detectable serum drug levels and serious adverse side effects are uncommon. This testing is indicated, however, if neonatal toxicity related to drug exposure is suspected. Infant serum monitoring is also indicated when the mother is nursing while taking lithium, valproic acid, or carbamazepine.

PSYCHIATRIC CONSULTATION AND POSTPARTUM PSYCHIATRIC ILLNESS

The postpartum period is considered a time of risk for the development of affective illness. Research has identified sub-groups of females at particular risk for postpartum worsening of mood. At the highest risk are women with a history of postpartum psychosis; up to 70% of women who have had one episode of puerperal psychosis experience another episode following a subsequent pregnancy.[64] Similarly, females with a history of postpartum depression are at significant risk, with rates of postpartum recurrence as high as 50%.[65] Women with BPD also appear to be particularly vulnerable during the postpartum period, with rates of postpartum relapse being greater than 30%, and they are significantly higher for cases in which mood-stabilizing medication was not maintained throughout pregnancy.[66] In all females (with or without a history of MDD), the emergence of depressive symptoms during pregnancy significantly increases the likelihood of postpartum depression.

Depression

Diagnosis

During the postpartum period, about 85% of females experience some mood disturbance. For most females the symptoms are mild; however, 13% to 19% of women experience clinically significant symptoms.[67] Postpartum depressive disorders are typically divided into three categories: postpartum blues, non-psychotic major depression, and puerperal psychosis. Because these three diagnostic sub-types overlap significantly, it is not clear if they represent three distinct disorders. It may be more useful to conceptualize these sub-types as existing along a continuum, in which postpartum blues is the mildest and postpartum psychosis the most severe form of puerperal psychiatric illness.

Postpartum blues does not indicate psychopathology; it is common and occurs in approximately 50% to 85% of females following delivery.[68] Symptoms, including reactivity of mood, tearfulness, and irritability are, by definition, time limited and typically remitted by the 10th postpartum day. Because postpartum blues are associated with no significant impairment of function and are time limited, no specific treatment is indicated. Symptoms that persist beyond 2 weeks require further evaluation and suggest an evolving depressive disorder. In women with a history of a recurrent mood disorder, the blues may herald the onset of postpartum MDD.

The signs and symptoms of postpartum depression usually appear over the first 2 to 3 months following delivery and are indistinguishable from the characteristics of MDD that occur at other times in a female's life. The presenting symptoms of postpartum depression often include depressed mood, irritability, and loss of interest in usual activities. Insomnia, fatigue, and loss of appetite are frequently described. Postpartum depressive symptoms also co-mingle with anxiety and obsessional symptoms, and females might present with generalized anxiety, panic attacks, or obsessive-compulsive symptoms.

Although it is sometimes difficult to diagnose depression in the acute puerperium given the normal occurrence of symptoms suggestive of depression (e.g., sleep and appetite disturbance, low libido), it is an error to dismiss neurovegetative symptoms (such as severely decreased energy, profound anhedonia, and guilty ruminations) as normal features of the puerperium. In its most severe form, postpartum depression can result in profound dysfunction. Risk factors for postpartum depression include prenatal depression, prenatal anxiety, and a history of depression.

Treatment

A wealth of literature on this topic indicates that postpartum depression, especially when left untreated, may have a significant impact on the child's well-being and development. In addition, the syndrome demands aggressive treatment to avoid the sequelae of an untreated mood disorder, such as chronic depression and recurrent disease. Treatment should be guided by the type and severity of the symptoms and by the degree of functional impairment. However, before initiating psychiatric treatment, medical causes for mood disturbances (e.g., thyroid dysfunction, anemia) must be excluded. Initial evaluation should include a thorough history, physical examination, and routine laboratory tests.

Non-pharmacologic therapies are useful in the treatment of postpartum depression, and various psychotherapy modalities including CBT and IPT have yielded encouraging results.[69,70] These non-pharmacologic interventions may be particularly attractive to patients who are reluctant to use psychotropic medications (e.g., females who are breast-feeding) or for patients with milder forms of depressive illness. Women with more severe postpartum depression will likely have the best clinical response to a combination of pharmacologic treatment and non-pharmacologic therapies.

To date, only a few studies have systematically assessed the pharmacological treatment of postpartum depression. Conventional antidepressant medications at standard antidepressant doses have shown efficacy in the treatment of postpartum depression. The choice of an antidepressant should be guided by the patient's prior response to antidepressants and a given medication's side-effect profile. SSRIs are ideal first-line agents because they are anxiolytic, non-sedating, and well tolerated; bupropion is another good option. TCAs are sometimes used, and because they tend to be more sedating, they may be more appropriate for females who have prominent sleep disturbances. Given the prevalence of anxiety in females with postpartum depression, adjunctive use of a benzodiazepine (e.g., clonazepam or lorazepam) may be very helpful.

Neurosteroids, brexanolone, and zuranolone, which are allopregnanolone analogs and positive allosteric modulators of gamma aminobutyric acid-A receptors, have emerged as novel treatments for postpartum depression. Brexanolone, FDA approved in 2019 for the treatment of postpartum depression, has demonstrated a rapid onset of action, with initial studies indicating remission of depressive symptoms within 24 to 48 hours after IV administration. Because of potentially serious adverse effects, specifically excessive sedation and loss of consciousness, the FDA requires a Risk Evaluation and Mitigation Strategies at facilities that administer brexanolone, which requires hospitalization and medical supervision. Zuranolone, an oral version of brexanolone, remains in clinical trials and has shown promise in the treatment of postpartum depression, albeit with a slower onset of action (3 days) than brexanolone.[71] Both options, however, are still much more rapidly acting than conventional antidepressants. Antidepressants are safe, well tolerated, and highly effective; they remain the clear first choice for females with postpartum depression.

In cases of severe postpartum depression, inpatient hospitalization may be required, particularly for patients who are at risk for suicide. In Great Britain, innovative treatment programs involving joint hospitalization of the mother and the baby have been successful; however, mother-and-infant units are much less common in the United States. Females with severe postpartum illness should be considered candidates for ECT. The option should be considered early in treatment because it is safe and highly effective. In choosing any treatment strategy, it is important to consider the impact of prolonged hospitalization or treatment of the mother on the infant's development and attachment.

Panic Attacks and Obsessive-Compulsive Disorder

Symptoms of postpartum generalized anxiety, panic attacks, and OCD are often included in the description of postpartum mood disturbance, and the relationship between postpartum depression and these anxiety symptoms is not fully understood. Co-morbid anxiety symptoms are particularly prominent in postpartum depression compared to non-postpartum MDD; one study demonstrated that 57% of women with post-partum-onset MDD reported obsessional thoughts compared with 36% of women with non-postpartum MDD, and that in postpartum females, obsessional thoughts were more frequent and more aggressive.[72] Postpartum OCD has also been described in the absence of co-morbid postpartum MDD. Symptoms often include intrusive obsessional thoughts to harm the newborn in the absence of psychosis. Treatment with anti-obsessional agents, such as fluoxetine or clomipramine, in addition to CBT, is often effective.

Psychosis

Postpartum psychosis is a psychiatric emergency. The clinical picture is most often consistent with mania or a mixed state consistent with an episode of BPD and can include symptoms of restlessness, agitation, sleep disturbance, paranoia, delusions, disorganized thinking, impulsivity, and behaviors that place the mother and the infant at risk. The typical onset is within the first 2 weeks after delivery, and symptoms can appear as early as the first 72 hours after delivery.

Although investigators have debated whether post-partum psychosis is a discrete diagnostic entity or a manifestation of BPD, treatment should follow the same algorithm to treat acute manic psychosis, including hospitalization and the potential use of mood stabilizers, antipsychotics, benzodiazepines, and ECT (although antidepressants should generally be avoided).

Prevention

It is difficult to predict reliably which women will experience a postpartum mood disturbance, but it is possible to identify sub-groups of females (e.g., females with a history of a mood disorder) who are more vulnerable to postpartum affective illness. Several investigators have explored the potential efficacy of prophylactic interventions for these females at risk.

For women with a history of postpartum depression, Wisner and colleagues have demonstrated in a double-blind, placebo-controlled study that there is a beneficial effect (lower rates of recurrent postpartum depression) from administering a prophylactic SSRI after delivery.[73] Several studies have demonstrated that women with a history of BPD or puerperal psychosis benefit from prophylactic treatment with lithium,

instituted either before delivery (at 36 weeks of gestation) or no later than the first 48 hours following delivery.[74] Prophylactic lithium appears to significantly reduce relapse rates and diminish the severity and duration of puerperal illness.

Other studies have demonstrated the efficacy of non-pharmacologic interventions in females at risk of postpartum mood disturbance. These include interventions ranging from targeted psychotherapy to coaching on infant behavioral interventions to reduce infant fussing and promote sleep.[75]

In summary, postpartum depressive illness may be conceptualized along a continuum, in which some females are at lower risk for puerperal illness and others are at higher risk. Although a less aggressive, wait-and-see approach is appropriate for women with no history of postpartum psychiatric illness, women with BPD or a history of postpartum psychiatric illness deserve close monitoring and specific prophylactic measures. All women should be screened for mood disturbance in the postpartum period and be referred for appropriate follow-up and treatment when indicated.

PERINATAL PSYCHIATRY: FROM SCREENING TO TREATMENT

Clinicians who manage the care of female psychiatric patients before, during, and after pregnancy may be called on to evaluate females who experience a broad spectrum of difficulties. Symptoms may be mild, although consultation is typically requested when symptoms become severe. It is not uncommon for women to present weeks or even months after the onset of psychiatric symptoms. Many women and their healthcare providers mistakenly believe that even serious mood symptoms are normal postpartum reactions, and many females may be afraid or embarrassed to disclose that they are suffering from depression. Psychiatric disorders may emerge anew during pregnancy, although more often clinical presentations represent persistence or exacerbation of an existing illness. Physicians therefore should screen more aggressively for psychiatric disorders either before conception or during pregnancy, integrating questions about psychiatric symptoms and treatment into the obstetric history. Identification of at-risk females allows the most thoughtful, acute treatment before, during, and after pregnancy and signals the opportunity to institute prophylactic strategies that prevent psychiatric disturbances in females during the childbearing years.

Even among females with identified psychiatric illness during pregnancy, definitive treatment is often lacking or incomplete. The extent to which women suffering from postpartum psychiatric illness are under-treated as a group is also very well described. Perhaps one of the reasons for the failure to treat women who have psychiatric disorders during pregnancy is the concern regarding fetal exposure to psychotropics. Many clinicians can conceptualize the need to weigh the relative risks of fetal exposure on the one hand versus the risk of withholding treatment on the other. However, given the inability to quantify these risks, clinicians often defer treatment entirely and consequently put patients at risk for the sequelae of untreated maternal psychiatric illness. Clinicians should realize that the process of managing psychiatric illness during pregnancy and the puerperium is not a process like threading a needle; it is not clear-cut, and much of the treatment described in the literature is not evidence based. However, thoughtful decisions can still be made with these patients as clinicians review available information with them and as clinician and patient realize that no decision is risk free, and no decision is perfect.

REFERENCES

1. Cohen LS, Altshuler LL, Harlow BL, et al. Relapse of major depression during pregnancy in women who maintain or discontinue antidepressant treatment. *JAMA*. 2006;295(5):499–507.
2. Viguera AC, Nonacs R, Cohen LS, et al. Risk of recurrence of bipolar disorder in pregnant and nonpregnant women after discontinuing lithium maintenance. *Am J Psychiatry*. 2000;157(2):179–184.
3. Viguera AC, Whitfield T, Baldessarini RJ, et al. Risk of recurrence in women with bipolar disorder during pregnancy: prospective study of mood stabilizer discontinuation. *Am J Psychiatry*. 2007;164(12):1817–1824. quiz 1923.
4. Wisner KL, Zarin DA, Holmboe ES, et al. Risk–benefit decision making for treatment of depression during pregnancy. *Am J Psychiatry*. 2000;157(12):1933–1940.
5. Kong L, Chen X, Liang Y, et al. Association of preeclampsia and perinatal complications with offspring: neurodevelopmental and psychiatric disorders. *JAMA Netw Open*. 2022 Jan 4;5(1):e2145719.
6. Leigh B, Milgrom J. Risk factors for antenatal depression, postnatal depression, and parenting stress. *BMC Psychiatry*. 2008;8:24.
7. Siu AL. The US Preventive Services Task Force (USPSTF). Screening for depression in adults: US Preventive Services Task Force recommendation statement. *JAMA*. 2016;315(4):380–387.
8. Flynn HA, Blow FC, Marcus SM. Rates and predictors of depression treatment among pregnant women in hospital-affiliated obstetrics practices. *Gen Hosp Psychiatry*. 2006;28(4):289–295.
9. Kim JJ, Silver RK, La Porte LM, et al. Suicide risk among perinatal women who report thoughts of self-harm on depression screens. *Obstet Gynecol*. 2014;123(suppl 1):60S.
10. Freeman M, Davis M, Sinha P, et al. Omega-3 fatty acids and supportive psychotherapy for perinatal depression: a randomized placebo-controlled study. *J Affect Disord*. 2008;110(1–2):142–148.
11. Wan Mohd Yunus WMA, Matinolli HM, Waris O, et al. Digitalized cognitive behavioral interventions for depressive symptoms during pregnancy: systematic review. *J Med Internet Res*. 2022 Feb 23;24(2):e33337.
12. Spinelli MG, Endicott J, Goetz RR, et al. Reanalysis of efficacy of interpersonal psychotherapy for antepartum depression versus parenting education program: initial severity of depression as a predictor of treatment outcomes. *J Clin Psychiatry*. 2016;77(4):535–540.
13. Anderson KN, Lind JN, Simeone RM, et al. Maternal use of specific antidepressant medications during early pregnancy and the risk of selected birth defects. *JAMA Psychiatry*. 2020;77(12):1246–1255. 10.1001/jamapsychiatry.2020.2453. https://jamanetwork.com/journals/jamapsychiatry/fullarticle/2769190.
14. U.S. Food and Drug Administration. FDA issues final rule on changes to pregnancy and lactation labeling information for prescription drug and biological products, *FDA News Release*; 2014. Available at: http://www.fda.gov/NewsEvents/Newsroom/PressAnnouncements/ucm425317.htm.
15. Kjaersgaard MI, Parner ET, Vestergaard M, et al. Prenatal antidepressant exposure and risk of spontaneous abortion – a population-based study. *PLoS ONE*. 2013;8(8):e72095.
16. Furu K, Kieler H, Haglund B, et al. Selective serotonin reuptake inhibitors and venlafaxine in early pregnancy and risk of birth defects: population-based cohort study and sibling design. *BMJ*. 2015;350:h1798.
17. Huybrechts KF, Palmsten K, Avorn J, et al. Antidepressant use in pregnancy and the risk of cardiac defects. *N Engl J Med*. 2014;370(25):2397–2407. https://doi.org/10.1056/nejmoa1312828.
18. Ankarfeldt MZ, Petersen J, Andersen JT, et al. Exposure to duloxetine during pregnancy and risk of congenital malformations and stillbirth: a nationwide cohort study in Denmark and Sweden. *PLoS Med*. 2021 Nov 22;18(11):e1003851.
19. Huybrechts KF, Bateman BT, Pawar A, et al. Maternal and fetal outcomes following exposure to duloxetine in pregnancy: cohort study. *BMJ*. 2020 Feb 19;368:m237.
20. Louik C, Kerr S, Mitchell AA. First-trimester exposure to bupropion and risk of cardiac malformations. *Pharmacoepidemiol Drug Saf*. 2014;23(10):1066–1075.
21. Gentile S. Tricyclic antidepressants in pregnancy and puerperium. *Expert Opin Drug Saf*. 2014 Feb;13(2):207–225. https://doi.org/10.1517/14740338.2014.869582. Epub 2014 Jan 3. PMID: 24383525.
22. Levinson-Castiel R, Merlob P, Linder N, et al. Neonatal abstinence syndrome after in utero exposure to selective serotonin reuptake

inhibitors in term infants. *Arch Pediatr Adolesc Med.* 2006;160(2): 173–176.

23. Huybrechts KF, Bateman BT, Palmsten K, et al. Antidepressant use late in pregnancy and risk of persistent pulmonary hypertension of the newborn. *JAMA.* 2015;313(21):2142. https://doi.org/10.1001/jama.2015.5605.

24. Suarez EA, Bateman BT, Hernández-Díaz S, et al. Association of antidepressant use during pregnancy with risk of neurodevelopmental disorders in children. *JAMA Intern Med.* 2022 Oct 3: e224268. https://doi.org/10.1001/jamainternmed.2022.4268. Epub ahead of print. PMID: 36190722; PMCID: PMC9531086.

25. Flynn HA, O'Mahen HA, Massey L, et al. The impact of a brief obstetrics clinic-based intervention on treatment use for perinatal depression. *J Womens Health (Larchmt).* 2006;15(10):1195–1204.

26. Lenze SH, Roders J, Luby J. A pilot, exploratory report on dyadic interpersonal psychotherapy for perinatal depression. *Arch Womens Ment Health.* 2015;18(3):485–491.

27. Cohen LS, Altshuler LL, Stowe ZN, et al. Reintroduction of antidepressant therapy across pregnancy in women who previously discontinued treatment. A preliminary retrospective study. *Psychother Psychosom.* 2004;73(4):255–258.

28. Krauer B. Pharmacotherapy during pregnancy: emphasis on pharmacokinetics. In: Eskes TKAB, Mieczyslaw F, eds. *Drug Therapy During Pregnancy.* Butterworths; 1985:9–31.

29. Jeffries WS, Bochner F. The effect of pregnancy on drug pharmacokinetics. *Med J Aust.* 1988;149(11–12):675–677.

30. Moses-Kolko EL, Bogen D, Perel J, et al. Neonatal signs after late in utero exposure to serotonin reuptake inhibitors: literature review and implications for clinical applications. *JAMA.* 2005;293 (19):2372–2383.

31. Anderson EL, Reti IM. ECT in pregnancy: a review of the literature from 1941 to 2007. *Psychosom Med.* 2009;71(2): 235–242.

32. Ward HB, Fromson JA, Cooper JJ, et al. Recommendations for the use of ECT in pregnancy: literature review and proposed clinical protocol. *Arch Womens Ment Health.* 2018;21:715–722. https://doi-org.treadwell.idm.oclc.org/10.1007/s00737-018-0851-0.

33. Patorno E, Huybrechts KF, Bateman BT, et al. Lithium use in pregnancy and the risk of cardiac malformations. *N Engl J Med.* 2017 Jun 8;376(23):2245–2254. https://doi.org/10.1056/NEJMoa1612222. PMID: 28591541; PMCID: PMC5667676.

34. Kaplan YC, Demir O. Use of phenytoin, phenobarbital, carbamazepine, levetiracetam, lamotrigine and valproate in pregnancy and breastfeeding: risk of major malformations, dose-dependency, monotherapy vs polytherapy, pharmacokinetics and clinical implications. *Curr Neuropharmacol.* 2021;19(11):1805–1824. https://doi-org.treadwell.idm.oclc.org/10.2174/1570159X19666210211150856.

35. Blotière PO, Raguideau F, Weill A, et al. Risks of 23 specific malformations associated with prenatal exposure to 10 antiepileptic drugs. *Neurology.* 2019;93(2):e167–e180. https://doi.org/10.1212/WNL.0000000000007696. Epub 2019 Jun 12. PMID: 31189695; PMCID: PMC6656651.

36. Wiggs KK, Rickert ME, Sujan AC, et al. Antiseizure medication use during pregnancy and risk of ASD and ADHD in children.

Neurology. 2020;95(24):e3232–e3240. https://doi.org/10.1212/WNL.0000000000010993. Epub 2020 Oct 28. PMID: 33115775; PMCID: PMC7836668.

37. Huybrechts KF, Hernández-Díaz S, Patorno E, et al. Antipsychotic use in pregnancy and the risk for congenital malformations. *JAMA Psychiatry.* 2016;73(9):938–946. https://doi.org/10.1001/jamapsychiatry.2016.1520. PMID: 27540849; PMCID: PMC5321163.

38. Andrade C. Major congenital malformations associated with exposure to second-generation antipsychotic drugs during pregnancy. *J Clin Psychiatry.* 2021;82(5): 21f14252.

39. Zhong QY, Gelaye B, Fricchione GL, et al. Adverse obstetric and neonatal outcomes complicated by psychosis among pregnant women in the United States. *BMC Pregnancy Childbirth.* 2018;18: 120. https://doi.org/10.1186/s12884-018-1750-0.

40. Rumeau-Rouquette C, Goujard J, Huel G. Possible teratogenic effect of phenothiazines in human beings. *Teratology.* 1977;15(1): 57–64.

41. Grigoriadis S, Graves L, Peer M, et al. Maternal anxiety during pregnancy and the association with adverse perinatal outcomes: systematic review and meta-analysis. *J Clin Psychiatry.* 2018;79: e1–e22.

42. Goodman JH, Chenausky KL, Freeman MP. Anxiety disorders during pregnancy: a systematic review. *J Clin Psychiatry.* 2014; 75(10):1153–1184.

43. Okun ML, Ebert R, Saini B. A review of sleep-promoting medications used in pregnancy. *Am J Obstet Gynecol.* 2015;212(4):428–441. https://doi.org/10.1016/j.ajog.2014.10.1106.

44. Enato E, Moretti M, Koren G. The fetal safety of benzodiazepines: an updated meta-analysis. *J Obstet Gynaecol Can.* 2011;33(1): 46–48.

45. Cohen LS, Sichel DA, Dimmock JA, et al. Postpartum course in women with preexisting panic disorder. *J Clin Psychiatry.* 1994;55(7):289–292.

46. Sichel DA, Cohen LS, Dimmock JA, et al. Postpartum obsessive-compulsive disorder: a case series. *J Clin Psychiatry.* 1993;54(4):156–159.

47. Goldstein H, Weinberg J, Sankstone M. Shock therapy in psychosis complicating pregnancy, a case report. *Am J Psychiatry.* 1941;98(2):201–202.

48. Kim DR, Snell JL, Ewing GC, et al. Neuromodulation and antenatal depression: a review. *Neuropsychiatr Dis Treat.* 2015;11: 975–982.

49. Sherer DM, D'Amico LD, Warshal DP, et al. Recurrent mild abruption placentae occurring immediately after repeated electroconvulsive therapy in pregnancy. *Am J Obstet Gynecol.* 1991;165(3):652–653.

50. Huybrechts KF, Bröms G, Christensen LB, et al. Association between methylphenidate and amphetamine use in pregnancy and risk of congenital malformations: a cohort study from the International Pregnancy Safety Study Consortium. *JAMA Psychiatry.* 2018;75(2):167–175.

51. Kolding L, Ehrenstein V, Pedersen L, et al. Associations between ADHD medication use in pregnancy and severe malformations based on prenatal and postnatal diagnoses: a Danish registry-based study. *J Clin Psychiatry.* 2021;82(1): 20m13458.

52. Newport DJ, Hostetter AL, Juul SH, et al. Prenatal psychostimulant and antidepressant exposure and risk of hypertensive disorders of pregnancy. *J Clin Psychiatry*. 2016;77(11):1538–1545.

53. Stowe Z. The pharmacokinetics of sertraline excretion into human breast milk: determinants of infant serum concentrations. *J Clin Psychiatry*. 2003;64(1):73–80.

54. Suri R, Stowe Z, Hendrick V, et al. Estimates of nursing infant daily dose of fluoxetine through breastmilk. *Biol Psychiatry*. 2002;52(5):446–451.

55. Epperson N, Czarkowski KA, Ward-O'Brien D, et al. Maternal sertraline treatment and serotonin transport in breast-feeding mother–infant pairs. *Am J Psychiatry*. 2001;158(10):1631–1637.

56. Birnbaum CS, Cohen LS, Bailey JW, et al. Serum concentrations of antidepressants and benzodiazepines in nursing infants: a case series. *Pediatrics*. 1999;104(1):e11.

57. Kelly LE, Poon S, Madadi P, et al. Neonatal benzodiazepines exposure during breastfeeding. *J Pediatr*. 2012;161(3):448–451.

58. Viguera AC, Newport DJ, Ritchie J, et al. Lithium in breast milk and nursing infants: clinical implications. *Am J Psychiatry*. 2007;164(2):342–345.

59. Liporace J, Kao A, D'Abreu A. Concerns regarding lamotrigine and breast-feeding. *Epilepsy Behav*. 2004;5(1):102–105.

60. Goldsmith D, Wagstaff A, Ibbotson T, et al. Spotlight on lamotrigine in bipolar disorder. *CNS Drugs*. 2004;18(1):63–67.

61. Oles KS, Gal P. Stevens–Johnson syndrome associated with anticonvulsant therapy in a neonate. *Clin Pharm*. 1982;1(6):565–567.

62. Frey BS. Transient cholestatic hepatitis in a neonate associated with carbamazepine exposure during pregnancy and breast-feeding. *Eur J Pediatr*. 1990;150(2):136–138.

63. Merlob P, Mor N, Litwin A. Transient hepatic dysfunction in an infant of an epileptic mother treated with carbamazepine during pregnancy and breastfeeding. *Ann Pharmacother*. 1992;26(12):1563–1565.

64. Davidson J, Robertson E. A follow-up study of postpartum illness. *Acta Psychiatr Scand*. 1985;71(5):451–457.

65. Kupfer DJ, Frank E. Relapse in recurrent unipolar depression. *Am J Psychiatry*. 1987;144(1):86–88.

66. Wesseloo R, Kamperman AM, Munk-Olsen T, et al. Risk of postpartum relapse in bipolar disorder and postpartum psychosis: a systematic review and meta-analysis. *Am J Psychiatry*. 2016;173(2):117–127.

67. Shorey S, Chee CYI, Ng ED, et al. Prevalence and incidence of postpartum depression among healthy mothers: a systematic review and meta-analysis. *J Psychiatr Res*. 2018;104:235–248. https://doi-org.treadwell.idm.oclc.org/10.1016/j.jpsychires.2018.08.001.

68. O'Hara MW, Wisner KL. Perinatal mental illness: definition, description and aetiology. Best practice & research. *Clin Obstet Gynaecol*. 2014;28(1):3–12. https://doi-org.treadwell.idm.oclc.org/10.1016/j.bpobgyn.2013.09.002.

69. Ngai FW, Wong PW, Leung KY, et al. The effect of telephone-based cognitive-behavioral therapy on postnatal depression: a randomized controlled trial. *Psychother Psychosom*. 2015;84(5):294–303.

70. O'Hara MW, Stuart S, Gorman LL, et al. Efficacy of interpersonal psychotherapy for postpartum depression. *Arch Gen Psychiatry*. 2000;57(11):1039–1045.

71. Deligiannidis KM, Meltzer-Brody S, Gunduz-Bruce H, et al. Effect of zuranolone vs placebo in postpartum depression: a randomized clinical trial. *JAMA Psychiatry*. 2021 Jun:30.

72. Wisner KL, Peindl KS, Gigliotti T, et al. Obsessions and compulsions in women with postpartum depression. *J Clin Psychiatry*. 1999;60(3):176–180.

73. Wisner K, Perel JM, Peindl KS, et al. Prevention of postpartum depression: a pilot randomized clinical trial. *Am J Psychiatry*. 2004;161(7):1290–1292.

74. Cohen LS, Sichel DA, Robertson LM, et al. Postpartum prophylaxis for women with bipolar disorder. *Am J Psychiatry*. 1995;152(11):1641–1645.

75. Werner EA, Gustafsson HC, Lee S, et al. PREPP: postpartum depression prevention through the mother–infant dyad. *Arch Womens Ment Health*. 2016;19(2):229–242.

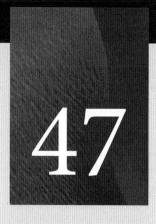

47 CULTURE AND PSYCHIATRY

NHI-HA TRINH, MD, MPH ■ ADERONKE BAMGBOSE
PEDERSON, MD ■ JUSTIN A. CHEN, MD, MPH ■
ALBERT S. YEUNG, MD, SCD

OVERVIEW

Race, ethnicity, and culture may all exert a tremendous impact on medical diagnosis, treatment, and outcomes. This is especially true in psychiatry, given the prominent role that culture plays in patients' interpretation and management of symptoms that fall within the affective, behavioral, and cognitive domains. Behaviors that appear bizarre in one cultural context may be perfectly acceptable in another. Although an in-depth understanding of every culture is impossible, familiarity with some fundamental principles will help minimize cultural clashes and reduce the risk of compromised medical care.

Understanding a patient's culture can support the delivery of high-quality and equitable care. However, a little knowledge can also be a dangerous thing. Variability among individuals is inevitable; a particular patient may not fit into a clinician's preconceived notion of the patient's culture. Thus the clinician must probe for clues regarding the patient's background, while also remaining flexible enough to recognize when a patient's behaviors and clinical presentation do not necessarily match what is expected. The clinician should be aware of their own feelings, biases, and preconceptions about other cultures. In addition, the consulting psychiatrist must assess the impact of the hospital environment, the attitudes of the medical and ancillary care teams, and the patient's experience within the healthcare system. Mistrust of the healthcare system is common and may influence a patient's behavior, level of cooperation, and adherence to treatment. Furthermore, disparities in healthcare delivery have been well documented and are influenced by factors such as sex, race, ethnicity, and culture.

The role of culture in health care has become a topic of increasing importance due to rapid demographic changes in the United States. Although the US population already exhibits tremendous racial and ethnic diversity, projections expect this pattern to become further magnified in the coming decades. By 2044 non-Hispanic/Latinx White population will be outnumbered by Black, indigenous, and people of color (BIPOC) in the United States, and by 2060 nearly one in five of the nation's total population is projected to be foreign-born.[1] Most BIPOC groups are projected to experience growth between 2014 and 2060, with the largest rates of growth projected for Hispanic/Latinx, Asians, and non-Hispanic/Latinx of two or more races.[1]

CULTURE AND PSYCHIATRY

Culture is the collected body of beliefs, customs, and behaviors that a group (or people) acquire socially and transmit from one generation to another through symbols, shared meanings, teachings, and life experiences. It provides the tools by which members of a given society adapt to their physical environment, their social environment, and one another. It organizes groups with ready-made solutions to common problems and challenges.

Physical culture—as exemplified by art, literature, architecture, tools, machines, food, clothing, and means of transportation—can be observed directly through the five senses, and through items collected in a museum or recorded on film. Ideological culture refs to aspects of culture that must be observed indirectly, usually through specific behaviors and customs. These include beliefs and values, the reasons for considering some things sacred and other things ordinary, the characteristics and events of which a society is proud or ashamed, and the sentiments that underlie patriotism or chauvinism. Religion, philosophy, psychology, literature, and the meanings that people give to symbols are all part of the ideological aspect of culture. The physical level of culture yields more easily to change and adaptation than does the ideological level, but without some understanding of the ideological aspect of culture, it is difficult to understand the meaning of a group purely at the physical level.

Each society establishes its own criteria regarding which forms of behavior are acceptable or abnormal, and which represent a medical problem. Learning more about an individual's culture and/or working with bilingual and bicultural interpreters can help to clarify normal and abnormal behaviors. It is also important to recognize that an individual may be influenced by multiple cultures or subcultures. The consulting psychiatrist must often employ the skills of a detective in a culturally sensitive manner to verify whether a patient's statements or beliefs are consistent with a patient's environment, heritage, and culture.

Cultural Differences in Illness Presentation

Cultural differences in the presentation of psychiatric illnesses abound. For example, a female originally from South Korea may present with chief complaints of dizziness, fatigue, and back pain, while she may not report other neurovegetative symptoms of depression, and she may not describe feelings of dysphoria. Mental healthcare clinicians in the United States are generally unfamiliar with various non-European cultural syndromes and culturally specific meanings attributed to certain symptoms.[2-4] For example, the Laotian way of describing feeling "tense" is feeling "like a balloon blown up until it is about to burst." Westermeyer,[5] in a case-controlled study in Laos, documented the general inability of psychiatrists with Eurocentric training to recognize the Laotian symptoms of depression. On the other hand, common American expressions, such as "feeling blue," cannot be readily translated into many other languages. A Cambodian clinician will ask Cambodian patients if

they "feel blue" by using Khmer terms, which literally translate as "heavy, overcast, gloomy."

Similarly, the phenomenology of panic disorder may vary among BIPOC groups within the United States. Compared with their White peers, for example, some Black people with panic disorder report more intense fears of dying or going crazy, as well as higher levels of numbing and tingling in their extremities and exhibit higher rates of co-morbid post-traumatic stress disorder (PTSD) and depression. Black people also use somewhat different coping strategies (e.g., religious practice and "counting one's blessings"), and endorse less self-blame. Cambodian populations may understand panic-like symptoms as *khyâl cap* (literally, "wind attacks") caused by *khyâl*, a wind-like substance, rising in the body and causing a range of serious effects, including compressing the lungs or entering the cranium.[6]

Accurate evaluation of the meaning and significance of seemingly bizarre beliefs, hallucinations, and psychotic-like symptoms among diverse populations remains a clinical challenge. For example, a Puerto Rican female who acknowledges hearing the voices of her ancestors may not be psychotic, as this phenomenon is relatively common among Caribbean Latinos in the absence of a thought disorder.[7] In many traditional, non-Western societies, spirits of the deceased are regarded as capable of interacting with, and possessing, those still alive. It may be difficult for the clinician to determine whether symptoms are bizarre enough to yield a diagnosis of a primary psychotic disorder without an adequate understanding of a patient's sociocultural and religious background and consideration of other salient clinical features, for example, a decline in function accompanied by cognitive changes. On the other hand, caution must be taken not to assume that bizarre symptoms are culturally appropriate, when in fact they are a manifestation of psychiatric illness. A culture may interpret abnormal behavior as relating to some kind of voodoo or anger and therefore regard the symptoms as normal, even though they are consistent with a primary psychotic disorder. The use of bilingual and bicultural interpreters, along with the search for information from other sources from the individual's community (e.g., family, community leaders, religious officials), as well as attention to other more objective features of psychiatric illness (e.g., poor self-care, impaired functioning, deterioration of personal and professional relationships), may help determine whether an individual's behavior is culturally acceptable or evidence of a psychiatric illness.

Clinicians who search only for physiologic explanations for somatic complaints (such as back pain, tinnitus, headaches, palpitations, and dizziness) may miss depression or anxiety. Afflicted patients are often prescribed meclizine for dizziness and analgesics for pain by their primary care providers when an antidepressant or anxiolytic would have been most appropriate. The appropriate diagnosis and treatment will only be elucidated if sufficient time and attention are spent understanding the cultural factors affecting an individual's distress, a process that is described further in the following section.

Cultural Assessment for Clinicians

The *Diagnostic and Statistical Manual of Mental Disorders, 5th edition* (DSM-5)[8] introduced several conceptual innovations regarding the role of culture in psychiatric diagnosis and treatment. These included direct cross-referencing of multi-cultural explanations for clusters of symptoms within the descriptions of each DSM-5 disorder, more detailed and structured information about cultural concepts of distress, and expanded clinical interviewing tools to facilitate person-centered and culturally focused assessments. In addition, DSM-5 went further than any previous versions of the manual in its explicit assertion that "all forms of distress are locally shaped, including the DSM disorders."[8]

DSM-5 and the subsequent text revision DSM-5-TR[9] provide clinicians with two practical tools to help clinicians produce a nuanced cultural assessment: the Outline for Cultural Formulation (OCF) and the Cultural Formulation Interview (CFI), both of which bear further description here, given this chapter's focus on the role of culture in psychiatry.

The *Outline for Cultural Formulation* describes five distinct domains, shown below, that can be used to describe an individual's ethnic and cultural context as related to psychiatric illness.

Cultural Identity of the Individual

The multiplicity of an individual's ethnic and cultural references are all critical to understanding that individual's identity. Clinicians should delve into this topic using open-ended questions with reference to cultural and social context, recognition of the hybrid nature of cultures, and the possibility of change over time.[10] For instance, an Asian American male who grew up in the Southern United States may exhibit patterns, behaviors, and views of the world that are more consistent with those of a White Southerner. Attention to language abilities and preferences must also be addressed. Other important aspects of cultural identity may also include religious affiliation, socioeconomic background, sexual orientation, sexual identity, country of origin, and migration history.

Cultural Conceptualizations of Distress

How an individual understands and experiences their symptoms are often communicated through cultural syndromes and idioms of distress (e.g., nervios/"nerves," possession by spirits, somatic complaints, misfortune). Individuals may also make sense of their experience in terms of a specific sequence of events or prior episodes of illness.[10] Thus the meaning and severity of an illness in relation to one's culture, family, community, and personal history should be elicited. The resultant explanatory model, in conjunction with past and current expectations of care, may prove extraordinarily helpful when developing an interpretation of symptoms, a diagnosis, and a treatment plan.

Psychosocial Stressors and Cultural Features of Vulnerability and Resilience

Culture impacts the psychosocial environment—for example, religion, family, social circle—and also significantly influences the interpretations of stress, social support, and level of disability versus ability to function. It is the physician's responsibility to determine a patient's level of functioning, resilience, and disability in the context of their cultural reference groups.[10]

Cultural Features of the Relationship Between the Individual and the Clinician

Clinicians should consider the cultural factors that affect both their relationship with the patient and the treatment itself. These could include difficulties with language (e.g., language discordance between the treater and the patient), establishing rapport, and eliciting symptoms or understanding their cultural significance. The consulting psychiatrist must also attend to the specific hospital environment in which the patient is receiving treatment. Interventions focused on these factors may improve the comfort of patients and providers as well as the quality of care more than any somatic intervention.

Overall Cultural Assessment

The formulation concludes with a summary of the implications of each component outlined above for psychiatric diagnosis, treatment, and other clinically relevant issues. This step directly acknowledges the fact that each society establishes its own criteria regarding which forms of behavior are acceptable, and which behaviors represent a medical problem.

The DSM-5 also includes the CFI, which consists of 16 questions that physicians can use in a more structured manner to assess the impact of culture on an individual's clinical presentation and care. The CFI focuses on four domains: cultural definition of the problem; cultural perceptions of the cause, context, and support of the problem; cultural factors affecting self-coping and past help seeking; and cultural factors affecting current help seeking. The interview aims to avoid stereotyping, as it centers on the individual and incorporates the cultural knowledge of the patient as well as the social context of their illness experience. Ideally the CFI is employed with every patient; it may also be utilized specifically when physicians experience difficulties in diagnostic assessments due to cultural differences, difficulties in determining illness severity or impairment, disagreements with patients regarding the course of treatment, or difficulties engaging patients in treatment.

Cultural Concepts of Distress

The previous version of the DSM, the DSM-IV-TR,[11] included a list of 25 "culture-bound syndromes" (also known as culture-specific syndromes or folk illnesses), defined as a combination of psychiatric and somatic symptoms considered to be a recognizable disease within a specific society or culture (i.e., not a voluntary behavior or false claim), not recognized as a disease in other cultures, and not associated with objective biochemical or structural alterations of body organs or functions. Examples of such syndromes include well-known entities such as *ataque de nervios*, *dhat syndrome*, and *shenjing shuairuo*.

The concept of culture-bound syndromes has been eliminated in the DSM and replaced with three related concepts: *cultural syndromes*, *cultural idioms of distress*, and *cultural explanations or perceived causes*.[8,9] The rationale for this change is that focusing on culture-bound syndromes "overemphasized the local particularity and limited distribution of cultural concepts of distress."[8,9] Additionally, the term "culture-bound syndrome" does not take into account that some "syndromes" are variations in ways people experience distress rather than distinct collections of symptoms (e.g., *nervios*), while others are causal explanations for a range of symptoms (e.g., *dhat* syndrome).

Cultural syndromes are clusters of symptoms that occur among individuals in specific cultural groups or communities. *Cultural idioms of distress* are shared ways of experiencing, communicating, and expressing personal or social concerns. *Cultural explanations or perceived causes* are labels, attributions, or features that indicate causation of symptoms, illness, or distress. As an example, depression fulfills the criteria for all three concepts. Western clinicians understand major depressive disorder as a "syndrome," or a cluster of symptoms that often appear together. Depression is also a cultural idiom of distress that is commonly used to talk about a certain clustering of physical and emotional symptoms. Finally, as a cultural explanation of distress or a perceived cause, the term "depression" helps imbue a set of behaviors with meaning and an associated etiology.

Despite these conceptual and semantic changes, DSM-5 continues to acknowledge the well-accepted place of culture-bound syndromes in psychiatric nosology and practice and includes a glossary of some of the most well-recognized "cultural concepts of distress," summarized in Table 47.1.

Acculturation and Immigration

As mentioned above, by 2060 nearly one in five of the nation's population is projected to be born outside of the United States.[1] Recent immigrants or refugees often arrive in the United States with a host of psychosocial challenges. Clinicians should ask about, and make an effort to understand, the circumstances surrounding immigration. An individual may have been

TABLE 47.1
Cultural Concepts of Distress

Syndrome	Populations
Ataque de nervios	Caribbean, Latin American, and Latin Mediterranean groups
Dhat syndrome (*semen loss*)	Southeast Asia
Khyâl cap	Cambodia
Kufungisisa	Shona of Zimbabwe
Maladi moun	Haiti
Nervios	Hispanic/Latinx in the United States, Mexico, Central America, and South America
Shenjing shuairuo (neurasthenia)	China; Traditional Chinese Medicine
Susto (fright or soul loss)[17]	Hispanic/Latinx in the United States, Mexico, Central America, and South America
Taijin kyofusho	Japan

a political prisoner or a victim of trauma and torture, or he or she may have been separated suddenly from family members. Under these circumstances, the level of depression and PTSD symptoms may be high. There is abundant literature documenting the contribution of acculturative stresses to the emergence of mental symptoms and disorders, including depression, anxiety, "culture shock," and PTSD.[12]

The trauma and torture experienced by many refugees are unfamiliar to most American practitioners.[3] While limited research does exist on refugee trauma and trauma-related psychiatric disorders and social handicaps, along with numerous reports of the concentration camp experiences in Cambodia, the sexual abuse of Vietnamese boat women, and the serious emotional distress associated with escape, refugee camps, and resettlement experiences, much more research is needed in this area.[13,14]

Impact of Race/Ethnicity on Psychiatric Diagnosis and Treatment

In the United States, race and ethnicity have a significant impact on psychiatric diagnosis and treatment.[15,16] The need to reduce disparities in the access to, and quality of, mental health care of racial and ethnic minorities was powerfully asserted by the Supplement

on Culture, Race, and Ethnicity to the US Surgeon General's landmark 2001 Report on Mental Health,[17] yet such disparities continue to persist. For example, Black and Hispanic/Latinx patients are disproportionately diagnosed with psychotic disorders compared to their White counterparts; parallel findings are documented in other countries globally when comparing immigrant BIPOC patients to the majority race.[18]

The reasons for misdiagnosis are complicated. They include the fact that individuals from some ethnic or cultural backgrounds may present to the medical system later in the course of their illness than White individuals, resulting in the perception of a more severe illness.[18] The late presentation itself may be related at least in part to mistrust of the healthcare system and challenges with healthcare access. Language barriers and unfamiliarity with cultural norms can contribute to misinterpretation and misattribution of patients' symptoms. Physician biases also play a major role in misdiagnosis. Psychiatric diagnoses are generally established by eliciting symptoms from patients; these symptoms are then interpreted by a clinician. Different disorders have overlapping symptoms that can be used to support one diagnosis or disregard another, depending on the clinician's bias or initial impression. In the case of Black people, affective symptoms are frequently ignored and psychotic symptoms are emphasized. This pattern has also been seen in other populations, including Hispanic/Latinx, Asians, and the Amish in the United States.[19]

Moreover, treatment decisions may also be affected by race. Black patients are more likely to receive higher doses of antipsychotic medications, to be prescribed first-generation or depot preparations of antipsychotics, to have higher rates of involuntary psychiatric hospitalizations, and to undergo seclusion and physical restraint while in psychiatric hospitals.[16,17,20,21] One interpretation of these statistics is that medical practitioners tend to over-sedate Black patients to reduce their perceived risk of violence despite, in some cases, little evidence that such a risk existed.

WORKING WITH INTERPRETERS

Miscommunication is common even between clinicians and patients who speak the same language and come from similar socioeconomic backgrounds. Therefore it is not difficult to imagine the challenges and obstacles that arise when patients exhibit low or limited English proficiency (LEP) and exhibit some of the cultural variations in behavior and symptom expression described above. Misunderstandings may lead to misdiagnosis and result in unnecessary or inappropriate treatment.[22] Patients, in turn, may feel frustrated, discouraged, or dissatisfied, leading them to refuse treatment or avoid care altogether.[23] Fortunately, skillful use of an interpreter can help bridge at least some of the communication gap between doctors and non-English-speaking patients and is essential to providing high-quality care to patients from non-English-speaking backgrounds.[24,25]

Many states now have laws that require federally funded medical facilities to provide interpreters for their non-English-speaking patients. While most medical interpreters must be trained and certified to work with healthcare providers, interpreting within a psychiatric context poses several unique challenges. Some of the common issues include the following:[26]

- Clinicians may feel they have less control over their work because their direct contact with the patient is decreased by the presence of the interpreter.
- Clinicians may feel uncertain about their role when working with interpreters who are more active and involved in the treatment process.
- Clinicians may have transference issues toward the interpreter.
- Conflicts may arise when clinicians and interpreters hold opposing views on a patient's diagnosis and treatment plans.
- Clinicians may feel frustrated when they cannot verify what is being said to the patient.
- Clinicians may feel left out if the patient appears to have more of a connection with the interpreter.
- Interpreters may feel uncomfortable when asked to translate certain issues (e.g., sexual history or childhood abuse).

Recommendations When Working With Interpreters

Clinicians must consider the qualifications of interpreters. Does the interpreter have experience working with mental health clinicians? How much does the interpreter know about psychiatric disorders and their treatment? What are the interpreter's personal views about mental illness? Interpreters who come from cultures in which mental illness is highly stigmatized may bring those biases or beliefs into the therapeutic process. Clinicians should meet with the interpreter briefly before each session to discuss expectations and clarify any issues or points that the clinician would like to address during the session.[26,27]

Clinicians should avoid using family members or friends as interpreters.[27,28] Patients may be unwilling to disclose sensitive information in front of these individuals, and it may be too distressing for a young child to hear details about a parent's symptoms. Family members have been known to omit or alter information they feel is too embarrassing or inappropriate to reveal to a clinician. Janitors and clerical staff have been used as interpreters in the medical setting, a practice that is strongly discouraged due to concerns about the adequacy of their knowledge of medical or mental health terminology.

Trained interpreters should be treated as professional colleagues by clinicians.[27] Most interpreters can offer important cultural knowledge that can help promote the clinician-patient relationship and facilitate a deeper understanding of the patient's culture, religion, and worldview. However, some clinicians prefer to use interpreters as word-for-word translation machines with no additional attempts to interpret or filter the meaning behind the patient's statements. Although such an approach allows the clinician to maintain their role as the primary caregiver and an illusion of control over what is being said to the patient, using direct translations can often lead to misunderstandings and confusion for both patients and clinicians alike. Literal translations from one language to another are often inaccurate and inappropriate. Certain words or concepts, such as depression and mental health, may not exist in the patient's native language. In addition, certain issues may be culturally inappropriate to discuss with a patient. For example, many females from Asian backgrounds feel uncomfortable when asked directly about certain topics, such as sexual abuse or family discord. Interpreters can be used as cultural consultants to help clinicians navigate these more complex issues. Allowing interpreters the freedom and flexibility to re-phrase or summarize what is being said can help prevent misunderstandings and improve the exchange between the clinician and the patient.

Time is a crucial factor when interpreters are involved. Interpreters must often explain psychiatric concepts to the patient, a process that may require more time than expected. Clinicians must be patient, bearing in mind that it may take 10 minutes to translate a single word. Patients do not get as much time with the clinician when communication must be accomplished through an interpreter, and clinicians may feel frustrated by the perceived inefficiency of the process. Clinicians should maximize their time with the patient by deferring any discussions with interpreters that can wait until after the session.

Clinicians should always remember to introduce the interpreter to the patient at the start of the session if they have not met. This is also a good time to reaffirm issues of confidentiality.[26,27] Because many ethnic communities are small and close-knit, patients may fear that the interpreter will divulge their private information to others and therefore be less willing to speak candidly. If possible, clinicians should try to use the same interpreter over time to help build trust and ensure continuity of care for the patient.[28]

During the session, the clinician should face and speak directly to the patient rather than the interpreter to facilitate connection through eye contact, gestures of acknowledgment, and other non-verbal behaviors.[29] The clinician should speak slowly, pause often, and avoid long sentences and technical jargon. It is important for both the clinician and interpreter to feel comfortable asking for clarification. Two-way conversations should be avoided. Tension may arise when someone in the group feels left out.

After each session, the clinician should encourage the interpreter to give their impression of the session. The interpreter can often provide important observations and feedback about cultural and non-verbal factors that may not have been apparent based solely on the patient's spoken responses.[24] Clinicians can use this time to learn more from the interpreter about the patient's culture. In sum, good communication, trust, and teamwork between the clinician and interpreter are essential when caring for patients with low or LEP.

THE "MEDICAL OMBUDSMAN" ROLE

In 1988 Pasnau[30] enumerated six fundamental functions of the consultation-liaison psychiatrist, including the role of "medical ombudsman" for the patient. Although the use of this term did not catch on, it signified the need for medical and surgical teams to be reminded of the unique human nature of each patient in their care. Racial, ethnic, and cultural factors are important characteristics in this regard. Psychiatrists in the general hospital can pay attention to these factors in their consultations and, as a result, enrich patient care.

ETHNICITY, CULTURE, AND PSYCHIATRIC MEDICATIONS

There is a large and growing body of research on ethnopsychopharmacology, or the study of racial and ethnic differences in how individuals respond to medications. In addition, several non-biological cultural factors are known to significantly affect BIPOC patients' relationship to, and use of, psychotropic medications. A familiarity with the basic principles in both these areas is necessary for effectively treating diverse populations.

Cultural Factors in Psychotropic Medication Usage

Culturally shaped beliefs play a major role in determining whether a particular explanation about an illness and recommended treatment plan (explanatory model) will make sense to a patient; for example, Hispanic/Latinx and Asian patients often expect rapid relief with treatment. Chinese and Vietnamese patients often express significant concerns about the addictive and toxic potential of Western medications and are reluctant to rely on these for extended periods. Many immigrant East and South Asian populations prefer traditional approaches to address their symptoms (e.g., Traditional Chinese Medicine, Ayurvedic medicine, or *kampo*), each of which may rely on a mixture of herbal medicines. Adherents to these traditions may believe that polypharmacy is more effective.

The use of herbal medicines carries with it the risk of medication interactions and medical or psychiatric side effects or toxicity. The US Food and Drug Administration has issued several warnings on herbal products, including the most popular weight loss products containing *Ephedra sinica* (*ma huang*), which is the main plant source of ephedrine and has been reported to cause mania, psychosis, and sudden death.

The Japanese herbs *Swertia japonica* and *Kamikihi-to*, and the Cuban *Datura candida*, have anticholinergic properties that may interact with tricyclic antidepressants (TCAs) or with low-potency neuroleptics. South American holly, *Ilex guayusa*, has a high caffeine content. The Nigerian root extract of *Schumanniophyton problematicum* (used to treat psychosis) is sedating and may interact with neuroleptics and with benzodiazepines. The Chinese herbs *Fructose schisandrae*, *Corydalis bungeana*, *Kopsia officinalis*, *Clausena lansium*, *muscone*, ginseng, and *Glycyrrhiza* increase the clearance of many psychotropic medications by stimulation of cytochrome P450 (CYP) enzymes. Oleanolic acid in *Swertia mileensis* and *Ligustrum lucidum* inhibits CYP enzymes.

On the other hand, for some patients and certain conditions, herbal remedies may produce significant benefits. Clinicians should not foreclose discussion of complementary and alternative treatments through judgmental or disparaging comments but rather use these topics to open a discussion about the patient's illness explanatory model and preferred treatment. The Engagement Interview Protocol (EIP) can facilitate a culturally respectful negotiation when the patient's and clinician's explanatory models differ.[31]

Communication difficulties and divergence between a patient's and a clinician's explanatory model can lead to treatment impasses. The EIP offers a systematic approach to exploring patient beliefs to improve communication, adherence, and outcomes.

Patient adherence may be affected by medication side effects, incorrect dosing due to differences in pharmacokinetics (see next section), and polypharmacy. Other factors include a poor therapeutic alliance; a lack of community support, money, or transportation; and concerns about the addictive potential of a medication.

Understanding and addressing each patient's social support system is crucial. Family interactions and functioning may have a significant impact on psychiatric treatment. For example, some Hispanic/Latinx patients may be accustomed to relying on extended family for medical decision-making and may become demoralized if their relatives are not involved in their treatment. Hispanic/Latinx and Asian patients have been described as relying on "closed networks" consisting of family members, kin, and intimate friends.

Biological Aspects of Psychopharmacology

Pharmacokinetics deals with absorption, distribution, metabolism, excretion, and blood levels of medications. Pharmacokinetics can be influenced by biochemical processes (such as conjugation, plasma protein binding, and oxidation by the cytochrome [CYP]P450 isoenzymes) as well as by characteristics of the individual (including genetics, age, sex, total body weight, and medical co-morbidities). Environmental factors that affect pharmacokinetics include dietary factors, sex hormones, and the use of caffeine, tobacco, alcohol, herbal medicines, and steroids, as well as ingestion of other prescription or illicit drugs.

The baseline activity of CYP liver enzymes is determined genetically, although environmental factors can alter their activity. Understanding how pharmacokinetic and environmental factors interact in different populations can help clinicians predict side effects, blood levels, and potential drug-drug interactions. For example, CYP2D6 is the isoenzyme that metabolizes many antidepressants (including the tricyclic and heterocyclic antidepressants and the selective serotonin reuptake inhibitors [SSRIs]); SSRIs can inhibit this enzyme, leading to the accumulation of other substrates. CYP2D6 also plays a role in metabolizing antipsychotics (such as clozapine, haloperidol, perphenazine, risperidone, thioridazine, and sertindole). Although much emphasis has been placed on CYP2D6's metabolism of psychotropic medications, it is also a major enzyme for the metabolism of numerous non-psychotropic medications. This fact, which is often ignored clinically, can have a significant effect on the tolerability or toxicity of a wide range of medications.

The incidence of poor metabolizers at the CYP2D6 isoenzyme ranges from 3% to 10% in White people; 1.9% to 7.3% in Black people; 2.2% to 6.6% in Hispanic/Latinx populations; and approximately 0% to 4.8% in Asians.[32,33] Another genetic variation of the metabolizer gene leads to "intermediate metabolizers" or individuals who exhibit CYP2D6 activity that is between poor (little or no CYP2D6 function) and extensive metabolizers (normal CYP2D6 function). Approximately 18% of Mexican Americans and 33% of Asian Americans and Black people have this gene variation. This may help explain ethnic differences in the pharmacokinetics of neuroleptics and antidepressants. Although these individuals are not as likely to experience toxicity at extremely low doses (e.g., poor metabolizers), they are likely to experience significant side effects at lower doses. These individuals may be mistakenly classified as "difficult patients" because they complain of side effects at unexpectedly low doses.

CYP2D6*4 (CYP2D6B) appears to be responsible for poor metabolizers in those who are White. CYP2D6*17 and CYP2D6*10 are found in individuals of Black and Asian origin, respectively, and are responsible for lower enzyme activity (intermediate or slow metabolizers). Individuals from these backgrounds are at great risk for toxicity, even when medications are used at low doses. For instance, a female who develops hypotension and a change in mental status several days after starting 20 mg of the TCA, nortriptyline, may be found to have toxic blood levels and require cardiac monitoring. Table 47.2 lists medications that are metabolized through different CYP enzyme systems.

Finally lithium appears to be a medication with significant differences in dosing and tolerability across populations. Black people are more likely to experience lithium toxicity and delirium compared with White counterparts (likely related to a slower lithium sodium pathway and connected to higher rates of hypertension). Individuals from East Asian backgrounds with bipolar disorder may respond to lower doses of lithium as compared with their White counterparts, with literature suggesting they can be successfully maintained at lower serum levels (0.4–0.8 mEq/L).[34]

The choice of medications, particularly atypical antipsychotics, should be tempered by an understanding of individual and population risk factors for medical morbidities (e.g., obesity, hypertension, diabetes mellitus, cardiovascular disease). For instance, many of the reports of diabetic ketoacidosis secondary to atypical antipsychotics have been in Black people, who are at higher risk for diabetes.[35,36]

Case 1

Mrs. E, a 30-year-old female with obsessive-compulsive disorder (OCD) originally from China, was recovering in the post-partum unit of a general hospital after giving birth to a healthy baby boy. She reported suicidal ideation and psychiatry was consulted. On interview, Mrs. E told the psychiatrist that since giving birth, she had experienced increasingly violent and ego-dystonic intrusive thoughts that she might harm her son and her husband, for example, by stabbing them with a knife. These thoughts were so distressing that she felt she would be better off dead rather than expose her family to her potentially violent actions.

Recognizing the potential significance of cultural factors in this case, the psychiatrist made sure to request the same Mandarin-speaking interpreter whenever possible when interacting with Mrs. E. She devoted some time to getting to know the interpreter and learned that the interpreter had a good grasp of psychiatric illnesses and did not consider them shameful or representative of individual weakness. The psychiatrist also adopted an attitude of cultural humility and spent more time than she usually would have to elicit Mrs. E's beliefs surrounding her symptoms and treatment. The psychiatrist learned that Mrs. E had a long history of being bullied and treated as an outcast with regard to her long history of OCD due to the stigmatization of mental illness in Chinese culture and that she was reluctant to take psychiatric medications due to fears of addiction and toxicity. She also learned from the interpreter that suicide may be seen as a viable option for some Chinese patients when confronted with insurmountable odds or shameful feelings.

In her treatment plan, the psychiatrist focused on psychoeducation about OCD and attempting to reduce feelings of stigma and shame. She allied with the patient's desire to be a good mother and convinced her to initiate treatment for her symptoms with an SSRI, taking extra time to address the patient's concerns about potential side effects, and agreeing to start at a lower dose and increase slowly per the patient's wishes. She also utilized cognitive-behavioral therapy techniques to gently challenge the patient's obsessions as well as her belief that suicide would result in a better future for her family. The patient felt understood and validated by the psychiatrist. Her suicidal ideation and obsessions gradually diminished with a combination of medications and psychotherapy, and she was ultimately discharged from the hospital with appointments for outpatient mental health follow-up.

TABLE 47.2

Common Cytochrome P450 Isoenzymes, Substrates, Inhibitors, and Inducers

CYP	CYP1A2	CYP2C9/10	CYP2C19	CYP2D6	CYP2E1	CYP3A3/4
Inhibitors	Fluvoxamine	Fluvoxamine	Fluoxetine	Bupropion	Diethylithiocarbamate (disulfiram)	Fluoxetine
	Moclobemide	Disulfiram	Fluvoxamine	Fluoxetine		Fluvoxamine
	Cimetidine	Amiodarone	Imipramine	Fluvoxamine		Nefazodone
	Fluoroquinolones	Azapropazone	Moclobemide	Hydroxybupropion		Sertraline
	Ciprofloxacin	D-Propoxyphene	Tranylcypromine	Paroxetine		Diltiazem
	Norfloxacin	Fluconazole	Diazepam	Sertraline		Verapamil
	Naringenin (grapefruit)	Fluvastatin	Felbamate	Moclobemide		Dexamethasone
	Ticlopidine	Miconazole	Phenytoin	Fluphenazine		Gestodene
		Phenylbutazone	Topiramate	Haloperidol		Clarithromycin
		Stiripentol	Cimetidine	Perphenazine		Erythromycin
		Sulfaphenazole	Omeprazole	Thioridazine		Troleandomycin
		Zafirlukast		Amiodarone		Fluconazole
				Cimetidine		Itraconazole
				Methadone		Ketoconazole
				Quinidine		Ritonavir
				Ritonavir		Indinavir
						Amiodarone
						Cimetidine
						Mibefradil
						Naringenin (grapefruit)
						Isoniazid
Inducers	Tobacco	Barbiturates		Rifampin		Ethanol
	Omeprazole	Phenytoin				Carbamazepine
		Rifampin				Barbiturates
						Phenobarbital
						Phenytoin
						Dexamethasone
						Rifampin
						Troglitazone

(Continued)

TABLE 47.2

Common Cytochrome P450 Isoenzymes, Substrates, Inhibitors, and Inducers—Cont'd

CYP	CYP1A2	CYP2C9/10	CYP2C19	CYP2D6	CYP2E1	CYP3A3/4
Substrates						
	Tertiary amine TCAs	THC	Citalopram	Fluoxetine	Ethanol	Carbamazepine
	Clozapine	NSAIDs	Moclobemide	Mirtazapine	Acetaminophen	Alprazolam
	Olanzapine	Phenytoin	Tertiary amine TCAs	Paroxetine	Chlorzoxazone	Diazepam
	Caffeine	Tolbutamide	Diazepam	Venlafaxine	Halothane	Midazolam
	Methadone	Warfarin	Hexobarbital	Secondary and tertiary amine TCAs	Isoflurane	Triazolam
	Tacrine	Losartan	Mephobarbital	Trazodone	Methoxyflurane	Buspirone
	Acetaminophen	Irbesartan	Omeprazole	Clozapine	Sevoflurane	Citalopram
	Phenacetin		Lansoprazole	Haloperidol		Mirtazapine
	Propranolol		Phenytoin	Fluphenazine		Nefazodone
	Theophylline		S-Mephenytoin	Perphenazine		Reboxetine
	Warfarin		Nelfinavir	Risperidone		Sertraline
			Warfarin	Sertindole		Tertiary amine TCAs
				Thioridazine		Sertindole
				Codeine		Quetiapine
				Dextromethorphan		Ziprasidone
				Hydrocodone		Diltiazem
				Oxycodone		Felodipine
				Mexiletine		Nimodipine
				Propafenone (IC antiarrhythmics)		Nifedipine
				β-Blockers		Nisoldipine
				Donepezil		Nitrendipine
				D-Fenfluramine		Verapamil
						Acetaminophen
						Alfentanil
						Codeine
						Fentanyl
						Sufentanil
						Ethosuximide
						Tiagabine
						Warfarin

CYP3A3/4 (continued): Amiodarone, Disopyramide, Lidocaine, Propafenone, Quinidine, Erythromycin, Androgens, Dexamethasone, Estrogens, Astemizole, Loratadine, Terfenadine, Lovastatin, Simvastatin, Atorvastatin, Cerivastatin, Cyclophosphamide, Tamoxifen, Vincristine, Vinblastine, Ifosfamide, Cyclosporine, Tacrolimus, Cisapride, Donepezil, Lovastatin, Protease inhibitors, Sildenafil, Disopyramide, Losartan

NSAID, Non-steroidal anti-inflammatory drug; *TCA,* tricyclic antidepressant; *THC,* tetrahydrocannabinol.

RECOMMENDATIONS FOR OPTIMIZING CLINICAL CARE OF DIVERSE POPULATIONS

Helpful Techniques

Certain techniques may help to avoid misdiagnosis, mistreatment, and cultural clashes. The first moments of an encounter are often crucial. A clinician must be mindful of maintaining a respectful attitude and may find it particularly useful to address patients from different ethnic backgrounds more formally (e.g., Mr., Ms., or Mrs.). In some cultures, an informal introduction is considered disrespectful and may have a lasting impact on the physician-patient relationship.

Forging an alliance with patients from diverse backgrounds may be more complex and require more time. It may also take extra time and effort to assure patients about confidentiality, to provide psychoeducation about mental illness to counteract cultural stigmas and to work with interpreters. If the diagnosis is unclear or affected by ethnicity or culture, the clinician should consider utilizing a structured diagnostic interview (e.g., the tools from DSM-5, such as the OCF or the CFI) to reduce the possibility of misdiagnosis, and should consider seeking consultation from other members of the patient's community regarding which aspects of the presentation might be culturally influenced as opposed to representing pathology (taking care, of course, to protect the patient's privacy in the process). The services of a trained medical interpreter should be utilized whenever possible.

Moving Beyond Cultural Competence and Toward Cultural Humility

The idea of "cultural competence" has been challenged on both conceptual and semantic grounds. The term has been noted to be problematic in its implication that culture can be reduced to "a technical skill for which clinicians can be trained to develop expertise."[37] Further, a focus on attaining "cultural competence" has been criticized as reinforcing the notion of culture as a static and categorical "other" to be mastered, which may reduce a patient's cultural background to a stereotyped core set of beliefs and values that may trivialize the role of culture in medical illness and treatment.[38]

Instead of striving for "competence," an alternative framework is that of "cultural respect" or "cultural humility." Cultural humility has been defined as the "ability to maintain an interpersonal stance that is open in relation to aspects of cultural identity that are most important to the patient."[39] The culturally humble physician is able to express respect and a lack of superiority with regard to the patient's culture and does not assume competence in terms of working with a particular patient simply based on prior experience working with other patients from a similar population or cultural background.

REFERENCES

1. Colby SL, Ortman JM. *Projections of the Size and Composition of the U.S. Population: 2014 to 2060.* Current Population Reports: U.S. Census Bureau; 2015.
2. Espí Forcén F, Velez Florez MC, Bido Medina R. Deconstructing cultural aspects of mental health care in Hispanic/Latinx people. *Psychiatr Ann.* 2023;53(3):127–132. https://doi.org/10.3928/00485713-20230215-02.
3. Mollica RF, Wyshak G, Lavelle J. The psychosocial impact of war trauma and torture on Southeast Asian refugees. *Am J Psychiatry.* 1987;144(12):1567–1572.
4. Mollica RF, Lavelle J. Southeast Asian refugees. In: Comas-Díaz L, Griffith EEH, eds. *Clinical Guidelines in Cross-Cultural Mental Health.* Wiley; 1988:262–304.
5. Westermeyer J. Lao folk diagnosis for mental disorders: comparison with psychiatric diagnosis and assessment with psychiatric rating scales. *Med Anthropol.* 1981;5:425–443.
6. Hinton DE, Otto MW. Symptom presentation and symptom meaning among traumatized Cambodian refugees: relevance to a somatically focused cognitive-behavior therapy. *Cogn Behav Pract.* 2006;13(4):249–260.
7. Geltman D, Chang G. Hallucinations in Latino psychiatric outpatients: a preliminary investigation. *Gen Hosp Psychiatry.* 2004;26(2):153–157.
8. American Psychiatric Association. *Diagnostic and Statistical Manual of Mental Disorders.* 5th ed. American Psychiatric Association; 2013.
9. American Psychiatric Association. *Diagnostic and Statistical Manual of Mental Disorders, Text Revision (TR).* 5th ed. American Psychiatric Association; 2022.
10. Lewis-Fernández R, Aggarwal NK, Bäärnhielm S, et al. Culture and psychiatric evaluation: operationalizing cultural formulation for DSM-5. *Psychiatry.* 2014;77(2):130–154.
11. American Psychiatric Association. *Diagnostic and Statistical Manual of Mental Disorders.* 4th ed. American Psychiatric Association Publishing; 1994.
12. Koneru VK, Weisman A, Flynn P, et al. Acculturation and mental health: current findings and recommendations for future research. *Appl Prev Psychol.* 2007;12(2):76–96.
13. Murray KE, Davidson GR, Schweitzer RD. Review of refugee mental health interventions following resettlement: best practices and recommendations. *Am J Orthopsychiatry.* 2010;80(4):576–585.

14. Mollica RF, Caridad KR, Massagli MP. Longitudinal study of posttraumatic stress disorder, depression, and changes in traumatic memories over time in Bosnian refugees. *J Nerv Ment Dis.* 2007;195(7):572–579.

15. Kales HC, Blow FC, Bingham CR. Race, psychiatric diagnosis, and mental health care utilization in older patients. *Am J Geriatr Psychiatry.* 2000;8(4):301–309.

16. Mallinger JB, Fisher SG, Brown S, et al. Racial disparities in the use of second-generation antipsychotics for the treatment of schizophrenia. *Psychiatr Serv.* 2006;57(1):133–136. https://doi.org/10.1176/appi.ps.57.1.133. PMID: 16399976.

17. Opolka JL, Rascati KL, Gibson PJ. Ethnicity and prescription patterns for haloperidol, risperidone, and olanzapine. *Psychiatr Serv.* 2004;55(2):151–156.

18. United States Public Health Service. *Mental Health: Culture, Race, and Ethnicity: A Supplement to Mental Health: A Report of the Surgeon General.* Office of the Surgeon General, U.S. Public Health Service; 2001.

19. Schwartz RC, Blankenship DM. Racial disparities in psychotic disorder diagnosis: a review of empirical literature. *World J Psychiatry.* 2014;4(4):133–140.

20. Rayburn TM, Stonecypher JF. Diagnostic differences related to age and race of involuntarily committed psychiatric patients. *Psychol Rep.* 1996;79(3 Pt 1):881–882.

21. Kuno E, Rothbard AB. Racial disparities in antipsychotic prescription patterns for patients with schizophrenia. *Am J Psychiatry.* 2002;159(4):567–572.

22. Drennan G, Swartz L. The paradoxical use of interpreting in psychiatry. *Soc Sci Med.* 2002;54(12):1853–1866.

23. Marcos L. Effects of interpreters on the evaluation of psychopathology in non-English speaking patients. *Am J Psychiatry.* 1979;136(2):171–174.

24. Bauer AM, Alegría M. The impact of patient language proficiency and interpreter service use on the quality of psychiatric care: a systematic review. *Psychiatr Serv.* 2010;61(8):765–773.

25. Karliner LS, Jacobs EA, Chen AH, et al. Do professional interpreters improve clinical care for patients with limited English proficiency? A systematic review of the literature. *Health Serv Res.* 2007;42(2):727–754.

26. Tribe RRH, ed. *Working With Interpreters in Mental Health.* Brunner-Routledge; 2003.

27. McPhee SJ. Caring for a 70-year-old Vietnamese woman. *JAMA.* 2002;287(4):495–504.

28. Juckett G, Unger K. Appropriate use of medical interpreters. *Am Fam Physician.* 2014;90(7):476–480.

29. Peterson DE, Remington PL, Kuykendall MA. Behavioral risk factors of Chippewa Indians living on Wisconsin reservations. *Public Health Rep.* 1994;109(6):820–823.

30. Pasnau RO. Consultation–liaison psychiatry: progress, problems, and prospects. *Psychosomatics.* 1988;29(1):4–15.

31. Yeung AS, Trinh NH, Chang TE, et al. The Engagement Interview Protocol (EIP): improving the acceptance of mental health treatment among Chinese immigrants. *Int J Cult Ment Health.* 2011;4(2):91–105.

32. Shimizu T, Ochiai H, Asell F, et al. Bioinformatics research on inter-racial difference in drug metabolism I. Analysis on frequencies of mutant alleles and poor metabolizers on CYP2D6 and CYP2C19. *Drug Metab Pharmacokinet.* 2003;18(1):48–70.

33. Bertilsson L, Dahl ML, Dalén P, et al. Molecular genetics of CYP2D6: clinical relevance with focus on psychotropic drugs. *Br J Clin Pharmacol.* 2002;53(2):111–122.

34. Pi EH, Zhu W. Cross-cultural psychopharmacology: a review. *Ann Gen Psychiatry.* 2010;9(suppl 1):S82.

35. Henderson DC. Clinical experience with insulin resistance, diabetic ketoacidosis, and type 2 diabetes mellitus in patients treated with atypical antipsychotic agents. *J Clin Psychiatry.* 2001;62(suppl 27):10–14, discussion 40–41.

36. Henderson DC. Atypical antipsychotic-induced diabetes mellitus: how strong is the evidence? *CNS Drugs.* 2002;16(2):77–89.

37. Kleinman A, Benson P. Anthropology in the clinic: the problem of cultural competency and how to fix it. *PLoS Med.* 2006;3(10):23.

38. Kumagai AK, Lypson ML. Beyond cultural competence: critical consciousness, social justice, and multicultural education. *Acad Med.* 2009;84(6):782–787.

39. Hook JN, Davis DE, Owen J, et al. Cultural humility: measuring openness to culturally diverse clients. *J Couns Psychol.* 2013;60(3):353–366.

48

LEGAL ASPECTS OF PSYCHIATRIC CONSULTATION

CELESTE PEAY, MD, JD ■ RONALD SCHOUTEN, MD, JD ■
REBECCA WEINTRAUB BRENDEL, MD, JD

OVERVIEW

Legal issues are common and acknowledged, though rarely welcomed, aspects of modern medicine. Physicians respond to these issues in various ways, such as by denying their existence, resenting the perceived intrusion into patient care that they can create, and obsessing about them, which can ultimately interfere with providing good clinical care.

Although legal issues are ever-present and at times are the dominant concerns of patients and providers, for the most part, they exist in the background of care. When specific legal issues do arise, medical and surgical physicians often turn to the consultation psychiatrist for assistance, perhaps because the most common legal issues that arise—decision-making capacity and treatment refusal—have to do with mental functions and abnormalities of behavior. Whatever the reason, the psychiatric consultant may be drawn into a turbulent atmosphere when medical and surgical staff are confronted with a legal issue. A well-prepared consultant can be invaluable in these matters.

The first and perhaps most important service provided by the consultant is to remind the consultee that the physician's safest havens within the law are the principles of good faith, common sense, and good clinical care. To be of maximum assistance, consultants should be familiar with relevant legal concepts and use this knowledge to diminish consultees' anxiety and help them perform their jobs. The challenge for the psychiatric consultant is to ease the burden on the consultee by providing clinical insights and legal information and to know when and how to use the input of the hospital's attorney.

Medicine advanced rapidly in the 20th century and continues to do so in the 21st, giving rise to an evolving array of medico-legal issues. These issues are reflected in questions asked by residents and staff alike: *How do I determine whether a patient is incompetent? If the patient is competent and making an irrational decision, does that decision have to be honored? What is my liability exposure as a consultant? If a managed care organization refuses to pay for continued hospitalization or for a patient's admission to a psychiatric facility, can the physician be held liable if the patient commits suicide? If the patient has expressed a desire to hurt someone else, what are my obligations to that third party? What obligations do I have if my patient is human immunodeficiency virus (HIV)-positive and refuses to inform their sexual partner?*

This chapter cannot provide definitive answers to these and all the other medico-legal questions faced by general hospital psychiatrists. Rather, this chapter outlines general principles that apply in almost all jurisdictions. Because state statutes and case law vary considerably on these medico-legal matters, hospital counsel and legal representatives of medical organizations and insurers should be consulted. They are excellent sources of information about the legal aspects of general hospital psychiatry.

PHYSICIANS' RIGHTS AND OBLIGATIONS

Malpractice Liability

Malpractice, negligence, and *liability* are three terms that engender great concern and are often misunderstood. Malpractice law is a type of personal injury or tort law that concerns itself with injuries allegedly caused by the negligent treatment activities of professionals. To establish a claim of malpractice, a plaintiff (the complaining party) must prove four things. First, it must be proven that the defendant physician owed a duty to the injured party. Where the injured party is the patient, the duty is to perform up to the standards of the average physician in the community practicing in that specialty. Failure to practice in accordance with that standard, unless there is some justification, constitutes the second element: negligence. The third and fourth elements are closely tied to the first two: the negligent behavior must be shown to have been the direct cause of actual damages. If all four elements are proved, the defendant may be held liable (responsible for the damage) and ordered to compensate the plaintiff, either directly or through their insurer.[1-5] The four elements of malpractice are often summarized as the four Ds: duty, dereliction of duty, direct causation, and damages.

Malpractice liability exposure can be a concern for psychiatric consultants as well as other clinicians. Treating clinicians have the primary duty of care for the patient. Consultants, who are brought in to advise the treating clinicians, do not have the same duty to the patient. The consultant's duty of reasonable care is owed to the consultee, not the patient. This rule does not hold, however, where the consultant steps out of the purely consultative role and assumes direct responsibility for some aspect of the treatment relationship. For example, the consultant who evaluates a patient and then recommends to the treating physician that a course of antidepressant treatment is appropriate is not liable for an adverse outcome from the treatment. If, however, the consultant writes the prescription and monitors the treatment course, he or she has assumed the status of the "treating physician" and may be held responsible for any adverse outcomes.

Liability and Managed Care

Managed care and liability for injury when coverage is denied have been important issues since managed care arrived on the healthcare scene. The basic problem can be seen in this hypothetical example.

Case 1

Mr. A was admitted to the trauma unit after leaping off a bridge into a river. After undergoing an open reduction and internal fixation of his bilateral femoral fractures, the psychiatric consultant saw him. Mr. A was found to be suffering from major depression as well as an alcohol use disorder. He was believed to be at a moderate-to-high risk for suicide, and suicide precautions were instituted on the floor. Mr. A was started on an antidepressant, but it had not yet begun to work when he was deemed surgically ready for discharge. The consultant recommended transfer to an inpatient psychiatry unit where Mr. A could undergo treatment for both his depression and substance use disorder. Mr. A's mental health coverage had been carved out of his medical-surgical coverage. The utilization reviewer for his medical-surgical coverage insisted that he be discharged from the hospital and scheduled for outpatient physical therapy with visiting nurse coverage. The mental health management company sent its psychologist reviewer to evaluate Mr. A. The reviewer agreed that Mr. A was depressed but denied authorization for psychiatric hospitalization. The reviewer opined that Mr. A was not acutely suicidal, did not need inpatient substance abuse treatment, and could be managed as an outpatient. He was given the names of the three psychiatrists in his town who were authorized under his plan and was able to get an appointment scheduled for 2 weeks after discharge. Mr. A was discharged from the hospital, over the objections of the consultant. The consultant had found that the patient was still significantly depressed and at risk of drinking again but not committable because he was not imminently suicidal. Ten days later, the visiting nurse found him hanged in his apartment. The death was ruled a suicide. Mr. A's family brought a malpractice action against the hospital, the treating physicians, the consultant, and the managed care company.

What liability does the managed care company have in cases like Case 1, in which the denial of care results in harm to the patient? Would the managed care company's liability supersede that of the physicians? The answers to these questions are still unclear. There have been a series of legal cases addressing these issues, and the law is still evolving. At present, there is a possibility that managed care companies may be held liable in these situations if the company exerted such control over the decision-making process that the physician's judgment was over-ridden. In other words, for the physician to avoid liability, they must protest the denial of care, appeal it to the highest level that the insurer provides, and take other reasonable steps to ensure the patient's safety. Depending on the facts, the liability may be assigned entirely to the managed care company, to the physician, or shared.[6-8] At present, treating physicians are regarded as independent contractors and therefore bear separate and often sole responsibility. There are policy arguments against that model, which may lead to future changes.[8]

Whatever the policy arguments, under federal law, there are specific limits on managed care companies' liability for denial of care. Most often, decisions made by managed care organizations to limit care are subject only to limited legal remedies under the Employee Retirement Income Security Act (ERISA) of 1974. ERISA limits most employees of private companies to use their health plans for the cost of the care denied by the managed care organization only, and not for the recovery of losses that result from the denial of care or for punitive damages. ERISA's protection of managed care plans from liability for the consequences of their decisions is increasingly seen as unfair given the level of control over treatment decisions exercised by some plans. As a result, several federal court cases have eroded the prohibition on damages under the law, but these cases represent only small gains, the trend in cases has appeared to have come to a halt, and there is no indication that lawmakers will amend ERISA to eliminate the preemption clause, and the Supreme Court continues to protect employer-sponsored plans from state requirements. In addition, state law efforts to hold managed care companies liable for damages have been largely unsuccessful. For the time being, in the face of bad outcomes, patients may try to shift liability to physicians and hospitals to recover losses.

Confidentiality and Privacy

Confidentiality is the clinician's obligation to keep matters revealed by a patient from the ears of third parties.[2] It is usually demanded and protected by statute and custom. A variety of exceptions to confidentiality exist, usually where the courts or the legislature determine that maintenance of confidentiality will result in

more harm than good from a societal standpoint. This rationale provided the basis for the California court's decision in *Tarasoff v. Board of Regents*,[9] in which the court held that psychotherapists must act to protect third parties where the therapist knows or should know that the patient poses a threat of serious risk of harm to the third party.[10]

Although not all states have adopted this view, the majority have. Several states have enacted statutes dealing with this fertile area of malpractice liability and either limited or eliminated the duty.[11] The consultant should be familiar with the relevant statutory and case law concerning this issue in their jurisdiction. In addition, a small number of states, including Massachusetts, have held that a physician may be held liable for injuries to a third person that result from the failure to warn a patient about the side effects of medications, such as when a patient falls asleep at the wheel of a car and was not warned of the sedating effects of medication.

Although infectious disease has been the subject of duty to protect cases in the past, infection with HIV has been treated somewhat differently than other infectious diseases. Controversy persists about the obligation of a physician to warn the partner of an HIV-positive patient when the patient refuses to do so. Many states have statutes that address this issue, with varied approaches, adding to the confusion and highlighting the controversial nature of the issue. The psychiatric consultant should learn the requirements of the jurisdiction in which they practice. Several articles and book chapters have addressed this controversial issue, some of which are cited in the references for this chapter.[12,13]

In addition to situations in which disclosure is mandated to protect a third party, such as in *Tarasoff* and infectious disease situations, other breaches of confidentiality may be mandated by statute or case law to protect vulnerable third parties. For example, all 50 states in the United States have statutes that require specific individuals, including physicians, to report suspected child abuse or neglect to state social service agencies.[14]

Many states also require that known or suspected abuse or neglect of the elderly or the disabled be reported. Failure to comply with these requirements can result in substantial penalties. More recently, some states have begun requiring physicians and others to report known or suspected cases of domestic violence to law enforcement or designated agencies. Mandatory reporting statutes serve an important societal purpose, but they are not without controversy. Every clinician should become aware of the specific requirements in their jurisdiction.

Patient health information is also subject to regulation under a federal law known as the Health Insurance Portability and Accountability Act (HIPAA) of 1996. As of mid-2003, institutions and individual providers are required to comply with HIPAA rules. HIPAA has affected hospital practice by requiring the distribution, in writing, of the institution's privacy policy to all patients and by mandating physicians to undergo training on privacy and disclosure provisions. The rules are too complex to review in full here; however, several salient points stand out for psychiatrists.

Among the most relevant provisions of HIPAA are the treatment of medical records and the distinction between general psychiatric records and psychotherapy notes. Patients are entitled to a copy of their medical records; they also have the explicit right to request changes in the record. Whether or not the applicable staff person amends the contested information, the involved correspondence becomes part of the record. Although HIPAA affords special status to psychotherapy notes and allows psychiatrists not to disclose these notes to patients, this exception is narrow. To qualify for protection under the psychotherapy notes provision, the notes must be kept separate from the patient's medical record. Specific types of information contained in psychotherapy notes are not subject to the psychotherapy notes exclusion; these include medications prescribed, test results, treatment plans, diagnoses, prognosis, and progress to date.[15-17] It should be noted, however, that notes falling within the HIPAA psychotherapy notes exception are considered to be part of the medical record if a subpoena is received for medical records.

The practical implication of HIPAA regarding psychiatric record-keeping is that psychiatric records, whether in an outpatient clinic or contained in a medical chart from a non-psychiatric hospitalization, are broadly accessible to patients or anyone they authorize to access their records. Therefore, consulting psychiatrists should be careful in the documentation of sensitive therapy material because it will be treated like the rest of the medical record unless the psychotherapy notes are kept in a separate file. Even more, it is now commonplace for patients to have legal access to their electronic medical records, including open notes for mental health treatment.[18]

As for patients, health insurance companies' access to psychotherapy records is restricted. Health insurance companies cannot demand access to information contained in psychotherapy notes as a requirement of payment for care. If, in a particular circumstance, psychotherapy notes are released to an insurance company, written consent from the patient is required under HIPAA. This consent requirement is in sharp contrast to the disclosure rules for the general medical and general psychiatric record for insurance purposes; HIPAA does not require consent for disclosure of this information to insurance companies to obtain payment for treatment—medical or psychiatric. HIPAA also does not require specific consent for the release of information for treatment or healthcare operations purposes (quality assurance, licensing, and accreditation). There are 11 additional circumstances in which disclosure is permitted without patient consent, including emergencies and mandated reporting situations, such as child abuse—which are generally considered to be a part of current medical practice. But other situations, including exceptions for law enforcement and attorney requests, may be more concerning.[15-17]

Refusal to Treat Patients

Refusal to treat patients, in or out of the hospital, is a right that is rarely invoked by physicians. The physician-patient relationship is contractual. Both parties have the same right to enter, or to refuse to enter, the relationship as they do with other contracts. Once the physician offers to treat and the patient accepts, the contract is established, and the physician's right to refuse or withdraw is limited in certain ways. For example, maintaining a walk-in clinic or emergency department (ED) can be construed as an implicit offer to treat on an emergent basis. The patient's presentation at the clinic or ED is an acceptance of the offer, creating a contract. It does not necessarily create an obligation to provide ongoing care, so long as the walk-in or emergency nature of the services is clear and appropriate information is provided regarding ongoing care.

In a situation in which a prospective patient discusses their history with a physician, it may be difficult to assert that no relationship has been established, particularly if the patient is under the impression that a treatment relationship exists. Physicians should clarify at the outset of the treatment encounter that they may or may not accept a case. It is usually helpful to explain at the first visit that this is an initial evaluation to determine whether it is appropriate for the physician to take this individual as a patient. The terms of an individual physician's relationship with the employing clinic can make it difficult to exercise this option. This principle does not include the emergent, or even urgent, medical problem, which imposes an obligation to provide care sufficient to stabilize the patient's condition. If no physician-patient relationship has been created in the initial contact, referral of the patient to a healthcare facility, such as a walk-in clinic, demonstrates concern for the patient without necessarily creating an obligation to treat.[19,20]

When the physician elects not to treat an individual, the physician should make every effort to provide an alternative course to avoid claims of abandonment.[1-3] Abandonment is the unilateral severance of the relationship by the physician, leaving the patient without needed medical care. The optimal care of the patient is the first consideration. Whenever a physician desires to transfer the patient to another physician, the transferring physician must take steps to ensure continuity of care by making a specific arrangement with the physician who is going to treat the patient. The physician may terminate the treatment relationship with a patient for a variety of reasons, including non-payment, repeated failure to keep appointments, or threatening behavior. In such cases, the patient should be notified of the decision, the available treatment options (including a specific referral, if possible), and the available sources of emergency care. The course pursued and the reasons and indications for the transfer or termination should be documented in the medical record.[2,3]

The physician's right to refuse to provide care for patients may be restricted where the refusal is based on the patient's specific illness or inherent characteristics. The refusal to care for patients of certain races, religions, ethnic origins, or disease types (e.g., acquired immunodeficiency syndrome) raises significant ethical concerns as well as potential liability under Title VII of the Civil Rights Act of 1964 and the Americans with Disabilities Act. These are beyond the scope of this chapter. The general rule, however, is that physicians and other clinicians may be charged with unethical conduct and, in some situations, with violation of patients' civil rights when treatment is refused on a discriminatory basis.[19,20]

The issue of terminating the physician-patient relationship usually arises when some conflict has developed between physician and patient throughout treatment or because of non-compliance.[21] Knowing about the physician's right not to treat is important for consultants. Often the knowledge that a physician can stop treating a particular patient allows enough "give" in a confrontation so that the consultee's anxiety diminishes, and negotiation can begin.

End-of-Life Care and Advance Directives

Care of dying and hopelessly ill patients continues to generate difficult questions, staff conflicts, and requests for help from physicians who find themselves faced with these clinical, ethical, and legal dilemmas.[22,23] Controversy and turmoil are generated when the patient loses the capacity to participate in the decision-making process. The decision of a competent patient to refuse life-sustaining treatment yields similar results. The general rule is that every competent adult has the right to make their own decisions about medical care based on personal preference, even if that choice conflicts with what most people would choose under similar circumstances. An important distinction must be drawn between the competent patient's request that treatment be withheld or withdrawn and requests that the physician take some active, independent step to terminate the patient's life. The former is generally regarded as being within the realm of the patient's right to make treatment decisions. The original illness, rather than the withholding or withdrawal of treatment, is regarded as the cause of death in such situations. Active steps taken to end a patient's life are considered euthanasia; in many states, the complying physician could be subjected to criminal prosecution.[23-25] In two 1997 cases, the Supreme Court of the United States upheld two state laws prohibiting physician-assisted suicide after physicians challenged the constitutionality of the laws.[26,27] However, the Supreme Court of the

United States has also limited the ability of the federal government to prevent states from allowing physician-assisted suicide. Specifically, in 2006, the Court ruled against the federal government when it attempted to use federal law to block the ability of Oregon physicians to prescribe controlled substances for physician-assisted suicide.[28] For more than a decade, Oregon was the only state that legalized physician-assisted suicide. As of this writing, Oregon, Washington, Montana, Vermont, Colorado, California, New Mexico, Hawaii, New Jersey, Maine, and Washington, DC, have passed physician-assisted dying statutes.

The treatment requests of the dying patient have not always been taken seriously, especially when the patient's choice is to terminate care. Physicians struggle when faced with a patient who refuses further treatment, especially when there is some hope for improvement. Physicians often find it difficult to give up the fight, even at the request of the patient. Consulting psychiatrists in such circumstances should be concerned with determining whether the patient's request to forego heroic efforts stems from a condition that can be reversed or mitigated, such as depression or pain, and whether the patient can understand the nature of the request. In other words, is the patient's refusal of further treatment informed? If it is, the next challenge is working with the treatment team so that they can accept the patient's decision.

When minor children suffer terminal conditions, in the absence of any over-riding legal requirements, parents are generally permitted to make decisions regarding the continuation of extraordinary efforts.[24,29,30] The consulting psychiatrist is urged to seek the advice of the hospital's general counsel when confronted with these issues. The maze of governmental regulations, statutes, and case law in this area, combined with the emotionally charged nature of the situation, demands expert legal input. Nevertheless, the larger challenge for the consultant and the treatment team lies in helping the child's parents with the turmoil at hand and the grief ahead.

The psychiatrist should do what they can to ensure the comfort of the patient, such as seeing that treatment of clinical depression and alleviation of tractable pain are not overlooked given the anxiety that surrounds the dying patient. Development and documentation of written guidelines for the management of these difficult situations can help ensure rational constancy in approach. Such attention to the relief of suffering decreases conflict between patient, family, and staff. In turn, this helps avoid legal involvement in the situation.

The status of the patient's right to refuse life-sustaining treatment varies among the states. In 1990 the Supreme Court of the United States handed down its opinion in *Cruzan v. Director, Missouri Department of Public Health*.[31] The Court held that all competent individuals have a constitutionally protected right to refuse life-sustaining treatment. When a patient cannot make their own decisions, however, the court held that the state can assert its interest in preserving life and require clear and convincing evidence of the now-incapacitated patient's preferences in such matters before a surrogate decision-maker will be allowed to refuse the treatment on the patient's behalf. In most jurisdictions, surrogate decision-makers, whether family members or guardians, are allowed greater freedom in concluding the patient's preference.

Many states have statutes that allow individuals to issue advance directives concerning future medical care in these situations. All states have statutes providing for durable powers of attorney, an instrument that can be used to delegate decision-making authority to another person in the event of incapacity, although they do not uniformly allow the durable power of attorney to be used for some specific, or even all, healthcare decisions. All physicians should be aware of what prior directives are valid in their jurisdictions and encourage their patients to explore these issues with them and with their legal representatives. Under the Patient Self-Determination Act of 1990, all healthcare facilities, nursing homes, and health maintenance organizations must inquire on admission or enrollment whether a patient has an advance directive. If not, the patient must be offered information on the subject and an opportunity to create a directive.[32-34] Nonetheless only a minority of Americans have executed an advance directive.

RIGHTS OF PATIENTS

It is no news that the relationship between physician and patient has changed considerably over the years. The pendulum has swung between the extremes of paternalism and total patient autonomy. More recently, the impact of restrictions on patient choice imposed by managed care has been added to the equation. Most physicians and their patients operate on some middle ground between the extremes of complete patient autonomy and medical paternalism. The fundamental principle is that the patient, not the physician, makes the ultimate choice regarding treatment. This ethical concept has been operationalized by legal decisions and legislation. Although some physicians still view these changes as dangerous to patient care and as intrusions into their domain of clinical judgment, they are part of an ever-shrinking minority, as more and more physicians have come to accept the idea of greater patient autonomy.[35]

Informed Consent and Evaluation of Decision-Making Capacity

Informed consent issues and the evaluation of decision-making capacity (commonly referred to as competency) are major components of the medico-legal workload. Informed consent has been an essential feature of medical practice since the 1960s. It is a process by which the patient agrees to treatment, in which the consent is based on adequate information, and it is voluntarily given by a patient who is competent to do so.[36] The term *informed consent* is somewhat misleading; we are as concerned with informed refusal as we are with informed consent. Bowing to convention, the term *informed consent* is used with the understanding that the same standards apply to informed refusal.

Informed consent is required before the initiation of any medical treatment, but exceptions do exist. Informed consent need not be obtained in an emergency in which delay would seriously threaten the well-being of the patient. In such cases, the physician is under an obligation to use their best judgment and to act in good faith. Such behavior is unlikely to result in litigation if the physician documents (immediately after the emergency passes) the events and the reasons for the steps taken, and that those steps were reasonable. Other exceptions to informed consent have been found where the patient waives the right to receive information, where the patient cannot make decisions, or where providing the information needed for informed consent would cause the patient's physical or mental health to deteriorate (known as therapeutic

privilege). The therapeutic privilege is problematic; it is mentioned here because it has been invoked in the past and was for many years a mainstay of medical paternalism (e.g., patients who were treated for carcinoma without being told the diagnosis for fear it "would just upset them" and worsen their overall condition). Situations in which the therapeutic privilege can be justifiably invoked are rare. The fact that providing the information might lead the patient to refuse treatment or would cause the patient considerable anxiety does not justify invoking therapeutic privilege. The situation must be one in which the informed consent process itself would cause a risk of grave harm. The physician who forgoes the informed consent process in the name of therapeutic privilege does so at their own risk.[36-38]

An essential feature of modern consent is that it is informed. Simple consent, in which the patient gives the physician blanket permission to take care of medical problems, is not deemed adequate, unless the patient has made a specific decision to waive informed consent. The amount and type of information to be provided to the patient or the surrogate decision-maker vary somewhat among jurisdictions.[2] The two basic standards are the professional standard and the patient-oriented standard. In the former, the physician is required to give that amount of information that the average physician in that specialty would provide under the circumstances. In other words, it looks to the standard of care. In other states, the amount of information to be provided is determined by what the patient would require to make an informed decision. This is also known as the materiality standard. In some states, the materiality standard is applied based on what the average patient would require to make a decision, whereas in other states it is assessed in terms of what the specific patient would require. In either case, the physician who covers the following information, taken from a leading Massachusetts case,[39] with the patient will generally be held to have provided adequate information:

- The diagnosis and condition to be treated,
- The nature of the proposed treatment,
- The nature and probability of the material risks of the treatment,

- The benefits that may be expected from the treatment,
- The inability of the physician to predict results,
- The irreversibility of the procedure, if that is the case,
- The likely results of forgoing treatment, and
- The likely results, risks, and benefits of alternative treatments.

The second requirement for informed consent is that the consent be given voluntarily. Coercion is often in the eye of the beholder; the fact that coercion ostensibly occurs in the service of the best interests of the patient does not justify it from an ethical standpoint or qualify it as an element of informed consent. The line between persuasion and coercion often appears to be both narrow and vague. If some negative contingency (including an exaggerated prediction of a poor prognosis) is attached to the patient's refusal of treatment, there is coercion, and any subsequent consent is technically invalid.

The presence of decision-making capacity, commonly referred to as competency, is the threshold issue in the informed consent process. The term *competency* is familiar to all physicians, but it is used imprecisely in the clinical setting. Competency is defined as the legal capacity of an individual to perform either a specific function or a wide range of functions; before such a determination by a judge, all adults are presumed to be competent. Only a judge can declare a person incompetent for specific functions or for all activities (global incompetence). The psychiatric consultant can only make a clinical assessment of the patient's capacity to function in certain areas. That assessment is usually, but not always, accepted by the court in its determination of incompetence.[2,36] What then to the numerous requests received by the consultation psychiatrist to determine the competency of medical and surgical patients? The use of competency as a shorthand term is justifiable, so long as the consultant and the consultee are clear that the most the consultant can do is to assess the patient's capacity to engage in the decision-making process in question. The change in the patient's legal status must be left to a judge. Just to add to the semantic confusion, the modern trend in the law is to forego the term *competency* and instead refer to a person's *capacities*. A person who lacks capacity may be referred to by the court as "the incapacitated person" rather than "the incompetent individual." This trend is not yet complete, and we mention it here in anticipation that this change in terminology will spread.

Capacity is usually task-specific and defined in relation to a specified act: to make a will (testamentary capacity), to testify in court (testimonial capacity), to consent or to refuse treatment (decision-making capacity), etc. Having the capacity to perform one act does not mean that one necessarily can perform another. Hence, the consultant called to evaluate a patient's "competency" must first determine the specific type(s) of capacity in question and be aware of the applicable judgment criteria. Once the consultant has determined the type of capacity in question, the judgment hinges on how well the patient meets the criteria. For example, regarding the capacity to make treatment choices, we look to the patient's understanding of three things: the illness (that something is wrong and to some degree how wrong); the treatment (what is proposed and why it is relevant to what is wrong); and the consequences of the decision. Although a variety of means of assessing decision-making capacity have been proposed, Appelbaum[40] has suggested the following four criteria that are particularly useful and straightforward:

1. Does the patient manifest a preference? A patient who is unable or unwilling to express a preference cannot presumably make a choice. It does not necessarily follow, however, that a patient who expresses a choice is competent.
2. Is the patient capable of attaining a factual understanding of the situation (nature of the illness, treatment options, prognosis with and without treatment, the risks and benefits of treatment, and so on)? The patient need not possess this level of understanding at the time of admission; he or she need only be able to receive the information and retain it in some reasonable form during the decision-making process.
3. Does the patient have an appreciation of the significance of the facts presented? Appreciation, in contrast to factual understanding, indicates a broader level of understanding related to the significance of the facts presented and the implications these facts hold for the patient's future.

4. Is the patient able to use the information presented rationally to reach a decision, that is, to weigh the facts presented in a logical manner? The focus here is not on the rationality of the ultimate decision, but on the rationality of the thought processes leading to the decision.

When a substitute decision-maker is deciding on behalf of an incapacitated patient, the same elements of capacity to decide apply. The patient's healthcare agent has the responsibility to express the patient's choice, with an awareness of the facts and appreciation for their significance, logically thinking through the material before deciding.

Capacity is not an all-or-nothing proposition, and the same level of capacity is not required for all medical decisions. Most experts agree that the strictness of the capacity test should vary as the risk/benefit ratio changes. In essence, there is a sliding scale for the level of capacity needed to make informed medical decisions.[40,41] The more favorable the risk-benefit ratio, the lower the standard for capacity to consent and the higher the standard for capacity to refuse. For example, the patient who agrees to accept incision and drainage of an obvious wound abscess would not have their capacity subjected to rigorous assessment. Refusal could not be taken so lightly; the more serious the abscess, the more intense the examination of capacity would have to be. If the risk-benefit ratio were unfavorable to the patient (e.g., extensive surgery to remove a slow-growing brain tumor in a 94-year-old), refusal would not have to be examined as meticulously as would consent. Although some criticize this approach as being too open to manipulation by a paternalistic physician, it accurately reflects professional obligations to ensure that patients make a truly informed decision, based on a rational weighing of the risks and benefits involved. A similar approach was endorsed by the President's Commission for the Study of Ethical Problems in Medicine and Biomedical and Behavioral Research.[42,43]

Dementia, delirium, and psychosis are the conditions most often cited as causes of incapacity.[44-47] The consultant should always consider the possibility of a mood disorder as a basis for impaired competence in making medical decisions. The following example demonstrates some of the complexities of these evaluations.

Case 2

A psychiatric consultant was asked to assess the decision-making capacity of Mr. B, a 62-year-old man who presented to the ED with a massive subdural hematoma that he had suffered in repeated falls owing to bradycardia. He had a profound expressive aphasia; despite the size of the subdural hematoma, Mr. B was medically stable and intermittently lucid. Nevertheless, neurosurgical staff were anxious to evacuate the subdural hematoma for fear of increased intracranial pressure. During his lucid intervals, the patient was verbally abusive to his physicians and the consultant, stated clearly that he did not want surgery, and demanded to be discharged. The limited duration of his lucid intervals and his general irritability prevented the consultant from conducting a more complete mental status examination and determining the degree of his cognitive impairment, if any. An interview with his family members revealed that he had been drinking and becoming more depressed, with marked suicidal ideation, in the previous weeks. He had refused to see a physician about his bradycardia, stating that he would prefer to die. Based on this information, his mental status examination, and the risk-benefit ratio of the proposed treatment, the consultant determined that the patient likely lacked the capacity to give an informed refusal. Out of an abundance of caution, an emergency court hearing was held with an "on-call" judge. The judge ruled that the patient lacked the capacity to refuse the planned procedure and appointed a family member to be his guardian. The guardian then consented to the evacuation of the subdural. The patient tolerated the procedure well; on recovering from surgery and anesthesia, he informed the staff in a clear voice that he was going to sue all of them. The appointment of a guardian and his informed consent, along with the excellent clinical outcome, eliminated the basis for a malpractice action.

Although depression must be considered as a possible cause of impaired judgment and incapacity, caution must be exercised. Just as a patient with schizophrenia is not automatically considered to lack capacity, a patient with major depression may also retain the ability to make rational decisions. Studies have found that medical decision-making capacity is impaired by severe depression but not by depression of lesser severity.[48]

Patients may make decisions in one moment and change those decisions minutes or hours later. This can cause significant disruption in treatment for the patient and others. Frequent shifts in patient choice can be the basis for questioning the patient's decision-making capacity. Ideally, the patient makes an informed choice at full capacity before suffering a shift in mental status. Family members should be included in this process so they can assist the treatment team in the event of a subsequent change in the patient's decision.

The cause of incapacity may be treatable. Intense pain may lead a patient to refuse a needed procedure; treatment with adequate doses of analgesics may resolve the problem. Treatment of depression, when it is a factor, may be attempted with psychostimulants, which may act within 1 to 2 days. This can restore the patient's perspective so that the decision to refuse or accept is competently made. Delirium and agitation often interfere with treatment decisions and should be treated with an antipsychotic if no specific cause of the confusional state can be found. The consultant should not determine that the patient is permanently incapacitated until these medications have been given an adequate trial, and other potential causes of the confusional state have been addressed. It must be remembered that even psychotic patients may have clear, rational, reasons for refusing treatment. Conversely, the refusal may be the result of voices telling the patient to leave the hospital, that they do not deserve treatment, or that the surgeon is a Federal Bureau of Investigation agent sent to spy on them.[49]

To give consent, the patient must be able to make an informed judgment on the matter at hand. Patients with deficits in this area, owing to communication difficulties (e.g., foreign language, deafness, or aphasia) or ignorance of important aspects of their care, cannot technically give consent. The physician who performs a procedure on a passive, confused, or fearfully mute patient who seems compliant or willing, does so at their peril; the physician risks a suit for battery. There is little protection in the ancient maxim *Qui tacet consentire videtur* ("silence gives assent").

The patient's capacity to give consent, understanding, and judgment should be documented in the chart or the office notes of the physician, along with the mental status examination and any specific questions asked about the proposed treatment. Impairment of intellect, memory, attention, or consciousness can limit the patient's understanding; impairment in reality testing, sense of reality, impulse control, and formal logic can influence judgment. The presence or absence of any or all of these should be documented clearly in the chart, along with their relationship to the illness and the decision-making process. Many states provide standardized forms that must be completed by a physician or other clinicians when medical guardianship is pursued in court.

The general rule for obtaining consent for the treatment of minor children is that parents have both the obligation to provide care and the right to make treatment decisions. However, there are several complicating issues in this area. First, the age of majority varies by state. Second, minors' rights and the legal ability to consent vary according to the type of treatment being contemplated. Massachusetts, for example, permits minors to give consent for the treatment of drug addiction and sexually transmitted diseases without seeking parental authorization. Virginia allows minors to consent to psychotherapy without parental consent. Third, the law is open to the examination of the reason for the parents' denial of consent, rather than upholding it automatically. Denial of life-saving treatment for a child because of the parents' religious beliefs will not be upheld by a court. Finally, the law recognizes the concept of the emancipated minor. This is a minor child who is free of parental control and dominance and is therefore deemed legally competent to consent in the eyes of the law, regardless of age. Informed consent by an emancipated minor, carefully documented in the record, usually protects the physician's action from criticism by the parent or guardian of that minor, so long as there is evidence of emancipation. Treating clinicians and consultants should learn the rules of their specific states concerning consent by minors.

New drugs, treatments, and procedures should not be used without informed consent by patients (or the appropriate surrogate decision-maker) and proper authorization from hospitals and government agencies. Although physicians have generally been given considerable freedom in prescribing medications and in doing procedures for off-label use (not approved by the US Food and Drug Administration [FDA] for the intended purpose), this freedom is constrained by federal and state regulations, the standard of care (enforced through malpractice actions), and the patient's right to be informed about the proposed treatment. The use of carbamazepine for the treatment of bipolar disorder is a common example of this. As a matter of policy, patients should be informed that the medicine prescribed has not been given FDA approval for that particular purpose and informed about the rationale for prescribing it.

Civil Commitment and Restraint

Civil commitment and physical restraint are commonly encountered but poorly understood by patients and many non-psychiatric physicians. Civil commitment is a process by which the power of the state is used to remove an individual from society and place them in an institutional setting. Historically, people with a mental illness were confined to institutions to protect the rest of society. As the approach toward mental illness became more enlightened, the goal of confinement was to provide treatment and protection. Under this approach, the state was fulfilling its role as protector of its citizens, much as a parent would act on behalf of a child. Hence, this is known as the state's *parens patriae* interest. With the blossoming of the civil liberties movement in the 1970s and the emphasis on individual autonomy, the individual's interest in personal freedom and privacy was given priority over the state's *parens patriae* interest. During the 1970s, the best interest or *parens patriae* approach to civil commitment was replaced by the dangerousness approach in most jurisdictions. This approach, based on the state's police powers, allows an individual to be involuntarily committed to a mental institution only if the individual poses a danger to himself or herself through direct injury, if there is a direct threat of physical harm to others, or if the individual is gravely disabled and unable to care for himself or herself in the community.[2,50]

In a general hospital, if a medical or surgical patient is psychiatrically committable but requires further medical or surgical treatment, the wisest course is to initiate commitment procedures and request that a local mental health facility accept the patient but allow the patient to remain in the general hospital for care. Budgetary concerns, insurance issues, and the general reluctance of both state and private psychiatric hospitals to take medically ill patients often make it difficult to place such patients. The prudent consultation psychiatrist should learn to anticipate the need for further psychiatric care and begin the search early. The need for commitment should be reassessed throughout this process and the process halted if appropriate.

The search for inpatient psychiatric placement increasingly requires negotiation with managed care companies to obtain permission for hospitalization. Often, the interaction with health insurance companies occurs through the process of pre-certification, which requires the transferring hospital to gain approval for transfer and inpatient care from the insurer before the patient can be transferred and admitted to the receiving psychiatric facility. Because of frequent differences in general medical and psychiatric benefits within health plans, the same pre-certification process may be required even when a patient is transferred from a medical ward to a psychiatric unit in the same hospital. It is now commonplace for insurance plans to "carve out" or sub-contract mental health benefits to a subsidiary or a different company with procedures and guidelines distinct from those of the parent company.

The psychiatric consultant often encounters questions regarding the restraint of patients on medical and surgical floors. Delirium, dementia, acute or chronic psychosis, or severe anxiety or panic can lead a patient to assault staff, wander off the ward, or fall. The suicidal patient being treated on an unlocked medical floor poses the risk of elopement and successful fulfillment of suicidal urges. Many hospitals have policies that allow the patient to be restrained before the psychiatric consultant is called. When this occurs, the role of the consultant is to provide management recommendations and approval for the restraint. Usually, the psychiatric consultant is asked to decide whether the restraints can be discontinued.

The legal aspects of restraint for patients on a medical or surgical ward vary among jurisdictions.[4,51] Generally speaking, a patient may be restrained to protect the patient or other patients and staff, to allow examination during an emergency, or for treatment in situations in which the patient appears to lack the capacity to make treatment decisions and is refusing care. In this latter situation, no forced treatment should be initiated in the absence of an emergency unless surrogate consent has been obtained. In handling these situations, physicians and staff are required to use the least restrictive alternative available. For example, where a sitter or observer is available for a potentially suicidal patient, that option is more appropriate than four-point restraints. Family members often ask whether they can substitute for a sitter. Although this may be possible in some situations, it requires careful clinical judgment that considers the type of pathology, the degree of impulsivity, the overall degree of risk, and the relative ability of the sitter to act objectively. Restraint is uncomfortable for the staff, as well as for the patient and family, and there may be a tendency to avoid it whenever possible for some types of patients and a tendency to overuse it with others. Again, careful clinical assessment is essential so that protection is provided for those patients who need restraint without zealously over-protecting and restricting those who do not. The justification for restraint, including history and formal mental status examination, should be documented in the medical record, along with the psychiatric differential diagnosis, treatment, and management recommendations.

The restraint of patients gives rise to two potential sources of liability: battery and false imprisonment.[1] A battery is defined as the touching of another person without their consent (expressed or implied) or justification. False imprisonment may be charged where an individual is denied the right to move about freely by real or perceived methods of confinement. Failure to restrain a patient with a tendency to wander, who is subsequently injured, may result in a charge of professional negligence.

Malpractice claims based on battery or false imprisonment are rarely successful if the use of restraint is reasonable under the circumstances, the reasons for the measures are documented in the medical record, proper technique is used, and hospital policies are followed. Failure to restrain when indicated and improper restraining techniques carry greater risks of harm to the patient and of malpractice claims.

Right to Refuse Treatment

The right to refuse a specific form of treatment or procedure has a long history and is firmly established in medicine. This right, based on the philosophical principle of autonomy, has been operationalized through the common law (case law), by legislation, and in state and US constitutions.[52-55] Although widely acknowledged, the right to refuse treatment is not absolute. It may be limited when it conflicts with legitimate state interests of preserving life, preventing suicide, protecting the interests of third parties, or protecting the integrity of the medical profession.[56] Generally, the decision of a patient who possesses the decision-making capacity to end treatment presents a dilemma for the treatment team. If the issue ever reaches court, the competent patient's preference is rarely over-ridden. With the advent of advance directives (e.g., healthcare proxies and durable powers of attorney), the wishes of the patient, expressed when competent, can be honored after the onset of incompetence. The path to this conclusion is not as smooth as this might suggest. Consider the following example.

Case 3

Ms. C, a 22-year-old woman, was admitted to the hospital after sustaining severe head injuries in a motor vehicle accident. After the emergency evacuation of a subdural hematoma, her condition stabilized. She was unresponsive to verbal stimuli, did not track, but did withdraw from pain. She showed decorticate posturing. The treatment team urged aggressive measures, arguing that the injury was recent and the ability to predict ultimate outcomes was limited. Tube feedings were begun, and early pneumonia was treated with antibiotics. The patient's family told the treatment team that the patient would never want to be kept alive under such circumstances. The patient's mother explained that the patient's cousin had been in a motor vehicle accident 5 years earlier and had lingered in a persistent vegetative state for 3 years until her death. The family had to engage in a costly legal battle to get permission to terminate supportive care. When this occurred, the patient (who was a nursing student at the time) vowed that she would never allow this to happen to her or her family. She told her family that she would want to be free of life-sustaining measures in the event of a serious injury if there was "no chance of recovery." In addition, she executed a healthcare proxy naming her mother as her agent for medical decision-making in the event of her incapacity. Her mother believed that the patient would have refused care if able to do so and insisted that the tube feedings be stopped. The treatment team resisted, arguing that there was hope for some recovery. After a series of meetings, the family acquiesced to the recommendations of the team, and the patient was transferred to a rehabilitation facility, still posturing and not responding. Two weeks after the transfer, she returned to the hospital with septicemia. This time the treatment team yielded to the family's preferences, and the patient died peacefully.

As Case 3 suggests, there are often no perfect answers to these problems. Both the treatment team and the family were well-meaning and tried to do what they believed was right for the patient. Meetings between the treatment team and the family, facilitated by the consultants to the unit, allowed a process to develop that gave the patient some chance at early recovery and for nature to take its course. Although difficult, the decision-making process was conducted with dignity to maintain the patient's autonomy and ensure that the decision was informed and with concern for the ethical integrity of her caretakers. In a more contentious setting, the family could have charged the treatment team with battery. Under the law in that state, the agent appointed by the healthcare proxy (the mother in this case) had the same authority to make decisions as the patient would have if competent, including refusal of permission for further treatment. The treatment team could have raised legal challenges to the exercise of the proxy, arguing that it was not evident that there was "no chance of recovery." In some states, an argument would be made that shutting off the life support constituted murder or assisted suicide or that the state's interest in preserving life and preventing suicide outweighed the individual's expressed wish. The likelihood of such arguments being made or succeeding is much lower considering the Cruzan decision.[31] Finally if the physicians or the institution had been ethically opposed to the termination of treatment, the request might have been denied and the patient transferred to the care of another physician or facility. The best solution to these challenging problems lies in the sharing of information and concerns between the family and the treaters. Immediate resort to legal posturing hardens positions and shuts off communications in most cases, to the detriment of all concerned.

The requirement of informed consent and the right to refuse treatment do not automatically apply in emergencies. In emergencies that appear to endanger the patient, or in acute situations that threaten the safety of the staff and other patients, the physician who acts in good faith while administering a treatment or procedure is generally not liable for failure to obtain informed consent. Good faith is in doubt, however, when the patient has made their preferences regarding treatment in the event of an emergency clearly known before the emergency and the physician chooses to disregard these preferences. For example, the physician who agrees to perform surgery on a Jehovah's Witness with the stipulation that there be no transfusions, even in an emergency, is hard pressed to plead good faith should he or she violate that agreement in the event of a sudden hemorrhage. Some institutions have adopted policies specific to such situations. In the case of chronic medical conditions, ongoing situations, and prolonged heroic measures to sustain life, the emergency exception loses its applicability, and decisions regarding treatment must be returned to the competent patient or an appropriate surrogate.

Leaving treatment against medical advice (AMA) is the prerogative of any competent, non-consenting patient.[57] The threat to leave AMA, like most other medico-legal conflicts, usually represents a clinical problem disguised as a legal dispute. The consultant called to evaluate the patient threatening to leave AMA must evaluate whether the patient can make that decision. During the evaluation, it is common to find that the patient is angry over a perceived lack of care or dissatisfaction with the amount of information provided by the treating physician. The consultant who can restore communication between physician and patient may be successful in getting the patient to complete the course of treatment. If the patient does leave, the consultant may then have to calm the staff in preparation for the patient returning later.

From a legal standpoint, if patients possess the capacity to make decisions and do not pose a risk of harm to themselves or others, they cannot be held against their will. A patient requesting to sign out AMA may be deemed to have the requisite capacity to do so if he or she understands the nature of the illness, the recommended treatment, the alternative treatments available, and the prognosis with or without treatment and can rationally use this information to reach a decision. If the patient meets these criteria, he or she can leave against advice, whether or not the form is signed. The discussions before release and the fact that the patient refused to sign the form should be documented in the medical record. If the patient refuses to sign the form, that documentation should suffice.

CONCLUSION

This chapter began with a discussion of the role of the psychiatric consultant in helping consultees deal with medico-legal issues. It is appropriate to close it with a few cautionary words about the temptations encountered by those who undertake this task. Consultants are often tempted to meet the needs of their consultees by telling them what they want to hear. Nowhere is this truer than in the assessment of a patient's capacity to consent to, or to refuse, treatment. This is compounded by the consultant's own bias, as a physician, to seek an outcome that is in the best clinical interests of the patient. In performing capacity assessments and other consultations on medico-legal issues, such temptations must be resisted. The role of the consultant is to be objective and focused on the issue at hand, rather than on what the consultant or consultee sees as the best overall clinical outcome. Such isolation of purpose is often difficult, but it is essential if the consultant is to serve the consultee and the patient. The consultant must also keep in mind that they are just that: a consultant whose job it is to advise, not to make treatment decisions. The treating physician may choose to disregard the consultant's assessment that a patient cannot make treatment decisions and proceed with treatment. The treating physician assumes both the legal and moral liability of their actions. The consultant can serve only as a guidepost and only then by being both knowledgeable and objective. This task is made easier by taking the following approach to consultation on these highly charged medico-legal issues:

1. Know what you are being asked to do. That is, understand both the overt request and any covert agenda that may exist.
2. Know the clinical facts of the consultation.
3. Know, or find out, the salient legal requirements involved.

4. Determine the presence of any apparent conflict between good clinical care and the law.
5. Get to know the hospital attorney, share information, and attempt to develop a multidisciplinary team approach to patient care.
6. Try to move all parties away from a crisis mentality to gain some time to resolve conflicts and encourage compromise. Avoid ultimatums. Pushing back deadlines for procedures, treatment, leaving the hospital AMA, etc., decreases time pressures and allows people to think more clearly.
7. Understand the personalities of the physician and the patient.
8. Know the patient's next of kin, their understanding, fears, biases, personalities, and the probabilities of obtaining informed consent from them.
9. Act as a go-between to diminish anxiety and communication gaps among physician, patient, and family and try to find areas for compromise and agreement.
10. Search out covert disagreements and hidden fears in the physician and patient; try to find commonsense measures that would remedy these, and search for loopholes and areas in which conflicts can be mended or avoided.
11. Provide detailed documentation in the patient's medical record (or chart) of the patient's understanding, judgment, capacity to give consent, and clinical and psychiatric status, as well as the course pursued.
12. Maintain an objective point of view while remaining mindful that the consultant's responsibility is to assess as accurately as possible the patient's capacity to give informed consent and that truth is a higher goal than scheduling concerns of the consultee and ward staff.
13. Use such consultations to teach physicians that they have little to fear from the law and to teach patients that they have little to fear from their physicians.

REFERENCES

1. Keeton WP, Keeton DB, Keeton RE, et al. *Prosser and Keeton on Torts.* 5th ed. West Publishing; 1984.
2. Schouten R, ed. *Mental Health Practice and the Law.* Oxford University Press; 2017.

3. Schouten R, Brendel RW, Edersheim JG, et al. Malpractice and boundary violations. In: Stern TA, Fava M, Wilens TE, eds. *Comprehensive Clinical Psychiatry*. 2nd ed. Mosby/Elsevier; 2016: 1165–1175.

4. Garrick TR, Weinstock R. Liability of psychiatric consultants. *Psychosomatics*. 1994;35:474–484.

5. Schouten R. Malpractice in medical-psychiatric practice. In: Stoudemire A, Fogel BS, eds. *Medical-Psychiatric Practice*, Vol. 2. American Psychiatric Association Publishing; 1993.

6. Hall RC. Social and legal implications of managed care in psychiatry. *Psychosomatics*. 1994;35:150–158.

7. Schouten R. Legal liability and managed care. *Harv Rev Psychiatry*. 1993;1:189–190.

8. Arlen J, MacLeod WB. Torts, expertise, and authority: liability of physicians and managed care organizations. *Rand J Econ*. 2005;36:494–519.

9. Tarasoff v. Board of Regents of the University of California, 1976; *17 Cal. 3d 425*.

10. Hemlinski F. Near the conflagration: the wide duty to warn. *Mayo Clin Proc*. 1993;68:709–710.

11. Soulier MF, Maislen A, Beck JC. Status of the psychiatric duty to protect, circa 2006. *J Am Acad Psychiatry Law*. 2010;38:457–473.

12. Rosmarin D. *Legal and ethical aspects of HIV disease. A Psychiatrist's Guide to AIDS and HIV Disease*. American Psychiatric Association Publishing; 1990.

13. Brendel RW, Cohen MA. Ethical issues, advance directives, and surrogate decision-making. In: Cohen MA, Gorman J, eds. *Comprehensive Textbook of AIDS Psychiatry*. Oxford University Press; 2015:577–584.

14. Schouten R. Legal responsibilities with child abuse and domestic violence. In: Jacobson JL, Jacobson AM, eds. *Psychiatric Secrets*. Hanley & Belfus; 1995.

15. Appelbaum PS. Privacy in psychiatric treatment: threats and responses. *Am J Psychiatry*. 2002;159:1809–1818.

16. Maio JE. HIPAA and the special status of psychotherapy notes. *Lippincotts Case Manag*. 2003;8:24–29.

17. Brendel RW, Bryan E. HIPAA for psychiatrists. *Harv Rev Psychiatry*. 2004;12:177–183.

18. O'Neill S, Blease C, Delbanco T. Open notes become law: a challenge for mental health practice. *Psychiatr Serv*. 2010;18: 353–358.

19. American College of Physicians Ethics manual. I. History of ethics, the physician and the patient, the physician's relationship to other physicians, the physician and society. II. Research, other ethical issues, recommended readings. *Ann Intern Med*. 1984;101: 129–137. 263–274.

20. Emanuel EJ. Do physicians have an obligation to treat patients with AIDS? *N Engl J Med*. 1988;318:1686–1690.

21. Appelbaum PS, Roth LH. Patients who refuse treatment in medical hospitals. *JAMA*. 1983;250:1296–1301.

22. Gostin L. The care of the dying: a symposium on the case of Betty Wright. *Law Med Health Care*. 1989;17:205–264.

23. Brendel RW, Schouten R. Legal concerns in psychosomatic medicine. *Psychiatr Clin North Am*. 2007;30:663–676.

24. Weinstock R, Leong GB, Silva JA. Competence to terminate life-sustaining care. *Am J Geriatr Psychiatry*. 1994;2:95–105.

25. Brendel RW, Epstein L, Cassem NH, et al. Care at the end of life. In: Stern TA, Fava M, Wilens TE, eds. *Massachusetts General Hospital Comprehensive Clinical Psychiatry*. 2nd ed. Mosby/ Elsevier; 2016:821–827.

26. Washington v. Glucksberg, 1997; *521 U.S. 702*.

27. Vacco v. Quill, 1997; *521 U.S. 793*.

28. Gonzales v. Oregon, 2006; *546 U.S. 243*.

29. Lahaie M, Kinscherff R. Juveniles and the Law. In: Schouten R, ed. *Mental Health Practice and the Law*. Oxford University Press; 2017.

30. Schouten R, Duckworth KS. Medicolegal and ethical issues in the pharmacologic treatment of children. In: Werry JS, Aman MG, eds. *Practitioner's Guide to Psychoactive Drugs for Children and Adolescents*. Plenum Medical; 1993.

31. Cruzan v. Director Missouri Department of Public Health, 1990 *110S. Ct. 2841*.

32. Emanuel EJ, Emanuel LL. Proxy decision-making for incompetent patients. *JAMA*. 1992;267:2067–2071.

33. Emanuel LL, Emanuel EJ. The medical directive: a new and comprehensive advance care document. *JAMA*. 1989;261: 3288–3293.

34. White BD, Siegler M, Singer PA, et al. What does Cruzan mean to the practicing physician? *Arch Intern Med*. 1991;151: 925–928.

35. Kilbride MK, Joffe S. The new age of patient autonomy. *JAMA*. 2018;320(19):1973–1974.

36. Appelbaum PS, Lidz CW, Meisel A. *Informed Consent: Legal Theory and Clinical Practice*. Oxford University Press; 1987.

37. Schouten R. Informed consent: resistance and reappraisal. *Crit Care Med*. 1989;17:1359–1361.

38. Drane JF. Competency to give an informed consent. *JAMA*. 1984;252:925–927.

39. Harnish v. Children's Hospital Medical Center, 1982; *387 Mass 152, 439 NE 2d 240*.

40. Appelbaum PS. Assessment of patients' competence to consent to treatment. *N Engl J Med*. 2007;357:1834–1840.

41. Roth LH, Meisel A, Lidz CW. Tests of competency to consent to treatment. *Am J Psychiatry*. 1977;134:279–284.

42. US Government *President's Commission for the Study of Ethical Problems in Medicine and Biomedical and Behavioral Research: Deciding to Forego Life-Sustaining Treatment*. US Government Printing Office; 1983.

43. US Government *President's Commission for the Study of Ethical Problems in Medicine and Biomedical and Behavioral Research: Making Health Care Decisions: A Report on the Ethical and Legal Implications of Informed Consent in the Patient–Practitioner Relationship*. US Government Printing Office; 1982.

44. Appelbaum PS, Roth LH. Clinical issues in the assessment of competency. *Am J Psychiatry*. 1981;138:1462–1467.

45. Mujic F, Von Heising M, Stewart RJ, et al. Mental capacity assessments among general hospital inpatients referred to a specialist liaison psychiatry service for older people. *Int Psychogeriatr*. 2009;21:729–737.

46. Ganzini L, Lee MA, Heintz RT, et al. The effect of depression on elderly patients' preferences for life-sustaining therapy. *Am J Psychiatry*. 1994;151:1631–1636.

47. Gutheil TG, Bursztajn H. Clinicians' guidelines for assessing and presenting subtle forms of patient incompetence in legal settings. *Am J Psychiatry*. 1986;143:1020–1023.

48. Sullivan MD, Youngner SJ. Depression, competence, and the right to refuse life-saving medical treatment. *Am J Psychiatry*. 1994;151:971.

49. Moye J. A conceptual model and assessment template for capacity evaluation in adult guardianship. *Gerontologist*. 2007;47:591–603.

50. Orlando J. Involuntary civil commitment and patients' rights. OLR Research Report 2013-R-0041. 2013

51. Glezer A, Brendel RW. The use of physical restraints in medical and psychiatric settings. *Harv Rev Psychiatry*. 2010;18:353–358.

52. Ende J, Kazis L, Ash A, et al. Measuring patients' desire for autonomy: decision-making and information-seeking among medical patients. *J Gen Intern Med*. 1989;4:24–30.

53. Massachusetts General Laws: Section 70E: Patients' and residents' rights, amended [Chapter 111]. 1989.

54. Sprung CL, Winick BJ. Informed consent in theory and practice: legal and medical perspectives on the informed consent doctrine and a proposed reconceptualization. *Crit Care Med*. 1989;17:1346–1354.

55. Swartz M. The patient who refuses medical treatment: a dilemma for hospitals and physicians. *Am J Law Med*. 1985;11:1–46.

56. Wear AN, Brahams D. To treat or not to treat: the legal, ethical and therapeutic implications of treatment refusal. *J Med Ethics*. 1991;17:131–135.

57. Albert HD, Kornfeld DS. The threat to sign out against medical advice. *Ann Intern Med*. 1973;79:888–891.

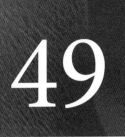

49

APPROACHES TO COLLABORATIVE CARE AND BEHAVIORAL HEALTH INTEGRATION

BJ BECK, MSN, MD, BFA, MFA ▪ MIRZA BAIG, MD ▪ JUSTIN A. CHEN, MD, MPH ▪ ALBERT S. YEUNG, MD, SCD ▪ CHRISTOPHER M. CELANO, MD

OVERVIEW

Historical trends in the research, education, and clinical practice of psychiatry[1] over the last century mirrored concerns and developments in the more general United States healthcare system[2] that called for system redesign to provide safe, personal, cost-effective, and high-quality health care. This included innovative approaches to the psychiatric care of patients in the general medical setting, where most patients still prefer to receive care and where it is the only available resource for many. Advances in psychopharmacology greatly facilitated the development of such models, which were designed to address quality, cost containment, and allocation of limited resources. Psychiatric consultation and care provided to medically ill patients was primarily hospital based, but ever-shorter inpatient stays increasingly shifted these services to outpatient settings. This paralleled the trend for shorter inpatient psychiatric hospitalizations (without increased community mental health resources),[3] which left primary care providers (PCPs) to treat more acute psychiatric illnesses in their outpatient practices. Innovative psychiatrists heeded the mandate to collaborate with their medical colleagues to develop and implement pragmatic, cost-effective, outpatient models of high-quality psychiatric care that could be delivered in the primary care setting.

Limited healthcare resources and the rapid escalation of healthcare expenses also contributed to a change in the focus from individual- to population-based care.[4] Although inherently painful in our individualistic society, this transition exposed the tremendous fiscal burden of psychiatric morbidity. The psychiatrically disordered population experiences increased *physical* healthcare utilization, work absenteeism, unemployment, subjective disability,[5-7] and mortality rates. Although more difficult to demonstrate, there is also a cost-offset of appropriate and timely psychiatric treatment.[8-10]

Changes in healthcare reimbursement resulted in conflicted PCP incentives.[11] On the one hand, capitated programs, such as health maintenance organizations (HMOs), revealed the costly use of general medical services by patients with untreated or poorly managed psychiatric illnesses, creating an incentive for PCPs to initiate treatment for the more common psychiatric problems seen in primary care. On the other hand, the PCP gate-keeper system, which evolved to manage the expense of specialty care, created a disincentive to address more serious mental illness (SMI) (or any psychiatric condition the PCP was not comfortable treating). Limited formularies, varying by plan, with onerous, time-consuming prior authorization requirements further complicated and deterred treatment initiation. Managed care organizations (MCOs) often carved out the management of substance use and mental health (collectively called behavioral health [BH]) benefits for managed BH organizations (MBHOs),[12] some with limited referral networks not inclusive of the PCP's psychiatric colleagues. This was not only a major referral disincentive but also complicated future communication and collaboration between BH and physical health providers. While many MBHOs have spearheaded initiatives to promote primary care treatment of common psychiatric problems, most do not credential or contract with non-psychiatric physicians, so this essentially cost shifted expense from the MBHO to the [medical] MCO.

Passage of the 2010 healthcare reform legislation (Patient Protection and Affordable Care Act) pushed the envelope to create more inclusive, accessible, coordinated, and integrated care systems[13] and to achieve the "triple aim" (of improved quality, improved outcomes, and reduced total healthcare cost).[14] Featured initiatives include the patient-centered medical home, the health home, accountable care organizations, and integrated programs for "dual eligible" populations (i.e., those eligible for both Medicare and Medicaid, including the elderly and/or disabled poor).[15] There is an important and recognized role for psychiatric consultants in each of these initiatives.[16] Medical and health homes share some features, but have notable differences, as summarized in Table 49.1.[13] Health homes specifically focus on care for patients with certain chronic conditions, recognizing that care for patients with multiple chronic illnesses is seven times as costly as the care of patients with only one such condition. SMI is one of the identified chronic conditions because two-thirds of affected adults have other medical conditions, and they die, on average, 25 years earlier than those in the general population, primarily from preventable medical issues. Collaborative care for this population has been shown to improve outcomes for both physical and psychiatric conditions.[17] Health homes are required to offer six core services, listed in Box 49.1, designed to integrate physical health care, BH care, and social services.[13]

EPIDEMIOLOGY

The Epidemiologic Catchment Area Study, conducted in the early 1980s, attempted to quantify the prevalence of psychiatric problems among community residents of the United States. Within 6 months, roughly 7% of the study sample sought help for a BH problem. Of these, more than 60% never saw a BH professional, but sought care in a medical setting (e.g., in an emergency department [ED] or PCP's office).[18] Even among those

TABLE 49.1

How Are Health Homes Different From Patient-Centered Medical Homes?[13]

Category	Health Homes	Medical Homes
Population served	Individuals with approved chronic conditions	All populations served
Staffing	May include primary care practices, community mental health centers, federally qualified health centers, health home agencies, and ACT teams	Are typically defined as physician-led care practices, but also mid-level practitioners
Payers	Currently are a Medicaid-only construct	In existence for multiple payers: e.g., Medicaid, commercial insurance
Care focus	Strong focus on behavioral health (including substance use treatment), social support, and other services (including nutrition, home health, coordinating activities)	Focused on the delivery of traditional care: e.g., referral and lab tracking, guideline adherence, electronic prescribing, provider-patient communication
Technology	Use of IT for coordination across the continuum of care, including in-home solutions such as remote monitoring in patient homes	Use of IT for traditional care delivery

ACT, Assertive community treatment; *IT*, information technology.
From Morgan L. Health homes vs. medical homes: big similarities and important differences. *OPEN MINDS Management Newsletter*; April 2012. http://www.openminds.com/market-intelligence/premium/2012/040112/040112f.htm?.

BOX 49.1
CORE SERVICES OF HEALTH HOMES[13]

1. Comprehensive care management
2. Care coordination and health promotion
3. Comprehensive transitional care from inpatient to other settings, including appropriate follow-up
4. Individual and family support
5. Referral to community and social support services
6. Use of health information technology to link services

who met the full criteria for a diagnosable psychiatric disorder, 75% were seen only in the general medical (rather than BH) setting.[19] About half of the general medical outpatients had some psychiatric symptoms. Psychiatric distress, therefore, was exceedingly common among primary care populations. The use of structured diagnostic interviews detected a prevalence of 25% to 35% for diagnosable psychiatric conditions in this patient population. However, roughly 10% of primary care patients had significant psychiatric distress without meeting the diagnostic criteria for a psychiatric disorder.[20] Most of the diagnosable disorders were mood disorders (80%), with depression being the most prevalent (60%), and anxiety was a distant second (20%). The more severe disorders (e.g., psychotic disorders) were more likely to be treated by BH professionals.[19]

The National Comorbidity Survey (NCS; conducted between 1990 and 1992), demonstrated a 50% life-time prevalence of one or more psychiatric disorders in US adults, with a 30% 1-year prevalence of at least one disorder.[21] Alcohol use disorder and major depressive disorder (MDD) were the most common disorders.

A rigorous replication of the NCS (NCS-R), in 2001 to 2002, also measured severity, clinical significance, overall disability, and role impairment.[22] The NCS-R found the risk of MDD was relatively low until early adolescence, when it began to rise in a linear fashion. The slope of that line has increased (i.e., becoming steeper) for each successive birth cohort since World War II. The life-time prevalence of significant depression was 16.2%; the 12-month prevalence was 6.6%. Two findings were of particular interest. First, 55.1% of depressed community respondents seeking care received that care in the BH sector. The other significant finding, attributable to advances in pharmacotherapy and educational efforts, was that 90% of respondents treated for depression in any medical setting received psychotropic medication. While this suggested improved community depression treatment, that finding was tempered by the fact that only 21.6% of patients received what recent, evidence-based guidelines (American Psychiatric Association, Agency for Healthcare Research and Quality) considered minimally adequate treatment (64.3% of those treated by BH providers and 41.3% of those treated by general

medical providers), and almost half (42.7%) of patients with depression still received no treatment.[22]

Older studies documented PCPs' failure to diagnose over half of the full criteria mental disorders of their patients,[23,24] but later studies demonstrated that PCPs recognized their more seriously depressed[25] or anxious[26] patients. These studies also demonstrated that higher-functioning, less severely symptomatic primary care patients had relatively good outcomes, even with short courses of relatively low doses of medications. This highlights the diagnostic difficulty of PCPs. Primary care patients are different from those who seek specialty care (i.e., the population in whom most psychiatric research is done). Primary care patients may seek treatment earlier in the course of their illness, since they have an established relationship with their PCP that is not dependent on their having a psychiatric disorder. They frequently present with somatic complaints, rather than with psychiatric symptoms. Since the soma is the rightful domain of the PCP, this further obscures the diagnosis. Primary care patients often present with acute psychiatric symptoms that clear quickly (i.e., before therapeutic medication levels are reached), suggesting that they might benefit as much from watchful waiting and the empathic support of their PCP. There is a high noise-to-signal ratio in psychiatrically distressed primary care patients: that is, as many as one-third of these patients have subsyndromal disorders that fail to meet the full criteria for a diagnosable mental disorder. This diagnostic ambiguity, coupled with relatively good outcomes after brief trials of sub-therapeutic medication doses,[23,27] is cause to reconsider the significance of the PCP's "failure" to diagnose. Much primary care patient angst resolves spontaneously, either with the resolution of an initiating event, expressed caregiver concern, or the placebo effect of a few days of medication. It may be attributable to an adjustment disorder.

COMPLEXITIES OF EVALUATION AND CARE: A CLINICAL VIGNETTE

Case 1

Ms. T, a 26-year-old single woman, moved to the area to start a post-doctoral fellowship. On her first visit with her new PCP, a screening Patient Health

Questionnaire-9 (PHQ-9) was elevated (with a score of 16) suggesting moderate depressive symptoms. Although records sent to her new PCP from her prior PCP had not described a history of mental health treatment, Ms. T explained that she had received psychiatric care and psychotherapy at a separate clinic whose records were not accessible to or routinely shared with her PCP. Indeed, Ms. T acknowledged her previous reluctance to have her mental health treaters communicate with her other medical treaters. Her new PCP discussed some of the advantages of greater integration of her psychiatric and general health care, took a careful history of depressive symptoms and an initial history that suggested prior trauma, and determined that there were no imminent safety concerns. She recommended re-starting citalopram, which the patient endorsed as having been helpful in the past, and suggested that Ms. T meet with the practice's care manager who would also work closely with a consulting psychiatrist. The practice care manager reviewed plans for medication dose escalation, created a safety plan in the event of worsening symptoms or suicidality, and introduced Ms. T to an online cognitive-behavioral therapy (CBT) resource. The practice care manager subsequently reviewed Ms. T's history and presentation with the consulting psychiatrist who agreed with the plan.

During a scheduled follow-up call with the care manager 1 week later, Ms. T endorsed increasing, but passive, suicidal thoughts. The PCP consulted with the practicing psychiatrist and contacted the patient with the recommendation that she be evaluated in the Psychiatry Urgent Care Clinic the following day. The evaluation confirmed the diagnosis of major depressive disorder with a history of prior trauma, and the PHQ-9 remained high, at 18. An initial safety plan was developed with Ms. T's input. Along with the recommendation to continue titration of citalopram from 20 to 40 mg, the previously effective dose, the Urgent Care psychiatrist determined that Ms. T had not accessed the online CBT resource as suggested. Given this finding, and her long-standing difficulties with distress tolerance and struggles with self-injurious urges, the Urgent Care psychiatrist conferred with the PCP and referred Ms. T to group and individual dialectical-behavioral therapy (DBT).

During the 2-week interim for these appointments, Ms. T had a weekly visit with the Urgent Care social worker and phone check-ins with the care manager.

Over the ensuing weeks, Ms. T continued to maintain regular contact with the care manager and PCP and worked closely with her DBT team whose electronic health records were readily available to the PCP, care manager, and psychiatrist. When she was feeling better but still suffering some residual symptoms, the consultant psychiatrist recommended the addition of low-dose aripiprazole, which had been effective for her in the past. The PCP prescribed the atypical antipsychotic and initiated enhanced metabolic screening while she was on the medicine. By the third month of treatment, Ms. T was feeling substantially better (back to herself) and was thriving in her post-doctoral program. With the help of the care manager, a plan for follow-up was coordinated with the PCP, psychiatrist, DBT therapists, and Ms. T.

Barriers to Treatment

Symptom recognition is necessary but not sufficient to ensure primary care treatment of psychiatric problems.[28] Even when PCPs are informed of standardized screening results, they may not initiate treatment. PCP, patient, and system factors collude to inhibit the discussion necessary to promote treatment ("don't ask/don't tell").[29]

Physician factors ("don't ask") include the failure to take a social history or to perform a mental status examination.[30] This may be attributed to deficits in the training of medical students and residents,[31] to time and productivity pressures, and to personal defenses (e.g., identification, denial,[32] isolation of affect). PCPs are more experienced and comfortable addressing physical complaints. Like many patients, the PCP may not believe treatment will help. Not having a ready response or approach is a major deterrent to the identification of a new problem within the context of a 15-minute primary care visit. Denial or avoidance may prevail when the time-pressured PCP feels unsure of how, or whether, to treat or to refer.

Stigma, prevalent among patients and providers, is a major patient deterrent to bringing up psychiatric symptoms. Often patients "don't tell" because of shame or embarrassment. Patients may not know they have a diagnosable or treatable BH disorder.[33] They may equate psychiatric problems with personal weakness, and assume their PCP shares that view. For these and other reasons, primary care patients frequently present with physical complaints, increasing diagnostic complexity[34] since medical disorders may simulate psychiatric disorders, psychiatric disorders contribute to physical symptoms, and psychiatric and medical disorders frequently co-exist.

System factors include the ever-changing healthcare finance and reimbursement climate (e.g., managed care, "carve-outs," provider risk, capitation, fee-for-service, coding nuances, differential formularies, prior authorization) contributing to financial imperatives to contain cost and to increase efficiency. This systemic instability, confusion, and administrative time-creep easily dwarfs the impulse to pursue the treatment of a possibly self-limited condition. BH carve-outs have complicated the possibility of reimbursing PCP treatment of BH disorders, while pre-paid plans (e.g., HMOs) decrease incentives to offer anything "extra."[35] The necessity to increase productivity has applied time pressure to the "routine visit," now often less than 15 minutes, while the excessive burden of required documentation further erodes clinically available time. Although the electronic medical record (EMR) has standardized and improved screening, documentation, and follow-up,[36] it is also a major contributor to clinical time pressures and dissatisfaction among mental healthcare providers. The care-promoting advent of new, safer, more tolerable psychotropic medications has been offset by soaring pharmacy costs and by restrictive (and possibly short-sighted[37]) formularies.

THE GOALS OF COLLABORATION

Now that effective, evidence-based treatments exist, access and quality of care remain significant issues, best addressed through the collaboration of psychiatry and primary care. The four major goals of collaboration are to improve access, treatment, outcomes, and communication.

Access

Collaborative care in the primary care setting addresses both physician and patient factors that limit the patient's access to appropriate assessment and treatment. Most patients are familiar with the general medical setting and feel more comfortable and less stigmatized there. Conversely, they may believe the mental health clinic is for "crazy people," not a (perceived) clientele with whom they identify. Even a defined BH unit in the primary care setting may be stigmatizing and thus a barrier to treatment access. Most patients do not know of a psychiatrist or how to access care from one and may not feel certain that they need one. The unaided decision to foray into the BH arena may be fraught with shame and anxiety, powerful deterrents to making that first call. Calling the PCP's office and making an appointment for fatigue, sleep problems, weight loss, or palpitations is infinitely less threatening.

An established relationship between the PCP and a trusted, accessible psychiatric consultant eases the burden of recognizing, treating, or referring patients with mental disorders. PCPs more readily identify psychiatric distress and initiate treatment when they have expert clinical back-up available.

Treatment

Historically, PCPs often prescribed insufficient doses of medications (e.g., amitriptyline 25 mg) for MDD.[38] Since the advent of safer, well-tolerated medications (e.g., selective serotonin reuptake inhibitors), PCPs' prescriptive choices have improved,[39,40] although the doses used often remain suboptimal. Benzodiazepines have been prescribed by PCPs more frequently than any other class of psychotropic medication, even for MDD,[41] but they now are appropriately surpassed by antidepressant prescriptions.[40] Collaboration with a consultation psychiatrist can improve the choice, dose, and management of psychotropic medications. Collaboration is also helpful when the PCP's preferred medication is off-formulary for a given patient. Such a treatment deterrent may instead become an opportunity for brief, pragmatic education.

Outcomes

Several studies have demonstrated better outcomes for seriously depressed primary care patients treated collaboratively by their PCP and a psychiatrist.[42-44] Cost-offset, however, is difficult to demonstrate because of the hidden costs of psychiatric disability.[6,45,46] Nonetheless, there is evidence for decreased total healthcare spending when BH problems are adequately addressed.[10] There is some evidence for the cost-effectiveness of collaborative care.[8,47–51] In addition, care for the patient's psychiatric problem is more cost-effective than spending the same amount of money addressing the often non-responsive, somatic complaints of high-utilizing medical patients.

Communication

Collaboration ends the PCP's justifiable complaint of the "black box" of psychiatry because communication is implicit in these care models. Information must flow in both directions to assist the psychiatrist and the PCP in the provision of quality care. Referrals by PCPs provide pertinent information and state the clinical question. In addition to the target psychiatric symptoms, the PCP has, and provides, important information about the medical history, allergies, treatments, and medications. The collaborating psychiatrist shares findings, diagnostic impressions, and treatment recommendations. Information about referrals and consultations should be written, and, whenever possible, provided verbally to ensure an understanding between collaborating care providers. Secure e-mail, EMR staff messaging, or other information technology (IT) solutions may also provide nearly instantaneous feedback and focus on pertinent details for the busy PCP.

Patients, of course, must be aware of the collaborative relationship between the PCP and the psychiatrist, as well as their shared communication.

ROLES, RELATIONSHIPS, AND EXPECTATIONS

Successful collaboration requires a clear understanding and definition of roles. All parties, including the patient, should recognize the PCP's responsibility for the patient's overall care. The PCP is the broker and overseer of all specialty services. The psychiatrist is a consultant to the PCP, and sometimes a co-treater, depending on the model. Collaboration does not breach patient confidentiality because the PCP and the psychiatrist are now within the circle of care, and the patient is informed of this relationship.

This free flow of communication and documentation has reasonable limitations. If a patient asks that certain details not be placed in his or her general medical record and these details do not directly affect

the patient's medical care (e.g., a history of childhood incest), it is reasonable to respect this wish. The pertinent information (e.g., the experience of childhood trauma) can be expressed in more general terms. If, however, information could affect medical treatment (e.g., current or past substance use disorder [SUD]) or safety (e.g., suicidal or homicidal intent, or previous suicide attempt), such information cannot be withheld from the PCP, and the patient should be so informed.

When the PCP refers the patient to the psychiatrist, the patient should understand what to expect from the visit. It is also the psychiatrist's responsibility to clearly describe the parameters of the contact (e.g., whether it will be a one-time consultation, with or without the possibility of medication follow-up, or possible referral for therapy). If the psychiatrist sees the patient more than once, the relationships (i.e., between the PCP and the psychiatrist, as well as between the patient and the psychiatrist) may need to be reiterated. The clarity of the providers' roles and relationships serves to spare the patient a sense of abandonment, either by the PCP when the patient is referred to the psychiatrist, or by the psychiatrist when the patient is returned to the PCP for ongoing psychiatric management.

In collaborative models of care, it is common for psychiatric notes to be placed in the general medical record, which may raise issues of confidentiality and privacy. Most states require a specific release for mental health or substance use treatment records. BH notes in the general medical record should be color coded or otherwise flagged, so they can be removed when records are copied for general medical release of information. With an EMR, there may be software coding solutions to avoid the inadvertent release of this information. (As BH issues are increasingly treated by PCPs, the question of how to document and protect such information is a growing concern, preferably to be addressed in a way that does not further complicate and deter such treatment.)

MODELS OF TREATMENT AND COLLABORATION

Collaborative treatment models differ in terms of where the patient is seen, whether there is a single medical record, how providers communicate, whether the psychiatrist recommends or initiates treatment, and whether the psychiatrist sees the patient (at all, once, more than once), or is an ongoing treater. Another important variable is whether both providers belong to the same medical staff and how available (physically, electronically, or telephonically) the psychiatrist is to the PCP. Table 49.2 summarizes the different outpatient models of psychiatric treatment.

General Outpatient Psychiatry Clinics

In outpatient psychiatry clinics, patients are typically referred (by PCPs, other providers, or themselves) to obtain psychiatric care that may be more difficult to deliver in a primary care setting (e.g., treatment of bipolar disorder or schizophrenia). Depending on the setting or the system, one medical record may be shared (this is now generally the norm), or providers may maintain separate records and share pertinent information. Outpatient psychiatry clinics affiliated with a medical center or primary care clinic may differ from those of private psychiatrists, who oftentimes

do not document care in a shared EMR and who may have limited contact with PCPs.

Specialty Psychiatric Clinics

Specialty psychiatric clinics (e.g., eating disorder clinics, substance use clinics), usually in teaching hospitals or tertiary care centers, generally require patients to be seen in the psychiatric clinic. They may or may not utilize a shared medical record with PCPs. Patients typically need to have well-defined problems to get referred. Although stigma may interfere with patient adherence to such a referral, one major advantage of such clinics is the expert, multi-disciplinary approach they provide for patients with complex psychiatric and medical problems.

Outpatient Psychiatric Consultations

Consultation psychiatrists[52,53] may render a one-visit opinion in the primary care clinic (or in the consultant's office, as is done for other specialty consultations).

TABLE 49.2
Outpatient Psychiatry Collaborative Models of Treatment

Model	Characteristics	Types of Disorders Typically Treated
Collaborative Care	Care is coordinated by a care manager (e.g., nurse, social worker) who monitors psychiatric symptoms, delivers brief psychological interventions, and coordinates psychiatric care between the PCP and a consulting psychiatrist. Collaborative care is characterized by a population health management approach, the use of screening tools to monitor symptom severity, and continued treatment until a target level of response is achieved.	Uncomplicated depression and anxiety disorders
Co-located Psychiatric Care	A psychiatrist is located within the primary care clinic. The psychiatrist may perform electronic "curbside" consultations, complete in-person consultations for diagnostic clarification or to make treatment recommendations, collaboratively manage patients temporarily (with a plan for the PCP to take over care when the patient is stabilized), or follow patients longitudinally.	Depression and anxiety disorders not responding to initial treatment; ADHD; mild to moderate bipolar disorder or mild SUDs.
General Outpatient Psychiatry Clinics	Care is delivered in a psychiatric clinic separate from primary care. Psychopharmacology and psychotherapy can be performed. In some instances, a medical record is shared with primary care, which facilitates collaboration.	A wide range of psychiatric disorders, including mood, anxiety, substance use, and psychotic disorders.
Specialty Psychiatry Clinics	Care is provided by mental health professionals with expertise in a particular type of psychiatric disorder. Psychiatrists may have insights into the management of illnesses refractory to treatment, and there may be availability of individual and group psychotherapy tailored to a particular illness. Levels of collaboration and shared medical records vary.	Treatment-refractory mood and anxiety disorders; specific other disorders, such as eating disorders, psychotic disorders, SUDs, and PTSD.

ADHD, Attention-deficit hyperactivity disorder; *PCP*, primary care provider; *PTSD*, post-traumatic stress disorder; *SUDs*, substance use disorders.

Patients are often referred for a one-time consultation in the setting of diagnostic uncertainty or when a specific treatment recommendation is needed. Like inpatient consultation, the consultation request and report are included in the primary care record. In outpatient consultations, the psychiatrist does not initiate treatment; instead, the psychiatrist provides clear diagnostic impressions and treatment recommendations to the PCP, delivered verbally or electronically. These communications should be performed in as timely a manner as possible to maximize the benefits to the PCP and expedite treatment initiation. The role of the PCP and its occurrence in the primary care setting enhances patient participation and decreases stigma. This model also promotes opportunities for ongoing informal education between the PCP and the consultant.

Co-located Psychiatric Care

When a psychiatrist is co-located within a primary care clinic or health center, there are enhanced possibilities for collaboration and shared care. This PCP-psychiatrist proximity facilitates communication, formal and informal education, immediate access to curbside consultation, and heightened PCP awareness of psychiatric problems in their patients. This arrangement can also provide an excellent opportunity for training both psychiatric and primary care residents. Patients also may appreciate being seen in the more familiar primary care setting, and they may feel less stigmatized.

A psychiatrist embedded in a primary care clinic may provide several different types of psychiatric services:

1. *Electronic "curbside" consultation.* PCPs may be comfortable managing some psychiatric conditions (e.g., MDD, generalized anxiety disorder) but may have questions about medication choices, management of side effects, or diagnostic clarification. In certain instances, an electronic consultation can be placed with a psychiatrist. The psychiatrist will review the patient's medical record and address the consultation question without evaluating the patient in person. These recommendations will be communicated electronically or verbally and may be made part of the patient's medical record.

2. *In-person psychiatric consultation.* One-time psychiatric consultations may be helpful when a patient's diagnosis is unclear, when a patient is not responding to treatment as expected, or when a specific treatment recommendation would be beneficial for a patient who will be managed by the PCP. The presence of a psychiatrist in the primary care clinic has several benefits. For instance, with a previously established agreement, the consultant may initiate the recommended treatment. The consultation psychiatrist may offer clinically relevant suggestions during case conferences or discussions with more complex patients. The psychiatrist may also see the patient with the PCP during the primary care visit, capitalizing on the PCP's extensive knowledge of, and long-term relationship with, the patient to provide more timely treatment recommendations.

3. *Collaborative management of psychiatric conditions.*[43,54] In collaborative management,[43,54] the patient alternates visits between the psychiatrist and the PCP in the primary care setting during the initiation of treatment (i.e., the first 4–6 weeks). The PCP then assumes responsibility for the patient's continued psychopharmacological treatment. Patients are typically engaged in collaborative management when they have failed an initial trial of a medication prescribed by a PCP; however, the goal is for treatment to be managed by the PCP. Implicit in this type of treatment are certain underlying assumptions. Collaborative management assumes that PCPs can initiate appropriate treatment for depression, manage the care of patients stabilized on antidepressant medications, and better care for more seriously depressed patients with the collaboration of an embedded psychiatric consultant.[55] This model also assumes that such collaboration begins with PCP education and training. In addition, PCPs participate in regular teaching conferences. A psychoeducational module for patients is also an integral part of the treatment (see Box 49.2).

4. *Parallel treatment of psychiatric illness.* An embedded psychiatrist may choose to care for a subset of patients—typically those with more complex illnesses, such as treatment-resistant

depression or bipolar disorder—seen in primary care. Such services may be particularly useful for individuals with mental illness and substantial medical illnesses that may require close follow-up in primary care. Unfortunately, the psychiatric capacity of primary care clinics that offer these services is often inadequate to meet the needs of the total clinic patient population; therefore, a specific system to triage patients to either this type of treatment or referral to an outpatient psychiatry clinic should be in place. Criteria might consider diagnosis, available community resources, language requirements, or payment sources.

One specific type of care within the framework of embedded psychiatric care is the primary care–driven model.[56] This model evolved from the practical necessity to assist PCPs in the provision of quality psychiatric care for their primary care patients with limited psychiatric resources. This model incorporates elements of consultation and collaborative management, with the goal of maximizing the treatment of appropriate primary care patients, in the primary care setting. Established criteria are used for triage, with the appropriateness of PCP management being the first consideration. When psychiatric assistance is needed,

the PCP creates a referral request that details the clinical issue to be addressed.

Within the primary care–driven model, an array of psychiatric services is available, including formal evaluation with stabilization over several visits and return of the patient to the PCP's care, electronic "curbside" consultation with the PCP, brief consultation with the patient and the PCP during the patient's primary care visit, or behavioral treatment planning for the difficult-to-manage patient. Non-psychiatric providers, such as social workers, mental health clinicians, or care managers, may provide additional services, such as short-term psychotherapy or care management services. Finally, when a patient does not meet the criteria for in-house treatment, the psychiatrist may recommend (and may facilitate) referral to appropriate outside services (e.g., a community mental health center, private psychiatrist, or therapist).

A premise of the primary care–driven model is that not all patients are appropriate for PCP management. The psychiatrist may help the PCP recognize which patients are better served by ongoing specialty care and assist with appropriate referrals. Patients not recommended for PCP management include those with thoughts of suicide (or high-risk factors for suicide), severe personality disorders, primary SUDs, inherently unstable conditions (e.g., psychotic disorders, bipolar disorder), or complicated medication regimens that require close monitoring.

Collaborative Care

"Collaborative care" refers to a specific, formalized model of consultative care that utilizes a care manager to coordinate psychiatric care between a PCP and a mental health specialist. It was developed initially by Katon and colleagues[43] and has several distinct characteristics. Specifically, collaborative care is: (1) team-driven, (2) population focused, (3) measurement guided, and (4) evidence based.[57] In this context, team-driven care refers to a multi-disciplinary group of healthcare professionals providing care and implementing treatment plans. In collaborative care, care managers interview patients independently to measure clinical progress, deliver targeted psychotherapy interventions, assess treatment adherence, and explore treatment preferences. The care managers then periodically discuss their patients with a consulting psychiatrist, who offers treatment recommendations that

---

BOX 49.2
UNDERLYING ASSUMPTIONS OF THE PRIMARY CARE–DRIVEN MODEL

1. Collaboration begins with the education of primary care providers (PCPs) and psychiatrists.
2. Patients' psychiatric needs should be met in the primary care setting when consistent with good care.
3. PCPs can manage the care of patients stabilized on psychiatric medications.
4. PCPs can initiate appropriate treatment for some psychiatric disorders.
5. PCPs can better care for the psychiatric needs of more patients with the collaboration of in-house psychiatric consultations.
6. Some patients and some disorders are unlikely to be stable enough for PCP management.
7. Responsibility for total care requires communication between the PCP and any other involved care provider or consultant.

are conveyed to the PCP (either directly by the psychiatrist or through the care manager). Additionally, collaborative care is population focused. During collaborative care case reviews, the team focuses on those individuals with more severe and treatment-refractory illnesses to maximize the impact of the intervention on the population. Collaborative care providers also may use the information from their case reviews to identify trends across the clinic population and advocate for system-wide interventions. Finally, formal collaborative care is measurement guided and evidence based, in that it involves the use of systematic, disease-specific, patient-reported outcome measures (e.g., symptom rating scales) to inform clinical decision-making. These characteristics help to ensure that patients continue to receive targeted psychotherapy interventions and ongoing adjustments to pharmacotherapy until specific treatment goals are reached.

Collaborative care has been implemented in a wide array of clinical settings and scenarios, including for the treatment of depressive disorders,[58] anxiety disorders,[59,60] and post-traumatic stress disorder (PTSD),[61] among others. It also has been utilized in outpatient general pediatric settings with adolescent populations.[62] More recently, collaborative care has been used in academic centers to provide psychiatric care to patients with cardiac co-morbidities, such as a recent history of a coronary artery bypass graft[63] or other acute cardiac events.[64-66] In several programs, care managers involved in the collaborative care teams contact and meet with patients while they are still hospitalized, thereby providing a bridge between an acute medical event that led to hospitalization and appropriate psychiatric follow-up.[65,66] In nearly all instances and treatment settings, collaborative care appears to be effective at improving targeted psychiatric symptoms, such as depression and anxiety.[58-67]

"Blended collaborative care" is a specific type of collaborative care in which a care manager (often a nurse) works with patients to coordinate care between PCPs and specialists for the management of both a mental illness (e.g., depression) and a medical condition (e.g., type 2 diabetes).[17,68] In a randomized controlled trial of blended collaborative care intervention for the management of depression, type 2 diabetes, and coronary artery disease, blended collaborative care led to significantly greater improvements in depressive symptoms,

hemoglobin A1C, low-density lipoprotein cholesterol, and systolic blood pressure, compared to usual care.[17] In a more recent trial of a blended collaborative care intervention for individuals with heart failure and depression, blended collaborative care was associated with greater improvements in mental health–related quality of life and mood—but not physical health–related quality of life or function—than usual care.[68] Although further work is needed, these studies provide preliminary support for the use of blended collaborative care as a way to improve depressive symptoms in individuals with both depression and chronic medical illnesses.

CHOOSING THE RIGHT MODEL

The choice of model depends on a variety of practice factors, such as patient population, payer mix, range of available community resources, and the location, type, and size of the practice. Patients with higher educational or socioeconomic status may feel less stigmatized and be more able and willing to seek and pay for outside psychiatric services.[69] Some patients feel more comfortable in private practice settings that allow the greatest possible privacy. BH problems are less acceptable or even shameful in some cultures. These patient populations will favor a more integrated and "invisible" system within the primary care setting. Capitation would most clearly demonstrate the cost-offset and cost-effectiveness of in-house, collaborative models. The primary care–driven model requires adequate community resources to refer patients not considered appropriate for primary care management. Suburban or rural areas that lack these resources are better served by parallel, or shared, care models. Small groups or solo practitioners may favor consultation models, either with a part-time but regularly scheduled consultant or through access to an outside consultant, as needed. Large practices, and especially training facilities, will benefit most from the full range of in-house consultative and collaborative services that include formal education, case conferences, curbside consultation, and collaborative care management. The current Affordable Care Act promotion of integrated care will likely employ or enhance some of these same features, and hopefully provide the necessary and sustainable funding for their continued success.

CONCLUSION

PCPs have held (and will continue to hold) an important front-line position in total healthcare, population-based care, and all levels of prevention.[70] Although mandated by changes in the healthcare system, collaborative models serve to increase access and improve treatment for patients who would be unable or unlikely to receive psychiatric care outside of the primary care setting. Several considerations determine the best model for a given practice setting. Such factors include size, patient population, available community resources, payer mix, and other reimbursement sources. To remain viable, high-quality and cost-effective models will need to adapt and evolve with the changing healthcare system. Psychiatrists and PCPs will need to be flexible and innovative in their approaches to patient care and to be diligent in the documentation of cost-offset to encourage payers to reimburse their services.[71,72] Medical,[73] psychiatric, and patient education will need to reflect these changes in caregiver roles and expectations.

REFERENCES

1. McKegney FP. After a century of C-L psychiatry, whither goest C-L in the 21st? *Psychosomatics.* 1995;36:202–203.
2. Committee on Quality Health Care in America, Institute of Medicine. *Crossing the Quality Chasm: A New Health System for the 21st Century.* National Academy Press; 2001.
3. Leslie DL, Rosenheck R. Shifting to outpatient care? Mental health care use and cost under private insurance. *Am J Psychiatry.* 1999;156(8):1250–1257. https://doi.org/10.1176/ajp.156.8.1250.
4. Katon W, Von Korff M, Lin E, et al. Population-based care of depression: effective disease management strategies to decrease prevalence. *Gen Hosp Psychiatry.* 1997;19(3):169–178. https://doi.org/10.1016/S0163-8343(97)00016-9.
5. Broadhead WE, Blazer DG, George LK, et al. Depression, disability days, and days lost from work in a prospective epidemiologic survey. *JAMA.* 1990;264(19):2524–2548. https://www.ncbi.nlm.nih.gov/pubmed/2146410.
6. Johnson J, Weissman MM, Klerman GL. Service utilization and social morbidity associated with depressive symptoms in the community. *JAMA.* 1992;267(11):1478–1483. https://www.ncbi.nlm.nih.gov/pubmed/1538538.
7. Wells KB, Stewart A, Hays RD, et al. The functioning and well-being of depressed patients. Results from the Medical Outcomes Study. *JAMA.* 1989;262(7):914–919. https://www.ncbi.nlm.nih.gov/pubmed/2754791.
8. Katon WJ, Roy-Byrne P, Russo J, et al. Cost-effectiveness and cost offset of a collaborative care intervention for primary care patients with panic disorder. *Arch Gen Psychiatry.* 2002;59(12):1098–1104. https://doi.org/10.1001/archpsyc.59.12.1098.

9. Katon WJ, Russo JE, Von Korff M, et al. Long-term effects on medical costs of improving depression outcomes in patients with depression and diabetes. *Diabetes Care.* 2008;31(6):1155–1159. https://doi.org/10.2337/dc08-0032.
10. Simon GE, Khandker RK, Ichikawa L, et al. Recovery from depression predicts lower health services costs. *J Clin Psychiatry.* 2006;67(8):1226–1231. https://doi.org/10.4088/jcp.v67n0808.
11. Pincus HA. Assessing the effects of physician payment on treatment of mental disorders in primary care. *Gen Hosp Psychiatry.* 1990;12(1):23–29. https://doi.org/10.1016/0163-8343(90)90034-a.
12. Frank RG, Huskamp HA, McGuire TG, et al. Some economics of mental health "carve-outs". *Arch Gen Psychiatry.* 1996;53(10):933–937. https://doi.org/10.1001/archpsyc.1996.01830100081010.
13. Morgan L. Health homes vs. medical homes: big similarities and important differences. http://www.openminds.com/market-intelligence/premium/2012/040112/040112f.htm.
14. Berwick DM, Nolan TW, Whittington J. The triple aim: care, health, and cost. *Health Aff (Millwood).* 2008;27:759–769.
15. Neuman P, Lyons B, Rentas J, et al. Dx for a careful approach to moving dual-eligible beneficiaries into managed care plans. *Health Aff (Millwood).* 2012;31:1186–1194.
16. Katon W, Unutzer J. Consultation psychiatry in the medical home and accountable care organizations: achieving the triple aim. *Gen Hosp Psychiatry.* 2011;33(4):305–310. https://doi.org/10.1016/j.genhosppsych.2011.05.011.
17. Katon WJ, Lin EH, Von Korff M, et al. Collaborative care for patients with depression and chronic illnesses. *N Engl J Med.* 2010;363(27):2611–2620. https://doi.org/10.1056/NEJMoa1003955.
18. Regier DA, Narrow WE, Rae DS, et al. The de facto US mental and addictive disorders service system. Epidemiologic catchment area prospective 1-year prevalence rates of disorders and services. *Arch Gen Psychiatry.* 1993;50(2):85–94. https://doi.org/10.1001/archpsyc.1993.01820140007001.
19. Shapiro S, Skinner EA, Kessler LG, et al. Utilization of health and mental health services. Three epidemiologic catchment area sites. *Arch Gen Psychiatry.* 1984;41(10):971–978. https://doi.org/10.1001/archpsyc.1984.01790210053007.
20. Barrett JE, Barrett JA, Oxman TE, et al. The prevalence of psychiatric disorders in a primary care practice. *Arch Gen Psychiatry.* 1988;45(12):1100–1106. https://doi.org/10.1001/archpsyc.1988.01800360048007.
21. Kessler RC, McGonagle KA, Zhao S, et al. Lifetime and 12-month prevalence of DSM-III-R psychiatric disorders in the United States. Results from the National Comorbidity Survey. *Arch Gen Psychiatry.* 1994;51(1):8–19. https://doi.org/10.1001/archpsyc.1994.03950010008002.
22. Kessler RC, Berglund P, Demler O, et al. The epidemiology of major depressive disorder: results from the National Comorbidity Survey Replication (NCS-R). *JAMA.* 2003;289(23):3095–3105. https://doi.org/10.1001/jama.289.23.3095.
23. Ormel J, Koeter MW, van den Brink W, et al. Recognition, management, and course of anxiety and depression in general practice. *Arch Gen Psychiatry.* 1991;48(8):700–706. https://doi.org/10.1001/archpsyc.1991.01810320024004.
24. Zung WW, Magill M, Moore JT, et al. Recognition and treatment of depression in a family medicine practice. *J Clin*

Psychiatry. 1983;44(1):3–6. https://www.ncbi.nlm.nih.gov/pubmed/6822483.

25. Coyne JC, Schwenk TL, Fechner-Bates S. Nondetection of depression by primary care physicians reconsidered. *Gen Hosp Psychiatry.* 1995;17(1):3–12. https://doi.org/10.1016/0163-8343(94)00056-j.

26. Roy-Byrne PP, Katon W, Cowley DS, et al. Panic disorder in primary care: biopsychosocial differences between recognized and unrecognized patients. *Gen Hosp Psychiatry.* 2000;22(6):405–411. https://doi.org/10.1016/s0163-8343(00)00101-8.

27. Tiemens BG, Ormel J, Simon GE. Occurrence, recognition, and outcome of psychological disorders in primary care. *Am J Psychiatry.* 1996;153(5):636–644. https://doi.org/10.1176/ajp.153.5.636.

28. Shapiro S, German PS, Skinner EA, et al. An experiment to change detection and management of mental morbidity in primary care. *Med Care.* 1987;25(4):327–339. https://doi.org/10.1097/00005650-198704000-00006.

29. Eisenberg L. Treating depression and anxiety in primary care. Closing the gap between knowledge and practice. *N Engl J Med.* 1992;326(16):1080–1084. https://doi.org/10.1056/NEJM199204163261610.

30. Schwab JJ. Psychiatric illness in medical patients: why it goes undiagnosed. *Psychosomatics.* 1982;23(3):225–229. https://doi.org/10.1016/S0033-3182(82)73413-9.

31. Weissberg M. The meagerness of physicians' training in emergency psychiatric intervention. *Acad Med.* 1990;65(12):747–750. https://doi.org/10.1097/00001888-199012000-00009.

32. Ness DE, Ende J. Denial in the medical interview. Recognition and management. *JAMA.* 1994;272(22):1777–1781. (https://www.ncbi.nlm.nih.gov/pubmed/7966927).

33. Karlsson H, Lehtinen V, Joukamaa M. Psychiatric morbidity among frequent attender patients in primary care. *Gen Hosp Psychiatry.* 1995;17(1):19–25. https://doi.org/10.1016/0163-8343(94)00059-m.

34. Bridges KW, Goldberg DP. Somatic presentation of DSM III psychiatric disorders in primary care. *J Psychosom Res.* 1985;29(6):563–569. https://doi.org/10.1016/0022-3999(85)90064-9.

35. Wells KB, Hays RD, Burnam MA, et al. Detection of depressive disorder for patients receiving prepaid or fee-for-service care. Results from the Medical Outcomes Study. *JAMA.* 1989;262(23):3298–3302. https://www.ncbi.nlm.nih.gov/pubmed/2585674.

36. Gill JM, Dansky BS. Use of an electronic medical record to facilitate screening for depression in primary care. *Prim Care Companion J Clin Psychiatry.* 2003;5(3):125–128. https://doi.org/10.4088/pcc.v05n0304.

37. Hamel MB, Epstein AM. Prior-authorization programs for controlling drug spending. *N Engl J Med.* 2004;351(21):2156–2158. https://doi.org/10.1056/NEJMp048294.

38. Katon W, von Korff M, Lin E, et al. Adequacy and duration of antidepressant treatment in primary care. *Med Care.* 1992;30(1):67–76. https://doi.org/10.1097/00005650-199201000-00007.

39. Olfson M, Marcus SC, Druss B, et al. National trends in the outpatient treatment of depression. *JAMA.* 2002;287(2):203–209. https://doi.org/10.1001/jama.287.2.203.

40. Pincus HA, Tanielian TL, Marcus SC, et al. Prescribing trends in psychotropic medications: primary care, psychiatry, and other medical specialties. *JAMA.* 1998;279(7):526–531. https://doi.org/10.1001/jama.279.7.526.

41. Wells KB, Katon W, Rogers B, et al. Use of minor tranquilizers and antidepressant medications by depressed outpatients: results from the medical outcomes study. *Am J Psychiatry.* 1994;151(5):694–700. https://doi.org/10.1176/ajp.151.5.694.

42. Druss BG, Rohrbaugh RM, Levinson CM, et al. Integrated medical care for patients with serious psychiatric illness: a randomized trial. *Arch Gen Psychiatry.* 2001;58(9):861–868. https://doi.org/10.1001/archpsyc.58.9.861.

43. Katon W, Von Korff M, Lin E, et al. Collaborative management to achieve treatment guidelines. Impact on depression in primary care. *JAMA.* 1995;273(13):1026–1031. https://www.ncbi.nlm.nih.gov/pubmed/7897786.

44. Robinson P. Integrated treatment of depression in primary care. *Strategic Med.* 1997;1:22–29.

45. Greenberg PE, Kessler RC, Birnbaum HG, et al. The economic burden of depression in the United States: how did it change between 1990 and 2000? *J Clin Psychiatry.* 2003;64(12):1465–1475. https://doi.org/10.4088/jcp.v64n1211.

46. Stewart WF, Ricci JA, Chee E, et al. Cost of lost productive work time among US workers with depression. *JAMA.* 2003;289(23):3135–3144. https://doi.org/10.1001/jama.289.23.3135.

47. Katon WJ, Schoenbaum M, Fan MY, et al. Cost-effectiveness of improving primary care treatment of late-life depression. *Arch Gen Psychiatry.* 2005;62(12):1313–1320. https://doi.org/10.1001/archpsyc.62.12.1313.

48. Smith GR Jr, Rost K, Kashner TM. A trial of the effect of a standardized psychiatric consultation on health outcomes and costs in somatizing patients. *Arch Gen Psychiatry.* 1995;52(3):238–243. https://doi.org/10.1001/archpsyc.1995.03950150070012.

49. Sturm R, Wells KB. How can care for depression become more cost-effective? *JAMA.* 1995;273(1):51–58. https://www.ncbi.nlm.nih.gov/pubmed/7996651.

50. Bosanquet K, Adamson J, Atherton K, et al. CollAborative care for Screen-Positive EldeRs with major depression (CASPER plus): a multicentred randomised controlled trial of clinical effectiveness and cost-effectiveness. *Health Technol Assess.* 2017;21(67):1–252. https://doi.org/10.3310/hta21670.

51. Richards DA, Bower P, Chew-Graham C, et al. Clinical effectiveness and cost-effectiveness of collaborative care for depression in UK primary care (CADET): a cluster randomised controlled trial. *Health Technol Assess.* 2016;20(14):1–192. https://doi.org/10.3310/hta20140.

52. Kates N, Craven MA, Crustolo AM, et al. Sharing care: the psychiatrist in the family physician's office. *Can J Psychiatry.* 1997;42(9):960–965. https://doi.org/10.1177/070674379704200908.

53. Nickels MW, McIntyre JS. A model for psychiatric services in primary care settings. *Psychiatr Serv.* 1996;47(5):522–526. https://doi.org/10.1176/ps.47.5.522.

54. Katon W, Von Korff M, Lin E, et al. Stepped collaborative care for primary care patients with persistent symptoms of depression: a

randomized trial. *Arch Gen Psychiatry.* 1999;56(12):1109–1115. https://doi.org/10.1001/archpsyc.56.12.1109.

55. Simon GE. Can depression be managed appropriately in primary care? *J Clin Psychiatry.* 1998;59(2):3–8.

56. Pirl WF, Beck BJ, Safren SA, et al. A descriptive study of psychiatric consultations in a community primary care center. *Prim Care Companion J Clin Psychiatry.* 2001;3(5):190–194. https://doi.org/10.4088/pcc.v03n0501.

57. American Psychiatric Association and Academy of Psychosomatic Medicine. Dissemination of integrated care within adult primary care settings: the collaborative care model. <https://www.psychiatry.org/File%20Library/Psychiatrists/Practice/Professional-Topics/Integrated-Care/APA-APM-Dissemination-Integrated-Care-Report.pdf.

58. Unutzer J, Katon W, Callahan CM, et al. Collaborative care management of late-life depression in the primary care setting: a randomized controlled trial. *JAMA.* 2002;288(22):2836–2845. https://doi.org/10.1001/jama.288.22.2836.

59. Rollman BL, Herbeck Belnap B, Abebe KZ, et al. Effectiveness of online collaborative care for treating mood and anxiety disorders in primary care: a randomized clinical trial. *JAMA Psychiatry.* 2018;75(1):56–64. https://doi.org/10.1001/jamapsychiatry.2017.3379.

60. Roy-Byrne P, Craske MG, Sullivan G, et al. Delivery of evidence-based treatment for multiple anxiety disorders in primary care: a randomized controlled trial. *JAMA.* 2010;303(19):1921–1928. https://doi.org/10.1001/jama.2010.608.

61. Fortney JC, Pyne JM, Kimbrell TA, et al. Telemedicine-based collaborative care for posttraumatic stress disorder: a randomized clinical trial. *JAMA Psychiatry.* 2015;72(1):58–67. https://doi.org/10.1001/jamapsychiatry.2014.1575.

62. Asarnow JR, Jaycox LH, Duan N, et al. Effectiveness of a quality improvement intervention for adolescent depression in primary care clinics: a randomized controlled trial. *JAMA.* 2005;293(3):311–319. https://doi.org/10.1001/jama.293.3.311.

63. Rollman BL, Belnap BH. The Bypassing the Blues trial: collaborative care for post-CABG depression and implications for future research. *Cleve Clin J Med.* 2011;78(suppl 1):S4–12. https://doi.org/10.3949/ccjm.78.s1.01.

64. Davidson KW, Rieckmann N, Clemow L, et al. Enhanced depression care for patients with acute coronary syndrome and persistent depressive symptoms: coronary psychosocial evaluation studies randomized controlled trial. *Arch Intern Med.* 2010;170(7):600–608. https://doi.org/10.1001/archinternmed.2010.29.

65. Huffman JC, Mastromauro CA, Beach SR, et al. Collaborative care for depression and anxiety disorders in patients with recent cardiac events: the Management of Sadness and Anxiety in Cardiology (MOSAIC) randomized clinical trial. *JAMA Intern Med.* 2014;174(6):927–935. https://doi.org/10.1001/jamainternmed.2014.739.

66. Huffman JC, Mastromauro CA, Sowden G, et al. Impact of a depression care management program for hospitalized cardiac patients. *Circ Cardiovasc Qual Outcomes.* 2011;4(2):198–205. https://doi.org/10.1161/CIRCOUTCOMES.110.959379.

67. Davidson KW, Bigger JT, Burg MM, et al. Centralized, stepped, patient preference-based treatment for patients with post-acute coronary syndrome depression: CODIACS vanguard randomized controlled trial. *JAMA Intern Med.* 2013;173(11):997–1004. https://doi.org/10.1001/jamainternmed.2013.915.

68. Rollman BL, Anderson AM, Rothenberger SD, et al. Efficacy of blended collaborative care for patients with heart failure and comorbid depression: a randomized clinical trial. *JAMA Intern Med.* 2021;181(10):1369–1380. https://doi.org/10.1001/jamainternmed.2021.4978.

69. Simon GE, VonKorff M, Durham ML. Predictors of outpatient mental health utilization by primary care patients in a health maintenance organization. *Am J Psychiatry.* 1994;151(6):908–913. https://doi.org/10.1176/ajp.151.6.908.

70. Druss BG, Mays RA, Edwards VJ, et al. Primary care, public health, and mental health. *Prev Chronic Dis.* 2010;7(1):A04. www.cdc.gov/pcd/sissues/2010/jan/09_0131.htm.

71. Pincus HA, Zarin DA, West JC. Peering into the "black box". Measuring outcomes of managed care. *Arch Gen Psychiatry.* 1996;53(10):870–877. https://doi.org/10.1001/archpsyc.1996.01830100016003.

72. Smith GR Jr, Hamilton Ge Jr. The importance of outcomes research for the financing of care. *Harv Rev Psychiatry.* 1995;2(5):288–289. https://doi.org/10.3109/10673229509017148.

73. Cole SA, Sullivan M, Kathol R, et al. A model curriculum for mental disorders and behavioral problems in primary care. *Gen Hosp Psychiatry.* 1995;17(1):13–18. https://doi.org/10.1016/0163-8343(94)00057-k.

50 COMMUNITY PSYCHIATRY

BJ BECK, MSN, MD, BFA, MFA ■ HYUN-HEE KIM, MD ■ ALEX S. KEUROGHLIAN, MD, MPH

OVERVIEW

A broad historical context is necessary to comprehend the evolution of the complex array of discontinuous services now under the rubric of "community psychiatry." This sociopolitical system, the third psychiatric revolution[1] (the first two revolutions being moral treatment and psychoanalysis, respectively), has variously followed the doctrines of public health, prevention, population-based care, and social activism. In the United States, the history of community psychiatry is a tale of decremental finances and shifting priorities (e.g., mental health for all versus focused resources for the seriously mentally ill; mainstream patients in the community versus remove and contain them in institutions) driven by surges of public outrage and activist reform, followed by ebbs of denial and neglect. The survival of community psychiatry, given the degree and rate of change in resources and mandates, has demanded a sustained and unparalleled creative effort.

TERMS AND DEFINITIONS

Because of this evolution, an appreciation for community psychiatry requires working knowledge of terms common to disciplines as disparate as sanitation and managed care. There are subtle differences in related, but not synonymous, fields that illustrate the lack of cohesive theory and practice. Formative social and public health policies and tenets have also played an important role. Economic, political, and systemic oversight developments continue to direct the future purview and practice of community psychiatry.

Beyond clinical terminology, each of these factors has its lexicon.

Related Fields

Various and possibly confusing terms are (imprecisely) used interchangeably with the term *community psychiatry* (e.g., *social psychiatry, community mental health [CMH], public psychiatry,* and *population-based psychiatry*). The theory of social psychiatry accentuates the sociocultural aspects of mental disorders and their treatments. Research to advance this theory views psychiatry and psychological features as variables to predict, describe, and mediate the expression of social problems. Community psychiatry is a clinical application of this theory with the mandate to develop an optimal care system for a given population with finite resources. Goal achievement entails working with individuals, groups, and systems, but that is the extent of agreement (in the field and over time) on the appropriate emphasis, boundaries, core services, and guiding principles of community psychiatry.[2] The following quoted definitions hint at this lack of consensus:

> …*the body of knowledge, theories, methods and skills in research and service required by psychiatrists who participate in organized community programs for the promotion of mental health and the prevention, treatment and rehabilitation of the mental disorders in a population.*[3]
>
> …*focusing on the detection, prevention, early treatment, and rehabilitation of emotional disorders and social deviance as they develop in the community rather than as they are encountered at large, centralized psychiatric facilities.*[4]

...subspecialty area in which psychiatrists deliver mental health services to populations defined by a common workplace, activity, or geographical area of residence.[5]

...responsible for the comprehensive treatment of the severely mentally ill in the community at large. All aspects of care—from hospitalization, case management, and crisis intervention, to day treatment, and supportive living arrangements—are included.[6]

CMH, as defined by the Community Mental Health Center (CMHC) Acts of 1963 (Public Law 88-164) and 1965 (Public Law 89-105), was envisioned to be an inclusive, multi-disciplinary, systemic approach to publicly funded mental health services provided for all in need, residing in a given geographical locale (i.e., a catchment area), without consideration of ability to pay. *Catchment* (from sanitation engineering: a cistern into which the sewage of a defined area is dumped) refers to a CMH service area with a population of 75,000 to 200,000.[7] Public psychiatry, a system of government-funded inpatient and outpatient services also initially conceived to meet the needs of all, has narrowed its focus on the seriously mentally ill who are unable to access appropriate services in the "private" sector (e.g., as fee-for-service or as paid by third-party insurance). A trend to privatize (i.e., to put out to private sector bid with government oversight) the public sector services threatens to further confuse the definition and blur the public/private distinction. In population-based psychiatry, the population may be defined by geography, or by several other attributes (e.g., payer, employer, guild, or care system). No matter how the population is defined, the system (e.g., a health maintenance organization [HMO]) is accountable for all members, as well as for an individual seeking treatment.

Social and Public Health Terms

Deinstitutionalization was a sociopolitical and economic trend to discharge long-term psychiatric inpatients to live and receive services in the community. More appropriately called de*hospitalization*[8] (or tran*s*institutionalism[2]), patients were merely maintained in non-hospital institutional settings. This trend was evident, however, long before the term (and such associated terms as *policy* or *movement*) ever appeared in the psychiatric literature, which suggests the convergence

of multiple precipitants, but no formal, purposeful, or driving policy.

The public health model describes three levels of prevention.[9] Primary prevention is concerned with measures to decrease the new onset (incidence) of disease (e.g., causative agent eradication, risk factor reduction, host resistance enhancement, and disease transmission disruption). Such measures, highly effective in the realms of infectious disease, toxins, deficiency states, and habit-induced chronic illnesses (e.g., lung and heart diseases), are less efficacious in the psychiatric realm, where the non-intervention outcome is less predictable. Nonetheless, putative programs and clinical activities of primary prevention include anticipatory guidance (e.g., for parents with young children), enrichment and competence-building programs (e.g., Head Start, Outward Bound), social support or self-help programs for at-risk individuals (e.g., bereavement groups), and early or crisis intervention following trauma (e.g., on-site student counseling after a classmate's suicide). Secondary prevention is concerned with measures to decrease the number of disease cases in a population at a given point in time (prevalence) through early discernment (case finding) and timely treatment to shorten the course and minimize residual disability. An educational campaign and screening for peripartum depression would be a psychiatric example of secondary prevention. Tertiary prevention is concerned with measures to decrease the prevalence and severity of residual disease-related defects or disabilities. Because optimal function in the setting of serious psychiatric illness is so allied with treatment adherence, examples of tertiary prevention in psychiatry would include case management and other measures to promote continuous care and treatment.

Case, or care, managers (usually social workers or mental health clinicians) assist in the patient's negotiation of a fragmented, complex system of agencies, providers, and services, with the goal of care being continuity and coordination through better inter-provider communication.[10] Obviously, patients with more, and more complex, needs also require more intensive care management. The greater the intensity of the management needs, the fewer cases a manager can adequately handle.[11] The care manager is the member of the treatment team who follows the patient through all care levels (e.g., inpatient, aftercare, residential), types (e.g., mental health, substance use, physical health), and agencies or services (e.g., housing, welfare, public entitlements).

Terms of Managed Care

Not to be confused with care management, managed care, primarily a cost-containment strategy, manages payment for care of a population through monitoring of services allocated to members of the specified population. Prior authorization, primary care provider (PCP) specialty referral (i.e., a gatekeeper system), and concurrent (or utilization) review are strategies commonly employed to manage healthcare expenditure. They are also increasingly recognized as vehicles to coordinate care, gather evidence for best practices, promote the development of alternative levels of care, and monitor treatment outcomes. Managed care organizations (MCOs) have proliferated to provide this service for public and private insurers under a neoliberal economic policy of the last four decades in the United States, promoting "free market" solutions to social inequities. Contracts between insurers and MCOs may include penalties for exceeding the service budget or financial incentives to hold service payments within a fixed budget. Healthcare costs have long been a concern of both providers and recipients of health care, but managed care has imposed the third-party payer's interests into the doctor-patient relationship, while failing to contain healthcare costs over the last 40 years in the United States. Proponents believe MCOs have promoted greater transparency, standardization, and evidence-based care (and possibly paved the way for numerous pay-for-performance [P4P] initiatives[12]).

HMOs, a type of MCO, generally contract for global healthcare services for a specified population by paying the provider a set amount, based on a rate (i.e., cap) per member, per month (i.e., capitation). Capitation plans have spurred initiatives to develop coordinated and collaborative systems of cost-effective, high-quality care, to maintain a high standard of overall health for the entire (covered) population. However, some MCOs, including capitated plans, separate the benefit management of physical health from mental health and substance use (i.e., "behavioral health [BH]") services, i.e., such plans "carve-out" BH benefit management. Companies that manage only these carved out

benefits are called managed behavioral health organizations (MBHOs). The advent of carve-outs set the stage for *cost shifting*, which is changing the care site (e.g., medical unit versus psychiatric unit) and thereby shifting the cost of care (e.g., from the physical health capitation pool to the mental health capitation pool).[13] This may or may not affect the overall quality or cost of the care, but it shifts the financial burden from (in this example) MCO to MBHO. This split-pot arrangement is antithetical to the collaborative efforts incentivized by single (i.e., global) cap programs. Cost shifting also occurs between other care/payer systems, such as state and federal (e.g., moving patients from state-funded hospitals to the community where they are eligible for federal subsidies and entitlements), public and private (e.g., privatization shifts the risk for burgeoning BH care costs from states to MCOs or MBHOs), and mental health to physical health (e.g., when patients bypass the mental health system and seek services in the physical healthcare system either for their mental health problems or for vague somatic complaints). Some also argue that cost shifting occurs from BH to the correctional system because the disenfranchised (e.g., the seriously mentally ill, the dually diagnosed, and substance users) may receive consistent care only when incarcerated.[14]

A cadre of oversight and accrediting agencies has evolved to ensure that MCOs balance their focus on cost containment with quality of care. The National Committee for Quality Assurance (NCQA), the largest such accrediting body for MCOs, includes accreditation standards for MBHOs, as well as for the BH portion of non-carve-out MCOs.[15] NCQA standards address accessibility and availability of appropriate, culturally sensitive services, coordination between BH and physical healthcare services, communication between all care providers, and disease management/preventive health services. Both over- and under-utilization of services must be managed to ensure that patients receive care appropriate to their needs. MCOs are also required to have a straightforward grievance and appeal process for patients when the MCO (or its MBHO) initially denies a request for care or particular services, though very few patients file for appeals[16] and the administrative complexity related to billing, prior authorizations, and appeals has been noted to be the greatest contribution to wasted dollars in American health care.[17] Another form of oversight, the Federal Interim Final Rule Under the Paul Wellstone and Pete Domenici Mental Health Parity and Addiction Equity Act of 2008 (Interim Final Rule on Parity) states, in general terms, that BH benefits may not be managed more restrictively than a plan's physical health benefits, "except to the extent that recognized clinically appropriate standards of care may permit a difference."[18] To the extent that NCQA appreciates the difference between BH and physical health care, entities that meet NCQA standards should also continue to meet the requirements of the Parity Law.

HISTORICAL BACKGROUND

The history of community psychiatry is a saga of alternating reform and neglect best understood within the political, economic, and sociocultural context of the times. Table 50.1 is a historical timeline of key events. Table 50.2 recaps the legislative acts that have affected the system in the United States.

The Age of Enlightenment

The "first psychiatric revolution" occurred late in the 18th century when French alienist (i.e., psychiatrist), Philippe Pinel, endorsed physical work and fresh air to return the mentally ill to a state of mental health and well-being.[19] Moral treatment dawned as Pinel released the insane from their shackles.[20] By the early 19th century, the movement had found its way to the United States, where Dorothea Dix promoted the development of village-style asylums for the mentally ill to retreat from the stresses of daily living.[21] The government-funded construction of institutions for the behaviorally deviant and mentally ill.[22]

By the end of the century, however, these institutions and asylums were hopelessly run-down and overcrowded.[23] In concert with the Industrial Revolution (focused on organization and productivity), moral treatment was replaced by custodial care and regimentation, and a wave of neglect. Even worse, however, was the onslaught of unproven, unbeneficial, and possibly harmful somatic therapies.[24,25] Among these "scientific" treatments, only two were found to have merit for select patients. Many institutionalized patients suffered from the general paretic form of tertiary neurosyphilis,[26] which was found to resolve with

the high fevers of malaria.[27] Patients with conversion (and possibly other) disorders were helped by Freud and his disciples, who used psychological understanding in their treatment.

Early 20th-Century Awareness

Urbanization of the Industrial Revolution spurred the preventive, public health movement, a necessity for sanitation and infection control. This was paralleled by the mental hygiene movement promoted by the writings of Adolph Meyer on prevention and the social context of mental illness. In 1908, Clifford Beers exposed the deplorable conditions inside mental institutions in his first-person account of living in one.[28] Beers joined forces with Meyer and William James to create the National Association for Mental Health in 1909.[29,30] The mental hygiene movement advocated for smaller hospitals and the establishment of community-based outpatient evaluation clinics. These clinics (variously viewed as the forerunners or beginnings of community psychiatry[2]) were less stigmatizing than large state hospitals, and they concentrated on evaluation, prevention, and the differentiation between persistent and acute disorders. They also emphasized inter-disciplinary training, affiliation with medical schools and mainstream medicine, and the use of applied psychodynamic theory and principles.

An extension of the mental hygiene movement, the child guidance movement proposed to apply psychodynamic theory in childhood to prevent the development of adult pathology.[3] However, such assumptions proved difficult to substantiate, leading to apathy and discouragement. This wave of neglect coincided with the Great Depression. Along with dwindling funds, professional infighting, and long waitlists, rigid acceptance criteria led to disillusionment and abandonment of these programs.

Mid-20th Century

The confluence of military experience, pharmacological breakthroughs, and epidemiological research provided the platform for mental health legislation to both advance knowledge and improve care. During World War II, the armed services had difficulty filling the ranks as new recruits were outnumbered by those either rejected or removed from service because of psychiatric casualties. In response, military psychiatrists

TABLE 50.1
Historical Development of Community Psychiatry

The Age of Enlightenment

Late 18th century: Pinel removes the shackles: advent of moral treatment

Early 19th century: United States-funded institutions

- Dorothea Dix: village-type asylums

Late 19th century: Industrial Revolution: productivity and organization

- Custodial care and "scientific" somatic therapies

Early 20th-Century Awareness

Adolph Meyer: mental hygiene movement

Clifford Beers: *A Mind That Found Itself*

Beers, Meyer, and William James: National Association for Mental Health

Child Guidance movement

The Great Depression

Mid-20th Century

World War II

1946: The National Mental Health Act

1949: National Institute of Mental Health

1954: Chlorpromazine released

1955: Pinnacle of custodial care: expository works in poor conditions

- Mental Health Study Act: Joint Commission on Mental Illness and Health

Late 1950s: Deinstitutionalization: revolving door policy

- Epidemiological studies: symptoms and impairment common

1961: Joint Commission recommendations: improve the public hospitals

- Focus on serious, persistent mentally ill

Birth of US Community Mental Health Movement

1963: First-ever presidential address on mental health and retardation

- Community Mental Health Center (CMHC) Acts: 1963 funds construction; 1965 funds staffing
- President Kennedy assassinated

Late 1960s: Funds dwindle, few centers built, fewer staffed

Late 1970s: First grant cycle ends

1975: Congressional Act: partially revitalizes, adds services

1977: President Carter's Commission on Mental Health

1979: National Alliance for the Mentally Ill: self-help movement in CMH

1980: Mental Health Systems Act

1981: Reagan Administration repeals 1980 Act: block grants replace categorical funding

Late 20th Century

Early 1980s: Privatization

1984: Epidemiologic Catchment Area Study: primary care practitioner "de facto" mental health system

- Managed care, carve-outs, cost shifting

1992: National Comorbidity Survey

Early 21st Century

2002: National Comorbidity Survey Replication

- Depression on the rise; more being seen in the mental health system
- Most who seek care in a medical setting receive medication

2008: Mental Health Parity and Addiction Equity Act

Current:

- Managed care networks approximating CMHC vision
- Promotion of accountable care organizations, Health Homes, and Medical Homes
- Cautious development of "Dual Eligible" programs: limited, combined funding

TABLE 50.2
US Legislation Affecting Community Mental Health

1946: The National Mental Health Act
1949: National Institute of Mental Health
1955: Mental Health Study Act: Joint Commission on Mental Illness and Health
1963: Community Mental Health Center (CMHC) Act: fund construction
1965: CMHC Act: fund staffing
1975: CMHC Amendments: partially revitalize, add essential services
1977: President's Commission on Mental Health
1979: National Alliance for the Mentally Ill
1980: Mental Health Systems Act
1981: Reagan Administration repeals Mental Health Systems Act; block grants replace categorical funding
2008: Mental Health Parity and Addiction Equity Act

were urged to lower acceptance standards and to move treatment interventions to the battlefield to reduce the number of psychiatric evacuees. Coupled with the post-war optimism, three central tenets of community psychiatry were culled from this experience: immediacy, proximity, and expectancy.[31] Briefly stated, treatment should occur without delay, on-site, and with the expectation of improvement/resolution. Treatment in, or near, the patient's usual environment decreased the likelihood of secondary gain and the development of avoidance. Far from being custodial, the care system was to support the concept of recovery and to promote the expectation that the patient would return to baseline function.

While the United States failed to pass a comprehensive universal healthcare system in the post-war era due to the efforts of the American Medical Association, the fledgling pharmaceutical lobby, and Cold War era politics, there was a massive expansion of employer-provided health insurance[32] and several landmark pieces of legislations on healthcare reform. In 1946, at the pinnacle of custodial care, with over 550,000 state hospital inpatients, Congress passed the National Mental Health Act, approving federal funds for mental health training and research. This Act also founded the National Institute of Mental Health in 1949. Shortly thereafter, chlorpromazine (Thorazine)[33] was first used in the United States, with a concomitant decrease in

psychotic symptoms and behavioral problems in long-institutionalized state hospital patients. More patients could now be treated at home with chlorpromazine, and they had far superior outcomes (e.g., symptomatic relief, improved cognition, overall function).[34] Also in the mid- to late-1940s, several expository works[35,36] heightened recognition of the apathy and other damaging effects of prolonged institutional living (e.g., poor social function and self-care skills). The depiction of overcrowded, dehumanizing conditions in large state institutions inspired another surge of public outrage. In 1955 the Mental Health Study Act established the Joint Commission on Mental Illness and Health, providing funds to assess the nation's available treatment services for the mentally ill. By the end of the decade, deinstitutionalization was in full swing, state hospital beds had dwindled to 100,000, and the insufficiency of community resources had become glaringly obvious. Long-hospitalized patients, often estranged from their families, lacked the coping and social skills to manage and advocate for themselves outside of the institution. Eighty percent were re-hospitalized within 2 years, a phenomenon called the revolving door policy.[6]

The Joint Commission reported in 1961 on its nationwide assessment,[37] and it recommended smaller hospitals with greater resources, and funds targeted to improve services for the most severely ill patients (i.e., patients with psychosis and major mental illness). Around this time, several epidemiological studies exposed the prevalence of psychiatric symptomatology and impaired function, pervasive across rural,[38] urban,[39] and suburban populations. At least one study also demonstrated that the population in greatest need had the least access to mental health services.[40]

Birth of the American Community Mental Health Movement

By 1963 political and social optimism were ripe for the first-ever presidential address to Congress regarding mental health and retardation (now called intellectual disability).[41] In this address, President Kennedy voiced his opposition to the prevailing institutional system and his conviction (in opposition to the Joint Commission recommendations) that more funding for this system would not improve the quality of care. He called for a "bold new approach," relying on new pharmacology and knowledge, to treat the mentally ill in their home communities, where they would be "returned to a useful place in society." Kennedy foresaw a "new type of health facility," the CMHC, as part of a comprehensive community care system, to improve quality and "return mental health care to the mainstream of American medicine." Within weeks of signing the CMHC Act, President Kennedy was assassinated.

The CMHC Acts of 1963 and 1965 provided for the funding of CMHC buildings and staff, respectively. Each CMHC was to provide five essential services: four levels of care (inpatient, outpatient, partial hospital, and emergency) and consultation/education. The goal was to use the public funds to build and staff 2000 centers by 1980, and to have fees and private insurers fund continued services. With the rise of neoliberalism in the late 1960s, however, both state and federal funds for health and welfare programs began to diminish. Even as the center was under construction, staff funding was decreased or withdrawn. Far from the projected number, fewer than 800 centers were built, many without adequate staff funding. This obvious failure to meet public expectations also fueled criticism and conflict about the role of community psychiatrists. Some believed psychiatrists valued social activism over the treatment needs of the mentally ill. By the mid-1970s, the imminent end of the first grant cycle funding CMHC staff, the mentally ill were generally not paying fees, insurers were also not supporting CMHC services, demand was overwhelming, and state hospital capacity was less than a fifth of what it had been. The severely mentally ill were flooding communities without adequate services in place.

Amidst an economic crisis with declining worker productivity, stagnant wages, and an unprecedented wave of corporate financial influence via political action committees, the national discourse on health care turned from aspirations of a universal health system to that of cost containment.[32] Cost control became bipartisan consensus as another wave of reforms and community activism followed the 1975 Congressional Act[42] to partially fund and revitalize the CMHCs (with a less idealistic mandate than Kennedy's vision), to target services for those who most perturbed the community, and to increase the essential services accordingly (i.e., to include specialized programs for children and the elderly, direct mental health screening services for the courts, follow-up care and transitional housing for the deinstitutionalized, and specialized drug and alcohol programs).[43] In 1977, President Carter established the President's Commission on Mental Health to launch another nationwide assessment of mental health services. The self-help movement in CMH was also gaining momentum, as mothers of mentally ill children began the National Alliance for the Mentally Ill (NAMI), in 1979. In 1980, Congress passed the Mental Health Systems Act (Public Law 96-398), which included some of the Joint Commission's recommendations from their nationwide assessment. With the intent to fund services for the most underserved populations (i.e., the old, the young, the seriously mentally ill, and minorities), the bill had provisions to build new CMHCs, to improve the coordination of total health care by linking mental and physical healthcare providers, and to fund essential, non-revenue-producing services (i.e., consultation, education, coordination of care, and CMHC administration).

In what can only be viewed as a major setback, 18 years of categorical federal funding for CMH disintegrated in 1981, when the Reagan Administration repealed the 1980 Mental Health Systems Act before it was implemented. The inadequate funds for substance use and mental health services were placed in block grants and left to the will of the individual states.

Late 20th Century

The retraction of federal funds and oversight resulted in 50 discontinuous state programs with insufficient resources to care for the most seriously mentally ill in the community. Early in the 1980s, the early 1980s privatization trend, and exemption from the Diagnosis-Related Groups legislation, encouraged the expansion of private, for-profit, psychiatric, and substance use hospitals. The Epidemiologic Catchment Area study of 1984 quantified the marked prevalence of psychiatric symptomatology and disorder in general community populations. The study determined that the preponderance of symptomatic community residents never sought care in the mental health system. Rather, they accessed the general medical system, dubbed the "de facto" mental health system.[44]

Early-1990s healthcare cost escalation spurred an explosion of managed care initiatives in both public and private sectors. Another epidemiological study, the National Comorbidity Survey (NCS, 1990–92), reiterated the high lifetime prevalence (50%) and 1-year incidence (30%) of mental disorders in community respondents (depression and alcohol use disorder being most prevalent).[45] The growth of private psychiatric hospitals, and the lack of treatment guidelines, standards, or criteria for levels or types of care, made mental health an easy target. While not generally embraced by clinicians, managed care had the potential to coordinate care, gather evidence for best practices, promote the development of alternative levels of care, and monitor treatment outcomes. However, it also set the stage for BH carve-outs, and the resultant cost-shifting strategies (to benefit the bottom line of the specific MCO or MBHO) that frequently created conflict between BH and physical health providers (and payers), without adequate consideration of the patient's best interest. Carve-outs have further fragmented the healthcare system, as medical colleagues have not been able to refer to in-house BH providers if they are not in the carve-out network (and there is an inverse relationship between the difficulty and likelihood of appropriate referral). This systemic convergence of decreased federal funding and oversight, healthcare cost escalation, privatization, managed care, carve-outs, and cost shifting further entrenched this complex and discontinuous system, which was increasingly difficult to access by the most vulnerable and disenfranchised (i.e., the poor, homeless, non-English speaking, uninsured, and deinstitutionalized).

Start of the 21st Century

The rigorous replication of the NCS (NCS-R, 2001–02) focused on severity, clinical significance, overall disability, and role impairment. NCS-R had several significant findings about depression, the disorder was again found to be the most prevalent. First, the prevalence of depression has increased in each birth cohort since World War II. Second, slightly more than half of depressed community respondents seeking care now receive that care in the mental health sector. The other significant finding, attributable to advances in pharmacotherapy and educational efforts, was that 90% of respondents treated for depression in any medical setting received medication. However, only about one in five of these respondents treated for depression received what would be considered minimally adequate treatment by current standards (and almost half of depressed community residents still received no treatment).[46]

Early in the 21st century, the CMH system remains substantially unchanged from that of the late 1990s. However, there is a focus on training and collaboration with PCPs to improve treatment (mostly of depression) for those who access care in the primary care sector (largely through funding mandates to federally qualified community health centers).[47-52] This has done little to improve the quality of life or care for the more seriously mentally ill, and others beyond the expertise of PCPs. For this population, the CMH "system" remains discontinuous, and includes the revolving door policy, now often on acute, rather than state hospital, inpatient units.

UNDERLYING PRINCIPLES OF COMMUNITY MENTAL HEALTH

The principles central to CMH are summarized in Table 50.3.

Population Responsibility

President Kennedy's vision, and the initial CMHC Acts of 1963 and 1965, mandated meeting the mental health

---

TABLE 50.3
Principles of Community Psychiatry

Population Responsibility
- Services for entire catchmented population
- Allocation of limited resources
- Clinically and culturally appropriate services

Prevention
- Decrease incidence (primary)
- Decrease prevalence (secondary)
- Decrease residual disability (tertiary)

Community-based Care (Proximity)
- Maintain family, social supports
- Avoid geographical isolation
- Promote patient's functional role in community

Citizen Involvement
- Community boards: set priorities, policies
- Patient input and feedback
- Lay-provider partnerships
- Political advocacy

Continuity of Care
- Ideal: seamless circle of care across all levels of treatment
- Reality: case managers coordinate fragmented services, facilitate communication between providers

needs of an entire, geographically defined (catchment area) population, regardless of ability to pay. No population member could be denied service. Defined catchment areas covered resident populations of 75,000 to 200,000. Population responsibility requires planning for the optimal use of limited resources to develop the most favorable system to meet the population's care needs. Services developed should match the patients' needs, not be tailored to treat the masses more economically (e.g., groups offered when clinically and culturally appropriate, not as cost-saving alternatives).

Prevention

Community psychiatry, like public health, should focus on prevention to decrease the incidence, prevalence, and disability of mental illness or disorders. However, limited resources largely restricted the focus to tertiary prevention[31] (i.e., rehabilitation to limit disability in the seriously mentally ill).

Community-Based Care

Both services and advocacy occur in the patient's home community. This proximity obviates the downfalls of geographical isolation, promotes the maintenance of family and social support, and encourages the patient's continued social role in their community. Patients with serious mental illness (SMI) have been shown to retain better social and self-care skills when treated in their communities. A variety of services have been developed to help patients access care and remain safely in the community, rather than in restrictive, long-term, custodial care.

The 1909 partnership of Beers and Meyer to form NAMI initiated lay-professional collaboration and citizen involvement in the CMH system. Community boards and BH professionals work together to establish priorities and develop policies. Involved community members also become powerful advocates to campaign for necessary continued resources.

Continuity of Care

The initially conceived CMHCs were to provide comprehensive care (i.e., across all levels and intensity of services) as well as coordination of services across the continuum. With all levels of care (e.g., outpatient, inpatient, partial hospital, crisis stabilization, day treatment, and residential) within the circle of care,

the information flow would follow the patient without hindrance, and providers would have unimpeded communication to facilitate the development and consistency of comprehensive treatment plans. Unlike the current discontinuous reality, there would be no place for cost shifting in an ideal, comprehensive system.

COMPONENTS AND SERVICES OF COMMUNITY MENTAL HEALTH SYSTEMS

The components of the ideal CMH system are summarized in Table 50.4. The reality is that each of these services may not be available in a given community, and those that are will likely span more than one agency.

Inpatient Care

Hospitalization remains a necessary resource, although reserved for the more acutely and seriously ill. Acute hospitalization is an active, intense level of evaluation, care, and safe containment, with scarce resemblance to bygone custodial care. General hospital and private psychiatric hospital beds are now more plentiful, and less stigmatizing, for brief, intense stays. Most units are now locked because most payers will only cover inpatient care when patients meet commitment standards (e.g., being suicidal, homicidal, or unable to care for themselves due to mental illness), even when patients sign in voluntarily. Financial constraints, the development of less restrictive care settings, and legal protection of the civil liberties of the mentally ill have made long-term, inpatient care largely a thing of the past. The revolving door (multiple, brief admissions) has

TABLE 50.4
Components of Community Mental Health

- Inpatient care
- Partial hospitalization
- Outpatient services
- Emergency services
- Community consultation/education
- Case management
- Homeless outreach
- Disaster or trauma response
- Evaluation and research

replaced extended hospitalization for many of the seriously mentally ill.

Partial Hospitalization

For patients with stable living situations, the less restrictive partial hospital program offers a helpful step-down, or diversion, from inpatient care. Patients have the structure of the hospital-based treatment program during the day, and they return home in the evening. This gradual return to, or maintenance in, the community with continued hospital support is an attempt to combat the inevitability of the revolving door.

Outpatient Services

Extensive outpatient service options promote effective community treatment for more seriously ill patients. Such services may include, but are not limited to, those listed in Table 50.5. Besides the common modalities (e.g., medication management; individual, group, or family therapy; substance use treatment), outpatient services also encompass transitional housing (e.g., half-way houses, group homes, supervised boarding rooms), day treatment, and specialized services for children and the elderly.

Emergency Services

Twenty-four-hour coverage by crisis teams, or crisis clinicians in emergency departments (EDs), allows

TABLE 50.5
Outpatient Community Services

Medication Management
Therapy
    Individual
    Group
      ■ Psychoeducation
      ■ Skills training
      ■ Self-help
    Family
Day Treatment
Transitional Housing
    Half-way houses
    Supervised boarding rooms
    Group homes
Specialized children's services
Specialized elderly services
Alcohol and drug use treatment programs

patients to be screened before hospitalization for crisis intervention, assessment for level of care, and immediate access to appropriate care.

Community Consultation/Education

Such non-reimbursable activities dwindled with decreased federal funds, although partially revitalized by the primary care "gatekeeper" system. As primary care patients tend to present with somatic complaints (rather than mood, anxiety, or substance use problems), and PCPs are increasingly encouraged (e.g., by managed care, global capitation, or federal mandate) to treat the less complicated mental disorders in their practices, they look to community psychiatrists to assist with appropriate diagnosis, treatment, or referral.

Case Management

Considered essential in the conception of the seamless CMH system, case (or care) management is an absolute necessity in the current, fragmented, care system. Care managers remain the liaison between care providers, although appropriate releases are now required to permit this important communication.

Homeless Outreach

The most disenfranchised, the growing numbers of the mentally ill homeless do not seek or access the services they need, for multiple reasons, including negative past experiences, lack of insight, and fear. By meeting them where they are, outreach workers must be adaptable to establish credibility, work in non-traditional settings, and bring services to this disadvantaged population.

Disaster or Trauma Response

The lessons from military psychiatry, bolstered by the post-9/11 events, have prompted some agencies to develop immediate-response teams for on-site assessment and treatment of disaster victims, to mitigate post-traumatic syndromes and residual disabilities.

Evaluation and Research

The push to develop evidence-based treatment guidelines in psychiatry and CMH aligns with mainstream medical trends. The major impetus toward program evaluation, or "outcomes research," however, has been the need to contain cost and to identify cost-effectiveness. In the community, true cost-effectiveness research must span multiple departments, agencies, and services. Cost-offset from one program to another (e.g., improved, but more costly, BH services, decrease the overall cost by relatively larger decreases in the expense of general medical care; increased pharmacy or crisis team expense results in greatly decreased inpatient expense) is particularly difficult to identify in this diffuse system. In contrast to the cost-shifting obfuscation of carve-out BH management, the inclusive responsibility of global capitation will promote and require total systems research to identify cost-offset and cost-effectiveness.

TRENDS

Disenfranchisement

The current minimalist patchwork of community services prioritizes the most severely mentally ill. This has both increased the stigma and failed to adequately meet the needs of the targeted population. As services diminish and barriers to access increase, progressively more of those with serious mental illness (SMI) are homeless, chemically dependent, or imprisoned.

Managed Care: The "Fourth Psychiatric Revolution?"

Most MCOs have now moved beyond the initial mandate for cost containment to concerns for quality and cost-effectiveness. Early cost savings from decreased hospital days were not the total means to functionally maintain this population in the community. In what might be considered convergent evolution, MCOs (or MBHOs, in the case of carve-out management) have pushed the public and private sectors to develop networks of closely affiliated services that span the levels of progressively less intensive and restrictive care, with intensive clinical managers to assist patients through these timely transitions and ensure communication between (serial and parallel) treaters. This push has included the development of alternative (previously unavailable) levels of care. These networks have been developed with much the same mandate and fiscal constraint as the 1960s CMHCs they resemble (i.e., to provide coordinated continuity of quality care, for a given population, with finite resources). Progressive MCOs solicit member and provider input through satisfaction surveys and advisory committees (like the CMHC community boards), to ensure relevant, culturally appropriate programs and user-friendly service. These more inclusive networks facilitate data collection and tracking so that progressive MCOs can now use data to inform policy. In this way, they have set standards for communication with PCPs, timely access to care, coordination of services, correlation of symptoms and function to level of care, treatment planning, monitoring, and recording.

Despite some of these improvements, healthcare costs in the United States have continued to rise far beyond the per capita spending of comparable developed countries[53] yet lag in almost every measure of health, access, and quality.[54] The interests of a profit-generating (or cost-saving) corporation remain fundamentally in contradiction with those of the patients they are supposed to serve, and the fiduciary duty of clinicians. Such external constraints, which have failed spectacularly to reduce healthcare costs for patients but have generated incredible returns for shareholders, have contributed significantly to the burnout of healthcare workers in medicine and allied fields.[55-57] Additionally, the trend toward privatization has significantly impacted financing for hospitals, especially safety net hospitals which are less attractive to MCOs.[58] In attempting to address perverse incentives of fee-for-service structures, the shifting institutional focus on clinician "productivity" has created clinic policies (such as no-show policies) that have disproportionately negative impacts on the already vulnerable working class and underserved patient populations.[59] While the proliferation of private MCOs has often been justified using the neoliberal language of competition and consumer choice, this has also served to deflect blame from such organizations failing to provide adequate coverage onto patients as expert consumers who have simply failed to select the "right" plan.[60]

Primary Care

Once the "de facto" system, the promotion of primary care management (i.e., by gatekeeper and global capitation systems, or by federal mandate) of subsyndromal BH problems in the community has progressed to include treatment of more SMI. Provider groups at financial risk for the total care of their patient population have spurred the development of innovative programs to integrate and coordinate physical and mental health services.

Creative Solutions

Among the multi-disciplinary innovations to keep the seriously mentally ill functioning well in their home communities, Community Treatment Teams,[61,62] or Assertive Community Treatment (ACT),[63,64] attempt to engage them in treatment where they live. Team members meet patients in their homes, boarding rooms, or shelters to organize a flexible range of services (e.g., medication management, activities of daily living, social skills training) and to incorporate the patient's family or social supports into the treatment. This enhances monitoring and facilitates the timely offer of more intense services when needed. ACT has kept the seriously mentally ill from falling between the (service) cracks. The presence and discontinuation of ACT have been linked, respectively, to the fall and rise in hospital admission rates. Unfortunately, ACT and other non-traditional programs have not been matched by equally flexible funding or reimbursement structures. Public and private plan administrators require a broad view that spans systems, agencies, disciplines, and funding streams to meet and drive innovation to safely maintain the most vulnerable in the community.

Current initiatives (e.g., accountable care organizations, health homes, medical homes) that address care integration (and eliminate cost shifting) require the inclusion of (or built-in access to) BH services within the primary care setting (or, less frequently, the inclusion of primary care in the CMH setting).[65] Federal and state policymakers are also focusing on the "dual eligible" population (i.e., qualifying for Medicare and Medicaid benefits). These diverse and complex populations (i.e., the elderly indigent or the under-65, poor, and disabled) utilize a disproportionate share of healthcare services and epitomize the high cost and poor care coordination of both discontinuous services and separate funding sources. Unfortunately, the ostensibly inadequate combined funding proposed for these programs threatens to meet neither the targeted population's service needs nor the extensive development and implementation costs of participating health plans, causing some plans and states to preemptively opt out.[66]

Telemedicine

While advances in communication technology have long shaped the practice of medicine and dissemination of information, the widespread and near-immediate adoption of telemedicine across the United States during the first weeks of the coronavirus disease 2019 (COVID-19) pandemic has been the most dramatic example in recent memory.

Heliographs, smoke signals, drums, signal flags, and other forms of communication at a distance have been used for the transmission of information about epidemics, and to announce health information, such as births or deaths, for thousands of years.[67] As medicine progressed, practitioners corresponded with each other regarding cases, provided consultations, and disseminated scientific discoveries and public health information.[68] Professionalization and specialization of medicine increasingly necessitated access to expert opinion and diagnostic technology, with examples of diagnosis and treatment at a distance dating back to the 17th century[67]; however, until the advent of electronic communications technology, treatment at a distance was substantially limited by distance and time. Recognizably modern forms of synchronous telemedicine began in the late 1800s, with a case published in the *Lancet* on the diagnosis of croup via telephone in 1879.[67] One notable early American example of the adoption of this technology in psychiatry was in 1959, between the University of Nebraska and Norfolk State Hospital, where two-way closed circuit television was used to provide neurological and psychiatric consultations for a remote hospital facility.[69] Through the 1960s and 1970s, the National Aeronautics and Space Administration pioneered the further development of telemedicine services via satellite technology through rural pilot programs.[70]

Telemedicine has been long marketed for its ability to bring care to populations with various barriers, whether for rural populations or for those with limited mobility or lacking transportation. For psychiatry, where the diagnosis is largely based on patient interviews rather than on a physical exam, and while facing significant workforce shortages and uneven distribution of specialists, telemedicine has been an especially attractive modality for the provision of psychiatric care. Before the COVID-19 pandemic, however, its use was significantly limited by a lack of reimbursement and by widely varying state-level regulations. In 2015, telemedicine reimbursement represented less than 0.01% of Medicare healthcare expenditures.[71]

As of 2020, Medicare provides telemedicine visits to beneficiaries at the same rates as in-person visits, and Medicaid provides reimbursement for live-video telemedicine visits in all 50 states, and several states now require telemedicine reimbursement to be on par with reimbursement for in-person services.[72]

Aside from the obvious geographic convenience, telemedicine can have significant economic advantages for patients. Compared to other on-demand services, telemedicine visits can produce cost savings by diverting care from more expensive settings, such as EDs,[73] by reducing travel,[74] or by reducing times away from work for caregivers[75] which may be especially important for hourly workers without sufficient leave time. Although some clinicians have expressed concerns about the acceptability of such a platform for patients with delusions and thought disorders, studies so far show that telemedicine is viewed as acceptable by most patients with schizophrenia for general outpatient psychiatric treatment.[76]

While telemedicine's efficacy has been well-established for general outpatient level of care, its adoption for more intensive levels of care, such as partial hospitalization programs, is a much newer phenomenon since the start of the COVID-19 pandemic. So far, the results seem promising, and comparable to traditional partial hospitalization programs,[77-79] although many of the current findings are based on sequential cohorts since the beginning of the pandemic rather than on patients randomized to concurrent virtual or in-person programs. As with other telemedicine services, the adoption of the telemedicine format has the potential to expand access for patients who would otherwise be physically unable to attend. Long, intensive therapy, programs, however, may come with challenges around engagement. It may not always be suitable for all patients, especially younger patients. One study of a pediatric partial hospitalization program noted that some patients were "noticeably disengaged, logged onto other devices simultaneously, were inactive during in-group meetings, turned off their videos, or logged off from the groups," and such difficulties were more pronounced for younger participants.[80] As with any group modality, dynamics among participants can be highly variable and difficult to manage, and there was a noticeable "contagion effect for disengagement."[80] Additional supports, such

as parents implementing rewards at home for attendance, and providing technical troubleshooting, were necessary for proper engagement with treatment,[80] which may present significant challenges for caregivers who also need to work full-time during program hours.

Telemedicine, despite its many advantages, has not been able to overcome all barriers to care. Despite many positive studies of the overall efficacy of telemedicine, many patients simply prefer in-person visits. Qualitative studies have found that some patients take visits "more seriously" in person,[81,82] and in some cases, the act of leaving the home for an appointment may have therapeutic benefits or may explicitly be a part of the treatment (as in exposures for anxiety). Additionally, telemedicine may amplify existing disparities. While the urban-rural digital divide continues to close, patients who are most in need of appropriate medical care—poor, rural, older patients—are still most likely to lack sufficiently fast internet connections and technology needed for telemedicine.[72] As of 2021 approximately 15% of rural Americans lack broadband access.[83] Continuation of governmental programs for subsidized internet and devices, which were started during the COVID-19 pandemic, may be necessary for patients to have equitable access to telemedicine services. Patients with limited English proficiency may have difficulty in accessing appropriate interpretation services (particularly with less common languages or using American Sign Language interpreters on a poor-quality video connection) and may have difficulty using apps or websites necessary for telemedicine if instructions are only provided in English.[84] In addition to the technological infrastructure necessary for telemedicine visits, a private space in which to participate in sessions is often an explicit requirement for partial hospitalization programs, but it may not be available for many patients and families. Patients may censor themselves due to perceived or actual risk of being overheard in telemedicine visits.[81] Adapting art, music, or play therapy for telemedicine may require significant planning and delivery of materials that would be otherwise easily available in a therapist's office.[85] The above factors underscore the importance of addressing underlying socioeconomic disparities, regardless of technological advancements in care delivery.

CONCLUSION

Revolution, the overthrow of tradition, implies radical change: from shackles to moral treatment, to psychoanalysis, to the community mental health movement. Revolution, cycles of rotation, implies repetition: from neglect to reform to neglect, and so on. History has also vacillated on the focus of CMH, whether inclusive (services available to every member of the population) or prioritized for the most seriously mentally ill (and most objectionable to the community). If only for fiscal reasons, the community will likely remain the locus of treatment (as opposed to more restrictive institutional settings), although there are multiple other reasons why this is preferable. Revolution, coming full circle, may hold promise as managed care increases the system of services to resemble the comprehensive system of President Kennedy's vision. What follows managed care may well determine the future turn of the CMH cycle, along with advances in pharmacology, evidence-based care, social activism, creativity, and legislation. The challenge for community psychiatry is to know enough history to not repeat the mistakes, hold on to the gains, and develop viable systems that are not only dynamic, responsive, and collaborative, but politically influential to garner the necessary resources to care for their most vulnerable populations.

REFERENCES

1. Bellak L, ed. Community Psychiatry: The Third Psychiatric Revolution. Handbook of Community Psychiatry and Community Mental Health. Grune & Stratton; 1963.
2. Talbott JA. Has academic psychiatry abandoned the community? Acad Psychiatry. 1991;15:106–114.
3. Rubin B. Community psychiatry: an evolutionary change in medical psychiatry in the United States. Arch Gen Psychiatry. 1969;20:497–507.
4. Stedman's Medical Dictionary, 24th ed. Williams & Wilkins; 1982:163.
5. Borus JF. Community psychiatry. In: Nicholi AM, ed. The New Harvard Guide to Psychiatry. Harvard University Press; 1988.
6. Kaplan HI, Sadock BJ, Grebb JA, eds. Kaplan and Sadock's Synopsis of Psychiatry: Behavioral Sciences, Clinical Psychiatry. 7th ed. Williams & Wilkins; 1994.
7. Sharfstein SS. Whatever happened to community mental health? Psychiatr Serv. 2000;51:616–620.
8. Geller JL. The last half-century of psychiatric services as reflected in psychiatric services. Psychiatr Serv. 2000;51:41–67.
9. Barton PL. Understanding the U.S. Health Services System. Health Administration Press; 1999:264–266.
10. Kantor J. Clinical case management: definition, principles, components. Hosp Comm Psychiatry. 1989;40:361–368.
11. Dieterich M, Irving CB, Park B, et al. Intensive case management for severe mental illness. Cochrane Database Syst Rev. 2010;10(10). Art No. CD007906. https://doi.org/10.1002/14651858.CD007906.pub2.
12. Van Herck P, De Smedt D, Annemans L, et al. Systematic review: effects, design choices, and context of pay-for-performance in health care. BMC Health Serv Res. 2010;10:247. http://www.biomedcentral.com/1472-6963/10/247.
13. Christensen RC. The ethics of cost shifting in community psychiatry. Psychiatr Serv. 2002;53:921.
14. Domino ME, Norton EC, Morrissey JP, et al. Cost shifting to jails after a change to managed mental health care. Health Serv Res. 2004;39:1379–1402.
15. Alter CL. New NCQA Standards: An Opportunity to Lead. Special Report. Academy of Psychosomatic Medicine. <www.apm.org/papers/ncqa.shtml>.
16. Pollitz K, Rae M, Mengistu S. Claims Denials and Appeals in ACA Marketplace Plans in 2020. Kaiser Family Foundation. <https://www.kff.org/private-insurance/issue-brief/claims-denials-and-appeals-in-aca-marketplace-plans/>; 2022.
17. Shrank WH, Rogstad TL, Parekh N. Waste in the US health care system: estimated costs and potential for savings. JAMA. 2019;322:1501–1509.
18. Interim Final Rules Under the Paul Wellstone and Pete Domenici Mental Health Parity and Addiction Equity Act of 2008; Final Rule. 26 CFR54.9812 (c)(4)(i); 29 CFR 2590.712(c)(4)(i); 45 CFR 146.135(c)(4)(i).
19. Weiner DB. Philippe Pinel's "Memoir on Madness" of December 11, 1794: a fundamental text of modern psychiatry. Am J Psychiatry. 1992;149:725–732.
20. Moral treatment in America's lunatic asylums. Hosp Comm Psychiatry. 1976;27:468–470.
21. Wilson DC. Stranger and Traveler. Little, Brown; 1975.
22. Dix LD. Crusader on behalf of the mentally ill. Hosp Comm Psychiatry. 1976;27:471–472.
23. Asylum: a late 19th century view. Hosp Comm Psychiatry. 1976;27:485–489.
24. Phrenology comes to America. Hosp Comm Psychiatry. 1976;27:484.
25. Braslow J. Mental Ills and Body Cures: Psychiatric Treatment in the First Half of the Twentieth Century. University of California Press; 1997.
26. Duffy JD. General paralysis of the insane: neuropsychiatry's first challenge. J Neuropsychiatry. 1995;7:243–249.
27. Austin SC, Stolley PD, Lasky T. The history of malariotherapy for neurosyphilis. Modern parallels. JAMA. 1992;268:516–519.
28. Beers CW. A Mind That Found Itself. 4th ed. Plimpton Press; 1917.
29. Beers C. A man for a cause. Hosp Comm Psychiatry. 1976;27:493–494.
30. Meyer A. Studying the whole of man. Hosp Comm Psychiatry. 1976;27:492–493.
31. Housman W, Rioch DK. Military psychiatry: a prototype of social and preventive psychiatry in the United States. Arch Gen Psychiatry. 1967;16:727–739.

32. Gaffney A. The neoliberal turn in American health care. *Int J Health Serv.* 2015;45:33–52.

33. The introduction of chlorpromazine. *Hosp Comm Psychiatry.* 1976;27(7):505.

34. Passamanick B, Scarpitti FR, Dinitz S. *Schizophrenics in the Community.* Appleton-Century-Crofts; 1967.

35. Deutsch A. *The Shame of the States.* Harcourt Brace; 1948.

36. Ward MJ. *The Snake Pit.* Random House; 1946.

37. Joint Commission on Mental Health and Mental Illness. *Action for Mental Health.* Basic Books; 1961.

38. Leighton DC, Harding JS, Macklin DB, et al. Psychiatric findings of the Sterling County Study. *Am J Psychiatry.* 1963;119:1021–1026.

39. Strole L, Langner TS, Michael ST, et al. Mental health in the metropolis: the Midtown Manhattan Study. In: Rennie TAC, ed. *Series in Social Psychiatry,* vol. 1. McGraw-Hill; 1962.

40. Hollingshead AB, Redlich FC. *Social Class and Mental Illness.* John Wiley; 1958.

41. Kennedy JF. Message from the president of the United States relative to mental illness and mental retardation to the 86th Congress. Document No. 58. Washington, DC; 1963.

42. Public Law 94-63: Community Mental Health Centers Amendments of 1975.

43. Sharfstein SS, Wolfe JC. The community mental health centers program: expectations and realities. *Hosp Comm Psychiatry.* 1978;29:46–49.

44. Regier DA, Narrow WE, Rae DS, et al. The de facto US mental and addictive disorders system. *Arch Gen Psychiatry.* 1993;50:85–94.

45. Kessler RC, McGonagle KA, Nelson CB, et al. Lifetime and 12-month prevalence of DSM-III-R psychiatric disorders in the United States. *Arch Gen Psychiatry.* 1994;51:8–19.

46. Kessler RC, Berglund P, Demler O, et al. The epidemiology of major depressive disorder: results from the National Comorbidity Survey Replication (NCS-R). *JAMA.* 2003;289:3095–3105.

47. Nickels MW, McIntyre JS. A model for psychiatric services in primary care settings. *Psychiatr Serv.* 1996;47:522–526.

48. Kates N, Craven MA, Crustolo A, et al. Sharing care: the psychiatrist in the family physician's office. *Can J Psychiatry.* 1997;42:960–965.

49. Katon W, Von Korff M, Lin E, et al. Stepped collaborative care for primary care patients with persistent symptoms of depression. *Arch Gen Psychiatry.* 1999;56:1109–1115.

50. Pirl WF, Beck BJ, Safren SA, et al. A descriptive study of psychiatric consultations in a community primary care center. *Primary Care Companion J Clin Psychiatry.* 2001;3:190–194.

51. Oxman T, Dietrich AJ, Williams JW, et al. A three-component model for reengineering systems for the treatment of depression in primary care. *Psychosomatics.* 2002;43:441–450.

52. Unutzer J, Katon W, Callahan CM, et al. Collaborative care management of late-life depression in the primary care setting, a randomized controlled trial. *JAMA.* 2002;288:2836–2845.

53. Wagner E, Ortaliza J, Cox C, Peterson KFF. *How Does Health Spending in the US Compare to Other Countries?* <https://www.healthsystemtracker.org/chart-collection/health-spending-u-s-compare-countries-2/#Average%20annual%20growth%20rate%20in%20health%20consumption%20expenditures%20per%20capita%202000%20through%202020,%20U.S.%20dollars,%20PPP%20adjusted%C2%A0>; 2022.

54. Schneider EC, Shah A, Doty MM, et al. Mirror, mirror, 2021. In: *Reflecting Poorly: Health Care in the U.S. Compared to Other High-income Countries.* The Commonwealth Fund; 2021.

55. Brody DS, Brody P. Managed care and physician burnout. *AMA J Ethics.* 2003:371–375.

56. Snibbe JR, Radcliffe T, Weisberger C, et al. Burnout among primary care physicians and mental health professionals in a managed health care setting. *Psychol Rep.* 1989;65:775–780.

57. Acker GM. The challenges in providing services to clients with mental illness: managed care, burnout and somatic symptoms among social workers. *Community Ment Health J.* 2010;46:591–600.

58. Zwanziger J, Khan N. Safety-net activities and hospital contracting with managed care organizations. *Med Care Res Rev.* 2006;63:90S–111S.

59. Horton S. The double burden on safety net providers: placing health disparities in the context of the privatization of health care in the US. *Soc Sci Med.* 2006;63:2702–2714.

60. Maskovsky J. "Managing" the poor: neoliberalism, Medicaid HMOs and the triumph of consumerism among the poor. *Med Anthropol.* 2000;19:121–146.

61. Arana JD, Hastings B, Herron E. Continuous care teams in intensive outpatient treatment of chronically mentally ill patients. *Hosp Comm Psychiatry.* 1991;42:503–507.

62. Teague GB, Drake RE, Ackerson TH. Evaluating the use of continuous treatment teams for persons with mental illness and substance abuse. *Psychiatr Serv.* 1995;46:689–695.

63. Dincin J, Wasmer D, Witheridge TF, et al. Impact of assertive community treatment in the use of state hospital inpatient bed-days. *Hosp Comm Psychiatry.* 1993;44:833–838.

64. McGrew JH, Bond CR, Dietzen L, et al. A multisite study of client outcomes in assertive community treatment. *Psychiatr Serv.* 1995;46:696–701.

65. Morgan L. Health homes vs. medical homes: big similarities and important differences. *OPEN MINDS Management Newsletter* <http://www.openminds.com/market-intelligence/premium/2012/040112/040112f.htm?>; April 2012.

66. Neuman P, Lyons B, Rentas J, et al. Dx for a careful approach to moving dual-eligible beneficiaries into managed care plans. *Health Aff.* 2012;31:1186–1194.

67. Nesbitt TS, Katz-Bell J. History of telehealth. In: Rheuban KS, Krupinski EA eds. Understanding Telehealth. New York: McGraw-Hill Education. Accessed 16.05.24.

68. Steinke H, Stuber M. Medical correspondence in early modern Europe. An introduction. *Gesnerus.* 2004;61:139–160.

69. Wittson CL, Benschoter R. Two-way television: helping the medical center reach out. *Am J Psychiatry.* 1972;129:624–627.

70. Freiburger G, Holcomb M, Piper D. The STARPAHC collection: part of an archive of the history of telemedicine. *J Telemed Telecare.* 2007;13:221–223.

71. Mahar JH, Rosencrance JG, Rasmussen PA. Telemedicine: past, present, and future. *Cleve Clin J Med.* 2018;85:938–942.

72. Kichloo A, Albosta M, Dettloff K, et al. Telemedicine, the current COVID-19 pandemic and the future: a narrative review and

perspectives moving forward in the USA. *Fam Med Community Health*. 2020;8(2).e0005. https://doi.org/10.1136/fmch-2020-00053.

73. Nord G, Rising KL, Band RA, et al. On-demand synchronous audio video telemedicine visits are cost effective. *Am J Emerg Med*. 2019;37:890–894.

74. Spaulding R, Belz N, Delurgio S, et al. Cost savings of telemedicine utilization for child psychiatry in a rural Kansas community. *Telemed J E Health*. 2010;16:867–871.

75. McConnochie KM, Wood NE, Kitzman HJ, et al. Telemedicine reduces absence resulting from illness in urban child care: evaluation of an innovation. *Pediatrics*. 2005;115:1273–1282.

76. Sharp IR, Kobak KA, Osman DA. The use of videoconferencing with patients with psychosis: a review of the literature. *Ann Gen Psychiatry*. 2011;10:14.

77. Bulkes NZ, Davis K, Kay B, et al. Comparing efficacy of telehealth to in-person mental health care in intensive-treatment-seeking adults. *J Psychiatr Res*. 2022;145:347–352.

78. Hom MA, Weiss RB, Millman ZB, et al. Development of a virtual partial hospital program for an acute psychiatric population: Lessons learned and future directions for telepsychotherapy. *J Psychother Integr*. 2020;30:366–382.

79. Zimmerman M, Ward M, D'Avanzato C, et al. Telehealth treatment of patients with borderline personality disorder in a partial hospital setting during the COVID-19 pandemic:

80. Baweja R, Verma S, Pathak M, et al. Development of a child and adolescent tele-partial hospitalization program (tele-PHP) in response to the COVID-19 pandemic. *Prim Care Companion CNS Disord*. 2020;22 (5):20m02743.

81. Barney A, Mendez-Contreras S, Hills N, et al. Telemedicine in an adolescent and young adult medicine clinic: a mixed methods study. *BMC Health Serv Res*. 2022;23(1):680.

82. Cerretier E, Bastide M, Lachal J, et al. Evaluation of the rapid implementation of telehealth during the COVID-19 pandemic: a qualitative study among adolescents and their parents. *Eur Child Adolesc Psychiatry*. 2022:1–11.

83. Federal Communications Commission. Fourteenth Broadband Deployment Report. Inquiry Concerning Deployment of Advanced Telecommunications Capability to All Americans in a Reasonable and Timely Fashion. 2021.

84. Katzow MW, Steinway C, Jan S. Telemedicine and health disparities during COVID-19. *Pediatrics*. 2020;146(2):e20201586. https://doi.org/10.1542/peds.2020-1586.

85. Sasangohar F, Bradshaw MR, Carlson MM, et al. Adapting an outpatient psychiatric clinic to telehealth during the COVID-19 pandemic: a practice perspective. *J Med Internet Res*. 2020; 22:e22523.

comparative safety, patient satisfaction, and effectiveness of in-person treatment. *J Pers Disord*. 2022;36:277–295.

51

GLOBAL PSYCHIATRY AND MENTAL HEALTHCARE DELIVERY

GIUSEPPE J. RAVIOLA, MD, MPH ■ MARIA C. PROM, MD ■
RAHEL BOSSON, MD ■ ZEINA CHEMALI, MD, MPH ■
NKECHI T. CONTEH, MBBS, MPH ■ BIZU GELAYE, PHD, MPH ■
GREGORY L. FRICCHIONE, MD

OVERVIEW

This chapter describes the evolving field of global psychiatry and mental healthcare delivery in the context of global health, global mental health, and public health in the United States for clinicians. Neuropsychiatric disorders, both common and severe, account for approximately 16% of the global burden of disease, with the burden doubling in the quarter century before coronavirus disease 2019 (COVID-19) and compounded by the pandemic; yet, health resources devoted to mental health around the globe have remained disproportionately small, with innovative approaches to care informed by the field of global mental health now a significant area of social innovation. From a health system–strengthening perspective, global psychiatry can contribute to global health, global mental health, and the field of psychiatry by ensuring that attention is paid to complexity, co-morbidities, and quality of care as part of "task-shared," comprehensive, collaborative, community-based efforts. Psychiatrists can serve as leaders in clinical care delivery, training, education, research, and advocacy to address the urgent need to expand access to mental health care and to integrate mental health into primary care, systems and communities. This includes utilizing clinical approaches as well as expanding engagement in supporting prevention and promotion through efforts to integrate mental health care outside of the health sector in every country, while being mindful of local contexts. Values grounded in diversity, equity, inclusion, de-coloniality, and confronting social determinants of health directly help to ensure that providers working in the post-pandemic

period can better recognize, affirm, and respond to the specific needs of socially, culturally, and medically under-resourced groups, practicing structural competency and humility. These values apply to "local" contexts in the United States as well as "global" environments, and are important in contextualizing the integration and adaptation of mental health interventions to enhance resilience of communities in anticipation of future health and humanitarian crises. Global psychiatry requires an inter-disciplinary approach that integrates broad clinical excellence, knowledge of specific core topic areas in global mental health, engagement with concerns relating to health equity and social justice leadership, adaptability to working in complex and unfamiliar environments with people who may be marginalized or less advantaged in their community or society, and appreciation of the value of local conceptualizations of illness and healing as well as the limitations of biomedical approaches.

In this chapter, the terms "developing" or "third world" are not used to describe countries, and the terms "low-, middle-, and high-income countries" are used with reservation because the terms convey a homogeneity of experience that does not often reflect local realities.[1] A domestic community or "global-local" paradigm serves as a subtext to the contents of this chapter, with an emphasis on the opportunity to learn bidirectionally (i.e., global work can inform domestic community work, and domestic community work can inform global work).[2] The benefits of this perspective are numerous and include enhancing the opportunity to improve culturally humble, proficient, and safe care across contexts.[2] Specifically, this chapter aims to provide a foundational introduction to the field of global psychiatry for clinicians.

GLOBAL PSYCHIATRY FROM A CLINICAL AND PUBLIC HEALTH PERSPECTIVE

The Global Burden of Illness and the Mental Health Services Gap

The World Health Organization (WHO) has described mental health as "a state of well-being in which every individual realizes [their] own potential, can cope with the normal stresses of life, can work productively and fruitfully, and is able to make a contribution to [their] community."[3] Mental disorders currently represent the greatest collective cause of disability worldwide. Despite the global burden of illness attributed to mental disorders being approximately 16% of total disability-adjusted life years (DALYs), governments globally have under-funded new mental health services; roughly 2% of governmental budgets globally are allocated for mental health spending.[4,5] *Service gaps* refer to poor treatment coverage as well as to a limited range and quality of services, particularly in low- and middle-income countries (LMICs); for example, 71% of people with psychosis do not receive mental health services.[6] The WHO's 2020 Mental Health Atlas, which included data from 171 countries, highlighted the ongoing need for investments in mental health care that strengthen health systems and the capacity to deliver formal mental health services, as well as investments for the prevention of illness and promotion of care early in life. This is reinforced by our understanding that 50% of mental disorders are noted by the age of 14 years, and 75% are evident by the age of 24 years (Fig. 51.1).[7,8]

Global Healthcare Delivery and the Practice of Psychiatry

Global health prioritizes improving health and achieving health equity for people around the globe.[9] Over the past three decades, *global mental health* has focused on reducing mental health disparities between and within nations, and seeking innovative community-based, systemic solutions to increase access to care.[10] Since the conceptualization of the *disability-adjusted life year lived with disability* (DALY) and *years lived with disability* (YLD) measures in 1990, mental disorders have been identified as the leading causes of the global health-related burden. From 1990 to 2019, the burden of disease secondary to mental disorders worldwide increased significantly.[11] A field of global mental health has applied new scientific knowledge

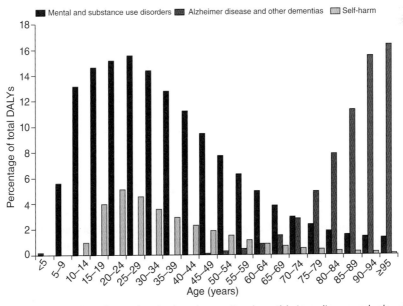

Fig. 51.1 ◼ The global burden of mental and substance use disorders, Alzheimer disease and other dementias, and suicide (self-harm) in disability-adjusted life years (DALYs) across the life span (Patel et al., 2018).[7]

regarding the global burden of illness to advocate for a world in which mental health services are valued, funded, implemented, and sustained equally to other major concerns in global health and development. Work in the field has been represented by four major discourses: (1) as research supporting evidence-based practices and implementation science that addresses the burden of illness and requires a globally led response that engages local stakeholders and informs practice and policy, (2) as implementation of services that de-emphasize institutional approaches to treatment and move toward community-based care, (3) as engagement of policies from a human rights perspective to prioritize and protect individuals living with *serious mental illness* (SMI), and (4) as advancement of global research and educational partnerships from LMICs as opportunities for creativity, innovation, and greater health equity, so as not to perpetuate or reinforce colonial practices.[6] Over the past decade the field has moved increasingly toward integrating mental health into the Sustainable Development Goals (SDGs) and paying increased attention to the *social determinants* of mental disorders.[12]

Global health delivery describes the practice of implementing interventions to improve healthcare delivery in low-resource settings, with attention to epidemiology, pathophysiology, culture, economics, politics, and social determinants as well as clinical care.[13,14] By extension, *global mental health delivery* refers to the implementation of effective, evidence-based, timely, accessible, and affordable mental health care in settings with limited formal mental health services, with attention paid to clinical and social dimensions, and consistent with the practices of global health delivery. With climate change and COVID-19 has come a growing emphasis on responses to humanitarian crises in the context of conflict and displacement. Over the past decade the field of global health has integrated the concepts of Mental Health and Psychosocial Support (MHPSS), which refers to any type of local or outside support that seeks to protect or promote psychosocial well-being and to prevent or treat mental disorders, particularly in the context of emergency responses.[15]

Psychiatry, as a branch of medicine, has focused on the diagnosis, treatment, and prevention of mental, emotional, and behavioral disorders. The field also plays an important role in global mental health and in

contributing to addressing the growing burden of mental disorders in locations with few formal services, or where access to services is poor.[16] This includes care in high-income countries (HICs), where significant disparities exist and where access to care is challenging. Psychiatrists have an essential role to play as leaders and clinical experts supporting the integration of *task-sharing* of psychosocial, psychological, and psychiatric interventions in collaboration with existing primary care resources, leveraging their experience and expertise in supervising, training, and mentoring general health workers and community providers, as well as improving care environments and advocating for action in other environments, such as homes, schools, and workplaces.[16] Psychiatrists treat patients with patients with complex mental health conditions, bringing their knowledge of medicine, neuroscience, psychiatric, psychological, and social approaches to those who live with myriad mental disorders. Psychiatric disorders are heterogeneous, often highly co-morbid, and require expertise to prioritize and address them sequentially and comprehensively. Psychiatrists have a unique perspective on patients, services, and systems; moreover, they often work in settings where support systems for people who live with mental disorders are inadequate. Although psychiatrists across global contexts often manage urgent clinical concerns, they also address mental health and illness from a *public health* perspective, attending to the social determinants of mental disorders.

Psychiatrists are therefore well-positioned to work as leaders in clinical care delivery, training, education, research, and advocacy to address and expand access to mental health care across all contexts and aspiring to a "global" scope of practice. Beyond the provision of care that draws from diverse clinical expertise (e.g., in emergency psychiatry, consultation-liaison psychiatry, inpatient care, adult community psychiatry, child and adolescent psychiatry, geriatric psychiatry, perinatal psychiatry, addiction psychiatry, human immunodeficiency virus [HIV] psychiatry, disaster psychiatry, psychotherapy), global psychiatrists benefit from knowledge of social and structural determinants of mental health, cultural aspects of mental health, health systems, humanitarian and psychosocial response to crises, resource allocation of mental health services, health equity, ethical practices of global health, history of psychiatry, quality improvement, and research in global mental health.[17] This includes using clinical approaches and expanding engagement to support prevention and promotion efforts inside and outside of the health sector. It also builds on the concepts of *structural competency and humility*, both in psychiatry and in global health, while integrating values of diversity, equity, inclusion, and de-coloniality; describing the functions and impacts of social structures in maintaining inequities; and recognizing structural interventions for addressing them.[18,19] The terms structural competency and humility refer to the capacity of health care professionals to "understand knowledge and practice gaps vis-à-vis structures, partner with other stakeholders to fill these gaps, and engage in self-reflection throughout the process."[20]

Non-Communicable Diseases, Neuropsychiatry, and Brain Health

Neuropsychiatric and non-communicable diseases (NCDs) are the leading causes of mortality and morbidity, and the largest contributors to DALYs worldwide. Over the past three decades, these numbers have continued to rise. Increasing life expectancies, sedentary lifestyles, unhealthy diets, cigarette smoking, and the harmful use of alcohol and other drugs have contributed to the growing incidence of NCDs. In LMICs, this rise has been especially problematic. With increasing population sizes, stalling economies, and stifled care delivery, many countries have been unable to keep pace with the rising need for neuropsychiatric care. Furthermore, in countries with more resource-constrained health systems, resources for brain care are extremely limited, making primary and secondary prevention critical to reducing the disease burden. Even with the best of intentions, countries lack the human resources and educational infrastructure to create change. Given the large gaps in education and services, there is a dire need to scale up capacity building and population-level interventions to address NCDs, educate healthcare workers, combat stigma, and improve access to appropriate treatment. Brain health is essential for general health; therefore, physicians require training to become brain specialists. This will reap major economic and educational benefits associated with improved mental health for all.

Integration of Categorical and Dimensional Approaches to Care and Support

While the United States has 52,000 psychiatrists and 8000 child psychiatrists, access to psychiatrists in the United States remains a significant challenge. Mental health service delivery in HICs stands to benefit from the lessons drawn from the delivery of community-based mental health services in lower-resource settings. In most global locales, psychiatrists are scarce. The global average is 3.96 psychiatrists per 100,000 population (1 in 27,000), a figure that is inadequate in all settings, particularly given the general lack of community-based services (Table 51.1).[21]

Even in HICs with many psychiatrists, a substantial proportion of their population lacks access to mental health care because of in-country health inequities. The lack of equitable access and availability to mental health care represents a failure of care delivery systems as well as inadequate human resources.

Psychiatrists can work collaboratively as part of a broader continuum of service providers and services across a range of allied mental health and non-specialist professions.[16] Depending on the context, services may be organized differently; however, the aim of *decentralization*—the elaboration of services increasingly from psychiatric facilities and institutions to general hospitals to health centers in urban and rural areas to community-based supports—represents an ongoing, shared global aspiration.[22] In addition to a need for more human resources for mental health, *quality of care* globally remains an additional concern. According to the WHO, "Quality encompasses the achievement of equitable care that is evidence-based and is cost-effective. To achieve optimal quality, the systems for delivering mental health care must be conducive to treatment and recovery. This requires the alignment of policy and commitment of key partners, alignment of funding, accreditation procedures for services, development and application of service standards, and ongoing routine quality improvement."[23]

Advancing a public health approach to mental health in concert with the clinical approach will require psychiatrists to accept and endorse current consensus regarding an ideal integration of both dimensional (emphasizing public health-oriented prevention, promotion and recovery) and categorical (emphasizing clinical diagnosis

TABLE 51.1
Numbers of Psychiatrists per 100,000 Population

Country	Number of Psychiatrists (Approximate)	Psychiatrists per 100,000 Population (2015–16 Estimate)
Norway	1050	48
New Zealand	550	28.5
Finland	1800	23.6
Argentina	4500	21.7
France	15,500	20.9
United Kingdom	12,700	19
Canada	4800	14.7
Australia	3500	13.5
Germany	18,200	13.2
Japan	13,000	11.9
United States	52,000	10.5
Ukraine	3500	10
Russian Federation	12,000	8.5
Italy	10,000	6.0
Mexico	5000	3.4
Brazil	6000	3.2
Peru	600	2.9
China	40,000	2.2
Colombia	900	1.8
Egypt	1000	1.6
United Arab Emirates	400	1.6
South Africa	700	1.5
Saudi Arabia	700	1.3
Lebanon	60	1.2
Cambodia	60	0.4
Myanmar	89	0.4
Syrian Arab Republic	80	0.4
Iraq	100	0.3
Indonesia	1000	0.3
India	9000	0.3
Afghanistan	60	0.2
Kenya	100	0.2
Nigeria	250	0.2
Bangladesh	260	0.16
Ghana	39	0.1
Yemen	46	0.1
Rwanda	13	0.1
Lesotho	1	0.04
Sierra Leone	3	0.03
Somalia	3	0.03
Ethiopia	85	0.08
Zimbabwe	15	0.01

Developed with information from the World Health Organization: https://www.who.int/data/gho/data/indicators/indicator-details/GHO/psychiatrists-working-in-mental-health-sector-(per-100-000) and treatment) approaches to mental health, on a continuum from well-being to distress, to the development of a disorder, to longer-term disability (Fig. 51.2). The dimensional approach integrates the concept of *well-being*—the subjective evaluation of life satisfaction.

Taken together, these perspectives invite psychiatrists to work at multiple levels, improving the quantity and quality of specialist services and engaging in broader-scale efforts to increase the use of community-based approaches that support prevention and promotion, as well as supporting recovery. As it has related to the practice of psychiatry, the WHO has encouraged a mix of community mental health services, including general hospital services, clinical care and support, psychosocial rehabilitation, and residential services, to extend care and support to people's homes and public spaces (Fig. 51.3).[6]

For the past two decades, the WHO has recommended a range of components of *formal and informal community mental health services* that can be built in communities and outside of facilities (Box 51.1).[22] In essence this means integrating the categorical and dimensional approaches to care and support.

The United Nations Special Rapporteur on the right to health has expressed concern about the dominance of the biomedical paradigm, power asymmetries that impact all levels of decision-making in mental health policies and services (including the exclusion of service users in the design, implementation, and delivery and evaluation of mental health services, systems and policies), and the biased use of evidence in mental health, particularly regarding the use of psychotropics.[24] This highlights the ongoing need to protect the

dignity and human rights of those with lived experience of mental disorders, to expand community efforts and de-emphasize institutional approaches.

Efforts to engage, include, and empower people with lived experience are informing this movement toward systems reform. *Stigma*, the prejudice and discrimination directed toward people living with mental disorders, continues to impact access to care and the outcomes of care.[25] The WHO QualityRights initiative was designed to improve the quality of care in mental health and related services and to promote the rights of people with psychosocial, intellectual, and cognitive disabilities.[26] *Psychosocial disability* refers to impairments related to mental disorders, with an interaction between these impairments and societal barriers combining to limit the ability to participate fully in social and community life. *Psychosocial rehabilitation* promotes personal recovery, gaining and retaining hope, successful community integration, and a satisfactory quality of life for persons who have a mental illness or a mental health and/or substance use concern.[27] The United Nations Convention on the Rights of Persons with Disabilities, adopted in 2006, is an international human rights treaty that serves as a cornerstone for the contemporary disability movement.[28] A more recent movement to integrate concepts of *neurodiversity* and *neurodivergence* for describing challenges of human cognition (such as autism, attention-deficit hyperactivity disorder, and dyslexia), represents an ongoing evolution toward greater de-medicalization, greater inclusion in society outside of health systems,

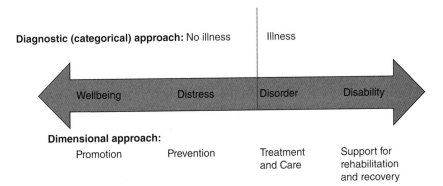

Fig. 51.2 ■ Global approaches to developing collaborative, comprehensive, community-based mental health services seek to integrate diagnostic (categorical, and clinical) and dimensional approaches, within and outside of health systems.

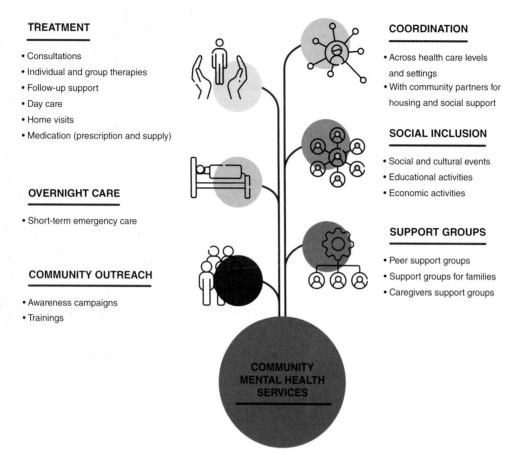

TREATMENT

- Consultations
- Individual and group therapies
- Follow-up support
- Day care
- Home visits
- Medication (prescription and supply)

OVERNIGHT CARE

- Short-term emergency care

COMMUNITY OUTREACH

- Awareness campaigns
- Trainings

COORDINATION

- Across health care levels and settings
- With community partners for housing and social support

SOCIAL INCLUSION

- Social and cultural events
- Educational activities
- Economic activities

SUPPORT GROUPS

- Peer support groups
- Support groups for families
- Caregivers support groups

COMMUNITY MENTAL HEALTH SERVICES

Fig. 51.3 ■ Guidance on community mental health services from the 2022 WHO World Mental Health Report.

BOX 51.1
COMPONENTS OF MENTAL HEALTH SERVICES

THE MENTAL HEALTH SYSTEM
- Mental hospital institutional services
  - Specialist institutional mental health services
  - Dedicated mental hospitals
- Mental health services in primary care
  - Mental health services in general hospitals
  - Mental health services in primary health care
- Community-based mental health services
  - Formal community mental health services
  - Informal community mental health services

EXAMPLES OF FORMAL COMMUNITY MENTAL HEALTH SERVICES
- Rehabilitation services
  - Community mental health centers and outpatient clinics

- Clubhouses
- Day care centers
- Drop-in centers
- Support groups
- Employment and rehabilitation workshops
- Sheltered workshops
- Supervised work placements
- Cooperative work schemes
- Supported employment programs
- Hospital diversion programs and mobile crisis teams
  - Mobile services for crisis assessment and treatment operating from community mental health centers or outpatient clinics
- Crisis services
  - Ordinary houses in neighborhood settings with 24-hour care given by mental health professionals

> ## BOX 51.1
> ## COMPONENTS OF MENTAL HEALTH SERVICES—CONT'D
>
> - ■ Support staff with mental health training and knowledge who can stay in a patient's own home overnight to provide support and supervision during a period of crisis
> - ■ Crisis centers
> - ■ Therapeutic and supervised residential services
>   - ■ Apartment buildings for persons in recovery (unsupervised)
>   - ■ Scattered apartments each occupied by two or three residents (unsupervised)
>   - ■ Group homes (staffed and unstaffed)
>   - ■ Hostels
>   - ■ Halfway houses
>   - ■ Psychiatric agricultural rehabilitation villages
>   - ■ Ordinary housing
> - ■ Home health services
>   - ■ Assessment, treatment, and management coordinated by a home care clinician from a community mental health center
>   - ■ Case management and assertive community treatment
>   - ■ Domiciliary (home-based) support centers
>
> - ■ Others
>   - ■ Clinical services in educational, employment, and correctional settings
>   - ■ Telephone hotline services
>   - ■ Trauma relief programs in refugee camps and community settings
>   - ■ Digital services
>
> **EXAMPLES OF INFORMAL COMMUNITY MENTAL HEALTH SERVICES**
>
> - ■ Traditional healers
> - ■ Village or community health workers
> - ■ Family members
> - ■ Self-help and user groups
> - ■ Advocacy services
> - ■ Lay volunteers providing parental and youth education on mental health issues and screening for mental disorders (including suicidal tendencies) in clinics and schools
> - ■ Religious leaders providing health information on trauma reactions in complex emergencies or retired members of local communities
> - ■ Humanitarian workers in complex emergencies
>
> Adapted from World Health Organization. *Organization of Services for Mental Health. Mental Health Policy and Service Guidance Package.* WHO; 2003.[22]

and a stronger focus on strength-based attitudes and approaches to care and support that is increasingly oriented toward equity.[29]

ACTIONS TO MEET THE GLOBAL HEALTH CHALLENGES OF THE FUTURE

Support and Capacity Building of Clinical Programs to Care for the Mentally Ill

Through Strengthening of Bi-directional Training and Collaboration in Education

Addressing the significant global burden of mental illness and inequities in mental healthcare access requires the sustainable development of local systems and services.[5] *Capacity building* is at the core of sustainable mental healthcare program development and scaling of care, research, and policy, especially as it relates to strengthening human resources.[30] This cannot be accomplished without a focus on training and education in many contexts, across a range of content areas.

In global health education, there is new momentum to teach de-coloniality and to promote practices of deep self-reflection and examination of existing structures of oppression and empowerment.[31] In psychiatry, an increased focus on social determinants of mental health has led to initiatives that seek to prepare trainees to understand and work at the systems levels to eliminate the structural causes of illness in their clinical training by increasing their understanding of patients' experiences of illness in the context of structural factors (e.g., unstable housing and violent neighborhoods leading to anxiety and trauma-related disorders); intervening to address structural factors at institutional levels (e.g., to work with community groups to promote recovery, to collaborate with schools and law enforcement to divert symptomatic people from arrest to clinical care, or to testify to city and state legislatures on the association between housing availability and mental health); and, developing community connectivity and *structural humility*, a posture of collaboration with community leaders and with other disciplines, and patience with the slow pace of structural change.[32] These efforts represent a new emphasis on transforming education in global health, global mental health, and psychiatry, to be more attentive to human rights, equitable partnerships, strengthening of existing structures and supports in communities, greater inclusiveness and use of person-centered approaches in the care of patients, and improvements in professional opportunities for over-burdened, under-paid front-line providers working in low-resource settings. Workforce diversity, structural inclusion, and investment in faculty from under-represented populations, and development of new curricula focused on *mental health equity*, in global psychiatry and global mental health are all necessary institutional commitments for the future.[33] These efforts by extension will support the development of *anti-racist* practitioners of psychiatry who will understand their own cultural identities; respect all cultures; seek out each patient's cultural identification; create culturally comfortable environments; conduct culturally sensitive evaluations; elicit patient and family expectations, preferences, and prior attempts to get help; adapt treatment techniques to the cultural values of the patient; understand broader societal influences on cultural groups; and advocate for institutional policies and practices of cultural humility, proficiency, and safety.[34]

This serves as a foundation for global mental health training in both LMICs and HICs, which should be approached jointly with an emphasis placed on bi-directional training, multi-specialty training, collaboration, and resource sharing between high-resource and under-resourced settings.[35] Training should encompass multiple areas essential to mental healthcare system development, including service delivery, quality improvement, research methods (qualitative and quantitative), policy development, advocacy, and leadership. Thoughtful bi-directional mental health training must also be critical of itself and build on a foundation of sociocultural humility and de-colonization.[36] It is essential to include training that is focused on nurses, midwives, healthcare workers, social workers, and rehabilitation specialists because they are in direct contact with the community and may be the first groups to be involved in patient care given the scarcity of physicians.

Addressing human resource inequities in under-resourced settings requires the training of mental health professionals who can lead program development and the sustainable training and ongoing supervision of non-mental health professionals.[35] As such, they can support innovative strategies for addressing mental healthcare access gaps, such as task sharing, integrating mental health care, and engaging in innovative digital

mental health initiatives. HIC psychiatry training programs can themselves benefit from incorporating global mental health concepts (such as global health disparities, humanitarian response, and sociocultural competency) into general curricular development. They can develop global training pathways that incorporate both local and international training and global partnerships, collaboration, and capacity building.[37,38] Academic institutions can trans-nationally collaborate to support bi-directional global mental health training through the development of professional career trajectories within the field of global mental health, as well as building supportive international collaborations.[35] For this to happen, there should be government policies that facilitate obtaining visas for an international healthcare force to shadow and train in the United States, Europe, and Canada for several months while healthcare workers from these regions travel to LMICs to learn what is feasible within a certain context, and hone cultural and structural humility.

With this background, various trans-national collaborations have focused on capacity by building psychiatry residency training programs, as well as to mid-level workers' community health curricula in neurology and psychiatry in various LMIC contexts. Government ministries of health have at times lacked trained personnel capable of effectively designing, implementing, managing, and evaluating programs that target brain health care needs of under-resourced populations. Education programs have turned out to be major hubs for collaboration with local universities and for increasing the delivery of clinical services. These programs have been met with daily challenges from logistics to analytics. To add to the challenges, although health services are delivered by public, private, and non-governmental organizations, comprehensive databases providing an accurate view of health needs or emerging diseases in several global regions are lacking. The key initial step to fostering a successful capacity-building program is to outline brain health and training needs by government, academic, and clinical leaders in the country, followed by field studies to examine the mental and brain health challenges and existing capacity for care for the region, with engagement of key stakeholders. Strategic plans should always be developed in close partnership with regional and national counterparts. Drawing on past collaborations from neighboring countries is valuable when it comes to overcoming the myriad challenges faced by the launch and sustained continuation of educational programs.

Challenges and limitations are not only met at the educational and clinical levels. Rigorous research is lacking, and there is an urgent need for high-quality studies to delineate disease prevalence and the resources needed to tackle them. Ideally, planning should seek to progress simultaneously in education and clinical delivery of services, as well as populating the literature with strong research. More sustainable healthcare infrastructure, from hospitals and intensive care units to personnel and staff, as well as policies aimed at education, clinical training, preventative care, and research are critical to delivering successful in-country programs and reducing overall disease and health burden.

Increasing Access to and Quality of Mental Health Care Through Task Sharing, MHPSS Response in Crises, and Strengthening of Community-Based Care

Key strategies to increase access to, and the quality of, mental health care in global settings include integrating mental health into primary care, increasing clinical care capacity by training non-specialized health workers (task shifting), and using technological tools to expand mental health coverage.[39] A significant contribution of the field of global mental health has been the identification and scale-up of cost-effective evidence-supported interventions, particularly psychological and psychosocial ones, and task sharing of such intervention delivery approaches to mental health–trained non-specialist providers or lay health workers.[40] This is a practice adapted from decades of community-based global health initiatives for care of those with HIV infection and tuberculosis (TB), involving the training of non-specialist or lay health providers, with little or no prior formal training or a background in mental health care, to deliver mental health care.[41] These health supporters and providers without specialized training have been known by a variety of names in various contexts, including community health workers (CHWs), lay health workers, midwives, nurses, primary care providers, village health workers, lady health workers, health promotors," auxiliary health staff, complementary alternative health providers, natural helpers,

helpers, paraprofessionals, frontline health workers, teachers, religious and traditional healers, community members, and non-specialist providers.[42]

The most fundamental research finding of the field of global mental health has been that non-specialist or lay providers working in low-resource settings can effectively deliver psychosocial interventions and components of psychological interventions, along the dimensional continuum, primarily for mild-to-moderate symptoms of depression and anxiety. Significant research has evaluated interventions and systems to address the global mental health treatment gap around this kind of work, and to build momentum toward identifying cost-effective, evidence-supported practices and services that could be made more feasible and widely available to low-income countries. The WHO became an important implementation partner to this research, developing guidelines (such as the *Mental Health Gap Action Programme [mhGAP] Intervention Guide* on clinical best practices for generalist physicians who operate without specialists), and adapting research findings into intervention packages that could be widely disseminated.[43] Guidance has been offered by the WHO, other multi-lateral organizations, and various other players in the field, including research teams and non-governmental organizations, on how to implement such task-shared programs. Utilizing the principle of task sharing, there can be a temporal progression in the development of services (starting with task sharing of MHPSS response in locales in which there are few formal services, and where complex humanitarian crises demand emergency responses) to more formal organization of services, if there are resources and political will to build sustained services. This progression is represented by the IASC Guidelines, and the WHO Pyramid Framework/Optimal Mix of Services pyramid for the Mental Health and Addiction Workforce, which de-emphasize specialist care, and prioritize non-clinical services, self-care, and community support (Fig. 51.4).

Many of task-shared psychosocial interventions have been derived from manualized psychological treatments, such as interpersonal therapy and cognitive-behavioral therapy, with research efforts also focused on identifying common elements of these approaches that could be simplified for use in communities without formal mental health care, as well as

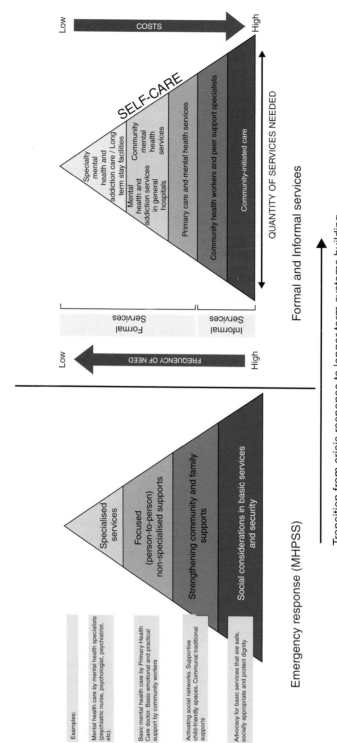

Fig. 51.4 ■ On the left is the Inter-Agency Standing Committee Intervention pyramid for mental health and psychosocial support (MHPSS). On the right is the WHO Pyramid Framework/Optimal Mix of Services pyramid for the Mental Health and Addiction Workforce. Both emphasize the development of programs and services at the bottom of each pyramid. [44,45]

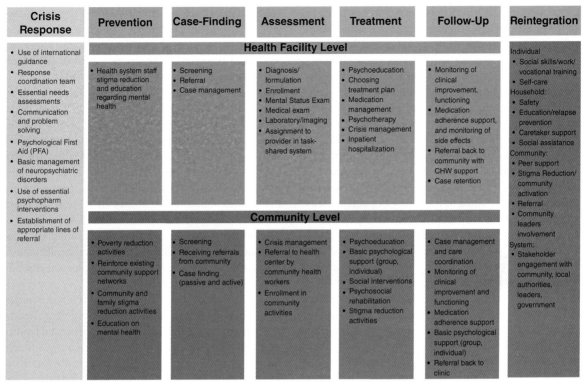

Crisis Response	Prevention	Case-Finding	Assessment	Treatment	Follow-Up	Reintegration
	Health Facility Level					Individual • Social skills/work/ vocational training • Self-care
• Use of international guidance • Response coordination team • Essential needs assessments • Communication and problem solving • Psychological First Aid (PFA) • Basic management of neuropsychiatric disorders • Use of essential psychopharm interventions • Establishment of appropriate lines of referral	• Health system staff stigma reduction and education regarding mental health	• Screening • Referral • Case management	• Diagnosis/ formulation • Enrollment • Mental Status Exam • Medical exam • Laboratory/imaging • Assignment to provider in task-shared system	• Psychoeducation • Choosing treatment plan • Medication management • Psychotherapy • Crisis management • Inpatient hospitalization	• Monitoring of clinical improvement, functioning • Medication adherence support, and monitoring of side effects • Referral back to community with CHW support • Case retention	Household: • Safety • Education/relapse prevention • Caretaker support • Social assistance Community: • Peer support • Stigma Reduction/ community activation • Referral • Community leaders involvement
	Community Level					System: • Stakeholder engagement with community, local authorities, leaders, government
	• Poverty reduction activities • Reinforce existing community support networks • Community and family stigma reduction activities • Education on mental health	• Screening • Receiving referrals from community • Case finding (passive and active)	• Crisis management • Referral to health center by community health workers • Enrollment in community activities	• Psychoeducation • Basic psychological support (group, individual) • Social interventions • Psychosocial rehabilitation • Stigma reduction activities	• Case management and care coordination • Monitoring of clinical improvement and functioning • Medication adherence support • Basic psychological support (group, individual) • Referral back to clinic	

Fig. 51.5 ■ A service delivery value chain that shows essential elements of care across non-specialist and specialist providers in a collaborative, comprehensive care delivery system linking communities to health centers in global mental health delivery. (Adapted from Mental Health Value Chain. *Partners In Health*. Available at: <https://www.pih.org/mental-health/pih-mental-health-value-chain>.[49])

the community components within which functional practices can be embedded.[42,46] In 2022, the WHO and UNICEF introduced the Ensuring Quality in Psychological Support (EQUIP) program to increase the quality of psychological support by improving the competence of helpers and the consistency and quality of training and service delivery.[47] The EQUIP platform makes freely available competency assessment tools and e-learning courses to support governments, training institutions, and non-governmental organizations, both in humanitarian and development settings, to train and supervise the workforce to deliver effective psychological support to adults and children.[47] It is important to note that most of the research and thus the implementation experience in using available tools, guidance, and intervention packages in global settings has been in the care and support of common mental disorders, with a greater emphasis and effort needed on meeting the needs of people with SMI through task sharing.[48]

Task sharing of psychosocial interventions to communities benefits greatly from the strengthening of primary care–delivered mental health services at health centers. Psychiatrists can work as part of local teams to elaborate comprehensive, community-based models, and systems of care delivery, adapting available international guidance within efforts led by local partners and teams. Implementation support tools foster the development of collaborative, comprehensive, health center- and community-linked mental health systems by providing roadmaps for front-line implementation teams. For example, the non-governmental organization International Medical Corps has developed a toolkit for the integration of mental health into general health care in humanitarian settings, and Partners In Health has developed a clinical care delivery value chain that describes the key system elements essential for the highest quality of care and value to patients that can be useful for service and program implementers (Fig. 51.5).[49,50] Practitioners of global mental health delivery can use tools such as these to apply their expertise, support local teams, and build and strengthen clinical capacities and health systems both in response to crises as well as for the long term.

During humanitarian crises, clinicians can support existing primary health care workers and provide clinical support, and they can support community members in strengthening community resources, applying principles from the *Inter-Agency Standing Committee (IASC) Guidelines* in context, and seeking an appropriate balance between clinical services and community-based supports. This means placing a strong emphasis on social considerations in basic services and security and strengthening community and family supports while providing clinical expertise. Efforts during crises can serve as a foundation for longer-term services through the task-sharing model. Psychiatrists can work in support of primary health care workers to address mental health in emergencies and contexts with minimal formal services and can apply several core skills, optimizing existing resources and deferring to local priorities (Box 51.2).[51,52]

Although each context is different, the skill sets of providers and their inter-relationships in an optimal continuum of care can be viewed as a framework for guiding front-line teams in implementing services based on various global experiences to date (Fig. 51.6). Principles underlying the development of collaborative, comprehensive, and community-based care in lower-resource settings include: evidence-based practice; a collaborative, stepped care approach at all stages of mental health; family-based care across the life cycle; integration of MHPSS into community-based services; the central role of primary health care providers; dedicated local mental health workers treating multiple and co-morbid conditions; support of people living with illness and families in clinical decision-making; engaging persons with lived experience as providers; providing workforce care, maintenance and development; addressing severe mental health conditions; and supporting those with intellectual disabilities and developmental disorders.[52]

The relevance of efforts to strengthen task-sharing in global public mental health has been amplified by the pandemic, the transition to remote mental healthcare delivery globally, and innovation in *digital mental health platforms*. Much attention and effort since the pandemic began has subsequently gone to seeking

---

BOX 51.2
ESSENTIAL SKILLS FOR PRIMARY HEALTHCARE WORKERS TO ADDRESS MENTAL HEALTH IN LOW-RESOURCE CONTEXTS

COMPETENCIES FOR PRIMARY HEALTHCARE WORKERS IN CRISIS RESPONSE
- Communication skills
- Basic problem-solving skills
- Refer to Inter-Agency Standing Committee Guidelines
- Psychological First Aid
- Use WHO mhGAP Intervention Guide and Humanitarian Intervention Guides
- Recognition and front-line management of mild, moderate, and severe neuropsychiatric disorders in adults and children including:
  - Acute and chronic psychosis
  - Epilepsy
  - Alcohol and substance misuse
  - Intellectual disability
  - Severe emotional disorders
  - Common mental disorders
- Simple cognitive-behavioral techniques, and interpersonal psychotherapy group or individual approaches

- Proper use of essential psychotropic medications to assist with autonomic hyperarousal and other immediate effects of exposure to stressful events
- Values of health equity, cultural humility, proficiency, and safety
- Trauma-informed care, spiritual care

MESSAGES DELIVERED BY PRIMARY HEALTHCARE WORKERS REGARDING CLINICAL CARE, WHEN INDICATED, FOR LONGER-TERM CARE (WITH THE SUPPORT OF PSYCHIATRISTS)
- Do no harm
- Protect individual autonomy and confidentiality while honoring collective culture and community norms
- Maintain therapeutic boundaries with the person, with attention to culture, class, and resource constraints
- Obtain a good history of the presenting problem (Use the ETHNICS mnemonic)
- Perform an adequate medical evaluation before a psychiatric diagnosis is made (ex: rule out delirium and other infectious or other medical illnesses)

BOX 51.2
ESSENTIAL SKILLS FOR PRIMARY HEALTHCARE WORKERS TO ADDRESS MENTAL HEALTH IN LOW-RESOURCE CONTEXTS—CONT'D

- Prioritize, where possible the least restrictive means for providing treatment
- Provide the person and family with clear information about diagnosis, recommended treatments, and treatment alternatives if they exist in context

MESSAGES DELIVERED BY PRIMARY HEALTHCARE WORKERS REGARDING TREATMENT, WHEN INDICATED, FOR LONGER-TERM CARE (WITH THE SUPPORT OF PSYCHIATRISTS)

- Both psychosocial and psychopharmacologic treatments can be effective, depending on the problem, using the medical approach; the medical approach is intended to be complementary to traditional and spiritual approaches
- Mild symptoms can often be treated with social or psychosocial interventions, or psychotherapy alone (collaborative, stepped care), as well as traditional and spiritual approaches
- Moderate and severe symptoms can be treated with a combination of psychosocial support, psychotherapy, and medication
- A family-based approach to mental health-related problems often can yield the greatest benefits
- Strength-based and preventive approaches delivered by peers can be highly effective, depending on the problem, whether illness is present and/or experienced by the person, and contextual realities (ex: limited health system resources)

COMPLIMENTARY FUNCTIONS OF EACH PROVIDER CADRE IN AN EVOLVING TASK-SHARED MODEL OF CARE THAT IS COLLABORATIVE, COMPREHENSIVE, AND COMMUNITY BASED

- Community psychosocial workers
  - Provide psychoeducation; teach basic coping
  - Provide social services and support
  - Refer to primary healthcare workers
  - Conduct community visits; foster social connectedness

- Primary healthcare workers
  - Assess individuals using mhGAP; manage common and severe disorders
  - Prescribe medications
  - Refer to community psychosocial workers and primary mental health counselors, depending on acuity
  - Receive back-referrals from hospital-based providers and specialized mental health services providers
- Primary mental health counselors
  - Provide psychotherapeutic interventions
  - Develop intervention plans that engage the family if appropriate
  - Act as case managers
  - Supervise community psychosocial workers
- Hospital-based providers (physicians and nurses in inpatient and outpatient secondary care facilities)
  - Diagnose and confirm mental and physical diagnoses
  - Make use of full-time inpatient acute monitoring that uses the least restrictive means
  - Provide pharmacology, psychological, and social support as needed
  - Manage discharge to the community
- Specialized mental health services providers (psychiatrists, psychologists, and psychiatric nurses affiliated with psychiatric hospitals or in private practice)
  - Receive referrals for the most complex clinical problems
  - Consult on care
  - Implement evidence-based strategies to improve care
  - Function in settings with extremely limited specialist services; provide remote support to local workers with attention to empathetic listening and communication, psychoeducation; be supportive, give hope, encourage basic problem solving; mobilize social support, grounding techniques, relaxation and breathing exercises, behavioral activation, and simple cognitive-behavioral or interpersonal techniques (delivered to individuals or to groups)

---

mhGAP, Mental health Gap Action Programme; WHO, World Health Organization.
Adapted from Jones L, Asare JB, El Masri M, et al. Severe mental disorders in complex emergencies. *Lancet.* 2009;374:654–661.[51]
Adapted from Bolton P, West J, Whitney C, et al. Expanding mental health services in low- and middle-income countries: a task-shifting framework for delivery of comprehensive, collaborative, community-based care. Global Mental Health. Accepted January 2023.[52]

new digital and technological avenues for the implementation of psychosocial interventions delivered by lay health workers and the potential applications of these practices to higher-income settings such as the United States, where, despite significantly greater human resources for mental health as compared to LMICs, ongoing significant barriers to effective care delivery remain that leave a significant percentage of the population without access to effective care. Across global settings, digital technologies can effectively support data collection, outcome tracking, health worker training, coordination of referrals, and improvement of communication among health workers and patients.[53]

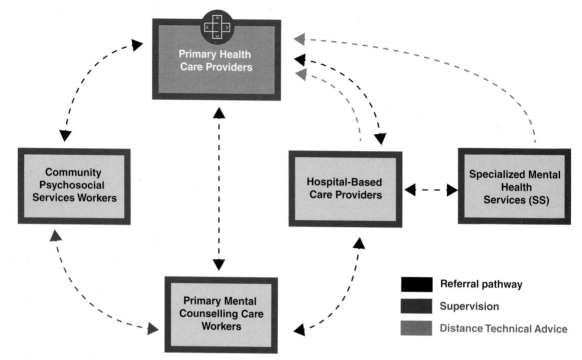

Fig. 51.6 ■ Complementary roles of five categories of workers delivering components of mental health care in a comprehensive, collaborative, community-based system. (Adapted from Bolton P, West J, Whitney C, et al. Expanding mental health services in low- and middle-income countries: a task-shifting framework for delivery of comprehensive, collaborative, community-based care. *Global Mental Health.* Accepted January 2023.[52])

Link Strengthening of Community-Based Care to Policy Change

The 2020 to 2023 COVID-19 *pandemic* exacerbated the global challenge of mental health and highlighted pre-existing inequities in the availability of mental health services for those with fewer financial resources, raising awareness about the urgent need for functional and accessible systems of care delivery. Global locations hit hardest by the pandemic had the greatest increases in the prevalence of major depressive disorder (MDD) and anxiety disorders, which disproportionally affect young people and females.[54] In the United States, the mental health crisis was combined with more frequent accounts of intimate partner violence, substance use, and exacerbation and complications of pre-existing medical and psychiatric problems (caused by delayed care for urgent and chronic co-morbid conditions); this has collectively been referred to as "pandemics within the pandemic." COVID-19 ushered in a new era of "polycrisis," a cross-cutting, cascading set of global challenges that span pandemic, climate (e.g., droughts,

floods, mega-storms, wildfires, extreme heat and cold) and by extension driving human migration and growing refugee emergencies, conflict over resources, and unstable political and national actors; it is now an era defined by growing complexity and uncertainty.[55]

As a result, the urgency of recommendations for restructuring the mental health workforce and other policy reforms by governments has only increased. A 2018 Lancet Commission on Sustainable Development and Mental Health, integrating a greater focus on actions relatetd to social determinants, suggested key messages and recommendations to advance mental health globally which are equally relevant in the post-pandemic period.[7] A 2020 report from the Pan American Health Organization made additional health policy recommendations for strengthening societal mental health responses (Box 51.3).[56]

Clearly, in under-resourced areas, site-specific priorities that are based on the advice and priorities of local and regional experts, and an inventory of existing resources and systems, must be enacted thoughtfully.

BOX 51.3
HEALTH POLICY RECOMMENDATIONS FOR GLOBAL MENTAL HEALTH DELIVERY AND PROGRAM IMPLEMENTATION

THE LANCET COMMISSION ON GLOBAL MENTAL HEALTH AND SUSTAINABLE DEVELOPMENT (2018)

- *Mental health needs to be re-framed within the sustainable development framework*
  - Mental health is a global public good and should be accessible to all people.
  - Mental health is the unique outcome of the interaction of environmental, biological, and developmental factors across the life course, with a unique trajectory for each person.
  - As mental health is not included in the basic healthcare package offered to people in most countries, mental health is a fundamental human right, with an equity perspective suggesting that priority should be given to vulnerable populations.
- *Mental health care is an essential component of universal health coverage*
  - The call for action to scale up services for mental disorders should be sustained with greater urgency.
  - Anticipating and counteracting threats to mental health is necessary, as demographic change, increasing social inequities, unplanned urbanization, changing family structures, and economic and employment uncertainties, coupled with large-scale migration due to war and climate change, will put increased demands on mental health and related social care services, and each pose their challenges to global mental health.
  - Embracing technological solutions will be helpful, for training and supporting providers, monitoring care practices, strengthening information systems, and promoting self-help, and should be used as an additional tool, rather than as a substitute for traditional approaches to mental health care, so as not to promote inequities.
- *Protecting mental health with public policies and development efforts*
  - Actions on social determinants of mental health are crucial through programs that promote mental health and well-being, and advance prevention and treatment of mental and substance use disorders.
  - Actions should target developmentally sensitive periods early in the life course that promote early identification of vulnerabilities to mental health and delivery of evidence-based interventions, such as life-skills curricula, parenting interventions, whole-school programs, and protection from neglect and violence.
- *Strengthening public awareness and engagement of people with mental disorders*
  - Engagement of civil society with mental health should be increased, especially for people with lived experience of mental disorders, to enhance both self-help and demand for services.

- *Investments for mental health should be enhanced*
  - National financing of mental health care should be increased.
  - International development assistance should prioritize mental health.
  - A partnership for financing and investing in mental health is urgently needed that engages UN agencies and development banks, academic institutions with expertise in implementation and prevention relevant to mental health, the private sector (for example, technology and pharmaceutical industries), civil society organizations representing the voices of people with lived experience of mental disorders, and policy-makers from national and international agencies.
- *Innovation and implementation should be guided by research*
  - Research investments should be increased and coordinated across a broad array of disciplines and funders to continue the creation of valuable knowledge.
- *Strengthening monitoring and accountability for global mental health*
  - A comprehensive monitoring mechanism for indicators of mental health should be implemented.
  - Accountability frameworks for mental health should be put in place, linked to the WHO World Mental Health Action Plan.

THE PAN AMERICAN HEALTH ORGANIZATION ACTIONS FOR STRENGTHENING MENTAL HEALTH RESPONSES TO COVID-19 (2020)

- *Scale up emergency mental health and psychosocial support (MHPSS)*
  - Build on services that address population needs.
  - Integrate into systems such as primary care, education, social services, and community support systems, to reach more people and reduce stigma.
  - Train front-line workers in WHO's Mental Health Gap Programme (mhGAP) Intervention Guide, mhGAP Humanitarian Intervention Guide, and other psychosocial interventions such as Psychological First Aid.
- *Improve and scale up tele-mental health*
  - Build infrastructure, develop policy frameworks and legislation, and facilitate relevant workforce training while striving to minimize inequities.
- *Reach populations shown to be in greater need of mental health support*
  - Front-line and healthcare workers, children, and adolescents, females, people with pre-existing mental health conditions, racial and ethnic minorities, and indigenous peoples
- *Increase social protections*
  - Economic support, food and housing assistance, livelihood protection, and childcare as essential to minimize

---

BOX 51.3
HEALTH POLICY RECOMMENDATIONS FOR GLOBAL MENTAL HEALTH DELIVERY AND PROGRAM IMPLEMENTATION—CONT'D

risk factors for mental health conditions for groups in situations of vulnerability
- *Develop communication materials*
  - Promote psychosocial well-being and connect people to appropriate MHPSS services that are adapted to reach at-risk groups.
- *Implement the strategies recommended by the 2018 Lancet Commission on Global Mental Health and Sustainable Development*
- *Advance the transition from mental health care in psychiatric hospitals to community-based care*

- Develop and strengthen mental health services in the community and reduce the number of long-stay beds in psychiatric institutions.
- *Implement a whole-of-society approach to MHPSS*
  - Provide multi-sectoral responses that include not only health care, but collaboration with other sectors including education, employment, housing, and social welfare to tackle mental health risk factors exacerbated by an emergency.
- *Actively work to incorporate MHPSS into all existing and future national emergency and disaster plans*
  - All emergency phases (preparedness, response, and recovery).

COVID-19, Coronavirus disease 2019; *WHO*, World Health Organization. Delivery and Program Implementation
Adapted from: (1) Patel V, Saxena S, Lund C, et al. The Lancet Commission on global mental health and sustainable development. *Lancet.* 2018;392:1553–1598.[7] and (2) Tausch A, Oliveira e Souza R, Viciana CM, et al. Strengthening mental health responses to COVID-19 in the Americas: a health policy analysis and recommendations. *The Lancet Regional Health—Americas* 2022;5:100118.[56]

RE-FRAMING MENTAL HEALTH CARE TO BETTER SERVE DISADVANTAGED COMMUNITIES

View Mental Health Through the Lens of Diversity, Equity, Inclusion, and De-coloniality

Individual practitioners of global mental health often gain comfort when they embark on a lifelong process of examining one's own beliefs and cultural identities, with the aim of engaging with concepts of cultural humility, proficiency, and safety. *Global health equity* refers to a vision of a world in which everyone can achieve the highest attainable level of health and no one is prevented from achieving this potential because of social position or any other socially, economically, demographically, or geographically defined circumstance or physical condition.[57] Although the pandemic caused irreversible damage in terms of morbidity and mortality, it created opportunities to re-shape the everyday functioning of contemporary society, shifting our understanding of the structuring of contemporary socioeconomic arrangements and other privileges in the United States and globally, and further clarifying the state of our psychosocial contract and social safety net.[58]

This has allowed providers to better recognize, affirm, and respond to the specific needs of socially and medically vulnerable groups, currently and in anticipation of new health crises and humanitarian disasters. Lessons from the pandemic have led investigators to take a closer look at inequities in public health, academic medicine, global health, and psychiatry, highlighting the need to develop a shared language of the values and definitions that can inform intentional *social justice and health equity leadership*.

De-colonization not only refers to the undoing of the historical control of powerful nations over weaker nations but also refers more generally to redressing inequity and imbalances of power in local contexts, including in the practice of psychiatry in the United States. In 2021 the American Psychiatric Association issued a formal apology for structural racism in psychiatry, a field which has experienced a significant shortage of clinicians of color, subsequently pledging to enact corresponding anti-racist activities.[59] Globally, the field of psychiatry has been subject to criticism for the perpetuation of institutional care, the continuation of practices of coercion and restraint, and the over-medicalization of everyday experience. Global mental health has been encouraged to prioritize local knowledge and traditional modalities of healing rather than primarily Western psychological models, to avoid over-prescription of pharmaceuticals, and to better encourage community-driven efforts.[40] Additional critiques have suggested that both psychiatry and the field of global mental health can do better to advance public mental health measures that target the structural and political determinants of mental health that lead a significant percentage of individuals to not seek services (rather than suffering from a "treatment gap").[60]

With the pandemic, prior experience and lessons learned from global health in LMICs could have informed a more effective response to the pandemic in the United States. The lessons from global health have included a focus on public health and inequity by linking development efforts with health, investing in reaching people where they are, focusing care delivery on the most marginalized people, investing in universal health care, making medicine affordable, and providing effective leadership.[61]

The practice of global health equity seeks to address and remove social factors as barriers to access to higher quality health care and to place local practitioners and their patients in the community at the center. A *social medicine* approach, informed by the fields of history, anthropology and sociology, has also been used to describe constructs in global health that inform our understanding of how social forces impact global health and the attainment of more equitable and accessible care. Kleinman described four social theories for global health: (1) *the unintended consequences of purposive (or social) action* (often applicable in the context of mental health and psychosocial response when describing response to disasters and humanitarian crises, but applicable in many situations of service, including in the practice of psychiatry), (2) the *social construction of reality* (such as relating to the stigma and fear related to mental disorders, as well as to the definition of mental disorders themselves), (3) *social suffering* (caused by the illness experience, socioeconomic and sociopolitical forces, the structural violence of deep poverty, as well as the ways in which institutions and health care bureaucracies that are developed to respond to suffering can also make suffering worse), and (4) *biopower* (described as the many ways in which political and economic governance exert control over bodies and populations, on example being the global pharmaceutical market).[62]

The past decade has brought a closer examination of systemic racism and the roles of global health practitioners from the "global north" as leaders and experts, as opposed to, in particular, Black, Indigenous, and other people of color, as well as women, as the leaders of global

health engaged at the frontline in their own communities.[63] It has been noted that the overuse of the term "LMICs," although intended to serve as a lens to understand global phenomena, can itself represent a form of structural racism when it serves to position innovation, knowledge, practices, and other important social goods, as the products of "HICs," marginalizing or silencing the contributions of those people originating from, living in, and working in the countries.[64] Global health equity can also more deliberately inform intentional actions by institutions to support and enhance local leadership, including directly funding organizations and institutions in local settings without pass-through funding to high-income country-based institutions; ensuring that decision-making on interventions and partnerships rests locally; transitioning from disease eradication to health system strengthening; moving toward reduction and the ending of short-term medical mission trips that perpetuate ethnocentrism; and actively monitoring progress in developing more equitable collaborations.[65]

Incorporate Inter-sectionality and Trauma-Informed Approaches

The US Substance Abuse and Mental Health Services Administration (SAMHSA) defines *trauma* as a widespread, harmful, and costly public health problem that occurs as a result of violence, abuse, neglect, loss, disaster, war, and other emotionally harmful experiences.[66] Individual trauma results from an event, series of events, or set of circumstances that is experienced by an individual as physically or emotionally harmful or life threatening and that has lasting adverse effects on the individual's functioning and mental, physical, social, emotional, or spiritual well-being.[66] *Inter-sectionality* refers to the social, personal, and political context where trauma is experienced, and to the complex and cumulative ways that multiple forms of discrimination combine, overlap, and intersect, especially in the experiences of marginalized individuals or groups.[58] *Inter-sectional trauma* refers to the psychosocial marginalization of individuals across multiple axes of identity, including race, ethnicity, sex, nativity status, religion, sexual orientation, mental health status, first language, immigration status, and body size.[58] The inter-sectionality of trauma requires inter-disciplinary, collaborative, action by psychiatrists as leaders in local and global contexts.

Trauma plays a significant role in mental and substance use disorders (SUDs) and it should be systematically addressed in prevention, treatment, and recovery settings, including in global and public health. Trauma is not confined to the behavioral health specialty service sector but is integral to other systems (e.g., child welfare, criminal justice, primary health care, peer-run, and community organizations) and is often a barrier to effective outcomes in each of these systems.[58] Aside from their clinical manifestations in forms that are consistent with the *Diagnostic and Statistical Manual of Mental Disorder,* Fifth Edition (DSM-5), trauma can be encompassed within various forms of depression, anxiety, somatoform conditions, SUDs, and other mental disorders. *Embodied trauma* was described by O'Brien and Charura as "the whole body's response to a significant traumatic event, where mental distress is experienced within the body as a physiological, psychological, biological, cultural, or relational reaction to trauma. Embodied trauma may include psychosomatic symptoms alongside the inability to self-regulate the autonomic nervous system and emotions, resulting in states of dissociation, numbing, relational disconnection, changed perceptions, or non-verbal internal experiences which affect every-day functioning."[67]

Trauma-informed care and a trauma-informed approach can strengthen the capacity of organizations to support people at risk in any setting. SAMHSA recommends that "A program, organization, or system that is trauma-informed realizes the widespread impact of trauma and understands paths for recovery; recognizes the signs and symptoms of trauma in clients, families, staff, and others involved with the system; and responds by fully integrating knowledge about trauma into policies, procedures, and practices, and seeks to actively resist re-traumatization."[66]

Embed Humanitarian Mental Health Crisis Response Capacity Across Sectors and Address Refugee Mental Health

Climate change poses an under-appreciated threat to mental health and emotional well-being, which it can impact through multiple pathways.[68] Humanitarian emergencies may cause social issues (such as family separation, destruction of community structures and social networks, and psychological issues), including depression, grief, anxiety, and stress-related conditions related to exposure to trauma and displacement. The relationship of climate change to natural disasters and other crises speaks to an increasing need for the embedding of MHPSS interventions across all sectors of society and to strengthening the resilience of communities through various approaches. The field of MHPSS emphasizes *functioning*: the ability of an individual to complete daily tasks (including self-care; fulfilling relevant social roles, as a member of a household, family and community; and taking part in activities, such as attending religious events and providing support for community members). It also highlights the overlap across sectors, including protection concerns (such as sexual or sex-based violence, and child abuse).

Refugees, migrants, and internally displaced people are living on the frontline of the climate catastrophe.[69] The experiences of these populations also inform our understanding of the practice of psychiatry in areas of conflict. In 2022, 89.3 million people were living forcibly displaced lives worldwide, with 83% hosted in LMICs, and 72% hosted in neighboring countries.[70] Roughly two-thirds (69%) of displaced persons in 2022 originated from five countries: the Syrian Arab Republic (6.8 million), Venezuela (4.6 million), Afghanistan (2.7 million), South Sudan (2.4 million), and Myanmar (1.2 million).[70]

Refugees often face stressors and traumas at different phases of displacement: *pre-migration* (i.e., war, famine, torture, job and property loss, rape), *during transit or migration* (i.e., family separation, physical and sexual assault, extortion, lack of access to services for basic needs), and *post-migration* (i.e., discrimination, acculturation shock, separation from family, detention, poor living conditions, barriers to accessing care).[71] The stressors can also be organized in terms of *traumatic experiences, re-settlement, acculturation,* and *isolation.*[72] These complex experiences are attributable to individual factors, social considerations, and political contexts, and they can have severe and long-term mental health consequences; it is important to understand mental health needs at each stage.[30] In the context of re-settlement, one can envision a multitier MHPSS model consistent with the IASC Guidelines, to support trauma-informed and culture-informed care that includes community-based and community-partnered interventions (Fig. 51.7).[73]

More specialized mental health care and treatment can be embedded within an integrated, inter-disciplinary

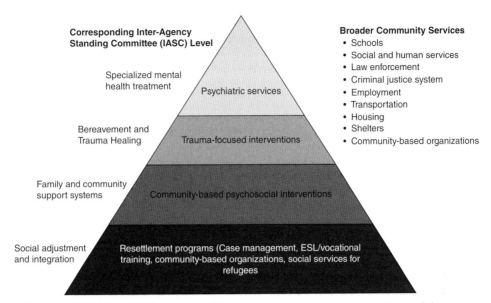

Fig. 51.7 ■ A multitier model of refugee MHPSS in the context of re-settlement. *ESL*, English as a second language; *MHPSS*, mental health and psychosocial support. (Adapted from Im H, Rodriquez C, Grumbine JM. A multitier model of refugee mental health and psychosocial support in resettlement: toward trauma-informed and culture-informed systems of care. *Psychol Serv*. 2020. https://doi.org/10.1037/ser0000412.[73])

primary care setting that includes primary care doctors, mental health providers, nurses, case managers, social workers, peer navigators, interpreters, and "cultural brokers" who can develop treatment plans that integrate refugees' cultural narrative, moral frameworks, and intersectional identities.[71] Evaluation should integrate the use of practices that specifically engage individuals around cultural and spiritual concerns. The *ETHNICS mnemonic* can be useful in providing culturally responsive care and treatment (Box 51.4).[74]

With regard to bereavement and the healing of trauma, although various clinical concerns should be addressed, including those related to autonomic hyperarousal and sleep disturbances, it is important to consider that refugees and other displaced persons are confronted with diverse, overlapping symptom constellations, as well as broader existential concerns that relate to adapting to the long-term erosion of psychosocial systems and institutions that in stable societies support psychological well-being and mental health.[75] Programs, such as the US Government Welcome Corps, enable all citizens, including providers, to engage in the process of supporting re-settlement for refugees.[76]

Comprehensively Address Maternal Mental Health and Early Child Development

Although the physical health of females and children has been emphasized, the mental aspects of their health are often ignored by maternal and child health programs, especially in LMICs.[77] Globally, in women of childbearing age, depression accounts for the largest proportion of the burden associated with mental or neurological disorders.[77] Regarding the global burden of disease, the prevalence of depression is higher in women than in men, with alternative epidemiological explanations related to stigma and culture. In 2010, for example, the global annual prevalence rates of major depressive disorder were 5.5% in women and 3.2% in men.[78]

This gap in prevalence rates has persisted over the years and has been exacerbated by the pandemic. Furthermore, multiple factors have been implicated in developing this disparity, including socioeconomic factors and biological vulnerabilities. In recent times, because of the pandemic and accompanying societal impacts, women were more likely to experience job insecurity, increased caregiver responsibilities, financial constraints, and exposure to intimate partner violence.

BOX 51.4
THE ETHNICS MNEMONIC

Explanation   Direct question: *"Why do you think you have this...?"* (use the patient's phrase for their symptom/illness/condition/problem)

Probe questions: *"What do friends, family, and others say about these symptoms? Do you know anyone else who has had or who has this kind of problem? Have you heard about/read/seen it on television/radio/newspaper/internet?"* (If the patient cannot explain, ask what concerns them about their problems).

Treatment   Direct question: *"What have you tried for this...?"* (use the patient's phrase for their symptom/illness/condition/problem)

Probe questions: *"What kind of medicines, home remedies or other treatments have you tried for this illness? Is there anything you eat, drink, or do (or avoid) on a regular basis to stay healthy? Tell me about it. What kind of treatments are you seeking from me?*

Healers   Direct question: *"Who else have you sought help from for this...?"* (use the patient's phrase for their symptom/illness/condition/problem)"

Probe question: *"Have you sought help from alternative or folk healers, friends, or other people who are not doctors for help with your problems?"*

Negotiate   Direct question: *"How best do you think I can help you?"*

Try to find options that will be mutually acceptable to you and your patient and that incorporate your patient's beliefs rather than contradicting them.

Intervention   Direct statement: *"This is what I think needs to be done now."*

Determine an intervention (e.g., diagnostic, pharmacological, psychosocial, educational) with your patient that may also incorporate alternative treatments, spirituality, healers, and other cultural practices (e.g., foods eaten or avoided in general and when sick).

Collaborate   Direct question: *"How can we work together on this and with whom else?"*

Collaborate with the patient, family members, healers, and community resources.

Spirituality   Direct question: *"What role does faith/religion/spirituality play in helping you with this ...?"* (use the patient's phrase for their *symptom/illness/condition/problem*)?

Probe question: Tell me about your spiritual life. How can your spiritual beliefs help you with this?

Adapted from Kobylarz FA, Heath JM, Like RC. The ETHNICS(s) mnemonic: a clinical tool for ethnogeriatric education. *J Am Geriatr Soc.* 2002;50:1582–1589.[74]

The lack of telepsychiatric opportunities in resource-limited settings has further exacerbated healthcare disparities, and disadvantaged populations have been more likely to report higher rates of perinatal mental healthcare disruption.[79] In addition, several studies have demonstrated a deterioration in maternal-infant bonding due to the pandemic and the limits on the usual mechanisms of social support in the hospital having a deleterious impact on maternal mental health, resulting in higher rates of traumatic birth experiences and birth-related post-traumatic stress disorder.[80,81]

Post-partum depression rates vary across countries.[82] In HICs, the rates are between 10% and 15%. In lower-income countries, the rates are as high as 18%, with the highest rates reported in Southern Africa (39.6%).[82]

Factors such as income, educational level, breastfeeding status, marital status, and social support services, are predictors of post-partum depression globally.[82] In LMICs, health status and economic factors significantly affect the development of post-partum depression rates.[83] Access to contraception and healthcare facilities plays a role in improving overall well-being. Cultural and religious acceptance also plays a major role. In many countries, taking medications during pregnancy or breastfeeding is frowned on, and females may be advised or pressured to stop psychiatric medications during pregnancy. Post-partum depressive symptoms may also be undetected or attributed to religious or supernatural causes. Cultural practices such as child marriage and teen pregnancy are associated with a two- to threefold higher risk of perinatal depression, which is depression during pregnancy and the post-partum period.[84] Children and adolescents are also at higher risk of obstetric fistulas with the accompanying sequelae of stigmatization, social isolation, chronic urinary or fecal incontinence, and maternal mortality.[85]

Prevention and treatment of post-partum depression should be individualized or tailored to the target population. Identification of at-risk individuals is paramount as the responsibility of screening clinicians to prevent further stigmatization of vulnerable patients. Sociocultural risk factors warrant special attention as this may influence participation in care beyond the peripartum period. Other risk factors, such as unplanned pregnancy and substance use should be addressed using a multi-disciplinary approach. Both behavioral and pharmacological interventions should be used as needed. Psychotherapeutic practices have been the preferred modality in most countries because they are cost-effective, often culturally acceptable, and associated with minimal to no risk.[86] Models of care include *integrated or collaborative care models*, in which team-based systems comprising obstetricians, midwives, and pediatricians cooperate to ensure continuity of care and a holistic approach to health care. Across all global settings CHWs and traditional midwives should be taught how to screen for depression and undertake preliminary preventive health measures based on research regarding the effectiveness of interventions, especially those that can be delivered by non-specialists.[87] Treatments should include a review of complementary and alternative healthcare practices that may be more culturally acceptable or preferred in the community, such as yoga, acupuncture, and meditation. Practical support (such as lactation assistance, transportation, and doula services) should be readily available and supported by local authorities and state or national policies. New models of care should be examined for cultural appropriateness and adapted for use in communities (such as telepsychiatry and virtual depression care managers).

Regarding pharmacological treatment, different ethnic and racial groups metabolize medications differently; attention should be given to considerations of ethnicity and psychobiology.[87] Attention should be paid to the risk of adverse effects to both mothers and children, and the acceptability of medication use. Long-acting injectable medications may reduce the stigma of daily pill use and should be offered when pills are not feasible. Discussions around medications and treatment methods should be explained, and screening tools and medication instructions should be written in the patient's preferred language.

Broadly, attention to early child development concerns is critical and is an egregiously under-supported area of global health that requires action.[88] Poor beginnings can include delivery by an unskilled attendant in the home, infections (such as malaria), diarrhea, inadequate micro-nutrients (such as iron and iodine), and inadequate psychosocial stimulation.[89] Rapid brain development in the first 3 years of life combined with greater neuroplasticity as a window of opportunity implies that it is important to start early; support both children and caregivers; and provide multiple protective inputs to promote *nurturing care*, including parenting support, promotion of attachment and bonding, support of breastfeeding, micronutrients and children feeding, prevention of child maltreatment, out-of-home interventions (such as early learning programs and nurturing environments); social safety net interventions (such as cash transfer programs and social protection efforts); and coordinated services across sectors.[90] The Nurturing Care Framework for Early Child Development promotes five key components of nurturing care: good health, adequate nutrition, responsive caregiving, safety and security, and opportunities for early learning.[91] The WHO has developed a training program for caregivers of children with developmental disabilities, including autism.[92]

Prioritize Action on Mental Health of Young People

Perhaps the greatest challenge facing global mental health in the coming decade will be the mental health of young people.[93] A 2021 UNICEF report, "On My Mind: The State of the World's Children, called on government leaders to promote, protect, and care for the mental health of the world's children through investment, combating stigma, advancing programs for prevention and promotion, supporting parents and caregivers, addressing poverty and mental health, addressing inequities of gender, and generating interventions across systems and sectors.[94] Globally, there is a paucity of child and adolescent psychiatrists to support the development of programs to meet the clinical and public health need. For care providers who work to provide quality clinical care in challenging circumstances in all contexts, including in the United States, it is important for psychiatrists to address the problems directly by considering action on the social determinants themselves on behalf of children and adolescents.[95] Clinicians can advocate for investments and programming for children, adolescents, and their families, for example for trauma-informed schools based on SAMHSA recommendations. Clinicians can also seek ways to act beyond the clinic on the promoters of structural inequities, in context (Box 51.5).[95]

CONCLUSION

What greater honor is there than having people share their greatest intimacies with you as a physician? And a physician has a special privilege of not only feeling wanted, but also needed. The physician has the opportunity to do good in a concentrated fashion.

Chester M. Pierce, MD

BOX 51.5
SOCIAL DETERMINANTS OF MENTAL HEALTH FOR CHILDREN AND ADOLESCENTS AND EXAMPLES OF HOW MENTAL HEALTH PROFESSIONALS CAN ADDRESS THEM IN THE CLINICAL SETTING

Economic instability

Food insecurity
- Compile a list of local food banks
- Advocate for policies that address food insecurity, that is, Supplemental Nutrition Assistance program

Housing insecurity
- Screen using the IHELLP tool. The American Academy of Pediatrics has a list of screening tools for social determinants of health that can be accessed at the Bright Futures Toolkit
- Partner with local legal aid programs

Parental unemployment
- Refer parent to an employment program
- Support the development, implementation, or enhancement of local JOBS program

Household income
- Create a local resource list for families experiencing financial hardship
- Encourage legislators to support a living wage

Education

Educational inequality
- Advocate for access to early childhood education programs for all children
- Refer to tutoring and other academic assistance programs
- Engage with local Parent to Parent chapter

Language and literacy
- Refer to literacy programs for child and/or guardian

Parental education
- Compile a list of free/reduced-cost adult education programs

Social and Community Context

Discrimination
- Use the *Diagnostic and Statistical Manual of Mental Disorder*, Fifth Edition (DSM-5) cultural formulation interview
- Hire people who reflect the diversity of the patient population

Immigration status
- Use the DSM-5 cultural formulation interview
- Refer to local immigration support services

Social isolation
- Refer to local parent and family support groups

Mental health stigma
- Consider providing mental health education to local schools and employers

Health and health care

Access to health care
- Consider expanding appointments and offering non-traditional hours (i.e., some evening or weekend hours)
- Partner with pediatricians to provide integrated health services

Quality of health care
- Use evidence-based care in all interactions
- Explore unconscious biases and potential impact on care using the Implicit Association Test at Project Implicit

BOX 51.5
SOCIAL DETERMINANTS OF MENTAL HEALTH FOR CHILDREN AND ADOLESCENTS AND EXAMPLES OF HOW MENTAL HEALTH PROFESSIONALS CAN ADDRESS THEM IN THE CLINICAL SETTING—CONT'D

Health literacy: parental and youth	▪ Use patient-friendly, developmentally appropriate language ▪ Encourage patients and families to ask questions about their care
Neighborhood and environment	
Condition of housing	▪ Encourage your practice to partner with a community health worker who can complete in-home assessments ▪ Advocate at local housing policy meetings
Community violence	▪ Support efforts and policies that reduce community violence ▪ Talk with legislators about the link between exposure to violence and youth mental health
Residential segregation	▪ Encourage efforts to enforce existing antidiscrimination laws in the housing market ▪ Learn about Purpose-Built Communities
Lack of childcare	▪ Advocate for policy that decreases the cost of day care and ensures access to preschool within the public school system
Access to transportation	▪ Support policies that promote the creation and maintenance of transportation services accessible to all neighborhoods ▪ Provide transportation support (e.g., bus fare, ride share) for patients attending clinic appointments
Access to emerging technologies, that is, Wi-Fi, cell phone	▪ Explore local programs for low-cost internet access, supplemental support for cell phones, and other technological resources
Parental psychosocial factors and adverse childhood experiences	
Witnessing interpersonal violence	▪ Screen for adverse childhood experiences (ACES) using the ACES score calculator
Child abuse	▪ Report suspected abuse to child protective services ▪ Encourage legislators to allocate funding for child welfare services with a particular emphasis on prevention
Parental substance use disorder	▪ Screen using the ACES score calculator ▪ Refer to local addiction resources
Parental depression	▪ Refer guardian to local adult mental health resources

Adapted from Cotton NK, Shim RS. Social determinants of health, structural racism, and the impact on child and adolescent mental health. *J Am Acad Child and Adolesc Psychiatry*. 2022;61(11):1385–1387.[95]

Founder, The Massachusetts General Hospital Division of Global Psychiatry

This chapter has presented the evolving field of global psychiatry in the context of global health and global mental health, and regarding public health in the United States, using a "global-local" paradigm, for clinicians. The doctor-patient relationship and the psychiatric interview serve as the foundational elements of a comprehensive understanding of, and engagement with, people living with problems related to mental illness. A collaborative, person-centered approach in which the preferences and values of the persons receiving care are honored and given precedence informs the attainment of optimal healing environments for individuals in their own cultural context. In many contexts, however—in the United States as well as globally—profound structural challenges and systemic gaps remain in under-resourced settings that prevent the preparation of optimal health environments for mental healthcare delivery. Developing a practice of *social justice leadership*, informed by the understanding that the inter-sectionality of race, class, and trauma amplify the marginalization of many people living in less advantaged communities, supports the implementation of structural changes that can enhance practice in any context.[91] The field of global psychiatry, informed by diverse other fields as well as by the clinical practice of psychiatry, stands to strengthen the quality and practice of clinical care in any context, as practitioners of psychiatry are today "global psychiatrists" wherever they work. The integration of global mental health concerns enhances the capacity of the field of psychiatry to most effectively act to confront urgent global challenges to public mental health, as well as to address structural challenges within the field of psychiatry itself, across all contexts.

REFERENCES

1. Khan T, Abimbola S, Kyobutungi C, et al. How we classify countries and people—and why it matters. *BMJ Global Health*. 2022;7:e009704.
2. Korte KJ, Hook K, Levey EJ, et al. A global-local paradigm for mental health: a model and implications for addressing disparities through training and research. *Acad Psychiatry*. July 2022. https://doi.org/10.1007/s40596-022-01695-0.
3. World Health Organization. *Comprehensive Mental Health Action Plan 2013–2020*. World Health Organization; 2013.
4. Arias D, Saxena S, Verguet S. Quantifying the global burden of mental disorders and their economic value. *eClinicalMedicine*. 2022;54:101675.
5. World Health Organization. *Mental Health Atlas 2020*. WHO; 2021.
6. World Health Organization *World Mental Health Report: Transforming Mental Health for All*. World Health Organization; 2022.
7. Patel V, Saxena S, Lund C, et al. The lancet commission on global mental health and sustainable development. *Lancet*. 2018;392:1553–1598.
8. Kessler RC, Berglund P, Demler O, et al. Lifetime prevalence and age-of-onset distributions of DSM-IV disorders in the National Comorbidity Survey Replication. *Arch Gen Psychiatry*. 2005;62(6):593–602.
9. Koplan JP, Bond TC, Merson MH, et al. Towards a common definition of global health. *Lancet*. 2009;373:1993–1995.
10. Patel V., Prince M. Global mental health: a new global health field comes of age. *JAMA*. 1976-1977; 303.
11. Ferrari AJ, Santomauro DF, Herrera AMM, et al. Global, regional, and national burden of 12 mental disorders in 204 countries and territories, 1990–2019: a systematic analysis for the Global Burden of Disease Study 2019. *Lancet Psychiatry*. 2022;9:137–150.
12. Lund C, Brooke-Sumner C, Baingana F, et al. Social determinants of mental disorders and the Sustainable Development Goals: a systematic review of reviews. *Lancet Psychiatry*. 2018;5:357–369.
13. Harvard University. Harvard Medical School. *Introduction to Global Health Care Delivery*. Available at: <http://ghsm.hms.harvard.edu/education/courses/global-health-delivery>.
14. Farmer P, Kim JY, Kleinman A, et al. *Chapter 1: Introduction: A Biosocial Approach to Global Health. Reimagining Global Health: An Introduction*. University of California Press; 2013:12.
15. United Nations High Commission for Refugees (UNHCR). *Mental Health and Psychosocial Support. UNHCR Emergency Handbook*. Available at: <https://emergency.unhcr.org/entry/49304/mental-health-and-psychosocial-support>.
16. Kestel D. Transforming mental health for all: a critical role for specialists. *World Psychiatry*. 2022;21(3):333–334.
17. Rajabzadeh V. Burn E, Sajun SA, et al. Understanding global mental health: a conceptual review. *BMJ Global Health*. 2021 6e004631.
18. Metzl JM, Hansen H. Structural competency and psychiatry. *JAMA Psychiatry*. 2018;75(2):115–116.
19. Harvey M, Neff J, Knight KR, et al. Structural competency and global health education. *Global Public Health*. 2022;17(3):341–362.
20. Davis S, O'Brien AM. Let's talk about racism: strategies for building structural competency in nursing. *Acad Med*. 2020;95: S58–S65.
21. World Health Organization. *Psychiatrists Working in Mental Health Sector (per 100,000)*. Available at: <https://www.who.int/data/gho/data/indicators/indicator-details/GHO/psychiatrists-working-in-mental-health-sector>-(per-100-000).
22. World Health Organization, Organization of Services for Mental Health. *Mental Health Policy and Service Guidance Package*. WHO; 2003.
23. Funk M, Lund C, Freeman M, et al. Improving the quality of mental health care. *Int J Qual Health Care*. 2009;21(6):415–420.
24. United Nations General Assembly. *Report of the Special Rapporteur on the Right of Everyone to the Enjoyment of the Highest Attainable Standard of Physical and Mental Health. Human Rights Council. Fourty-Fourth Session. 6-23 June 2017. Agenda Item 3*. Available at: <https://www.ohchr.org/en/stories/2020/07/overuse-biomedical-interventions-ignores-humans-emotional-complexity-says-un-experthttps://www.ohchr.org/en/special-procedures/sr-health/right-mental-health>.
25. Pescosolido BA, Halpern-Manners A, Luo L. Trends in public stigma of mental illness in the US, 1996-2018. *JAMA Network Open*. 2021;4(12):e2140202.
26. *WHO Quality Rights*. Available at: <https://www.who.int/teams/mental-health-and-substance-use/policy-law-rights/qr-e-training>.
27. Psychosocial Rehabilitation Canada. Available at: <https://www.psrrpscanada.ca/what-psychosocial-rehabilitation>.
28. United Nations. *Convention on the Rights of Persons With Disabilities*. Available at: <https://www.ohchr.org/en/instruments-mechanisms/instruments/convention-rights-persons-disabilities>.
29. Doyle N. Neurodiversity at work: a biopsychosocial model and the impact on working adults. *Br Med Bull*. 2020;135(1): 108–125.
30. Kakuma R, Minas H, Dal Poz MR, et al. Strategies for strengthening human resources for mental health. In: Patel V, Minas H, Cohen A, eds. *Global Mental Health: Principles and Practice*. Oxford University Press; 2014.

31. Ratner L, Sridhar S, Rosman SL, et al. Learner milestones to guide decolonial global health education. *Ann Global Health*. 2022;88:99, 1–8. < https://doi.org/10.5334/aogh.3866>.

32. Hansen H, Braslow J, Rohrbaugh RM. From cultural to structural competency—training psychiatric residents to act on social determinants of health and institutional racism. *JAMA Psychiatry*. 2017;75(2):117–118.

33. Jordan A, Shim RS, Rodriguez CI, et al. Psychiatry diversity leadership in academic medicine: guidelines for success. *Am J Psychiatry*. March 2021;178(3):224–228.

34. Moreno F. Justice, equity, diversity and inclusion in psychiatric education, research and practice. *Presentation at the 60th Annual Meeting of the American College of Psychiatrists*. February, 2023.

35. Fricchione GL, Borba CPC, Alem A, et al. Capacity building in global mental health: professional training. *Harv Rev Psychiatry*. 2012;20(1):47–57.

36. Akomolafe AC. Decolonizing the notion of mental illness and healing in Nigeria, West Africa. *Ann Rev Crit Psychol*. 2013;10:726–740.

37. Griffith JL, Kohrt BA, Dyer A, et al. Training psychiatrists for global mental health: cultural psychiatry, collaborative inquiry, and ethics of alterity. *Acad Psychiatry*. 2016;40(4):701–706.

38. Wang M, Katz C, Wiegand J. Global mental health as a component of psychiatric residency training. *Psychiatr Q*. 2012;83:75–82.

39. Rebello TJ, Marques A, Gureje O, et al. Innovative strategies for closing the mental health treatment gap globally. *Curr Opin Psychiatry*. 2014;27(4):308–314.

40. Whitley R. Global Mental Health: concepts, conflicts and controversies. *Epidemiol Psychiatr Sci*. 2015;24:285–291.

41. Callaghan M, Ford N, Schneider H. A systematic review of task-shifting for HIV treatment and care in Africa. *Hum Resour Health*. 2010;8(8):1–9.

42. Singla DR, Kohrt BA, Murray LK, et al. Psychological treatments for the world: lessons from low- and middle-income countries. *Annu Rev Clin Psychol*. 2017;13(1):149–181.

43. World Health Organization. *mhGAP Intervention Guide for Mental, Neurological and Substance Use Disorders in Non-specialized Health Settings: mental health Gap Action Programme (mhGAP) – Version 2.0*. 2016.

44. Inter-Agency Standing Committee (IASC). *IASC Guidelines on Mental Health and Psychosocial Support in Emergency Settings*. IASC; 2007. http://www.who.int/mental_health/emergencies/guidelines_iasc_mental_health_psychosocial_june_2007.pdf.

45. World Health Organization. *Service Organization Pyramid for an Optimal Mix of Mental Health Services. Organization of Services for Mental Health: Mental Health Policy and Service Guidance Package*. WHO; 2003. Visual from 2009; https://apps.who.int/iris/bitstream/handle/10665/44219/9789241598774_eng.pdf.

46. Kohrt BA, Asher L, Bhardwaj A, et al. The role of communities in mental health care in low- and middle-income countries: a meta-review of components and competencies. *Int J Environ Res Public Health*. 2018;15(1279):1–31.

47. World Health Organization. *Ensuring Quality in Psychological Support (EQUIP)*. Available at: <https://www.who.int/teams/mental-health-and-substance-use/treatment-care/equip-ensuring-quality-in-psychological-support>; 2021.

48. Hanlon C. Next steps for meeting the needs of people with severe mental illness in low- and middle-income countries. *Epidemiol Psychiatr Sci*. 2017;26:348–354.

49. Mental Health Value Chain. *Partners In Health*. Available at: <https://www.pih.org/mental-health/pih-mental-health-value-chain>

50. International Medical Corps. *Toolkit for the Integration of Mental Health Into General Healthcare in Humanitarian Settings*. Available at: <https://www.mhinnovation.net/collaborations/IMC-Mental-Health-Integration-Toolkit>.

51. Jones L, Asare JB, El Masri M, et al. Severe mental disorders in complex emergencies. *Lancet*. 2009;374:654–661.

52. Bolton P, West J, Whitney C, et al. Expanding mental health services in low- and middle-income countries: a task-shifting framework for delivery of comprehensive, collaborative, community-based care. *Global Mental Health*. 10(e16), 2022, 1–14.

53. Raviola G, Naslund NA, Smith SL, et al. Innovative models in mental health delivery systems: task-sharing care with non-specialist providers to close the mental health treatment gap. *Curr Psychiatry Rep*. 2019;21(44):1–13.

54. Santomauro DF, Herrera AMM, Shadid J, et al. Global prevalence and burden of depressive and anxiety disorders in 204 countries and territories in 2020 due to the COVID-19 pandemic. *Lancet*. 2021;398:1700–1712.

55. Janzwood S., Homer-Dixon T. What is a global polycrisis? Discussion Paper 2022–4. Cascade Institute. Available at: <https//cascadeinstitute.org/technical-paper/what-is-a-global-polycrisis/>.

56. Tausch A, Oliveira e Souza R, Viciana CM, et al. trengthening mental health responses to COVID-19 in the Americas: a health policy analysis and recommendations. *Lancet Reg Health Am*. 2022;5:100118.

57. Centers for Disease Control. *Global Health Equity*. Available at: <https://www.cdc.gov/globalhealth/equity/home.html>.

58. Ezell JM, Salari S, Rooker C, et al. Intersectional trauma: COVID-19, the psychosocial contract, and America's racialized public health lineage. *Traumatology*. 2021;27(1):78–85.

59. *APA's Apology to Black, Indigenous and People of Color for its Support of Structural Racism in Psychiatry*. Available at: <https://www.psychiatry.org/newsroom/apa-apology-for-its-support-of-structural-racism-in-psychiatry>; 2021.

60. Roberts T, Esponda GM, Torre Costanza, et al. Reconceptualizing the treatment gap for common mental disorders: a fork in the road for global mental health? *Br J Psychiatry*. 2022;221:553–557.

61. Holmes CB, Goosby EP. How lessons from global health can improve health and the response to COVID-19 in the US. *Health Affairs Forefront: Global Health Policy*. Available at: <https://www.healthaffairs.org/do/10.1377/forefront.20200806.949101/full/>; 2020.

62. Kleinman A. Four social theories for global health. *Lancet*. May 1, 2010;375:1518–1519.

63. Abimbola S, Pai M. Will global health survive its decolonization? *Lancet*. November 21, 2020;396:1627–1628.

64. Lencucha R, Seupane S. The use, misuse and overuse of the 'low-income and middle-income countries' category. *BMJ Global Health*. 2022;7:e009067.

65. Foretia DA. To decolonize surgery and global health we must be radically intentional. *Am J Surg*. October 14, 2022. https://doi.org/10.1016/j.amjsurg.2022.10.015.

66. Substance Abuse and Mental Health Services Administration. *SAMHSA's Concept of Trauma and Guidance for a Trauma-Informed Approach. HHS Publication No. (SMA) 14-4884*. Substance Abuse and Mental Health Services Administration; 2014.

67. O'Brien CV, Charura D. Refugees, asylum seekers, and practitioners' perspectives of embodied trauma: a comprehensive scoping review. *Psychological Trauma: Theory, Research, Practice, and Policy*. August 1, 2022.

68. Lawrance E, Thompson R, Fontana G, et al. *The impact of climate change on mental health and motional wellbeing: current evidence and implications for policy and practice. Grantham Institute Briefing Paper No. 36*. Institute for Global Health Innovation. Imperial College; May 2021:1–36.

69. United Nations High Commission for Refugees (UNHCR). *Climate Change and Disaster Displacement*. Available at: <https://www.unhcr.org/en-us/climate-change-and-disasters.html>.

70. United Nations High Commission for Refugees (UNHCR). *Global Trends Forced Displacement in 2021*. Available at: <https://www.unhcr.org/en-us/publications/brochures/62a9d1494/global-trends-report-2021.html>; 2022.

71. Mattar S, Gellatly R. Refugee mental health: culturally relevant considerations. *Curr Opin Psychol*. 2022;47(101429):1–5.

72. Boston Children's Hospital Trauma and Community Resilience Center. *Refugee and Immigrant Core Stressors Toolkit*. Available at: <https://www.childrenshospital.org/programs/trauma-and-community-resilience-center>.

73. Im H, Rodriquez C, Grumbine JM. A multitier model of refugee mental health and psychosocial support in resettlement: toward trauma-informed and culture-informed systems of care. *Psychol Serv*. 2020. https://doi.org/10.1037/ser0000412.

74. Kobylarz FA, Heath JM, Like RC. The ETHNICS(s) mnemonic: a clinical tool for ethnogeriatric education. *J Am Geriatr Soc*. 2002;50:1582–1589.

75. Jou YC, Pace-Schott EF. Call to action: addressing sleep disturbances, a hallmark symptom of PTSD, for refugees, asylum seekers, and internally displaced persons. *Sleep Health*. 2022;8(6):593–600.

76. Welcome Corps. Available at: <https://welcomecorps.org>.

77. Atif N, Lovell K, Rahman A. Maternal mental health: the missing "m" in the global maternal and child health agenda. *Semin Perinatol*. 2015;39:345–352.

78. Whiteford HA, Degenhardt L, Rehm J, et al. Global burden of disease attributable to mental and substance use disorders: findings from the Global Burden of Disease Study 2010. *Lancet*. 2013 Nov 9;382(9904):1575–1586. https://doi.org/10.1016/S0140-6736(13)61611-6. Epub 2013 Aug 29. PMID: 23993280.

79. Shuffrey LC, Thomason ME, Brito NH. Improving perinatal maternal mental health starts with addressing structural inequities. *JAMA Psychiatry*. 2022;79(5):387–388. PMID: 35262622; PMIDC: PMC9081213.

80. Mayopoulos GA, Ein-Dor T, Dishy GA, et al. COVID-19 is associated with traumatic childbirth and subsequent mother-infant bonding problems. *J Affect Disord*. 2021;282:122–125. https://www.sciencedirect.com/science/article/pii/S0165032720331918. doi: 10.1016/j.jad.2020.12.101.

81. Diamond RM, Colaianni A. The impact of perinatal healthcare changes on birth trauma during COVID-19. *Women Birth*. 2022 Sep;35(5):503–510. https://doi.org/10.1016/j.wombi.2021.12.003. Epub 2021 Dec 11. PMID: 34924337; PMCID: PMC8678623.

82. Kessler RC, Bromet EJ. The epidemiology of depression across cultures. *Annu Rev Public Health*. 2013;34:119–138. https://doi.org/10.1146/annurev-publhealth-031912-114409. PMID: 23514317; PMCID: PMC4100461.

83. Wang Z, Liu J, Shuai H, et al. Mapping global prevalence of depression among postpartum women. *Transl Psychiatry*. 2021;11:543. https://doi.org/10.1038/s41398-021-01663-6.

84. Burgess RA, Jeffery M, Odero SA, et al. Overlooked and unaddressed: a narrative review of mental health consequences of child marriages. *PLOS Glob Public Health*. 2022;2(1):e0000131. https://doi.org/10.1371/journal.pgph.0000131.

85. Swain D, Parida SP, Jena SK, et al. Prevalence and risk factors of obstetric fistula: implementation of a need-based preventive action plan in a South-eastern rural community of India. *BMC Women's Health*. 2020;20:40. https://doi.org/10.1186/s12905-020-00906-w.

86. McHugh RK, Whitton SW, Peckham AD, et al. Patient preference for psychological vs. pharmacological treatment of psychiatric disorders: a meta-analytic review. *J Clin Psychiatry*. 2013;74:595.

87. Burroughs VJ, Maxey RW, Levy RA. Racial and ethnic differences in response to medicines: towards individualized pharmaceutical treatment. *J Natl Med Assoc*. 2002 Oct;94(10 suppl):1–26. PMID: 12401060; PMCID: PMC2594139.

88. Richter L, Black M, Britto P, et al. Early childhood development: an imperative for action and measurement at scale. *BMJ Global Health*. 2019;4:i154–i160. https://doi.org/10.1136/bmjgh-2018-001302.

89. Aboud FE, Yousafzai AK. Global health and development in early childhood. *Annu Rev Psychol*. 2015;66:433–457.

90. Britto PR, Lye SJ, Proulx K, et al. Nurturing care: promoting early child development. *Lancet*. 2017;389:91–102.

91. The Nurturing Care Framework for Early Child Development. Available at: <https://nurturing-care.org>.

92. World Health Organization. *Training for Caregivers of Children With Developmental Disabilities, Including Autism*. Available at: <https://www.who.int/teams/mental-health-and-substance-use/treatment-care/who-caregivers-skills-training-for-families-of-children-with-developmental-delays-and-disorders>.

93. McGorry PD, Mei C, Chanen A, et al. Designing and scaling up integrated youth mental health care. *World Psychiatry*. 2022;21:61–76.

94. United Nations Children's Fund. *The State of the World's Children 2021: On My Mind—Promoting, Protecting and Caring for Children's Mental Health*. UNICEF, October 2021.

95. Cotton NK, Shim RS. Social determinants of health, structural racism, and the impact on child and adolescent mental health. *J Am Acad Child Adolesc Psychiatry*. 2022;61(11):1385–1387.

52

CARE OF LGBTQIA+ PATIENTS

HYUN-HEE KIM, MD ■ ALEX S. KEUROGHLIAN, MD, MPH

OVERVIEW

The clinical care and health research into lesbian, gay, bisexual, transgender, queer, intersex, and asexual (LGBTQIA+) people have expanded tremendously in recent decades. This chapter provides a brief and broad overview of LGBTQIA+ health topics relevant to psychiatric practice.

HISTORICAL CONTEXT WITHIN PSYCHIATRY

Same-sex desires and sexual behaviors, non-dichotomous gender roles, and gender-expansive people are not simply modern-day phenomena; they have been observed across history in many different human societies around the globe (see Table 52.1 for the definitions of common terms). Gender roles and sexual norms are culturally specific and thus they vary among cultures and throughout time. The rigidly enforced binary gender paradigm and the promotion of a procreative nuclear family with which we may recently be most familiar are intimately tied to the development of capitalism and imperialism in the modern era.[1] In medicine, the conceptualization of both non-heterosexual behaviors and gender diversity has broadly fallen into three camps since the 1800s: (1) sexual and gender diversity as natural variation and thus not a manifestation of psychopathology; (2) sexual and gender diversity as pathology (e.g., due to inadequate parenting, in utero hormone exposures, or abuse) and a defect to be avoided; or (3) sexual and gender diversity as a normative stage

in development that may present as immaturity or stunted growth but not a particularly negative or pathological outcome.[2]

Medicine plays an important role in reinforcing social norms and potentially contributing to the marginalization and stigmatization of individuals who deviate from the idealized standards of their time, whether in anatomy or behaviors. Although Freud famously advised a mother that her son's homosexuality was "nothing to be ashamed of, no vice, no degradation," and that it "could not be classified as an illness," for much of the duration of modern psychiatry, homosexuality was indeed considered an illness. Homosexuality was retained in the *Diagnostic and Statistical Manual of Mental Disorders* (DSM) until 1974, with ego-dystonic homosexuality finally being removed in 1987.[3] In a similar vein, various gender-related diagnoses were entered into and phased out of the DSM, for example, transsexualism and gender identity disorder in DSM-III became gender dysphoria in DSM-5.[4] Diagnoses are neither neutral nor objective descriptions of natural phenomena, but rather concepts arrived at by consensus, shaped by material realities of the time (e.g., retention of any gender diagnosis was partly out of concern that, without a specific billable diagnosis in the United States, transgender patients might lose access to gender-affirming medical care) and the proactive efforts of practicing clinicians, academics, and activists (e.g., removal of homosexuality as a diagnosis would not have been possible without the gay liberation movement of the 1970s and the activism of psychiatrists within the American Psychiatric Association).[2]

901

	TABLE 52.1
	Definitions of Terms Related to LGBTQIA+ Issues

Terms	Definitions
Sex or gender assigned at birth	Gender presumed at birth, most commonly based on physical sex characteristics, such as external genitalia and chromosomes
Intersex	Variations in physical sex development that do not fit traditional notions of female/XX or male/XY bodies
Gender identity	An individual's inner sense of their own gender (e.g., boy/man, girl/woman, both, beyond, no gender, or any number of culturally specific identities)
Cisgender person	An individual whose gender identity aligns with societal expectations based on the sex assigned at birth
Transgender person	An individual whose gender identity does not align with societal expectations based on the sex assigned at birth
Two spirit	Modern term encompassing non-dichotomous gender identities among North American Indigenous people.
Sexual orientation identity	An individual's own experience of their emotional, romantic, or physical attachments, or lack thereof (e.g., asexual or aromantic persons), to other people. This cannot be assumed based on sexual behaviors (e.g., not all men who have sex with other men identify as gay, bisexual, or queer, and they may identify as straight).
Gender expression	External signifiers of an individual's gender, such as speech, gait, voice, clothing, and hairstyle. This may or may not align with cultural expectations for someone's current gender identity, or sex assigned at birth.

LGBTQIA+, Lesbian, gay, bisexual, transgender, queer, intersex, and asexual.

Perhaps even now, the presence of a chapter entitled "Care of LGBTQIA+ Patients" may imply that caring for patients is somehow different from that for general (i.e., cisgender, heterosexual) patients. Indeed, the foundation of good patient care requires balancing respect for autonomy, beneficence, non-maleficence, and justice, which should not change regardless of a patient's gender identity, sexual orientation, or sex development. Given that many LGBTQIA+ patients, however, have been traumatized in clinical settings, denied appropriate care, and excluded from our fields, they are often understandably wary of psychiatry. Given our historical role as gatekeepers who have pathologized gender and sexual diversity, specific education of clinicians about LGBTQIA+ mental health care is warranted.

MINORITY STRESS MODEL

Many health inequities have been documented among LGBTQIA+ patients. These are best understood in a culturally specific context that normalizes cisgender and heterosexual identities. Under the Minority Stress Model,[5] LGBTQIA+ people experience higher rates of depression and anxiety, not due to an inherent pathology attributable to being LGBTQIA+, but rather to minority stress experienced by gender and sexually diverse people. These stressors may be external, distal stressors (such as outright violence targeting LGBTQIA+ people), or internal proximal stressors (such as internalized negative beliefs).[6] Although some have criticized the Minority Stress Model for its emphasis on an individual's response to a societal-level process and for neglecting the root causes of such stressors, it is nevertheless a helpful lens to de-pathologize gender and sexual diversity.

Gender identity and sexual orientation identity are not the only salient facets of a person's lived experience. Ability, age, citizenship, class, ethnicity, language, race, religious/spiritual identities, and any number of other characteristics may be relevant for clinical formulation. These other aspects of a person's identity may interact with gender identity and sexual orientation identity regarding how gender and sexual norms are experienced, reinforced, or rejected. Patients may experience stressors along multiple axes of identity, and different aspects of their identities may lend different degrees of resilience to stress. It is important to understand that these different facets of identity are not simply additive but can interact in complex ways.[7] While LGBTQIA+ people experience greater rates of depression, anxiety, and thoughts of suicide compared to their cisgender and heterosexual counterparts, and American people of color (POC) are less likely to access mental health services, these are not necessarily additive. LGBTQIA+ POC do not necessarily experience worse mental health outcomes compared to their White counterparts despite experiencing minority stress along multiple axes of their identity. Despite the common perception that religion and internalized homophobia or transphobia are closely linked, religiosity is not a consistent risk factor for worse mental health outcomes of LGBTQIA+ people. Clinicians should understand internal and external conflicts as relevant to the individual patient rather than imposing preconceived notions or assumptions.

RISK FACTORS, RESILIENCE FACTORS, AND INTERSECTIONALITY

Both risk and resilience factors can be conceptualized as individual-, family-, and community-level factors.[5] Risk factors are associated with negative outcomes, while resilience or protective factors may be associated with positive outcomes or may buffer against negative outcomes.[8] Patients should not be defined solely by their risk factors, nor should their resilience be measured in metrics of capitalist success or based on an ability to adapt maximally to an oppressive environment. Nevertheless, an understanding of risk and resilience factors may provide helpful points for potential interventions.

Minority stress can lead to significant disparities that may greatly compound over the course of a lifetime. LGBTQ+ adults are more likely to have experienced adverse childhood experiences (ACEs) as children,[9] and studies of LGBTQ+ youth noted a much higher likelihood of having the highest number of ACEs (four or more) compared to non-LGBTQ+ youth.[9] The impact of ACEs has been well documented in the general population as a significant risk factor for numerous physical and mental health consequences.[10] LGB youth who experienced more than 2 ACES had over 10 times the odds of suicidal ideation and suicide attempts compared to non-LGB youth who had not experienced any ACEs.[11] LGB status seems to specifically increase the potential risk of ACEs and similar lifetime trauma, as LGB youth are more likely to experience abuse than their non-LGB siblings, and LGB adults are more likely to report psychological maltreatment and intimate partner violence.[12]

Overall, LGBTQ+ youth are at higher risk for suicidal thoughts, self-harm, depression, anxiety, and substance use.[13] Transgender youth are more likely to have been psychiatrically hospitalized.[14] LGBTQ+ patients are at higher risk of disordered eating.[15] Transgender youth experiencing gender dysphoria may be especially vulnerable to disordered eating when unable to access other medically monitored means of gender affirmation. Transgender elders are much more likely to be in overall poor physical health and more likely to experience disability, depression, and higher levels of perceived stress.[16]

In addition to the many risk factors and health disparities noted above, LGBTQ+ patients have been noted to be much less likely to endorse protective factors. LGBTQ+ patients are less likely to be insured, less likely to have a doctor, or to have received appropriate preventative care.[17] LGBTQ+ young adults who also identify as a racial or ethnic minority are more likely to lack a regular source of care.[18]

LGBTQIA+ patients commonly experience workplace discrimination and housing discrimination, and transgender POC are particularly vulnerable to such discrimination.[19] Beyond the immediate economic harms, experiences of discrimination against LGBTQ+ people have been consistently linked to worse mental health and increased thoughts of suicide.[20]

RESILIENCE FACTORS FOR LGBTQIA+ PATIENTS

In terms of protective factors (see Table 52.2), high self-esteem and self-forgiveness are associated with decreased shame, anxiety, an earlier age of recognition of LGBTQIA+ identity, and outness.[21] Identity pride and self-esteem have been consistently associated with positive mental health and positive health-promoting behaviors.[21] Family acceptance is a crucial protective factor, especially for LGBTQIA+ youth, and it is associated with higher self-esteem. Family rejection and social isolation are consistent risk factors for a greater risk of depression and suicidal behavior.[22] For patients without ties to biological kin, chosen families and other support networks may be crucial. Connections to a greater community help patients develop a sense of solidarity and belonging and may help patients contextualize their individual experience of marginalization

TABLE 52.2
Resilience Factors for LGBTQIA+ Patients

Individual	Family	Community/Societal
Positive self-regard	Family acceptance	Social connectedness
Identity-based pride	Family connectedness and support	Anti-discrimination legislation
Health-promoting behaviors		Anti-bullying/anti-discrimination school policies
Proactive coping styles		Gender-Sexuality Alliance (GSA) groups
Cognitive ability to mediate stress		
Spirituality		

LGBTQIA+, Lesbian, gay, bisexual, transgender, queer, intersex, and asexual.

into a larger historical context and develop a sense of solidarity and belonging rather than despair.

Not all protective factors are equally protective for all patients. Although school connectedness and the presence of supportive adults were protective for white transgender youth, this was not found to be a protective factor for Black or Latine transgender youth.[23] In a study of adult men, connection to the LGBTQ+ community had a stronger role in mediating the relationship with stress for white respondents compared to the POC respondents surveyed in the study.[24] Despite this potential lack of protective effects conferred by connection to LGBTQIA+ community, LGBTQIA+ POC are not more likely to experience negative mental health outcomes compared to their white peers, suggesting that POC may acquire factors for resilience earlier in life related to their experience of being an ethnic or racial minority, which helps adults cope with stressors experienced later in life related to their LGBTQIA+ identities.[24]

Although LGBTQIA+ patients face numerous challenges, there can also be protective sociopolitical factors and policies. LGB youth attending schools with Gender-Sexuality Alliance (GSA) groups, and protective policies around anti-bullying and anti-discrimination, were significantly less likely to attempt suicide than students attending schools without GSA groups or such policies.[25] LGB residents of states without legal protections for sexual minorities were more likely to

endorse symptoms of depression and anxiety compared to those residing in states with such protections.[26]

Resilience factors are not static, but rather qualities that may be actively cultivated, social connections that may be built, and policies that may be advocated for. By taking an actively affirming stance, clinicians can challenge internalized homophobia or transphobia, counter negative stereotypes about being LGBTQIA+, encourage connection to the greater community, and help foster self-esteem and identity pride. Clinicians and institutions can also advocate for public health policies and protections for LGBTQIA+ patients that will help to create a more equitable and safer environment for all patients.

LGBTQIA+ AFFIRMATIVE CARE

Given the centrality of risk and resilience factors to a patient's overall well-being, an LGBTQIA+ affirmative stance is a crucial part of working with LGBTQIA+ patients (see Table 52.3). LGBTQIA+ affirmative care does not mean prioritizing a patient's gender identity or sexual orientation identity at the expense of the patient's other identities, nor does it imply conceptualizing the totality of a patient's difficulties through the lens of gender- and sex-related factors. Clinicians should seek to cultivate a nuanced understanding of how a person's gender identity, sexual orientation, and sex development may play an important role in their life and may interact with other aspects of their identity, sometimes in ways that may produce conflicts. The patient must ultimately work to resolve these conflicts and to integrate each part of themselves into a cohesive whole and need not "take sides" regarding their own lived experience.

LGBTQIA+ affirmative mental health care aims to counteract the ubiquitous and life-long anti-LGBTQIA+ messages a patient may have internalized.[27] LGBTQIA+ affirmative therapy is not in contradiction to an integrative, or person-centered approach to therapy. Both therapeutic approaches, however, stand in contrast to controversial efforts to change gender identity or sexual orientation ("reparative therapy" or "conversion therapy"). Such efforts are opposed by most medical and professional groups and illegal in clinical settings in many US jurisdictions, although they occur with a high prevalence, particularly for transgender adults across the country.[28,29]

TABLE 52.3
Strategies for Affirming Mental Health Care

Affirming Mental Health Care for LGBTQIA+ People

Clinician-Level Interventions:
- Use the correct name and pronouns
- Use non-judgmental language
- Avoid making assumptions (e.g., gender-inclusive language instead of "wife/husband"—spouse/partner(s)/significant other; instead of "mother/father"—parents, caregivers, or guardians; not assuming specific family structures)

System-Level Interventions:
- Create welcoming healthcare environments (e.g., with signs, pins, artwork, and diverse representation in photography)
- Provide inclusive forms for demographic information and collections of sexual orientation and gender identity data: pronouns, affirmed name, sex assigned at birth, gender identity, sexual orientation, organ inventories, etc.
- Use correct names on all patient-facing documentation (including meal tickets, medication administration, wristbands)
- Provide the uninterrupted continuation of gender-affirming hormones (e.g., administration of gonadotropin-releasing hormone analogs, estradiol, testosterone if not on hospital formulary then mechanisms for administration of home medications)
- Provide LGBTQIA+-specific training and support for staff and trainees
- Create and disseminate anti-discrimination policies for sexual orientation, gender identity, and gender expression

Community-Level Interventions:
- Partner with LGBTQIA+ community organizations
- Involve community and patient representatives as stakeholders in assessing and meeting clinical needs
- Advocate for the health needs of LGBTQIA+ patients in public health policy

LGBTQIA+, Lesbian, gay, bisexual, transgender, queer, intersex, and asexual.

While patients and families should be advised on the negative impact of change efforts, which cause significant psychological harm,[27,28,30] including increased risk of suicide,[28] clinicians should understand that patients and families often seek such services with good intentions. Many patients and families experience genuine distress when grappling with sexual orientation or gender identity, particularly in the early phases of identity development. Patients cite deeply held religious beliefs that they believe conflict with their sexual orientation or gender identity and that are often not adequately addressed in secular settings, such as traditional psychotherapy. POC, immigrants,[31] and patients and families of lower socioeconomic status are more likely to have sought out change efforts,[32] likely due in part to the historical mistrust of medical institutions, a lack of familiarity with counselors or physicians, and a lack of access to appropriately affirming care due to economic factors, such as a lack of insurance.[33] Patients often cite seeking acceptance, connection, and a sense of belonging during change efforts, due to their isolation from their faith

communities or their families; however, benefits that patients perceive in change efforts, such as a sense of community, can be provided more effectively and sustainably in an identity-affirming context. Patients may find it helpful to explore options outside of therapy with affirming congregations or clergy, with other LGBTQIA+ POC, and with LGBTQIA+ people of faith to find positive examples of peers who have navigated similar identity conflicts.

SPECIFIC POPULATIONS
Working With Youth and Families

All families have an enormous influence on the health and well-being of their children. This includes nuclear families comprised of biological parents and siblings, and extended kin relationships (such as aunts, uncles or grandparents, adoptive families, and non-kin guardians). For LGBTQIA+ youth, as family acceptance can be a significant protective factor against depression, suicide, and high-risk behaviors (such as substance use disorders),[34] direct clinical care with family systems merits special mention. Working with families is integral to the care of pediatric patients and may also be important for many young adults who remain on their parents' insurance, reside with family members, or have impairments in their capacity to provide informed consent for gender-affirming care. In the treatment of adult patients, working with intimate partners may also be relevant to care.

Most common clinical dilemmas arise when the patient and the family are at odds about the patient's LGBTQIA+ identity. Clinicians can help bridge this gap by facilitating communication and providing education (particularly in countering misinformation about being LGBTQIA+). Even affirming families, however, may have complex feelings and understandable concerns that require support. Separate sessions for the patient and the family can be helpful to provide family members with their own dedicated time to process feelings and address their concerns more frankly, without subjecting one another to questions that may seem invalidating or rejecting. Parents of LGBTQIA+ youth are also at risk of rejection and stigma from their extended family members and community at large; thus, they may also benefit from support from parent peers through organizations such as their local Parents, Families, and Friends of Lesbians and Gays (PFLAG) chapter.

LGBTQIA+ ELDERS

In the United States, there are over 2.7 million adults aged 50 years or older who identify as LGBTQIA+. LGBTQIA+ seniors have endured a lifetime of marginalization and continue to face many challenges in meeting their needs. This is particularly reflected in the economic disparities experienced by many LGBTQIA+ seniors: 40% of LGB+ seniors and nearly 50% of transgender adults above the age of 50 live at or below 200% of the federal poverty line.[35] With same-sex unions only recently being legalized, LGBTQIA+ older adults also experience significantly lower rates of marriage[36] and are more likely to age alone compared to heterosexual seniors,[37] which puts them at greater risk of social isolation and economic distress. Housing and long-term care placement are an area of significant concern for LGBTQIA+ adults, to the point that a survey of transgender adults noted respondents

who reported they were planning to take their own life before reaching old age.[38]

For same-sex couples whose partners died before same-sex marriage was legalized, the surviving partner is not eligible to receive Social Security Survivor benefits and is often ineligible for their partner's retirement or other survivor's benefits or inheritance. LGBTQIA+ seniors, like younger adults, often avoid seeking care altogether due to concerns about poor treatment or lack of expertise and die at younger ages compared to their heterosexual and cisgender counterparts.[37] Although chosen families and friendships are undoubtedly important, LGBTQIA+ seniors may be at greater risk of social isolation than their married, heterosexual, and cisgender peers. Even for seniors with strong chosen families and social networks, as friends tend to age simultaneously, they may be unable to care for one another as they age. Additionally, friends and non-married partners typically lack the benefits of a legally recognized kin relationship (such as family leave, shared health insurance plans and benefits, and proxy decision-making powers).

LGBTQIA+ education is as pertinent for geriatric and adult psychiatrists as it is for child and adolescent psychiatrists, and many surveys note concerns about a lack of training and familiarity as a major reason for which LGBTQIA+ seniors may decline medical care. In addition to providing LGBTQIA+-affirming psychiatric care in all age settings, clinicians should help facilitate social connections, particularly with other LGBTQIA+ seniors, advocate for LGBTQIA+-affirming services in nursing homes and long-term facilities, and expand age-appropriate programming for LGBTQIA+ seniors.

PATIENTS RECEIVING GENDER-AFFIRMING MEDICAL AND SURGICAL TREATMENTS

Being transgender and accessing medical or surgical affirmations are not synonymous, nor are medical or surgical affirmations universally desired by all transgender and gender-diverse patients. Gender-affirming medical and surgical treatments (GAMST), however, may be an important part of the affirmation process for many transgender and gender-diverse patients. Gender-affirming care includes pubertal suppressants (i.e., gonadotrophin-releasing hormone agonists—GnRHAs), hormones (e.g., estradiol, testosterone, progestins), and a variety of procedures that include chest surgery, phalloplasty, vaginoplasty, and many more. There is no set sequence for gender affirmation, which should be tailored to the individual's gender embodiment goals.

Although medications used for gender-affirming hormone therapy (GAHT) do not have a specific FDA indication for gender affirmation, they have been safely used with cisgender patients for a variety of indications for many years (see Table 52.4). Appropriately monitored GAMST has been shown to be safe and effective. Severe side effects and serious adverse events are very rare.[39] GAMST is also linked with numerous benefits and improvements in health outcomes. GAMST has been associated with many positive outcomes across the lifespan for people who can access it, including improvements in global functioning,[40] decreased depression and anxiety,[41] decreased suicidality,[42,43] improved body image,[44] and decreased behavioral dysregulation.[45] Given the many demonstrated benefits of gender affirmation for those patients who seek it, delaying care should not be seen as a neutral choice.

POTENTIAL PSYCHIATRIC IMPACTS OF GAHT

The current literature indicates that the impact of GAHT on psychological functioning is generally positive. Psychiatric diagnoses should not be interpreted as contraindications for GAHT unless the condition is impairing the person's capacity to provide informed consent (e.g., a patient who is acutely psychotic or manic and unable to engage in a meaningful informed consent discussion). Psychiatric co-morbidities should be treated concurrently with gender affirmation, rather than being a barrier to accessing gender affirmation.

Estrogen: Patients may report transient mood changes with the initiation of GAHT, though it should be noted that this is usually not perceived negatively.[46] Patients should be advised to remain consistent with their estradiol adherence. It may be helpful to adjust to a daily patch or oral dosing rather than relying on estradiol injections if mood fluctuations seem to consistently correlate with injection schedules.

Progesterone: Progesterone is at times assumed to negatively impact mood; however, this has not been consistently shown in prospective, randomized controlled trials.[47] For most cisgender patients taking exogenous progesterone, there is no conclusive link between progesterone and negative psychiatric effects, although some patients may be more sensitive to certain types of progestins (e.g., androgenic progestins, different formulations).[48]

Testosterone: Past versions of the World Professional Association for Transgender Health's (WPATH) Standards of Care (SOC) listed mania/hypomania or psychotic symptoms as a "possibly increased risk" for those patients on testosterone-based GAHT with underlying psychiatric disorders. This has been removed from the newest SOC,[49] as this initial risk was linked to supraphysiologic doses of testosterone. Medically monitored GAHT and testosterone

TABLE 52.4
Gender-Affirming Hormonal Therapies and Procedures

Gender-Affirming Hormone Therapy	Gender-Affirming Surgeries/Procedures
GnRHAs: may be used for pubertal suppression with children and adolescents at Tanner stage 2 or in adults as an anti-androgen (e.g., histerelin, leuprolide, goserelin)	Facial surgeries (e.g., brow reconstruction, rhinoplasty, genioplasty, lip/cheek fillers)
Estradiol, testosterone: major sex hormones used to induce desired changes in secondary sex characteristics	Chondrolaryngoplasty ("tracheal shave")
	Chest surgery/mastectomy or breast augmentation ("top surgery")
Progesterones: used alone in patients assigned female sex at birth for menstrual suppression (e.g., norethindrone) or as adjunctive therapy with estradiol	Phalloplasty, metoidioplasty, vaginoplasty, vulvoplasty ("bottom surgery")
	Orchiectomy, hysterectomy/oophorectomy
Spironolactone: a commonly used anti-androgen in North America	Body contouring
	Hair removal (e.g., needed for phalloplasty, vaginoplasty/vulvoplasty)

replacement therapy for hypogonadal cisgender males consist of testosterone doses within the physiological range.[41] The prior concern originated in part from cases of exogenous testosterone use, violence, and psychiatric symptoms, which typically involved regimens that included multiple synthetic anabolic steroids at more than 10 times the physiologic dose.[50] There does not appear to be a consistent relationship between serum testosterone levels among transgender and gender-diverse patients and anger, or even necessarily a prior psychiatric diagnosis.[51]

The impact of hormones—whether endogenous or exogenous—on mental health is undoubtedly complex. Additionally, such changes may be driven at least in part by cultural expectations, gender norms, and social stress commonly experienced by patients at the beginning of the affirmation process. For most patients, mood fluctuations appear to be transient and most noticeable at the beginning of treatment and may be addressed by changing GAHT dosing or intervals.[41]

GnRHAs: In both children with central precocious puberty and gender dysphoria, the use of GnRHAs generally has not been shown to increase behavioral or emotional issues. For children with gender dysphoria, the use of GnRHAs has been linked with improved behavioral dysregulation. Similarly, in a study of transgender adults receiving GnRHAs and estrogen, none of the participants reported depression as a side effect.[52]

POTENTIAL MEDICATION INTERACTIONS FOR GAHT

Both testosterone and estradiol are primarily metabolized by CYP 3A4.[53,54] Medications that induce or inhibit CYP 3A4 may cause unexpected changes to serum hormone levels. Enzyme-inducing anti-epileptic drugs (AEDs) can induce hepatic metabolism and increase serum levels of sex hormone–binding globulins,[55] which can potentially decrease the proportion of bioactive-free hormone and may decrease the efficacy of GAHT. Estradiol increases hepatic glucuronidation and can decrease levels of serum lamotrigine.[56]

Estradiol, testosterone, and GnRHAs are all associated with changes in body composition and metabolism (see Tables 52.5 and 52.6). Both estrogen and testosterone are associated with an increase in total body weight: estrogen is associated with increased

TABLE 52.5
Medications That Affect Hormone Levels

Medications That May Increase Testosterone or Estradiol Levels	Medications That May Decrease Testosterone or Estradiol Levels	Other Interactions
CYP 3A4 Inhibitors Fluvoxamine Nefazodone Suboxone	**CYP 3A4 Inducers** Modafinil St. John wort Tobacco Topiramate **Enzyme-Inducing AEDs** Carbamazepine Oxcarbazepine Topiramate Phenobarbital	**Lamotrigine:** Level decreased by estrogen and some progestins **Lithium:** Level increased by spironolactone

body fat percentage and decreased lean body mass, while testosterone is associated with decreased body fat and increased lean body mass.[57] GnRHAs have been linked with weight gain among transgender and gender-diverse youth,[58] although this effect may be at least in part due to the body composition of transgender and gender-diverse youth compared to cisgender peers of their affirmed gender. Typically children assigned male sex at birth tend to have lower body fat percentages than those assigned female sex at birth.[59] Transgender boys experience a decrease in their body fat percentage with initiation of GnRHAs (while cisgender boys typically remain stable); transgender girls tend to gain more body fat than cisgender girls.[59] In addition to the potential metabolic and body composition changes due to GAHT, transgender and gender-diverse patients are less likely to meet the recommended daily minimum for exercise,[60,61] due to both internal factors (such as dysphoria) and external factors (such as a lack of inclusive and safe facilities). Clinicians should be aware of the potential metabolic impacts of psychiatric medications and help counsel patients on addressing modifiable risk factors and reducing polypharmacy whenever possible.

For testosterone, transient elevations in liver enzymes can be quite common, though serious hepatotoxicity is rare.[62] Of the psychiatric medications, antipsychotics can similarly cause a benign elevation

TABLE 52.6
Overlapping Side Effect Profiles of GAHT and Psychiatric Medications

Estrogen-Based Regimens

Adapted From WPATH SOC8		Psychiatric Medications
Likely increased	Venous thromboembolism (VTEs) Hypertriglyceridemia Weight gain	Antipsychotics—VTEs, dyslipidemia, weight gain Amitriptyline, mirtazapine, paroxetine—weight gain Lithium, valproic acid—weight gain
Likely increased with additional risk factors	Cerebrovascular disease Cardiovascular disease Polyurea/dehydration (spironolactone) Cholelithiasis	Lithium—polyurea Clonidine, guanfacine, propranolol—decreased blood pressure
Possibly increased	Hypertension Erectile dysfunction	SSRIs, SNRIs, antipsychotics—erectile dysfunction, sexual side effects
Possibly increased with additional risk factors	Lower bone mass density (BMD)/osteoporosis Hyperprolactinemia	Antipsychotics—lower BMD, elevated prolactin

Testosterone-Based Regimens

Adapted From SOC8		Psychiatric Medications
Likely increased	Polycythemia Acne Hypertension Sleep apnea Weight gain Decreased high-density lipoprotein, increased low-density lipoprotein	Antipsychotics—VTEs, dyslipidemia, weight gain Amitriptyline, mirtazapine, paroxetine—weight gain Lithium, tricyclic antidepressants, SSRIs, quetiapine—acne
Possibly increased with additional risk factors	Type 2 diabetes	Antipsychotics—elevated risk of type 2 diabetes
Other	Elevated liver enzymes	Antipsychotics—elevated liver enzymes

GAHT, Gender-affirming hormone therapy; SOC, standards of care; SNRIs, serotonin-norepinephrine reuptake inhibitors; SSRIs, selective serotonin reuptake inhibitors; WPATH, World Professional Association for Transgender Health.

in liver enzymes. Carbamazepine, valproic acid, and lamotrigine have all been linked with various hepatic effects, such as elevated liver enzymes, hyperammonemia, and rare cases of liver failure.[63]

While testosterone typically increases libido and sexual satisfaction in transgender and gender-diverse patients, those on estrogen-based regimens for GAHT may experience lowered libido and erectile dysfunction.[64] Both are common side effects of many psychiatric medications, particularly selective serotonin reuptake inhibitors (SSRIs)/serotonin-norepinephrine reuptake inhibitors (SNRIs) and antipsychotics.[65] Patients taking spironolactone as their anti-androgen may require additional monitoring for blood pressure with clonidine, guanfacine, propranolol, and

antipsychotics, particularly clozapine, chlorpromazine, and quetiapine.[66]

LETTERS OF SUPPORT FOR GENDER-AFFIRMING SURGERIES

Historically, psychiatrists and other mental health professionals have been gatekeepers to GAMST, a role that has been viewed as mostly harmful and unnecessary by patients. Mental health assessments were intended to prevent regret, particularly about irreversible surgical procedures. Current studies of transgender adults undergoing gender-affirming surgery show rates of regret are very low, and that cessation of gender-affirming care is most often due to external factors, such as discrimination and rejection.[67] The most recent WPATH guidelines reflect the shift toward a patient-centered, informed consent approach to gender-affirming surgeries, and recommend that if a letter is required to recommend such treatment, only one should be required.[49] Nevertheless, many health insurances in the United States still require letters for reimbursement of gender-affirming surgery and may remain an insurance requirement for the foreseeable future, given the challenge of disseminating the WPATH SOC8 for widespread uptake and adoption by third-party payors and surgical practices. These assessment sessions may be less aversive and more helpful to the patient if the clinician adopts an autonomy- and informed consent-based approach, which focuses not on establishing that the patient is transgender or gender diverse or that they meet an arbitrary level of suffering or distress, but rather on helping the patient understand the benefits and risks of the desired procedure, whether it would be a realistic way to achieve the patient's gender embodiment goal, and helping the patient begin to plan for a major surgical procedure that will likely necessitate significant dedication of their time, energy, social supports, and resources. Such an approach allows for more frank discussions of the patient's concerns and feelings (including ambivalence), rather than incentivizing the patient to try to fit the clinician's preconception of the normative transgender experience to achieve clearance as a surgical candidate (see Table 52.7).

Most patients report improved quality of life and satisfaction with gender-affirming surgery procedures,[68,69] though specific rates of complications vary by procedure. Clinicians writing letters of support should become familiar with the procedure requested by the patient and the general risks and complications. Patients may wish to pursue fertility preservation

---

TABLE 52.7
Clearance for Surgical Candidacy

Areas of Assessment	Relevance
Medical history/family history	Identification of potential medically complicating factors (e.g., bleeding, clotting disorders)
Surgical history	Knowledge of past reactions to anesthesia and surgery, ability to cope with physical distress
Psychiatric history	Identification of potentially psychiatrically complicating factors in informed consent (e.g., cognitive disorders, psychosis, mania) Knowledge of the potential for exacerbation in stressful post-operative period Identification of mental health supports and treatment team (if needed)
Gender embodiment goals/current dysphoria	Enhancement of the understanding of the patient's current goals, wishes for their body
Substance use history	Facilitating quitting of smoking for optimal healing Identification of post-operative withdrawal risk, potential medication interactions
Understanding the risks of surgery	Helping to educate the patient on the specific risks of surgery Empowering the patient to request further information from the surgeon (e.g., rates of specific complications, typical recovery course)
Social history – Finances – Insurance coverage – Time off work/school – Supports	Helping the patient plan for affording surgery, time off to recover Ensuring consistent insurance coverage through the post-operative period Identification of social supports to help with activities of daily living, emotional supports, transportation to/from hospital or clinic post-operatively Planning for activity restrictions
Patient's concerns, feelings of loss/ grief, ambivalence	Exploring the patient's worries about the procedure and the potential outcomes and help to communicate with the surgeon about these concerns Although regret is rare, there can be feelings of loss or grief Anticipating transiently worsening dysphoria in the context of physical changes and healing, or when complications occur, or pre-operatively if needing to stop GAHT

GAHT, Gender-affirming hormone therapy.

before gonadectomies. Given the importance of after-care and post-surgical follow-up, clinicians should help patients plan as thoroughly as possible, especially if traveling long distances for gender-affirming surgeries.

LGBTQIA+ RESOURCES

Given the numerous socioeconomic and health disparities experienced by LGBTQIA+ patients, clinicians may find that they often need to help connect patients to community resources to meet their needs.

While local resources are likely the most important and helpful daily, however, these are less feasible to compile in a general textbook. Fortunately, most major cities have at least one LGBTQIA+ community center, which is generally an excellent starting point for accessing or learning about local formal and informal resources, such as lists of LGBTQIA+ health clinics and individual-practice clinicians, inclusive shelters/housing, intimate partner violence resources, affirming clothing closets, and mutual aid organizations, to name a few. These centers may also provide health services themselves, such as testing for sexually transmitted infections, preventative health screenings, and support groups.

On the national level, the National Center for Transgender Equality has excellent guides for name and gender marker changes, and LGBTQIA+ legal issues (https://transequality.org/). Trevor Project offers a 24/7 crisis line for LGBTQIA+ youth and a safe social media space (https://www.thetrevorproject.org). Trans Lifeline is a trans-led and staffed hotline that does not practice non-consensual rescue (https://translifeline.org) and can help patients feel much more at ease about utilizing a hotline.

CONCLUSION

The term LGBTQIA+ encompasses numerous complex and varied gender identities, sexual orientation identities, and sex development experiences of people with diverse socioeconomic, cultural, racial, and ethnic backgrounds, and should not be considered a monolith. Such a broad term to describe a vast range of people potentially runs the risk of flattening individual lived experience to one facet of identity held in common, defined against culturally normalized heterosexual and cisgender identities. Nevertheless, it is still a helpful

term to conceptualize psychiatric care for gender and sexually diverse people who experience similar and overlapping marginalization and oppression. This is far from an exhaustive resource on LGBTQIA+ psychiatry. Much more research remains to be done to improve the quality of care for our LGBTQIA+ patients on the nuances and long-term outcomes of GAMST, psycho-pharmacological studies for patients on concurrent GAHT, application, and modification of psychotherapy for LGBTQIA+ patients, inclusive and accurate training of students and clinicians, and quality improvement to make mental healthcare systems more equitable. We hope this chapter serves as a starting point for clinicians who provide mental health care that affirms LGBTQIA+ people, with an aspiration toward liberation.

REFERENCES

1. Engels F. *Origin of the Family, Private Property, and the State.* Marx/Engels Internet Archive; 1884.
2. Drescher J. Queer diagnoses: parallels and contrasts in the history of homosexuality, gender variance, and the diagnostic and statistical manual. *Arch Sex Behav.* 2010;39(2):427–460.
3. Drescher J. Out of DSM: depathologizing homosexuality. *Behav Sci.* 2015;5(4):565–575.
4. Beek TF, Cohen-Kettenis PT, Kreukels BP. Gender incongruence/gender dysphoria and its classification history. *Int Rev Psychiatry.* 2016;28(1):5–12.
5. Testa RJ, Habarth J, Peta J, et al. Development of the gender minority stress and resilience measure. *Psychol Sex Orientat Gend Divers.* 2015;2(1):65–77.
6. Mongelli F, Perrone D, Balducci J, et al. Minority stress and mental health among LGBT populations: an update on the evidence. *Minerva Psichiatr.* 2019;60(1):27–50.
7. Cyrus K. Multiple minorities as multiply marginalized: applying the minority stress theory to LGBTQ people of color. *J Gay Lesbian Mental Health.* 2017;21(3):194–202.
8. Colpitts E, Gahagan J. The utility of resilience as a conceptual framework for understanding and measuring LGBTQ health. Int J Equity Health. 2016;15(60):1–8. https://www.ncbi.nlm.nih.gov/pmc/articles/PMC4822231/
9. Craig SL, Austin A, Levenson J, et al. Frequencies and patterns of adverse childhood events in LGBTQ+ youth. *Child Abuse Negl.* 2020;107:104623.
10. Kalmakis KA, Chandler GE. Health consequences of adverse childhood experiences: a systematic review. *J Am Assoc Nurse Pract.* 2015;27(8):457–465.
11. Clements-Nolle K, Lensch T, Baxa A, et al. Sexual identity, adverse childhood experiences, and suicidal behaviors. *J Adolesc Health.* 2018;62(2):198–204.
12. Balsam KF, Rothblum ED, Beauchaine TP. Victimization over the life span: a comparison of lesbian, gay, bisexual, and heterosexual siblings. *J Consult Clin Psychol.* 2005;73(3):477–487.

13. Russell ST, Fish JN. Mental health in lesbian, gay, bisexual, and transgender (LGBT) youth. *Annu Rev Clin Psychol*. 2016;12:465–487.

14. Reisner SL, Vetters R, Leclerc M, et al. Mental health of transgender youth in care at an adolescent urban community health center: a matched retrospective cohort study. *J Adolesc Health*. 2015;56(3):274–279.

15. Parker LL, Harriger JA. Eating disorders and disordered eating behaviors in the LGBT population: a review of the literature. *J Eat Disord*. 2020;8:51.

16. Fredriksen-Goldsen KI, Cook-Daniels L, Kim HJ, et al. Physical and mental health of transgender older adults: an at-risk and underserved population. *Gerontologist*. 2014;54(3):488–500.

17. Dilley JA, Simmons KW, Boysun MJ, et al. Demonstrating the importance and feasibility of including sexual orientation in public health surveys: health disparities in the Pacific Northwest. *Am J Public Health*. 2010;100(3):460–467.

18. Macapagal K, Bhatia R, Greene GJ. Differences in healthcare access, use, and experiences within a community sample of racially diverse lesbian, gay, bisexual, transgender, and questioning emerging adults. *LGBT Health*. 2016;3(6):434–442.

19. Kattari SK, Whitfield DL, Walls NE, et al. Policing gender through housing and employment discrimination: comparison of discrimination experiences of transgender and cisgender LGBQ individuals. *J Soc Social Work Res*. 2016;7(3):427–447.

20. Sutter M, Perrin PB. Discrimination, mental health, and suicidal ideation among LGBTQ people of color. *J Couns Psychol*. 2016;63(1):98–105.

21. Perrin PB, Sutter ME, Trujillo MA, et al. The minority strengths model: development and initial path analytic validation in racially/ethnically diverse LGBTQ individuals. *J Clin Psychol*. 2020;76(1):118–136.

22. Yadegarfard M, Meinhold-Bergmann ME, Ho R. Family rejection, social isolation, and loneliness as predictors of negative health outcomes (depression, suicidal ideation, and sexual risk behavior) among Thai male-to-female transgender adolescents. *J LGBT Youth*. 2014;11(4):347–363.

23. Vance SR Jr, Boyer CB, Glidden DV, et al. Mental health and psychosocial risk and protective factors among Black and Latinx transgender youth compared with peers. *JAMA Netw Open*. 2021;4(3):e213256.

24. McConnell EA, Janulis P, Phillips 2nd G, et al. Multiple minority stress and LGBT community resilience among sexual minority men. *Psychol Sex Orient Gend Divers*. 2018;5(1):1–12.

25. Hatzenbuehler ML. The social environment and suicide attempts in lesbian, gay, and bisexual youth. *Pediatrics*. 2011;127(5):896–903.

26. Hatzenbuehler ML, Keyes KM, Hasin DS. State-level policies and psychiatric morbidity in lesbian, gay, and bisexual populations. *Am J Public Health*. 2009;99(12):2275–2281.

27. Tozer EE, McClanahan MK. Treating the purple menace: ethical considerations of conversion therapy and affirmative alternatives. *Couns Psychol*. 1999;27(5):722–742.

28. Turban JL, Beckwith N, Reisner SL, Keuroghlian AS. Association between recalled exposure to gender identity conversion efforts and psychological distress and suicide attempts among transgender adults. *JAMA Psychiatry*. 2020;77(1):68–76.

29. Turban JL, King D, Reisner SL, Keuroghlian AS. Psychological attempts to change a person's gender identity from transgender to cisgender: estimated prevalence across US states, 2015. *Am J Publ Health*. 2019;109(10):1452–1454.

30. Haldeman DC. Therapeutic antidotes: helping gay and bisexual men recover from conversion therapies. *J Gay Lesbian Psychother*. 2002;5(3-4):117–130.

31. Ryan C, Toomey RB, Diaz RM, et al. Parent-initiated sexual orientation change efforts with LGBT adolescents: implications for young adult mental health and adjustment. *J Homosex*. 2020;67(2):159–173.

32. Meanley S, Haberlen SA, Okafor CN, et al. Lifetime exposure to conversion therapy and psychosocial health among midlife and older adult men who have sex with men. *Gerontologist*. 2020;60(7):1291–1302.

33. Hipp TN, Gore KR, Toumayan AC, et al. From conversion toward affirmation: psychology, civil rights, and experiences of gender-diverse communities in Memphis. *Am Psychol*. 2019;74(8):882–897.

34. Katz-Wise SL, Rosario M, Tsappis M. Lesbian, gay, bisexual, and transgender youth and family acceptance. *Pediatr Clin North Am*. 2016;63(6):1011–1025.

35. SAGE MAP. *Understanding Issues Facing LGBT Older Adults*. Available at: <https://www.lgbtmap.org/policy-and-issue-analysis/understanding-issues-facing-lgbt-older-adults>; 2017.

36. Houghton A. *Maintaining Dignity. A Survey of LGBT Adults Age 45-plus*. 2018. AARP. https://www.aarp.org/dignitysurvey.

37. Ware S. Health care inequalities surrounding LGBTQ elder care. *J Adv Gen Soc Work Pract*. 2020;15(1):1–14.

38. Ward R, Rivers I, Sutherland M. *Lesbian, Gay, Bisexual, and Transgender Ageing: Biographical Approaches for Inclusive Care and Support*. Jessica Kingsley Publishers; 2012.

39. Mahfouda S, Moore JK, Siafarikas A, et al. Gender-affirming hormones and surgery in transgender children and adolescents. *Lancet Diabetes Endocrinol*. 2019;7(6):484–498.

40. Nguyen HB, Chavez AM, Lipner E, et al. Gender-affirming hormone use in transgender individuals: impact on behavioral health and cognition. *Curr Psychiatry Rep*. 2018;20(12):110.

41. Davis SA, St. Amand C. Effects of testosterone treatment and chest reconstruction surgery on mental health and sexuality in female-to-male transgender people. *Int J Sexual Health*. 2014;26(2):113–128.

42. Allen LR, Watson LB, Egan AM, et al. Well-being and suicidality among transgender youth after gender-affirming hormones. *Clin Practice Pediatr Psychol*. 2019;7(3):302–322.

43. Turban JL, King D, Carswell JM, Keuroghlian AS. Pubertal suppression for transgender youth and risk of suicidal ideation. *Pediatrics*. 2020;145(2):e20191725.

44. Grannis C, Leibowitz SF, Gahn S, et al. Testosterone treatment, internalizing symptoms, and body image dissatisfaction in transgender boys. *Psychoneuroendocrinology*. 2021;132(10):53–58.

45. de Vries AL, Steensma TD, Doreleijers TA, et al. Puberty suppression in adolescents with gender identity disorder: a prospective follow-up study. *J Sex Med*. 2011;8(8):2276–2283.

46. Randolph JF. Gender affirming hormone therapy for transgender females. *Clin Obstetr Gynecol.* 2018;61(4):705–721.

47. Prior JC. Progesterone is important for transgender women's therapy-applying evidence for the benefits of progesterone in ciswomen. *J Clin Endocrinol Metab.* 2019;104(4):1181–1186.

48. Standeven LR, McEvoy KO, Osborne LM. Progesterone, reproduction, and psychiatric illness. *Best Pract Res Clin Obstet Gynaecol.* 2020;69:108–126.

49. Coleman E, Radix AE, Bouman WP, et al. Standards of care for the health of transgender and gender diverse people, Version 8. *Int J Transgend Health.* 2022;23(suppl 1):S1–S259.

50. Johnson JM, Nachtigall LB, Stern TA. The effect of testosterone levels on mood in men: a review. *Psychosomatics.* 2013;54(6):509–514.

51. Defreyne J, Kreukels B, T'Sjoen G, et al. No correlation between serum testosterone levels and state-level anger intensity in transgender people: results from the European Network for the Investigation of Gender Incongruence. *Horm Behav.* 2019;110:29–39.

52. Dittrich R, Binder H, Cupisti S, et al. Endocrine treatment of male-to-female transsexuals using gonadotropin-releasing hormone agonist. *Exp Clin Endocrinol Diabetes.* 2005;113(10):586–592.

53. Kuhl H. Pharmacology of estrogens and progestogens: influence of different routes of administration. *Climacteric.* 2005;8(suppl 1):3–63.

54. Usmani KA, Tang J. Human cytochrome P450: metabolism of testosterone by CYP 3A4 and inhibition by ketoconazole. *Curr Protocols in Toxicol.* 2004;20(1):4.13.1–9.

55. Isojarvi JIT, Tauboll E, Herzog AG. Effect of antiepileptic drugs on reproductive endocrine function in individuals with epilepsy. *CNS Drugs.* 2005;19(3):207–223.

56. Johnson EL, Kaplan PW. Caring for transgender patients with epilepsy. *Epilepsia.* 2017;58(10):1667–1672.

57. T'Sjoen G, Arcelus J, Gooren L, et al. Endocrinology of transgender medicine. *Endocr Rev.* 2019;40(1):97–117.

58. Jensen RK, Jensen JK, Simons LK, et al. Effect of concurrent gonadotropin-releasing hormone agonist treatment on dose and side effects of gender-affirming hormone therapy in adolescent transgender patients. *Transgend Health.* 2019;4(1):300–303.

59. Klaver M, de Mutsert R, Wiepjes CM, et al. Early hormonal treatment affects body composition and body shape in young transgender adolescents. *J Sex Med.* 2018;15(2):251–260.

60. Lee JY, Finlayson C, Olson-Kennedy J, et al. Low bone mineral density in early pubertal transgender/gender diverse youth: findings from the Trans Youth Care Study. *J Endocr Soc.* 2020;4(9):bvaa065.

61. Alzahrani T, Nguyen T, Ryan A, et al. Cardiovascular disease risk factors and myocardial infarction in the transgender population. *Circ Cardiovasc Qual Outcomes.* 2019;12(4):e005597.

62. Velho I, Fighera TM, Ziegelmann PK, et al. Effects of testosterone therapy on BMI, blood pressure, and laboratory profile of transgender men: a systematic review. *Andrology.* 2017;5(5):881–888.

63. Sedky K, Nazir R, Joshi A, et al. Which psychotropic medications induce hepatotoxicity? *Gen Hosp Psychiatry.* 2012;34(1):53–61.

64. Holmberg M, Arver S, Dhejne C. Supporting sexuality and improving sexual function in transgender persons. *Nat Rev Urol.* 2019;16(2):121–139.

65. Smith S. Drugs that cause sexual dysfunction. *Psychiatry.* 2007;6(3):111–114.

66. Turban JL, Kamceva M, Keuroghlian AS. Psychopharmacologic considerations for transgender and gender diverse people. *JAMA Psychiatry.* 2022;79(6):629–630.

67. Wu CA, Keuroghlian AS. Moving beyond psychiatric gatekeeping for gender-affirming surgery. *JAMA Surg.* 2023;158(3):231–232.

68. Akhavan AA, Sandhu S, Ndem I, et al. A review of gender affirmation surgery: what we know, and what we need to know. *Surgery.* 2021;170(1):336–340.

69. Almazan AN, Keuroghlian AS. Association between gender-affirming surgeries and mental health outcomes. *JAMA Surg.* 2021;156(7):611–618.

53

BUILDING INTERDISCIPLINARY COLLABORATIONS ACROSS HEALTHCARE SETTINGS

VICTORIA A. GRUNBERG, MS, PHD ■ KATHERINE A. McDERMOTT, PHD ■ HEENA R. MANGLANI, PHD ■ CHRISTINA L. RUSH, PHD ■ JULIA E. HOOKER, PHD ■ KATE N. JOCHIMSEN, PHD, ATC ■ ANA-MARIA VRANCEANU, PHD

BACKGROUND

The biopsychosocial model of disease is a guiding framework for contemporary health care.[1] This model of care requires healthcare professionals (e.g., physicians, nurses, physical/occupational therapists, clinical psychologists, social workers, chaplains) to work together to treat the whole person—that is, their physical, psychological, social, and spiritual health.[2] Because people are living longer with more chronic conditions, this interdisciplinary approach (also known as integrated or interprofessional care) is needed to address the highly co-morbid physical (e.g., pain, illness), psychological (e.g., stress, depression, health behavior attitudes, adherence) and social challenges that patients and their families experience across the lifespan.[3] In addition to treating disease, interdisciplinary teams can help patients cope with a new diagnosis, adhere to treatment, prevent and manage symptoms, promote healthy living, and engage with resources and support.[2] Interdisciplinary care has been associated with better treatment engagement, improved patient outcomes, fewer medical visits, and lower healthcare costs across primary care settings,[4,5] pediatric units,[6] gastrointestinal clinics,[7] and rehabilitation centers.[8]

For decades, research has demonstrated that psychological (affective, behavioral, and cognitive) and social factors impact the development and management of disease. It is well established that behavioral lifestyle factors (e.g., smoking, diet, exercise, sleep) can increase the risk for chronic illnesses and shorten life expectancy.[9,10] In addition, emotional distress (e.g., depression, anxiety) has been linked to poorer medical adherence, increased healthcare utilization, worse physical functioning, and lower health-related quality of life.[11–14] Cognitive (e.g., beliefs, attitudes) and social factors (e.g., relationships, resources) can also influence risk for, and prognosis of, medical conditions, such as cancer, cardiovascular disease, chronic pain,[15] diabetes, and neurological diseases.[1] Together, this work has helped inform the development of behavioral health interventions for medical populations[16–18]—that have been shown to improve health outcomes and reduce hospital utilization (~2.5 days) and costs (saving $2205/person).[19]

Despite the clear need, interdisciplinary care has yet to be fully adopted across healthcare settings, such as acute and surgical medical units[20] and community health settings. To implement interdisciplinary models of care, we need to use theories to inform practice, relationships to promote collaborations, science to demonstrate value and cost-effectiveness, and education to promote interprofessional teamwork. In this chapter, we outline current barriers to the implementation of interdisciplinary care. We also discuss general and specific approaches to building interdisciplinary collaborations. Finally, we conclude with lessons learned.

BARRIERS TO INTERDISCIPLINARY CARE

Several barriers can impede the implementation of interdisciplinary care. First, there is a clear gap between theory and implementation. Although many integrated care frameworks have been developed, few have been applied and tailored to practice. Second, interdisciplinary care requires a shift in healthcare organization and culture. Given how specialized health care has become, silos among disciplines need to be bridged to provide team-based care. Third, healthcare funding is currently based on pathological diagnoses.[21] Therefore, funding often poses a challenge and may require support from leadership. We describe each barrier in more detail below.

Theory to Implementation Gap

Thirty-seven integrated care theoretical frameworks have been developed, yet only 6% have led to clinical initiatives.[22] Without clinical application, it is difficult to evaluate the efficacy of these models and determine how to tailor them to different populations and settings. Because there is no "one-size-fits-all" solution, interdisciplinary care models need to be tailored to specific populations, teams, units, and systems.[23] Each organization needs to determine: (1) team member roles and responsibilities, (2) ways to effectively and efficiently communicate, (3) procedures for treatment decision-making and delivery, (4) strategies for sharing resources, (5) governance structure for interprofessional coordination, (6) implementation strategies that overcome administrative, social, and financial barriers to integrating clinical and research initiatives, and (6) methods for the evaluation or assessment of such initiatives. Clear and agreed-on procedures—that are informed by a strong framework yet tailored to the population and setting—can help ensure that care is coordinated and cohesive.

A Paradigm Shift

Implementation requires a paradigm change in how we view and deliver health care.[24] Our healthcare system has become focused on treating patients with a certain condition and training providers in specialties. This approach has created a fragmented system; unfortunately, a lack of coordination leads to inefficient allocation of resources—which negatively impacts healthcare quality, cost, and outcomes.[25] A cultural shift in how we approach healthcare service and education is needed to fully adopt interdisciplinary approaches.

At the educational level, the performance of teams (rather than individuals) and collaboration and communication skills need to be taught and rewarded appropriately. In addition, education and training should be geared toward the prevention of illness and promotion of health, rather than only treating disease.[25] At the service level, endorsement and reinforcement of team-based approaches from leaders of hospitals, departments, and units is essential.[25] Leaders can help by promoting shared values and goals, mutual trust, and systems to assess and evaluate team efficiency and efficacy. They also need to ensure that all team members understand the value of integrating care and are aware of, and educated on each other's roles and responsibilities. For example, behavioral health providers have historically been considered an 'ancillary' or 'dispensable' service in medical settings. Team members need to know that behavioral health providers can help reduce patients' risk for morbidities and rehospitalizations, promote treatment adherence, improve staff-patient-family communication, and address staff distress.[26] Mutual understanding and respect for each team members' roles and contributions are necessary for effective collaboration.

Need for Resources

Infrastructure and resources are needed to build and sustain interdisciplinary care. To be successful, a long-term plan for sharing resources and allocating funding is important. However, existing reimbursement models do not adequately support team-based care. In the United States, the dominant fee-for-service (FFS) billing model is tied to the volume of procedures provided directly to the patients.[21] Given that team-based models combine services with activities (e.g., referrals, documentation) and collaborations (e.g., care coordination, meetings, consultations), it is difficult to bill for these services in the FFS model.[21] Alternative models, such as bundled rates or per-member-per-month payments, may help make team-based care sustainable.[21,27] Grant, foundation, or philanthropic funding can also help develop, assess, and refine integrated care models. However, they are competitive and may not necessarily lead to sustainable changes in clinical care. Given these challenges, advocacy, policy changes, and research demonstrating the cost-effectiveness will help incentivize interdisciplinary models of care.

AN APPROACH TO MOVE TOWARDS INTERDISCIPLINARY CARE

Although the above-mentioned barriers may require structural or socio-political changes, having research and clinical services demonstrate the benefit of inter-disciplinary care is a valuable first step. To facilitate these collaborations, it is important to build trust and relationships among professionals, create a team vision and goals, communicate frequently, and share resources (e.g., personnel, space). Integrating psychosocial care also requires interdependence, newly created professional activities, flexibility, collective ownership of goals, and a reflective process.[28]

At the Massachusetts General Hospital (MGH) Center for Health Outcomes and Interdisciplinary Research (CHOIR), the goal is to break silos and promote interdisciplinary care across medical and community settings. We develop, test, and implement psychosocial interventions for medical populations across the lifespan. Currently, our interdisciplinary team (e.g., clinical psychologists, psychiatrists, athletic trainers) is building collaborations across diverse healthcare settings (e.g., neurology, orthopedics, geriatrics, pediatrics, community health care, skilled nursing facilities). We use clinical, research, and/or education to address the unique needs of varied populations and units. This tailored approach can offer a roadmap for building mutually beneficial and sustainable collaborations, integrating psychosocial providers into clinic workflows, and using research to promote biopsychosocial care.

Below, we describe a general framework for how we have integrated psychosocial care into healthcare units or clinics. Then, we offer specific examples that illustrate the development and implementation of clinical research that meets the unique needs of each setting.

General Framework for Integrating Psychosocial Care

Assessment is a crucial first step for evaluating needs and establishing "buy-in" from all partners, including leadership, providers, staff, and patients/families. Needs assessments (e.g., informal meetings, interviews with staff or patients, self-report surveys) can help gather information on the clinical needs of patients, staff, and the unit. They can provide information related to

(1) psychosocial challenges of patients, families, and/or staff, (2) current clinical services and research projects, (3) gaps in care, (4) barriers and facilitators to providing biopsychosocial care, and (5) resources needed to integrate care. This information can inform the services (e.g., higher level psychosocial care), key personnel (e.g., clinical psychologists, social workers), procedures (e.g., warm handoff to clinical psychologists and outpatient therapists), and outputs (e.g., intervention programs, pre-/post-treatment data).

Qualitative data (e.g., focus groups, interviews) can provide in-depth information on challenges faced by patients, family members, and staff, as well as processes for implementing care. Further, patient-reported outcome measures (PROMs, e.g., depression, anxiety) using electronic health record systems (e.g., EPIC) can be a valuable way to assess biopsychosocial functioning. Clinicians and researchers can also brainstorm ways to embed PROMs within clinical visits to serve as pilot data for grant submissions. Grants can help support personnel and allocate the time needed for program development, refinement, and evaluation.

Next, personnel need to be integrated into the clinic flow. This requires an understanding of daily operations/meetings, what services the clinician could offer and to whom, and the timing of care. For example, a psychologist may offer individual, dyadic, or group therapy programs for patients and families, support groups to staff, and "on-the-fly" consultations to teams. After establishing services, it is important to tailor them to the needs of the unit.

Finally, services should be assessed at regular intervals. This can inform the adaptations needed to optimize them and adjust based on socio-contextual factors (e.g., COVID-19). For example, after implementing a screening initiative, clinics may recognize that triage systems are needed to ensure that patients receive adequate and efficient care. In addition, informal and formal feedback on such initiatives can enhance feasibility, patient engagement, and interprofessional teamwork.

EXAMPLES OF INTERDISCIPLINARY COLLABORATIONS

Interprofessional partnerships, clinical assessments, clinical and research interdisciplinary initiatives, evaluation of such initiatives, and flexible adaptations can help inform and sustain interdisciplinary models of care. To help illustrate how interdisciplinary collaborations can be developed, we present examples from the MGH's CHOIR. Below, we describe several successful interdisciplinary initiatives and those that are underway.

Neurosciences Intensive Care Unit

The Neuroscience Intensive Care Unit (Neuro-ICU) provides 24-hour neurocritical care to individuals who have experienced life-threatening neurological injuries or illnesses (e.g., stroke, traumatic brain injury). This hospitalization can be traumatic for patients and their families (e.g., caregivers). About 20% to 40% of patients experience depression, anxiety, and post-traumatic stress during and after hospitalization.[29] This unit is also stressful for staff—with up to 50% reporting burnout.[30] Despite this need, psychosocial services are limited.

Nearly a decade ago, the MGH Neuro-ICU clinic staff observed high levels of stress among patients and families. This stress negatively impacted staff burnout, morale, and turnover. To improve the unit, the Neuro-ICU Chief contacted the CHOIR Founding Director (Vranceanu), a clinical health psychologist who develops resiliency interventions for medical populations. Together, they developed an ongoing interdisciplinary partnership. Our integration was successful because of shared goals, mutual trust, accountability, and shared responsibilities and resources.[22,31,32] Fig. 53.1 presents our framework for this integration.

We began by offering clinical psychosocial services to patients, families, and staff. A part-time embedded clinical psychologist (0.2 full-time equivalent or ~1 day/week) conducted bedside assessments, delivered psychotherapy to patients and/or families, provided consultation for psychosocially complex patients, and led support sessions for staff.

Dr. Vranceanu and colleagues secured funding to conduct research to develop psychosocial programming. We conducted a prospective survey to better understand the risk and resiliency factors associated with emotional distress among patients and families. Next, we conducted qualitative interviews with staff to learn their perspectives on treatment needs and the preferences of patients, families, and staff. These data

helped inform the Recovering Together (RT) intervention, a six-session, skills-based resiliency intervention for patients with acute neurological illnesses and their informal caregivers (i.e., "dyads") to prevent chronic emotional distress.[29,33] We conducted a single-blind randomized clinical trial (RCT), comparing RT with an attention-matched educational control in the Neuro-ICU to test for feasibility. RT was feasible, acceptable, and exhibited preliminary efficacy.[29] Simultaneously, we started the training component. The part-time embedded psychologist spent 2 to 4 hours/week training clinical psychology fellows. Having trainees deliver the intervention allows us to offer more services to the unit, support the research, and help them build clinical, research, and collaboration skills necessary for their training.[32]

Currently, with National Institutes of Health funding and trainee support, we are testing RT in a fully powered efficacy-effectiveness RCT (Fig. 53.1; years 9+). We have recruited 102 dyads (of 200) and will analyze outcomes both individually and dyadically.[34] If it is effective, we hope to disseminate RT to other ICUs to enhance healthcare outcomes. We hope that RT and this framework (Fig. 53.1) can serve as a model for sustainable psychosocial care in acute medical settings.

Neonatal Intensive Care Unit

The Neonatal Intensive Care Unit (NICU) provides critical care to babies who were born preterm (before 37 weeks gestation) and/or experienced complex medical complications (e.g., respiratory distress syndrome, intraventricular hemorrhage, necrotizing enterocolitis).[35] As babies fight for their lives, parents are fearful and anxious about their future, grieving the loss of their expected childbirth experience, and feeling guilty and helpless about how to care for their baby. The stressful milieu of the NICU is evidenced by the fact that ~50% of parents experience depression, anxiety, and post-traumatic stress[36] and up to 50% of staff report burnout.[37]

A clinical psychologist at CHOIR (Grunberg) whose work is focused on NICU families sought out a collaboration with the Chief of the Mass General for Children's Newborn Medicine. This interdisciplinary partnership has set the foundation for building psychosocial research, care, and training in this setting.

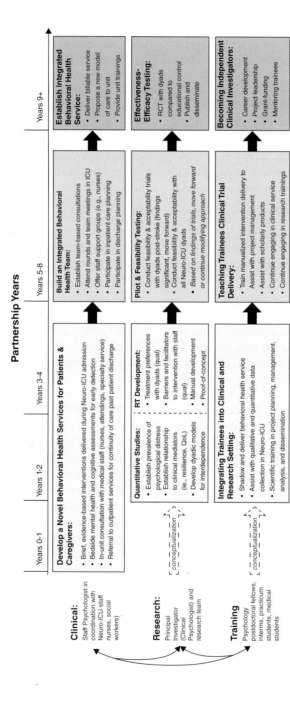

Fig. 53.1 ■ Clinical, research, and training (CRT) framework for recovering together (RT) initiative. *ICU*, Intensive care unit; *QoL*, quality of life; *RCT*, randomized clinical trial.

This integration has been successful because of leadership support, shared goals and vision, mutual trust, frequent informal and formal communication, and shared resources. To build the infrastructure, we conducted preliminary studies to assess the need (via a prospective mixed-methods survey); hired a full-time research coordinator to support this and other research in the unit; built relationships with multidisciplinary staff; and secured federal funding to build a resiliency intervention for parent couples in the NICU. This work is underway and has the potential to improve the standard of NICU family-centered care.[38]

Orthopedic Clinics

About half of orthopedic patients develop chronic pain after traumatic injuries (e.g., fractures, joint dislocations).[39] Psychosocial health factors including pain catastrophizing (ruminating and magnifying pain they feel helpless to overcome), pain anxiety (excessive pain-related worry and attention), and activity avoidance (forgoing participating in valued life activities) are key predictors of chronic pain.[39] Given the psychosocial needs of this population, Dr. Vranceanu developed research collaborations with several orthopedic units across the United States.

Vranceanu and colleagues[39,40] developed the Toolkit for Optimal Recovery (TOR), a four-session, virtual program that aims to reduce the risk for chronic pain. In this program, patients learn psychoeducation about pain and skills, such as relaxation techniques (e.g., mindful awareness of pain, body scanning), adaptive thinking and restructuring, physical activity pacing, and strategies to promote value-based living. In single site[39] and multi-site[41] feasibility trials, TOR exceeded feasibility benchmarks and demonstrated preliminary efficacy in preventing chronic pain. Having a cohesive interdisciplinary team (clinical psychologists, rehabilitation providers, surgeons, and nurses) helped translate this research into practice. However, the successful implementation of TOR required multiple iterations and ongoing collaboration.

In the early stages of developing TOR, several factors interfered with implementing psychosocial care in this setting. These included the biomedical focus of orthopedic care, limited time with patients, and lack of training and comfort in addressing psychosocial factors by providers.[40,41] We conducted focus groups to develop strategies to overcome these barriers to implementation.[40] We learned several key strategies that helped promote feasibility: (1) having a clinical research coordinator embedded in the clinic helped to streamline recruitment and reduce the burden on staff, (2) offering TOR virtually helped increase access for patients, and (3) having study champions (e.g., orthopedic surgeons), incentive structures, and regular check-ins helped promote staff buy-in. Future multi-site trials will test the efficacy and effectiveness of TOR in promoting physical function following orthopedic trauma.

ALS Clinic

Amyotrophic lateral sclerosis (ALS) is a devastating, progressive, terminal illness. About 50% of patients and their care partners endorse clinically significant distress.[42] To address this need, a clinical psychology investigator at CHOIR (Rush) developed a research and clinical collaboration with the Sean M. Healey & AMG Center for ALS at MGH.

In the initial stages of this partnership, the focus was on understanding the clinic's needs and flow. Through informal meetings with leadership, focus groups with staff, and interviews with patients and their families, Dr. Rush gathered information about patient and family mental health challenges, gaps in care, and strategies for successful implementation. In addition, it has been important to understand and integrate into the unit. We shadowed providers, delivered talks to the department and clinic, met with leadership monthly to discuss the clinic status (e.g., hiring waves, provider load, adjustments desired to the recruitment process, education on ALS), and disseminated this work in collaboration with ALS providers. Dr. Rush also secured research funding to support the assessment and preliminary development of a psychosocial intervention for patients with ALS and their care partners. In addition, a clinical service is actively being established. To create such a service, strategies to overcome barriers are key (e.g., insurance requirements, protected effort for therapists, in-clinic versus virtual care, establishing a referral and waitlist process). This partnership has flourished because of the flexibility, collaboration, and persistence of interdisciplinary providers and researchers working together to address gaps in psychosocial care.

MS Clinic

Multiple sclerosis (MS) is a progressive neurological disease that increases the risk of depression, anxiety, fatigue, pain, and sleep difficulties.[43] To address these challenges, a CHOIR clinical psychologist specializing in MS (Manglani) built a clinical and research collaboration with the MGH MS Clinic. First, Dr. Manglani conducted a needs assessment and learned that there was a long waitlist for psychosocial care. She then developed a proposal for the clinic, which included purposes, goals, clinical services, research studies, resources, and funding. Initially, the MS clinic director helped fund this initiative. Shortly thereafter, they were able to secure philanthropy funding to support this work. Currently Dr. Manglani provides brief (six to eight sessions), individual, dyadic, and group psychotherapy to patients and their families. This service has helped increase access to psychosocial care and improve the efficiency of clinical operations. Dr. Manglani is also leading mixed-methods research that can help evaluate and inform new programming. As more clinics seek to embed psychosocial care, it is important to balance clinical efforts with research—it can help assess, inform, and enhance clinical care. It is important to note that when Dr. Manglani started this collaboration, she was a trainee, and therefore her time and effort were supported by the MS clinic. Since becoming licensed, she has been able to bill insurance for her services. This process demonstrates how interdisciplinary collaborations can support training and help create sustainable interdisciplinary care.

COMMUNITY PRIMARY CARE

Chronic pain is most prevalent and disabling among older, underserved adults in the community, yet our pain interventions have largely been developed in affluent, mostly White samples. Seeking to bridge this gap between existing research and clinical need, we partnered with MGH-Revere HealthCare Center (RHC) to develop an intervention (Improving Health for Older Adults with Pain through Engagement) to improve health and well-being among older adults with chronic pain.

RHC is a primary care clinic that provides healthcare services (e.g., internal medicine, physical therapy, mental health) to an economically and ethnically diverse population of patients. The study team, led by Drs. Ana-Maria Vranceanu (CHOIR) and Christine Ritchie, connected with the RHC medical director, who identified a need for psychosocial programming for patients with chronic pain. To address this need, we adapted a mind-body intervention for chronic pain (GetActive) for this setting. GetActive is a group intervention that teaches mind-body skills (e.g., deep breathing, mindfulness, cognitive restructuring, quota-based pacing) to increase engagement in physical activity. Groups are facilitated by a mental health provider (psychologist or social worker) and a nurse practitioner (NP). In addition to co-leading the group, the NP provides brief medical check-ins either individually (for English-speaking groups) or collectively (for Spanish-speaking groups). We used this shared medical visit model so that psychoeducation, skills, and medical treatment could be presented in one setting. Shared medical visits improve social connection and reduce costs by integrating care.

When building this collaboration, the first step was to connect with the clinic's medical staff to learn about current programming and patient needs. However, the demands of this setting made it difficult to meet regularly. Therefore we needed to be flexible and adjust our approach to integration. For example, we conducted focus groups and interviews with staff during existing meetings and encouraged them to come and go as needed. We also met with primary care physicians, nurses, physical therapists, mental health providers, and medical interpreters whenever we fit into their schedules. Meeting with staff was key because they provided insight into barriers and facilitators that would impact integrated programming. They described barriers, such as limited training and time more stress, and lower health literacy among patients. They also shared facilitators, such as the importance of integrating into the clinic flow, using existing referral systems, social connection with both patients and providers and being flexible in delivery (e.g., encouraging group attendance regardless of homework completion).

This information helped inform an open pilot of GetActive+ for both English and Spanish-speaking older adults. Support from clinic champions (primary care physicians) has helped encourage providers to refer patients to this program. Buy-in for this work has also been strengthened by the positive feedback that patients have shared with their providers. Providers have also been encouraged by the program after seeing this benefit for their patients—especially those who typically lack access to psychosocial care.

LESSONS LEARNED

Our experiences building interdisciplinary collaborations have emphasized the importance of: (1) building relationships, (2) ongoing communication, (3) identifying the unique needs of the setting, (4) working within existing clinic structures, (5) being flexible and pragmatic, and (6) combining the utility of research and clinical work to enhance patient care.

Success across these settings has been possible because of relationships and communication. Support from clinic leadership was important for establishing projects, including access to protected time and resources. Further, connections with clinical staff have been crucial for integration (e.g., providing feedback and referrals). Having a member of the study staff embedded in the medical setting or clinic staff to champion the study helped enable recruitment and retention.

We also learned the importance of conducting needs assessments and/or using qualitative methods to understand the unique needs, barriers, and facilitators to integrated care in each setting. Involving stakeholders early in the process helps ensure that the interventions are tailored to clinic needs and can be integrated into the existing clinic flow. For example, Neuro-ICU (RT) and NICU staff highlighted that support from the clinical team has been key for integrating into such fast-paced, high-acuity settings. The ALS and MS collaborations created psychosocial clinics that could offset clinical burdens and continue to grow research that can help inform new interventions. Providing services to the clinic helps build trust and cohesion among teams, enabling a pathway for formal and informal communication, and helping to inform research and, in turn, funding sources to further integrate care.

Flexibility and pragmatism were key across all settings. For example, in the orthopedic and community clinics, provider time was limited. As a result, we had to work within existing meeting schedules or conduct meetings and interviews with providers at varying times. We also adapted our interventions depending on staff input and clinic needs. For example, community clinic providers shared that they had limited time to provide education or skills; therefore we increased the psychoeducation component of our intervention to support both patients and staff.

CONCLUSIONS

To fully adopt the biopsychosocial model of care, we need interdisciplinary teams to work together to treat the whole person. Given the current limitations in reimbursement models, structural changes are needed to promote this approach. However, systemic changes to healthcare require changes across all levels—individual, team, and system. To move towards this model, we described specific strategies for building individual and team interdisciplinary collaborations across diverse settings. Future work is needed to examine the efficacy, efficiency, and cost-effectiveness of such programs. We encourage researchers, clinicians, and administrators to work together to enhance the quality and accessibility of interdisciplinary health care.

REFERENCES

1. Bolton D, Gillett G. *The biopsychosocial model 40 years on. The Biopsychosocial Model of Health and Disease.* Springer International Publishing; 2019:1–43. https://doi.org/10.1007/978-3-030-11899-0_1.
2. Jansen L. Collaborative and interdisciplinary health care teams: ready or not? *J Prof Nurs.* 2008;24(4):218–227. https://doi.org/10.1016/j.profnurs.2007.06.013.
3. Zonneveld N, Driessen N, Stüssgen RA, et al. Values of integrated care: a systematic review. *Int J Integr Care.* 2018;18(4): Accessed January 21, 2024. https://www.ncbi.nlm.nih.gov/pmc/articles/PMC6251066/.
4. Lanoye A, Stewart KE, Rybarczyk BD, et al. The impact of integrated psychological services in a safety net primary care clinic on medical utilization. *J Clin Psychol.* 2017;73(6):681–692. https://doi.org/10.1002/jclp.22367.
5. Godoy L, Long M, Marschall D, et al. Behavioral health integration in health care settings: lessons learned from a pediatric hospital primary care system. *J Clin Psychol Med Settings.* 2017;24(3-4):245–258. https://doi.org/10.1007/s10880-017-9509-8.
6. Shafran R, Bennett SD, McKenzie Smith M. Interventions to support integrated psychological care and holistic health outcomes in paediatrics. *Healthcare.* 2017;5:44.
7. Lores T, Goess C, Mikocka-Walus A, et al. Integrated psychological care reduces health care costs at a hospital-based inflammatory bowel disease service. *Clin Gastroenterol Hepatol.* 2021;19(1):96–103.

8. Shields GE, Wells A, Doherty P, et al. Cost-effectiveness of cardiac rehabilitation: a systematic review. *Heart*. Available from: <https://heart.bmj.com/content/early/2018/04/13/heartjnl-2017-312809.info?versioned=true>. Published online 2018.

9. Li Y, Pan A, Wang DD, et al. Impact of healthy lifestyle factors on life expectancies in the US population. *Circulation*. 2018; 138(4):345–355. https://doi.org/10.1161/CIRCULATIONAHA.117.032047.

10. Li Y, Schoufour J, Wang DD, et al. Healthy lifestyle and life expectancy free of cancer, cardiovascular disease, and type 2 diabetes: prospective cohort study. *BMJ*. 2020:368. https://www.bmj.com/content/368/bmj.l6669.short.

11. Cook JA, Grey D, Burke J, et al. Depressive symptoms and AIDS-related mortality among a multisite cohort of HIV-positive women. *Am J Public Health*. 2004;94(7):1133–1140. https://doi.org/10.2105/AJPH.94.7.1133.

12. Carney RM, Freedland KE, Miller GE, et al. Depression as a risk factor for cardiac mortality and morbidity: a review of potential mechanisms. *J Psychosom Res*. 2002;53(4):897–902.

13. McLaughlin TP, Khandker RK, Kruzikas DT, et al. Overlap of anxiety and depression in a managed care population: prevalence and association with resource utilization. *J Clin Psychiatry*. 2006;67(8):1187–1193.

14. Katon WJ, Rutter C, Simon G, et al. The association of comorbid depression with mortality in patients with type 2 diabetes. *Diabetes Care*. 2005;28(11):2668–2672.

15. Goudman L, Vets N, Jansen J, et al. The association between bodily functions and cognitive/emotional factors in patients with chronic pain treated with neuromodulation: a systematic review and meta-analyses. *Neuromodulation Technol Neural Interface*. 2023;26(1):3–24. https://doi.org/10.1016/j.neurom.2021.11.001.

16. Tsai AC, Morton SC, Mangione CM, et al. A meta-analysis of interventions to improve care for chronic illnesses. *Am J Manag Care*. 2005;11(8):478.

17. Viswanathan M, Golin CE, Jones CD, et al. Interventions to improve adherence to self-administered medications for chronic diseases in the United States: a systematic review. *Ann Intern Med*. 2012;157(11):785. https://doi.org/10.7326/0003-4819-157-11-201212040-00538.

18. Feliu-Soler A, Cebolla A, McCracken LM, et al. Economic impact of third-wave cognitive behavioral therapies: a systematic review and quality assessment of economic evaluations in randomized controlled trials. *Behav Ther*. 2018;49(1):124–147.

19. Wilson DK, Sweeney AM. The role of behavioral medicine in integrated healthcare. In: Duckworth MP, O'Donohue WT, eds. *Behavioral Medicine and Integrated Care*. Springer International Publishing; 2018:9–27. https://doi.org/10.1007/978-3-319-93003-9_2.

20. Wade DT, Halligan PW. The biopsychosocial model of illness: a model whose time has come. *Clin Rehabil*. 2017;31(8):995–1004. https://doi.org/10.1177/0269215517709890.

21. *Reimbursement Mechanisms Challenges*. Available from: <https://aspe.hhs.gov/sites/default/files/documents/2e04001edc7cdbf57e00766c149bb100/reimbursement-mechanisms-challenges-brief.pdf>

22. Peterson K, Anderson J, Bourne D, et al. Health care coordination theoretical frameworks: a systematic scoping review to increase their understanding and use in practice. *J Gen Intern Med*. 2019;34(suppl 1):90–98. https://doi.org/10.1007/s11606-019-04966-z.

23. Maruthappu M, Hasan A, Zeltner T. Enablers and barriers in implementing integrated care. *Health Syst Reform*. 2015;1(4): 250–256. https://doi.org/10.1080/23288604.2015.1077301.

24. O'Reilly P, Lee SH, O'Sullivan M, et al. Correction: assessing the facilitators and barriers of interdisciplinary team working in primary care using normalisation process theory: an integrative review. *PLoS One*. 2017;12(7):e0181893.

25. Enthoven AC. Integrated delivery systems: the cure for fragmentation. *Am J Manag Care*. 2009;15(12):S284.

26. Possemato K, Johnson EM, Beehler GP, et al. Patient outcomes associated with primary care behavioral health services: a systematic review. *Gen Hosp Psychiatry*. 2018;53:1–11.

27. Mose JN, Jones CB. Alternative payment models and team-based care. *N C Med J*. 2018;79(4):231–234.

28. Bronstein LR. A model for interdisciplinary collaboration. *Soc Work*. 2003;48(3):297–306. https://doi.org/10.1093/sw/48.3.297.

29. Vranceanu AM, Bannon S, Mace R, et al. Feasibility and efficacy of a resiliency intervention for the prevention of chronic emotional distress among survivor-caregiver dyads admitted to the neuroscience intensive care unit: a randomized clinical trial. *JAMA Netw Open*. 2020;3(10):e2020807. https://doi.org/10.1001/jamanetworkopen.2020.20807.

30. Bienvenu OJ. Is this critical care clinician burned out? *Intensive Care Med*. 2016;42(11):1794–1796. https://doi.org/10.1007/s00134-016-4497-y.

31. Lawrence PR, Lorsch JW. Differentiation and integration in complex organizations. *Adm Sci Q*. 1967;12(1):1–47. https://doi.org/10.2307/2391211.

32. Lester EG, Grunberg VA, Bannon SM, et al. The Recovering Together initiative: integrating psychosocial care into ICUs. *NEJM Catal*. 2022;3(8). https://doi.org/10.1056/CAT.22.0103.

33. Vranceanu AM, Woodworth EC, Kanaya MR, et al. The Recovering Together study protocol: a single-blind RCT to prevent chronic emotional distress in patient-caregiver dyads in the neuro-ICU. *Contemp Clin Trials*. 2022;123:106998. https://doi.org/10.1016/j.cct.2022.106998.

34. Cook WL, Kenny DA. The actor–partner interdependence model: a model of bidirectional effects in developmental studies. *Int J Behav Dev*. 2005;29(2):101–109. https://doi.org/10.1080/01650250444000405.

35. *Common Conditions Treated in the NICU*. Available from: <https://www.marchofdimes.org/find-support/topics/neonatal-intensive-care-unit-nicu/common-conditions-treated-nicu>.

36. Roque ATF, Lasiuk GC, Radünz V, et al. Scoping review of the mental health of parents of infants in the NICU. *J Obstet Gynecol Neonatal Nurs JOGNN*. 2017;46(4):576–587. https://doi.org/10.1016/j.jogn.2017.02.005.

37. Tawfik DS, Phibbs CS, Sexton JB, et al. Factors associated with provider burnout in the NICU. *Pediatrics*. 2017;139(5): https://publications.aap.org/pediatrics/article-abstract/139/5/e20164134/38839.

38. Grunberg VA, Vranceanu AM, Lerou PH. Caring for our caretakers: building resiliency in NICU parents and staff. *Eur J*

Pediatr. 2022;181(9):3545–3548. https://doi.org/10.1007/s00431-022-04553-1.

39. Vranceanu AM, Jacobs C, Lin A, et al. Results of a feasibility randomized controlled trial (RCT) of the Toolkit for Optimal Recovery (TOR): a live video program to prevent chronic pain in at-risk adults with orthopedic injuries. *Pilot Feasibility Stud.* 2019;5(1):30. https://doi.org/10.1186/s40814-019-0416-7.

40. Vranceanu AM, Bakhshaie J, Reichman M, et al. Understanding barriers and facilitators to implementation of psychosocial care within orthopedic trauma centers: a qualitative study with multidisciplinary stakeholders from geographically diverse settings. *Implement Sci Commun.* 2021;2(1):102. https://doi.org/10.1186/s43058-021-00208-8.

41. Bakhshaie J, Doorley J, Reichman M, et al. Optimizing the implementation of a multisite feasibility trial of a mind–body program in acute orthopedic trauma. *Transl Behav Med.* 2022;12(5):642–653. https://doi.org/10.1093/tbm/ibac004.

42. Fisher P, Dodd R, Barrow E, et al. Predictors of distress in amyotrophic lateral sclerosis: a systematic review. In: Rodriguez-Blazquez C, ed. *Cogent Psychol.* 2019;6(1):1608031. https://doi.org/10.1080/23311908.2019.1608031.

43. Hyarat SY, Subih M, Rayan A, et al. Health related quality of life among patients with multiple sclerosis: the role of psychosocial adjustment to illness. *Arch Psychiatr Nurs.* 2019;33(1):11–16. https://doi.org/10.1016/j.apnu.2018.08.006.

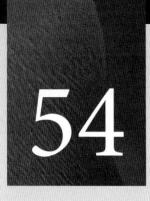

54

MANAGEMENT OF A PSYCHIATRIC CONSULTATION SERVICE

FELICIA A. SMITH, MD ■ JOHN B. TAYLOR, MD, MBA ■ THEODORE A. STERN, MD

OVERVIEW

This chapter aims to give inpatient consultation-liaison (C-L) practitioners an understanding of the complex business aspects of their work. Appropriately adhering to the often-confusing guidelines for reimbursement can be challenging for clinicians and expose them to time-consuming and stressful audits and substantial penalties, both personally and for their institutions. In this atmosphere, providing ethical, legal, and clinically astute services can be daunting. A fuller understanding of coding and billing will also help psychiatrists, C-L hospital-based programs, and hospital administrators collect the appropriate reimbursement for services rendered. In this chapter, we address principles of coding, billing, and documentation to improve medical documentation by C-L clinicians, as well as enhance clinical outcomes and economic benefits accrued by general hospitals due to smoothly running C-L services. Assessment, assurance, and improvement of the C-L service's quality will also be discussed.

DOCUMENTATION SHOULD REFLECT THE SERVICE PERFORMED

Successful C-L services rely on cooperative and collaborative relationships with medical colleagues. Hospital-based physicians are exposed to psychiatric co-morbidity daily. Consultations may be requested for guidance regarding the creation of differential diagnosis recommendations for evaluation and treatment or approaches to inpatient care when behavioral issues exist. The needs of a physician do not always mirror

the severity of the patient's medical condition. Billing, however, is geared to the patient's illness. Although a medical service may purchase a psychiatrist's time and involvement based on their expertise or to guarantee a readily available psychiatrist, the insurance company or other third-party payer is paying solely for a service provided to an individual patient (rather than purchasing a clinician's expertise).

BILL ONLY FOR SERVICES DOCUMENTED IN THE MEDICAL RECORD

The overriding principle for third-party reimbursement is to bill only for those services that are documented in the medical record. The charge for service and the reimbursement for that service are guided by definitions established by Current Procedure Terminology (CPT) codes. A brilliant, life-saving consultation that goes undocumented is not billable. Given the current healthcare landscape, significant pressure may be placed on clinicians to "maximize revenue" for the services they provide. "Up-coding" (i.e., charging for a more intensive service than delivered) is illegal and unethical. On the other hand, inadvertent "down-coding" on account of the complicated documentation and billing rules is also unfair and ultimately damages the ability of hospitals and providers to care for patients. While the effectiveness and expertise of the consultant are also of significant importance from a clinical perspective, understanding coding and billing requirements is an important, and practical, aspect of consulting work.

FOLLOW THE MEDICARE GUIDELINES FOR ALL ENTRIES IN THE MEDICAL RECORD

Medicare is the predominant insurance coverage in most general hospitals. CPT codes were developed by the American Medical Association (AMA) and adopted by the Health Care Financing Administration in the early 1990s. Current guidelines dictate that Evaluation and Management CPT codes (which are not specific to psychiatry but cover psychiatric hospital-based and outpatient encounters), along with the 10th revision of the International Statistical Classification of Diseases and Related Health Problems, are to be used for billing. These mandatory guidelines, established for Medicare and Medicaid billing, are essentially universal in that they apply to most insurance plans. More importantly, Medicare guidelines for reimbursement are the strictest among insurance plans. Adhering to the Medicare guidelines ensures that the provider will be following the requirements of all insurance plans for appropriate coding and reimbursement purposes.

Documentation requirements for inpatient psychiatric and consultation services are different (in form and content) from the documentation that might be employed in outpatient practices. Codes for billing inpatient or emergency department (ED) consultations are based on either Medical Decision-Making (MDM) or Time Based. A premium is paid for thoroughness and attention to the complexity of the problems being addressed, the data reviewed, and the risk of complications. The critical ingredients of a note that are congruent with an appropriate billing code will be addressed in the section on documentation and coding.

OBTAIN PREAUTHORIZATION FOR SERVICES WHENEVER NECESSARY

Although mental health parity was mandated by the 2010 Patient Protection and Affordable Care Act, mental health coverage is often governed by insurance carve-outs and may require prior authorization. Health insurance companies vary in their requirements for precertification (i.e., permission to provide a consultation before the service is delivered to enable payment for that service). Although Medicare does not require precertification, some carve-out behavioral

health organizations do. A patient may be authorized by the primary insurance carrier for medical admission, which authorizes payment for all physicians who perform medical consultations, save for the psychiatric team but requires specific and separate authorization from the carve-out company for payment for the psychiatric consultation. Critical to the financial viability of C-L services is the management and monitoring of the billing and collection of third-party claims and the understanding that the billing and authorization process for each payer is essential to receive payment for services rendered.

IDENTIFY THE PAYER

During the admission process, most hospitals will identify the patient's primary, secondary, and supplementary insurance coverage. The managers of a C-L service must understand how each type of insurance adjudicates claims for professional services. In many cases, health insurance claims for hospital services are separated into two components: the technical or hospital charges, and the professional or physician charges. Some insurers link these charges together, whereas others bill them separately. Payments for each component are based on a previously negotiated fee schedule or percentage of charges submitted. Managed care plans typically negotiate an all-inclusive fee for services rendered and will not pay for the professional charges separately, unless they are specifically contracted for, apart from the day-rate hospital charge.

When a patient is insured by a managed care plan, C-L services must be contracted separately to receive reimbursement beyond the all-inclusive rate that the hospital receives through the day rate. If the insurer carves out the management of its mental health and substance abuse benefits to a behavioral health subcontractor, separate professional bills must be submitted to the carve-out behavioral health subcontractor. The best method for ensuring that the correct payer is billed is to confirm with the medical insurer to determine whether the mental health benefit is carved out and, if so, to what organization. Ideally, a systematic method for navigating this system should be built into the consultation process through departmental or hospital-level billing/reimbursement staff with at least initial guidance, and periodic review, by the C-L administrator.

DEVELOP A STANDARD FORMAT FOR WRITING THE CONSULTATION NOTE

Several standards and guidelines collide when writing an efficient and effective consultation note. Standards established by the American Psychiatric Association (APA) Practice Guidelines for the Psychiatric Evaluation of Adults, Third edition,[1] address the content of an appropriate psychiatric examination; these standards should then be adapted to the special conditions of the consultative examination. As noted by the Academy of Psychosomatic Medicine (APM) Practice Guidelines for Psychiatric Consultation in the General Medical Setting,[2] the psychiatric consultation should also address the consultee-stated versus the consultant-assessed reason for referral, the extent to which the patient's psychiatric disturbance was caused by the medical or surgical illness, the adequacy of pain management, the extent of the psychiatric disturbance caused by medications or substance abuse, disturbances in cognition, the patient's character style, thoughts of dying, and psychiatric symptomatology. At the same time, those same APM guidelines stated that the "note is best if brief and focused on the referring physician's concerns."[2]

The consultation note should include the chief complaint, history of the present illness, medical and psychiatric history, social and family history, review of systems, mental status examination, as well as an impression and treatment plan. It should also include data to support the billing code for reimbursement; documentation should reflect the appropriate level of care provided. Given the proliferation of electronic medical record (EMR) systems, the creation of an electronic template that meets Medicare guidelines for billing and the practice guidelines outlined by the APA and APM (now called the Academy of Consultation-Liaison Psychiatry) will allow for quick, routinized documentation without worry about meeting billing and compliance standards. In addition, a template can facilitate more complete consultations, serve as a teaching tool for trainees, and catalyze research or internal review projects. Templates also lend themselves to inclusion in EMRs, prevent the loss of critical observations and recommendations that result from illegible notes, and decrease medical errors. With the developing capacity to import computerized (observational and laboratory) results, vital signs, recent laboratory values, medication orders, and drug administration, data can be more easily included in the consultation note. At the same time, care must be taken to keep computerized notes focused and helpful.[3] The ability, conferred by technology, to import information easily or cut and paste text can be more of a hindrance than a help if not coupled with actual human attention to what is pertinent and accurate.

BILL THE APPROPRIATE CODE

On November 1, 2019 the Centers for Medicare and Medicaid Services (CMS) finalized a provision in the 2020 Medicare Physician Fee Schedule Final Rule. This provision included revisions to the Evaluation and Management (E/M) office visit CPT codes, code descriptors, and documentation standards. To provide continuity, these revisions were broadened to extend to all other E/M categories (including consultation) in 2023. Inpatient consultations are reimbursable using codes 99222-99223 for initial consults, and 99231-99233 for subsequent visits. Of note, the older 99251-99255 initial consultation codes are out of date per CMS guidelines, and only payers who do not follow Medicare guidelines typically still accept these codes. Consultations in the ED are reimbursed using 99242-99245 for initial consultations. Consultation codes 99241 and 99251 have been deleted.

To use consultation codes properly, it must be made clear that the consultation is a service requested by another physician or another provider rather than by the patient or the patient's family. The requesting physician must enter a written or digital request for psychiatric consultation in the EMR. E/M levels are based on either Medical Decision-Making or may be Time Based. The extent of the history and physical examination performed is no longer required for selecting the level of service, although it is still important for these elements to be documented as medically appropriate. Services for initial consultations may be billed when the patient has not been consulted by a qualified healthcare professional from the exact same specialty during the same inpatient or observation admission. Subsequent services may be used when the patient has received these services during the current stay. Of note, when Advance Practice Providers (APPs) are working with physicians, they are considered as working in the exact same specialty as the physician. The specialty designation is determined by how a provider is enrolled with insurance companies.

Medical Decision-Making consists of the following three elements: the number and complexity of the problems being addressed during the encounter, the amount or complexity of the data to be reviewed and analyzed, and the risk of complications and morbidity or mortality associated with patient management. Four types of MDM are recognized: straightforward, low, moderate, and high; each has corresponding codes. Documentation of all work and the contributing thought process performed is key. The AMA published guidelines have descriptions of each level for reference purposes.[4] Time-based coding, on the other hand, is based on the total time spent on the date of service; it includes both face-to-face and non-face time personally spent by the clinician on the day of the encounter. This may include (but is not limited to) activities such as preparing to see the patient by obtaining a history or reviewing tests, performing a medically appropriate examination/evaluation, coordinating care, communicating recommendations to other team members, documenting clinical information in the record, and spending time with other physicians or APPs. Of note, the clinician's total time excludes general teaching time; it is limited to the management of the patient being seen as well as time spent by a resident or fellow alone with the patient. For this reason, MDM criteria may work best on teaching services when trainees are spending more time with patients than faculty. Time-based coding ranges from 35 to 80 minutes at the highest level. For services of 95 minutes or longer, there are prolonged service codes (e.g., 993X0) that may be used.[4] Engaging the assistance of a professional coder to perform periodic audits and training sessions for physicians is essential to remain abreast of changes in federal auditing guidelines. In addition, providing psychiatrists with simplified pocket billing guidelines and definitions of terms and selecting the appropriate CPT code can be helpful.

EVALUATE THE COSTS AND BENEFITS OF THE CONSULTATION SERVICE

C-L services are rarely lucrative cost centers.[5] Moreover, providing fee-for-service psychiatric consultation by independent practitioners is not often a financially viable service model. Meaningful consultation requires that clinicians expend significant time away from the bedside. Necessary tasks include the review of the medical record and case discussion before and after the consultation with the referring physician, nursing staff, and social service. Ancillary meetings with family members are often necessary to collect critical information that is not obtainable from a medically compromised patient. The new CPT initial consultation codes are meant to reflect this complexity.

In contrast to the preceding scenario, a "value accounting" methodology approaches the consultation service in a broader, systematic manner.[6] This methodology looks at cost, clinical outcome, and consumer satisfaction as interrelated domains. With a broader view, we can examine the impact of a C-L service on the care of the patient, the educational or academic mission of the hospital, and the financial function of the hospital. From a fiscal perspective, the availability of C-L services may result in decreased length of stay (LOS)[7] and recidivism rates, outcomes especially critical in a capitated, managed care environment. Decreasing the LOS lowers overall hospital costs; there is also evidence that effective consultations reduce the use of other medical services.[8] This additional revenue is separate from the financial savings in staff time expended while managing aggressive, confused, uncooperative, or "undesirable" patients; the costs of security; and the use of restraints and secondary problems of injuries and infections.

There is an emerging literature on proactive consultation services, in which a mental health professional reviews all admissions to a service and facilitates early consultation rather than waiting for the primary team to identify the need.[9] In one study, this resulted in a significant reduction in LOS (0.64 days in patients admitted for fewer than 31 days). This study also noted high satisfaction rates and expansion to units beyond those designated in the study. If C-L services can demonstrate their worth using the LOS as an indicator, the cost/benefit analysis may continue to tip in psychiatry's favor.

From a public health perspective, the involvement of the C-L psychiatrist may lead to improved disease-management protocols and best practices, helping patients understand and cope with chronic illness.

Enrolling patients in smoking cessation or weight-control programs may initiate or support their general health and wellness. Consider that 25% to 40% of patients in the general hospital are being treated for ailments secondary to alcohol use disorder and that the societal losses secondary to alcoholism may exceed $115 billion per year.[8,10]

For hospitals and healthcare systems, there is an increasing focus on assigned populations of patients through structures such as accountable care organizations. In this model, the individual patient and the assigned population of patients become simultaneous priorities, requiring resources to be allocated so that each of the assigned patients receives the necessary care. Although this can be done creatively (e.g., using electronic "virtual visits," via telepsychiatry, and others), reimbursement has not caught up in many instances—there is work still to be done in this arena to maximize the ability of consultation services to be compensated for innovations in this regard. Value-based purchasing has increasingly become a strategy for the buyers of care (e.g., government and insurers) to ensure that the care being provided is both high-quality and efficient with the insurers' and hospitals' goals aligned; as C-L psychiatry demonstrates its ability to decrease LOS and improve care in the hospital, its inclusion in value-based purchasing may be an area of future growth.

PROVIDE QUALITY ASSURANCE AND QUALITY IMPROVEMENT ON THE PSYCHIATRIC CONSULTATION SERVICE

Consensus has emerged that the overarching goals of health care, from provider to department to system, are "the triple aim:" improving the health of populations, improving the experience of care, and reducing healthcare costs.[11] The cost of health care and the rate of its growth as a percentage of gross domestic product is widely thought to be unsustainable. The government and insurers are increasingly demanding proof that the money being spent on health care is improving the outcomes of the patients that they insure. Transparency about outcomes has led to public reporting of success rates for some procedures, allowing patients to make better-informed decisions about where they will receive

their health care. Measures of quality are increasingly being tied to reimbursement, whether as part of pay-for-performance (i.e., increased reimbursement for better outcomes) or non-payment for so-called "never events" (e.g., medical errors, the development of decubitus ulcers, rapid readmission after discharge). Interestingly, though the care of proceduralists (e.g., surgeons) and hospitalists (e.g., internists) has come under the most scrutiny, quality of care measures have generally not been tied to reimbursement in the same way for consultants. This may change in the future.

UNDERSTAND DONABEDIAN'S MODEL

Donabedian was an epidemiologist and health services researcher who many consider to be the father of the modern healthcare quality movement. Among his contributions was a simplified model that identified three types of interconnected pieces of information (structure, process, and outcome) from which one could draw inferences about the quality of care delivered.[12]

By structure, he referred to both the material and human resources required to provide healthcare. By process, he referred to the activities that comprised care delivery. By outcome, he referred to a wide-ranging set of changes (positive or negative) in patients that could be attributed to the processes of care delivered. These three components are not attributes of quality per se, but rather windows through which the quality of care can be viewed and assessed.

The model is elegant in its simplicity; it has stood the test of time as a framework for the assessment of healthcare quality in several settings. Defining exactly how these general concepts apply to a specific aspect of health care (e.g., general hospital psychiatry) has proven more difficult. In addition, the hypothesized links between structure, process, and outcome may not always be robust causal connections. Nevertheless, this provides a reasonable frame for thinking about quality in any practice setting.

USE STRUCTURAL MEASURES OF CONSULTING QUALITY

A consultation service is only as good as the consultants who comprise it. Unlike other technical areas of medicine, psychiatric consultation is knowledge work, and, as such, the key measure of structural quality relates to the human resources (consultation psychiatrists) that form the team. In this regard, two questions need to be asked: (1) Is the team well-staffed? and (2) Is the team well-trained?

Staffing refers to the number of mental health providers (often including psychiatrists, psychologists, and APPs) who provide coverage to the general hospital (based on recruitment, retention, and full-time equivalents). The size of the roster will depend on multiple factors (e.g., the size of the hospital, the prevailing patient mix, the presence of trainees, the full-time/part-time status of staff, and the referral frequency). Defining "adequate coverage" is certainly up for discussion; no doubt there is a minimum threshold, below which the timeliness of consultations becomes an issue and the burden on individual practitioners is so substantial as to promote burnout. Beyond the raw number of staff on the service, the turnover rate of psychiatric consultants is another important structural measure of quality. One cannot underestimate the value of in-depth knowledge of the structure and culture of the specific setting in which one is employed; high rates of turnover make it difficult to develop this inside knowledge that is so critical to the framing of recommendations that are accepted.

Training refers both to the formal educational and training backgrounds of the providers and their clinical experience with general hospital psychiatry. The former would include measures such as the percentage of board-certified staff, the percentage of staff with subspecialty training in psychosomatic medicine, or the percentage of staff with formal subspecialty certification. The latter refers more to the years of experience, numbers of total cases seen, and markers of expertise in specific domains (such as the publication of peer-reviewed articles and chapters). There is evidence that both physician certification[13] and volume of cases seen[14] can be associated with clinical outcome, though to our knowledge, these relationships have not yet been established for psychiatry.

One final structural indicator relates to the degree of organizational learning that occurs with experience. This concept, sometimes referred to as "knowledge management," is an important aspect of major management consulting firms. How can the consultation

service use the combined wisdom and experience of thousands of cases seen over time and bring this to bear on the next consult request? Can the service itself have value beyond the sum of the individuals that comprise it? The answer is likely yes, but methods of knowledge management within hospital-based consultation services are at present rudimentary when compared with those used in business. This may improve with the more widespread use of EMRs for inpatient care. Until then, services might consider other aspects of knowledge management, such as the use of daily team rounding, the creation of an anonymous consult registry with "lessons learned," and the publication of important observations in peer-reviewed literature.

APPLY PROCESS MEASURES OF CONSULTING QUALITY

There is a core set of processes that make up the practice of "consultation psychiatry." These processes can be broadly construed under the categories of data gathering (speaking with the referring clinician, reviewing the chart, as well as interviewing and examining the patient); data integration (formulating a diagnosis and crafting a plan); and communication (writing and discussing impressions and recommendations). The skill with which these activities are carried out likely influences patient outcomes. It will also influence the service's reputation within the general hospital, in turn influencing the volume of referrals or high-performing consultation services; this can create a positive reinforcement loop in which a high-quality consult leads to high perceived value, which leads to increasing consultation requests, which leads to increased experience, which when captured leads to greater process skill, and so forth. Despite the widely acknowledged importance of process excellence in these three domains, they are only rarely, if ever, assessed once a physician has completed his or her postgraduate training. Unlike many other areas of the general hospital, there are no national standards for process quality in consultation psychiatry.

CONSIDER OUTCOME MEASURES OF THE CONSULTANT'S QUALITY

When a well-staffed and well-trained service implements high-quality processes, good outcomes are bound to occur. Donabedian identified seven domains of outcomes (Clinical, Physiological, Physical/Functional, Psychological, Social, Mortality/Longevity, and Patient Satisfaction) that ran the gamut from enhanced patient understanding of their condition to prolongation of life. Even a cursory glance at these items makes it clear that high-quality psychiatric consultation can have a substantial impact on many, if not all, of these outcomes.

In addition, several patient-safety issues could be addressed by timely and effective psychiatric consultation. Within-hospital suicides, suicide attempts, and staff assaults are a few dramatic and important examples. Other events may include the removal of intravenous lines, tubes, or wires by delirious patients. Tracking the frequency of these events on a hospital-wide basis may be a useful marker of the effectiveness of care implemented because of a psychiatric consultation. This requires a robust and reliable event-reporting system so that bad outcomes and "near misses" can be tallied and used as the basis for discussion.

FOLLOW THE GUIDING PRINCIPLES OF QUALITY MEASUREMENT

There is a benefit in measuring the structure, processes, and outcomes associated with a psychiatric consultation service. Through measurement, value can be identified that contributes to the mission of the general hospital, serving to justify the expense of maintaining this type of internal consultancy to hospital leadership. It may also enhance the standing of knowledge-based specialties in the eyes of healthcare purchasers and payers while working toward equilibrating reimbursement disparities that have long favored procedure-based specialties. Most of all, this type of measurement can provide the type of feedback needed to continually improve overall quality.

That said, attempts at measurement in and of themselves are potentially costly and time-consuming. All too many measurement efforts in today's healthcare landscape seem to be nothing more than costly box-checking exercises that do little to create practice change. There are three suggestions to avoid a similar fate:

1. Measurements should be devised, conducted, and reviewed by those on the front lines of care, sometimes called clinical microsystems.[15] In this way, those with the greatest knowledge of the care delivery processes and expected outcomes can play a central role in the measurement effort. This type of bottom-up effort is critical in the change process because it engenders "buy-in" from the beginning, rather than pushing mandates down the throats of providers in a top-down fashion.

2. Measurement cannot be considered a stand-alone process. It must be integrated with quality assurance and quality improvement activities. A quarterly report on the frequency of in-house suicide attempts is meaningless unless it is linked with careful efforts to reduce the rate of occurrence through root cause analysis of reported adverse events[16] and the implementation of rapid cycle change. In addition to formal quality assurance reviews and specific project-based quality improvement efforts, a wide variety of tools are available to promote change within the hospital setting. These include presentations at grand rounds, discussions at case conferences, systematic surveillance for complex cases with early intervention, and supervision with feedback for both trainees and staff.

3. The cost of measurement (in time and dollars) should be accounted for, and measurement efforts should be reassessed periodically to determine whether they are providing an adequate return on this investment. In this way, the hospital (or hospital microsystem, such as the consultation psychiatry service) can make certain that quality assessment enhances, rather than detracts from, the core capacity of the institution: to provide excellent clinical care.

CONCLUSION

Running a psychiatric consultation service requires both adherence to strict billing and documentation guidelines and maintenance of somewhat nebulous quality standards. Proving the service's worth to the general hospital can be challenging; however, it may require demonstrating cost offset and indirect means of value.

Over the past half-century psychiatric consultation in the general hospital has advanced from a novelty to a full-fledged medical subspecialty. As part of this coming of age, the time has come to not simply ask, "Do you have a psychiatric consultation service?" but rather "How good is the psychiatric consultation service at your institution?" This question is posed to initiate introspection by all who are involved in this field. A continuous examination of the consultation service's functioning is necessary to ensure that its practices are up to date and optimal.

REFERENCES

1. American Psychiatric Association. *Practice Guidelines for the Psychiatric Evaluation of Adults.* 3rd ed. American Psychiatric Association Publishing; 2016.
2. Bronheim HE, Fulop G, Kunkel EJ, et al. The Academy of Psychosomatic Medicine practice guidelines for psychosomatic consultation in the general medical setting. *Psychosomatics.* 1998;39(4):S8–S30.
3. Hartzband P, Groopman J. Off the record—avoiding the pitfalls of going electronic. *N Engl J Med.* 2008;358(16):1656–1658.
4. AMA CPT code and guideline updates. Available from: <https://www.ama-assn.org/system/files/2019-06/cpt-office-prolonged-svs-code-changes.pdf>; 2021
5. Goldberg RJ. Financial management challenges for general hospital psychiatry. *Gen Hosp Psychiatry.* 2001;23(2):67–72.
6. Butler SF, Docherty JP. A comprehensive system for value accounting in psychiatry. *J Ment Health Adm.* 1996;23:479–491.
7. Saravay SM, Lavin M. Psychiatric comorbidity and length of stay in the general hospital. *Psychosomatics.* 1994;35(3):233–252.
8. Hall RC, Rundell JR, Hirsch TW. Developing a financially viable consultation–liaison service. *Psychosomatics.* 1994;35(3):308–318.
9. Sledge WH, Gueorguieva R, Desan P, et al. Multidisciplinary proactive psychiatric consultation service: impact on length of stay for medical inpatients. *Psychother Psychosom.* 2015;84(4):208–216.
10. Schneekloth TD, Morse RM, Herrick LM, et al. Point prevalence of alcoholism in hospitalized patients: continuing challenges of detection, assessment, and diagnosis. *Mayo Clin Proc.* 2001;76(5):460–466.
11. Berwick DM, Nolan TW, Whittington J. The triple aim: care, health, and cost. *Health Aff.* 2008;27(3):759–769.
12. Donebedian A. *An Introduction to Quality Assurance in Health Care.* Oxford University Press; 2003.
13. Curtis JP, Luebbert JJ, Wang Y, et al. Association of physician certification and outcomes among patients receiving an implantable cardioverter-defibrillator. *JAMA.* 2009;301(16):1661–1670.
14. Begg CB, Reidel ER, Bach PB, et al. Variations in morbidity after radical prostatectomy. *N Engl J Med.* 2002;346(15):1138–1144.
15. Nelson EC, Godfrey MM, Batalden PB, et al. Clinical microsystems, part 1. The building blocks of health systems. *Jt Comm J Qual Patient Saf.* 2008;34(7):367–378.
16. Weiss AP. Quality improvement in healthcare: the six P's of root cause analysis [letter]. *Am J Psychiatry.* 2008;166(3):372–373.

INDEX

Page numbers followed by "*f*" indicate figures, "*t*" indicate tables, and "*b*" indicate boxes.

End-stage renal disease (ESRD) *(Continued)*
  movement disorder, 452–453
  psychiatric disorders in, 450–454
  psychiatric treatment considerations, 454
Enfuvirtide, for HIV infection, 494
Engagement Interview Protocol (EIP), 823
Enhanced autonomy, 13
Enkephalins, in pathophysiology of pain, 271
Entry inhibitors, for HIV infection, 494
Environmental factors
  in circadian rhythm, 390
  doctor-patient relationship and, 13–15
  gene interactions with, 579
  of psychiatric consultations, 4
Enzymes
  biological aspects of psychopharmacology, 823,
    825*t*–826*t*
  in gastrointestinal tract, 642
  hepatic, 641
  inhibitors and inducers, 643, 644*t*
Epidemiological Catchment Area (ECA) study
  collaborative care in, 846–847
  depression and, 105
Epidemiology, 846–847
  of anxiety in cardiac patients, 427–428
  of burnout, in physicians, 606–607
  of delirium in cardiac patients, 437
  in genetics of psychiatric disorders, 577–578,
    578*t*
  of HIV infection and AIDS, 491–492, 491*t*
  of neurocognitive disorders, 149–150
  of sexual dysfunction, 410–411
  of suicide, 740
Epilepsy, suicide and, 743
Epithelial sodium channels (ENaK), 446
Epworth Sleepiness Scale, 392, 392*t*
Erectile disorder, 415–416
Erectile dysfunction, 419–422
  first-line treatment for, 420*t*
  second-line treatment for, 421*t*
EROS-CTD, for female sexual dysfunction, 422
Erythrocyte sedimentation rate (ESR), elevated, in
    infectious or inflammatory encephalitis,
    356–357
Erythroxylum coca, 212–213
Escitalopram, for HIV infection, 505
EsDEPACS study, 433–434
Estimated glomerular filtration rate (eGFR), 455*t*
Ethical issues
  end-of-life care and, 794–796
  living organ donation, 478
Ethnicity
  psychiatric diagnosis and, 820
  psychiatric medications and, 822–827, 825*t*–826*t*
  "ETHNICS" mnemonics, 892–893, 894*b*
Euthanasia, 796
  medical aid, 796
Excretion, of drugs, 646–647
Executive function, 76–77, 77*t*
  in neurologic examination, 64
  neuropsychological assessment for, 75–77
Exercise, efficacy of, 698

F
Facial nerve, 60
Factitious disorders, 243–250
  clinical presentation, 245*t*
  clinical presentation of, 245*t*
  detection, 244–245
  diagnostic approach, 246–247
  DSM-5-TR, 246
  emergency departments (EDs), 247
  Munchausen syndrome, 245*t*
  with physical symptoms, in pain, 278–279
  primary and secondary gain, 243
Failure of treatment, 639–640
Failure, perception of, psychiatrists and, 608
Falls, in elderly, depression and, 106, 116
Family
  history
    neurocognitive disorders and, 156
    in psychiatric interview, 38
  members
    in end-of-life care, 793
    as interpreters, 821
    neurocognitive disorders and, 154
  of psychiatrists
    communication of anticipated unavailability to,
      for self-neglect, 616
    concerns in, 612
Fasciculations, in motor symptoms, 341*t*
Fatigue
  in cancer patients, 542–543
  in HIV infection, 499
Female sexual dysfunction, 422. *See also* Sexual
    dysfunction
Fetal alcohol syndrome, genetic factors of, 592–593
Fetal anomalies, during pregnancy, anticonvulsants
    and, 804
Fibromyalgia, 240
Financial stress, psychiatrists and, 609
Finger Localization Test, 81
Finger-Tapping Test, 81
Firearms, suicide and, 744
First-generation antipsychotics, 181–182
Flumazenil, for benzodiazepine overdose, 224
Fluorescence in situ hybridization (FISH),
    579–580
Fluoxetine, anticholinergic effects of, 116
Fluphenazine, for delirium, 141
Fluvoxamine, 186
Focal seizures, 304
  in motor symptoms, 341*t*
Focal unaware seizures, 306
Folate, 713–714
Folic acid, for mood disorders, 711
Folstein Mini-Mental State Examination (MMSE),
    6, 135–136
  for delirium, 135
  in psychiatric consultation, 6
Formal thought disorder, 171
Fostemsavir, 494
Fractional absorption, 641–642
Fragile X syndrome, 586–587
Frontal lobe function, in delirium, 137

Frontal lobe syndrome, 111
Frontotemporal neurocognitive disorder, 152–153
Functional neurologic symptom disorder (FND),
    in pain, 278
Functional neurological disorder (FND), 234–235
  prognosis and treatment of, 235–236
Functional somatic syndromes, 238–241, 239*t*
  anxiety disorders and, 237
  depressive disorders and, 236
  fibromyalgia and, 240
  irritable bowel syndrome and, 240–241
  personality disorders and, 238
  psychotic disorders and, 236
  substance use disorders and, 237
Funduscopy, in visual examination, 59
Fusion inhibitors, for HIV infection, 494

G
GABA$_B$R antigen, associated with autoimmune
    encephalitides, 359*t*–360*t*
GABAergic interneuron, 379
Gabapentin, 431, 483
  for alcohol use disorder, 211
  drug interactions of, 655
  for kidney disease, 457
GAD-65 antigen, associated with autoimmune
    encephalitides, 359*t*–360*t*
Gait, observation of, 67
Gait syndromes, 341*t*
Galantamine, for neurocognitive disorders, 162–163,
    162*t*
Gamma amino butyric acid (GABA), 390
Gaslight phenomenon, 3–4
Gastroesophageal reflux disease, 461
Gastrointestinal bleeding, SSRI-related, 469
Gastrointestinal disease, 460–474
  esophagus, stomach and upper, 460–464
    dysphagia, 460
    gastric bypass, 463
    gastroesophageal reflux disease, 461
    gastroparesis, 462–463
    globus hystericus, 460
    nausea and vomiting, 461–462
  liver disorders, 466–468
  lower, 464–466
    constipation, 464–466
    diarrhea, 464
    inflammatory bowel disease, 465–466
    irritable bowel syndrome, 464–465
  medication considerations in, 469, 470*t*, 471*t*
  pancreas, disorders of, 468–469
Gastrointestinal (GI) drug absorption, 641–642
Gastroparesis, 462–463
Gender dysphoria, 412, 417, 423
Gender identity disorder, 901
Gender-affirming hormonal therapies (GAHT)
  estrogen, 907
  GnRHAs, 908
  medications, 908–909, 908*t*
  procedures, 907*t*
  progesterone, 907